# MINIMALLY INVASIVE SURGERY OF THE HEAD, NECK, AND CRANIAL BASE

## *Associate Editors*

**PETER D. COSTANTINO, M.D.**

*Co-Director, Center for Cranial Base Surgery*
*Department of Otolaryngology*
*St. Lukes–Roosevelt Medical Center*
*New York, New York*

**WESLEY A. KING, M.D.**

*Associate Professor*
*Department of Neurosurgery*
*Mount Sinai School of Medicine*
*New York, New York*

**JAMES A. KOUFMAN, M.D., F.A.C.S.**

*Professor and Director, Center for Voice Disorders*
*Department of Otolaryngology*
*Wake Forest University School of Medicine*
*Winston-Salem, North Carolina*

**DENNIS S. POE, M.D.**

*Assistant Clinical Professor*
*Department of Otolaryngology and Laryngology*
*Harvard Medical School*
*Surgeon*
*Department of Otolaryngology*
*Massachusetts Eye and Ear Infirmary*
*Boston, Massachusetts*

**TIMOTHY L. SMITH, M.D., M.P.H.**

*Associate Professor and Chief*
*Division of Rhinology and Sinus Surgery*
*Department of Otolaryngology and Communication Sciences*
*Medical College of Wisconsin*
*Milwaukee, Wisconsin*

## *Illustrator*

**ROBERT E. FENN, C.M.I.**

*Medical Art Studios*
*Milwaukee, Wisconsin*

# MINIMALLY INVASIVE SURGERY OF THE HEAD, NECK, AND CRANIAL BASE


*Editors*

**PHILLIP A. WACKYM, M.D., F.A.C.S.**

*John C. Koss Professor and Chairman*
*Department of Otolaryngology and Communication Sciences*
*Medical College of Wisconsin*
*Milwaukee, Wisconsin*

**DALE H. RICE, M.D., F.A.C.S.**

*Tiber/Alpert Professor and Chairman*
*Department of Otolaryngology–Head and Neck Surgery*
*University of Southern California School of Medicine*
*Los Angeles, California*

**STEVEN D. SCHAEFER, M.D., F.A.C.S.**

*Professor and Chairman*
*Department of Otolaryngology*
*New York Medical College*
*Valhalla, New York*
*Director and Chairman*
*Department of Otolaryngology*
*New York Eye & Ear Infirmary*
*New York, New York*



LIPPINCOTT WILLIAMS & WILKINS

A **Wolters Kluwer** Company

Philadelphia • Baltimore • New York • London
Buenos Aires • Hong Kong • Sydney • Tokyo

*Acquisitions Editor:* James Merritt
*Developmental Editor:* Leah Ann Kiehne Hayes
*Production Editor:* Rosemary Palumbo
*Manufacturing Manager:* Tim Reynolds
*Cover Designer:* Mark Lerner
*Compositor:* Lippincott Williams & Wilkins Desktop Division


**530 Walnut Street**
**Philadelphia, PA 19106 USA**
**LWW.com**



Printed in China

---

**Library of Congress Cataloging-in-Publication Data**
Minimally invasive surgery of the head, neck, and cranial base / editors, Phillip A. Wackym, Dale H. Rice, Steven D. Schaefer.
p.; cm.
Includes bibliographical references and index.
ISBN 0-7817-2045-1
1. Head—Endoscopic surgery. 2. Neck—Endoscopic surgery. 3. Skull base—Endoscopic surgery. 4. Otolaryngology, Operative. I. Wackym, Phillip A. II. Rice, Dale H. III. Schaefer, Steven D., 1945–
[DNLM: 1. Head—surgery. 2. Endoscopy. 3. Neck—surgery. 4. Surgical Procedures, Minimally Invasive. WE 705 M665 2002]
RF51.M53 2002
617.5′1059—dc21

2001029500

---

Care has been taken to confirm the accuracy of the information presented and to describe generally accepted practices. However, the authors, editors, and publisher are not responsible for errors or omissions or for any consequences from application of the information in this book and make no warranty, expressed or implied, with respect to the currency, completeness, or accuracy of the contents of the publication. Application of this information in a particular situation remains the professional responsibility of the practitioner.

The authors, editors, and publisher have exerted every effort to ensure that drug selection and dosage set forth in this text are in accordance with current recommendations and practice at the time of publication. However, in view of ongoing research, changes in government regulations, and the constant flow of information relating to drug therapy and drug reactions, the reader is urged to check the package insert for each drug for any change in indications and dosage and for added warnings and precautions. This is particularly important when the recommended agent is a new or infrequently employed drug.

Some drugs and medical devices presented in this publication have Food and Drug Administration (FDA) clearance for limited use in restricted research settings. It is the responsibility of the health care provider to ascertain the FDA status of each drug or device planned for use in their clinical practice.

10 9 8 7 6 5 4 3 2 1

*To my wife Jeremy and my son Ashton, from whom I have stolen innumerable hours in pursuit of the highest standard of academic otolaryngology–head and neck surgery, and to Paul Ward–the teacher who has influenced me the most.*

P.A.W.

*To my wife Ann, my stepdaughters Katherine, Rebecca, and Hannah, and my son Zander.*

D.H.R.

*To my wife Phyllis and my daughter Jessica.*

S.D.S.

# CONTENTS

# CONTRIBUTING AUTHORS


**Ashraf S. Abou-Halawa, M.B.Bch., M.S.** Department of Otolaryngology, Massachusetts Eye and Ear Infirmary, Boston, Massachusetts

**Milan R. Amin, M.D.** Assistant Professor, Department of Otolaryngology/ Head & Neck Surgery, Medical College of Pennsylvania /Hahnemann School of Medicine; Director, Center for Voice & Swallowing Disorders, Hahnemann University Hospital, Philadelphia, Pennsylvania

**Thomas Balkany, M.D., F.A.C.S.** Hotchkiss Professor and Chairman, Department of Otolaryngology, University of Miami School of Medicine; Chief, Department of Otolaryngology, Jackson Memorial Hospital, Miami, Florida

**Fred G. Barker, M.D.** Assistant Professor, Department of Neurosurgery, Harvard Medical School; Attending Neurosurgeon, Massachusetts General Hospital, Boston, Massachusetts

**Minerva Becker, M.D.** Division of Diagnostic Radiology, Geneva University Hospital, Geneva, Switzerland

**Frederic Braccini, M.D.** Head and Neck Surgeon, Timone Hospital Center, Nice, France

**Daniel I. Branovan, M.D.** Assistant Professor, Division of Head and Neck Surgery, Department of Otolaryngology, New York Eye & Ear Infirmary, New York, New York

**Dan J. Castro, M.D., Ph.D.** Professor, Division of Head and Neck Surgery, University of California, Los Angeles School of Medicine, Los Angeles, California

**Peter D. Costantino, M.D.** Co-Director, Center for Cranial Base Surgery, Department of Otolaryngology, St. Lukes–Roosevelt Medical Center, New York, New York

**Robin T. Cotton, M.D.** Professor, Department of Otolaryngology–Head & Neck Surgery, University of Cincinnati College of Medicine; Director, Department of Pediatric Otolaryngology–Head & Neck Surgery, Children's Hospital Medical Center, Cincinnati, Ohio

**William T. Couldwell, M.D., Ph.D.** Professor and Chairman, Department of Neurosurgery, New York Medical College; Director, Department of Neurosurgery, Westchester Medical Center, Valhalla, New York

**Harel Deutsch, M.D.** Resident, Department of Neurosurgery, Mount Sinai School of Medicine, New York, New York

**Wolfgang Draf, M.D., Ph.D., F.R.C.S.** Chairman and Director, Department of Ear Nose and Throat Diseases, Head, Neck and Facial Plastic Surgery and Communication Disorders, University of Marburg, Fulda Hospital, Fulda, Germany

**Pavel Dulguerov, M.D.** Department of Otolaryngology–Head & Neck Surgery, University of Geneva Medical School, Geneva University Hospital, Geneva, Switzerland

**Charles N. Ford, M.D., F.A.C.S.** Professor and Chairman, Division of Otolaryngology, Department of Surgery, University of Wisconsin Hospital and Clinics, Madison, Wisconsin

**David R. Friedland, M.D., Ph.D.** Fellow, Department of Otolaryngology–Head and Neck Surgery, Johns Hopkins University, Baltimore, Maryland

**Michel Gagner, M.D.** Professor, Department of Surgery, Mount Sinai School of Medicine; Chief, Division of Laparoscopic Surgery, Mount Sinai Medical Center, New York, New York

**Julio F. Gallo, M.D., F.A.C.S.** Voluntary Instructor, Department of Otolaryngology, University of Miami School of Medicine, Miami, Florida; Simons Center for Nasal and Facial Plastic Surgery, North Miami Beach, Florida

**Richard E. Gliklich, M.D.** Associate Professor, Department of Otology and Laryngology, Harvard Medical School; Surgeon, Department of Otolaryngology, Massachusetts Eye and Ear Infirmary, Boston, Massachusetts

**Patricia A. Hudgins, M.D.** Professor, Section of Neuroradiology, Department of Radiology, Emory University School of Medicine; Director, Section of Neuroradiology, Department of Radiology, Emory University Hospital, Atlanta, Georgia

**Amin R. Javer, M.D.** Fellow, Georgia Rhinology and Sinus Center, Savannah, Georgia

**Gregg H. Jossart, M.D.** Division of Laparoscopic Surgery, Mount Sinai School of Medicine, New York, New York

**Joseph E. Kerschner, M.D.** Assistant Professor and Chief, Division of Pediatric Otolaryngology, Department of Otolaryngology and Communication Sciences, Medical College of Wisconsin; Children's Hospital of Wisconsin, Milwaukee, Wisconsin

**Wesley A. King, M.D.** Associate Professor, Department of Neurosurgery, Mount Sinai School of Medicine, New York, New York

**James A. Koufman, M.D., F.A.C.S.** Professor and Director, Center for Voice Disorders, Department of Otolaryngology, Wake Forest University School of Medicine, Winston-Salem, North Carolina

**Frederick A. Kuhn, M.D.** Director, Georgia Rhinology and Sinus Center, Savannah, Georgia

**Jeffrey T. Laitman, M.D.** Acting Chairman, Department of Cell Biology and Anatomy, Mount Sinai School of Medicine, New York, New York

**William Lawson, M.D., D.D.S.** Professor and Vice-Chairman, Department of Otolaryngology, Mount Sinai School of Medicine; Attending Physician, Department of Otolaryngology, Mount Sinai Medical Center, New York, New York

**Willy Lehmann, M.D.** Professor, Department of Ear, Nose, and Throat–Head and Neck Surgery, Cantonal University Hospital, Geneva, Switzerland

**Howard L. Levine, M.D.** Director, Cleveland Nasal Sinus and Sleep Center, Marymount Outpatient Care Center; Adjunct Staff, Department of Neurosurgery, Cleveland Clinic Foundation, Cleveland, Ohio

**Christopher J. Linstrom, M.D.** Associate Professor, Department of Otolaryngology, New York Medical College, Valhalla, New York; Director, Otology and Neurology, Department of Otolaryngology, New York Eye & Ear Infirmary, New York, New York

**Todd A. Loehrl, M.D.** Assistant Professor of Otolaryngology and Communication Sciences, Division of Rhinology and Sinus Surgery, Medical College of Wisconsin, Milwaukee, Wisconsin

**Francis Marchal, M.D.** Division of Head and Neck Surgery, Geneva University; Clinical Faculty, Department of Otolaryngology–Head and Neck Surgery, Cantonal Hospital, Geneva, Switzerland

**Samuel Márquez, M.D.** Faculty, Department of Cell Biology and Anatomy, Mount Sinai School of Medicine, New York, New York

**Kevin X. McKennan, M.D.** Assistant Clinical Professor, Department of Otolaryngology, University of California, Davis; Staff, Department of Otolaryngology, Sutter/Mercy General Hospital, Sacramento, California

**Ralph Metson, M.D.** Associate Clinical Professor, Department of Otology and Laryngology, Harvard Medical School; Surgeon, Department of Otolaryngology, Massachusetts Eye and Ear Infirmary, Boston, Massachusetts

**Glenn A. Meyer, M.D.** Professor, Department of Neurosurgery and Department of Otolaryngology and Communication Sciences, Medical College of Wisconsin; Senior Attending Physician, Department of Neurosurgery, Froedtert Memorial Lutheran Hospital, Milwaukee, Wisconsin

**Robert G. Ojemann, M.D.** Professor, Department of Neurosurgery, Harvard Medical School; Senior Attending Neurosurgeon, Massachusetts General Hospital, Boston, Massachusetts

**Marcos B. Paiva, M.D.** University of California, Los Angeles School of Medicine, Los Angeles, California

**Jerome Paris, M.D.** Resident, Department of Otolaryngology–Head and Neck Surgery, Marseille University, La Timone Hospital Center, Marseille, France

**Dennis S. Poe, M.D.** Assistant Clinical Professor, Department of Otolaryngology and Laryngology, Harvard Medical School; Surgeon, Department of Otolaryngology, Massachusetts Eye and Ear Infirmary, Boston, Massachusetts

**Gregory N. Postma, M.D.** Assistant Professor, Center for Voice Disorders, Wake Forest University School of Medicine; Assistant Professor, Baptist Medical Center, Winston-Salem, North Carolina

**Elie E. Rebeiz, M.D.** Associate Professor, Department of Otolaryngology, Tufts University School of Medicine; Chief, Department of Head and Neck Surgery, New England Medical Center, Boston, Massachusetts

**Anthony J. Reino, M.D.** Assistant Clinical Professor, Department of Otolaryngology, Mount Sinai School of Medicine; Assistant Attending Physician, Department of Otolaryngology, Mount Sinai Medical Center, New York, New York

**John S. Rhee, M.D.** Assistant Professor and Chief, Division of Plastic and Reconstructive Surgery, Department of Otolaryngology and Communication Sciences, Medical College of Wisconsin, Milwaukee, Wisconsin

**Dale H. Rice, M.D., F.A.C.S.** Tiber/Alpert Professor and Chairman, Department of Otolaryngology–Head and Neck Surgery, University of Southern California School of Medicine, Los Angeles, California

**Michael A. Rothschild, M.D.** Associate Professor, Departments of Otolaryngology and Pediatrics, Mount Sinai School of Medicine; Chief, Department of Pediatric Otolaryngology, Mount Sinai Medical Center, New York, New York

**Michael J. Rutter, M.D. F.R.A.C.S.** Assistant Professor, Department of Otolaryngology, University of Cincinnati; Assistant Professor, Department of Pediatric Otolaryngology, Children's Hospital Medical Center, Cincinnati, Ohio

**Ibrahim Sabit, M.D.** Resident, Department of Neurosurgery, Westchester County Medical Center, Valhalla, New York

**Mary J. Sandage, M.A., C.C.C.-S.L.P** Clinical Instructor, Department of Communicative Disorders, University of Wisconsin, Madison; Clinical Speech Pathologist, Division of Otolaryngology -Voice Clinic, University of Wisconsin Hospital, Madison, Wisconsin

**Romaine E. Saxton, Ph.D.** Adjunct Professor of Surgery and Radiological Sciences, Department of Surgical Oncology, University of California, Los Angeles School of Medicine, Los Angeles, California

**Steven D. Schaefer, M.D., F.A.C.S.** Professor and Chairman, Department of Otolaryngology, New York Medical College, Valhalla, New York; Director and Chairman, Department of Otolaryngology, New York Eye & Ear Infirmary, New York, New York

**Chandranath Sen, M.D.** Professor and Vice-Chairman, Department of Neurosurgery, Mount Sinai School of Medicine, New York, New York

**Brent A. Senior, M.D., F.A.C.S.** Associate Professor, Department of Otolaryngology–Head and Neck Surgery, University of North Carolina, Chapel Hill, North Carolina

**Stanley M. Shapshay, M.D., F.A.C.S.** Professor, Department of Otolaryngology–Head and Neck Surgery, Boston University School of Medicine and Boston Medical Center, Boston, Massachusetts

**Michelle M. Smith, M.D.** Associate Professor, Department of Radiology, Medical College of Wisconsin; Chief, Head and Neck Neuroradiology, Department of Radiology, Froedtert Memorial Lutheran Hospital, Milwaukee, Wisconsin

**Timothy L. Smith, M.D., M.P.H.** Associate Professor and Chief, Division of Rhinology and Sinus Surgery, Department of Otolaryngology and Communication Sciences, Medical College of Wisconsin, Milwaukee, Wisconsin

**Jean Marc Thomassin, M.D.** Professor, Department of Otolaryngology, University of Medecine; Chief, Department of Ear, Nose, and Throat, Timone Hospital Center, Marseille, France

**Elizabeth H. Toh, M.D.** Assistant Professor, Department of Otolaryngology, University of Pittsburgh School of Medicine; Assistant Professor, Department of Otolaryngology, Pittsburgh Eye and Ear Clinic, Pittsburgh, Pennsylvania

**Joseph G. Toner, M.D., F.R.C.S.** Clinical Lecturer, Department of Otolaryngology, Queens University, Belfast; Director, Department of Otolaryngology, Northern Ireland Cochlear Implant Centre, Belfast City Hospital, Belfast, Northern Ireland

**Robert J. Toohill, M.D.** Professor, Department of Otolaryngology and Communication Sciences, Medical College of Wisconsin; Senior Staff Physician, Department of Otolaryngology–Head and Neck Surgery, Froedtert Memorial Lutheran Hospital, Milwaukee, Wisconsin

**Phillip A. Wackym, M.D., F.A.C.S.** John C. Koss Professor and Chairman, Department of Otolaryngology and Communication Sciences, Medical College of Wisconsin; Medical Director of Otolaryngology, Audiology, and Speech Pathology, Children's Hospital of Wisconsin; Chief, Department of Otolaryngology–Head and Neck Surgery, Froedtert Memorial Lutheran Hospital, Milwaukee, Wisconsin

**Rainer Weber, M.D., Ph.D.** Professor, Department of Ear, Nose, and Throat, University of Magdeburg, Magdeburg, Germany; Chief, Department of Ear, Nose, and Throat–Head and Neck Surgery, Marien Hospital, Stuttgart, Germany

**Peak Woo, M.D.** Clinical Director, Grabscheid Voice Center, Department of Otolaryngology, Mount Sinai School of Medicine, New York, New York

**B. Tucker Woodson, M.D., F.A.C.S.** Associate Professor, Department of Otolaryngology and Communication Sciences, Medical College of Wisconsin; Director, Froedtert and Medical College Sleep Disorders Program, Milwaukee, Wisconsin

**Nathaniel W. Yang, M.D.** Clinical Associate Professor, Department of Otorhinolaryngology, University of the Philippines College of Medicine, Philippine General Hospital, Manila, Philippines; Visiting Consultant, Department of Otorhinolaryngology, The Medical City, Mandaluyong City, Philippines

**Steven M. Zeitels, M.D., F.A.C.S.** Associate Professor, Department of Otology and Laryngology, Harvard Medical School; Director, Division of Laryngology, Massachusetts Eye and Ear Infirmary, Boston, Massachusetts

# FOREWORD

There are many volumes in the medical literature which regurgitate information found in other sources. This book is uniquely different. Doctors Phillip Wackym, Dale Rice, and Steven Schaefer, along with the associate editors, Doctors Costantino, King, Koufman, Poe, and Smith, have brought together experts in endoscopy of the ear, nose, throat, head and neck, airway, and the upper digestive tract. This remarkable book, presented in an atlas format, provides comprehensive coverage of optics, operative techniques, and complications. This compendium is of great value to the subspecialists as well as general otolaryngologists serving the broader field.

These editors and authors are dedicated physicians and surgeons who have established credibility and senior status in our field. They have a perspective about endoscopy unique to their respective subspecialties, which allows them to elaborate upon the fine points in each of these surgical procedures. We applaud these outstanding otolaryngologists and head and neck surgeons in this landmark effort.

*Harold C. Pillsbury III, M.D., F.A.C.S.*
*Thomas J. Dark Distinguished Professor and Chairman*
*Department of Otolaryngology/Head and Neck Surgery*
*University of North Carolina School of Medicine*
*Chapel Hill, North Carolina*

*Paul H. Ward, M.D., F.A.C.S.*
*Emeritus Professor and Chief*
*Division of Head and Neck Surgery*
*Department of Surgery*
*University of California, Los Angeles School of Medicine*
*Los Angeles, California*

# PREFACE

During the past decade several excellent books have been published about endoscopic surgery of the paranasal sinuses. Incorporation of endoscopic techniques in all areas of surgery has revolutionized many surgical disciplines. There have also been significant applications of endoscopic techniques to all areas of otolaryngology–head and neck surgery. However, to date, no comprehensive book addresses the advances, treatment advantages, and limitations of endoscopic techniques in otolaryngology–head and neck surgery.

The purpose of this book is to provide a reference atlas that incorporates discussion of the advantages and disadvantages of each technique for subspecialists in otology, neuro-otology, and cranial base surgery; rhinology and sinus surgery; head and neck oncology and plastic and reconstructive surgery; and laryngology and bronchoesophagology. Most importantly, general otolaryngologists will be able to incorporate many of the techniques described. The multidisciplinary nature of the book is intended to provide cross-fertilization of the subspecialties.

Much of the book focuses on detailed methods that will facilitate the adoption of the techniques to the practice of otolaryngology–head and neck surgery. The advantages in adopting some of the methods described will range from better photodocumentation for teaching, medical-legal application, and patient outcome to minimally invasive techniques to decrease hospital stay and improve treatment outcomes.

The book contains 45 chapters and is divided into five sections ranging from general principles to subspecialty applications of endoscopic techniques. Intraoperative color endoscopic photographs, grayscale photographs, patient positioning photographs, and equipment photographs are used. Color illustrations have been used when black and white line drawings do not convey the necessary information. Robert Fenn, medical illustrator, worked with each author to provide continuity in style and precision in head and neck anatomy.

The strength of this book is the group of editors and associate editors. The full spectrum of the specialty of otolaryngology–head and neck surgery is represented with well-respected clinician-teachers, each an expert in their subspecialty. Each of the editors and associate editors provide a perspective that brings a well-matured synthesis of these endoscopic techniques to the book. Each of the contributing authors were selected with their level of clinical expertise and innovation, leadership, and diversity of training experiences in mind.

*Phillip A. Wackym, M.D., F.A.C.S.*
*Dale H. Rice, M.D., F.A.C.S.*
*Steven D. Schaefer, M.D., F.A.C.S.*

# ACKNOWLEDGMENTS

The following companies provided unrestricted educational grants to the publisher. Their contributions are greatly appreciated.

BrainLAB Inc.
100 Marine Parkway, Suite 305
Redwood City, California 94065
www.brainlab.com

Gyrus ENT (formerly Smith Nephew ENT)
2925 Appling Road
Bartlett, Tennessee 38133
www.gyrus-ent.com

Stryker-Leibinger
4100 East Milham Avenue
Kalamazoo, Michigan 49001-6197
www.leibinger.com

SECTION

I

# GENERAL PRINCIPLES

# 1

# OPTICS

## COMPARISON OF THE OPERATING MICROSCOPE WITH THE RIGID ENDOSCOPE

ELIZABETH H. TOH
JOSEPH E. KERSCHNER
PHILLIP A. WACKYM

---

The operating microscope and the rigid endoscope have become essential tools in the surgical armamentarium of the head and neck surgeon. The initial introduction of the binocular operating microscope launched a golden era of microsurgery, with options for adjustable magnification, wider fields of view, longer working distances, and concentric illumination of the operative field. The rigid endoscope, on the other hand, allowed magnified views of anatomic structures normally inaccessible to the operating microscope. The development and innovative application of surgical endoscopes in most surgical specialties have fueled major advances in minimally invasive keyhole surgery. This chapter reviews essential optical principles as they apply to the operating microscope and the rigid endoscope. Advantages, disadvantages, and general indications for the use of each of these systems are discussed.

## TERMINOLOGY

The following terms represent fundamental concepts to be familiar with prior to reviewing optical physics.

*Magnification:* The perceived size of any visualized object is related to the size of its retinal image. Magnification is the ratio of the retinal image of an object when seen through the naked eye to that seen through a magnifying glass at its intrinsic focal length.

*Field of view:* Refers to the diameter of the visualized operative field through the optical system employed.

*Viewing angle:* The angle subtended by the visual limits of the field of view and the tip of the optical system (Fig. 1.1).

*Direction of view:* The angle between the long axis of the endoscope or microscope head (i.e., optical axis) and the line joining the tip of this instrument to the center of the field of view. This corresponds to the bisection of the viewing angle (Fig. 1.1).

*Working distance:* Measured between the operative field and the distal end of the viewing system.

## OPERATING MICROSCOPE

The operating microscope is designed as a magnification tool that offers a range of working magnifications and fields of view for a specified working distance (Fig. 1.2). Conceptually, it represents a simple magnifying glass mounted serially on a galilean binocular system (1). The key optical components of any microscope assembly include an image transmission and a light transmission system. The modular design of the image transmission system offers tremendous versatility of use by allowing for the combination of various lens pieces within the basic microscope body (Figs. 1.3 and 1.4).

### Image Transmission System

#### *Objective Lens*

The objective lens is a simple magnifying lens mounted on the distal end of the microscope head. The focal length of the objective lens determines the working distance between the microscope and the patient. In the absence of an objective lens, the microscope focuses at infinity, much like field binoculars. Commercially manufactured lenses are available in focal lengths ranging from 100 to 400 mm at 25-mm increments. In selecting the appropriate objective lens, consideration should be given to the fact that a longer focal length offers more working distance and a larger field of view at the expense of decreased magnification and illumination. The recommended working lenses for most otolaryngologic–head and neck surgical applications range between 200- and 400-mm lenses, which offer comfortable working distances of 8 to 16 inches, respectively. Fine focusing of the image at focal length can be achieved using

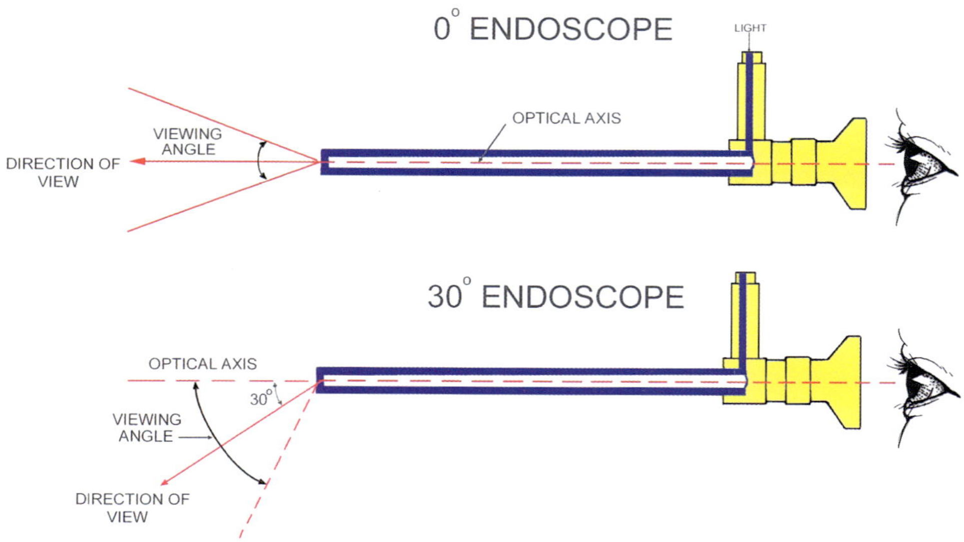


**FIGURE 1.1.** Comparison of 0° and 30° endoscopes demonstrates that the optical axis remains constant while the direction of view is shifted by a prism located at the tip of the rigid Hopkins rod-lens endoscope. The direction of view can be 30°, 45°, or 70°, depending on the specific prism used in the construction of the endoscope. The viewing angle is fixed for each endoscope.

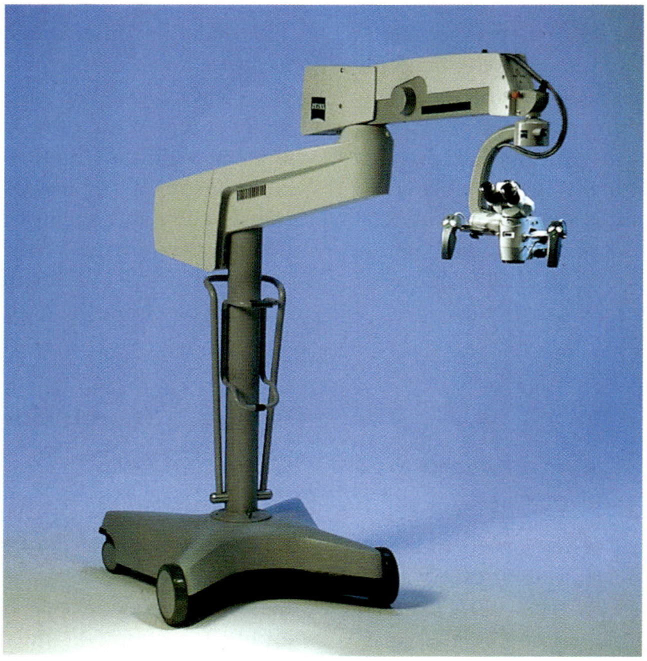

**FIGURE 1.2.** The Zeiss OPMI VARIO microscope has a variable focal length.

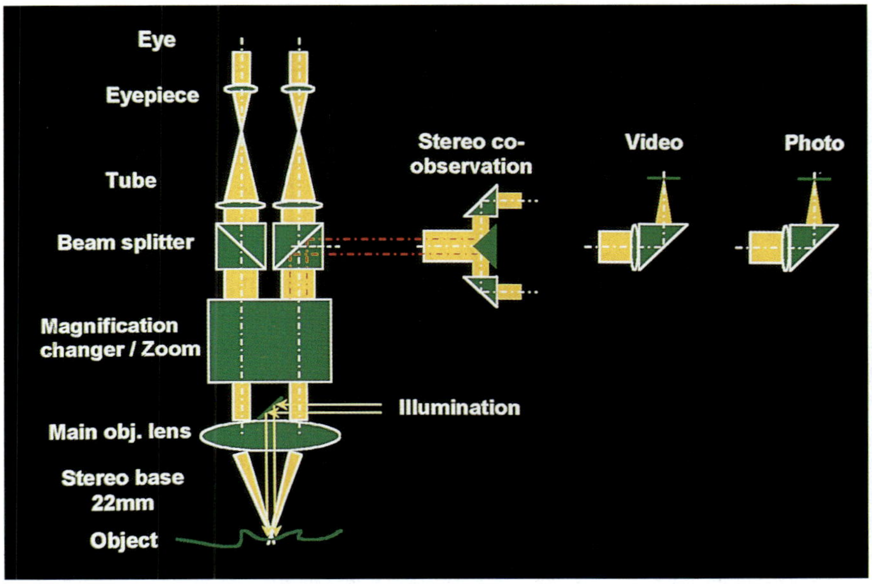


**FIGURE 1.3.** Schematic of the binocular microscope shows the illumination source, lens systems, and beam-splitter components. The beam splitters allow stereo coobservation, video, and photographic capabilities.

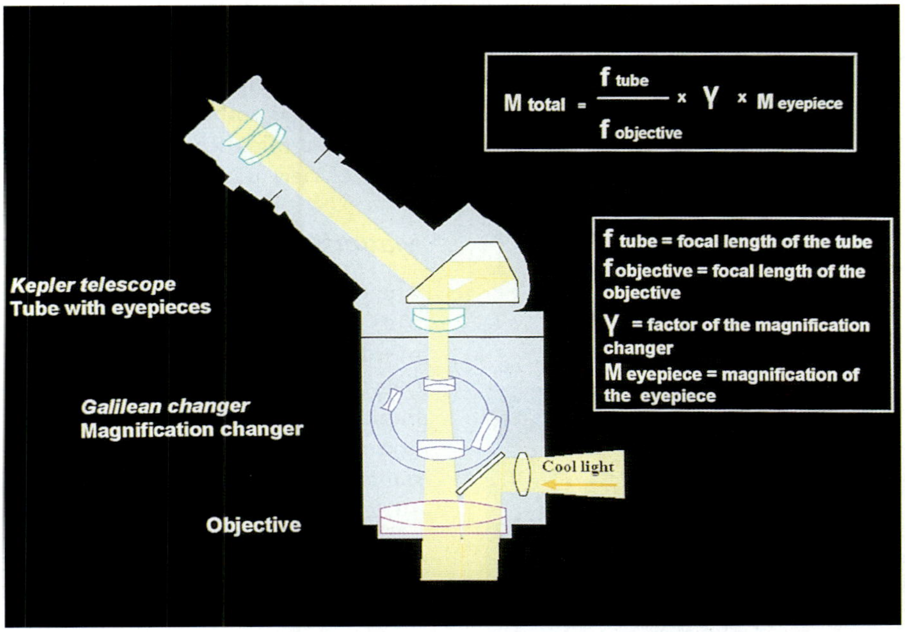


**FIGURE 1.4.** The traditional manual step changer drum for the operating microscope consists of two pairs of refractor lenses mounted on a rotating turret interposed between the objective lens and the binocular assembly.

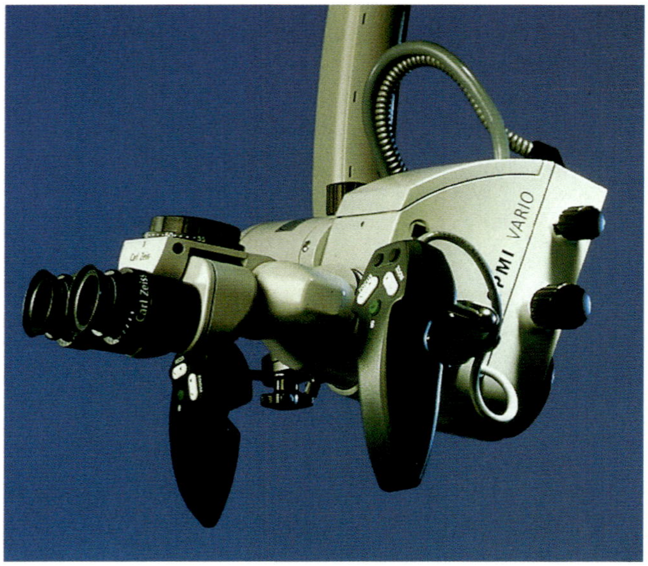


**FIGURE 1.5.** The variable focal length and magnification can be manipulated by hand controls, as shown here on the Zeiss OPMI VARIO microscope. Foot controls are also available and obviate the need to stop operating to adjust the focal length or the magnification.

manual or motorized control knobs located on the microscope head or foot pedal.

Variable focal length microscopes have been developed with built-in optical technology (e.g., Leica M500-N surgical microscope, Carl Zeiss OPMI VARIO microscope system), allowing for a variable working distance of 200 to 415 mm (Figs. 1.2, 1.5, and 1.6). These microscopes obviate the need for objective lens changes during the procedure as changes in working distance develop.

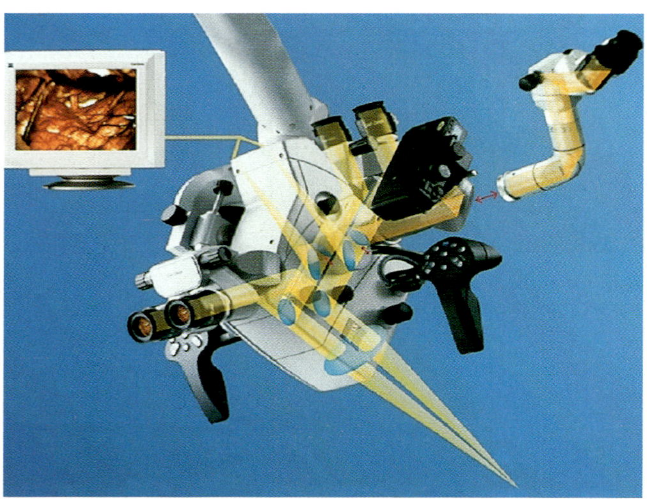

**FIGURE 1.6.** Beam splitters allow a video camera, a still camera, and a stereo coobserver side arm to be attached to the operating microscope, as shown here on a Zeiss OPMI VARIO microscope.

### Binocular Assembly

The binocular assembly comprises two eyepieces mounted on separate tubes. The binoculars split the light reflected from the operative field equally between the two eyes to provide stereoscopic vision for depth perception. These are available in the 125-mm and 160-mm focal lengths, and they can be mounted in a straight or inclined position relative to the axis of the microscope head to allow greater flexibility in viewing directions.

The eyepieces are a set of encased lenses available in increasing ocular powers of 10×, 12.5×, 16×, and 20×. Each eyepiece is further fitted with an adjustable diopter scale to correct for the viewer's refractive error.

The total magnification provided by any microscope is a combination of two magnification factors. *Base magnification* is provided by the objective lens and binocular assembly but is determined primarily by the focal length of the binocular tubes. Unlike the case of the objective lens, an increase in the focal length of the binocular tubes results in a linear increase in image magnification and decrease in field of view. Base magnification is therefore a fixed magnification factor, predetermined at the beginning of the procedure by the optical properties of any given combination of assembled components. Further *variable magnification* is provided by the magnification changer, which enables the operator to increase or decrease base magnification of the microscope assembly during use. As the overall magnification of the microscope is increased, the field of view and depth of view are correspondingly decreased.

### Magnification Changer

The traditional manual step changer drum consists of two pairs of refractor lenses mounted on a rotating turret interposed between the objective lens and binocular assembly (Fig. 1.4). When the traditional manual microscope is parfocaled, rotation of the drum gives five different magnification options at a constant working distance. Drum constants are numbered sequentially in the order of 6, 10, 16, 40, 25, and 16, representing a magnification (25×, 40×) or reduction (6×, 10×) in the objective lens image. At position 16, the drum channel is open, and therefore the image size is not influenced by the magnification changer.

The newer motorized power-zoom changers afford a continuous dynamic range of magnification by moving a series of lenses back and forth on a focusing ring. This adds considerable flexibility to the overall magnification of the microscope assembly (1.5× to 18×). This function is directed by manual control knobs on the microscope head (Fig. 1.5) or foot pedals.

## Light Transmission System

The light source for standard operating microscopes is derived from high-intensity xenon or quartz halogen bulbs.

This light is beamed through a series of lenses and prisms within the microscope head and exits through the objective lens onto the surgical field. From there, the light is reflected back through the optical components of the image transmission system into each eye separately (Figs. 1.3 and 1.4). This construction allows for coaxial illumination of the field of view and three-dimensional depth perception.

The intensity of light reflected back from the field is inversely related to the focal length of the objective lens. As the focal length increases, the diameter of the illuminated area increases, but the luminance per unit area decreases. Changes in the variable magnification of the microscope during use do not alter the area of illumination, but the associated reduction in field of view results in less light being reflected back through the eyepieces. Control of the aperture allows increased delivery of available light to the narrowed field of view when working at increased magnification.

Insertion of a beam splitter between the binocular assembly and magnification changer drum allows the reflected light beam to be split in fixed proportions between the operator and any optional auxiliary attachments, such as viewing tubes, cameras, or video recorders (2) (Figs. 1.3 and 1.6).

## RIGID ENDOSCOPE

Early prototypes of the rigid endoscope consisted of a series of small lenses separated by large air spaces within a closed tube and coupled to an external light source (3). This construction unfortunately suffered from limited viewing angles, poor image resolution and contrast, and inefficient light transmission. Although the basic design of the endoscope system has remained unchanged during the past century, significant modifications in the internal lens components have mostly overcome these shortcomings. The Hopkins rod-lens telescope represents the technologic standard after which all modern rigid endoscopes are modeled (4). As in the operating microscope, the functioning endoscope comprises image and light transmission systems.

### Image Transmission System

The essential difference between the Hopkins rod-lens system and the early endoscope is the replacement of small optical lenses with larger quartz rod lenses that are separated by small air spaces (Fig. 1.7). Because light transmission through glass is significantly more efficient than through air, the resulting image is markedly clearer and brighter.

Three lens systems—the objective lens, relay system, and eyepiece—are arranged sequentially from distal to proximal locations within the endoscope sheath. The intermediate image produced by the objective lens is reflected through a series of rod-lens inversion systems. Each inversion system inverts the optical image. An even number of inversion systems eventually produce an upright image at the proximal viewing end of the scope, which is then magnified and viewed through the eyepiece. This two-dimensional image is viewed monocularly and therefore does not offer the operator an appreciation for depth of field. The working image is usually displayed by means of a three-chip video camera onto a 19-inch or larger, high-resolution video monitor.

The eyepiece lens is the only intrinsic magnifying component of this optical system. It therefore provides a fixed base magnification factor unique to the specific endoscope. Additional variable magnification is provided by adjusting the working distance of the endoscope. These variables are inversely related, meaning that the closer the endoscope is placed to the object in view, the higher the magnification obtained.

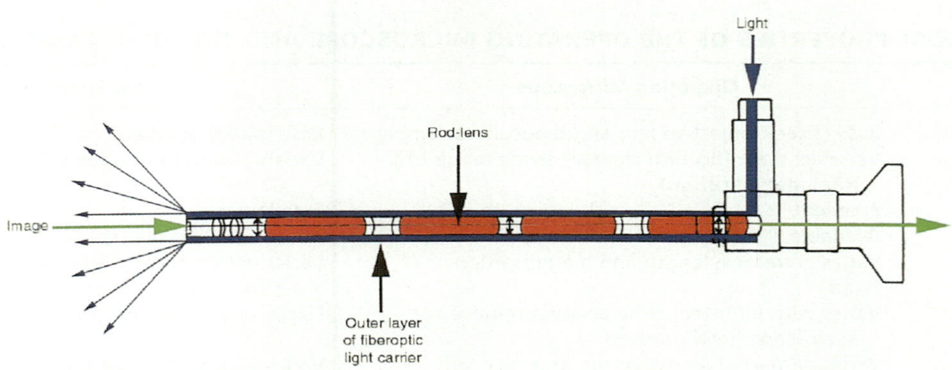


**FIGURE 1.7.** Schematic diagram of a Hopkins rod-lens–style rigid endoscope. Notice the air-filled spaces separated by quartz rod lenses, which are surrounded by the fiberoptic light carrier.

One of the distinct advantages of the rigid endoscope is the ability to see around corners and obstructing anatomic structures. This is achieved by reflecting the optical axis at the endoscope tip through a glass prism incorporated into the objective lens (Fig. 1.1). Using this principle, endoscopes with different viewing directions have been constructed to accommodate a variety of surgical accesses and procedures. The commonly used viewing directions in head and neck surgery include 0°, 30°, 45°, and 70°. The 0° telescope provides a constant panoramic view of the surgical field directed toward the front. The forward-oblique 30° telescope offers different views as the endoscope is rotated along its long axis, enabling the operator to see around corners. The 70° telescope allows lateral viewing, but because of an inherent inability to visualize the endoscope tip, it must be advanced only under direct vision. The recent addition of the 45° rigid endoscope (Smith Nephew Richards, Memphis, TN) provides a compromise between the 30° and 70° endoscopes while permitting a better forward view than the 70° endoscope. Another potential hazard associated with the use of angled telescopes is the loss of illumination, which may compound the confusion resulting from an already unfamiliar viewing direction. Training and experience are critical to be able to use the advantages of angled endoscopes without increasing operative morbidity.

### Light Transmission System

Endoscopic illumination is provided by an external light source coupled to the endoscope through a fiberoptic cable and carried to the tip of the endoscope through fiberoptics within the endoscope sheath. Projection of light concentrically through the endoscope tip provides coaxial illumination of the surgical field. A variety of light sources are available, including tungsten halogen, metal halide, and xenon short arc, with various degrees of brightness and whiteness of light. The intensity of the delivered light usually is greater than that provided by the surgical microscope. This is principally because of the large distance between the target object and the final lens with the microscope relative to the endoscope.

## ADVANTAGES, DISADVANTAGES, AND INDICATIONS FOR USE

The optical properties of the operating microscope and the rigid endoscope are compared in Table 1.1. With these key features understood, the overall advantages and disadvantages of each optical system are summarized, and general indications for the use of each system are offered.

### Operating Microscope

#### *Advantages*

- Magnification is easily adjustable before and during use of the microscope.
- Tremendous versatility of use results from the modular construction of the image transmission system.
- Stereoscopic view provides depth perception.
- Beam-splitting system allows concurrent direct monocular viewing through a side tube, video recording, digital image capture, and still photography. Selected microscopes offer a second beam-splitting system that provides a binocular view for the observer.
- An excellent range of instrumentation is available.
- Bimanual operative technique is the mainstay of microsurgery.

#### *Disadvantages*

- It can visualize structures beyond the line of vision.
- The system is bulky and relatively immobile compared with the maneuverability of an endoscope.

**TABLE 1.1. OPTICAL PROPERTIES OF THE OPERATING MICROSCOPE AND THE RIGID ENDOSCOPE**

| Optical Properties | Operating Microscope | Rigid Endoscope |
|---|---|---|
| Magnification | Base (fixed): objective lens and binocular assembly<br>Variable: magnification changer (wide range of total magnification) | Base (fixed): eyepiece<br>Variable: working distance |
| Image resolution | Excellent | Excellent |
| Stereoscopic vision | Available | Not available |
| Field of view | Varies with focal length and magnification | Varies with working distance |
| Viewing angle | Fixed | Fixed for each endoscope |
| Direction of view | Varies with binocular tube position relative to microscope head position | Fixed for each endoscope (0°, 30°, 45°, 70°) |
| Working distance | Varies with local length of the objective lens | Varies with endoscope position |
| Illumination | Varies inversely with magnification, modified by aperture in some microscopes | Fixed for specific endoscope, but overall reduced in angled endoscopes |
| Risk of thermal injury | Possible, desiccation of tissue | Possible, proportional to the proximity to tissue |

- Illumination and the viewing angle are limited by the size of surgical access.
- There is a relatively large distance between optics and focal point of surgical field.

### *Indications for Use*

- It is an indispensable workhorse instrument in the fields of otology and neuro-otologic skull base surgery, neurosurgery, and microvascular reconstructive surgery.
- It is used preferentially when binocular view and resulting depth perception plays a critical role in the operative technique.

## Rigid Endoscope

### *Advantages*

- It can be inserted through small surgical incisions and keyhole craniotomies, allowing for the possibility of decreased operative time, duration of hospitalization, and postoperative morbidity.
- It allows the surgeon visual access to anatomic locations normally obscured by intervening soft tissue or bone, obviating the need for removal or retraction of vital structures.
- The viewing angle is wider than that of the operating microscope because of the shorter focal length of the objective lens.
- Illumination and image detail are enhanced by the ability to position the endoscope in close to the visualized structure.

### *Disadvantages*

- It requires familiarity with relevant surgical anatomy and endoscopic techniques because of the increased technical difficulty of operating within a narrower field of view and modified viewing directions (i.e., 30°, 45°, or 70° endoscope).
- Poor depth perception results from the dual dimensionality of the endoscope image. This may be ameliorated in the future with the use of stereoscopic goggles and dual camera-endoscope systems.
- The proximity of endoscope to the surgical field results in frequent tip soiling and the need for intermittent cleaning of the endoscope tip. Irrigation systems that are available for selected endoscope applications resolve tip soiling without withdrawing the endoscope.
- The surgeon cannot operate bimanually unless the endoscope is secured to the patient's body or an external fixation device.
- A limited range of adjunctive endoscopic microinstruments is available for use in otologic and neuro-otologic skull base surgical procedures.
- There is a potential for thermal injury from the light source.

### *Indications for Use*

- Experienced surgeon
- Upper aerodigestive tract procedures, where access is limited by the natural size of the lumen or cavity
- Exploratory or second-look procedures (e.g., cholesteatoma)
- Minimally invasive neuro-otologic surgery (e.g., vestibular neurectomy)
- As an adjunct to microsurgery, with the explicit purpose of viewing around corners and improving image detail and illumination in cases involving minimal access surgery (5)
- Range of applications in the head and neck region that are highlighted throughout this textbook

## REFERENCES

1. Hoerenz P. The design of the surgical microscope, part I. *Ophthalmic Surg* 1973;4:40–45.
2. Rubinstein R. The anatomy of the surgical operating microscope and operating positions. *Dent Clin North Am* 1997;41:391–413.
3. Nitze M. Eine neue Beobachtung und Untersuchungsmethode d. Harnblase. *Wein Med Wochenschr* 1879;24:649–651.
4. Hopkins HH. Optical principles of the endoscope. In: Berci G, ed. *Endoscopy*. New York: Appleton-Century-Crofts, 1976:3–27.
5. Perneczky A, Fries G. Endoscope-assisted brain surgery, part 1: evolution, basic concept, and current technique. *Neurosurgery* 1998;42:219–225.

2

# DIGITAL IMAGE PROCESSING

PHILLIP A. WACKYM

The goal of this chapter is to provide the basic steps necessary to process digital images for publication. The underlying mechanisms of each step are explained so that surgeons can understand how each of these actions and variables can be manipulated to produce the highest-quality endoscopic images for presentation and publication.

## IMAGE ACQUISITION

A variety of methods are available to produce digital endoscopic images. The means of image acquisition and conversion to a digital file format are considered in this section. Table 2.1 summarizes some of the hardware and software resources that are available. There is a wide range in cost and quality of hardware; however, even with modestly priced equipment, it is a straightforward matter to produce high-quality endoscopic images for presentation and publication.

### Cameras

Two types of cameras are available for endoscopic surgery of the head, neck, and cranial base: one-chip and three-chip video cameras. These cameras use solid-state, light-sensitive receptors, called charge-coupled devices (CCDs) or "chips," that are able to detect brightness differences at different points throughout an image. A 3-CCD camera (Fig. 2.1) uses a beam splitter that separates the full color image into its red, blue, and green components. Reflection off of a color-selecting mirror, or passage through the mirror for one of the colors, in the beam splitter directs each of these three colors to one of the three dedicated CCDs. White is represented by the presence of all three colors, and black is represented by the absence of all three colors. These 3-CCD cameras provide the greatest resolution and light sensitivity; however, they are also the most expensive.

The 1-CCD cameras use a single CCD with an overlay of millions of colored filters. Electronics within the camera or camera control unit are able to determine what filter the light hitting a specific point in the CCD is passing through. It is therefore possible to produce a smaller and less expensive camera than a 3-CCD camera; however, resolution and light sensitivity are both compromised.

### Digital Capture

Although expensive, digital image capture systems offer the greatest ease in digital image acquisition and processing, as well as superb image quality (Fig. 2.2). In both of my endoscopy towers, I have Stryker Digital Capture systems (www.strykerendo.com). The latest model (SDC Pro, Stryker Endoscopy, Santa Clara, CA) uses a writeable CD-ROM drive to archive the digital images, whereas the initial model (SDC) used a Zip disk to store the images. Other custom systems can be assembled at a lower cost, but they require a laptop or dedicated personal computer (PC) and digital capture board placed in the endoscopic tower. We have used these custom systems in the private office setting where we have laptop computers with digital capture boards for endoscopic documentation.

**TABLE 2.1. SELECTED WEB SITES FOR IMAGE PROCESSING INFORMATION**

| Web Site | Materials and Service |
|---|---|
| **Photoshop Resources** | |
| www.photoshopcentral.com | Portal to multiple Photoshop resources |
| www.photoshopio.com | Photoshop training videotapes |
| www.idignet.com | Photoshop use and education |
| www.adobe.com | Maker of the Photoshop software |
| **Hardware** | |
| www.strykerendo.com | Digital Capture System, cameras |
| www.circoncorp.com | Cameras |
| www.karlstorz.com | Cameras |
| www.sony.com/medical | Digital video printers |
| www.tektronix.xerox.com | Dye sublimation printers |
| www.microtek.com | Flatbed scanners |
| www.umax.com | |
| www.hp.com | |
| www.nikonusa.com | Slide scanners |
| www.polaroid.com | Digital film recorders |

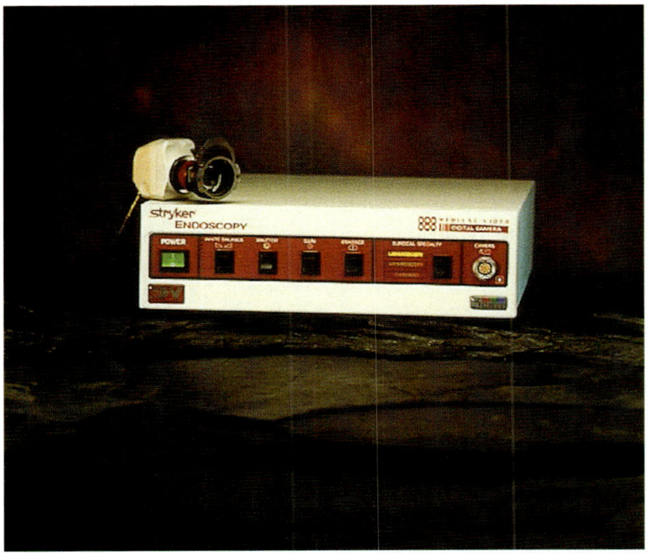


**FIGURE 2.1.** Three-chip digital video camera. This Stryker Endoscopy digital camera is an excellent three-chip charge-coupled device (3-CCD) endoscopic camera (www.strykerendo.com). These cameras use solid-state, light-sensitive receptors called CCDs, or chips, that are able to detect brightness differences at different points throughout an image. A 3-CCD camera uses a beam splitter that separates the full color image into its red, blue, and green components. Reflection off of a color-selecting mirror or passage through the mirror for one of the colors in the beam splitter directs each of these three colors to one of the three dedicated CCDs.

## Scanning Digital Prints

If a digital capture system is not available in the operating room, an alternative means of producing a digital endoscopic image is to scan a digital photographic print. Most operating rooms are equipped with endoscopic towers that contain a digital printer and a video recorder. One group of commonly encountered printers is the Sony dye transfer sublimation thermal printers (www.sony.com/medical). Depending on the model purchased, these printers (Fig. 2.3) are capable of producing 4.5 × 6 inch images with 310 dots per inch (dpi) and containing up to 16 million colors. The endoscopic image may be captured and printed during the surgery, or because these printers accept S-video and composite NTSC inputs, it is also possible to capture images at a later date from endoscopic video acquired during surgery. After selecting the prints to scan, a flatbed scanner (Fig. 2.4) can be used to convert

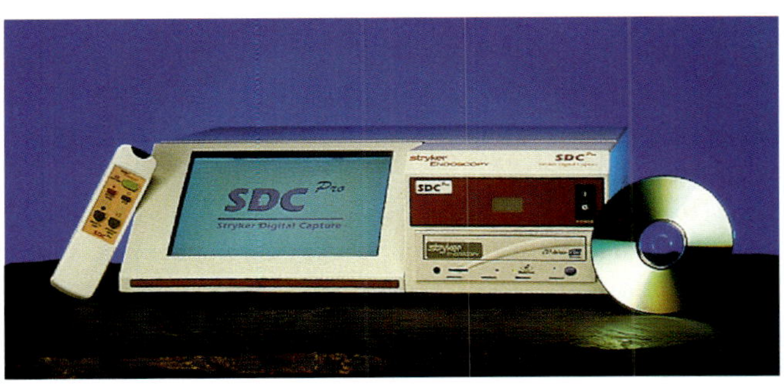


**FIGURE 2.2.** Digital image capture systems offer greater ease in digital image acquisition and processing, as well as superb image quality. This Stryker Digital Capture system (SDC Pro) (www.strykerendo.com) uses a writeable CD-ROM drive to archive the digital images. The initial model (SDC) used a Zip disk to store the images. Other custom systems can be assembled at a lower cost, but they require a laptop or dedicated personal computer and digital capture board placed in the endoscopic tower.

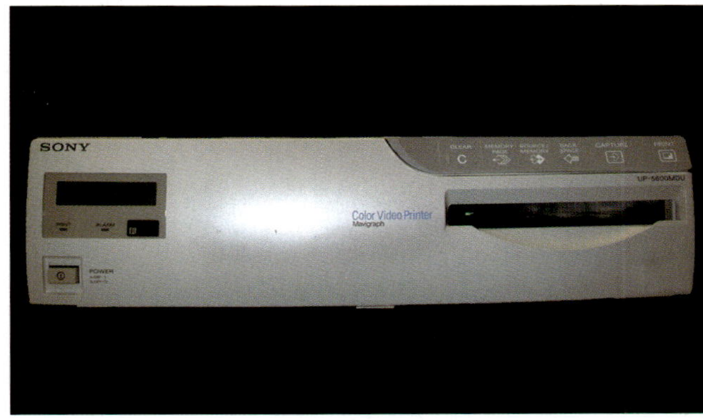


**FIGURE 2.3.** Sony dye transfer sublimation thermal printer (www.sony.com/medical). This printer is capable of producing 4.5 × 6 inch images with a resolution of 310 dots per inch and containing up to 16 million colors. The endoscopic image may be captured and printed during the surgery, or because these printers accept S-video and composite NTSC inputs, it is also possible to capture images at a later date from endoscopic video acquired during surgery.

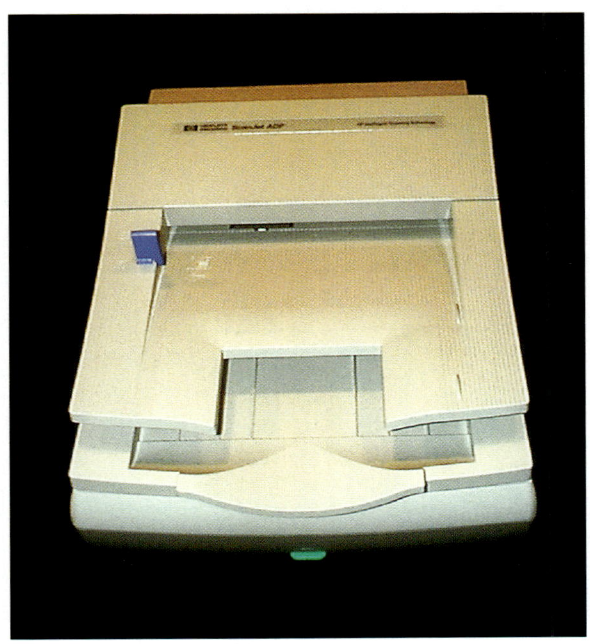

**FIGURE 2.4.** Flatbed scanner. Hewlett-Packard offers (www.hp.com) an inexpensive, high-quality flatbed scanner that can be used to produce a digital image file from an existing digital print.

these images into a digital format. It is important to scan the images at a resolution of at least 300 pixels per inch (ppi); however, I recommend scanning at a resolution of at least 600 ppi, so that if resampling or resizing is necessary, there will be no loss of resolution. These issues are addressed in detail later in this chapter. A wide variety of flatbed scanners are available (Table 2.1) and optical hardware scanning resolutions of up to 1,220 × 3,048 dpi (maximum interpolated resolutions of 12,192 × 12,192 dpi) are available.

### Scanning 35-mm Slides

If the surgical endoscope is coupled to a 35-mm camera and color slide film has been used for photodocumentation, a film scanner can be used to produce a digital image. This is a necessary hardware acquisition if magnetic resonance (MRI) or computed tomography (CT) images captured on slides or if preoperative, intraoperative, or postoperative patient images are to be used in illustrating endoscopic techniques, findings, or outcomes. There are several personal film scanners on the market; however, the Nikon Coolscan III is an outstanding and inexpensive unit (Fig. 2.5 and Table 2.1). I typically scan each 35-mm slide at an optical resolution of 1,350 ppi, which produces an adequately sized image at 300 ppi when resized and resampled. The Nikon Coolscan III is capable of scanning at an optical resolution of 2,700 ppi.

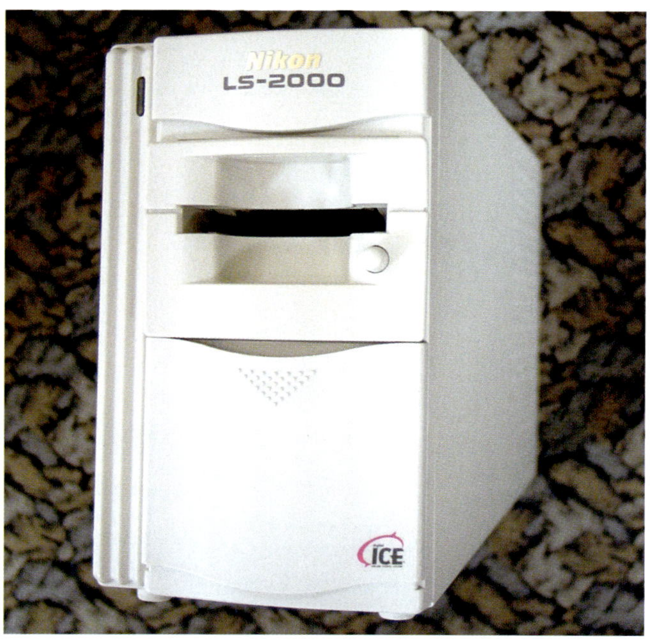


**FIGURE 2.5.** A 35-mm film scanner. This Nikon Coolscan III film scanner (www.nikonusa.com) is an inexpensive, high-quality scanner that is useful in producing a digital image file from a standard 35-mm slide.

## FILE FORMATS

At a minimum, the surgeon using Photoshop should become familiar with three file formats. These include the native Photoshop format (*.psd file extension), the JPEG format (*.jpg file extension), and the TIFF format (*.tif file extension). Each is considered here, and although many other file formats are available, I focus on these three because they are the most important for processing images for publication.

### Photoshop Format

Photoshop offers its own native format, and the greatest advantage of this format is that it is optimized for all of the program's functions and capabilities. Most importantly, it allows the use of layers, a subject that is considered later in this chapter. This format saves every feature of the application that has been used with the software, and the program saves more rapidly in this format than it does with other file formats. Although the Photoshop format allows file compression without loss of data, I usually do not use this feature.

The native Photoshop file format has two disadvantages. First, very few applications support it, and it is intended for use only with the extremely flexible Photoshop program. Second, most publishers do not accept this format when digital files are submitted with the manuscript. I usually submit individual files with the Photoshop format and the TIFF format so that the publisher has the flexibility of returning to the native Photoshop format to manipulate the image if necessary.

### JPEG Format

*Joint Photographic Experts Group* (JPEG) is the most efficient compression format available and serves as the industry standard. Unfortunately, it is a *lossy compression scheme*, and image quality is sacrificed to reduce file size. However, the degree of loss can be controlled during the save operation. When saving an image in the JPEG format, a dialog box offers a total of 11 compression settings, with the 0 setting producing the most severe compression and 10 producing the least compression. The low values compress the image to occupy the least space; however, there is more severe distortion of the image (Fig. 2.6). Because of these image distortion issues, I recommend using a quality setting of 8 or higher for digital endoscopic images.

Another important point regarding the use of JPEG in Photoshop is that it is a cumulative compression scheme. This means that Photoshop recompresses the image every time you save it in the JPEG format. Because JPEG works from the on-screen version of the file, there is no disadvan-

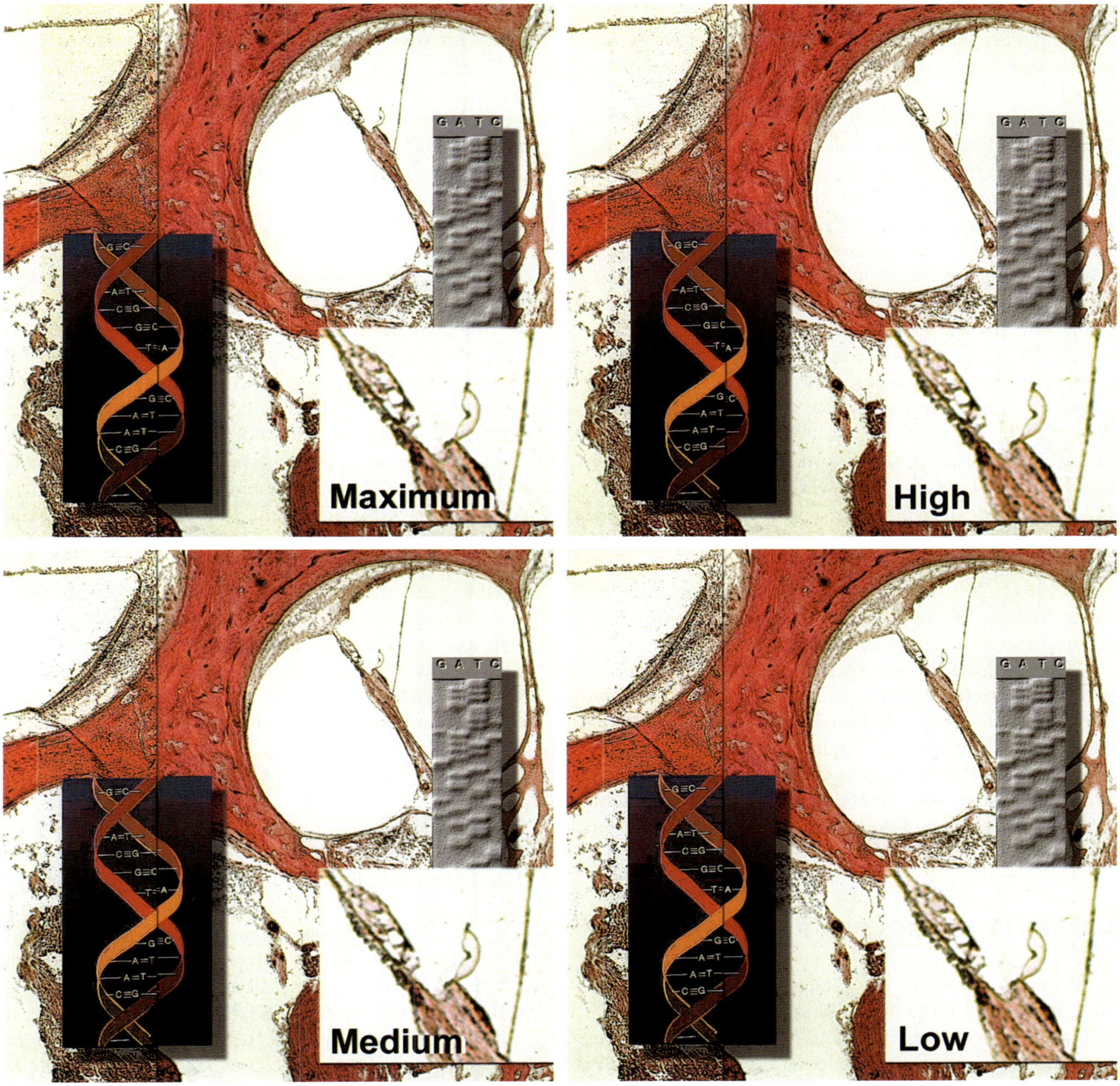


**FIGURE 2.6.** Joint Photographic Experts Group (JPEG) compression. This composite figure compares differences in the four JPEG compression settings, from maximum quality plus minimum compression *(top left)* to minimum quality plus maximum compression *(bottom right)*. A vertical strip of each original figure has been compressed and sharpened to demonstrate the subtle erosion of details. A rectangular segment has been enlarged to show a similar erosion of details.

tage in saving the image to the disk repeatedly during a single session; however, if you close an image, reopen it, and save it in JPEG format, there will be additional loss of image quality. If you choose to use the JPEG format, I recommend completing your image processing in the Photoshop format, flattening it and saving it once in the JPEG format.

## TIFF Format

The *Tag Image File Format* (TIFF) and JPEG formats serve as the industry standards for the management and manipulation of digital image files. Consequently, there is almost uniform support for these two file formats among graphics applications.

TIFF was developed by the Aldus Corporation (now Adobe Systems Inc., San Jose, CA) to standardize a burgeoning and diverse population of digital images early on when this technology was rapidly evolving. TIFF is the most widely supported image printing format across the Macintosh and PC platforms. It is principally for this reason that I use TIFF to save the initial raw digital images, to save the final processed and labeled figures for use in publication, or to import into PowerPoint to prepare slide presentations of my digital endoscopic images.

When saving a Photoshop file in the TIFF or JPEG format, remember that these formats do not support layers. Any labels, arrows, or other annotation marks are *irreversibly* flattened onto the digital endoscopic image. I therefore save a raw, unprocessed TIFF file and the processed Photoshop file before flattening the layered image into the final TIFF format. When saving a flattened Photoshop image in the TIFF format, Photoshop displays the TIFF options dialog box, which offers two options. First is the choice of Byte Order. The operator must choose between a PC or Mac Byte Order to use the PC or Mac variation of TIFF. Second is the option of using Lempel-Ziv-Welch (LZW) compression. The LZW compression strategy looks at the computer code that describes an image and substitutes frequently used codes with shorter equivalents. Because LZW substitutes strings of data, this strategy does not alter or lose a single pixel in the image. It is a *lossless compression strategy*. Although most image editing or desktop publishing software applications can import LZW compressed TIFF images, some do not, including applications used by some journal and textbook publishing companies. For this reason, I do not use the LZW compression option.

## PREPARING IMAGES FOR PUBLICATION

In this section, I describe the standard method used to prepare a raw digital image for publication using Photoshop. For more advanced techniques and for digital correction of the photographic flaws, there are several excellent books that should be consulted (1–4).

### Resolution, Size, and Storage Media

The ultimate use of the image dictates the required resolution and size. Typically, I process an image for publication, because this requires the greatest resolution, and then reduce the resolution and save this separate version of the file for use in preparing slides. Most publishers require the image resolution to be 300 ppi, and I usually construct the image's physical size to be the same as that of the published image. For files used for importation into PowerPoint for slides, I use a resolution of 150 or 200 ppi and save these as separate, flattened TIFF files.

Changing the resolution and size of an image affects the number of pixels. There are two ways to do this: resampling and cropping. Resizing also can be used, but with this option, the image is enlarged or reduced without changing the number of pixels (Fig. 2.7). Before resizing or resampling, I usually crop the image (i.e., *Image → Crop*) so that the desired features are included in the image.

#### Resizing

Choose *Image → Image Size* to access the control panel that allows the pixel dimensions and resolution of an image to be modified. The starting point of the raw image depends on how the digital image was acquired. As discussed in the Image Acquisition section of this chapter, the raw images captured with the Stryker Digital Capture system are 72 ppi at screen size (approximately 8.8 × 6.7 inches), and scanned digital photographic prints (Sony Electronics, Park Ridge, NJ) are 300 or 600 ppi, depending on what I selected when using the flatbed scanner. The Resample Image check box should be turned off to maintain a constant number of pixels in an image. The desired height or width should be typed in, and the corresponding width or height, respectively, is automatically calculated if the Constrain Proportions remains selected (recommended). Typically, this results in a raw image with more than 300 ppi and dimensions of 3 × 3 inches to 3 × 4 inches. After resizing has been completed, resampling can be performed to adjust the image to 300 ppi.

#### Resampling

Resampling an image means that it is scaled so that it contains a larger or smaller number of pixels. With resizing, there is an inverse relationship between size and resolution (Fig. 2.7), but resampling affects size and resolution independently. Figure 2.7 shows an image resized and resampled to 50% of its original dimensions. The original and resampled images have exactly the same resolution, whereas the resized image has twice the resolution of the other two images. Choose *Image → Image Size* to access the control panel that allows resampling of the image. The Resample Image check box should be turned on.

Resampling up adds pixels. When this action takes place, Photoshop makes up the information in the added pixels, and as expected, the new image does not look as good as the original. In contrast, resampling down smooths the pixelation of digital images, photographic grain, halftone patterns, and other scanning artifacts. This is why I typically scan digital prints at a high resolution (e.g., 600 or 1,200 ppi) and resample the scan down to 300 ppi. The size of the file decreases, requiring less storage space.

Because these image files are large, I use Zip disks as my working storage media. For long-term storage and submission of images for publication, I burn CD-ROM disks.

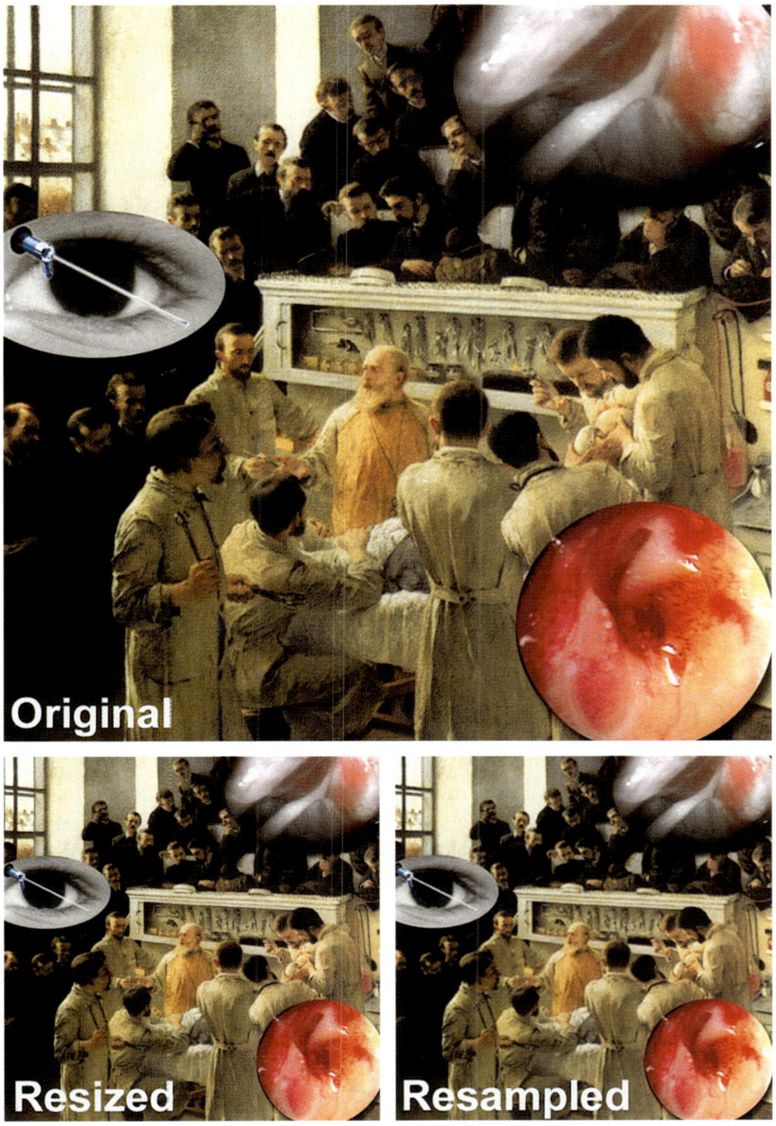


**FIGURE 2.7.** Resizing versus resampling. With resizing of the original image, the resolution has doubled as the dimensions have been cut in half. In contrast, with resampling of the image, the original and resampled images have exactly the same resolution as the dimensions have been cut in half.

## Layers

Layers add tremendous flexibility in processing digital endoscopic images for publication or presentation. Each layer is independent of the others, and this allows the user of Photoshop to change the labeling of an image at will. In contrast, if the image were flattened, the pixels would be merged, and if you wanted to remove a label or arrow, the basic image would not be left intact. This is illustrated later in this chapter. The following sections demonstrate the basic processing of an image using layers. Advanced texts should be consulted to resolve more complex image flaws (1–4).

## Preparing the Basic Image

After cropping, resampling, and resizing the image, I create an empty layer by choosing *Layer → New → Layer,* or I follow the parallel path from the Layers palette. Be sure to turn on the Group With Previous Layer check box. Next, in the Background Layer containing the original image, choose *Select → All* and then *Edit → Cut.* Select Layer 1 and then choose *Edit → Paste.* This action transfers the raw image to the new layer. The next step is to choose *Layer → Duplicate Layer* or to follow the parallel path in the Layers Palette. We are now ready to begin the corrective filtering stage of the digital image processing.

### *Corrective Filtering of Digital Images*

I routinely use a series of steps to clean up a digital image (Fig. 2.8). These measures firm the detail and smooth the color transitions by applying a combination of filters. These are, in order of use, Despeckle, Median, Gaussian Blur, and

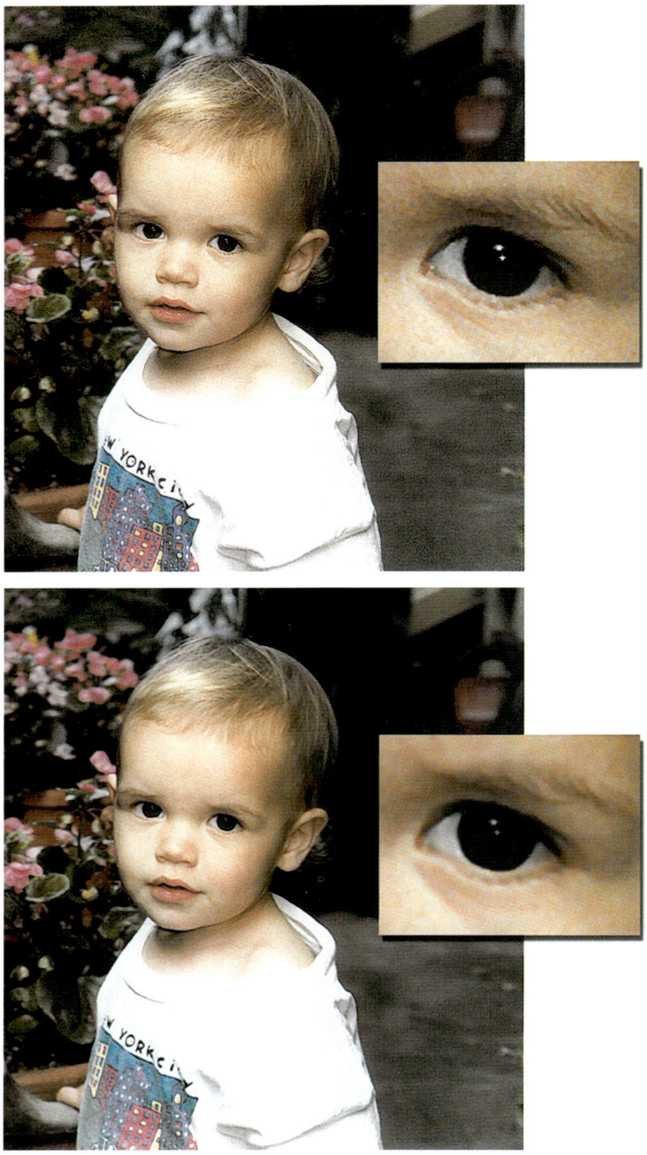

**FIGURE 2.8.** Corrective filtering of digital images. The difference is illustrated between directly filtering a digital image **(top)** and waiting to sharpen it until after preparing the image with Despeckle, Median, Gaussian Blur, and Unsharp Mask **(bottom)**.

Unsharp Mask. All of these steps are followed only in the Duplicate Layer.

1. Choose *Filter → Noise → Despeckle.* This filter blurs a selection while simultaneously preserving its edges. This has the effect of minimizing unwanted noise in the most noticeable area—the continuous regions of an image.
2. Choose *Filter → Noise → Median.* Median removes noise by averaging the colors in an image, 1 pixel at a time. I select a value of 2.0 pixels in the Radius options box. The filter averages the colors in the neighboring pixels that fall inside the specified radius, ignoring any pixels that are starkly different and thereby avoiding skewing the average, and it then applies the average color to the central pixel.
3. Choose *Filter → Blur → Gaussian Blur.* In contrast to Median, Gaussian Blur softens or destroys edges, depending on the pixel radius selected. I select a Radius value of 1.0 pixels to soften the edges that Median created. This blurs the detail slightly.
4. Choose *Filter → Sharpen → Unsharp Mask.* This step produces intense sharpening of the digital image. I use the maximum amount (500%) and a Threshold of 0 levels. It is important to match the radius used in the Gaussian Blur step (e.g., Radius of 1.0).
5. Lower the layer's opacity value. The visible layer, which is the uppermost layer containing the filter image in this case, becomes a little too smooth. The opacity can be adjusted in the Layers Palette, and the default level is always 100%. I decrease this to 50%, which allows the starker original digital image to have a semitransparent, smoother version superimposed on it.
6. Merge the image. Choose *Filter → Sharpen → Unsharp Mask* with a Radius of 1.0 pixel, Threshold of 0 levels, and an Amount of 200%. It is typically necessary to choose *Edit → Undo Unsharp Mask* and redo the Unsharp Mask filtering with a greater or lesser amount of unsharp masking until the desired appearance has been achieved. Figure 2.8 shows the difference between applying the Unsharp Mask filter to the original image (Fig. 2.8, top) and the filtered mixture (Fig. 2.8, bottom) resulting from these steps 1 through 6. The top figure shows a wealth of undesirable artifacts, whereas the bottom figure appears smooth and crisp.

### *Special Filtering*

There is another filter offered in the *Filter → Noise* submenu called Dust & Scratches. This filter is designed to remove dust particles, hairs, scratches, and other imperfections of a scan. Trial and error with the two options of Radius and Threshold produce the cleanest, most visually pleasing image.

### *Adjustment of Color, Brightness, and Contrast*

After completing the corrective filtering, I begin the process of adjusting the color and brightness. Choose *Image → Adjust → Variations*, and you can see a thumbnail or the Original Image, as well as a thumbnail image of the Current Pick, allowing easy comparison. Options for adjusting Shadows, Midtones, Highlights, or Saturation are available, and one of these should be selected first. I usually work with the Midtones. Options are then available to add more Green, Yellow, Cyan, Red, Blue, or Magenta. Multiple choices can be made, and the composite Current Pick can be compared alongside the Original Image. The image can also be made Lighter or Darker in this control panel. After the image has been adjusted in the control panel, the selections can be applied to the entire image. If dissatisfied, choose *Edit → Undo Variations* and begin again.

For more controlled changes of brightness and contrast, choose *Image → Adjust → Brightness/Contrast* and sliding scales for each are available in the control box. Checking the Preview box allows assessment of how each variable has affected the image.

Color correction is a huge topic, and Photoshop has a wide range of sophisticated tools to accomplish this. The reader is referred to a variety of texts that address these methods in great detail (1–4).

## Labeling

Annotation of the digital image often enhances the ability to clearly present anatomic information or a specific point in surgical technique. With Photoshop, these labels can be directly added to the digital image. By using layers, labels, lines, or arrows can be added without disturbing the original image.

### *Use of Layers*

Another tremendous advantage of Photoshop's layers is the ability to add a layer on top of the image and then apply labels or arrows without affecting the pixels of the image. These labels can be subsequently moved or removed without damaging the digital image. Choose *Layer → New → Layer* and then check the Group with Previous Layer option found in the control panel. You are now ready to begin annotating the image.

### *Develop Label File*

Using the Type Tool found on the Tool Bar, a control box will offer options of Font, Size, and Alignment. After typing the desired information, selecting OK places the text in the layer above the digital image. Arrows can be added using the Line Tool found on the Tool Bar; a control box offers options of Weight (i.e., thickness of the line) and whether the arrowhead is at the start or end of the line to be drawn. I recommend placing the arrowhead at the start so that precise placement relative to the image can be obtained. Options for the shape of the arrowhead are offered, and they include the Width, Length, and Concavity.

I have found it useful to create a separate file that contains labels, arrows, and arrowheads (Fig. 2.9).These have been constructed so that a black version of the letter or arrow is placed in an offset manner over a white version of the same letter or arrow and merged. Each of these can be copied by selecting the Rectangular Marquee Tool found on the Tool Bar, drawing a rectangle around the desired object,

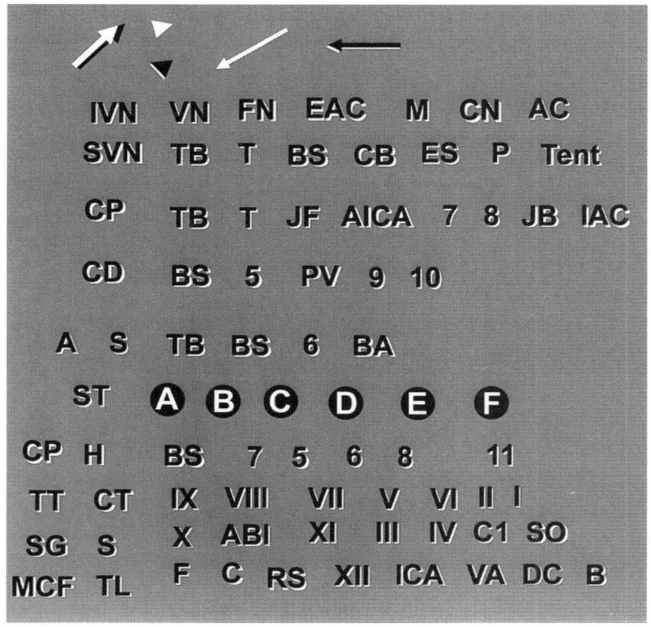


**FIGURE 2.9.** Label file. Creation of a separate file containing labels, arrows, and arrowheads is a useful and time-saving measure. Copying the desired label and pasting it into a new layer on top of the digital endoscopic image allows annotation without damage to the original image. Inversion before copying allows white-on-black labels, if this is more appropriate for the area of the endoscopic image to be annotated.

choosing *Edit → Copy*, and then after returning to the layer above the digital image, choosing *Edit → Paste*. The label or arrow can then be moved using the Move Tool found on the Tool Bar. For arrows or arrowheads, rotation to place the tip at the desired target can be accomplished by choosing *Edit → Free Transform* and rotating the selected arrow or arrowhead.

The black-on-white letters and arrows provide enhanced contrast and improve the ease of seeing the label over the digital endoscopic image. If a white-on-black label provides better contrast, then choose *Image → Adjust → Invert* in the Label File before starting the selection and then use the copy, paste, move, and transform sequence previously described.

After completing all of the labeling, I recommend merging all of the layers that contain labels into one layer; however, it is important *not* to merge this layer with the layer containing the endoscopic image. As discussed in the introductory paragraph discussing Layers, this allows the flexibility of changing your mind about the labeling in the future. The final Photoshop file is then saved. I then flatten the image by choosing *Layer → Save As*, and in the control panel, I select Save As TIFF and then select OK. At this point, I have a 300 ppi Photoshop file with the Layers intact and a TIFF file with the pixels merged. Next, I choose *Image → Image Size* and resample the image to decrease the resolution to 150 or 200 ppi while keeping the size constant. I then choose *File → Save As*, add 150 or 200 ppi to the file name, and save it as a separate TIFF file. This lower-resolution image occupies much less disk space and can be inserted into a slide using a presentation software program such as PowerPoint.

## SUBMISSION OF DIGITAL IMAGES FOR PUBLICATION

Most publishers prefer digital images be submitted as TIFF files with a resolution of 300 ppi. I also submit the Photoshop format file with the layers intact in case the production staff wish to change the labeling. Because of the file sizes, it is necessary to submit all of the files together on a Zip disk or as a CD-ROM. I also send digital prints from a dye sublimation printer or color slides so that the colors and image quality I was happy with at the time of submission can be faithfully reproduced during the production process.

### Color

An understanding of the differences between the RGB and CMYK color modes is necessary when finalizing the digital image for publication.

#### *Red, Green, and Blue Model*

RGB is the color mode of light and comprises three primary colors: red, green, and blue. Each of these three colors can vary among 256 levels of intensity and therefore can provide tremendous range in creating colors. The RGB model is an *additive primary model* because a color becomes lighter as you add higher levels of red, green, and blue light. All computer monitors, data projection systems, televisions, and movie projectors use the additive primary model. Unfortunately, the commercial printing industry cannot use this model. This means that it is necessary to print in the RGB mode using a high-resolution color printer, such as a dye sublimation printer or output the image on a film recorder. Both of these imaging instruments are briefly discussed later; however, it is important to submit color prints or slides so that the professionals can match the RGB colors as closely as possible using CMYK color correction.

#### *Cyan, Magenta, Yellow, and Black Model*

In contrast to the additive primary model, our eyes perceive pigments according to the *subtractive color model.* When white light is projected on an object, the object absorbs (i.e., subtracts) some of the light and reflects the rest. The reflected light is the color you see. Pigments on a sheet of paper work the same way. The subtractive primary colors used by commercial printers are cyan, magenta, and yellow (CMY). To accentuate shadows, deepen dark colors, and print true blacks, a fourth color is added—black (K).

Because of the huge range of colors available in RGB, it is possible to create colors that are vivid and cannot be produced in the CMYK mode. This is why, when you switch from RGB to CMYK, the colors appear duller. I provide the color RGB prints or color RGB generated slides to the printer so that the production department can perform the CMYK color correction.

### Printers

Ink jet and thermal wax printers are inexpensive color printers that can be useful in the assessment of various stages of digital image processing. However, they are unacceptable to produce photographic-quality prints. Dye sublimation printers can fulfill this need. Dye sublimation ink permeates the surface of the paper, literally dying it different colors. The cyan, magenta, yellow, and black pigments mix in various opacities from one dot to the next, resulting in a continuous tone image that appears nearly as smooth on the page as it does on the screen. I use a Tektronix Phaser 450 dye sublimation printer, which can print files in RGB or CMYK color formats. Additional information can be found in their web site (www.tektronix.xerox.com).

### Film Recorders

Film recorders transfer digital images to full-color 35-mm slides or to 4 × 5 inch transparencies in more expensive devices. Commercial printers can use the slides to create color separations. Further information about various film recorders can be found in several of the web sites listed in Table 2.1.

## CONCLUSIONS

This chapter outlined the basic steps of digital image processing. More advanced techniques are described in the references provided, and additional resources are available in the web sites provided in this chapter. However, there is much greater satisfaction in working with and experimenting with Photoshop.

## REFERENCES

1. McClelland D. *Photoshop 6 for Windows bible*. New York: Hungry Minds, 2000.
2. McClelland D, Eismann K. *Photoshop studio secrets*, 2nd ed. New York: Hungry Minds, 1999.
3. Evening M. *Adobe Photoshop 6 for photographers*. Woburn, MA: Focal Press, 2001.
4. Margulis D. *Professional Photoshop 5: the classic guide to color correction*. New York: John Wiley & Sons, 1998.

# 3

# COMPUTED TOMOGRAPHY- AND MAGNETIC RESONANCE-GUIDED IMAGING SYSTEMS FOR STEREOTACTIC SURGERY OF THE HEAD AND NECK

TODD A. LOEHRL
TIMOTHY L. SMITH
PETER D. COSTANTINO
PHILLIP A. WACKYM

The development of image-guidance systems has facilitated the expansion of minimally invasive approaches to complex surgical head and neck problems. Real-time stereotactic image-guided systems have been especially useful in endoscopic sinus surgery for minimally invasive surgical management of inflammatory and neoplastic disease and for skull base diseases involving the anterior, central, and lateral skull base. Computer-guided endoscopic surgery (CGES) allows the surgeon to localize an instrument in a head or neck cavity through the use of computerized stereotactic tracking systems. Such a system provides a real-time video display of instrument location on a preoperative computed tomography (CT) scan, based on the digital CT image data set resulting from the study. CGES is especially helpful in identifying spaces within the sinonasal cavity or skull base when previous surgery or disease processes have distorted the normal anatomic landmarks. This chapter reviews the role of CGES in the management of surgical head and neck diseases.

## IMAGE GUIDANCE SYSTEMS

Image guidance systems were initially developed for neurosurgical and neuro-otologic procedures using a stereotactic frame that required fixation of the patient's head (1). They were subsequently adapted for use in endoscopic sinus surgery. These systems assist the surgeon with intraoperative stereotactic anatomic localization through the use of computerized tracking devices. The tracking devices can localize the position of endoscopic instruments within the sinonasal cavity and depict them on a real-time video display of the preoperative CT scan using the digital data set of the imaging study.

Four types of technology allow intraoperative image guidance: electromechanical, electromagnetic, optical, and sonic. For practical purposes, electromagnetic and optical systems are the most useful for CGES. The sonic system is not widely available in the United States and is not discussed further in this chapter. An example of the electromechanical system was introduced by ISG Technologies (Mississauga, Ontario, Canada). It uses a mechanical arm, called a *wand*, for anatomic localization. Anon and colleagues reviewed their experience with this system in treating 70 patients. No complications were reported, and anecdotally, the investigators believed the system was useful for revision surgery, massive disease, frontal recess or sphenoid disease, and anatomic variants (2). However, this system requires preoperative placement of fiducials, repeat registration with intraoperative head movement, and a mechanical arm (3). With the early generations of these devices, these more complex systems were necessary for use with neuro-otologic skull base surgery applications, but with the advances described later, the electromagnetic and optical systems are the most commonly used for paranasal sinus surgery and neuro-otologic skull base surgery.

Visualization Technology, Inc. (Woburn, MA), introduced an electromagnetic system (InstaTrak) that relies on a radiofrequency transmitter mounted to a patient headset and an electromagnetic sensor incorporated in a handpiece (Figs. 3.1 and 3.2). The InstaTrak is a frameless, wandless system that uses preoperative CT images for three-plane, real-time intraoperative localization of curved and straight surgical aspirators (Fig. 3.3). The headset contains seven fiducial markers. Disadvantages of this system include the need to wear a headpiece during the preoperative CT scan and interference from metallic objects near the surgical field. Neumann and coworkers reviewed their experience using the electromagnetic InstraTrak system in 109 patients, 76 of whom had undergone previous surgery. The estimated accuracy was less than 3 mm in 106 (97.2%) patients, and in no patients did unacceptable intraoperative drift occur. Setup of the InstaTrak system, including headset placement, draping, calibration, and verifi-

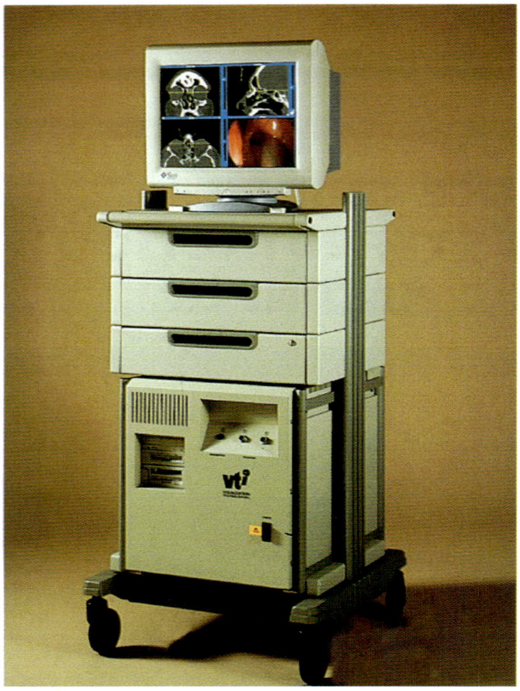

**FIGURE 3.1.** Electromagnetic image-guidance system (InstaTrak, Visualization Technology, Inc., Woburn, MA).

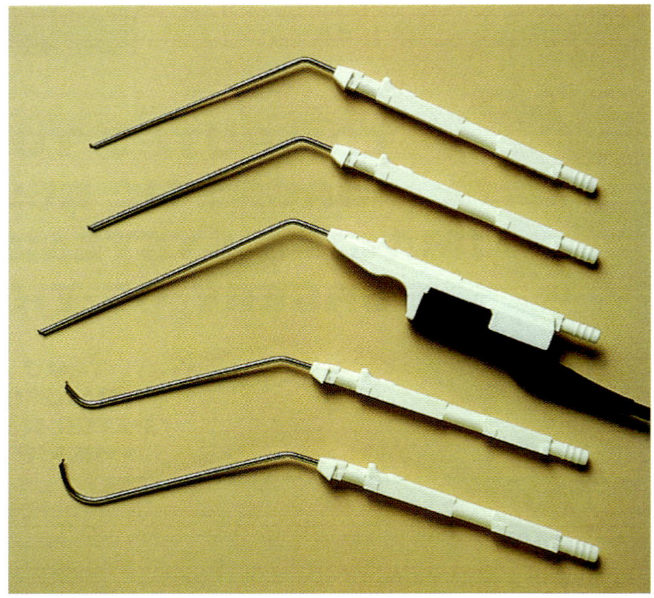

**FIGURE 3.3.** Integrated sinus instrumentation (Instatrak, Visualization Technology, Inc., Woburn, MA).

cation, took less than 5 minutes in all cases. Orbital fat exposure occurred in two patients and was the only reported intraoperative complication. Two patients developed cerebrospinal fluid leaks, but these were anticipated given the underlying pathology (i.e., osteoma and meningioma). Postoperative complications included persistent synechiae in four patients and epistaxis in one patient. These investigators concluded that the technology was useful for all patients undergoing revision sinus surgery, patients with skull base defects, those with paranasal sinus tumors, and patients with extensive disease undergoing primary surgery (4).

The optical-based image guidance system uses an infrared camera to monitor instrument and head positions. Light-emitting diodes (LEDs) are mounted on the surgical instrument and the headset worn by the patient, which are tracked by an infrared camera (Figs. 3.4 to 3.6). The tracking data is processed by an optical digitizer that displays the instrument location on reformatted and triplanar CT images (Fig. 3.7). Several investigators have evaluated the utility of this stereotactic system in neuro-otologic skull base surgery and in endoscopic sinus surgery (5–7). Metson and associates reviewed

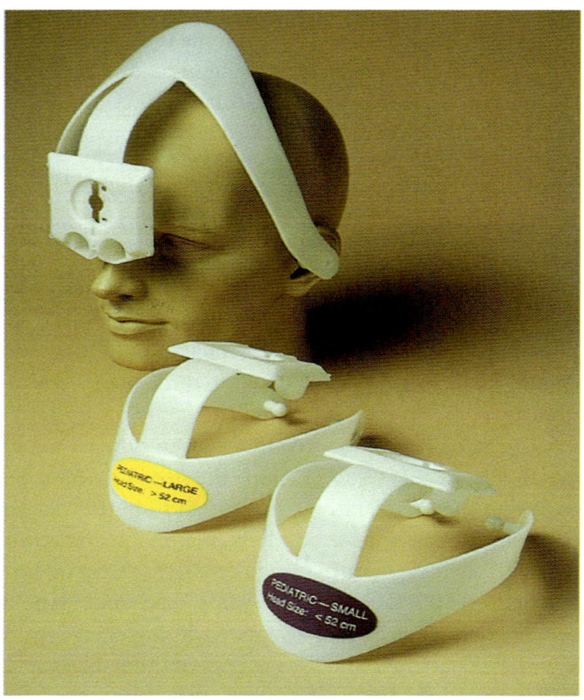

**FIGURE 3.2.** Autoregistration head sets (InstaTrak, Visualization Technology, Inc., Woburn, MA).

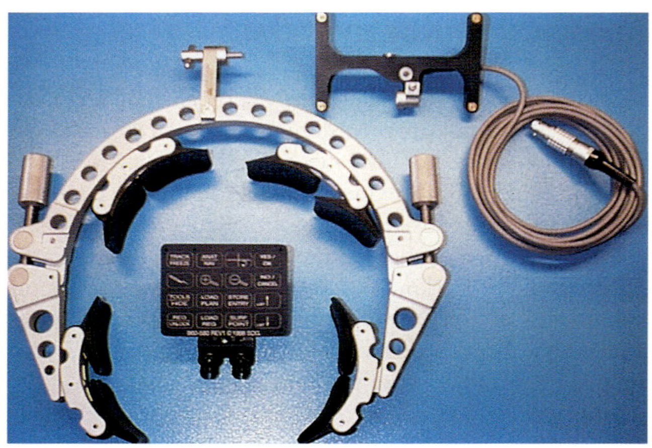

**FIGURE 3.4.** Infrared image-guidance system registration headset (Medtronic/LandmarX, Xomed, Inc., Jacksonville, FL).

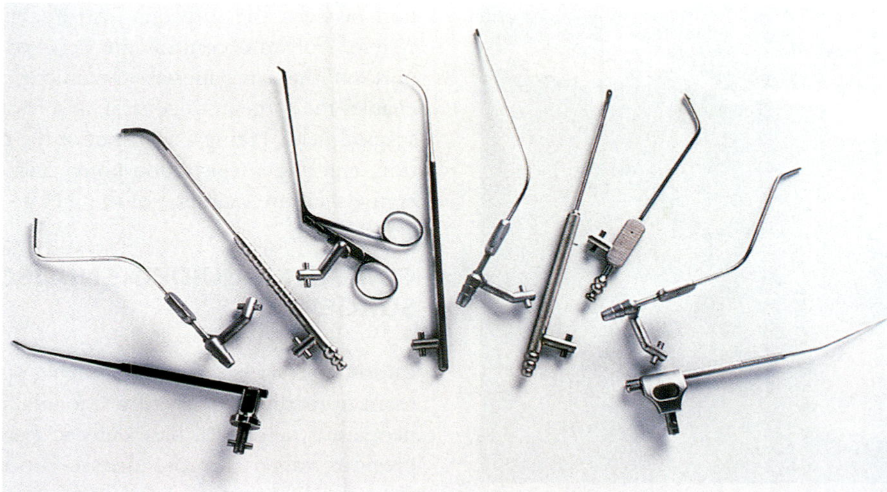

**FIGURE 3.5.** Integrated sinus instrumentation (Medtronic/LandmarX, Xomed, Inc., Jacksonville, FL).

754 consecutive patients undergoing computer-guided endoscopic sinus surgery (CGESS) by 34 physicians using the LandmarX system (Xomed, Inc., Jacksonville, FL). This wandless, frameless system does not require fiducial or headset placement for the preoperative CT scan. The mean accuracy of anatomic localization at the beginning of surgery was 1.69 ± 0.38 mm when five anatomic fiducials were used in the registration process. The use of the image guidance system was estimated to increase operating room time by 15 to 30 minutes for the first five cases each surgeon performed. With experience, surgeons required only 5 to 15 minutes of setup time. There were no intraoperative complications; however, three cases of epistaxis occurred within 1 week of surgery. The three cases of epistaxis were unrelated to CGESS. The mean follow-up time was 15 months, and the surgeons who used the system completed a questionnaire. The most common case in which CGES was used was revision sinus surgery. The major reported disadvantage was increased operating room time (71%), and the major advantage was an increased level of confidence during surgery (85%). The overall use of this system was rated "easy" (31.8%) or "very easy" (50%) by surgeons. Ninety-two percent of surgeons anticipated continued use at the same or increased frequency. The investigators conclude that an optical-based CGES can be successfully integrated into a busy operating room environment used by multiple sinus surgeons. When properly used, it may extend the limits of safe and effective sinus surgery, especially in patients with distorted anatomic landmarks (8).

BrainLAB, Inc. (Redwood City, CA), introduced two optical-based computer-guided imaging systems named VectorVision$^2$ (Fig. 3.8) and VectorVision Compact. Of the several novel features of these systems, most notable is that they are wireless and allow the calibration of any preexisting

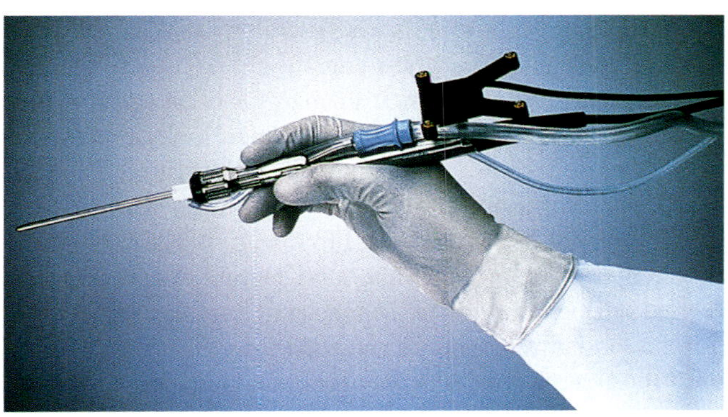

**FIGURE 3.6.** Integrated microdebrider (Medtronic/LandmarX, Xomed, Inc., Jacksonville, FL).

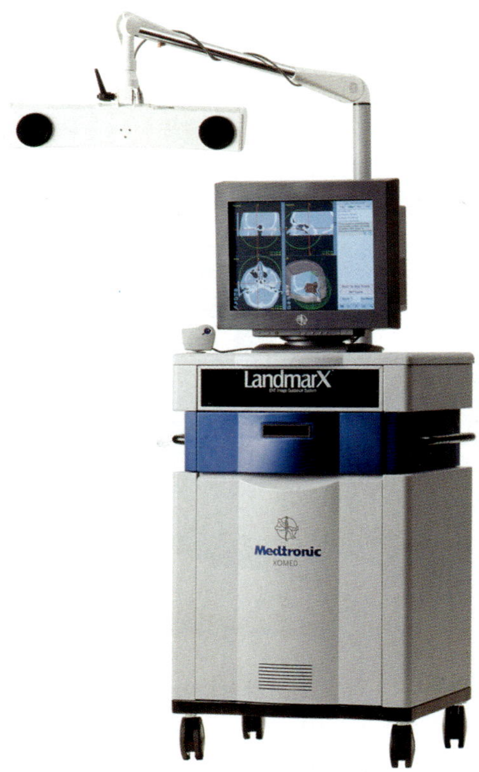


**FIGURE 3.7.** Infrared image guidance system (Medtronic/LandmarX, Xomed, Inc., Jacksonville, FL).

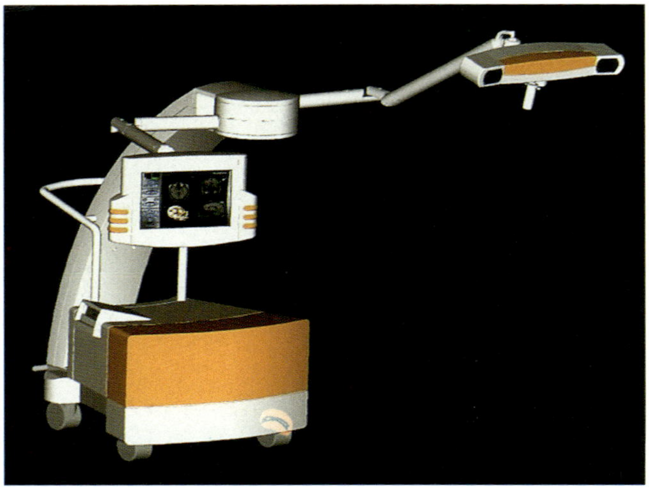

**FIGURE 3.8.** VectorVision² (BrainLAB, Inc., Redwood City, CA).

instrument within seconds through the use of passive markers that are clamped to the handle of the instrument. This system does not require fiducial markers, because registration can be accomplished with a computer comparison of intraoperative laser scanning of the head to the CT or MRI data set (or both data sets). Another advantage of this system is the flat panel monitor that uses a touch pad technology that obviates the need for a computer keyboard or a mouse.

Stryker Leibinger (Kalamazoo, MI) developed an optical-based image guidance system that uses wireless light emitting diodes. As is the case with the BrainLAB system, the Stryker Navigation system does not require fiducial or headset placement for preoperative imaging. The system uses wireless LEDs in the instrumentation and patient tracking systems (Fig. 3.9). The Stryker IGT camera incorporates an active communication between the surgeon's instrument and the navigational system. Software controls are accessed through an infrared port on the navigational instrument. This communication enables the surgeon to control all software functions from the surgical field. Taking a snapshot of the current operative position, entering a registration point, and changing the intraoperative view are examples of the remote software functions.

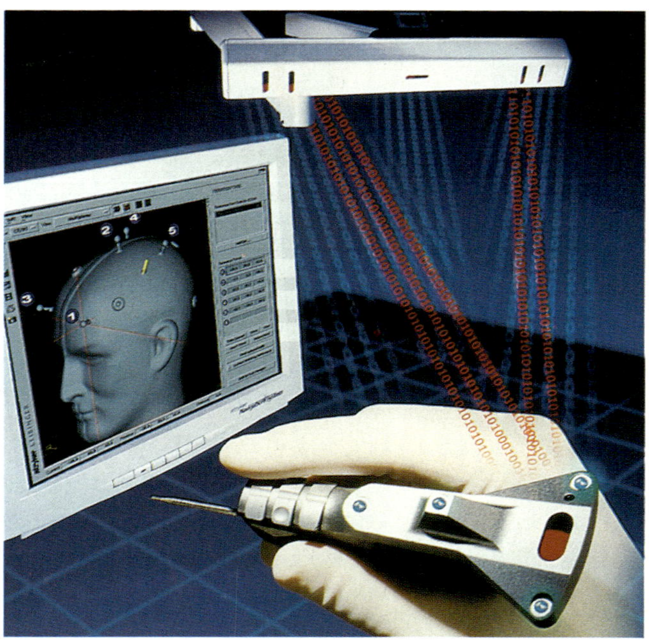

**FIGURE 3.9.** Stryker Navigational system (Stryker Leibinger, Kalamazoo, MI).

## COMPUTER-GUIDED ENDOSCOPIC SINUS SURGERY

Endoscopic sinus surgery is a viable option for the management of medically refractory sinonasal inflammatory disease, neoplasms, and skull base defects. However, in many cases, previous surgery or the disease process has distorted the anatomy. In cases of severe sinonasal inflammation or some tumors, bleeding can obscure the surgeon's view. This can make thorough removal of diseased tissue difficult and potentially hazardous to the patient. Given the close proximity of vital structures, including the intracranial contents and orbit, even minimal intraoperative disorientation can result in serious complications. In an attempt to improve the safety and efficacy of the endoscopic approach to sinonasal disease, image guidance systems were developed. Although several surgeons have reviewed their experience with different types of image guidance systems in the published literature, it is still unclear whether CGESS accomplishes these goals.

The ideal image guidance system allows for correlation of the patient's anatomy with the CT image to 2 mm or less. Intraoperative head movement should not affect the accuracy of the system. Other favorable characteristics include a frameless, wandless system; ease of setup and use; and lack of need for fiducial placement on skin. There are several drawbacks to using the skin fiducial method, including the need for placement of the fiducials and the CT scan the day before surgery. The fiducials may fall off and may move after the patient is anesthetized and the facial musculature relaxes.

One article reviewed the experience of two of the surgeons with optical- and electromagnetic-based systems in treating 79 patients. Both systems provided an accuracy of less than 2 mm at the start of surgery. However, by the completion of surgery, accuracy had deteriorated by an average of 0.89 mm because of anatomic drift. Even at this accuracy level, the surgeons thought both systems were useful because, when properly used, image guidance systems should be used to identify larger spaces, not to distinguish margins of safety at a millimeter level. Disadvantages of the system include increased operating room time and expense. CGES increased the mean total operating room time by 17.4 minutes. However, the actual surgical time was not prolonged because the time required to position, calibrate, and register the system was carried out before the start of surgery. This value represented a mean, and after operating room personnel became familiar with the system, this value was reduced to less than 10 minutes. The investigators calculated that use of CGESS increased total charges by $496 per case because of the increased operating room time. Because of the increased time and expense associated with CGESS, the investigators do not recommend it for routine head and neck cases (9).

At the Medical College of Wisconsin, an optical-based computerized image guidance system (Medtronic/Sofamor Danek Stealth Station, using the LandmarX software) is positioned, calibrated, and registered as follows (10). The patient undergoes a preoperative image-guided CT scan without fiducials. During the induction of anesthesia, the system is set up and the CT data loaded into the computer. After the patient is asleep, topical decongestants are placed in the sinonasal cavity. While waiting for decongestion to occur, the image-guided headset is placed. The patient is subsequently prepped and draped. The endoscopes and instrumentation are arranged for the procedure, and local anesthetic (i.e., 1% lidocaine and 1:100,000 epinephrine) is injected into the side to be operated on first. While allowing vasoconstriction to occur, the registration is carried out using six anatomic landmarks. After accurate registration is obtained (<2 mm), CGESS commences. In most cases, this takes less than 2 minutes to accomplish, and we wait another 3 to 5 minutes for vasoconstriction. Although it could be argued this process adds to operating room time, it is substantially less than 5 minutes of net additional time.

We have found the system to be most useful in cases requiring frontal sinus ventilation, revision surgery, repair of skull base defects, and resection of sinonasal tumors (11). The instrumentation, which can be integrated (Fig. 3.5), is particularly useful in the endoscopic approach to the frontal sinus. CGESS should be viewed as a means to help identify spaces within the sinonasal cavity, not to measure millimeter increments. It is not a replacement for sound surgical technique, anatomic knowledge, and experience. The following case report indicates how CGESS can be used to more thoroughly ventilate the frontal sinus.

*Case:* A 42-year-old, white woman presented with right frontal discomfort that she had experienced for the past 4 years. She had undergone bilateral functional endoscopic sinus surgery at an outside institution 5 years earlier. She denied nasal obstruction or purulence. She had failed to respond to medical attempts to ventilate her frontal sinus, including allergy evaluation, numerous courses of antibiotics, topical and systemic steroids, saline irrigations, and decongestants. She subsequently underwent right frontal sinusotomy [i.e., Draf II procedure (12)] with complete resolution of her symptoms (Figs. 3.10 to 3.12). She remains asymptomatic at 1 year after surgery with a widely patent frontal recess.

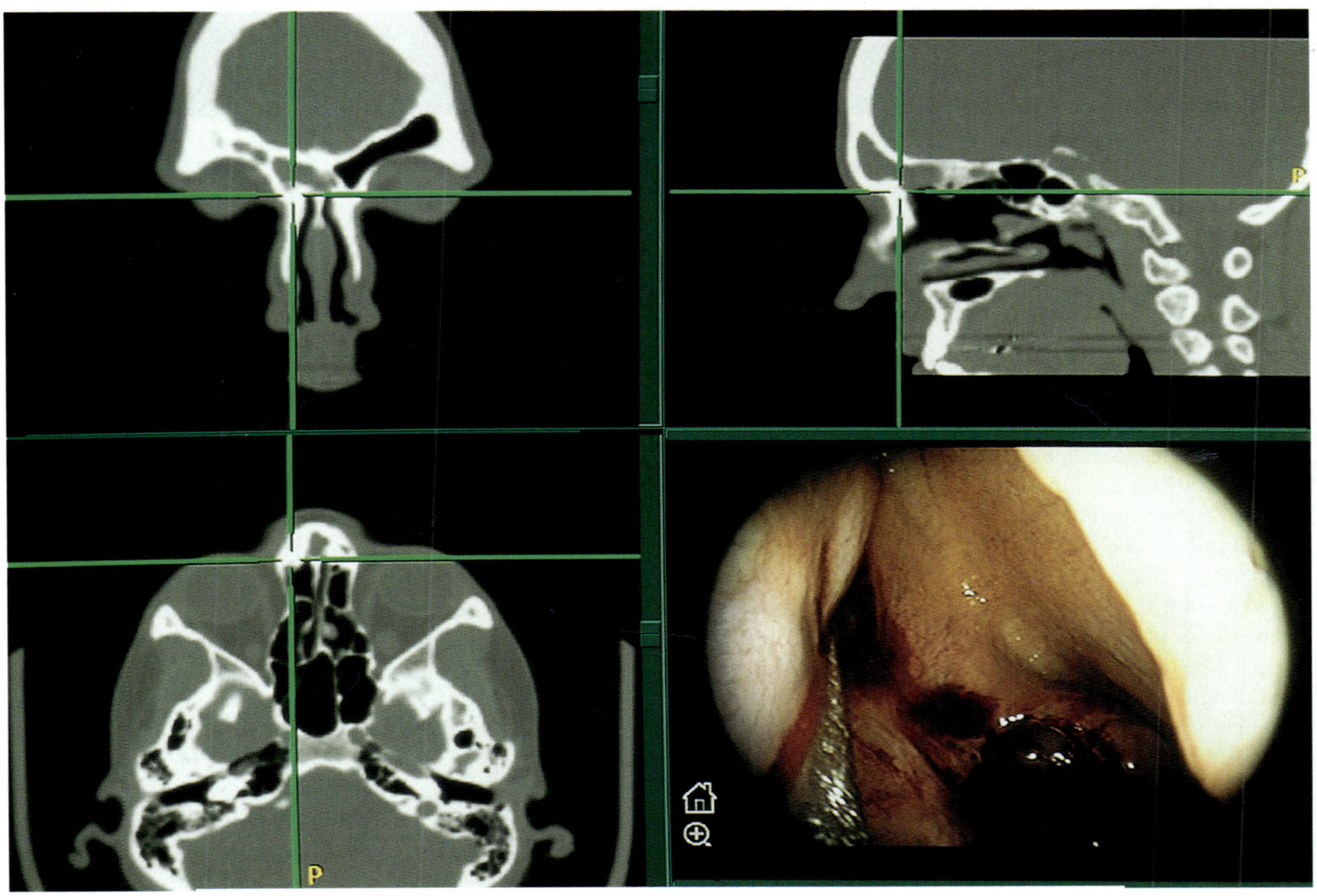


**FIGURE 3.10.** Intraoperative view before surgical manipulation of the right frontal recess. Notice the distorted surgical landmarks. The location of the instrument on the endoscopic and radiographic images helps confirm the surgeon's position relative to the right frontal recess.

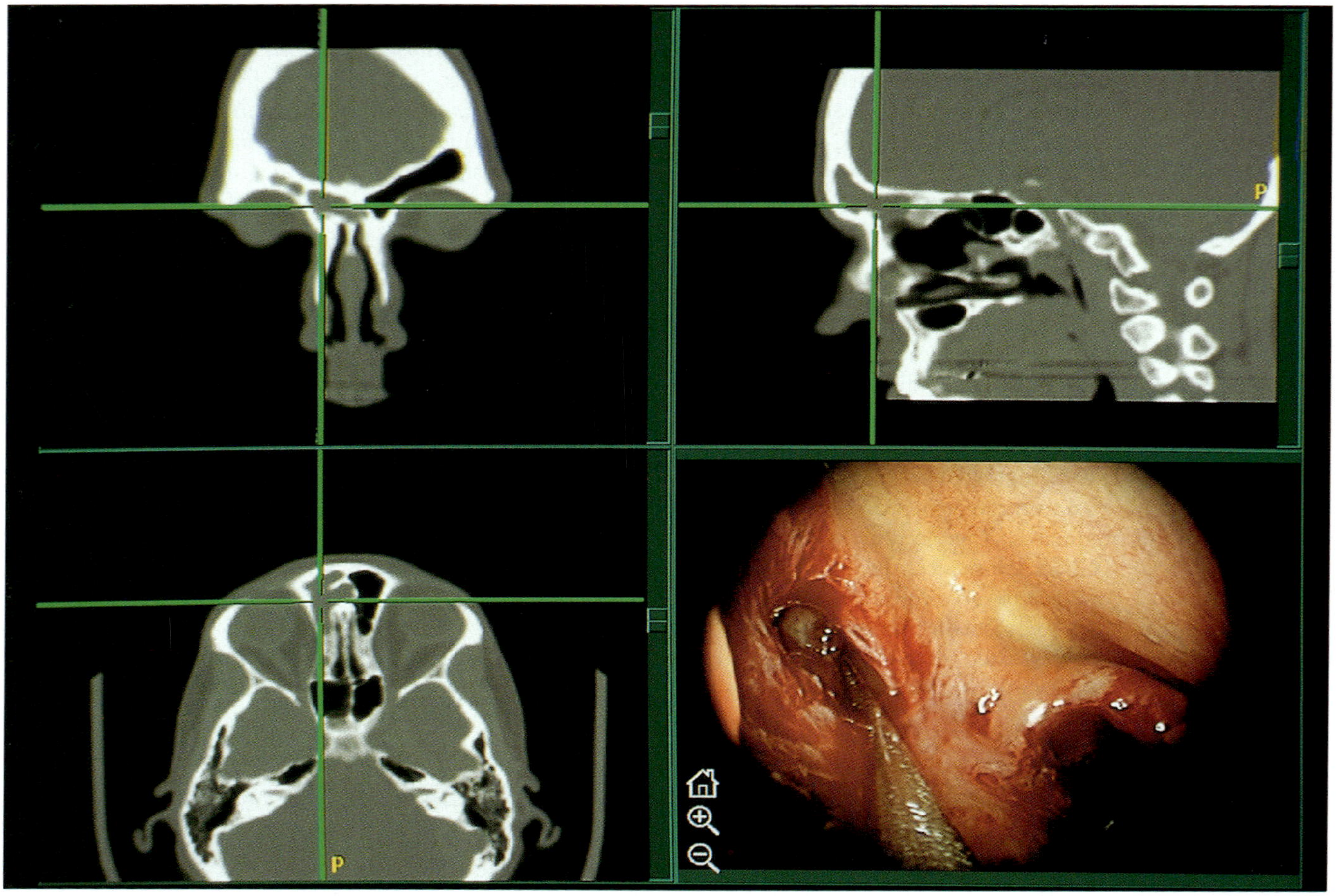

**FIGURE 3.11.** Computer-guided endoscopic sinus surgery, showing intraoperative localization after identifying and ventilating the lateral portion of the frontal recess.

## COMPUTER-GUIDED STEREOTACTIC NEURO-OTOLOGIC SKULL BASE SURGERY

At the Medical College of Wisconsin, we use a frame-based stereotactic system to perform endoscopic surgery for selected, complex skull base lesions. The Stealth Station (Sofamor Danek, Memphis, TN) with the Cranial Software is an optical-based, computerized image guidance system that can be coupled to a handheld probe and used with the surgical microscope or endoscope. The patient undergoes a preoperative image-guided CT scan with fiducial markers placed around the head and fixed with adhesive. This scan can be preformed the day before surgery or the morning of surgery. The disadvantage of the former is that it is possible for individual fiducial markers to fall off; the disadvantage of the latter situation is the additional 30 minutes required to acquire this data set. The data generated during the CT is saved on an optical disk and uploaded in the Stealth workstation at the time of surgery. During the induction of anesthesia, the Stealth workstation is set up and the CT data loaded into the computer. After the patient is asleep, the surgeon places the patient's skull in the head frame. The open-loop stereotactic ring is then attached to the head frame, and the blunt-tipped probe is used to register the fiducial markers. Visual confirmation of external landmarks (e.g., nasal tip) is then completed.

After accurate registration has been obtained (1 to 1.5 mm accuracy within a 3-cm target region), the stereotactic ring is removed. The patient is subsequently prepped and draped, and a sterile stereotactic ring is repositioned. The blunt-tipped probe is then used to confirm the reproducibility of the accuracy relative top the fixed reference post implanted earlier. In our experience, the first five cases required an additional 30 minutes to set up; however, we are now able to routinely accomplish this process in 15 to 20 minutes.

We have found the system to be most useful in the management of complex skull base tumors. The greatest advantage is in providing rapid orientation during the surgical approach that provides complementary information to visually identified landmarks. The stereotactic imaging system can be used with the surgical endoscope in one com-

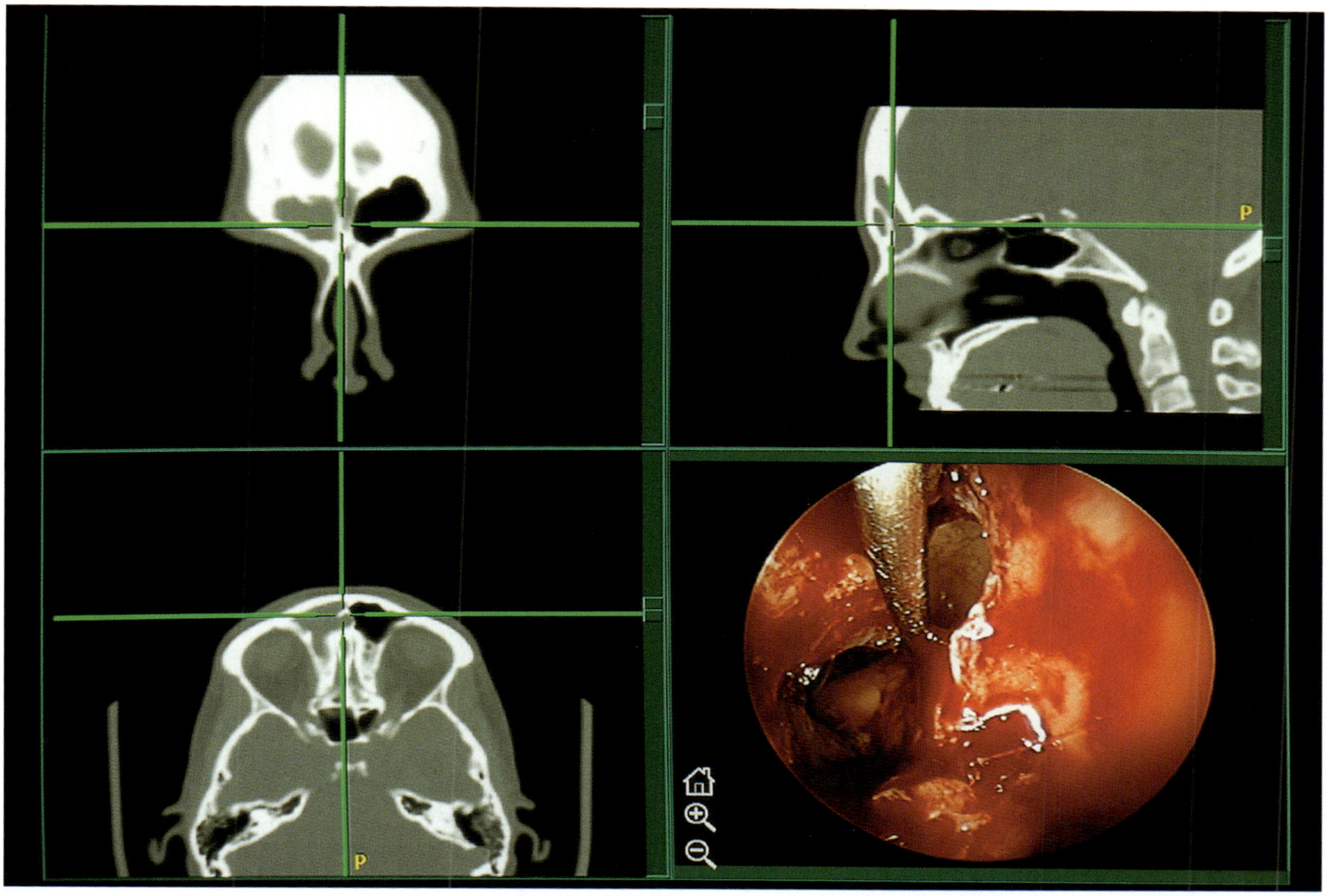


**FIGURE 3.12.** Computer-guided endoscopic sinus surgery after the medial and lateral portions of the right frontal sinus have been ventilated using a Draf type II procedure. A separate pocket of mucopurulence was identified in the medial portion of the frontal sinus with the aid of the image guidance system.

posite image (Fig. 3.13), providing the opportunity for three-dimensional stereotactic orientation while visualizing the anatomic structures adjacent to the top of the endoscope. As is the case with stereotactic endoscopic sinus surgery, this technique is not a replacement for sound surgical technique, anatomic knowledge, and experience.

## ENDOSCOPIC SURGERY WITH MAGNETIC RESONANCE IMAGING GUIDANCE

Endoscopic sinus surgery with magnetic resonance imaging guidance (MRIG) is still in the early phases of development, but it has been used in sinus surgery (13). The investigators reported their experience operating on 12 patients in a vertically open-configuration MRI unit (Signa SP, General Electric Medical Systems, Milwaukee, WI). The main advantage of MRIG is the opportunity to obtain real-time localization and visualization intraoperatively. MRI-updated images could be obtained in as little as 14 seconds so that soft tissue changes resulting from surgery could be monitored intraoperatively. All 12 operations were completed without complications, but the investigators found several limitations to MRIG. These include the lack of MR-safe instrumentation, need for a specialized MRIG suite, and inferior MR image quality. Although CT guidance is sufficient for most procedures, with improved technology, real-time MRIG will be advantageous, particularly in skull base tumor resection. MR incompatibilities, such as with pacemakers, joint replacements, or other metallic prosthesis, can limit use of this modality.

## CONCLUSIONS

Although all investigators agree that computer-guided stereotactic surgery of the head and neck is a helpful adjunctive tool, no study has examined the long-term out-

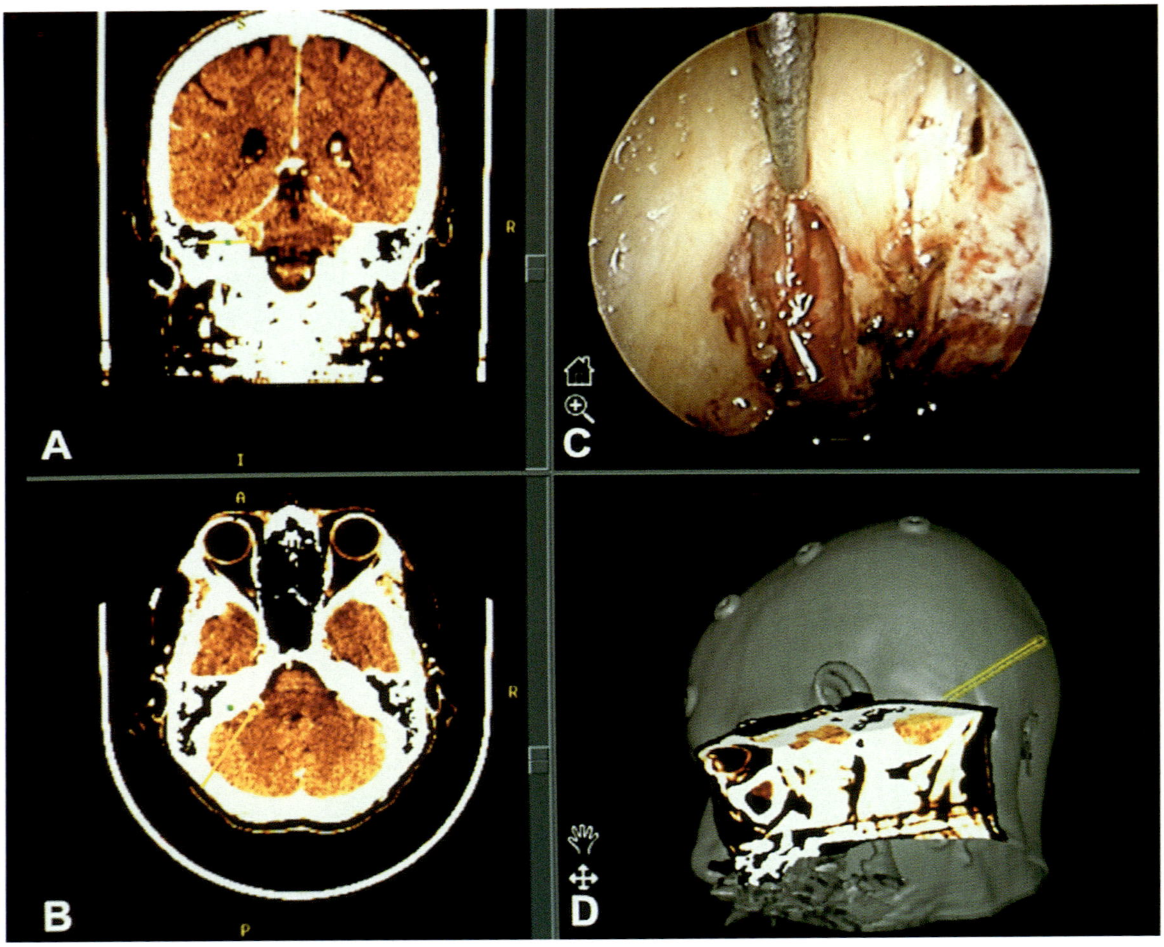


**FIGURE 3.13.** Computer-guided stereotactic endoscopic acoustic neuroma surgery with real-time viewing of the preoperative data set after registration of fiducial markers. The computer workstation formats the computed tomographic data and can display the coronal **(A)** and axial **(B)** images containing the contact point of the blunt-tipped probe *(green dot)*. Notice the left-right formatting convention. The window settings can be adjusted to emphasize bone when determining the lateral extent of internal auditory canal dissection relative to the posterior semicircular canal. A simultaneous operative image **(C)** using a 45° endoscope is also seen on the video monitor. Shown here is the blunt-tipped probe at the fundus of the opened internal auditory canal after a retrosigmoid resection of a left, 1.7-cm-diameter acoustic neuroma. A reconstructed image of the patient's head **(D)** demonstrates the adhesive fiducial markers on the head and the angle of surgical approach *(yellow pointer)*.

comes of the procedure. However, it is possible to surmise that accurate intraoperative anatomic localization should result in more thorough removal of obstructive tissue, neoplasms, or vascular lesions, reducing the need for revision surgery. The image guidance system is useful in surgically managing skull base defects, neuro-otologic skull base surgery, and maintaining orientation during endoscopic resection of sinonasal neoplasms. When properly applied, image guidance extends the limits of endoscopic surgery in the head and neck. However, computer-guided stereotactic surgery remains an adjunct to a thorough knowledge of anatomy, sound surgical technique, and experience.

## REFERENCES

1. Goerss SJ, Kelly PJ, Kall BA, et al. A computed tomographic stereotactic adaptation system. *Neurosurgery* 1982;10:375–379.
2. Anon JB, Lipman SP, Oppenheim D, et al. Computed-assisted endoscopic sinus surgery. *Laryngoscope* 1994;104:901–905.
3. Casiano RR. Intraoperative image-guidance technology. *Arch Otolaryngol Head Neck Surg* 1999;125:1275–1278.
4. Neumann AM, Pasquale-Niebles K, Bhuta T, et al. Image-guided transnasal endoscopic surgery of the paranasal sinuses and anterior skull base. *AJR Am J Roentgenol* 1999;13:449–454.
5. Sargent EW, Bucholz RD. Middle cranial fossa surgery with image-guided instrumentation. *Otolaryngol Head Neck Surg* 1997;117:372–379.

6. Goldsmith MM, Bucholz RD, Smith KR, et al. Clinical applications of frameless stereotactic devices in neurotology: preliminary report. *Am J Otol* 1995;16:475–479.
7. Anon JB, Lipman SP, Oppenheim D, et al. Computer-assisted endoscopic sinus surgery. *Laryngoscope* 1994;104:901–905.
8. Metson RB, Cosenza MJ, Cunningham MJ, et al. Physician experience with an optical image guidance system for sinus surgery. *Laryngoscope* 2000;110:972–976.
9. Metson R, Cosenza M, Gliklich RE, et al. The role of image-guidance in head and neck surgery. *Arch Otolaryngol Head Neck Surg* 1999;125:1100–1104.
10. Loehrl T, Toohill RJ, Smith TL. The use of computer-aided surgery for frontal sinus ventilation. *Laryngoscope* 2000;110: 1962–1967.
11. Smith TL, Loehrl T, Smith M. Surgery of the frontal recess and sinus: the utility of a CT image guidance system in selected cases. *Otolaryngol Head Neck Surg* 2001;12:7–12.
12. Draf W. Endonasal micro-endoscopic frontal sinus surgery: the Fulda concept. *Otolaryngol Head Neck Surg* 1991;2:234–240.
13. Fried MP, Topulos G, Hsu L, et al. Endoscopic sinus surgery with magnetic resonance imaging guidance: initial patient experience. *Otolaryngol Head Neck Surg* 1998;119:374–380.

# 4

# LASERS IN ENDOSCOPIC SURGERY

**TODD A. LOEHRL**
**PHILLIP A. WACKYM**

Lasers are useful tools in the treatment of a diverse array of head and neck disorders. A century ago, Albert Einstein developed several of the theories essential for the creation of the laser. Approximately 60 years later, the first laser was built using a ruby crystal and a flash lamp. Lasers have subsequently moved from the laboratory to the clinic after a series of improvements.

Several characteristics of lasers make them useful in the medical field. Current lasers may be used in conjunction with endoscopes for tissue vaporization, for blood vessel coagulation, and for use as a light scalpel. The specific endoscopic uses of lasers are highlighted in subsequent chapters. This chapter focuses on applicable physics, delivery mechanisms, tissue interactions, safety issues, and pulse structure to facilitate the proper selection and use of lasers in the treatment of patients.

## ADVANTAGES AND DISADVANTAGES OF ENDOSCOPIC LASER USE

The use of endoscopic techniques has revolutionized the management of a variety of surgical problems in numerous disciplines, including otolaryngology, neurosurgery, general surgery, orthopedic surgery, and cardiothoracic surgery. Endoscopes facilitate visualization by providing high magnification and illumination. In contrast to the operating microscope, endoscopic visualization (with angled or flexible endoscopes) is not limited to the linear line of sight, allowing the surgeon to "look around" obstructing anatomic structures. The use of endoscopes potentially enables the use of smaller incisions or avoidance of any incision and allows less collateral tissue manipulation or retraction, resulting in less postoperative discomfort, improved cosmesis, and an expedited recovery.

Endoscopic techniques do have disadvantages. When using endoscopes, the surgeon is essentially a one-handed surgeon, using the endoscope in one hand and an instrument in the other. Even minimal bleeding can result in a compromised view of the surgical field, especially when operating in a tight anatomic area. With the operating microscope, the surgeon can suction with one hand and manipulate tissue with the other. The development of proper surgical technique requires extensive training and practice before operating on patients. The attendance at a certified continuing education course addressing the surgeon's specific area of interest is the minimal requirement before operating on human patients. Ideally, participation in such a course involves supervised cadaver dissection as a part of the curriculum. Observation of experienced endoscopic surgeons and of individual cadaver dissection can further develop the surgeon's technical ability and knowledge.

The use of a thermal coagulating device, such as a laser, in conjunction with endoscopic visualization often enables the surgeon to take a less invasive approach to the patient's disease process than was previously possible. The laser's ability to provide hemostasis, to effect precise tissue ablation, and to incise tissue potentially enhance the surgeon's ability to proceed in a minimally invasive fashion. Continued development and analysis of surgical lasers have resulted in a better understanding of their potential uses and limitations in the treatment of patients. Improvements in surgical laser delivery mechanisms will increase flexibility further, resulting in an even wider variety of applications.

## OVERVIEW OF LASER FUNCTION

Laser is an acronym that stands for light amplification by the stimulated emission of radiation. A laser consists of three basic components: a lasing medium (e.g., a ruby crystal), an excitation source, and two parallel mirrors. The various materials used as a lasing medium are shown in Figure 4.1. The lasing medium is placed in a resonant cavity, which most commonly consists of two precisely aligned parallel mirrors. The lasing medium is then excited so that the molecules are promoted to an excited state. Excitation may be accomplished with flash lamps, continuous lamps, other lasers, or an electrical current. After the laser is excited

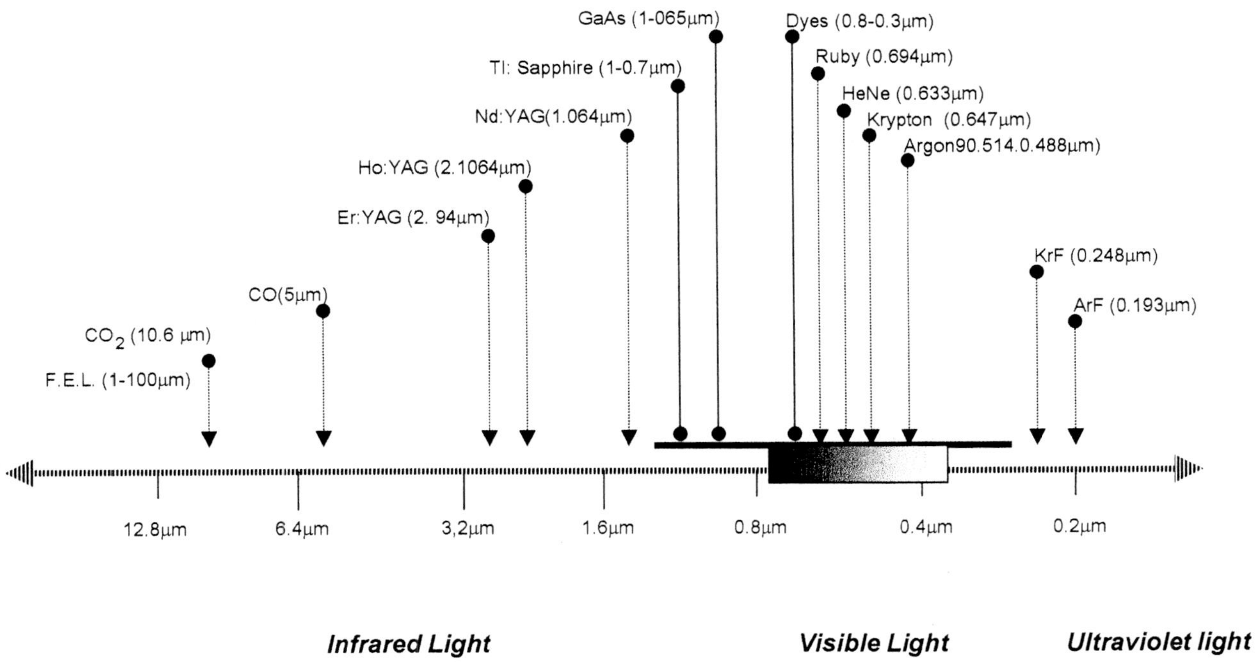


**FIGURE 4.1.** Various materials are used in producing laser light, and their respective wavelengths are shown.

to a higher state, a process referred to as *spontaneous emission* occurs. Spontaneous emission occurs when the excited atoms or molecules decay from their excited state to a lower energy state. The absorbed energy is randomly emitted in all directions. Some of the emission can be reflected back into the lasing medium, stimulating additional radiation. These waves of light continue to propagate through the lasing medium, resulting in a net amplification of the light. When more atoms are in the excited state than the ground state, the condition is called a *population inversion*.

The waves of light reach the front mirror, are reflected back through the lasing medium, and are emitted in the same direction as the incident light. All the waves of light are parallel. This process continues as long as the population inversion exists. A fraction of the laser light is emitted from the resonant cavity through a partially reflecting mirror. The remaining fraction continues to stimulate atoms into the excited state within the lasing medium.

Laser light is monochromatic, coherent, and collimated, and it has high power. These four properties make laser light distinct from a typical overhead light. The monochromatism, collimated nature, and high power of laser light are most important with regard to medical applications. When laser light is passed through a prism, one or a few distinct lines appear on the wall. In contrast, when light from a tungsten lamp is passed through a prism, a rainbow of colors is produced. When intensity versus wavelength is plotted, very high intensities at distinct, separate wavelengths are observed for laser light. The specific wavelength of the individual laser affects hemostasis, tissue absorption, and the zone of thermal necrosis (1).

The high power of laser light enables tissue ablation. When discussing power, the term *power density* (i.e., irradiance) should be used. Power density is intensity of the laser divided by the area of the light beam ($W/cm^2$). The operator also should be aware of the *fluence* of the light. Fluence refers to the energy density and corresponds to the power density multiplied times the exposure time in seconds ($J/cm^2$).

The collimated nature of laser allows the light to be focused to a small spot. The ability to focus the light to a small spot and achieve a high power density is the important factor in achieving tissue ablation.

The laser light can be continuous or pulsed, which affects the laser's interaction with tissue. The pulsed mode allows delivery of the same total amount of light energy per second to the tissue, but there is less thermal damage compared with the continuous mode. High peak intensity of light delivered in a short time interval allows for less thermal diffusion and tissue damage. The variability of the pulse duration can range from seconds to femtoseconds. Different mechanisms are required to achieve different pulse durations. A mechanical shutter is used to obtain pulses from 1 ms to 1 second. This method relies on obstructing the laser beam with a mechanical shutter. Pulses from 1 μs to 1 ms can be obtained using flash lamp–pumped lasers. The laser only emits light when the flash lamp (i.e., excitation source) is on.

Pulse lengths ranging from 10 ns to 10 μs are achieved by Q-switching. A Q-switched laser is a flash lamp–pumped laser with a very fast shutter that is formed by a polarizer and a Pockels cell (Cleveland Crystals, Inc., Cleveland, OH). A Pockels cell is a crystal that rotates the polarization of light when a high voltage is applied. A short, intense laser pulse can be obtained by turning on and off these high voltages very quickly. Electro-optic polarization rotators and acousto-optic beam deflectors are frequently used for Q-switching (2,3).

Most commercial lasers produce a laser beam with a gaussian profile. This is referred to as the fundamental mode or $TEM_{00}$ mode of the laser. This means that the intensity peaks at the center of the beam and falls off with a gaussian-type distribution, allowing a small focal point when the beam is focused through a lens. Some lasers operate in higher-order modes (e.g., $TEM_{01}$) that result in a higher intensity at the edges of the light beam, making them doughnut- or target-shaped beams. The ability to focus the spot size is limited with the higher-order modes (3).

## DELIVERY

Laser light can be delivered by four mechanisms, two of which are suitable for use in conjunction with endoscopes. Articulated arms use mirrors placed at 45° angles to tubes carrying the laser light. The tubes rotate about the normal axis of the mirrors, allowing flexibility in delivery of the laser light. Typically, this method is used for the delivery of carbone dioxide ($CO_2$) laser light. Disadvantages of this delivery mode include the articulating arms, which sometimes do not allow movement in a straight line, and a counterweight that may pull against the surgeon's hand. Despite these drawbacks, this continues to be a very important means of laser delivery.

The optical fiber is commonly used with visible and near-infrared lasers. It is composed of a thin core of glass (400 to 600 μm) that traps the light and allows it to propagate down through the fiber. This process is referred to as *total internal reflection*. In the process of delivery through the optical fiber, the laser light loses coherence and collimation. The loss of collimation limits the focal spot size.

The other two techniques for laser light delivery include handheld lasers and patient-to-laser methods. Because they are not feasible for endoscopic surgery, they are not discussed further in this chapter.

## LASER-TISSUE INTERACTION

The wavelength of the laser used determines the tissue effects produced by the radiant energy as each tissue type has its own absorption spectrum (4). Three processes play a role in the laser energy tissue effect. First, the laser energy is absorbed by chromophores within the tissue, resulting in the production of heat. Second, the radiant energy of the laser can stimulate specific molecules within a cell, causing a chemical reaction.

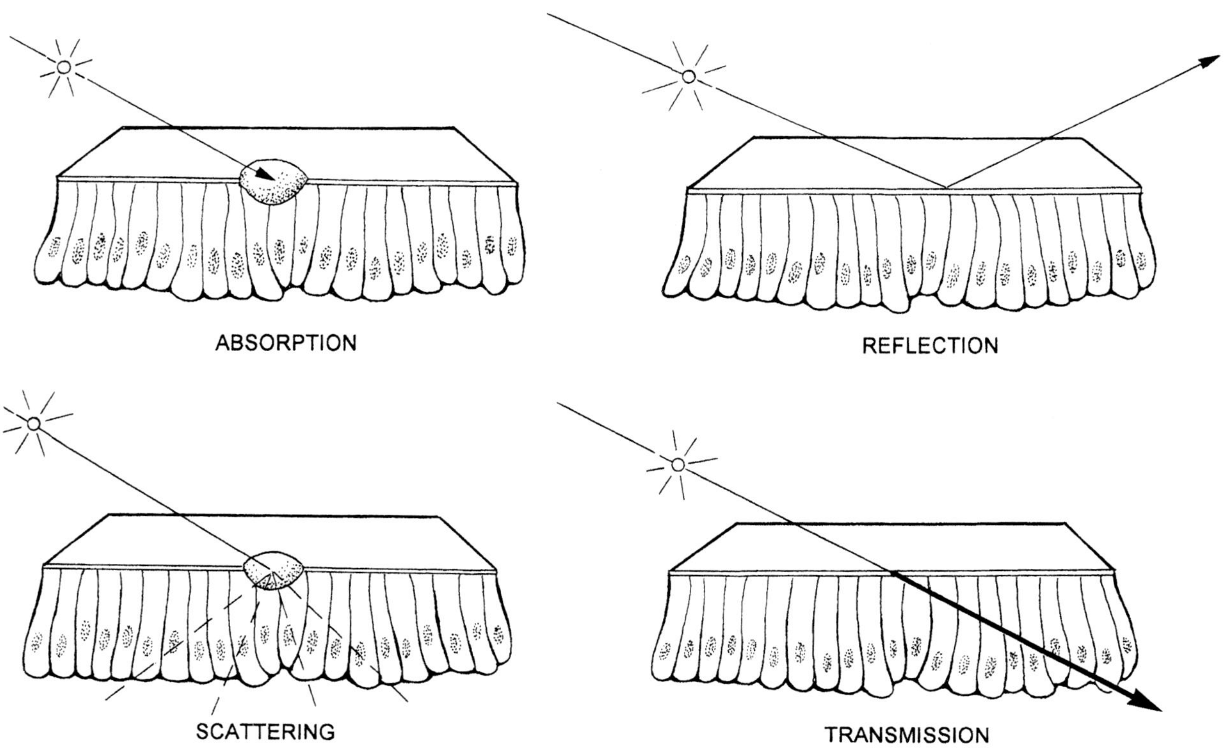


**FIGURE 4.2.** Light can interact with tissue in four ways: absorption, reflection, scatter, and transmission.

This photochemical process is the mechanism by which photodynamic therapy works. Third, short pulses of high energy disrupt cellular architecture because of the production of sound waves, a nonthermal tissue effect.

Light can interact with tissue by four mechanisms: scatter, reflection, absorption, and transmission (Fig. 4.2). Transmission refers to the process by which light passes through some tissues with minimal or no tissue injury. This is important in the treatment of retinal lesions in which the light transmits through the intraocular fluid to reach the retina. Another example is the transmission of light through the skin to reach the vascular tissue in a port-wine stain.

Light may also reflect off the surface of a tissue. The larger the angle of incidence, the greater is the amount of light reflected. It is best to minimize the reflection of light by keeping the laser perpendicular to the surface of the tissue. This approach maintains the intensity of light entering the tissue at a constant level.

The absorption of light follows Beer's Law of Absorption, or an exponentially decaying light intensity. The light is absorbed by molecules in the tissue and is transformed into heat. This results in vaporization of water and tissue ablation.

Light may interact with tissue through a mechanism referred to as *scattering*, which occurs when the incident light bounces around within the tissue. Scattering causes the beam to spread out, which irradiates a larger area of tissue than expected. The depth of penetration of the light is limited by its backward scatter (3).

## TISSUE ABLATION

The most common means of laser incision is photothermal ablation. The absorption of laser energy by the tissue is changed to heat energy. When the temperature in the tissue exceeds 100°C, water starts to vaporize, and the resultant steam causes vacuole formation, craters, and tissue shrinkage (Fig. 4.3). In the center of the wound is an area of tissue vaporization that is surrounded by a zone of thermal necrosis (about 100 μm wide). Within the zone of thermal necrosis, small vessels, nerves, and lymphatics are sealed. There is also a zone of thermal conductivity and repair (300 to 500 μm wide). A short laser pulse duration helps minimize the lateral thermal damage by reducing thermal diffusion.

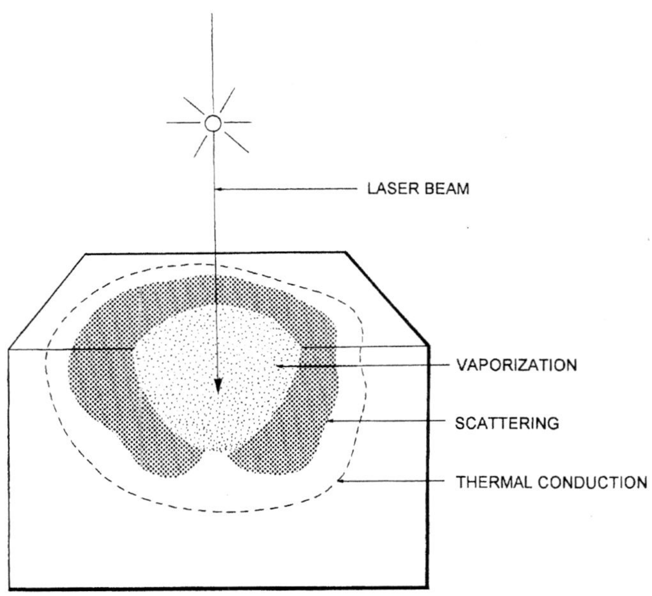


**FIGURE 4.3.** Laser tissue vaporization.

## TYPES OF LASERS AND THEIR APPLICATIONS

Several different lasers are available to the endoscopic surgeon. The surgeon should consider the precise tissue-absorptive characteristics and wavelength when choosing a laser for a specific use. An overview of the different laser types follows to facilitate proper selection. More detail regarding specific laser applications is provided in subsequent chapters.

### Argon Tunable Dye Laser

An argon laser produces a high-intensity beam that is focused on dye that is circulating in a second optically coupled laser. The second laser emits light at a longer wavelength than the pump beam, depending on the type of dye. The laser energy can be transmitted through flexible fiberoptic systems in conjunction with endoscopic visualization. It may also be inserted directly into tumors. The main use of this laser is with selective photodynamic therapy for malignant tumors that have been photosensitized with an intravenous injection of a hematoporphyrin derivative (5). It may also be considered for vascular malformations and hemangiomas of the airway, but the neodymium:yttrium-aluminum-garnet (Nd:YAG) laser is preferred in these cases (6).

### Carbon Dioxide Laser

Light from the $CO_2$ laser has a wavelength of 10.6 μm in the infrared (invisible) range of the spectrum. A coaxial helium neon laser is necessary as an aiming beam because the $CO_2$ laser light is invisible. The $CO_2$ laser radiant energy is absorbed strongly by water or tissue with a high water content and is independent of tissue color. Reflection and scatter are negligible, and the extinction length of the $CO_2$ laser beam is 0.03 mm. The thermal affects of this laser on surrounding tissue are minimal, making it a versatile laser for endoscopic surgery. The $CO_2$ laser light must be transmitted through an articulating arm to the desired tissue (7). It can be used in a freehand fashion, attached to the operating microscope for use through a laryngoscope, and used through an adapter coupled to the rigid bronchoscope (8).

The $CO_2$ laser is useful in a wide variety of otolaryngologic disorders that are managed endoscopically. In the sinonasal cavity, it has been used in treating choanal atresia (9), squamous papilloma, and hereditary hemorrhagic telangiectasia (10).

The $CO_2$ laser is frequently used in the endoscopic management of benign and malignant disease of the larynx, including papillomatosis, polyps, leukoplakia, laryngotracheal stenosis, and capillary hemangiomas. The properties of $CO_2$ laser light allow excellent precision, preservation of surrounding normal tissue, and minimal postoperative edema.

### Neodymium:Yttrium-Aluminum-Garnet Laser

Nd:YAG laser light has a wavelength of 1.064 μm in the invisible range of electromagnetic spectrum. Light absorption is slightly color dependent, with darkly pigmented tissues having increased absorption. Strong scattering occurs in forward and backward directions. Backward scatter can account for 40% of the total amount of scattering. The zone of damage produced by the Nd:YAG laser results in a homogenous zone of necrosis and thermal coagulation that extends up to 4 mm deep and lateral from the surface. The deeper penetration compromises laser precision, but the coagulation properties are superior.

Endoscopic applications of this laser include palliation of obstructive tracheobronchial or esophageal lesions (11,12). The Nd:YAG laser is particularly helpful in the management of vascular tracheobronchial lesions because of its deep penetration, which results in superior hemostasis. The laser light can be transmitted through a flexible fiberoptic delivery system that allows it to be used with a flexible fiberoptic endoscope or rigid bronchoscope. However, it is safer to use the rigid ventilating bronchoscope in the management of patients with lesions obstructing the tracheobronchial tree (12). Advantages of the rigid bronchoscope include ventilatory control of the compromised airway, palpation of the tumor-cartilage interface, and use of the bronchoscope tip for compression of a bleeding blood vessel. The flexible bronchoscope may be passed through the rigid bronchoscope for pulmonary suctioning and distal laser application after securing the airway.

### Potassium-Titanyl-Phosphate Laser

The potassium-titanyl-phosphate (KTP) laser emits light at 532 nm with scatter and absorption characteristics very similar to the argon laser. However, KTP laser light is more strongly absorbed by hemoglobin. The KTP crystal halves the wavelength (i.e., doubles the frequency) of the Nd:YAG laser; the output between the 532-nm KTP light and 1064-nm Nd:YAG can often be switched. Similar to the Nd:YAG laser, KTP laser energy is passes easily through clear solutions and is absorbed by pigment. In contrast to the Nd:YAG laser, it causes less collateral tissue damage because of less thermal transfer. However, transfer of thermal energy to surrounding tissue is still an issue especially as the tissue becomes charred. The laser is an optically pumped, solid-state instrument that produces emerald-green light (13).

The KTP laser is useful in the management of epistaxis associated with hereditary hemorrhagic telangiectasia (10). The optical fiber delivery system of the KTP laser light can be used in conjunction with endoscopic visualization of the sinonasal, middle ear, or intracranial cavities. The KTP laser is routinely used for stapedectomy in the United States. This laser can also be used for lesions of the tracheobronchial tree through a rigid ventilating bronchoscope as small as 3 mm in diameter (14).

### Diode Laser

Semiconductor diode lasers are inexpensive, their energy is fiber delivered, and they can be used in the continuous or pulsed modes. They are widely used for telecommunications, computers, and compact disc technology. Medical applications have been limited because power output has been limited to less than 100 mW, which is inadequate for tissue effects. Clinically available wavelengths range from 800 to 1,000 nm, which falls between the hemoglobin and water absorption peaks. Experimental work with the 810-nm diode laser revealed them to produce deep, extensive thermal damage because of unpredictable reflection or deep absorption with scatter resulting in widespread thermal injury (15). However, in a study designed to improve the techniques to perform a stapedotomy without prosthesis (i.e., stapedioplasty), an 812-nm diode laser was coupled with high-resolution small endoscopes. Both 100- and 300-μm contact tips were used for delivery, and temperature measurements were made within the vestibule. Using the 100-μm probe, all temperature elevations were considered clinically acceptable. The quality of the burns was very clean, with minimal char and tight, round craters. The investigators conclude that this technique shows promise for minimally invasive surgery of the stapes footplate (16).

## LASER SAFETY CONSIDERATIONS

When used properly, lasers can be a used to advantage in the management of a broad array of otolaryngologic problems. However, lasers are not without disadvantages and risks. The decision to use a laser and the selection of a particular laser must be backed by solid knowledge. Before granting laser privileges, most hospitals require participation in a hands-on laser training course that includes laser biophysics, tissue interactions, safety precautions, and hands-on training. It is also helpful to practice on animal or cadaver specimens before progressing to use in patients.

Most injuries associated with laser use are related to airway fires and ignition of the surgical drapes (17). Attention to detail and communication with the anesthesia team and laser personnel are the keys to preventing these potentially devastating complications. The laser personnel and anesthesia personnel should attend appropriate didactic sessions before participating in cases involving use of the laser (18). Laser personnel should adhere to a safety protocol, including protection of the skin and eyes of patients and operating room personnel, laser smoke evacuation, choice of anesthetic technique, endotracheal tube choice, and instrument selection. Adherence to a safety protocol has been shown to allow safe use of the laser with minimal risk to the patient and operating room personnel (19–21).

Depending on the wavelength of the laser used, different structures of the eye are at risk, including the cornea and retina. Retinal effects are associated with laser emission wavelengths in the visible and near-infrared range of the electromagnetic spectrum (0.4 to 1.4 μm). Laser radiation at this wavelength is focused to a small spot size and, if directed toward the eye, is absorbed by the retina, resulting in serious injury. Corneal injury results from light in the ultraviolet (<0.4 μm) or infrared range (>1.4 μm).

Minimizing the risk of ocular injury to operating room personnel requires proper selection of eye protection based on the wavelength of the laser in use. When a laser is to be used, a sign should be placed outside the operating room door warning all personnel entering the room to wear the appropriate protective eyewear. This eyewear should be conveniently placed outside the room so that it is readily available to additional personnel needing to enter. Protective glasses should also have side protectors. The operating room door should remain closed during $CO_2$ laser cases and locked during use of the Nd:YAG and argon lasers.

Patients undergoing endoscopic laser surgery should have a double layer of saline-moistened eye pads secured over the eyes with silk tape. Before placing the eye pads, the eyelids should be taped shut with silk tape to prevent corneal injury.

When using the microscope with the $CO_2$ laser, the operating surgeon does not need to wear protective eyewear because they are protected by the microscope optics (22). When using the Nd:YAG or KTP laser, all operating room personnel must wear wavelength-specific eye glasses. The surgical microscope can be equipped with an electronically controlled filter for use with the KTP laser. Although the beam direction and impact may appear to be confined to within the endoscope, the beam may be deflected because of poor contact, disruption of the delivery fiber, or disconnection between the fiber and the endoscope.

Great care should be taken to protect the patient's skin and mucous membranes. A carefully placed double layer of saline-soaked surgical towels is used to completely drape the patient's face while leaving the proximal lumen of the laryngoscope exposed. The towels must remain moist and properly positioned during the course of the procedure. If teeth are in the operating field, they should be protected with saline-saturated surgical sponges (22).

Rigid bronchoscopy is the preferred method, rather than using flexible fiberoptics, when using the laser in the tracheobronchial tree. If vigorous hemorrhage occurs, control with the flexible fiberoptic instrumentation is almost impossible. If necessary, two or three suction cannulas can be passed through a rigid bronchoscope to facilitate blood removal.

In general, instrumentation used with the laser should have minimal direct reflectance and large scattered reflectance to prevent unwanted tissue injury in case the laser beam inadvertently strikes the instrument. Plastic or flammable instruments should be avoided to prevent injuries caused by melting or fire.

It is important to minimize laser-induced smoke exposure to the patient, operating room personnel, and surgeon. Papillomavirus has been detected in the laser plume, although there are no reported cases of clinical transmission during a laser surgery (23). Another report suggests that $CO_2$ laser-induced smoke is mutagenic (24). To prevent laser-induced smoke inhalation during surgery with a closed anesthetic system, constant suctioning should be used. Two separate suctions should be available during laser surgery: one for clearing the field of blood and mucus and the other for laser smoke removal. Endoscopic equipment with built-in smoke-evacuating channels facilitate the removal of smoke from the operative field (25).

Most patients undergoing endoscopic laser surgery require general endotracheal anesthesia. The use of a small, cuffed endotracheal tube that creates a closed ventilatory system is preferable when the endotracheal tube does not obstruct the area to be operated on. The forced inspiratory oxygen level should be maintained at less than 30% using mixtures of helium or air plus oxygen. A forced inspiratory oxygen concentration of 30% helps to ensure adequate oxygenation of the patient while minimizing the risk of airway fire (6). Nonflammable anesthetics such as halothane or enflurane are commonly used. Muscle relaxation is necessary to prevent vocal cord motion during the procedure. Intravenous supplementation with small doses of narcotics or tranquilizers is helpful to shorten the emergence period after anesthesia.

If jet ventilation is selected, it is important to ensure preoperatively that the anesthesiologist is familiar with the technique. This technique is useful in selected patients, such as those with posterior glottic or subglottic lesions in whom even a small endotracheal tube would obscure the surgical field (26,27).

Endotracheal tube selection for cases involving laser surgery of the upper aerodigestive tract is important. There is no widely accepted endotracheal tube for these cases, but the traditional polyvinyl endotracheal tube should *not* be considered. This tube offers little resistance to penetration by the laser, the combustion products are toxic, and the associated tissue injury if a fire occurs is severe. The Roesch Red Rubber Tube (Hoffmann-LaRoche, Nutley, NJ) offers more resistance to laser penetration and causes less tissue damage if combustion occurs. If a laser beam strikes an unprotected, oxygen-carrying endotracheal tube, combustion can result in a catastrophic, blowtorch-type airway fire (28). The use of a red rubber endotracheal tube with U.S. Food and Drug Administration–approved reflective metallic tape diminishes the risk of this event if a wavelength-specific laser tube is not available. Silicone tubes are more resistant to laser penetration, but if a fire does occur, the residual silica ash may result in silicosis (19). Endotracheal tubes are available for the $CO_2$, argon, KTP, and Nd:YAG lasers. These tubes are wrapped with reflective tape (Xomed Treace Laser-Shield II, Xomed Treace, Jacksonville, FL) or made of reflective materials (Laser-Flex Tracheal Tube, Mallinckrodt, St. Louis, MO) that diminish the likelihood of endotracheal tube ignition and airway fire. The point should be made that, despite these precautions, if enough energy is transferred to the endotracheal tube by the laser, combustion can occur.

Care should be taken with the cuff of the endotracheal tube as well. Saline-saturated Cottonoids should be placed above the cuff to protect it from exposure to the laser light beam. It is important to keep these pledgets moist and clean to decrease their chances of ignition. The endotracheal tube cuff should also be inflated with methylene blue–tinted saline so that the surgeon is alerted by the Cottonoids turning blue if the cuff is penetrated (19). Another helpful technique involves use of the microlaryngeal operating platform. This instrument is placed in the subglottic larynx above the saline-saturated Cottonoids, protecting the Cottonoids, endotracheal tube, and cuff from laser light injury (29).

## REFERENCES


1. Fuller TA. The physics of surgical lasers. *Lasers Surg Med* 1980;1:5–14.
2. Ossoff RH, Reinisch L, Garrett GC. Laser surgery: basic principles and safety considerations. In: Cummings CW, Fredrickson JM, Harker LA, et al, eds. *Otolaryngology–Head and Neck Surgery*, 3rd ed. St. Louis: Mosby, 1998:197–215.
3. Reinisch L. Laser physics and tissue interactions. *Otolaryngol Clin North Am* 1996;29:893–914.
4. Waner M. Light-tissue interaction. *Facial Plast Surg Clin North Am* 1996;4:223–229.
5. Dougherty TJ, Kaufman JE, Goldfarb A, et al. Photoradiation therapy for the treatment of malignant tumors. *Cancer Res* 1978;38:2628–2635.
6. Courey MS, Ossoff RH. Laser applications in adult laryngeal surgery. *Otolaryngol Clin North Am* 1996;29:973–986.
7. Ossoff RH, Karlan MS. Laser surgery in otolaryngology. In: Ballenger JJ, ed. *Diseases of the nose, throat, ear, and neck.* Philadelphia: Lea & Febiger, 1985.
8. Ossoff RH, Karlan MS. Universal endoscopic coupler for carbon dioxide laser surgery. *Ann Otol Rhinol Laryngol* 1982;91:608–609.
9. Healy GB. Management of choanal atresia with the carbon dioxide laser. *Ann Otol Rhinol Laryngol* 1978;87:658–662.
10. Siegel MB, Keane WM, Atkins JF Jr, Rosen MR. Control of epistaxis in patients with hereditary hemorrhagic telangiectasia. *Otolaryngol Head Neck Surg* 1991;105:675–679.
11. Dumon JF, Shapsay S, Bourcereau J, et al. Principles for safety in application of neodymium-YAG laser in bronchology. *Chest* 1984;86:163–168.
12. Fleischer D. Endoscopic laser therapy for gastrointestinal neoplasms. *Surg Clin North Am* 1984;64:947–953.
13. Ossoff RH, Coleman JA, Courey MS. Clinical applications of lasers in otolaryngology–head and neck surgery. *Lasers Surg Med* 1994;15:217–248.
14. Ward RF. Treatment of tracheal and endobronchial lesions with the potassium titanyl phosphate laser. *Ann Otol Rhinol Laryngol* 1992;101:205–208.
15. Wyman DR, Schatz SW, Maguire JAC. Comparison of 810 nm and 1064 nm wavelengths for interstitial laser photocoagulation in rabbit brain. *Lasers Surg Med* 1997;21:50–58.
16. Poe DS. Laser-assisted endoscopic stapedectomy: a prospective study. *Laryngoscope* 2000;110:1–37.
17. Sliney DH. Laser safety. *Lasers Surg Med* 1995;16:215–225.
18. Spilman LS. Nursing precautions for $CO_2$ laser surgery. *Symposium proceedings, The Laser Institute of America.* 1983;37:63.
19. Ossoff RH, Duncavage JA, Eisenman TS, Karlan MS. Comparison of tracheal damage from laser-ignited endotracheal fires. *Ann Otol Rhinol Laryngol* 1983;92:333–336.
20. Healy GB, Strong MS, Shapsay S, et al. Complications of $CO_2$ laser surgery of the aerodigestive tract: experience 4416 cases. *Otolaryngol Head Neck Surg* 1984;92:13–18.
21. Ossoff RH. Laser safety in otolaryngology—head and neck surgery: anesthetic and educational considerations for laryngeal surgery. *Laryngoscope* 1989;99:1–26.
22. Ossoff RH, Hotaling AJ, Karlan MS, Sisson GA. $CO_2$ laser in otolaryngology—head and neck surgery: a retrospective analysis of complications. *Laryngoscope* 1983;93:1287–1289.
23. Abramson AL. Is papillomavirus detectable in the plume of laser-treated laryngeal papilloma? *Arch Otolaryngol Head Neck Surg* 1990;116:604–607.
24. Tomita Y, Mihashi S, Nagata K. Mutagenicity of smoke condensates induced by $CO_2$-laser irradiation and electrocauterization. *Mutat Res* 1981;89:145–149.
25. Ossoff RH, Karlan MS. Instrumentation for microlaryngeal laser surgery. *Otolaryngol Head Neck Surg* 1983;91:456–460.
26. Edelist G, Alberti PW. Anesthesia for $CO_2$ laser surgery of the larynx. *J Otolaryngol* 1982;11:107–110.
27. Williams SR, Van Hasselt CA, Aun CST. Tubeless anesthetic technique for optimal carbon dioxide laser surgery of the larynx. *Am J Otol* 1993;14:271–274.
28. Schramm VL, Mattox DE, Stool SE. Acute management of laser-ignited intratracheal explosion. *Laryngoscope* 1981;91:1417–1426.
29. Ossoff RH, Karlan MS. Instrumentation for $CO_2$ laser surgery of the larynx and tracheobronchial tree. *Surg Clin North Am* 1984;64:973–980.

SECTION

# II

# OTOLOGY, NEURO-OTOLOGY, AND CRANIAL BASE SURGERY

5

# ENDOSCOPIC SECOND-LOOK PROCEDURE IN CHOLESTEATOMA SURGERY

JEAN MARC THOMASSIN
FREDERIC BRACCINI
JEROME PARIS

Endoscopy gave new impetus to the surgery of the middle ear. For 50 years, the operating microscope enabled decisive progress in the surgery of auricular cavities, but its use was hampered by the existence of blind spaces, particularly the retrotympanum and epitympanum (1,2).

Despite the safe cholesteatoma excision that endoscopic techniques procure, most investigators consider that cholesteatoma surgery remains a two-stage operation. The second-look procedure should be performed 12 to 24 months after the first surgery.

During the first operative stage for cholesteatoma excision, the endoscopic procedure complements the classic operating microscope surgery. Endoscopically guided surgery with video monitoring constitutes a new concept for the second-look cholesteatoma operation. It allows a minimal cutaneous approach and provides better verification of possible residual cholesteatoma.

The second-look procedure can be performed under day-surgery conditions, and it is well accepted by patients with asymptomatic ears. The endoscopic second-look procedure for cholesteatoma surgery is performed in 80% of our patients through a minimal cutaneous approach, whatever the preoperative computed tomography findings are (3,4). If there is a major recurrence, we abandoned purely endoscopic surgery and enlarged the cutaneous approach, as in the classic approach, and use the operating microscope.

## EQUIPMENT

### Endoscopes

For otovideo-endoscopic surgery of the cavities of the middle ear, the surgeon should have at his disposal three optical systems whose technical characteristics give a full-screen image on the video monitor (1,2): 2.7-mm-diameter optical systems with angles of 0°, 30°, and 70° (i.e., Storz Teleotoscope). The 30° and 70° endoscopes can explore the retrotympanum to any depth (e.g., sinus tympani).

The endoscopes are arranged on the instrument table in a support to protect them from shocks. Each endoscope has a color code according to its angle of vision (Fig. 5.1). A demisting fluid is essential to clean the lenses before each use.

### Cold Light Source

A 300-W xenon cold light source provides excellent luminosity. Light transmission between the generator and endoscope is ensured by a 180-cm-long cold light cable.

### Microcamera

A microcamera should be connected to the end of the endoscope. It must be light and very sensitive, and it must have a zoom lens that gives an enlarged image on the monitor. For image acquisition, we use a three-chip charge-coupled device (3-CCD) video camera (Endovision Tricam, Storz Instruments, Tuttlingen, Germany). The video camera has to be watertight for decontamination process. However, if this is not the case, it should be wrapped in a sterile covering.

### Instruments for Microsurgery

Specific instrumentation is essential for retrotympanum surgery. The different regions of the retrotympanum axes perpendicular to the external acoustic meatus and are recessed relative to the bony margin of the tympanic membrane. Cholesteatoma excision in this region requires the use of microinstruments angled at 90°.

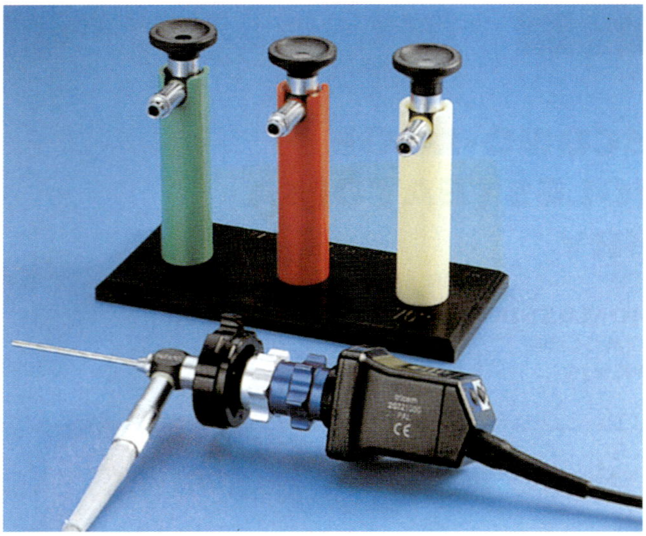

**FIGURE 5.1.** Otoendoscopes in their support to protect them from shocks. Each color indicates the angulation of the optical systems.

The Storz instrument set includes the following elements (Fig. 5.2):

- A double microdissector, with one end bent to the right and the other to the left
- A curved microhook, bent at 90°
- A microdissector, bent at 90° to the right and another one bent to the left
- A microrugine
- A support for the microsuckers
- Microsuckers with 0.6-, 0.8-, and 1-mm diameters
- Microforceps bent at 90° with hollow (punch) and grooved jaws

### Laser Instrumentation

Laser instrumentation includes two guide stems adaptable on the 0° and 30° endoscopes that have an operator canal allowing the introduction of the optic fiber. The fiber diameter can be 200 to 400 μm in diameter.

## VIDEO-ENDOSCOPIC SECOND-LOOK SURGERY

The video-endoscopic second-look surgery is performed under general anesthesia for most of our patients, but local anesthesia can be employed (4).

### Arrangement of the Operating Room and Patient

The patient is supine, in dorsal decubitus, with his head turned to the opposite side. The operating table must be in a 15° to 20° anti-Trendelenburg position to reduce preoperative bleeding in the operating field. The region of the external ear is placed directly under the vision of the surgeon, who is seated at the head of the table on the right or left side. The foot of the operating microscope is opposite the surgeon. The articulated arm is carried as a bridge over the head. The instrument nurse is at the head of the operating table, with the instrument table alongside. An instrument tray supported by a single leg is situated above the patient's abdomen. On it are arranged the microcamera; the optical support with endoscopes of 0°, 30°, and 70°; the cold light cable; and a small dish containing unwoven compresses with a demisting fluid. A video stand housing the video monitor is installed opposite the surgeon, next to the microscope.

A 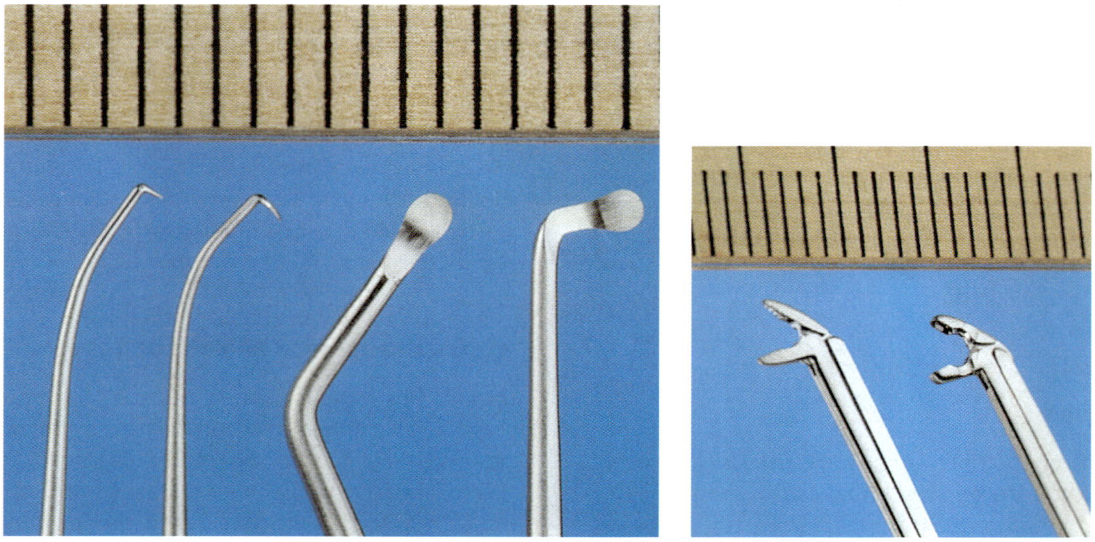 B

**FIGURE 5.2. A,B:** Set of instruments for microsurgery.

This arrangement enables a quick and easy change from the microscope to the endoscope, displacing sideways the arm of the microscope. An electronic control box with a simple switch allows transfer from the microcamera coupled to the endoscope to the camera of the operating microscope.

## Surgical Technique

The procedure begins with a lesional assessment (3,4). After cleaning the external auditory meatus through a speculum using the operating microscope, we insert an endoscope with a 0°-angle of vision and that is 2.7 or 4 mm in diameter for accurate assessment of the tympanic lesions. If there is a major perforation of the tympanic membrane, we make use of this aperture to insert an endoscope to visualize the ossicular chain and the tympanic cavity.

### *Minimal Posterior Approach*

A local anesthetic infiltration is made in the retroauricular region and the external auditory meatus before performing the skin incision with a no. 11 scalpel blade. We use a minimal retroauricular incision that is 1 to 1.5 cm long, situated in the retroauricular fold, and centered on the conchal part of the helix (Fig. 5.3). This approach incises the musculoperiosteal coat and deeper the mucosa lining the mastoid cavity while ensuring careful hemostasis with diathermy forceps (Fig. 5.4). We have reported few cases of children with mastoid reossification for whom limited burring of the mastoid bone allowed the introduction of optic and other instruments for microsurgery. A clawed, self-retaining retractor holds the skin edges apart. An otologic speculum supported by an articulated arm can be used to avoid soiling the lenses.

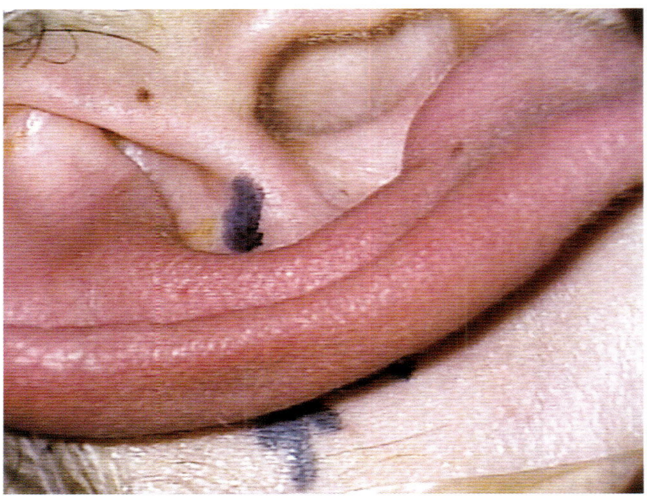

**FIGURE 5.3.** Right ear: line of a minimal retroauricular incision.

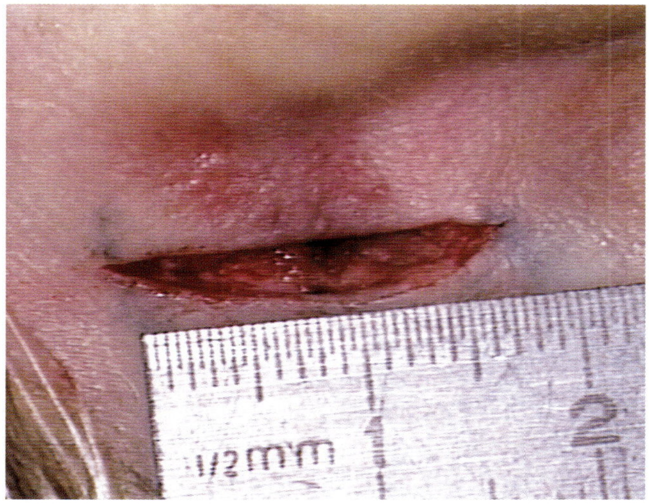

**FIGURE 5.4.** Right ear: minimal skin incision and section of the musculoperiosteal coat.

### *Posterior Cavities Inspection*

The check begins with inspection of the mastoid cavity. The 0° endoscope is held in the left hand of a right-handed operator and inserted into the mastoid cavity. There is always a mastoid felting, which is progressively dilacerated with microinstruments and a laser combined with the endoscope (Figs. 5.5 and 5.6). The laser provides careful hemostasis. The lens is moved with circular movements to sweep the mastoido-antro-epitympanic cavity in the direction of the tegmen antri. If a thick Silastic has been used during the first stage, it should be removed.

If a residual cholesteatoma pearl is in that region (Fig. 5.7), it should be easily seen, looking like a natural white pearl and illuminated by the cold light (Figs. 5.8 and 5.9). The laser can vaporize contact mucosa.

### *Inspection of the Epitympanum*

Inspection of the mastoid cavity is followed by inspection of the epitympanum. Residual cholesteatoma often occurs in the epitympanum, and this region should always be carefully inspected (Fig. 5.10). The exploration is pursued forward, where the operating microscope is hampered by blind angles and venous or meningeal prolapse.

The endoscope identifies the protrusion of the horizontal semicircular canal. During passage of the endoscope, the posterior tympanotomy window should be observed. A covering that is progressively opened by means of a microdissector or laser vaporization often obstructs this window. Through this window, the wide-angle lens system of the 0° scope reveals the superstructure of the stapes, medial wall of the tympanic cavity, and bulge of the second portion of the facial canal.

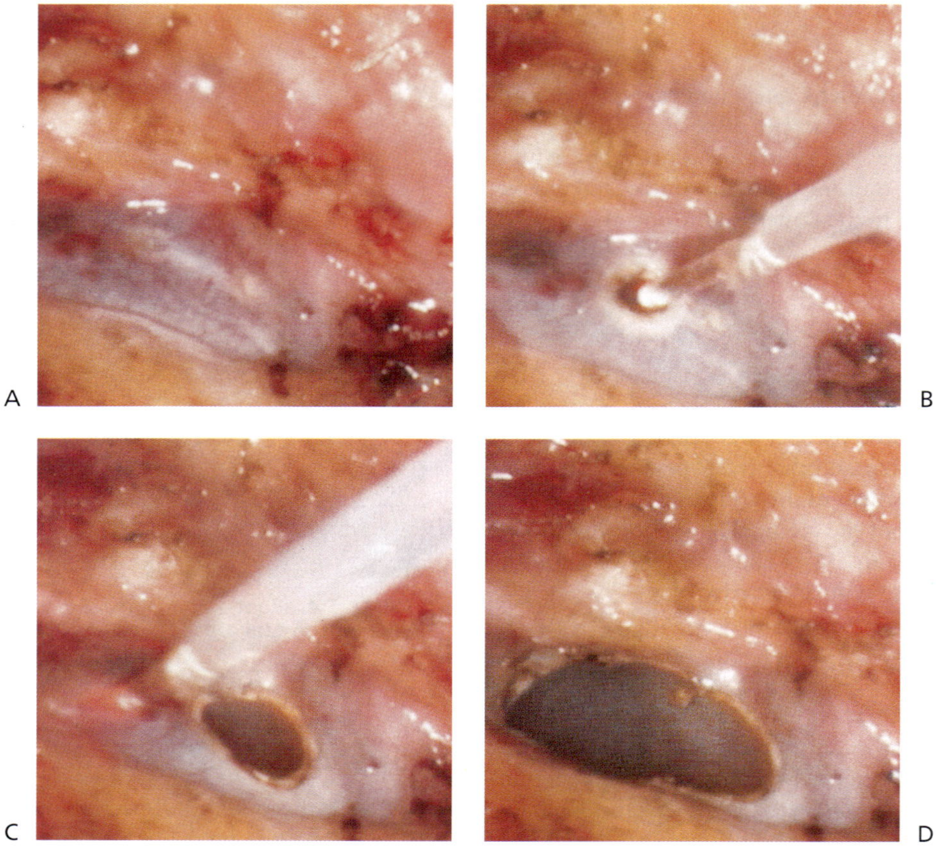

A B C D

**FIGURE 5.5. A–D:** Right ear: first case of mastoid felting laser vaporization.

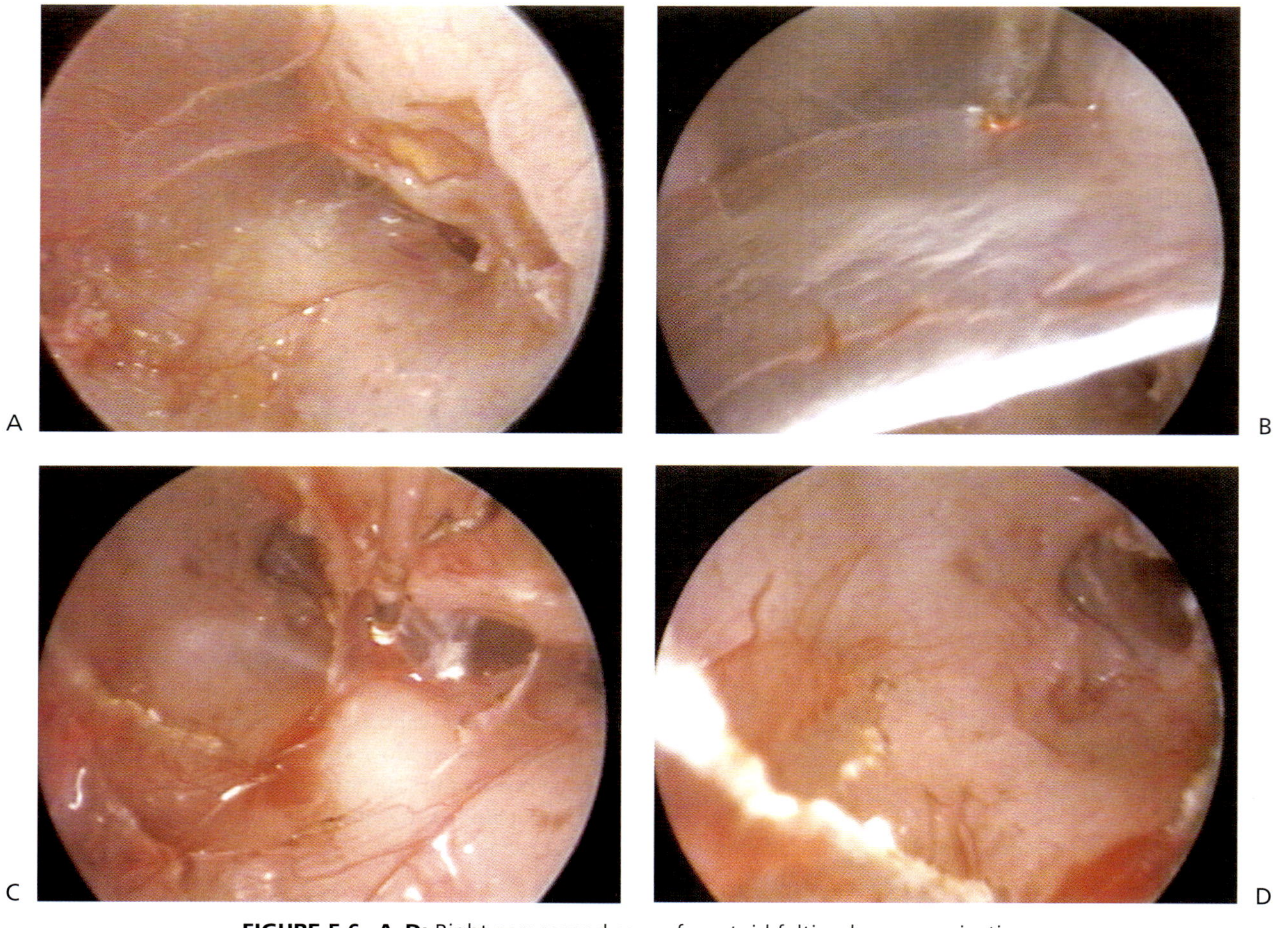

A B C D

**FIGURE 5.6. A–D:** Right ear: second case of mastoid felting laser vaporization.

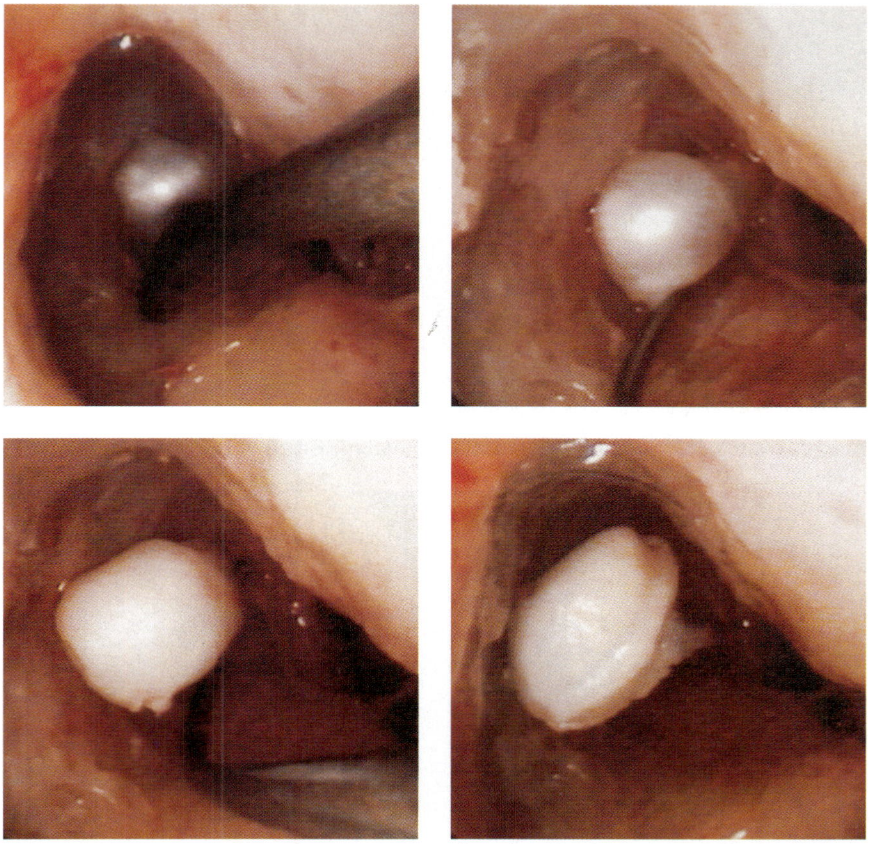

A B C D

**FIGURE 5.7. A–D:** Right ear: cholesteatoma pearl in the posterior cavity. Exeresis is performed under video control.

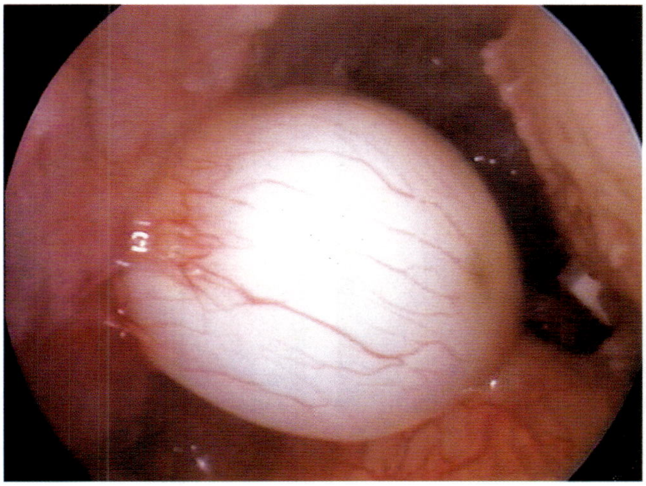

**FIGURE 5.8.** Right ear: cholesteatoma pearl in the epitympanum. Exeresis is performed under video control.

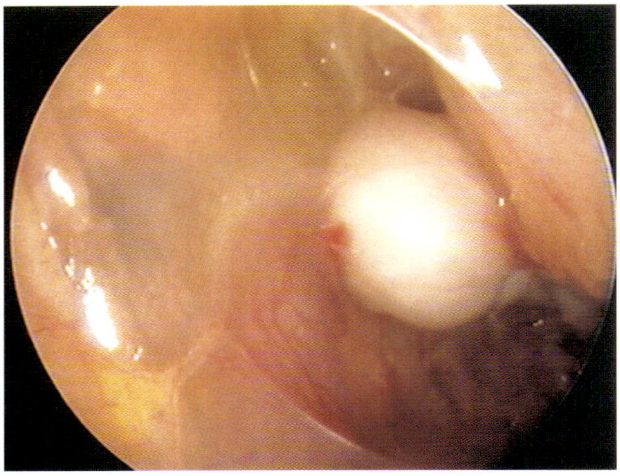

A

**FIGURE 5.9. A–E:** Right ear: two important cases of cholesteatoma pearls in the posterior cavities.

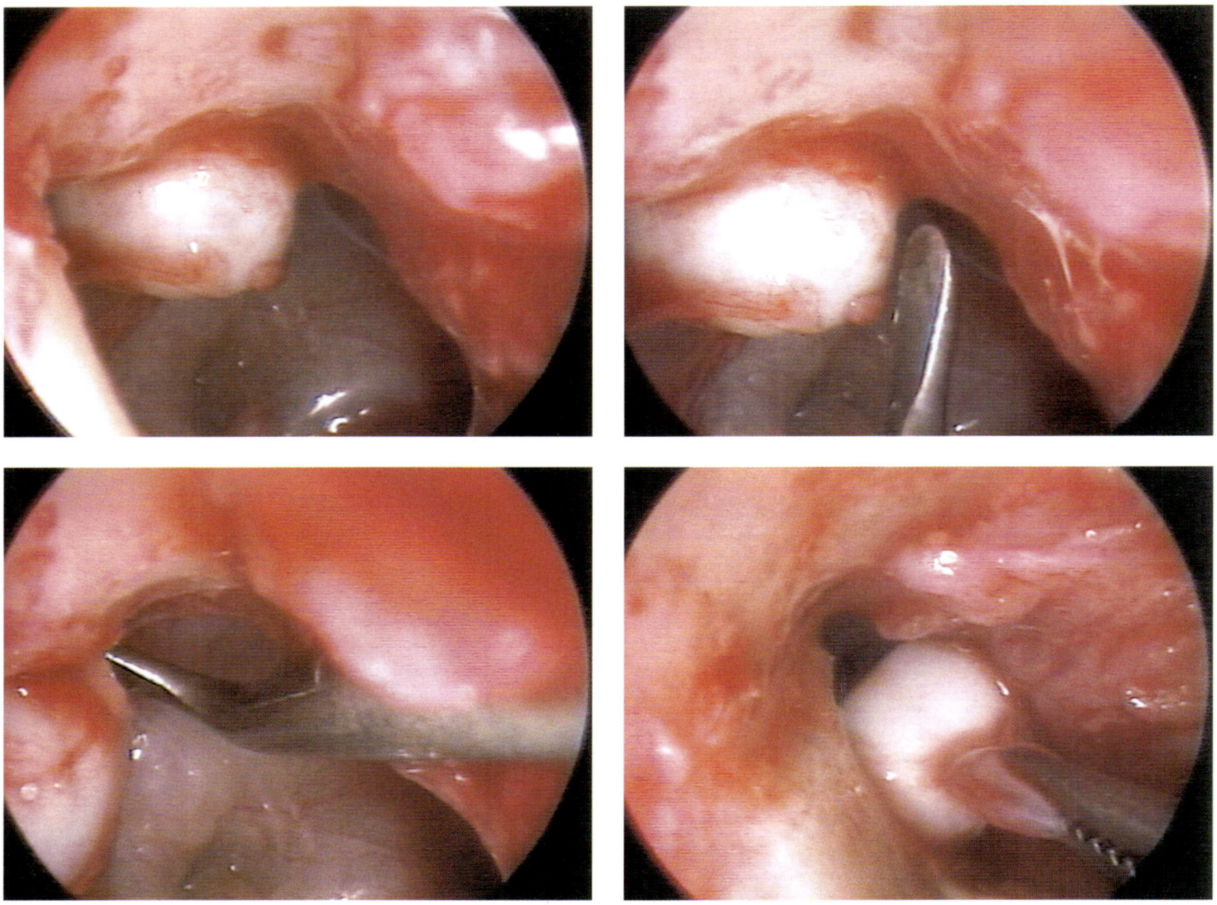

B C D E

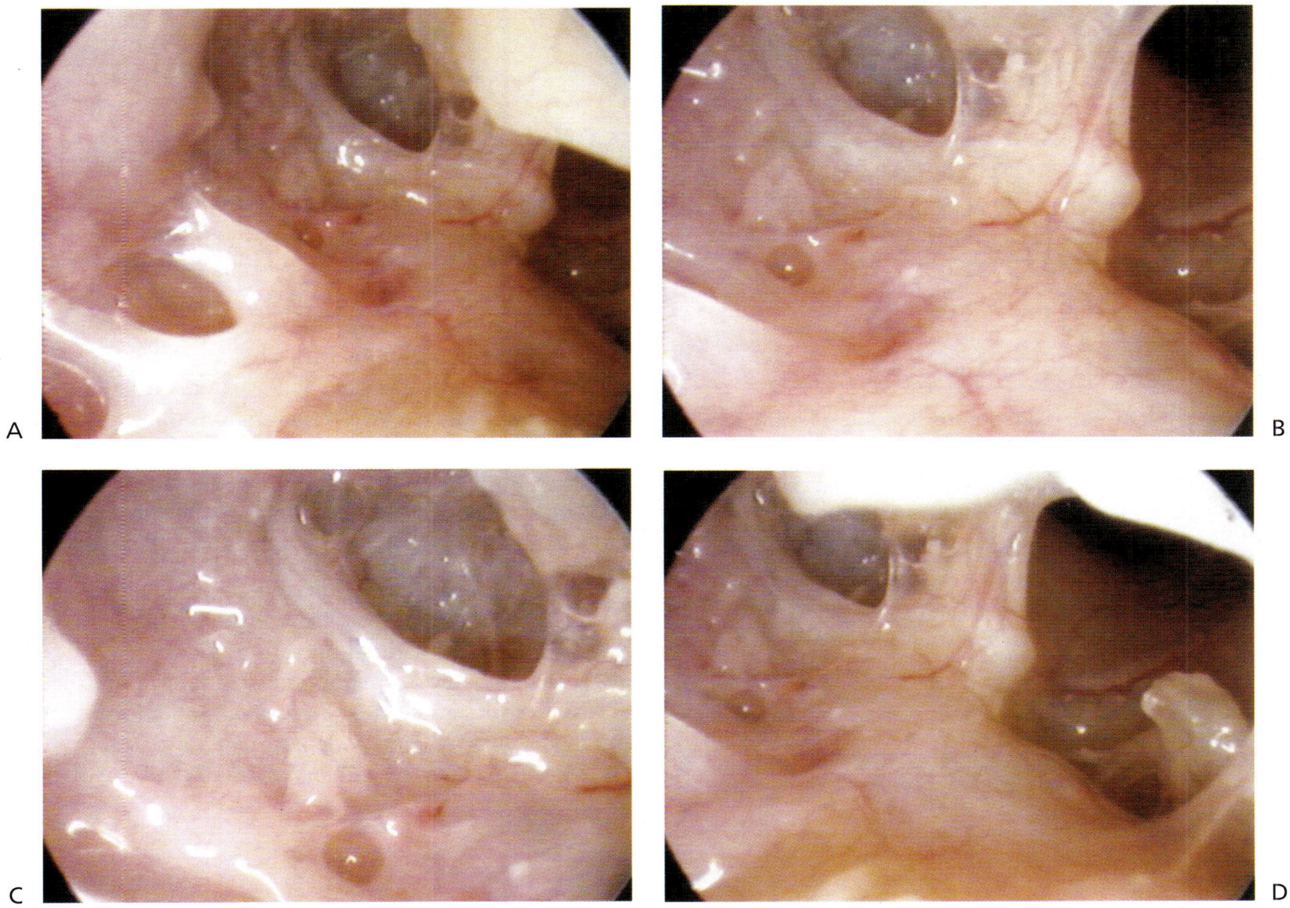

**FIGURE 5.10. A–D:** Right ear: endoscopic view of the disease-free cavity.

## *Inspection of the Tympanic Cavity*

A complete view of the inner tympanic cavity, with the exception of the internal retrotympanum, is obtained by insertion into the epitympanum of 30° and 70° endoscopes with a slight pivoting movement of the endoscope-camera system. This technique allows assessment of the inner tympanic membrane. A transmeatal route combined with a minimal posterior approach can be performed to inspect the retrotympanum or to perform an ossiculoplasty (Fig. 5.11). Residual cholesteatoma excision can be easily performed with the specific microinstruments designed by Thomassin. We end the procedure with an ossiculoplasty performed through the window of the posterior tympanotomy or, more often, by a transmeatal route.

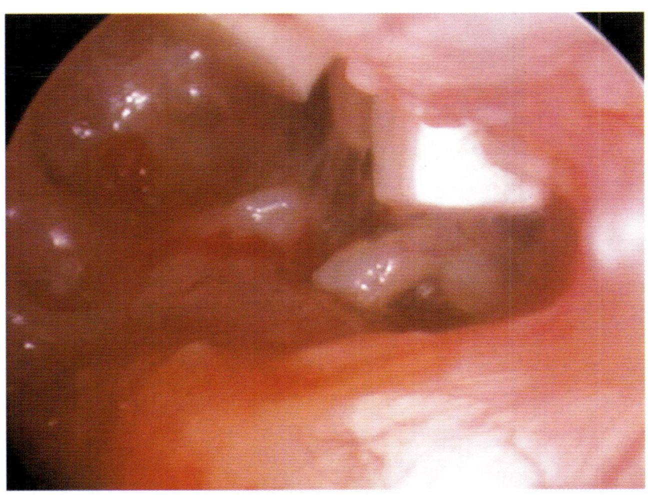

**FIGURE 5.11.** Right ear: ossiculoplasty is performed under endoscopic control.

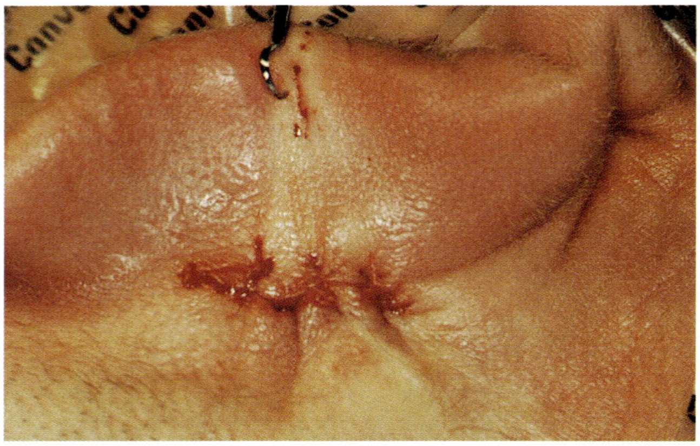

**FIGURE 5.12.** Right ear: skin closure is achieved with slowly absorbed sutures.

### *Closure*

Closure of the retroauricular skin incision is performed in two layers with slowly absorbed sutures (Fig. 5.12). The usual packing, such as Gelfoam and rolled Silastic, is placed in the external auditory canal in patients who underwent surgery using a transmeatal approach (Fig 5.13).

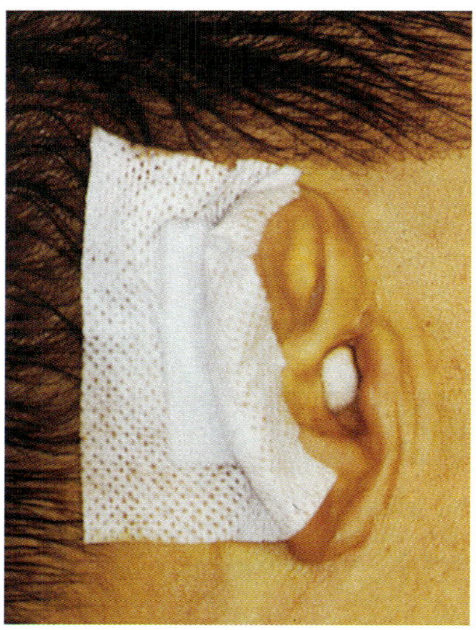

**FIGURE 5.13.** Right ear bandage.

## CONCLUSIONS

Endoscopic techniques have considerably changed cholesteatoma second-look surgery. In patients with asymptomatic ear disorders, most of the second-look procedures are performed through a minimal incision.

In patients with a tympanic retraction pocket before the second-look operation or with obvious recurrent cholesteatoma, the classic approach with an operating microscope should be employed. We achieved excision of residual cholesteatoma of the posterior part of the tympanic cavity in all patients using a minimal approach. This technique has multiple advantages:

- It permits complete verification of the mastoid cavities and epitympanic cavity accurately in its anterior region, such as the supratubal recess, with a better level of safety than obtained with an operating microscope.
- It reduces mucous membrane deterioration in the posterior cavities and can be performed under local anesthesia in ambulatory surgery departments.
- Minimally invasive surgery reduces the cost of treating these patients.

## REFERENCES

1. Thomassin JM, Duchon-Doris JM, Emram B, et al. Oto-chirurgie endoscopique, premier bilan. *Ann Otol Laryngol (Paris)* 1990;107: 564–570.
2. Thomassin JM, Korchia D, Duchon-Doris JM. Endoscopic-guided otosurgery in the prevention of residual cholesteatoma. *Laryngoscope*1993;103:939–943.
3. Thomassin JM, Korchia D. Retrotympanum endoscopic-guided surgery in the canal wall-up technique in cholesteatoma. In: *Proceedings of the Fourth International Conference on Cholesteatoma and Mastoid Surgery, Niigata, Japan.* Amsterdam: Kugler Publications, 1993:581–586.
4. Thomassin JM, Antoni Candela F, Decat M, et al. Surgery under oto-endoscopic control. *Rev Laryngol Otol Rhinol* 1996;117: 409–416.

# 6

# USE OF ENDOSCOPES IN TYMPANOMASTOID SURGERY

**KEVIN X. McKENNAN**

Operating microscopes furnish clear and relatively undistorted views of surgical anatomy. The binocular nature of these microscopes creates what is referred to optically as *depth of field*, which is a great advantage during dissection. Unfortunately, operating microscopes have certain limitations. Their size precludes direct insertion into the surgical field. From an optical standpoint, they have a linear (0°) field of view that causes potential blind areas at any angle off the 0° line of view. Endoscopes of various degrees produce an angled view of the surgical field and can be inserted directly into the surgical field (Fig. 6.1). However, monocular endoscopes have the serious limitation of lacking depth of field. The use of endoscopes and microscopes is complementary.

The otolaryngologic use of endoscopes began more than 30 years ago in laryngology and rhinology, but it has been only during the past decade that endoscopes have been employed in specific situations in otology and neuro-otology (1,2). Anticipated developments such as binocular endoscopes and laser attachments will make these instruments even more helpful and easy to use. Like many new technologies, it has specific uses and limitations. It requires a financial investment and a small time investment to learn its applications.

## INDICATIONS

An endoscope should be considered another tool in our armamentarium for the surgical treatment of cholesteatoma (Fig. 6.2). In nearly all cases, it *supplements* the view of the binocular microscope. In some ear operations, endoscopes are used for only a few minutes of operating time. The use of endoscopes in cholesteatoma surgery falls into two broad categories: second-look tympanomastoid surgery and intraoperative examination of areas that are blind to a binocular microscopic view (i.e., an alternative to microscopic mirrors). It also has other neuro-otologic applications.

Cholesteatomas can be treated with a closed (i.e., tympanoplasty with or without intact canal wall mastoidectomy) or an open (i.e., tympanoplasty with canal wall down) technique. The canal wall down technique rarely necessitates a second-look operation because the cholesteatoma is exteriorized out of the mastoid and epitympanum. There are no bony areas, such as the canal wall or scutum, behind which a cholesteatoma can recur. Cholesteatomas can redevelop within a reconstructed middle ear space, but the ramifications of this type of recurrence are less severe and more readily detected than if the canal wall is maintained. Unfortunately, the overall quality of life for patients with a canal wall down operation is considerably less than when the canal wall is left intact. Most mastoid bowls require some degree of maintenance for the rest of the patient's life. Certain athletic activities, such as swimming, are more difficult when there is a mastoid cavity. More importantly, the hearing results are generally better the more the middle ear anatomy is preserved, as in an intact canal wall procedure. As a result, most otologic surgeons perform an intact canal wall technique when the combination of anatomy and extent of disease permit it.

One major disadvantage of intact canal wall mastoidectomy is the potential for any missed matrix to redevelop into an entrapped cholesteatoma. Because the epitympanum and mastoid cavity are completely hidden from view, any recurrence can grow to large proportions before detection. Computed tomography (CT) scanning is not accurate enough to detect the residual cholesteatoma matrix (3). Studies have demonstrated that residual cholesteatoma occurs in 5% to 35% of patients whose cholesteatomas were removed using an intact canal wall technique (4,5). The consensus approach is to surgically explore these patients 9 to 12 months after the first surgery with a second-look procedure. Moreover, it is during this second-look operation that Silastic sheeting is removed, the ossicular chain is repaired, and any other refinements are performed. These

Endoscopes

- 4 mm 30°, 0°, 45°
- 2.7 mm 30°, 0°
- 1.5 mm 15°
- 1.2 mm 0°
- Fiberoptic 2.2, 1.6, and .8 mm scopes

**FIGURE 6.1.** Lenses in a variety of sizes and angles used during surgery.

patients are often ideal candidates in whom endoscopes are used during the second-look procedure. If the sole purpose of the operation is to exclude any residual cholesteatoma and remove Silastic sheeting, most of the operation can be done with an endoscope. If the ossicular chain is also in need of repair, the endoscope is used to supplement the binocular microscopic examination of the mastoid, epitympanum, and middle ear.

Another major use of an endoscope is during a primary cholesteatoma surgery when it may be impossible to view certain areas using only a binocular microscope. The two most common hidden areas are the epitympanum and the sinus tympani. Other troublesome areas include the facial recess, oval window niche, and hypotympanum. Mirrors are helpful in viewing these hidden areas but have several disadvantages compared with endoscopes. Endoscopes provide a clearer and more panoramic view than mirrors. In this application, an endoscope functions as a high-tech mirror.

What can you do?

- R/O residual cholesteatoma
- Remove residual pearls
- Remove silastic
- Excise air tract fibrosis that may lead to recurrent cholesteatoma
- Check ossiculoplasty

**FIGURE 6.2.** A limited number of maneuvers are possible endoscopically.

## CONTRAINDICATIONS

Because the endoscope is often an adjunct to the binocular microscope, there are no specific contraindications to its use in the traditional sense. Patients with significant middle ear cholesteatoma should not have the second-look operation confined only to the mastoid and epitympanum; the middle ear should be examined using a transcanal or postauricular tympanotomy.

## PREOPERATIVE EVALUATION

Standard preoperative studies of endoscopic candidates are few, as is the case for any other set of cholesteatoma patients. All patients require bone and speech audiometry and a careful in-office binocular microscopic examination. CT scanning of the temporal bone is used when unusual problems are suspected, such as brain herniation, labyrinthine fistula, facial paresis, or cerebrospinal fluid leakage. CT scans are often ordered for patients who have had prior operations. Temporal bone radiographs have been replaced by CT scanning in most otologic practices.

## CASE EXAMPLE

J.M. is a 42-year-old man who presented with a several-month history of recurrent otorrhea and one episode of spontaneous bleeding from the left ear but no hearing loss. In-office binocular microscopic examination revealed an epitympanic cholesteatoma with no obvious middle ear extension. In January 1997, he underwent a stage 1 (primary), intact canal wall mastoidectomy with cartilage tympanoplasty. At surgery, an epitympanic and antral cholesteatoma was excised in the standard fashion. The far reaches of the epitympanum, especially the medial wall of the scutum, were examined intraoperatively with a 4-mm, 30° endoscope. The scutum defect was repaired with a tragal cartilage graft. The malleus and incus had superficial erosion from the cholesteatoma, but the ossicular linkage was intact. A significant portion of the tegmen tympani and tegmen mastoideum was eroded by the cholesteatoma. The facial recess was widely opened to create an accessory air tract into the mastoid. After the first surgery, the tympanic membrane and scutum appeared anatomically normal. There was no significant conductive hearing impairment before or after surgery. Nine months after surgery, the only concern is whether any residual cholesteatoma matrix remained in the epitympanum and mastoid antrum. This patient is an ideal candidate to undergo an endoscopic second-look operation because he has no need for an ossicular reconstruction and there was no extension into the middle ear.

At the stage 2, second-look operation, a 1-cm postauricular incision was made. The prior mastoidectomy cavity was entered. The argon laser was used to burn through the fibrous adhesions to expose the entire surgical region. The Silastic sheeting, which had been inserted through the facial recess, was removed with a cup forceps, and the argon laser was used to trim away obstructing fibrous tissue. Through this stab incision, 4-mm, 30° and 70° endoscopes were used to examine the mastoid and epitympanum. There was no evidence of residual cholesteatoma. The surgical cavity was filled with saline, and the incision was closed with 4-0 absorbable suture and a bandage.

This case represents a common presentation and surgical treatment. The nonendoscopic procedure would require a longer postauricular incision and redrilling any reformed mastoid cortex. The endoscopic technique is more easily tolerated because it is minimally invasive.

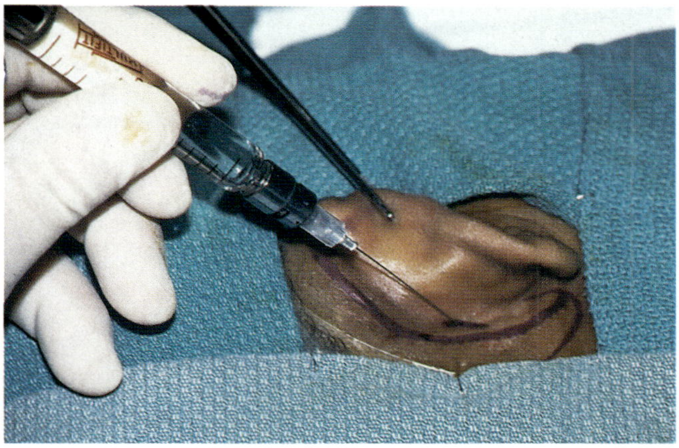

**FIGURE 6.3.** The anticipated site of entry is mapped out.

## INSTRUMENTATION

Three types of equipment are needed:

1. Endoscopes: standard adult (4-mm) and pediatric (2.7-mm) endoscopes are available from a large number of commercial venders. The most commonly used angles are 30° and 70°. A 0° endoscope can be used for orientation but is inferior to the 0° view that a binocular microscope furnishes.
2. Powerful light source
3. Argon or potassium-titanyl-phosphate (KTP) laser: a fiberoptically administered laser is essential to burn away fibrous adhesions that usually form after a stage 1 cholesteatoma surgery and to create a relative bloodless surgical field. Any active bleeding hampers the use of an endoscope or operating microscope.

## ANESTHESIA

General anesthesia is used in all primary cholesteatoma operations. General or local anesthesia with sedation is used for patients undergoing second-look procedures, depending on the preference of the patient and surgeon.

## OPERATIVE TECHNIQUE FOR SECOND-LOOK ENDOSCOPIC SURGERY

1. A 1-cm postauricular incision is made. It is best to center this just above the level of the meatus to facilitate entry into the epitympanum (Figs. 6.3 to 6.5).
2. Sharp dissection is carried out with a scalpel and small sharp scissors to enter and then define previous mastoid cavity.
3. Débridement of fibrous adhesions is achieved with a KTP or argon fiberoptically delivered laser. The laser preserves the maximum amount of mucosa that has relined the middle ear cleft. Silastic sheeting, when used during the first operation, is removed, and the laser is used to maximally reestablish the normal ventilatory air tracts. This reduces unnecessary removal of normal mucosa when a nonendoscopic technique is used.
4. Meticulous hemostasis is obtained with bipolar Bovie cautery, argon or KTP laser, topical 1 : 1,000 epinephrine and Gelfoam pledgets, and other methods.
5. A medium-large otic speculum is introduced through the postauricular incision (i.e., not into the ear canal).

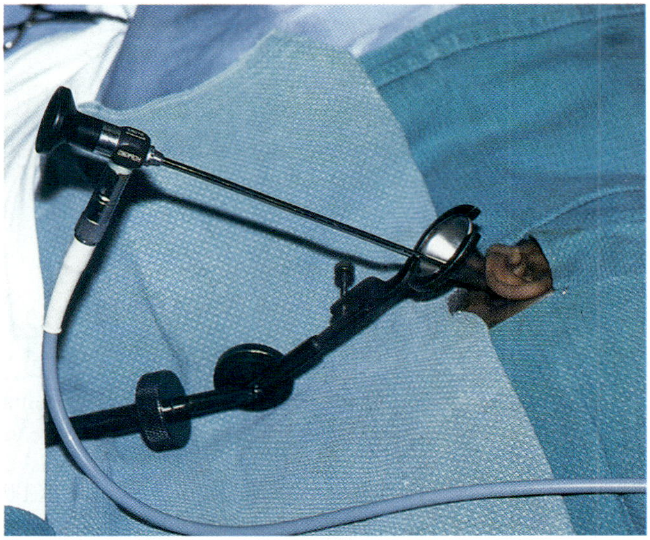

**FIGURE 6.4.** The path of passage of the endoscope is lined by a no. 3 optic speculum secured on a speculum holder.

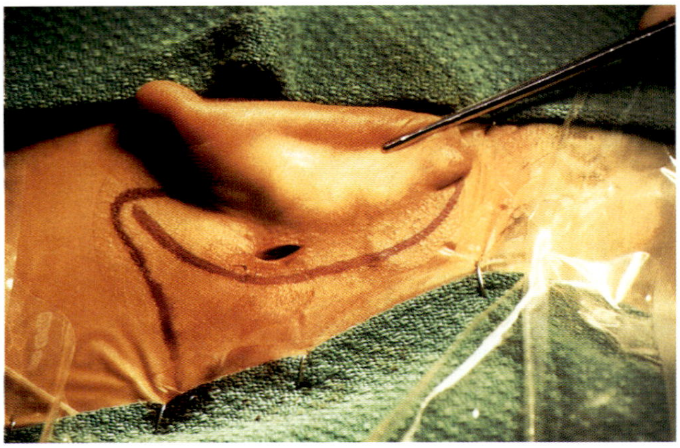

**FIGURE 6.5.** The incision is closed with an absorbable subcuticular suture.

The speculum is best immobilized with a speculum holder (Fig. 6.4). This permits the rapid passage of various-sized and -angled endoscopes into the mastoid cavity without staining the endoscopic lens with blood.

6. The mastoid cavity and epitympanum are examined.
7. Usually, a 2.7-mm endoscope can be passed entirely or partially through the facial recess to examine the middle ear, especially the facial recess, hypotympanum, and medial surface of the tympanic membrane. Available endoscopes do not have an angle obtuse enough to see into the sinus tympani through the facial recess. This area must be visualized through the ear canal by an exploratory tympanotomy if cholesteatoma matrix was removed from this area during the stage 1 operation.
8. Ossicular chain reconstruction is performed through an enlarged postauricular incision or through the canal, depending on the anatomy.
9. The incision is closed with one or two absorbable subcuticular sutures.
10. A small dressing, such as an adhesive bandage or small piece of gauze or Tegaderm, is applied.

## ADDITIONAL ENDOSCOPIC TECHNIQUES DURING PRIMARY CHOLESTEATOMA SURGERY

The use of endoscopes during primary cholesteatoma surgery is more straightforward because the exposure is larger than necessary. The most important prerequisite is to obtain meticulous hemostasis, for which the argon or KTP laser is invaluable. The endoscope should initially be introduced with both hands for better stability. Dissection of questionable tissue often is performed by alternating between the binocular microscope and the endoscope. In this use, the surgeon should consider the endoscope similar but superior to an operative mirror.

## POSTOPERATIVE CARE

The postoperative care of an endoscopically performed second-look operation is considerably easier than for the more traditional postauricular second-look mastoidectomy technique. Instead of a Glasscock plastic ear bubble or a mastoid dressing, a small piece of gauze or an adhesive bandage over the stab incision is all that is required. Usually, the dressing is removed the night of surgery or the next morning. Minimal pain medicine, usually acetaminophen or aspirin, is used. Showering the morning after surgery is encouraged, but water in the ear canal should be avoided if the tympanic membrane has been covered by packing or ointment.

## COMPLICATIONS

There have been no instances of significant endoscopic injury to the facial nerve, brain, dura, cochlea, semicircular canals, or ossicular chain in nearly 10 years of using this technique in hundreds of cholesteatoma surgeries, including second-look and during primary cholesteatoma operations. These complications can and do occur for various other reasons but not due exclusively to the endoscopic technique. Minor complications such as bruising of the mucosa on the cochlear promontory, ear canal hematomas, and bumping the ossicular chain are not uncommon but have little long-term adverse effects. Using a bimanual grasp of the endoscope, especially until the surgeon is familiar with the instrumentation, reduces major and minor complications.

## ADVANTAGES OF THE ENDOSCOPIC TECHNIQUE

The advantages of using the endoscopic technique are twofold. First, there is better visualization of pathology. The endoscope augments rather than replaces the binocular microscope. It allows the surgeon to see around corners and into areas that are at an acute or right angle. Second, there is less normal tissue distortion and damage.

## REFERENCES

1. McKennan KX. Endoscopic "second look" mastoidoscopy to rule out residual epitympanic/mastoid cholesteatoma. *Laryngoscope* 1993;103:810–814.

2. Takahashi H, Honjo I, Fujita A, et al. Transtympanic endoscopic findings in patients with otitis media with effusion. *Arch Otolaryngol Head Neck Surg* 1990;116:1186–1189.
3. Schindler RA, Lanser MJ. The surgical management of cholesteatoma—the contribution of the laser. In: Tos M, Thomsen J, Peitersen E, eds. *Proceedings of the Third International Conference on Cholesteatoma*. Amsterdam: Kugler & Ghedini Publications, 1988:769–778.
4. Shelton C, Sheehy JL. Tympanoplasty: review of 400 staged cases. *Laryngoscope* 1990;100:679–681.
5. Austin DF. Staging in cholesteatoma surgery. *J Laryngol Otol* 1989;103:143–148.

# 7

# PERILYMPHATIC FISTULA

**ASHRAF S. ABOU-HALAWA**
**DENNIS S. POE**

Middle ear endoscopy has been employed as a minimally invasive procedure in the diagnosis and management of cases of perilymph fistulas (PLFs). A PLF is an abnormal communication between the perilymphatic space and the middle ear, usually occurring in the region of oval or round windows. Temporal bone studies of patients with the diagnosis of PLF during their life showed patent fissula antefenestrae and microfissures filled with loose areolar tissue. The latter are usually found in the region between the round window and posterior semicircular canal ampulla. Congenital anomalies have been clinically associated with an increased incidence of fistulas (1).

Stapedectomy, head trauma, barotrauma, surgery of chronic ear disease, and physical exertion are the main predisposing factors for acquired PLF. However, in about 25% of cases, no such factors could be found. The designation spontaneous or idiopathic PLF is appropriate in these cases. However, the diagnosis and even the mere existence of spontaneous PLF are among the most controversial issues among otologists.

Despite the large case series and detailed case reports in the literature (2,3), some eminent otologists accept the possibility of perilymph leak after otologic surgery, significant head trauma, and congenital anomalies, but they question the so-called spontaneous PLF (4). Simmons (5) expressed the frustration of many otolaryngologists because of lack of firm guidelines for preoperative diagnosis of spontaneous PLF and questioned the indications for surgical exploration in such cases. There is general agreement that the signs and symptoms of PLF are variable, specific diagnostic tests are lacking, intraoperative diagnosis is fraught with artifactual errors, and uniform guidelines for PLF management are lacking.

## CLINICAL EVALUATION AND INVESTIGATIONS

Symptoms of PLF are nonspecific and may include a whole spectrum of hearing loss, tinnitus, vertigo, and aural fullness. Hearing loss may be sudden, profound, fluctuating, or progressive, and it is reported to some degree in more than 80% of patients. Fluctuation of word recognition scores alone occurs in 20% (6). Vestibular symptoms are not specific to PLF and include true vertigo, disequilibrium, lightheadedness, and motion intolerance. Ménière's disease, vestibular migraines, and other vestibular disorders must be considered in the differential diagnosis. Some patients have vertigo only with straining, exertion, or a Valsalva maneuver (2–6). A strong history of previous surgery, trauma, or barotrauma are the most suggestive historical factors for possible PLF.

The most commonly reported clinical test for a fistula is the *fistula test,* which involves sustained positive and negative pressure challenges to the tympanic membrane with pneumatic otoscopic or tympanometric equipment. The test is considered positive if deviation of the eyes is detected (i.e., objective response) or the patient reports the sensation of dizziness (i.e., subjective response) (6). Collective series report only 35% of patients with PLF as having a positive fistula test result, and different investigators use various techniques to enhance the test, such as doing the test with the patient standing (i.e., platform fistula test) or monitoring with electronystagmography (7). Conventional electronystagmography is frequently done but is neither sensitive nor specific for PLF. Neuro-otologic examination, laboratory, and imaging studies, as appropriate, should be done to investigate the possibility of other vestibular or neurologic disorders.

After the diagnosis of PLF has been entertained, the management is controversial. Acute PLF may be managed conservatively with light activity, bed rest, or acetazolamide, or it may be urgently explored. Failure of medical management for several days is a common indication for surgical exploration.

## SURGICAL EXPLORATION OF PERILYMPHATIC FISTULA

When the clinical history, examination, and diagnostic tests indicate a PLF, many investigators proceed to middle ear exploration, arguing that closure of the PLF can eliminate or improve the vestibular symptoms in most cases and stabilize hearing in many patients (2,3,6,7). Even when no fistula can be definitely confirmed, most otologists patch the oval and round windows with tissue grafts because of the possibility of a minute or intermittently patent fistula (8).

Confirmation of perilymph leak at the time of middle ear exploration depends on the repeated accumulation of fluid in the oval and round window niches. Observation for at least 5 minutes with very gentle suction to demonstrate the repeated collection of fluid is recommended (2,3,5–8). Intraoperative provocative measures to elevate venous and cerebrospinal fluid (CSF) pressure with a Trendelenburg position, compression of the jugular vein, Valsalva maneuver, or increased intrathoracic pressure may help detect a PLF. However, the local anesthetic solution injected during the operation or tissue transudates from the incisions may be mistaken for perilymph (9).

Locally injected anesthetic solution and tissue transudates from incisions pool in the dependently located oval and round window niches and may be easily mistaken for perilymph. Reaccumulation of these fluids after repeated aspiration looks identical to pooling because of a perilymphatic fistula. Repeated accumulation of fluids in the niches cannot be used as a true confirmation of PLF. It may be reasonably assumed that fluid artifacts have contributed to false-positive explorations reported in the literature, because it is nearly impossible to completely eliminate these unwanted fluid collections (9).

Fluorescein has been used intrathecally (10) and intravenously (11) to enhance detection of PLF during surgical exploration. Although intrathecal fluorescein may be useful as a tracer for the perilymph through the cochlear aqueduct, there may be complications related to its use (12). Intravenous fluorescein has not been found to accumulate in the inner ear of animal models and has no usefulness for PLF evaluation (13).

Protein electrophoresis may differentiate between perilymph and other clear fluids that may pool in the window area during exploration (14). $\beta_2$-Transferrin is found in perilymph and CSF but not in high concentrations in serum. Problems with the $\beta_2$-transferrin assay have prevented its adoption as a standard assay for PLF. It is difficult manage very small sample sizes. The assay requires time, and the results are received after surgery is completed. Western blot techniques for $\beta_2$-transferrin are highly specific for perilymph and CSF but unfortunately of low sensitivity because of dilutional artifacts with the very small sample size (15).

Until the development of sensitive biochemical assays, imaging techniques, or specific tracers, there is a need for a minimally invasive procedure in the diagnosis and management of suspected PLF. The senior author (A.S.A-H.) has used middle ear endoscopy for various otologic conditions, including suspected cases of PLF, since 1990. Endoscopy has the advantages of providing excellent views of the window niches without introducing the injection or transudate artifacts (16).

## INDICATIONS FOR MIDDLE EAR ENDOSCOPIC EXPLORATION FOR POSSIBLE PERILYMPHATIC FISTULA

Any patient who has a suspected PLF and is a candidate for open surgical exploration may be considered for an endoscopic exploration. The history in adults should include a strong association between a significant traumatic event (e.g., otologic surgery, head injury, barotrauma) and the onset of symptoms. The patient must have true vertigo, disequilibrium, or hearing loss. Most cases have vertigo with or without hearing loss. Exploration on the basis of hearing loss is done mostly in pediatric cases or highly suspicious adult cases. There may be a relationship between fluctuations in hearing or vertigo and straining, bending, lifting, or Valsalva maneuver, but careful questioning is needed to differentiate between a true association with elevated CSF pressure and head movement–induced vertigo. The physical examination should show no other obvious otologic or neurologic pathology. A positive subjective or objective fistula response should be elicited. Laboratory and imaging studies, if indicated, should be negative for other causes of hearing loss or vertigo.

Children may have additional compelling indications such as congenital anomalies and fluctuating or progressive sensorineural hearing loss (17). Children must be carefully evaluated for various pathologic conditions, with the child's parents actively participating in the management protocol.

In the event of noniatrogenic trauma, a few days of observation with light activities or bed rest may be tried before recommendation for exploration. The final decision for middle ear endoscopy or formal middle ear exploration is individualized, because there are no conclusive signs, symptoms, or testing on which to base and objective diagnosis. Appropriate informed consent for the procedure is obtained, including a discussion of the controversies surrounding fistula diagnoses and examinations.

## CONTRAINDICATIONS TO MIDDLE EAR ENDOSCOPY

Middle ear endoscopy as an office procedure is contraindicated for apprehensive patients and children. A narrow or tortuous external canal may make endoscopic examination difficult or impossible. Acute hemotympanum, middle ear effusion, and inflammation prohibit adequate examination of the window niches. A thick, scarred, or inflamed tympanic membrane can cause excessive bleeding during endoscopy, and objective assessments of fluid pooling in the window niches is then impossible. Any middle ear condition obscuring the windows, such as severe tympanosclerosis, prohibits adequate endoscopic examinations. Tympanic membrane atrophy is a relative contraindication, because the myringotomy incision may result in persistent perforation.

## INSTRUMENTATION

Endoscopy is performed with rigid Hopkins rod telescopes with diameters of 1.7 to 1.9 mm and a length of 10 to 12 cm (Karl Storz Endoscopy–America, Inc., Culver City, CA; Richard Wolf Medical Instruments, Rosemont, IL; Smith & Nephew, Inc., Memphis, TN). The telescopes have view angles of 0° to 5° for straightforward overall views and 25° to 30° for close-up detailed inspection of the window niches. Illumination may be done with as little as a 150-W halogen light source. Higher-intensity illumination is not routinely required unless 35-mm photography is desired, and a 300-W source with a synchronized strobe is then recommended. Examinations may be done viewing directly through the endoscopes or preferably with a video camera and high-resolution monitor. Video recorders are recommended to allow review of the examination after the endoscope is withdrawn. Examinations are done with an otologic speculum in the external auditory canal. The myringotomy is performed with an operating microscope, phenol USP topical anesthesia applied with a 20-gauge suction tip, and a myringotomy blade. Defogging agents are applied each time before introducing endoscopes into the middle ear.

## OFFICE PROCEDURE LAYOUT

The patient is placed in the supine position in the examination chair with the affected ear facing upward as for a routine myringotomy. The operating microscope is readily available so that alternating between endoscopes and the microscope may be done easily. The endoscopes and myringotomy instruments are arranged on an equipment table above and adjacent to the patient's head. The video equipment is immediately adjacent to the equipment table to so that the operator need not rotate her or his head more than 90 degrees from the operating field during endoscopy (Fig. 7.1).

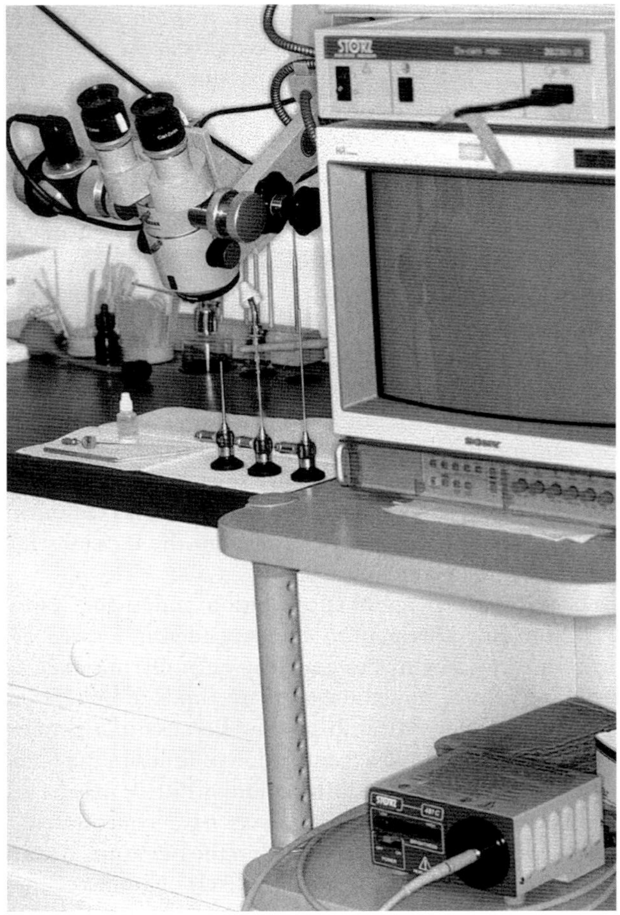

**FIGURE 7.1.** Endoscopic setup in the office.

## ANESTHESIA

Middle ear endoscopic examinations may be performed on awake patients in the office setting or as part of an exploration in the operating room before the open procedure. In either case, fluid artifacts are reduced to permit a more objective examination for fluid welling up in the window niches.

In the office, the patient is placed in the supine position. Under microscopic visualization through an otologic speculum, the tympanic membrane is inspected. A myringotomy is placed midway between the incus and round windows. If the location of the windows is not readily apparent, the incision should be made in the posterior-superior quadrant of the tympanic membrane along a radial line from the malleus umbo toward scutum at approximately 70° from the tympanic membrane's 12 o'clock position. A 20-gauge suction tip is connected to the suction tubing without turning on the suction and dipped into a small container of phenol USP solution. The container is immediately recapped to limit toxic fume exposure and the excess drops of phenol gently tapped off of the suction tip until a fine drop remains on the end of the tip. The tympanic membrane is visualized under the microscope again, and the suction tip is applied to the tympanic membrane along the radial line described previously from the umbo to nearly contacting the annulus at the scutum. The suction is then activated to remove any excess phenol. The patient usually experiences several seconds of burning sensation while the treated tympanic membrane blanches white. The anesthesia is then complete but only on the treated line. Phenol is the preferred anesthetic because it is also hemostatic and reduces transudates or blood from the incision. If the endoscopy is to be performed under general anesthesia, no topical treatment is needed.

## TECHNIQUE FOR MIDDLE EAR ENDOSCOPY

An otologic speculum is used that extends as far into the external auditory canal as possible, limiting possible discomfort or bleeding from inadvertent contact with the canal wall. The posterior-superior quadrant of the tympanic membrane is incised with a myringotomy blade along the radial line already anesthetized (Fig. 7.2). If using general anesthesia, the incision is made along the same line, but it may bleed. Gentle application of nasopharyngeal swabs or dry Gelfoam pledgets may aid in rapid hemostasis. The microscope is moved aside.

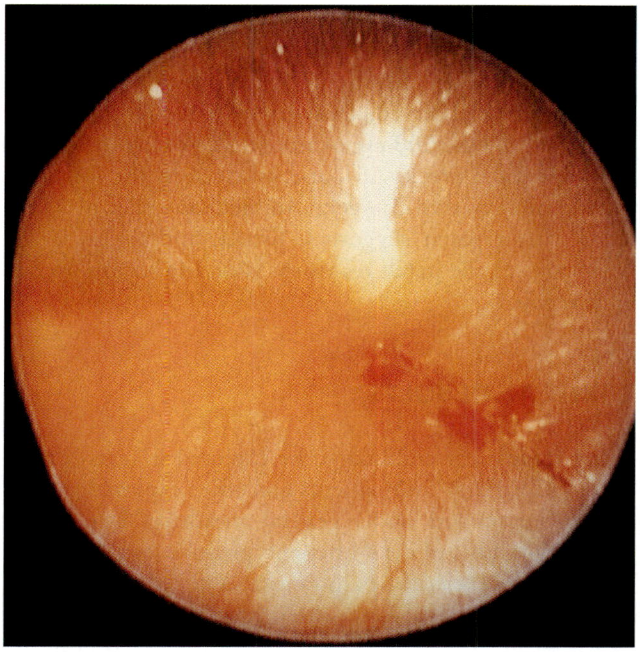

**FIGURE 7.2.** Tympanic membrane with myringotomy incision.

The patient is instructed to do several Valsalva maneuvers and hold each for several seconds. If the procedure is done under general anesthesia, the head is placed in a Trendelenburg position, and the intrathoracic pressure is elevated for several seconds.

The rigid telescope is inserted atraumatically into the middle ear space to visualize the oval and round window niches. A drop of defogging solution is placed on the endoscope tip. The nondominant hand holds the speculum in place, keeping the thumb and forefinger free to hold and guide the endoscope barrel. The main weight of the scope is held in the dominant hand, grasping it by the wider objective lens portion. The scope may be placed close to the myringotomy by looking along the scope's barrel and, once in position, viewing through the scope (Fig. 7.3).

Surgeons less familiar with endoscopic techniques find it easier to begin with a 0° or 5° forward-viewing scope and perform the examination looking directly through the endoscope. The 25° and 30° scopes are particularly disorienting because the view is angulated. It takes practice to be able to keep oriented using a camera and video monitor, but the image is superior. The straight-viewing endoscopes are useful only for examining the anatomic arrangement of the middle ear (Fig. 7.4).

The angled scope is introduced, and the oval window is examined first to confirm the location of the ossicles. The angled scope is rotated with the bevel directed superiorly (Fig. 7.5).The video camera stays in the same orientation throughout the examination. Only the endoscope is rotated. The scope is placed adjacent to the myringotomy, and looking at the monitor, it is then passed into the middle ear. Careful examination is performed to look for pooling or welling of perilymph. The endoscope is removed,

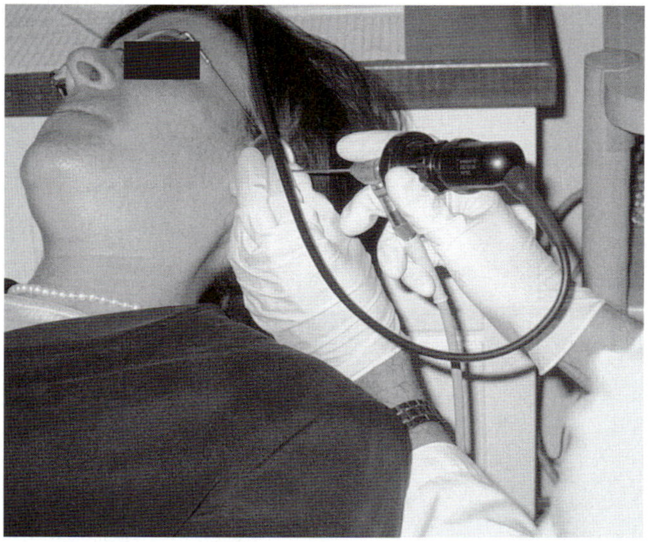

**FIGURE 7.3.** Introducing the endoscope into the middle ear.

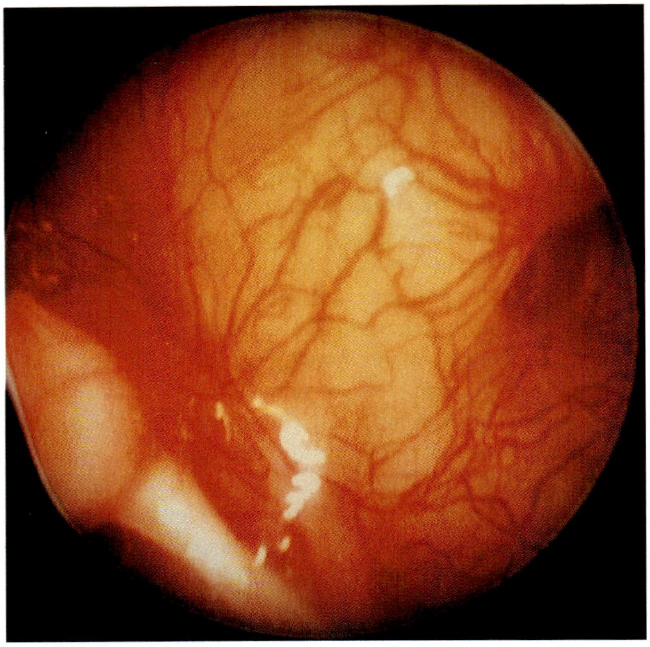

**FIGURE 7.4.** The 0° endoscopic view of a normal middle ear.

rotated to view the inferior mesotympanum, and replaced into the middle ear to inspect the round window (Fig. 7.6). Valsalva maneuvers are performed each time the scope is withdrawn, and several minutes are permitted to elapse for the potential accumulation of perilymph.

At the termination of the procedure, the myringotomy is reinspected under the microscope. If the myringotomy

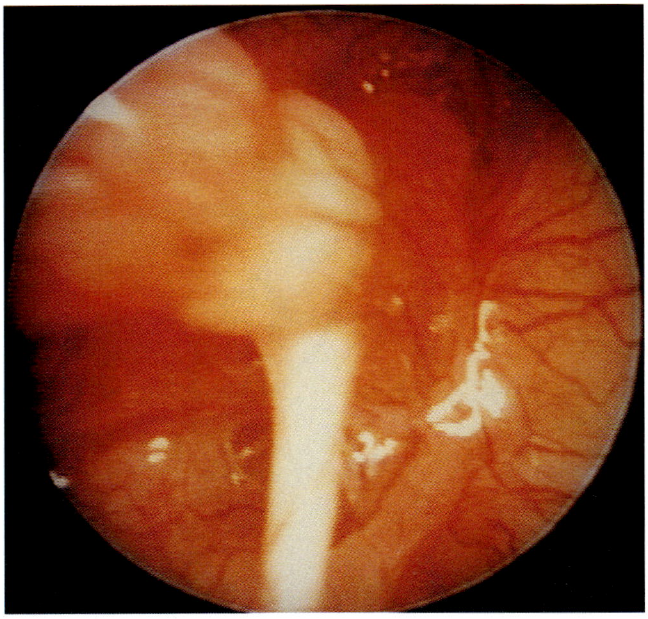

**FIGURE 7.5.** The 30° endoscopic view of the oval window in a normal middle ear.

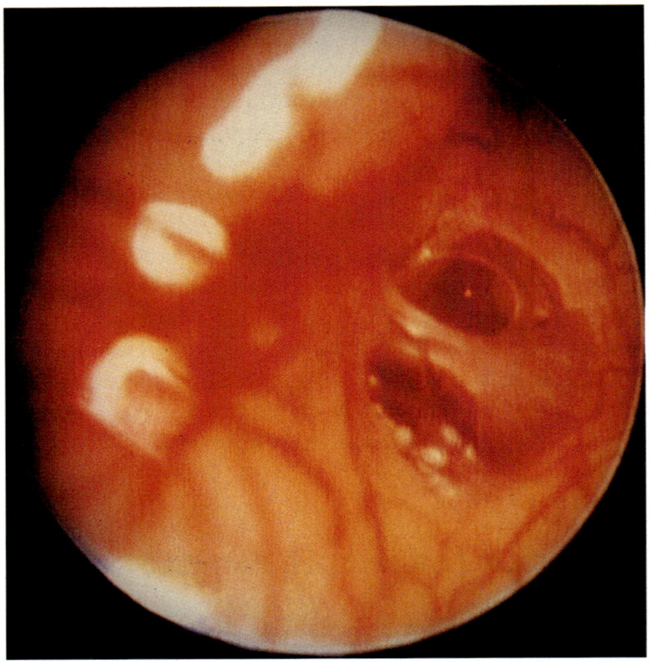

**FIGURE 7.6.** The 30° endoscopic view of the round window in a normal middle ear.

margins are widely separated, an adhesive Steri-Strip is placed over the defect, trimming a small circle and introducing it with an 18-gauge suction tip holding the nonadhesive surface.

If a fistula is observed or if it is suspected but not observed, an autologous blood patch may be introduced (18). It is delivered through the myringotomy with 27-gauge, 1.5-inch needle to fill the entire mesotympanum. The patient is kept supine until clotting of the blood in the syringe is observed. Patients with blood patches are instructed to take 500 mg of amoxicillin orally three times each day for 1 week. All patients are seen for follow-up examination within 3 weeks. Immediate relief of symptoms with a patch suggests a fistula, and return of the symptoms as the patch reabsorbs is an indication for surgical repair.

## CLINICAL RESULTS

Using middle ear endoscopy, we explored 67 ears for suspected PLF. Forty-four patients had office explorations, and 13 were examined under general anesthesia before open exploration. One of the 44 patients positive for a fistula had suffered a recent scuba barotrauma injury and was experiencing vertigo with head movements and straining. There had been no hearing loss. A thin membrane covering the round window niche was seen with yellow fluid filling the niche (Fig. 7.7). A blood patch produced immediate relief

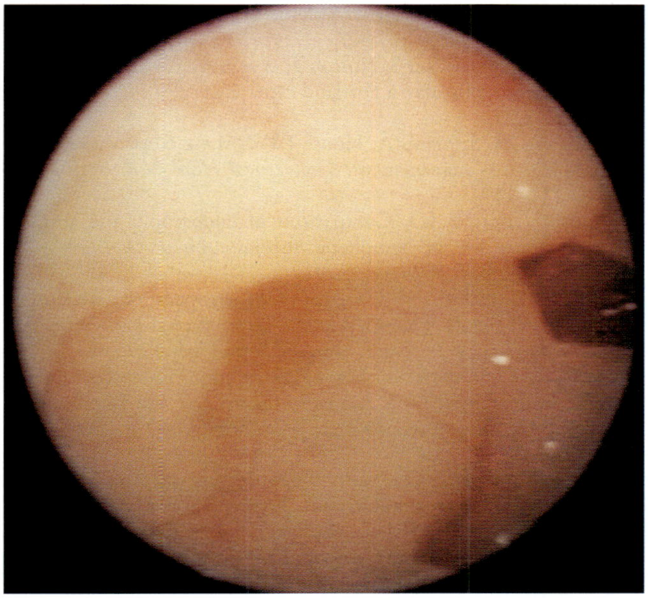

**FIGURE 7.7.** The 30° endoscopic view of a perilymphatic fistula in a round window.

of all vertigo. The vertigo began to return 1 week later but subsequently subsided.

In the general anesthesia group, the endoscopic examination was first completed, and 1 mL of lidocaine (1% solution) with 1 : 100,000 epinephrine then was injected into the external auditory meatus to compare with the endoscopic view. There were two identified fistulas (15%). Findings for 6 (46%) of the 13 cases were negative with the endoscopic exploration, but findings for the open examinations appeared to be positive, with clear fluid welling up in the oval or round window niches. It was concluded that the open examinations were seeing artifacts, because the immediately previous endoscopy was thorough and had completely negative results. There were five cases of inadequate examinations because of bleeding from lysis of adhesions in previously operated patients.

## SPECIAL POINTS

Of the 67 cases in our series, only three cases showed perilymph leak. Two of them were poststapedectomy cases, and the third was a scuba diver. We think that PLF is a rare clinicopathologic entity and that spontaneous PLF is unlikely in adults. This assessment agrees with the results of studies. Rosenberg (19) found no single case of perilymph leak in 13 middle ear endoscopies. Pyykkö (20) found only two cases as a result of exploration of 350 cases.

Patients with no detectable fluid leak during middle ear endoscopy may have Ménière's disease. We no longer recommend routine patching of the oval and round windows so that they may benefit from intratympanic injection of medications such as gentamicin if indicated in the future.

## POSTOPERATIVE CARE ISSUES

The ear is to be kept dry, and routine water precautions are recommended for 2 weeks. Nose blowing should be avoided. If a fistula was diagnosed, head elevation during sleep and no lifting of more than 15 kg are recommended actions for 4 weeks. A postoperative visit is usually scheduled 3 to 4 weeks later to ensure complete closure of the myringotomy.

## COMPLICATIONS

We have not had any complications with transtympanic middle ear endoscopy in 120 cases, including diagnoses other than PLF. There has been no persistent tympanic membrane perforation, hearing loss, infection, or vertigo. One patient who had a sudden hearing loss before the endoscopy continued to have progressive deterioration of speech discrimination score (SDS) after endoscopy, but by the end of 6 months, there was a definite improvement in his SDS. Different investigators have reported 1% to 2% rates of persistent drum perforation and middle ear infection. There have been anecdotal reports of dislocated ossicles from endoscopy, and care with the angled endoscopes is emphasized.

## ADVANTAGES OF MIDDLE EAR ENDOSCOPY AND LIMITATIONS

Middle ear endoscopy is a minimally invasive technique that reduces morbidity, anesthetic use, costs, and surgical artifacts. Visualization of the round and oval windows is comparable to the view with an operating microscope, and with an angled scope, it is possible to see areas in the window niches not visible with the microscope. Resolution is sufficient to detect fluid pooling in these areas. Middle ear endoscopy, however, needs much practice before mastering the technique and working off the monitor. In traumatic or postoperative cases, there may be adhesions and membranous obstructions that hinder the view or cause bleeding. The round window membrane or portions of the oval window may be covered with adhesions, but there is usually sufficient visualization to adequately inspect for accumulation of perilymph. Prolonged examinations (>1 minute in the middle ear) with a 300-W light source has created sufficient heating to induce a caloric response with vertigo and nystagmus. The effect subsides after removal of the endoscope.

## CONCLUSIONS

Transtympanic endoscopy of the middle ear is a useful technique for the evaluation of PLF. It has reduced the problems of intraoperative artifacts, improving the accuracy of fistula reporting. Since the use of endoscopy in our series and others, the rate of positive identifications has been markedly reduced from the rates in studies using open techniques. We must conclude from these data that open examinations for PLF include a significant number of false-positive findings and that observation of clear fluid welling up in the window niches in such cases is no longer an adequate standard for making the diagnosis. Specificity for a PLF is much improved endoscopically, but there still remains the challenge of identifying the source of fluid observed, even with an endoscope. Further work on assays of fluid samples and imaging, perhaps with spectroscopic analysis, may resolve some of these problems in the future.

## REFERENCES


1. Kohut RI, Hinojosa R, Thompson JN, et al. Idiopathic perilymphatic fistulas: a temporal bone histopathologic study with clinical, surgical, and histopathologic correlations. *Arch Otol Head Neck Surg* 1995;121:412–420.
2. Friedland DR, Wackym PA. A critical appraisal of spontaneous perilymphatic fistulas of the inner ear. *Am J Otol* 1999;20:261–279.
3. Weider DJ, Johnson GD. Perilymphatic fistula: a New Hampshire experience. *Am J Otol* 1988;9:184–196.
4. Shea JJ. The myth of spontaneous perilymph fistula. *Otolaryngol Head Neck Surg* 1992;107:613–616.
5. Simmons FB. PLF: some diagnostic problems. *Adv Otorhinolaryngol* 1982;28:68–72.
6. Seltzer S, McCabe BF. Perilymphatic fistula: the Iowa experience. *Laryngoscope* 1986;94:37–49.
7. Black FO, Pesznecker S, Norton T, et al. Surgical management of perilymphatic fistulas: a Portland experience. *Am J Otol* 1992;13:254–262.
8. Hughes GB, Sismanis A, House JW. Is there consensus in perilymph fistula management? *Otolaryngol Head Neck Surg* 1990;102:111–117.
9. Poe DS, Bottrill ID. Comparison of endoscopic and surgical exploration for perilymphatic fistulas. *Am J Otol* 1994;15:735–738.
10. Rauch SD. Intrathecal fluorescein for intraoperative detection of perilymph fistula. Presented at the International Perilymph Fistula Conference; Portland, Oregon; September 1990.
11. Syms CA, Atkins JS, Murphy TP. Intravenous fluorescein for the detection of perilymph fistulae. Presented at the International Perilymph Fistula conference; Portland, Oregon; September 1990.
12. Moseley JI, Carton CA, Stern WE. Spectrum of complications in the use of intrathecal fluorescein. *J Neurosurg* 1987;48:765–767.
13. Poe DS, Gadre AK, Rebeiz EE, Pankratov MM. Intravenous fluorescein for detection of perilymphatic fistulas. *Am J Otol* 1993;14:51–55.
14. Weber PC, Kelly RH, Bluestone CD, Bassiouny M. Beta-2-transferrin confirms perilymphatic fistula in children. *Otolaryngol Head Neck Surg* 1994;110:381–386.
15. Buchman CA, Luxford WM, Hirsch BE, et al. Beta-2-transferrin assay in the identification of perilymph. *Am J Otol* 1999;20:174–178.
16. Poe DS, Rebeiz EE, Pankratov MM. Evaluation of perilymphatic fistulas by middle ear endoscopy. *Am J Otol* 1992;13:529–533.
17. Supance JS, Bluestone CD. Sudden or fluctuating hearing loss and vertigo in children due to perilymph fistula. *Ann Otol Rhinol Laryngol* 1987;87:761–771.
18. Causse JB. Personal communication, 1991.
19. Rosenberg SI, Silverstein H, Wicox TO, Gordon MA. Endoscopy in otology and neurotology. *Am J Otol* 1994;15:168–172.
20. Pyykkö I, Selmani Z, Ramsay H. Middle ear imaging in neurotological work-up. *Acta Otolaryngol Suppl* 1995;520:273–276.

# 8

# EUSTACHIAN TUBE ENDOSCOPY

CHRISTOPHER J. LINSTROM

## INDICATIONS

The natural clinical course of chronic suppurative otitis media and cholesteatoma may best be understood in light of underlying eustachian tube dysfunction (1–7). The eustachian tube has been evaluated in an effort to correlate pathologic findings within the tube with medical and surgical treatment outcomes (1,2,5–9). Microendoscopy of the middle ear cleft has been well described, and various instruments for this technique are readily available (4,10–12). Previous work in the literature describes attempts to view the eustachian tube (13–16). Common themes among these investigators include the need for a small, flexible endoscope; the difficulty of retrograde (nasopharynx to middle ear cleft) intubation; and problems with instrument fit and with instrument breakage.

Endoscopy of the eustachian tube should be considered as an adjunct to other functional tests, such as tympanometry, manometry, and eustachian tube clearance tests. Endoscopy of the eustachian tube is largely a qualitative evaluation, although this technique is able to locate areas of expected narrowing such as the isthmus and other areas of obstruction. There does not appear to be a strict correlation between pathologic findings and functional outcome. However, it must be stressed that eustachian tube endoscopy is still in its formative stages, and conclusions cannot be drawn at this time about its efficacy.

Endoscopy of the eustachian tube may be indicated for the surgical patient with suspected or proven severe eustachian tube dysfunction, as evidenced by chronic suppurative otitis media, cholesteatoma, adhesive otitis media, or recurrent serous otitis media. However, it remains an investigative technique.

## CONTRAINDICATIONS

Contraindications to endoscopy of the eustachian tube are similar to those for endoscopy of the middle ear and mastoid, including lack of patient cooperation or tolerance, usually because of insufficient local anesthesia of the area to be examined; an anatomic misfit of the eustachian tube orifice; and evidence of instrument malfunction, especially of instrument breakage.

## PREOPERATIVE EVALUATION

The patient to be evaluated by endoscopy of the eustachian tube has clinical evidence of eustachian tube malfunction. These patients almost always have adhesive or chronic suppurative otitis media or cholesteatoma. Endoscopy should be viewed as an adjunct to the overall patient evaluation.

The patient requires a thorough history and physical examination, with careful attention to items in the history that would support eustachian tube dysfunction such as a cleft palate, seasonal allergies, a smoking history, or for an adult, a history of recurrent ear infections as a child. The otologic history should concentrate on recurrent ear infections with or without a perforation of the tympanic membrane and cholesteatoma formation. Most patients present with features of hearing loss and recurrent otorrhoea.

The physical examination of the ear should include all parts of the ear that can be examined, including the auricle and the complete tympanic membrane. If the ear is occluded with wax or debris, it must first be cleaned, preferably under a microscope with suction. Care is taken to examine *all* aspects of the pars tensa and pars flaccida. Any crusts are gently removed in the cooperative patient. These crusts often conceal perforations or cholesteatoma.

If the patient has a perforation, the examiner should consider the status of the middle ear mucosa, the thickness of it, and any accompanying polypoid formation or discharge. Sequestration of keratinous debris suggests cholesteatoma and should be looked for. The status of the ossicular chain is recorded. This may often be difficult in the patient with severe tympanosclerosis.

In the patient with clinical evidence of eustachian tube dysfunction, the nasopharynx should be examined through an indirect (mirror) examination or with a fiberoptic endoscope. The adenoid bed and the fossae of Rosenmüller should be carefully examined for evidence of anatomic obstruction. This is rarely found in the adult. If there is residual adenoid tissue, the surgeon may wish to perform an adenoidectomy before definitive otologic surgery. However, there is no proven medical or surgical means to restore function to the eustachian tube. Artificially stenting the eustachian tube has not provided enduring benefit to the patient.

The patient must have a reliable audiogram with measurements for each ear of pure tone and bone thresholds, speech reception threshold, and word discrimination. Immittance testing should include tympanometry, ipsilateral and contralateral reflex testing, and tests for acoustic reflex decay for each ear.

Most patients have computed tomography (CT) of the temporal bones without contrast before surgery. These studies should be done with edge enhancement and with thin cuts of 1.0 to 1.5 mm, and they should include bone windows in the axial and true coronal planes. Both planes must be imaged to adequately define the structures in question. Attention is given to areas of bony erosion, especially of the scutum, the horizontal canal, and the ossicular chain. The mastoid air cell system is evaluated for development and aeration. The course of the facial nerve is followed from its entrance within the internal auditory canal, through its intratympanic course, and through the stylomastoid foramen.

## CASE EXAMPLES

### Case 1

#### *History*

A 55-year-old man had chronic serous otitis media with pars tensa perforation of the right ear. The clinical classification was Bellucci type 3 (i.e., perforation of ear drum, usually moist; intervals of dryness) (1). The patient did not have a history of recurrent ear infections and had had no previous otologic surgery.

#### *Investigations*

**Audiometry**

Preoperatively, the patient was found to have moderate mixed hearing loss with a notch at 4 kHz. The A-B gap was 20 to 25 dB, with 50 dB at 4 kHz. The speech reception threshold showed a 40-dB hearing loss, and the speech discrimination score was 96%. The tympanogram was type B with absent ipsilateral reflexes.

**Eustachian Tube Function**

Preoperative tests of eustachian tube clearance, including the Toynbee (i.e., swallowing with oral and nasal occlusion) and Valsalva (i.e., forced expiration against a closed nose and mouth) maneuvers with impedance bridge measurement of pressure, were abnormal. The patient could not clear the middle ear cleft.

**Radiologic Studies**

A CT scan without contrast of the petrous temporal bones revealed a well-developed, opacified middle ear cleft and mastoid process with thinning of the tegmen tympani and mastoideum. Encephalocele of the temporal lobe was suspected. T1-weighted, T2-weighted, and flair magnetic resonance images with gadolinium enhancement failed to definitively diagnose an encephalocele.

**Surgical Findings**

A right tympanoplasty with mastoidectomy (canal wall up) was performed on December 12, 1998. The middle ear mucosa was normal. No cholesteatoma was seen. The ossicular chain was intact and mobile. A temporal lobe encephalocele extended from the tegmen tympani over the ossicular chain. It was resected and confirmed by frozen section to be brain tissue. It was repaired from below. Underlay grafting of the tympanic membrane was performed.

**Endoscopy**

A flexible, nonarticulating (0.5-mm) endoscope was used. There was complete passage and the eustachian tube mucosa was normal (Fig. 8.1). No anatomic obstruction was found.

**Postoperative Course**

The ear healed well with mild retraction of the graft. A postoperative audiogram on February 9, 1999, showed a

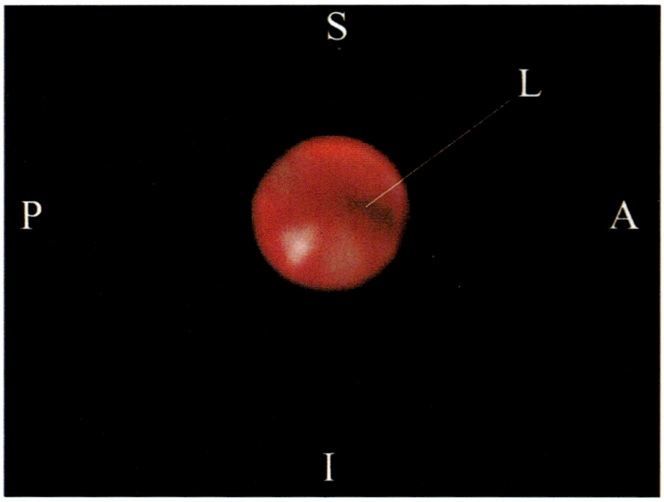


**FIGURE 8.1.** Right ear: chronic suppurative otitis media. The nonarticulating scope was used and passed to 6 mm (i.e., infundibulum). The mucosa is moderately thickened. *A,* anterior; *I,* inferior; *L,* lumen; *P,* posterior; *S,* superior.

10-dB improvement for the right ear, with a speech reception threshold of 35 dB and speech discrimination score of 100%. The tympanogram was type C with absent reflexes. Clinically, the patient is beginning to autoinsufflate the middle ear cleft with the Valsalva maneuver.

## Case 2

### History

A 49-year-old man had chronic suppurative otitis media of the right ear with perforation of the pars tensa. The Bellucci classification was type 2 (i.e., perforation of ear drum, usually dry; intervals of moisture).

### Investigations

**Audiometry**
Preoperatively, the patient has severe mixed hearing loss, with an A-B gap of 50 dB in low to middle frequencies. The speech reception threshold test showed a 70-dB hearing loss, and the speech discrimination score was 80%.

**Eustachian Tube Function**
Preoperatively, the patient had severe eustachian tube dysfunction. The tympanogram was flat, with an absent peak pressure and absent acoustic reflexes. Tests of eustachian tube clearance, including the Toynbee and the Valsalva maneuvers with an impedance bridge measurement, were flat, indicating a lack of clearance.

**Radiologic Imaging Studies**
A preoperative CT scan of the petrous temporal bones without contrast revealed a completely sclerotic mastoid and a large central perforation of the tympanic membrane with opacification of the middle ear space extending to Prussak's space, the fossa incudis, the oval window niche, and the hypotympanum. The manubrium of the malleus and the stapes were not well imaged. The structures of the otic capsule were normal.

**Surgical Findings**
No cholesteatoma was found. The middle ear mucosa was hypertrophic with polyp formation. Examination of the ossicular chain revealed an intact and mobile malleus and an intact and mobile stapes arch. There was incudostapedial arch erosion. A right tympanoplasty with mastoidectomy with incus interposition was performed.

**Endoscopy**
The articulating endoscope (1.0 mm diameter) was used to examine the middle ear cleft and the eustachian tube. The eustachian tube mucosa was moderately thickened at the orifice (Fig. 8.2). The endoscope passed easily through the eustachian tube to the nasopharynx. Nasal vibrissae could be seen clearly.

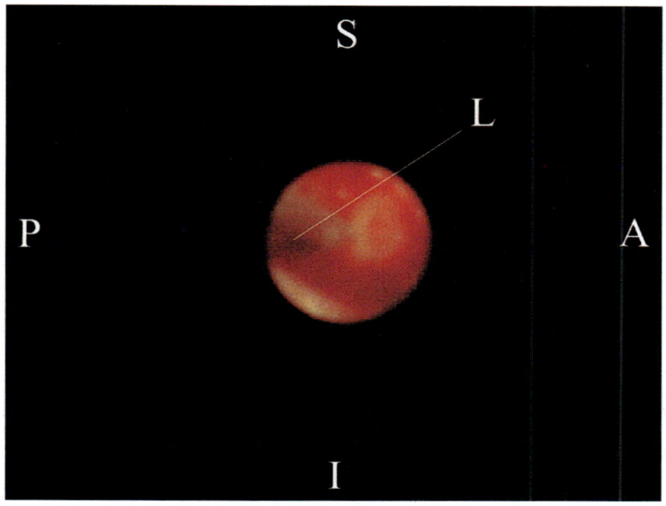


**FIGURE 8.2.** Right ear: intraluminal view of the eustachian tube. The nonarticulating scope used, with passage to 15 mm and showing hypertrophic eustachian tube mucosa. *A,* anterior; *I,* inferior; *L,* lumen; *P,* posterior; *S,* superior.

The postoperative audiogram performed on November 17, 1998, showed no significant change in the A-B gap. The speech recognition threshold test result was 65 dB with 96% discrimination. Immittance testing revealed a type C tympanogram with peak pressure of −140 daPa.

## INSTRUMENTATION

My colleagues and I have developed a small, nonarticulating endoscope (0.5 mm diameter, 3,000 pixels) (Fig. 8.3) and an articulating endoscope (1.0 mm diameter, 3,000 pixels) (Fig. 8.4) for the study of the eustachian tube (Ωmega Endoscopic Technologies, San Diego, CA). All commercially available articulating fiberoptic endoscopes that we tried were too large to pass into the eustachian tube.

The eustachian tube microendoscope is illuminated by a xenon light source and articulates with a digital video camera. The signal from this digital camera is then split and connected first to a digital picture-in picture (PIP) processor and then to a super VHS recorder (SVHS VCR) and into a video monitor. The second portion of the split signal is linked to a digital still recorder and then into the monitor. An outline of the instrument setup is provided in Fig. 8.5. A source list for components is provided in Table 8.1.

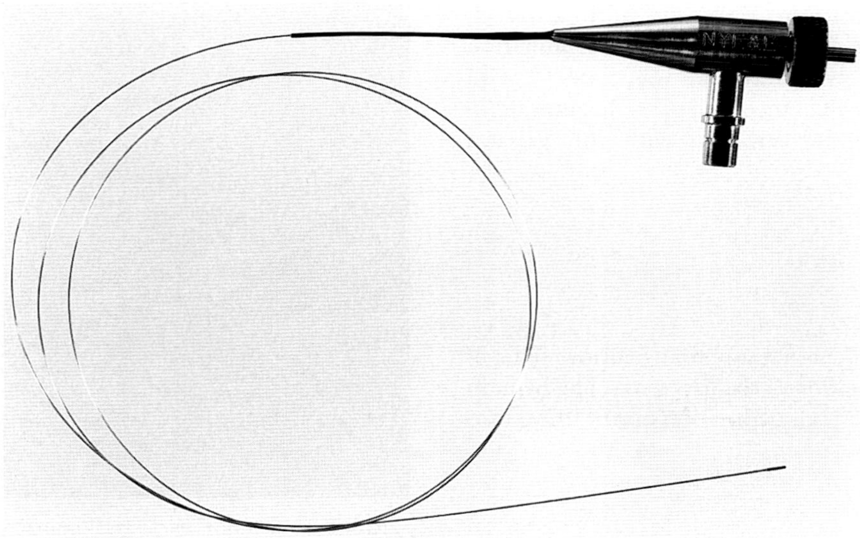

**FIGURE 8.3.** Nonarticulating endoscope (0.5-mm diameter; 3,000 pixels).

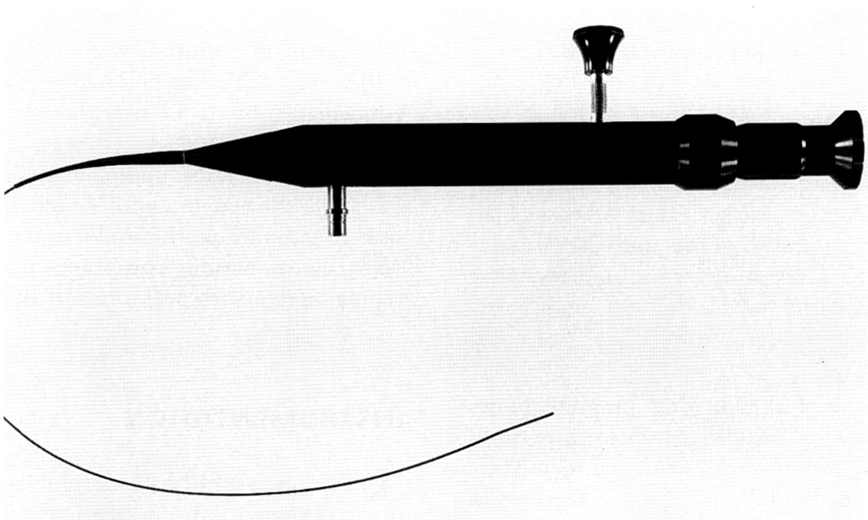

**FIGURE 8.4.** Articulating endoscope (1.0-mm diameter; 3,000 pixels). The endoscope articulates 180° in one direction only.

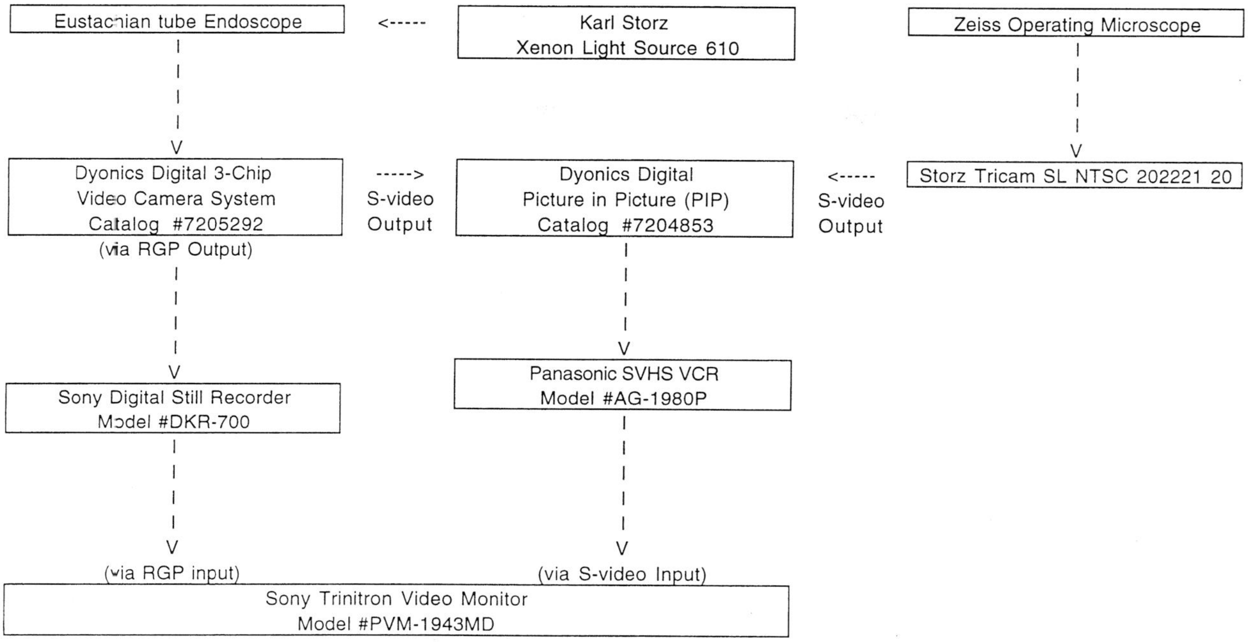


**FIGURE 8.5.** A scheme for all components of the imaging system.

## TABLE 8.1. COMPONENT SOURCE LIST

Ωmega Endoscopic Technologies, Inc.
4452 Conrad Avenue
San Diego, CA 92117
(619) 224-6946
(New York Eye and Ear Infirmary
Eustachian Tube Endoscope)

Panasonic, Inc.
Division of Matushita Electric of Puerto Rico, Inc.
San Global Industrial Park
65th Infantry Avenue, Km. 9.5
Carolina, P.R. 00630
(800) 524-0864
(Video SVHS Camera/Recorder,
Model: AG-1980P)

Sony Medical Systems
Sony Electronics, Inc.
3 Paragon Drive
Montvale, NJ 07645
(800) 686-7669
(Video Monitor and Digital Still Recorder
Model: DKR-700)

Karl Storz Endoscopy
91 Carpenter Hill Road
Charlton, MA 01507
(800) 421-0837
Xenon Light Source Model 610
and Tricam SL NTSC 20221-20 Camera)

Smith & Nephew Endoscopy
160 Dascomb Road
Andover, MA 01810
(800) 343-5717
(Dyonics Digital 3-Chip Camera #7205292
with Picture-in-Picture [PIP] #7204853)

Zeiss, Inc.
One Zeiss Drive
Thornwood, NY 10594
(800) 633-6610
(Zeiss Operating Microscope)

## OPERATING ROOM LAYOUT

The operating room is configured in the standard layout for otologic surgery. Ideally, the microscope lies at the head of the table, the surgeon sits on the side of the operated ear, and the nurse is positioned directly across the table from the surgeon. The anesthesiologist is positioned at the foot of the patient, on the side of the operated ear. A 65-cm-long inhalational circuit should be used to maximize the working room.

The monitoring equipment is best contained in a single, rolling unit, if this is possible. The monitor should be placed upwardmost within this unit or supported on a separate wall-mounted unit for easy viewing. The monitor should be able to be viewed by the surgeon, the scrub nurse, and all personnel within the room. Because part of the operating equipment remains sterile and part is not sterile, a working space must be left near the sterile field for the circulating nurse or nonsterile assistant to hand instruments onto the field. The circulating nurse or medical assistant must have sufficient room near the head of the patient to pass instruments toward the sterile field and assemble connecting cables to the monitoring equipment.

## ANESTHESIA

All of our cases have been performed under general endotracheal anesthesia as part of a larger otologic surgical procedure for perforation of the tympanic membrane, chronic suppurative otitis media, or cholesteatoma. Because intraoperative facial nerve monitoring is used during most of these cases, the patient may not be paralyzed during the entire procedure. Short-acting depolarizing agents or longer-acting agents that are reversed during the operation may be used. Other than this, there are no restrictions regarding the selection of inhalational anesthetic agents.

As with other forms of middle ear endoscopy, this technique lends itself to local anesthesia. The tympanic membrane may be anesthetized topically with 20% phenol or with a four-quadrant injection of the external auditory canal with local anesthetic. The middle ear mucosa may be easily anesthetized with a topical anesthetic agent such as lidocaine (Xylocaine) with or without epinephrine. This usually provides at least a half-hour's worth of anesthesia of the eustachian tube that is more than sufficient for its examination. The endoscopic equipment we employ is designed to be passed in an orthograde fashion (i.e., middle ear to nasopharynx) but may occasionally be passed in a retrograde fashion (i.e., nasopharynx to middle ear cleft). The nose should be anesthetized separately for the retrograde technique.

## OPERATIVE TECHNIQUE

Endoscopy of the eustachian tube is conducted under sterile conditions in an operating room as part of a larger surgical procedure. My colleagues and I do not perform eustachian tube endoscopy as a separate, outpatient procedure or as an office-based procedure.

Two flexible endoscopes have been employed in our studies. The first is a 0.5-mm flexible, *nonarticulating* endoscope. This is basically an angioscope that has been shortened to 40 cm to be manageable in and around the ear. The second is a flexible, *articulating* endoscope that is 1.0 mm in diameter. Both endoscopes have a ring for fine focus, a port for a halogen or xenon light source, and an end adapted for the television camera. Because the light cable is connected to a nonsterile light source, it is held by the nonsterile assistant. The camera and sterile endoscope may be handled by the surgeon or the scrub nurse.

Because of the small size necessary for the endoscope to pass through the eustachian tube, the number of pixels within the fiberoptic cable is limited to approximately 3,000. Likewise, the size of the picture on the television monitor is smaller than that obtained with a rigid endoscope. The viewer must prepare for these limitations that can be overcome in part by a doubling device within the camera or monitoring system. This enables a slightly larger picture to be presented, but it does not cover the entire screen.

The fiberoptic endoscope does not have the resolution power of a rigid endoscope. Middle ear structures, which are clearly seen with rigid endoscopy, appear somewhat fuzzy. This is the price of miniaturization and flexibility.

Before the surgeon passes the endoscope, it is important to defog it, usually with a liquid defogging agent or with warm saline, to white balance the system and to focus the endoscope. White balance is performed using a sterile white gauze. The instrument is fine focused by viewing any sterile object with printing on it, such as a suture package or a paper ruler. This is ordinarily easy to do. If the fine focus is especially difficult or impossible, the instrument is dirty or fogged over, or the fiberoptic cable is broken. The latter problem is a very real possibility with the articulating microendoscope. Every caution must be taken with these endoscopes to prevent internal breakage of the fiberoptic cable. Because of the small diameter, they are expensive and fragile.

After the instrument has been balanced, defogged, and focused, it is ready to be passed into the middle ear cleft. It is best to do this first under direct vision so that an important structure such as the ossicular chain is not inadvertently damaged.

As with any other surgical procedure, proper preoperative planning can maximize the efficient use of ancillary personnel and the yield of clinical information. An assistant familiar with all parts of the endoscopic equipment and setup must be present within the room to assist the scrub nurse and the surgeon. This individual may be the circulating nurse or a trained assistant. We employ a research assistant in this position. It is this individual's job to ensure that the patient has been adequately prepared for this part of this surgical procedure and that the endoscopic equipment is functional, that those parts touching the patient have been sterilized, that the video camera and recorder are prepared, and that the room has been properly prepared for the endoscopic procedure. By assigning these tasks to one individual, we have had no cancellations because of oversight. The research assistant also records pertinent data such as the status of the middle ear mucosa, the status of the ossicular chain, the length of passage of the endoscope within the eustachian tube, and other important points.

## SPECIAL POINTS

It must be stressed to all individuals involved in the procedure that the endoscopes are very fragile, expensive, and can be easily broken. They should be uncoiled gently and should never be pulled or subjected to any force. This inevitably leads to breakage of the fiberoptic cable. Simple care of a delicate instrument is the main factor for longevity of use. Despite this care, there is instrument breakage, especially of the articulated endoscopes. This breakage is usually discovered before the instrument is even placed into the ear. We have had no endoscopes break within a patient.

The surgeon should obtain a view of the entire middle ear cleft, first with the microscope and then through the endoscope on the monitor. To prevent instrument breakage and patient injury, it is important that the surgeon become familiar with looking back and forth between these two fields of view. This is easily done. After the middle ear cleft has been adequately evaluated, the endoscope is prepared for insertion into the eustachian tube orifice. It is important to observe the rules of any endoscopic procedure for endoscopy of the eustachian tube. The endoscope may only be passed where it can go. It is *never* forced or pushed within the eustachian tube, but rather it is guided through the orifice and eustachian tube if there is enough room for it to pass. Many adult eustachian tubes allow for at least partial passage of the nonarticulated microendoscope, at least to the area of the isthmus. It is important to observe as carefully on the way out of the eustachian tube as on the way in, because the lumen may be better viewed on withdrawal of the microendoscope than on the way in.

## POSTOPERATIVE CARE

Endoscopy of the eustachian tube requires no additional postoperative care than that for the underlying otologic surgery. The patient's postoperative instructions are based on the underlying surgery and not on the endoscopy. In most cases, the patient is asked to refrain from heavy lifting or vigorous nose blowing. The remainder of the postoperative care follows that dictated by the underlying ear surgery.

## COMPLICATIONS

The most serious complication is instrument breakage within the eustachian tube. This is unlikely as long as the fiberoptic instrument is used carefully and appropriately. The instrument is securely wrapped, and even if the fiberoptic cable were to break within the eustachian tube, it is unlikely that the entire cable would snap off. It is a diagnostic instrument, not a therapeutic one, and it must never be forced into a closed space. Even the smallest endoscope (0.5 mm) may occasionally not traverse the eustachian tube orifice. The examiner must stop at this stage. Likewise, if the endoscope cannot be withdrawn from a passage, it must not be forcefully removed, lest it break. In this case, sterile saline, water, or sterile mineral oil may be instilled near the endoscope to lubricate it and facilitate movement. This has not been a problem in our hands.

All endoscopes must be illuminated from a light source, which usually is very hot. Transilluminated heat is a potential source of soft tissue damage. The rigid endoscopes absorb more heat than the fiberoptic endoscopes, but both should be frequently monitored by the surgeon for excessive heating. The endoscope must be frequently wiped clean of debris and defogged. This is also an opportunity to periodically cool it. We have experienced no soft tissue injuries caused by heating.

The field of view should be cleared of fluid and blood, and the resolution of the endoscope must be optimal before a structure is viewed. Structures within the middle ear, such as the ossicular chain, may be damaged if inadvertently traumatized by an endoscope. The examiner may wish to place the instrument into the middle ear cleft under direct vision before looking through it, ensuring that the endoscope is not near a delicate structure. This is more of a potential problem with the rigid than fiberoptic endoscope. In all cases, the examiner must use common sense and not proceed with the endoscopy if there is an obstructed view. The precautions for the use of otologic endoscopes are identical to those for rigid or flexible esophagoscopes and bronchoscopes.

## ADVANTAGES AND LIMITATIONS OF THE ENDOSCOPIC TECHNIQUE

Until the underlying pathophysiologic dysfunction of the eustachian tube is better understood, chronic suppurative otitis media and acquired cholesteatoma will continue to be treated but not cured. Endoscopy of the eustachian tube offers several possible advantages, particularly the ability to image the structure that is thought to cause the patient's disease. Although still in its formative stages, endoscopy of the eustachian tube may offer insights into the treatment of this most difficult problem.

There are, however, significant limitations in the endoscopic evaluation of the eustachian tube that have slowed its development. Chief among them is the need for a flexible system of endoscopy. This immediately limits the power of resolution of the endoscope. The second is the need for a system small enough to pass through the eustachian tube orifice. For almost all individuals, an endoscope of 1.0 mm in its outer diameter is the absolute maximum width that can pass through the eustachian tube. For many patients, an outer diameter of 0.9 mm is still too large to pass through the orifice. With these requirements, the power of resolution and the flexibility are reduced. A flexible endoscope small enough to pass through the orifice contains approximately 3,000 pixels at most. With the need to bend the endoscope, resolution is sacrificed for flexibility. The number of pixels per endoscope must be reduced to allow for an articulating wire. For each direction of articulation (e.g., 180° upward only versus 180° upward and downward), an articulating wire must be wrapped within the endoscope. A working portal would further enlarge the outer diameter. If the outer diameter must be kept constant, each additional feature limits resolution, because the only variable in size is the number of pixels within the fiberoptic cable; hence, resolution is sacrificed for flexibility. Because of these limitations, we use two types of endoscopes:

- A 0.5-mm (outer diameter) nonarticulating endoscope
- 1.0-mm (outer diameter) articulating endoscope

Figures 8.1 and 8.2 show that the microendoscopes do not offer the same bright pictures as their rigid counterparts. This is not to say, however, that they offer no information. At this stage of development, the microendoscopes in most cases yield descriptive information about anatomic obstruction with precise location within the eustachian tube and can give information about the status of the mucosa within the eustachian tube.

## CONCLUSIONS

Microendoscopy of the eustachian tube, although described in the literature more than 10 years ago, is still a developing technique. It may offer insight into the underlying pathophysiology of eustachian tube dysfunction. It should be considered a developmental technique whose full application remains to be discovered.

With newer imaging modalities, especially with the development of flexible microendoscopes with optical systems able to enhance and enlarge a small picture, it is anticipated that endoscopy of the eustachian tube will yield new information regarding a most difficult problem in otology, eustachian tube dysfunction.

## ACKNOWLEDGMENTS

The author wishes to thank Carol A. Silverman, Ph.D., and Tina M. Presutti, B.Sc., for their assistance. This work was supported in part by grant no. C2017-2RA, Department of Veterans Affairs Medical Center, East Orange, New Jersey.

## REFERENCES

1. Bellucci RJ. Selection of cases and classification of tympanoplasty. *Otolaryngol Clin North Am* 1989;22:911–926.
2. Bluestone CS. Physiology of the middle ear and eustachian tube. In: Paparella MM, Shumrick DA, Gluckman JL, et al, eds. *Otolaryngology*, vol I. Philadelphia: WB Saunders, 1991:163–197.
3. Colletti V, Fiorino FG, Indelicato T. Surgery vs. the natural course of chronic otitis media: long-term hearing evaluation. *Acta Otolaryngol (Stockh)* 1991;111:762–768.
4. Edelstein DR, Magan J, Parisier SC, et al. Microfiberoptic evaluation of the middle ear cavity. *Am J Otol* 1994;15:50–55.
5. MacKinnon DM. Relationship of the pre-operative eustachian tube function to myringoplasty. *Acta Otolaryngol* 1970;69: 100–106.
6. Manning SC, Catekin EI, Kenna MA, et al. Prognostic value on eustachian tube function in pediatric tympanoplasty. *Laryngoscope* 1987;97:1012–1016.
7. Sato H, Nakamura H, Honjo I, et al. Eustachian tube function in tympanoplasty. *Acta Otolaryngol (Stockh)* 1990;471[Suppl]: 9–12.
8. Riedel CL, Wiley TL, Block MG. Tympanometric measures of eustachian tube function. *J Speech Hear Res* 1987;30:207–214.
9. Sheehy JL. Testing eustachian tube function. *Ann Otol Rhinol Laryngol* 1990;90:562–565.
10. Mer SN, Derbyshire AJ, Brushenko BE, et al. Fibreoptic endotoscopes for examining the middle ear. *Arch Otolaryngol* 1967;85: 61–67.
11. Poe DS, Rebeiz EE, Pankratov MM, et al. Transtympanic endoscopy of the middle ear. *Laryngoscope* 1992;102:993–996.
12. Poe DS, Rebeiz E, Pankratov MM, et al. Evaluation of perilymphatic fistulas by middle ear endoscopy. *Am J Otol* 1992;13: 529–533.
13. Conticello S, Saita V, LaMantia I, et al. Endoscopy of the eustachian tube: use of the fibrescope and telescope. *Arch Otorhinolaryngol* 1989;246:256–258.
14. Jaumann MP, Steiner W, Berg M. Endoscopy of the pharyngeal eustachian tube. *Ann Otol Rhinol Laryngol* 1980;89[Suppl 68]: 54–55.
15. Lavorato AS, Lindholm CE. Fibreoptic visualization of motion of the eustachian tube. *Otorhinolaryngol* 1977;84:534–541.
16. Yamashita K, Miyazaki T. Diagnostic significance of endoscopy of the eustachian tube. *Auris Nasus Larynx* 1985;12[Suppl I]:S55–S57.

# 9

# MINIMALLY INVASIVE COCHLEAR IMPLANTATION

JOSEPH G. TONER
NATHANIEL W. YANG
THOMAS BALKANY

During the past decade, cochlear implant technology has evolved in the direction of smaller and more powerful implantable cochlear stimulators. This has enabled smaller external incisions, smaller skin flaps, shortened surgical time, and faster healing. The rate of skin flap complications, previously the most common serious sequelae of cochlear implant surgery, have been drastically reduced. Similarly, current techniques in cochleostomy and electrode insertion have resulted in preservation of residual hearing in many cases after cochlear implantation. Unfortunately, peephole cochleostomy, sometimes called *soft surgery*, has occasionally led to misinsertion of electrodes into the scala media and vestibuli because of lack of visualization and control.

In this chapter, we review some of the methods designed to reduce the surgical trauma and healing time after cochlear implantation. A conservative cochleostomy technique, designed to allow appropriate access to the scala while minimizing intracochlear damage, is discussed. We also describe the technique of endoscopy of the cochlea that is used in cases of obstruction, dysplasia, and reimplantation.

## MINIMAL INCISIONS

The first cochlear implants used clinically in the United States were simple, hand-wound induction coils implanted behind the ear through a moderate-sized, C-shaped incision and flap. As implants became more complex and larger, the corresponding C-shaped incision (Fig. 9.1) became quite large, and the flap became a surgical problem. Up to 2.5% of postauricular C-shaped flaps developed complications (1). An optimal incision provides adequate exposure without unnecessary dissection and disruption to the blood supply. An inverted U-shaped incision used in Australia was adopted and then modified in the United States. Subsequently, reduction in the size of implantable receiver-stimulators has led to progressively smaller incisions with fewer complications and shorter healing times (2–4). A simple postauricular incision with a stepped pericranial layer is now widely employed and has been compared favorably with the earlier incisions in terms of flap related complications (5–7). Use of the extended postauricular incision (Fig. 9.2) requires an anteriorly based pericranial flap to provide an uninterrupted tissue layer at the point where the electrode crosses the skin incision. Use of the postauricular incision has allowed outpatient surgery for selected patients (7) and reduced the delay until initial stimulation from 6 weeks to 2 to 3 weeks.

## COCHLEOSTOMY

A peephole cochleostomy, sometimes called soft surgery, has been used in a variety of cochlear implantation centers. It consists of a very small cochleostomy that does not allow adequate visualization of the scala tympani. When used with relatively stiff, straight electrodes, it may result in poor control of the electrode and misinsertion into scala vestibuli or destruction of scala media (8). More severe damage, such as fracture of the osseous spiral lamina, has also occurred.

In contrast, we use an adequately sized cochleostomy in which 1.5 to 2 mm of bone is removed anterior and inferior to the round window membrane. The endosteum of the scala tympani is identified and preserved intact whenever possible. When all drilling has been completed, the entire operative area is carefully irrigated to remove all bone dust and meticulous hemostasis is obtained. Bone dust and blood may lead to osteoneogenesis and should be kept out of the scala.

The endosteum is then opened with a cataract knife and reflected using a right-angle pick, providing good visualization of the scala from the cochleostomy to the ascending turn. A lubricant such as hyaluronic acid or 50% glycerin may be used to aid in the insertion of the more difficult to insert electrodes (i.e., Nucleus 24 or Nucleus "Curly" elec-

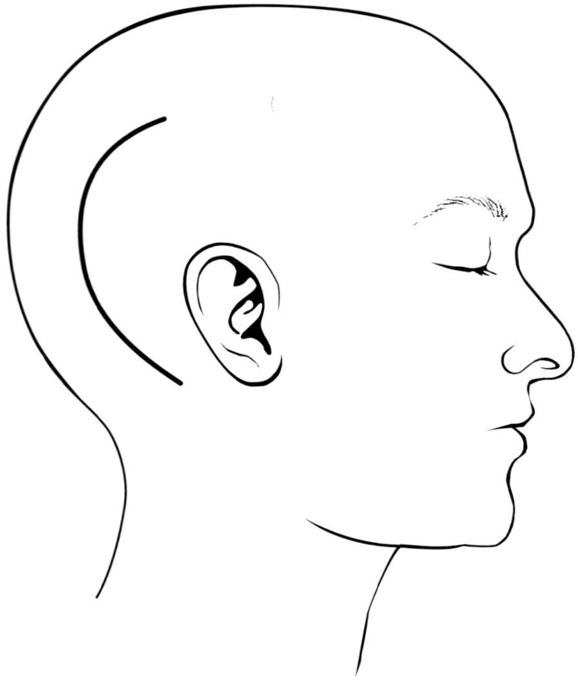

**FIGURE 9.1.** C-shaped incision.

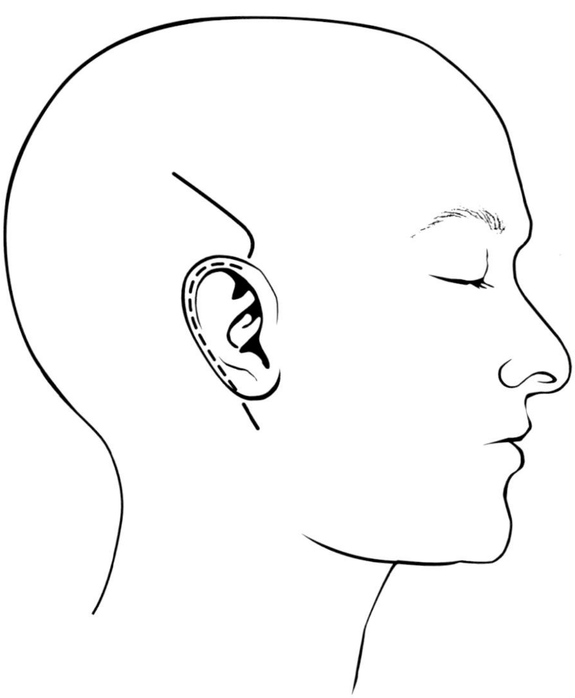

**FIGURE 9.2.** Extended postauricular incision.

trodes). The technique described allows adequate visualization for proper atraumatic insertion of electrodes while minimizing potential for osteoneogenesis.

## MINIMAL SURGERY FOR THE OSSIFIED COCHLEA

Profound sensorineural hearing loss may be associated with obstruction of the fluid spaces of the cochlea. This obstruction usually takes the form of new bone formation and has been associate with a variety of causes in patients undergoing cochlear implantation: meningitis, autoimmune diseases, ototoxicity, otosclerosis, congenital disorders, malignant otitis externa, and trauma. Temporal bone studies have shown that the most frequent location for the development of fibrosis and new bone formation is the scala tympani of the basal turn of the cochlea, regardless of the cause of hearing loss. However, the apical and middle turns of the cochlea may be more extensively involved by the process of ossification.

The use of high-resolution computed tomography (CT) has been helpful in determining the nature and extent of bony obstruction within the cochlea. Nonetheless, in many cases, it is impossible to ascertain the true degree of obstruction. False-normal high-resolution CT findings have been reported in up to 46% of cases of surgically demonstrated cochlear obstruction (9–12). Magnetic resonance imaging (MRI) has further enhanced the preoperative evaluation of cochlear patency. Improved resolution of scanners and more sophisticated software packages for image manipulation (particularly three-dimensional reconstruction) are increasingly available. These techniques have enabled the scala tympani and the scala vestibuli to be viewed separately and have provide more detailed information on cochlear patency (13,14). However, in a significant number of cases, obliteration is detected only at surgery.

In the past, radiographic evidence of ossification of the scala tympani was considered a contraindication for placement of multichannel cochlear implant electrodes. First, it was considered difficult or impossible to achieve safe electrode insertion in the face of bony obstruction. The electrode or the inner ear structures could be damaged. Second, the capacity to stimulate effectively surviving neural elements by multichannel format was questioned for patients with partially ossified cochleas. In such cases, a 4- to 6-mm tunnel drilled into the scala tympani for placement of a single electrode had been recommended. Studies of partially and fully obstructed cochleas have demonstrated reliable techniques for multichannel electrode insertion (15,16). Results in many cases have been the equivalent of those seen in nonobstructed cochleas (16,17).

The early techniques for implanting the ossified cochlea involved removal of the canal wall; the radical cavity created required obliteration with abdominal fat, closure of the eustachian tube, and blind sac closure of the external meatus (18). A "combined approach" with an intact canal wall allows the canal wall to be preserved while achieving full surgical access to the cochlea (19,20).

## SURGICAL TECHNIQUE

The usual aseptic preparations are performed for surgery, and the external canal is carefully débrided and filled with povidone iodine (21). A standard postauricular incision is made, ensuring good access to the external meatus (22). Cortical mastoidectomy and a facial recess approach enable an anteroinferior cochleostomy. Drilling of the basal turn is performed confirming complete obliteration to the level of the carotid canal. This confirms the requirement for total drill-out technique. A posterior or superior tympanomeatal flap is elevated, possibly requiring separation from the malleus to enhance visualization of the anterior mesotympanum. The incus, cochleariform process, tensor tympani tendon, and muscle are removed. The region of the carotid canal is identified inferior to the medial orifice of the eustachian tube. A 2-mm diamond burr is used to perform the drill-out within the limits of the dissection: the cochleostomy tunnel inferiorly, carotid canal anteriorly, tensor tympani semi-canal superiorly, and oval window posteriorly. The obliterative bone can often be identified by its lighter color and softer consistency. A trough is created around the modiolus, and the anterior segment of the original cochleostomy tunnel is unroofed. The electrode can then be inserted in the normal manner through the facial recess. The electrode is manipulated into the trough, and the electrode may be secured using the lenticular process and pieces of the long process of the incus. The tunnel is packed with fascia, and the cable is secured in the split bridge (23). The promontory is covered with temporalis fascia and held in position with Gelfoam filling the middle ear.

The intact canal wall total drill-out is a less invasive approach to the technical challenge of a completely ossified cochlea. It avoids the risk of blind sac closure and radical mastoidectomy but is more difficult, and care must be taken in avoiding complications, particularly in relation to the facial nerve. Alternative procedures are being tested using split electrode arrays and middle cranial fossa approaches to the cochlea.

## ENDOSCOPY OF THE COCHLEA

Cochlear endoscopy was first described by Balkany and colleagues (24), who employed a new generation of flexible fiberoptic miniendoscopes (0.7 to 1 mm in diameter). Endoscopy was found to be helpful in visualizing obstructed segments, confirming patency after removal of the obstruction. The efficacy of this technique was confirmed by temporal bone studies (25,26) that also determined the limit of safe insertion. This technique also enables the use of lasers to remove obstructed segments in the scala (27).

## INDICATIONS

In our experience, endoscopy of the cochlea during cochlear implantation has limited indications and equally limited efficacy, and we do not recommend its routine use during cochlear implantation. When cochlear obstruction is encountered during the procedure, the initial segment of obstruction may be removed with a drill, fine picks, or endoscope-guided laser. After the obstruction has been removed, endoscopy can confirm a smooth passageway for the electrode traversing the obstructed segment into the patent segment of the cochlea. This may be useful, because occasionally a good flow of perilymph is encountered, but the lumen may be seen endoscopically to remain too obstructed to safely pass an electrode, and further bone removal is necessary. During reimplantation, the endoscope can confirm that the fibrous tract of the previous electrode does not fully obstruct the scala and that insertion alongside of the previous electrode tract is possible. If endoscopy demonstrates that this is impossible, insertion within the previous fibrous tract becomes necessary (Fig. 9.3). Electrode insertion in cases of cochlear dysplasia may be facilitated using the endoscope. Confirmation that the electrode smoothly lies within the confines, especially of a common cavity deformity, is also helpful (Fig. 9.4).

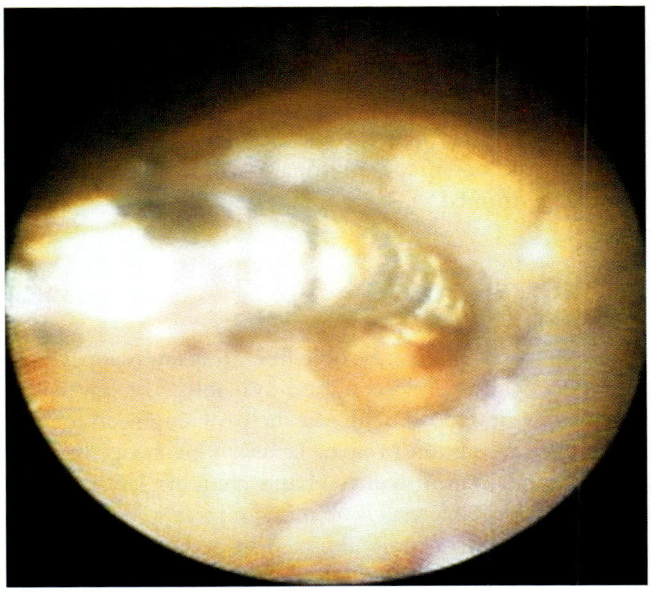

**FIGURE 9.3.** Cochlear implant electrode insertion within the previous fibrous tract.

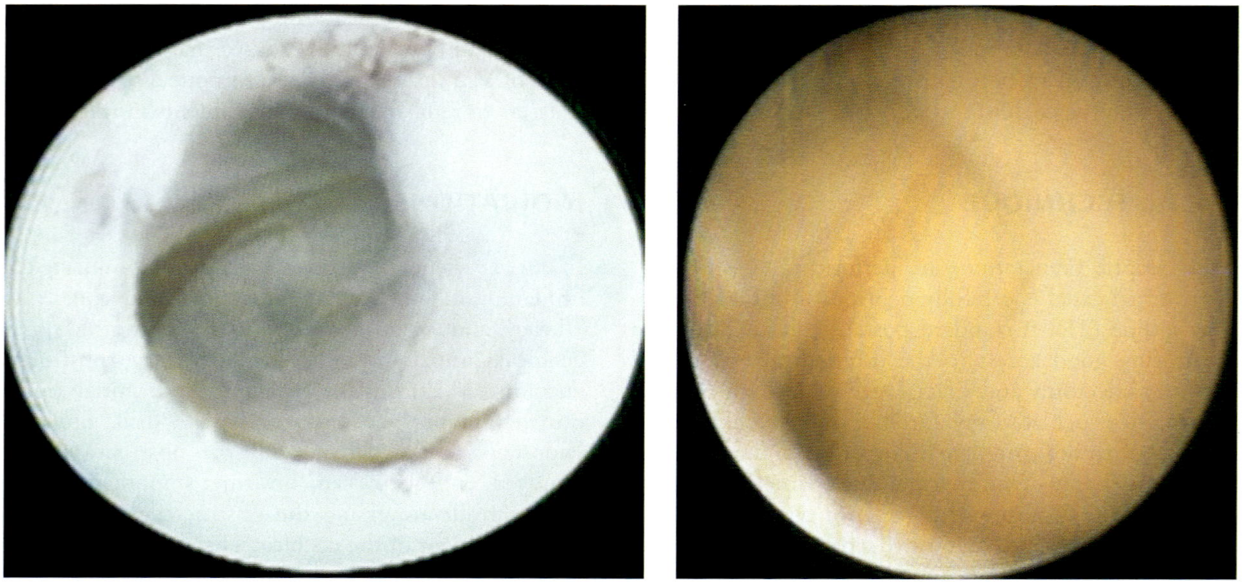

A B

**FIGURE 9.4. A,B:** Common cavity deformity.

## CONTRAINDICATIONS

No contraindications to routine flexible fiberoptic endoscopy performed during cochlear implantation have been identified. It has been used to visualize the cochlea in cochlear implant candidates with normal preoperative imaging studies and in cases of fibrosis, ossification, dysplasia, and reimplantation.

## PREOPERATIVE EVALUATION

Routine preimplantation evaluation is performed, including full audiologic assessment, imaging of the cochlea with high-resolution CT and MRI. Patient or parent counseling regarding the potential additional risks of implantation is likewise performed.

## INSTRUMENTATION

Several smaller-diameter flexible fiberoptic endoscopes suitable for cochlear endoscopy are available. We have used endoscopes developed with the help of engineers of the Machida Corporation (Tokyo, Japan). This device is made in 0.7- and 1.0-mm diameters and contains 1,600 quartz fibers. Its effective length is 60 mm, and it is well controlled with a pencil-grip handle designed to be held like an otologic instrument. The fiber bundles are strain relieved at the entrance and exit of the instrument handle. The back end is adapted for use with direct vision, video, or a 35-mm camera. The field of vision is 55°, with a depth of focus of 1 to 25 mm and magnification of 60×.

An 0.89-mm-diameter endoscope (OM3-080) from Omega (London, UK) is the smallest device with an active-steering flexible tip. It is also suitable for direct and video endoscopy. The field of vision is 70°, with a depth of focus of 2 to 20 mm and magnification of 50×. Endoscopes with diameters of 0.35 and 0.5 mm are also available from Omega. They do not have steering flexible tips, and they are very fragile and soft.

A 300-W, adjustable light source is used. Images can be recorded through attachments to standard videotape or 35-mm photographic film.

## OPERATING ROOM LAYOUT

The patient is placed in the supine position on the operating table with the head turned so that the ear to be implanted is upmost. The surgeon is seated on the patient's side, with the surgical nurse opposite the surgeon. The anesthesiologist is positioned at the patient's feet, with access to the controls for moving the table.

## ANESTHESIA

General endotracheal anesthesia using inhalational agents is routinely used. Short-acting muscle relaxants are used only in the induction period to allow intraoperative monitoring of facial nerve activity. We routinely administer perioperative antibiotics. Steroids are not routinely given.

## OPERATIVE TECHNIQUE

The surgeon's routine cochlear implant technique is used up to and including the cochleostomy. At that point, if endoscopy is indicated, the endoscope is advanced through the facial recess and to the cochleostomy using microscopic control. We then switch to a video projection of the endoscopic image rather than direct visualization. This keeps the endoscopist's head away from the operative site and allows recording. The endoscope is gently and slowly inserted into the cochlea under continuous visualization. Steerable endoscopes are preferred because they allow visualization around the ascending turn of the basal turn of the cochlea. Care is taken not to bump the tip of the electrode into the spiral ligament at the ascending turn.

Structures such as the osseous spiral lamina, basilar membrane, and spiral ligament are easily visualized. The endoscope is then carefully withdrawn under visual control, and the implantation procedure proceeds as usual.

## COMPLICATIONS

Insertional trauma is of concern with the use of cochlear endoscopes. A human temporal bone study using the 0.7- and 1.0-mm-diameter endoscopes demonstrated a mean insertion depth of 10 mm (25). At this point, the inherent stiffness of the endoscope caused the tip of the endoscope to impinge om the spiral ligament at the ascending turn. Histopathologic examination demonstrated tears in the spiral ligament at the point of impingement. We consider it imprudent to attempt to pass the device until resistance is met, as is done with multichannel electrodes, because of the potential for causing damage to the remaining inner ear structures.

A similar maximum insertion depth of 10 mm has been determined for the 0.89-mm, active-steering flexible endoscope, and the maximum insertion depth for the 0.35- and 0.5-mm endoscopes is 13 mm (28).

## ADVANTAGES AND LIMITATIONS OF ENDOSCOPIC TECHNIQUE

Flexible fiberoptic endoscopy during cochlear implantation allows evaluation of the extent and type of cochlear obstruction, as well as determination of cochlear patency after removal of the obstruction. Identification of normal and certain pathologic structures, such as otosclerosis and a fibrous sheath that remained in place after removal of an electrode during cochlear reimplantation, is possible.

Cochlear endoscopy is hampered only by the technologic limitations of the available devices. The inherent stiffness and lack of flexibility does not allow passage around the turns of the cochlea. This decreases the endoscope's effectiveness and increases its potential for causing damage to the remaining sensory apparatus within the inner ear. Although definite visualization of the intracochlear structures is achieved, the clarity of the images is somewhat marginal and less than ideal. Both problems await improvements in technology. The potential for endoscopy of the functioning cochlea for diagnostic or surgical purposes remains unknown.

## CONCLUSIONS

Cochlear implantation in the presence of obliteration remains one of the significant surgical challenges for the otologist. Preoperative evaluation with high-resolution CT scans and increasingly enhanced MRI with three-dimensional reconstruction can provide useful preoperative information. However, there are still cases of unexpected obliteration that strain the surgeon's skills. Cochlear endoscopy can enhance, with minimal additional trauma, the ability to evaluate the degree of obstruction and monitor its progressive removal.

## REFERENCES

1. Cohen NL, Hoffman RA. Complications of cochlear implant surgery in adults and children. *Ann Otol Rhinol Laryngol* 1991; 100:708–711.
2. Hoffman RA, Cohen NL. Surgical pitfalls in cochlear implantation. *Laryngoscope* 1993;103:741–744.
3. Telian Steven A, El-Kashlan H, Arts HA. Minimizing wound complications in cochlear implant surgery. Presented at the Vth International Cochlear Implant Conference; New York, NY; May 1–3, 1997.
4. Gerencer RZ, Oldring DJ. Cochlear implant flap complications. Presented at the Vth International Cochlear Implant Conference; New York, NY; May 1–3, 1997.
5. Gibson WP, Harrison HC, Prowse C. A new incision for placement of cochlear implants. *J Laryngol Otol* 1995;109:821–825.
6. Gibson WP, Harrison HC. Further experience with a straight, vertical incision for placement of cochlear implants. *J Laryngol Otol* 1997;111:924–927.
7. Toner JG, John G, McNaboe EJ. Cochlear implantation under local anesthesia, the Belfast experience. *J Laryngol Otol* 1998; 112:533–536.
8. Cohen NL. Cochlear implant soft surgery: fact or fantasy? *Otolaryngol Head Neck Surg* 1997;117:214–216.
9. Nikolopoulos TP, O'Donoghue GM, Robinson KL, et al. Preoperative radiologic evaluation in cochlear implantation. *Am J Otol* 1997;18(Suppl 6):S73–S74.
10. Wang G, Vannier MW, Skinner MW, et al. Spiral CT image deblurring for cochlear implantation. *IEEE Trans Med Imaging* 1998;17:251–262.

11. Frau GN, Luxford WN, Lo WN, et al. High-resolution computed tomography in evaluation of cochlear patency in implant candidates: a comparison with surgical findings. *J Laryngol Otol* 1994;108:743–748.
12. Dahm MC, Dietrich B, Reich A, et al. The accuracy of preoperative high-resolution computed tomography in predicting cochlear pathology. *Adv Otorhinolaryngol* 1995;50:25–30.
13. Ivers CR, Hans P, Jackson A, et al. 3D reconstruction of magnetic resonance images of the cochlea—clinical applications. Presented at the Vth International Cochlear Implant Conference; New York, NY; May 1–3, 1997.
14. Dahm MC, Mack MG, Tykocinski M, et al. Submillimeter imaging and reconstruction of the inner ear. *Am J Otol* 1997; 18[Suppl 6]:S54–S56.
15. Balkany TJ, Gantz BJ, Steenerson RL, et al. Systematic approach to electrode insertion in the ossified cochlea. *Otolaryngol Head Neck Surg* 1996;114:4–11.
16. Balkany TJ, Gantz BJ, Nadol JB Jr. Multichannel cochlear implants in partially ossified cochleas. *Ann Otol Rhinol Laryngol* 1988;97[Suppl 135]:3–7.
17. Cohen NC, Waltzman SB. Partial insertion of the nucleus multichannel cochlear implant: technique and results. *Am J Otol* 1993;14:357–361.
18. Gantz BJ, McCabe BF, Tyler RS. Use of multichannel cochlear implants in obstructed and obliterated cochlea. *Otolaryngol Head Neck Surg* 1988;98:72–81.
19. Balkany T, Bird PA, Hodges AV, et al. Surgical technique for implantation of the totally ossified cochlea. *Laryngoscope* 1998; 108:988–992.
20. Balkany T, Luntz M, Telischi FF, et al. Intact canal wall drill-out procedure for the totally ossified cochlea. *Am J Otol* 1997; 18(Suppl 6):S58–S59.
21. Balkany TJ, Berman SA, Watson WJ. Sterile preparation of the external auditory canal with povidone-iodine. *Otolaryngol Head Neck Surg* 1979;87:258–260.
22. Balkany TJ, Hodges AV, Luntz M. Update on cochlear implantation. *Otolaryngol Clin North Am* 1996;29:277–289.
23. Balkany TJ, Telischi FF. Fixation of the electrode cable during cochlear implantation: the spilt bridge technique. *Laryngoscope* 1995;105:217–218.
24. Balkany T. Endoscopy of the cochlea during cochlear implantation. *Ann Otol Rhinol Laryngol* 1990;99:919–922.
25. Balkany T, Fradis M. Flexible fiberoptic endoscopy of the cochlea: human temporal bone studies. *Am J Otol* 1991;12:46–48.
26. Balkany T, Hodges AV, Whitehead M, et al. Cochlear endoscopy with preservation of hearing in guinea pigs. *Otolaryngol Head Neck Surg* 1994;111:439–445.
27. Kautzky M, Susani M, Franz P, et al. Flexible fiberoptic endoscopy and laser surgery in obliterated cochleas: human temporal bone studies. *Lasers Surg Med* 1996;18:271–277.
28. Baumgartner WD, Franz P, Gstoettner W, et al. Cochlea endoscopy in vivo. *Adv Otorhinolaryngol* 1997;52:62–65.

# 10

# ENDOSCOPIC AUDITORY BRAINSTEM IMPLANTATION

DAVID R. FRIEDLAND
PHILLIP A. WACKYM

The restoration of hearing in individuals with clinically significant hearing loss from a wide range of causes has made dramatic strides over the past decades. Surgical intervention in the form of cochlear implants can provide useful auditory perception in individuals deriving little or no benefit from hearing aids; however, these auditory prostheses require an intact cochlear nerve to conduct these electrical signals to the brainstem. The restoration of auditory perception in individuals deafened by loss of the vestibulocochlear nerve is provided by auditory brainstem implants (ABIs).

The ABI is a device consisting of several electrodes placed on the brainstem surface to directly stimulate the cochlear nuclei (1–4) (Fig. 10.1). Peripherally, it is coupled with a digital speech processor similar to that of a cochlear implant. Studies have shown that such stimulation can provide useful perception of environmental sounds and even open-set speech comprehension (5–8).

The Cochlear Corporation's (Melbourne, Australia) ABI is approved by the U.S. Food and Drug Administration (FDA), and the Med-El Corporation's (Innsbrück, Austria) ABI remains an investigational device, currently used only in individuals 17 years or older with neurofibromatosis type 2 (NF2) undergoing resection of a vestibular schwannoma (i.e., acoustic neuroma) (9). Such individuals are often left with complete sensorineural deafness because of the sacrifice of both cochlear nerves during resection of bilateral tumors (10). Optimal placement of the electrode onto the cochlear nucleus is difficult because the operating microscope is unable to directly visualize this complex by means of the surgical approaches used to resect these tumors. However, the use of the endoscope in placement of an ABI electrode array has been explored to accomplish this goal (11). The endoscope has been employed successfully as an adjunct to resection of acoustic neuromas and surgery of the vestibular nerve (12–14).

This chapter describes the results of a cadaveric study on endoscope-assisted ABI placement and focuses on the neuroanatomic landmarks important for successful implantation. Detailed operative considerations are described in this chapter based on acoustic neuroma resection followed by ABI placement.

## AUDITORY BRAINSTEM IMPLANTS

Different ABIs are used in the United States and in Europe. The Cochlear Corporation's array is a 21-electrode device with the electrodes embedded in a Silastic paddle backed with Dacron mesh (Fig. 10.2). This device is also used intraoperatively as a stimulating electrode for evoked auditory brainstem response to help refine implant position (5). The speech processor currently in use is the Nucleus Spectra processor using the SPEAK coding strategy (5). The recommended protocol with this device uses a translabyrinthine approach to the tumor and subsequent implantation of the ABI (2). An FDA clinical trial of a new electrode array using a penetrating electrode is in preparation.

The second device has been designed and manufactured by the Med-El Corporation. This device uses two electrode arrays. The first is a four-electrode "positioning electrode" used for intraoperative electrophysiologic testing such as electrically evoked auditory brainstem responses or facial and glossopharyngeal nerve electromyography (Fig. 10.3). This array is used intraoperatively to identify the most effective placement for the ABI. After a location is determined, the positioning electrode is removed and replaced with the ABI. The actual implant is identical in size to the positioning electrode but has a Dacron mesh backing and contains 12 stimulating electrodes. The speech processor is likewise manufactured by the Med-El Corporation and uses a high-rate continuous interleaved sampling (CIS) coding strategy. A novel feature of the Med-El ABI electrode paddle is that it can be contoured to the surface topography of the brainstem (Figs. 10.4 to 10.6). The

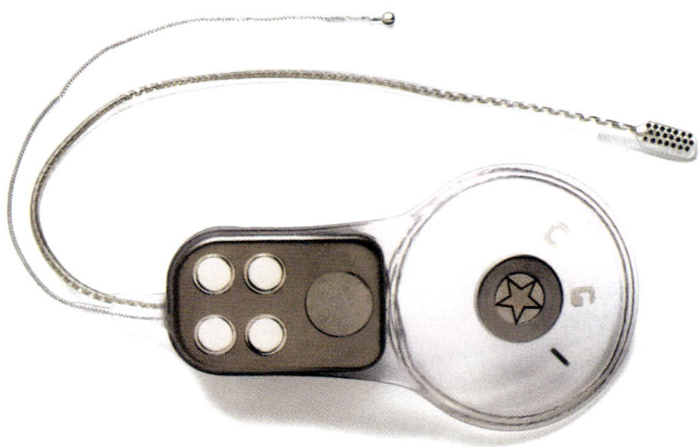

**FIGURE 10.1.** Cochlear Corporation (Melbourne, Australia) auditory brainstem implant: internal stimulator-receiver, electrode array, and reference electrode.

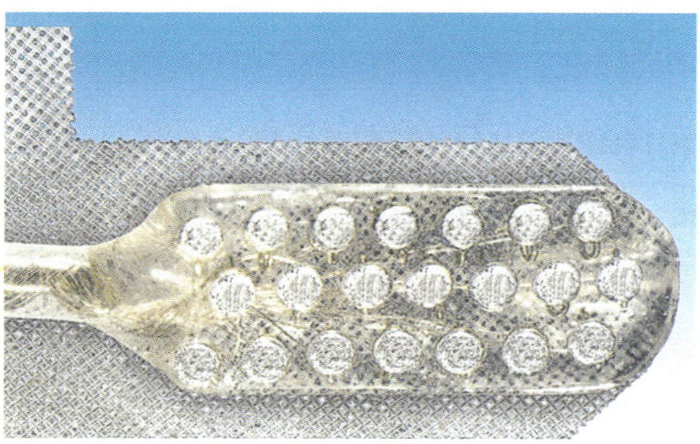

**FIGURE 10.2.** Detail of the 21-electrode paddle of the Cochlear Corporation (Melbourne, Australia) device. Notice the Dacron mesh backing and 21-electrode array.

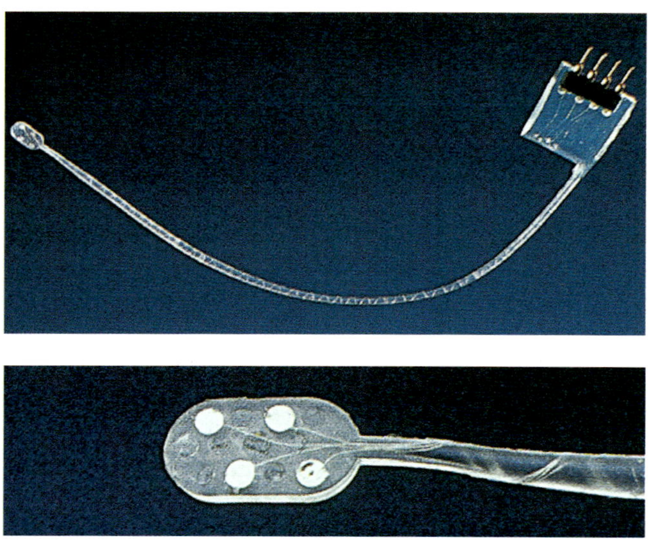

**FIGURE 10.3.** Med-El (Innsbrück, Austria) positioning electrode. This is a Silastic paddle consisting of four 1-mm electrodes.

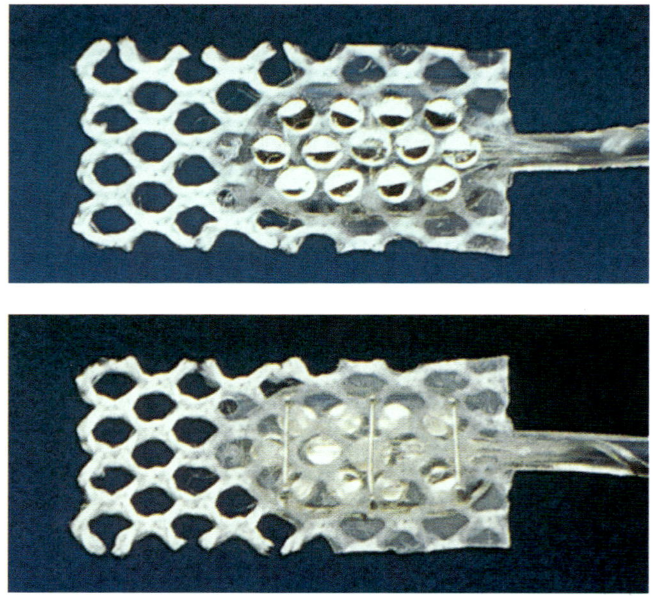

**FIGURE 10.4.** The Med-El (Innsbrück, Austria) implant electrode array contains 13 active electrodes and has a Dacron mesh backing to promote adhesion to the brainstem surface. Titanium bars allow bending of the electrode paddle to conform to the brainstem topography.

stimulator-receiver is positioned in the skull in the same manner as a cochlear implant (Fig. 10.7).

## ANATOMY OF IMPLANTATION

The ABI is placed directly on the surface of the brainstem with the goal of stimulating central auditory neurons. The ideal neurophysiologic site for implantation is over the ventral cochlear nucleus because it contains the spheroid cells thought to be the principal second-order afferent auditory neurons (15). However, clinical experience has made the dorsal cochlear nucleus the target of choice for two reasons (16). First, the inferior and middle cerebellar peduncles and a portion of the pons obscure the ventral cochlear nucleus, whereas the dorsal cochlear nucleus is relatively unobstructed (17–19). Second, ventral placement of the electrode array has produced extra-auditory stimulation, most notably of the facial nerve (7).

Localization of the brainstem surface overlying the dorsal cochlear nucleus is difficult. Brackmann and colleagues found that the dorsal nucleus in lower mammals forms a characteristic "bulge" on the brainstem surface that they had not observed in humans (16). Our cadaveric studies demonstrated a surface bulge in this region in several specimens when examined endoscopically, which may indicate that such a landmark is, at best, inconsistent and therefore unreliable (20).

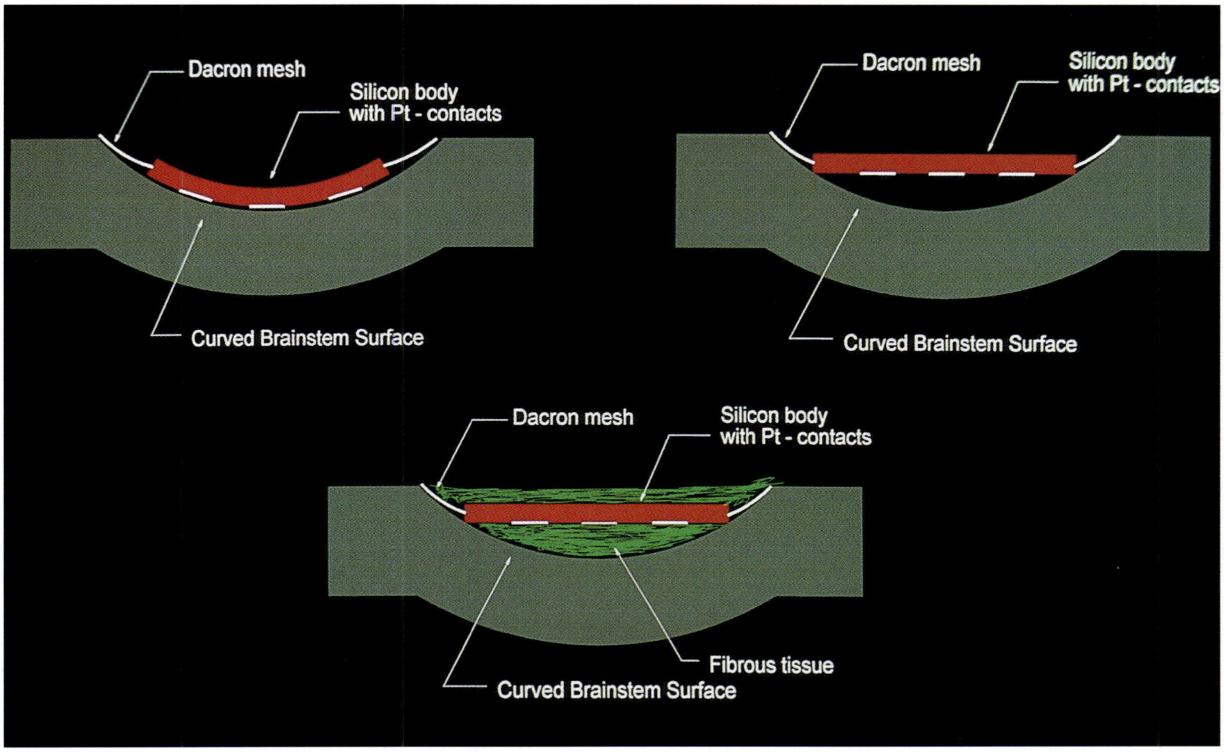


**FIGURE 10.5.** Variations of the cochlear nucleus brainstem surface are accommodated by conforming the Med-El (Innsbrück, Austria) electrode paddle to the surface topography using the titanium bars in the silicon body and platinum electrodes. Failure to conform the electrode array to the brainstem results in fibrous tissue deposition between the electrode paddle and the brainstem.

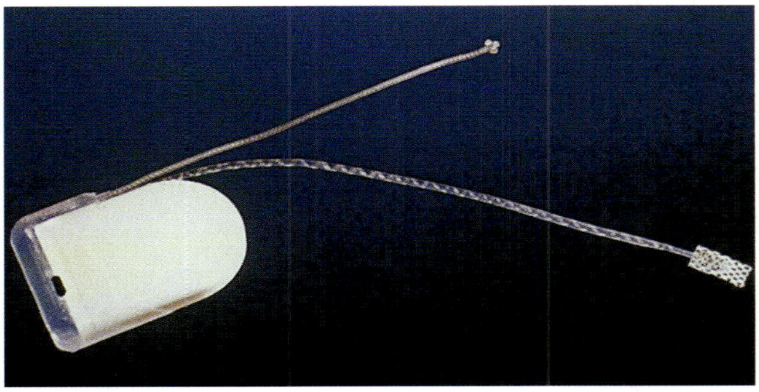

**FIGURE 10.6.** The Med-El Corporation (Innsbrück, Austria) auditory brainstem implant, internal stimulator-receiver, electrode array, and reference electrode.

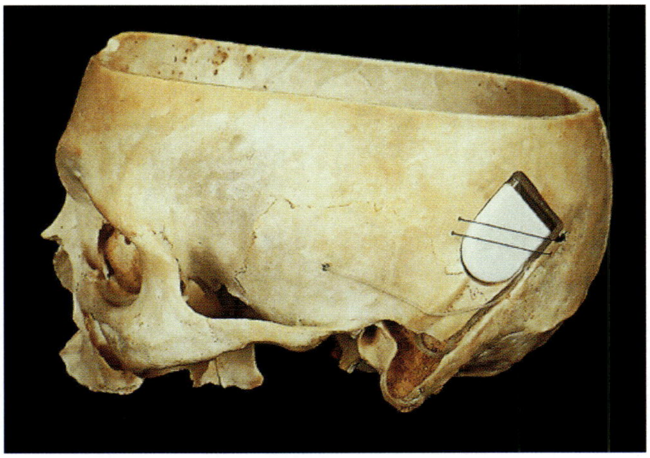

**FIGURE 10.7.** Internal cochlear stimulator-receiver is seen set in the skull. This is a Med-El (Innsbrück, Austria) device; however, the Cochlear Corporation device (Melbourne, Australia) is positioned in a similar manner.

Further complicating localization of the dorsal cochlear nucleus is its position within the lateral recess of the fourth ventricle, an area reported to be *not* directly visible within the standard translabyrinthine surgical field (21). Additional reports have likewise indicated that the site of implantation may be obscured in a translabyrinthine dissection (16,22). As such, this region is difficult to localize in a clinical setting, and the importance of surgical landmarks to guide the surgeon has been stressed (23). The advent of ABIs stimulated renewed interest in the anatomy of the cochlear nuclei and the cerebellopontine angle (18,19,22, 24–26).

The dorsal cochlear nucleus is near the brainstem surface at the lateral recess of the fourth ventricle. This portion of the fourth ventricle gives rises laterally to the foramen of Luschka. Within the recess and extending out through the foramen is the choroid plexus. The foramen is formed by the tela choroidea, often referred to as the rhomboid lip, and the surface of the brainstem. A thin layer of tissue, the taenia chordae, covers the foramen and the choroid plexus. The taenia has been reported to delineate the junction between the dorsal cochlear nucleus and the inferior ventral cochlear nucleus (16,18,19).

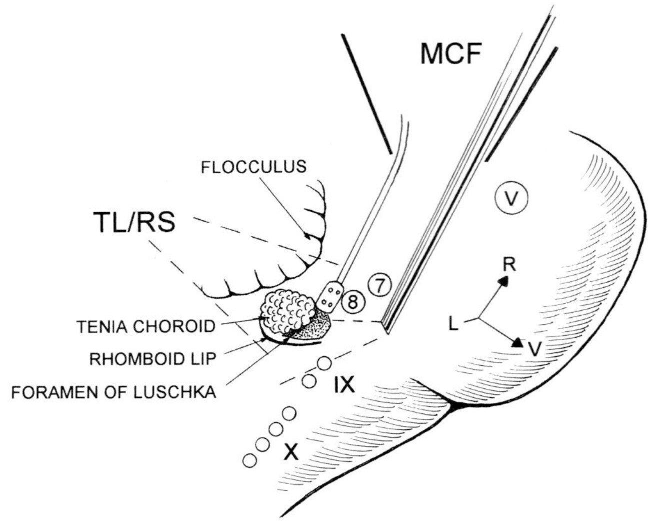


**FIGURE 10.9.** Schematic of the cerebellopontine angle. The lateral view of the region demonstrates landmarks for the localization of the lateral recess of the fourth ventricle and the brainstem surface overlying the dorsal cochlear nucleus. The endoscope is placed beyond the seventh and eighth nerve complex, and therefore these nerves are not in view when visualizing the cochlear nucleus through the middle cranial fossa *(MCF)* approach. *TL,* translabyrinthine approach; *RS,* retrosigmoid approach; circled *V,* trigeminal nerve; *X,* vagus nerve; *IX,* glossopharyngeal nerve; *L,* lateral; *R,* rostral; *V,* ventral; *7,* facial nerve; *8,* vestibulocochlear nerve.

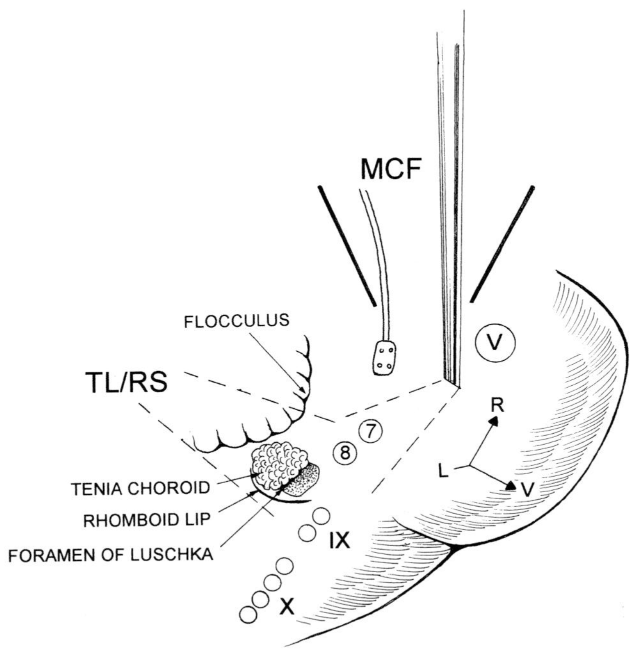


**FIGURE 10.8.** Schematic of the cerebellopontine angle. The lateral view of the region demonstrates landmarks for the localization of the lateral recess of the fourth ventricle and the brainstem surface overlying the dorsal cochlear nucleus, including the view from the retrosigmoid *(RS),* translabyrinthine *(TL),* and middle cranial fossa *(MCF)* approaches. The endoscopic view with a 30° endoscope is shown from the TL and RS approaches *(dotted lines)* and from the MCF approach *(dotted line)*. Notice the position of the endoscope tip in the MCF approach when the facial nerve is in view—the cochlear nucleus and the foramen of Luschka are blocked from view by the facial *(7)* and vestibulocochlear *(8)* nerves. Circled *V,* trigeminal nerve; *IX,* glossopharyngeal nerve; *X,* vagus nerve; *L,* lateral; *R,* rostral; *V,* ventral.

Additional landmarks directing the surgeon to the implant site include the root entry zones (REZs) of the vestibulocochlear and glossopharyngeal nerves. The dorsal cochlear nucleus is near the base of the cochlear nerve as it enters the brainstem along the pontomedullary junction. These structures are located just rostral to the flocculus, the lateral-most portion of the cerebellum. Figures 10.8 and 10.9 are schematic depictions of these landmarks and show their relation to the implant site within the lateral recess of the fourth ventricle.

## SPECIFIC INSTRUMENTS

Several instruments are required:

- The 0°, 30°, and 45° endoscopes (Smith Nephew Richards, Memphis, TN; Karl Storz, Culver City, CA)
- Three-chip video camera (Stryker Endoscopy, Santa Clara, CA; Karl Storz, Culver City, CA)
- A 19-inch video monitor (Sony Corp., Tokyo, Japan)
- S-VHS videotape recorder (Sony Corp., Tokyo, Japan)
- Digital capture system (Stryker Endoscopy, Santa Clara, CA)

- Fisch middle cranial fossa retractor (Leibinger, Dallas, TX)
- McCabe 22° and 45° angled flap knife (V. Mueller, Munich, Germany)
- Electrode claws for cochlear implant insertion: straight, forward, and reverse (Cochlear Corporation, Melbourne, Australia)
- Photoshop digital image processing software (Adobe Systems, Inc., San Jose, CA [www.adobe.com])
- Digital dye-sublimation printer (Tektronix Phaser 450, www.tek.com)

## SURGICAL APPROACHES

### Translabyrinthine Approach

The translabyrinthine dissection should be performed in standard fashion with operating microscope and basic otologic instruments. In brief, a complete mastoidectomy is performed, and the facial nerve and semicircular canals identified. The vestibular labyrinth is removed and the posterior and middle fossa dura exposed. Working from the superior canal ampulla, the internal auditory canal is skeletonized. The jugular bulb is identified and should be thoroughly decompressed to provide direct visualization of the rostral fibers of the glossopharyngeal nerve. This allows identification of an important landmark and provides access for the endoscope during implantation. The posterior fossa dura is then incised and reflected, exposing the cerebellum and flocculus (Figs. 10.10 and 10.11).

At this point, the tumor would be removed, but the following account describes ABI placement in an ideal (i.e., nonoperated, tumor-free) setting. Additional intraoperative challenges would result from the distortion of landmarks produced by tumor compression or by tumor extirpation. The use of landmarks is even more critical in such cases as a stepwise approach may allow identification of the implant site in a grossly distorted cerebellopontine angle.

A 0° endoscope is advanced into the operative field and used to identify the flocculus, vestibulocochlear, and glossopharyngeal nerves. In some individuals, the choroid plexus may be visible over or just inferior to the flocculus. The vestibulocochlear and glossopharyngeal nerves appear to converge behind the flocculus with the imaginary point of convergence near the dorsal cochlear nucleus. A 30° endoscope can be passed over (i.e., lateral to) the flocculus, allowing visualization of the choroid plexus, which can be traced medially to the rhomboid lip and foramen of Luschka (Fig. 10.12A).Use of the angled endoscope allows this to be accomplished with minimal retraction on the flocculus and helps to preserve the taenia chordae. The McCabe flap knife can be used under endoscopic visualization to gently retract the choroid and expose the surface of the brainstem and lateral recess of the fourth ventricle. The

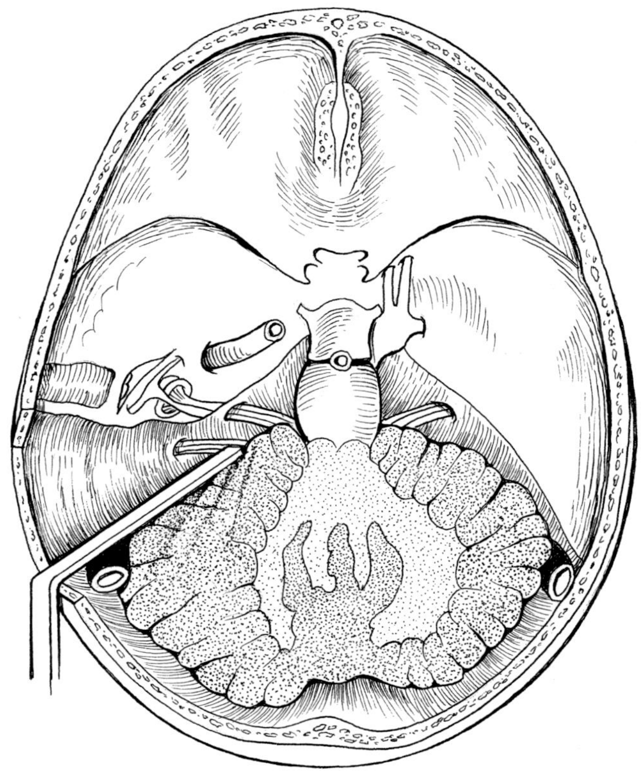

**FIGURE 10.10.** Overview of the translabyrinthine approach.

surface of the brainstem within the recess has a characteristic glistening appearance due to the overlying ependyma (Fig. 10.12A).

The endoscope should be stabilized at the periphery of the operative field to allow introduction and manipulation of the electrode and instruments. It can be positioned superiorly against the tegmen or inferiorly, against the bony ridge remaining over the tympanic and mastoid facial nerve. Decompression of the jugular bulb allows adequate space for the distal aspect of the endoscope to be maneuvered. Positioning of the endoscope is determined by the side of the patient being operated on and the handedness of the surgeon. There is a tendency for the temperature of the distal endoscope to increase, which can cause neural stimulation and potentially cause neural damage. Care must be taken in positioning the endoscope near the facial nerve and attention paid to intraoperative neurophysiologic monitoring.

The implant, or positioning electrode, is introduced into the site with electrode claw and the paddle directed into the foramen of Luschka with the flap knife (Fig. 10.12B). The angled endoscope allows visualization of the entire length of the electrode array, ensuring full contact with the brainstem (Fig. 10.13). The position of the implant can be recorded with digital image capture and intraoperative dye sublima-

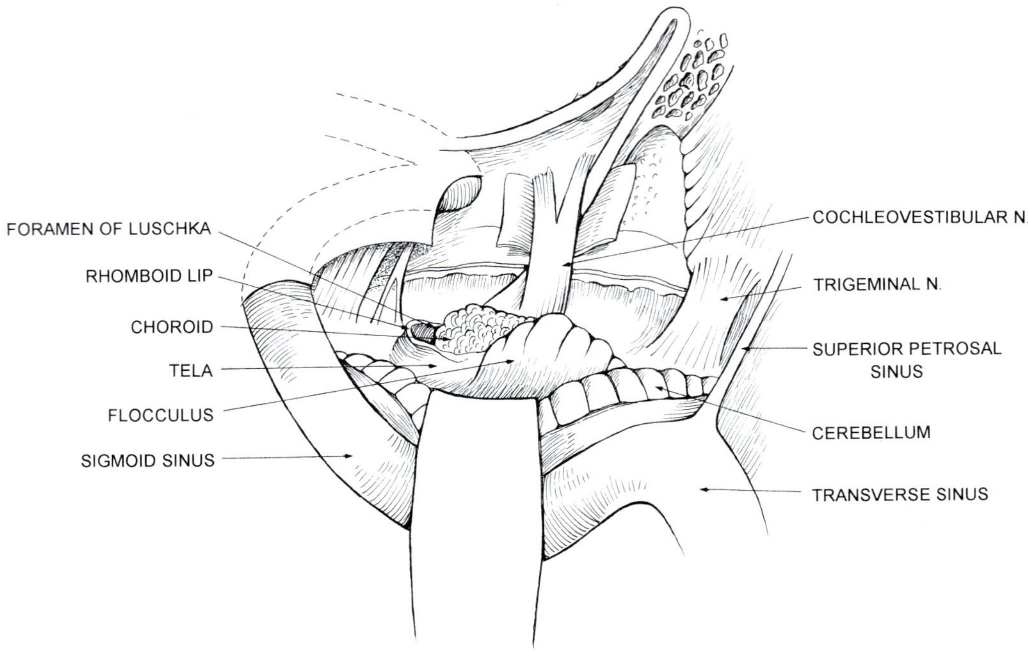


**FIGURE 10.11.** Detail of the landmarks visible near the cochlear nucleus by means of the translabyrinthine approach.

tion printing. This helps to correlate anatomy with the results of electrophysiologic testing. If the Med-El system is used, placement of the actual implant can be better achieved by comparison with photographic documentation of the positioning electrode.

The distal portion of the electrode extends through the surgical defect to the receiver-stimulator. This device is similar to that of a cochlear implant and is implanted identically. The defect is closed in standard translabyrinthine fashion, and routine postoperative management is followed.

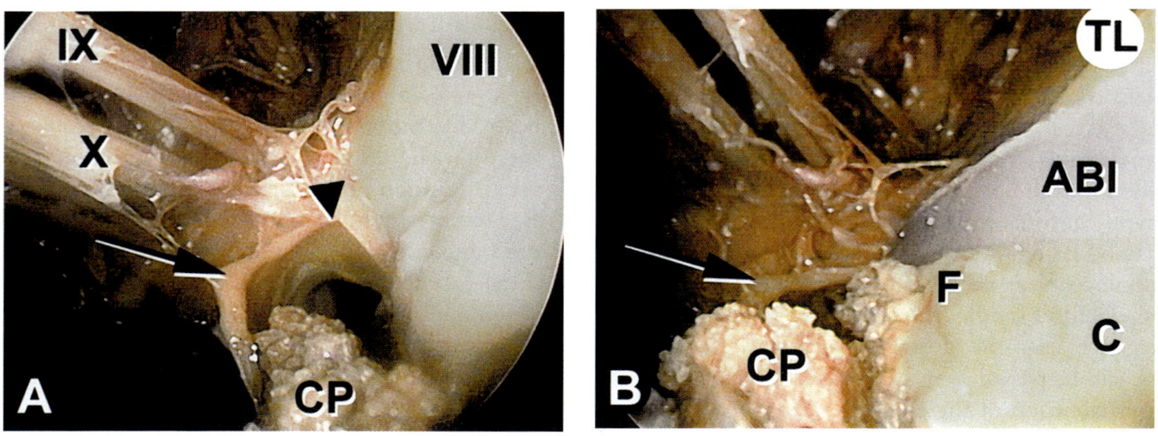


**FIGURE 10.12.** Endoscopic assisted auditory brainstem implantation. View of the lateral recess with a 30° endoscope using the translabyrinthine approach. Notice the excellent visualization of the lateral recess. The electrode paddle can be placed on the brainstem surface overlying the cochlear nucleus with visual endoscopic guidance. **A:** Surface topography of the cochlear nucleus. **B:** View with the electrode paddle in place over the cochlear nucleus. *VIII,* vestibulocochlear nerve; *IX,* glossopharyngeal nerve fibers; *X,* vagal nerve fibers; *CP,* choroid plexus; *F,* flocculus; *C,* cerebellum; *ABI,* auditory brainstem implant lead and paddle in the lateral recess; *arrow,* rhomboid lip; *arrowhead,* region of the cochlear nucleus.

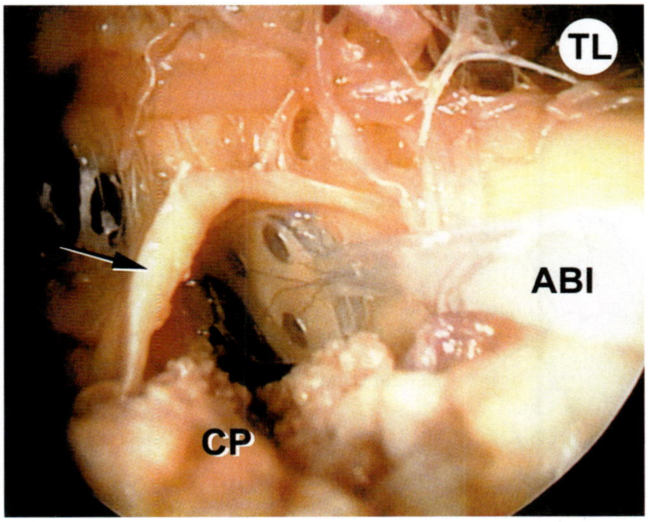


**FIGURE 10.13.** Endoscopic view of the positioning electrode in the lateral recess through the translabyrinthine approach. The full length of the paddle is visible, as are deeper aspects of the lateral recess. Using the endoscope, the electrode position can be easily assessed and repositioned. In this example, the distal electrode lost contact with the brainstem surface and overshot the cochlear nucleus. *ABI,* auditory brainstem implant lead and paddle in the lateral recess; *CP,* choroid plexus; *arrow,* rhomboid lip.

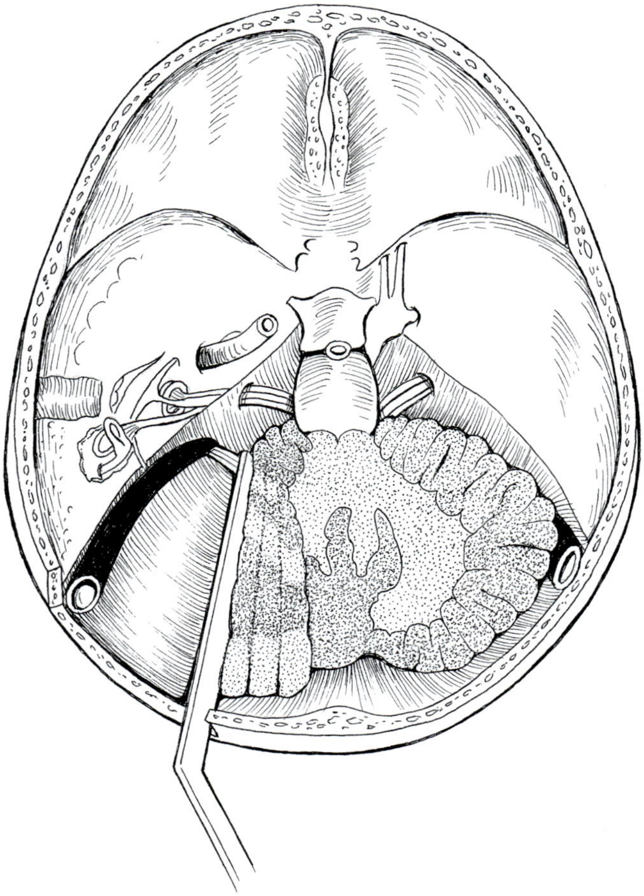

**FIGURE 10.14.** Overview of the retrosigmoid (suboccipital) approach.

## Retrosigmoid Approach

The retrosigmoid or suboccipital approach is performed in standard manner and should be of a size adequate for safe tumor extirpation (Figs. 10.14 and 10.15). The use of the endoscope allows a smaller craniotomy than would be needed with the operating microscope, but the optical modality used for tumor removal should take precedence and determine surgical approach. In our study, a 3 × 2 cm craniectomy over the posterior fossa, inferior to the transverse sinus and posteromedial to the sigmoid sinus, was completed. The dura was incised and reflected to expose the cerebellum. A cerebellar retractor was placed to provide access to the cerebellopontine angle. It is assumed that decompression by opening the lateral medullary cistern and drilling of bone over the internal auditory canal is done in the course of exposing the tumor. For endoscopic placement of the ABI, no drilling of the petrous temporal bone was necessary.

The principal criticism of the retrosigmoid approach for ABI placement is the need for extensive cerebellar retraction to expose the implant site (21,23). However, for endoscopic visualization of the lateral recess of the fourth ventricle, less retraction is necessary compared with the translabyrinthine approach. The 30° endoscope can be passed along the cerebellar retractor and "look" medially into the implant site, even though it may not be directly visible through the craniotomy (Fig. 10.16A).

The landmarks for the dorsal cochlear nucleus in the retrosigmoid approach are identical to those used in the translabyrinthine approach (Fig. 10.8). The perspective is slightly caudally shifted, however, and visualization of the surface of the brainstem within the recess is less oblique (compare Fig. 10.12A with Fig. 10.16A). As in the translabyrinthine approach, the 0° endoscope is introduced first to identify the flocculus and vestibulocochlear and glossopharyngeal nerves. The REZs of the eighth nerve are hidden behind the flocculus, but the entry of the glossopharyngeal rootlets may be apparent.

After orientation of the gross anatomy is considered, the 30° endoscope can be introduced to "look around" the flocculus (Fig. 10.16A). The REZs should be clearly visible, as is the choroid plexus emerging from the foramen of Luschka. The flocculus can be retracted with the McCabe flap knife, exposing the rhomboid lip, lateral recess, and glistening brainstem surface overlying the dorsal cochlear nucleus (Fig. 10.16A). A small amount of taenia chordae may be visualized, helping to further define the cochlear nuclear complex.

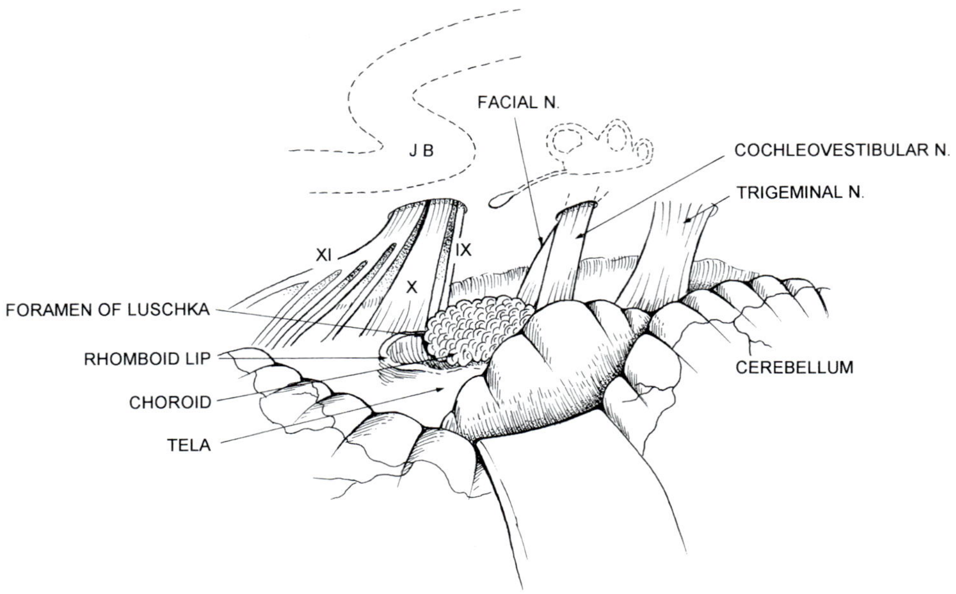


**FIGURE 10.15.** Detail of the landmarks visible near the cochlear nucleus through the retrosigmoid approach. *IX,* glossopharyngeal nerve fibers; *X,* vagal nerve fibers; *XI,* spinal accessory nerve fibers; *JB,* jugular bulb (ghosted in position).

The endoscope should be stabilized against the cerebellar retractor at the superior or inferior aspect of the field. The side of the operation and handedness of the surgeon determine the site. The ABI is advanced to the implant site, with electrode claw and maneuvered into the foramen of Luschka with the McCabe flap knife. We found that the 22° instrument combined with the less oblique approach to the brainstem made placement of the implant relatively easy. The position of the implant can be confirmed with the endoscope and electrophysiologic testing and documented with the digital video printer (Fig. 10.16B).

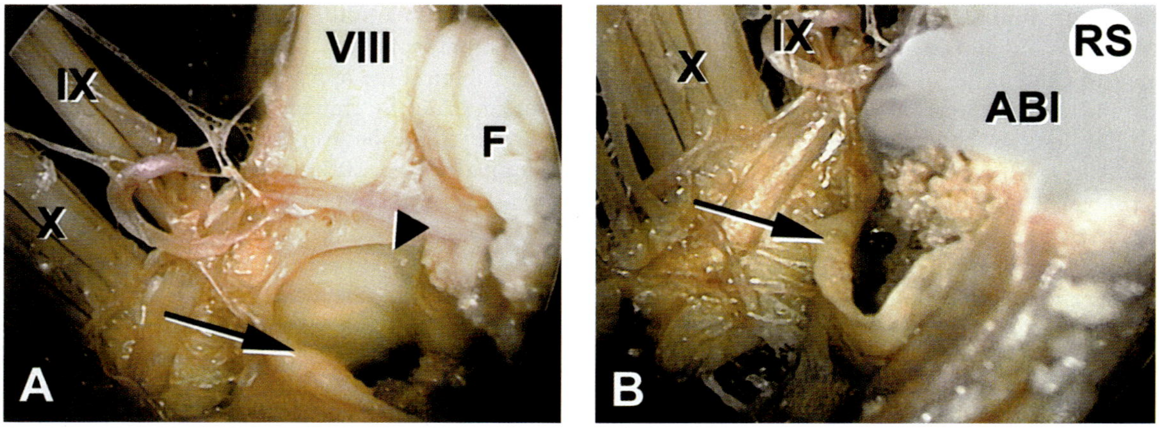


**FIGURE 10.16.** Endoscopic assisted auditory brainstem implantation. View of the lateral recess with a 30° endoscope using the retrosigmoid (*RS*) (suboccipital) approach. Notice the excellent visualization of the lateral recess. The electrode paddle can be placed on the brainstem surface overlying the cochlear nucleus with visual endoscopic guidance. **A:** Notice the more direct view of the cochlear nucleus relative to the translabyrinthine approach shown in Figure 10.12A and the choroid plexus adjacent to the flocculus. **B:** The electrode paddle can be seen to be in contact with the cochlear nucleus. *VIII,* vestibulocochlear nerve; *IX,* glossopharyngeal nerve fibers; *X,* vagal nerve fibers; *F,* flocculus; *ABI,* auditory brainstem implant lead and paddle in the lateral recess; *arrow,* rhomboid lip; *arrowhead,* region of the cochlear nucleus.

The implant would emerge through the craniotomy and is therefore secured in a bony pocket as for cochlear implant receiver-stimulators. The craniotomy is closed in the routine manner, and the usual postoperative intensive care unit monitoring and postoperative care is delivered.

## Middle Cranial Fossa Approach

A middle cranial fossa approach is performed as described by Fisch (27,28). Briefly, a 3 × 4 cm temporal craniotomy is made centered over the zygomatic root. A Fisch middle cranial fossa retractor is introduced to retract the dura and temporal lobe. The temporal bone is dissected anterior to the superior semicircular canal (SCC) within a 60° angle whose vertex is the SCC ampulla, and the internal auditory canal is skeletonized (Fig. 10.17). To provide adequate space for the endoscope and instrumentation to place the ABI electrode, the cochlea is identified and partially removed. The dura is then opened.

The 0° endoscope is introduced to identify the facial and vestibulocochlear nerves (Fig. 10.18). The glossopharyngeal rootlets are obscured by these nerves as the surgical approach is rotated superorostrally approximately 110° from that of the translabyrinthine and retrosigmoid approaches (Figs. 10.8 and 10.9). Initial identification of the facial nerve is critical, because the endoscope is placed rostral to this nerve and the implant caudally. The 30° endoscope is placed rostral to the facial nerve along the bony groove created by removal of the cochlea. Care must be taken to avoid undue contact of the warm endoscope tip with the facial nerve.

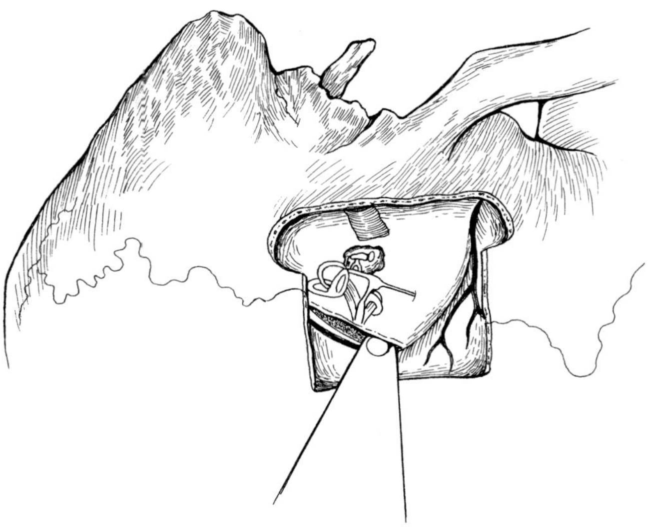

**FIGURE 10.17.** Overview of the middle cranial fossa approach.

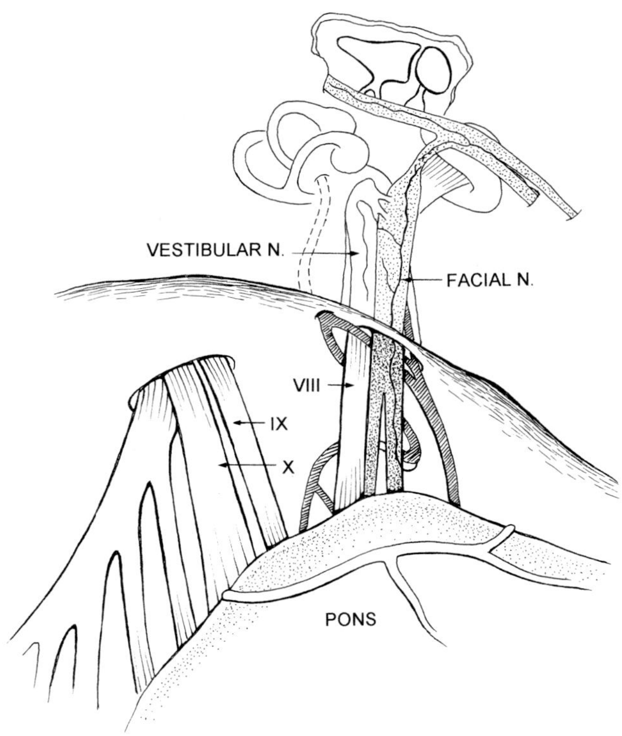


**FIGURE 10.18.** Detail of the landmarks visible at the brainstem (pons) near the root entry zone of the vestibulocochlear nerve using the middle cranial fossa approach. *VIII,* vestibulocochlear nerve; *IX,* glossopharyngeal nerve fibers; *X,* vagal nerve fibers.

Using the 30° endoscope, the glossopharyngeal rootlets can be identified (Fig. 10.19A). In the space between the eighth and ninth nerves is the implant site (Fig. 10.19A). The choroid plexus should be visible as it emerges from the foramen of Luschka. Likewise, the rhomboid lip helps to define the foramen. The implant is introduced in the posterior aspect of the surgical field and maneuvered with the electrode claw and flap knife caudal to the seventh and eighth nerves (Fig. 10.19B). The electrode claw was found to be most efficacious in manipulating the electrode into the lateral recess. By advancing and rotating the 30° endoscope, the lateral recess of the fourth ventricle and an extremely oblique view of the brainstem surface could be achieved (Fig. 10.20). This should be performed with caution to confirm or document electrode position, because the endoscope is in contact with or close to the facial nerve during this maneuver.

The proximal electrode extends through the temporal craniotomy, and the receiver-stimulator is placed in a bony recess. An extended postauricular incision may be necessary to provide an accessible and cosmetic site for the magnet and attachment of external processor. The craniotomy is closed, and standard postoperative care is provided.

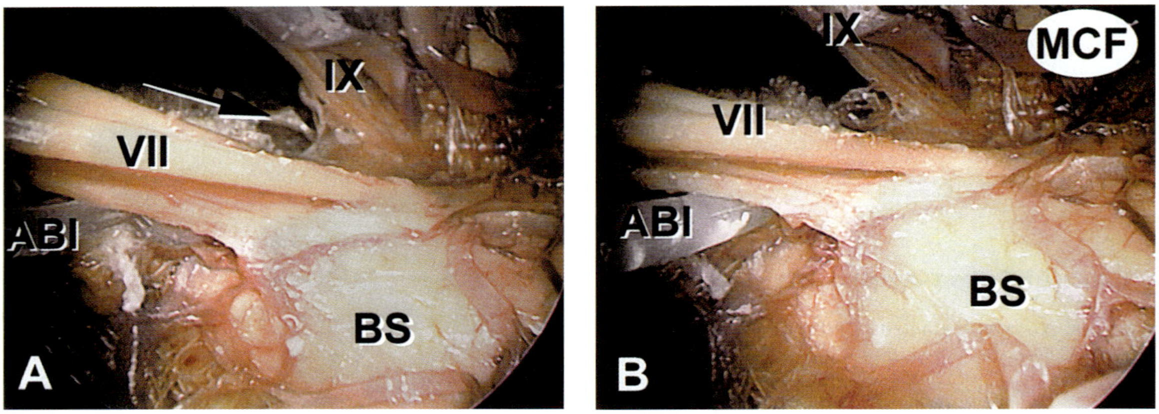


**FIGURE 10.19.** Endoscopic assisted auditory brainstem implantation. View of the lateral recess with a 30° endoscope using the middle cranial fossa *(MCF)* approach. Notice the excellent visualization of the brainstem *(BS)*. The electrode paddle cannot be placed on the brainstem surface overlying the cochlear nucleus with visual endoscopic guidance unless the endoscope tip is beyond the facial and vestibulocochlear nerve complex (see Figs. 10.8 and 10.9). **A:** The rhomboid lip is visible *(arrow)* as a landmark for the cochlear nucleus. **B:** The electrode array is placed against the vestibulocochlear nerve *(VII)* rather than the facial nerve. *IX,* glossopharyngeal nerve fibers; *ABI,* auditory brainstem implant lead and paddle in the lateral recess.

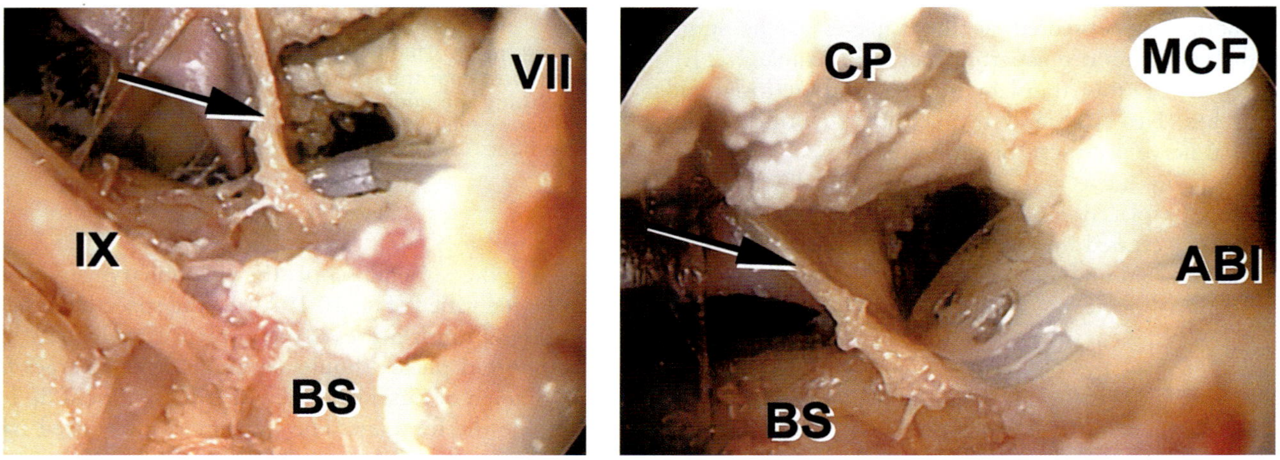


**FIGURE 10.20.** View of the foramen of Luschka from the middle cranial fossa *(MCF)* approach using a 30° endoscope. **A:** The endoscope has been advanced ventral (anterior) to the facial and vestibulocochlear nerves. **B:** By rotating the endoscope, the lateral recess and brainstem surface can be visualized. Care must be taken to avoid shaft-induced or heat-induced injury of the facial nerve. *VII,* facial nerve; *IX,* glossopharyngeal nerve fibers; *ABI,* auditory brainstem implant lead and paddle in the lateral recess; *BS,* brainstem; *CP,* choroid plexus; *arrows,* rhomboid lip.

## CONCLUSIONS

A systematic approach to finding the dorsal cochlear nucleus is necessary to appropriately position the ABI on the brainstem surface. This is particularly important when tumor or surgical extirpation has altered the normal appearance of the cerebellopontine angle. The 0° and 30° endoscopes provide high-resolution views of these landmarks and allow examination of the cerebellopontine angle with minimal retraction or manipulation. This enables preservation of delicate structures, which can further delineate the dorsal cochlear nucleus.

In the translabyrinthine, retrosigmoid, and middle cranial fossa approaches, identical landmarks are used and followed to localize the implant site:

- The flocculus and eighth and ninth cranial nerves are identified.
- The region between the REZs of these nerves and rostral to the flocculus contain the choroid plexus.
- The choroid plexus can be followed into the foramen of Luschka and the lateral recess of the fourth ventricle.
- The fold of tela choroidea forming the rhomboid lip further delineates the foramen of Luschka.
- The REZ of the eighth nerve "points" to the region of the cochlear nuclear complex.
- The taenia chordae, if preserved, attaches at the junction of the dorsal and inferior ventral cochlear nuclei.
- The brainstem surface in the recess over the cochlear nuclear complex has a glistening ependymal layer.
- The brainstem overlying the dorsal cochlear nucleus may have a slight bulge.

The endoscope can document electrode position and provide an anatomic correlation with electrophysiologic results. In the Med-El strategy of implantation, the endoscope in conjunction with video documentation allows accurate reproduction of the placement of the stimulating electrode after removal of the positioning electrode. With the Cochlear Corporation ABI strategy of implantation, the endoscope, in conjunction with electrically evoked auditory brainstem response can allow optimal placement of the electrode.

Specific details should be attended to with each approach:

| ***Surgical Approach*** | ***Important Technical Points*** |
|---|---|
| Translabyrinthine | Decompress the jugular bulb to provide access for the endoscope and surgical instruments. |
| Middle Cranial Fossa | The cochlea must be partially removed to allow access for the endoscope. The implant crosses caudal to the eighth and seventh nerves. The endoscope is close to the facial nerve and requires care to avoid neural injury. |
| Retrosigmoid | Less cerebellar retraction may be needed than with the operating microscope. The retractor can be used to stabilize the endoscope. |

The operative approach should be determined by the nature and extent of the primary lesion and by the optical modality used for tumor removal. Placement of the ABI should follow adequate and safe removal of tumor.

## REFERENCES


1. McElveen JT Jr, Hitselberger WE, House WF, et al. Electrical stimulation of cochlear nucleus in man. *Am J Otol* 1985; Nov(Suppl):88–91.
2. Edgerton BJ, House WF, Hitselberger W. Hearing by cochlear nucleus stimulation in humans. *Ann Otol Rhinol Laryngol Suppl* 1982;91:117–124.
3. Eisenberg LS, Maltan AA, Portillo F, et al. Electrical stimulation of the auditory brain stem structure in deafened adults. *J Rehabil Res Dev* 1987;24:9–22.
4. Hitselberger WE, House WF, Edgerton BJ, et al. Cochlear nucleus implants. *Otolaryngol Head Neck Surg* 1984;92:52–54.
5. Otto SR, Shannon RV, Brackmann DE, et al. The multichannel auditory brain stem implant: performance in twenty patients. *Otolaryngol Head Neck Surg* 1998;118:291–303.
6. Otto S, Staller S. Multichannel auditory brain stem implant: case studies comparing fitting strategies and results. *Ann Otol Rhinol Laryngol Suppl* 1995;166:36–39.
7. Shannon RV, Fayad J, Moore J, et al. Auditory brainstem implant: II. Postsurgical issues and performance. *Otolaryngol Head Neck Surg* 1993;108:634–642.
8. Laszig R, Sollmann WP, Marangos N. The restoration of hearing in neurofibromatosis type 2. *J Laryngol Otol* 1995;109:385–389.
9. Otto SR, Brackmann DE, Staller S, et al. The multichannel auditory brainstem implant: 6-month coinvestigator results. *Adv Otorhinolaryngol* 1997;52:1–7.
10. Miyamoto RT, Campbell RL, Fritsch M, et al. Preservation of hearing in neurofibromatosis 2. *Otolaryngol Head Neck Surg* 1990;103:619–624.
11. Friedland DR, Wackym PA. Evaluation of surgical approaches to endoscopic auditory brainstem implantation. *Laryngoscope* 1999; 109:175–180.
12. Tatagiba M, Matthies C, Samii M. Microendoscopy of the internal auditory canal in vestibular schwannoma surgery. *Neurosurgery* 1996;38:737–740.
13. Cohen AR, Perneczky A, Rodziewicz GS, et al. Endoscope-assisted craniotomy: approach to the rostral brain stem. *Neurosurgery* 1995;36:1128–1129; discussion 1129–1130.
14. Wackym PA, King WA, Barker FG, et al. Endoscope-assisted vestibular neurectomy. *Laryngoscope* 1998;108:1787–1793.
15. Dublin WB. Cytoarchitecture of the cochlear nuclei: report of an illustrative case of erythroblastosis. *Arch Otolaryngol* 1974;100: 355–359.
16. Brackmann DE, Hitselberger WE, Nelson RA, et al. Auditory brainstem implant: I. Issues in surgical implantation [See comments]. *Otolaryngol Head Neck Surg* 1993;108:624–633.
17. Terr LI. Cochlear nucleus stimulation [Letter, comments]. *Laryngoscope* 1992;102:724.
18. Terr LI, Edgerton BJ. Three-dimensional reconstruction of the cochlear nuclear complex in humans. *Arch Otolaryngol* 1985;111: 495–501.
19. Terr LI, Edgerton BJ. Surface topography of the cochlear nuclei in humans: two- and three-dimensional analysis. *Hear Res* 1985; 17:51–59.
20. Friedland DR, Meyer GA, Wackym PA. Anatomic basis for endoscope-assisted placement of auditory brainstem implants. *Neurosurgery* 2001 *(in press)*.
21. Kuroki A, Moller AR. Microsurgical anatomy around the foramen of Luschka in relation to intraoperative recording of auditory evoked potentials from the cochlear nuclei. *J Neurosurg* 1995;82:933–939.
22. Lejeune R, Vincent C, Louis E, et al. Anatomic basis for auditory brainstem implant. *Surg Radiol Anat* 1997;19:213–216.
23. Monsell EM, McElveen JT Jr, Hitselberger WE, et al. Surgical

approaches to the human cochlear nuclear complex. *Am J Otol* 1987;8:450–455.
24. McElveen JT Jr, Hitselberger WE, House WF. Surgical accessibility of the cochlear nuclear complex in man: surgical landmarks. *Otolaryngol Head Neck Surg* 1987;96:135–140.
25. Mobley JP, Huang J, Moore JK, et al. Three-dimensional modeling of human brain stem structures for an auditory brain stem implant. *Ann Otol Rhinol Laryngol Suppl* 1995;166:30–31.
26. Sinha UK, Terr LI, Galey FR, et al. Computer-aided three-dimensional reconstruction of the cochlear nerve root. *Arch Otolaryngol Head Neck Surg* 1987;113:651–655.
27. Wackym PA, Andrews JC. Middle cranial fossa approach. In: Samii M, Cheatham M, Becker D, eds. *Atlas of cranial base surgery*. Philadelphia: WB Saunders, 1995:26–31.
28. Fisch U, Mattox D. *Microsurgery of the skull base*. New York: Thieme Medical Publishers, 1988.

# 11

# ENDOSCOPY AND ENDOSCOPIC STEREOTACTIC SURGERY DURING ACOUSTIC NEUROMA RESECTION

**PHILLIP A. WACKYM**
**WESLEY A. KING**
**GLENN A. MEYER**
**ROBERT G. OJEMANN**
**FRED G. BARKER**
**DENNIS S. POE**

The morbidity associated with acoustic neuroma surgery has declined steadily since the first operation was performed more than 100 years ago (Figs. 11.1 and 11.2). Historically, facial nerve sacrifice was the rule, but postoperative facial nerve function is expected in most patients today. In selected patients, hearing can be maintained (1). Although the permanent complication rate is very low, cerebrospinal fluid (CSF) leakage can occur in up to 20% of patients, with most cases resulting from poor intraoperative identification of exposed air cells within the temporal bone (2–5). Incomplete tumor removal, especially within the internal auditory canal (IAC), does occur after retrosigmoid (suboccipital) resection (6) and rarely after translabyrinthine resection (7).

Endoscopic techniques have revolutionized the practice of surgery in a number of specialties (8,9). With several clinical applications, smaller incisions and exposures are possible, resulting in decreased postoperative pain, shorter recuperation, better cosmetic results, and shorter hospitalizations. Endoscopes have the ability to provide high magnification and illumination of the operative field, but unlike the operative microscope, they do not limit the surgeon's view to the linear line of sight. Using flexible or angled endoscopes (or both), the surgeon is able to look "around corners" past obstructing tissue and structures. Applications of the endoscope to vestibular neurectomy (10) and auditory brainstem implantation (11) have been reported, as well as the broad applications in neurosurgery (8) and otolaryngology (9). Preliminary reports of the series of 24 acoustic neuroma surgical cases operated by one of the neuro-otologist authors (D.S.P.) and the early series of 10 cases operated by the other neuro-otologist author (P.A.W.) using endoscopes have been published (5,12). The expanded clinical experience with the adjunctive use of endoscopes during 78 acoustic neuroma surgeries performed by the authors of this chapter has been published (13). Our hypothesis remains that, in specific clinical situations, endoscopes offer better visualization than the microscope during acoustic neuroma (vestibular schwannoma) surgery and can thereby decrease the incidence of the postoperative complications of CSF leakage and recurrence of tumor. Current work further supports this hypothesis and expands our clinical series. Clinical illustrations of the relevant information provided by the adjunctive use of endoscopes in acoustic neuroma surgery are provided. The application of stereotactic endoscopic surgery during acoustic neuroma resection is explored.

## PATIENTS AND METHODS

We prospectively studied all consecutive patients ($n$=73) undergoing a primary retrosigmoid (suboccipital) approach for resection of an acoustic neuroma between June 1993 and July 2000 by D.S.P. and all consecutive patients ($n$=55) undergoing a primary retrosigmoid (suboccipital), translabyrinthine, or middle cranial fossa approach for resection of an acoustic neuroma between January 1996 and July 2000 by P.A.W. All patients in this series ($n$=128) had the adjunctive use of endoscopy incorporated into their surgical procedures. The first 24 patients in the series of D.S.P. have been previously reported (5). The neuro-otologist–neurosurgeon teams, location, and number of tumors operated included D.S.P., R.G.O., or F.G.B. (Massachusetts General Hospital, Boston, MA, $n$=49), P.A.W. or W.A.K. (Mount Sinai Hospital, New York, NY, $n$=22), and P.A.W., G.A.M.,

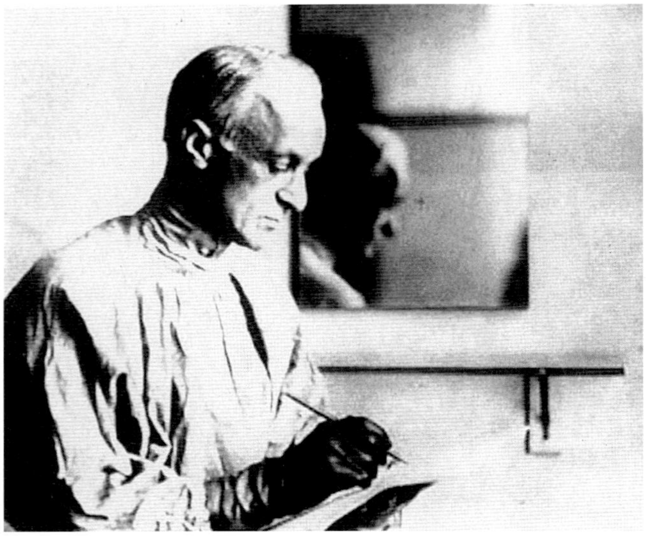

**FIGURE 11.1.** Harvey Cushing, M.D. (1869–1939). Cushing introduced several technical advances, reported between 1905 and 1932, that resulted in a reduction in the mortality rate from a high of 84% (Krause's series of 31 patients reported in 1913) to only 4% (Cushing's series of 50 patients reported in 1932). These included decompression of the posterior fossa; electrocautery, silver clips, and application of Horsley's bone wax to facilitate hemostasis; partial cerebellar resection; and subtotal tumor debulking to preserve brainstem vasculature and cranial nerve function. He emphasized meticulous surgical technique and gentle handling of tissues instead of operative speed.

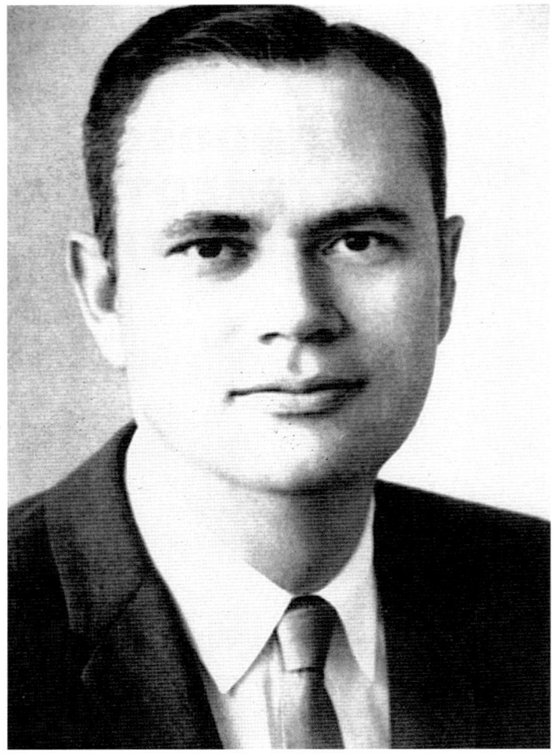

**FIGURE 11.2.** William F. House, D.D.D., M.D. (1923–). Many consider House to be the father of neuro-otology. He introduced the operating microscope and otologic techniques to the field of neurosurgery in reintroducing and refining the middle fossa approach and translabyrinthine approach for the treatment of acoustic neuromas. He also championed the concept of a neuro-otologist and neurosurgeon team for the microsurgical management of skull base tumors. Consequently, the mortality rate for acoustic tumor removal fell dramatically, and facial nerve preservation became the rule rather than the exception.

or P.R.W. (Froedtert Memorial Lutheran Hospital, Milwaukee, WI, *n*=33). All acoustic neuroma cases performed by P.A.W. with the other two neurosurgeons (Kalmon Post and Chandranath Sen) with whom he operated at the Mount Sinai Hospital were excluded because endoscopy was not performed. All translabyrinthine and middle cranial fossa approaches for resection of acoustic neuroma performed by D.S.P. were excluded from analysis because endoscopy was not used during these cases.

Every patient underwent magnetic resonance imaging (MRI) preoperatively. The tumor size was measured on the MRI scans and classified in one of four categories: intracanalicular, extracanalicular (≤1.5 cm), extracanalicular (1.6 to 3.0 cm), and extracanalicular (>3.0 cm). The diagnosis of acoustic neuroma was confirmed histologically in every case. The patients were divided into four groups: group 1 (*n*=73) contained cases using the retrosigmoid approach performed by D.S.P. and his neurosurgical colleagues; group 2 (*n*=35) contained cases using the retrosigmoid approach performed by P.A.W. and his neurosurgical colleagues; group 3 (*n*=17) contained cases using the translabyrinthine approach performed by P.A.W. and his neurosurgical colleagues; and group 4 (*n*=3) contained cases using the middle cranial fossa approach performed by P.A.W. and

**TABLE 11.1. DISTRIBUTION OF AGE, SEX, AND LATERALITY FOR PATIENTS UNDERGOING ACOUSTIC NEUROMA RESECTION**

| Group[a] | Mean Age (Range) | Female : Male Ratio (%) | Right : Left Ratio (%) |
|---|---|---|---|
| Group 1 (*n* = 73) | 49.7 (14–76) | 36 : 37 (49.3/50.7) | 32 : 41 (43.8/56.2) |
| Group 2 (*n* = 35) | 48.1 (17–81) | 17 : 18 (48.6/51.4) | 19 : 16 (54.3/45.7) |
| Group 3 (*n* = 17) | 54.4 (38–76) | 10 : 7 (58.8/41.1) | 9 : 8 (52.9/47.1) |
| Group 4 (*n* = 3) | 51.0 (46–58) | 1 : 2 (33.3/66.7) | 1 : 2 (33.3/66.7) |

[a]Group 1, retrosigmoid (D.S.P.); Group 2, retrosigmoid (P.A.W.); Group 3, translabyrinthine (P.A.W.); Group 4, middle cranial fossa (P.A.W.); the author-surgeon's initials are given for each group.

**TABLE 11.2. PREOPERATIVE TUMOR SIZE IN ENDOSCOPE-ASSISTED SURGERY GROUPS**

| | Tumor Size | | | |
|---|---|---|---|---|
| Group[a] | IC *n* (%) | EC ≤ 1.5 cm *n* (%) | EC 1.6–3.0 cm *n* (%) | EC > 3.0 cm *n* (%) |
| Group 1 (n = 73) | 5 (6.8) | 26 (35.6) | 36 (49.3) | 6 (8.2) |
| Group 2 (n = 35) | 2 (5.7) | 11 (31.4) | 16 (45.7) | 6 (17.1) |
| Group 3 (n = 17) | 5 (29.4) | 5 (29.4) | 7 (41.1) | — |
| Group 4 (n = 3) | 2 (66.7) | 1 (33.3) | — | — |

IC, intracanalicular; EC, extracanalicular.
[a]Group 1, retrosigmoid (D.S.P.); Group 2, retrosigmoid (P.A.W.); Group 3, translabyrinthine (P.A.W.); Group 4, middle cranial fossa (P.A.W.); the author-surgeon's initials are given for each group.

W.A.K. Table 11.1 compares the age, female to male ratios, and the laterality of the tumors in all four groups studied. Table 11.2 compares the preoperative tumor size in all four groups studied.

## ADJUNCTIVE ENDOSCOPY AND OPERATIVE TECHNIQUE

### Endoscopic Instrumentation

The rigid endoscope was used in this series of patients. The diameter of the endoscope was 2.7 or 4.0 mm, and both 0° and 30° (or 45°) endoscopes were used (Karl Storz America, Culver City, CA; Smith Nephew Richards, Memphis, TN; Codman Endoscopy, Randolph, MA). Illumination was provided by a xenon light source (e.g., Stryker Endoscopy, Santa Clara, CA). The patient position and equipment arrangement in the operating room is shown in Fig. 11.3. The endoscope was held by the operating surgeon, the co-surgeon, or attached to a rigid fixation device (Codman Endoscopy). A three-chip camera (Karl Storz America or Stryker Endoscopy) was attached to the lens of the endoscope and the picture was displayed on a 19-inch video monitor (Sony Electronics, San Jose, CA). The operative field was generously irrigated before inserting the endoscope to improve visualization. Endoscopy with a rigid glass lens endoscope was used during tumor removal to examine posterior fossa neurovascular structures and after tumor excision to inspect the internal auditory canal (IAC), inner ear, and middle ear, depending on the approach used. Digital capture of the image (Sony Electronics or Stryker Endoscopy) was completed for medical documentation purposes and to illustrate the anatomic relationships identified endoscopically. When possible, corresponding images through the operating microscope were captured for comparison.

### Retrosigmoid Approach

A retrosigmoid (suboccipital) transmeatal approach was performed in 108 patients (groups 1 and 2) using conventional technique and instrumentation. After the craniotomy or craniectomy was performed, the dura was opened parallel to the transverse and sigmoid sinuses or with a Y-shaped incision and secured to the adjacent soft tissue. The cerebellum was gently elevated to expose the lateral medullary cistern, which was opened to allow release of CSF. The cerebellum was then retracted medially to expose the cerebellopontine angle (CPA) and tumor.

In patients with a small or medium-sized tumor, an initial examination was performed with the endoscope. Specific attention was paid to cranial nerves IV through XI, the IAC, and the vascular anatomy. The intracanalicular portion of the tumor was exposed before tumor removal except when the lesion was large, in which case it was first internally debulked. The dura was incised and removed along the posterior lip of the IAC. Under continuous irrigation, the exposed bone was removed with an otologic drill (Med$^{next}$, Sofamor Danek, Memphis, TN). Bone dust was prevented from entering the subarachnoid space, and care was taken not to violate the labyrinth during the dissection of the IAC. When a tumor with lateral extension was approached through a retrosigmoid route, a 30° or 45° degree endoscope was used to monitor the lateral dissection so that the lateral limit (i.e., exposure of the intraosseous endolymphatic sac) could be identified before violation of the posterior semicircular canal. In several cases, computer-guided stereotactic endoscopic surgery was performed to determine the lateral extent of the internal auditory canal (Stealth, Sofamor Danek).

After the IAC was opened, the lateral extent of the tumor was dissected gently from the facial and cochlear nerves. This was accomplished with the Kartush stimulus-dissection instruments (Xomed, Jacksonville, FL) and facial nerve electromyography. The bulk of the tumor was removed in a standard fashion using a combination of blunt and sharp dissection, as well as ultrasonic aspiration for large tumors. After tumor removal, the IAC was inspected microscopically and endoscopically, looking for residual tumor at the fundus of the canal or air cells opened during the bony dissection. When residual tumor was identified, a

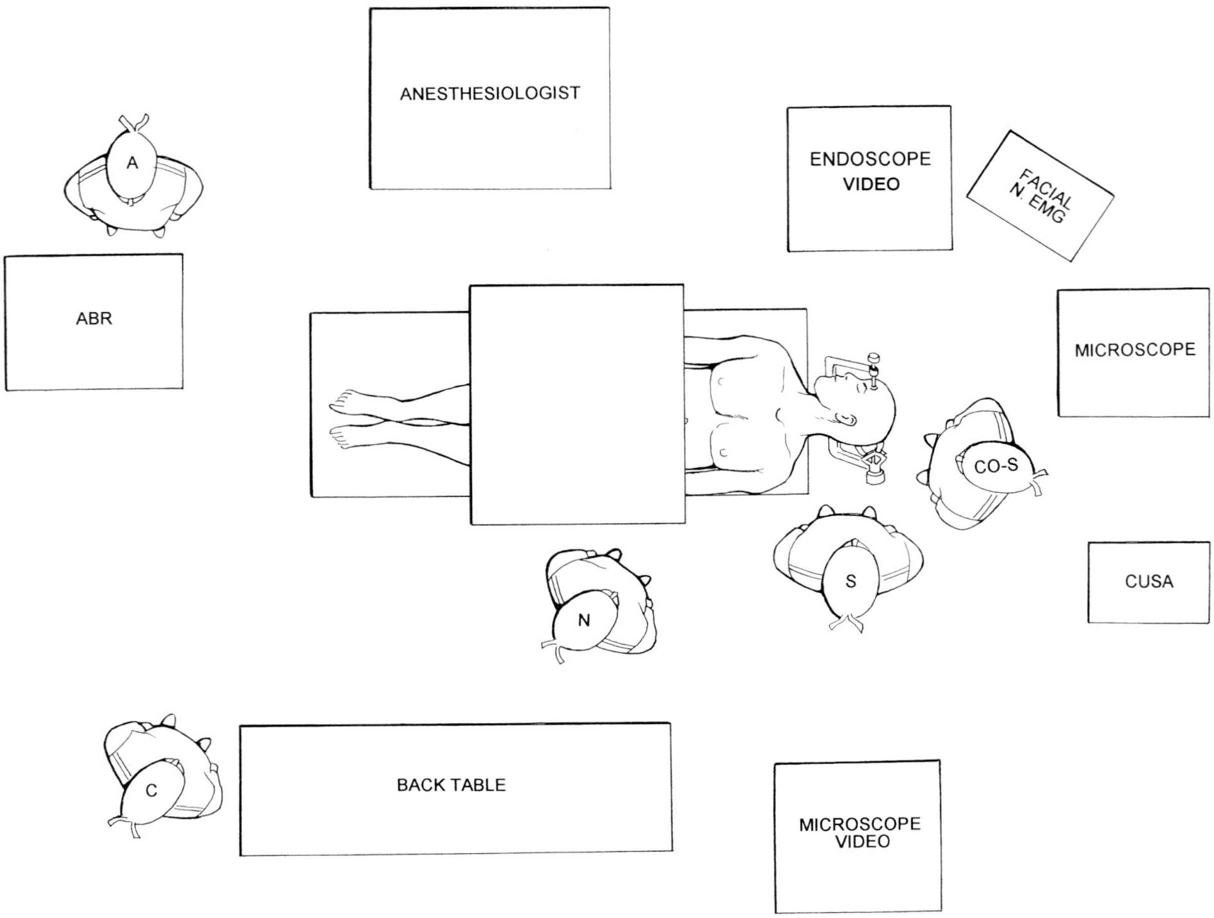


**FIGURE 11.3.** Patient position for microsurgical and endoscopic removal of an acoustic neuroma through the translabyrinthine approach. Notice the relationship between the video monitor and the surgeons *(S, CO-S)*. The Mayfield head holder is used to attach the endoscope holder. Intraoperative facial nerve electromyography is performed, and the ultrasonic aspirator *(CUSA)* is used to debulk large tumors. The computerized stereotactic navigational system can also be coupled with the endoscope for real-time determination of anatomic position within the internal auditory canal. When undergoing a middle cranial fossa approach for tumor resection, the patient remains supine, and the surgeon sits at the vertex of the head. For the retrosigmoid approach, the positions of the surgeon and equipment remain unchanged; however, the patient is placed in a lateral decubitus position with the operated ear uppermost. *A*, audiologist; *ABR*, auditory brainstem evoked response; *C*, circulator; *Facial n. emg*, facial nerve electromyography; *N*, nurse.

30° or 45° endoscope was used to examine the fundus and complete the tumor removal. Bone wax was applied to the identified air cells under direct or indirect vision, and the remaining defect was filled with a free muscle or fat graft harvested from the wound margin. The patients were monitored postoperatively for CSF leaks.

## Translabyrinthine Approach

A translabyrinthine approach and resection of the acoustic neuroma was performed in 17 patients (group 3) using conventional techniques and instrumentation. A 30° or 45° endoscope was used to visualize the undersurface of the stapes footplate to be certain that the stapes was not displaced from the oval window. The field of the bony dissection was inspected to determine if there were open air cells that had not been identified with the microscope and sealed with wax. After sealing all open air cells, the middle ear was partitioned from the mastoid and posterior fossa defect with fascia or Alloderm (LifeCell, The Woodlands, TX) and the defect filled with abdominal fat. The patients were monitored postoperatively for CSF leaks.

## Middle Cranial Fossa Approach

A middle cranial fossa approach and resection was performed in three patients using conventional techniques and instrumentation (group 4). The 0° and 30° (or 45°)

endoscopes were then used to visualize the neurovascular relationships of the cochlear and facial nerves within the IAC and extending medially to the brainstem. Digital photography documented the integrity of these cranial nerves. The floor of the middle cranial fossa and the opened IAC were inspected to determine if there were open air cells that had not been identified with the microscope and sealed with wax. After sealing all open air cells, the IAC was filled with a free muscle graft harvested from the temporalis muscle. Layers of temporalis fascia and bone, taken from the temporal craniotomy flap, were used to reconstruct the floor of the middle cranial fossa. The patients were monitored postoperatively for CSF leaks.

## RESULTS

There were no complications related to the use of the endoscopy. Rare complications not related to CSF leakage or residual tumor include failed hydroxyapatite cement (Bone Source, Leibinger, Dallas, TX) cranioplasty (group 2, $n$=1); local wound infection (group 3, $n$=1); chronic headache (group 1, $n$=1; group 3, $n$=1); meningitis (group 1, $n$=2); and focal cerebellar infarction (group 1, $n$=1). There were no deaths. The single case of failed hydroxyapatite cement cranioplasty occurred in a patient who, despite postoperative counseling, engaged in vigorous sexual intercourse during the first week postoperatively and noticed a popping sensation at the site of his craniotomy. The cranioplasty material had fractured and required removal with reconstruction using a polymer cranioplasty material.

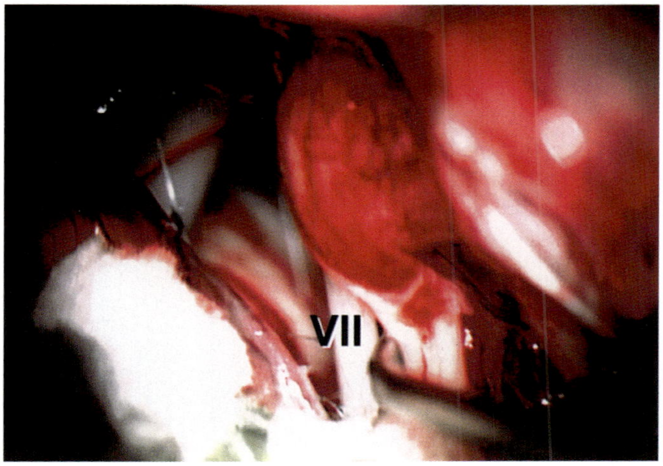


**FIGURE 11.5.** Microscopic view of a 1.2-cm acoustic neuroma in the right cerebellopontine angle. Gentle retraction with a Rhoton 6 dissector clearly shows the facial *(VII)* nerve ventral anterior to the vestibulocochlear nerve.

The endoscope was used to examine the tumor and neurovascular relationships before tumor removal in groups 1 and 2 (Figs. 11.4 to 11.23). Vascular loops and branches passing into the IAC were also better appreciated. In all cases (groups 1 through 4), this gave more information than was possible with the microscope alone.

During the surgical dissection of the IAC with the retrosigmoid approach, the use of 30° or 45° endoscopes allowed the maximum lateral extension of the exposure

*(text continues on page 92)*

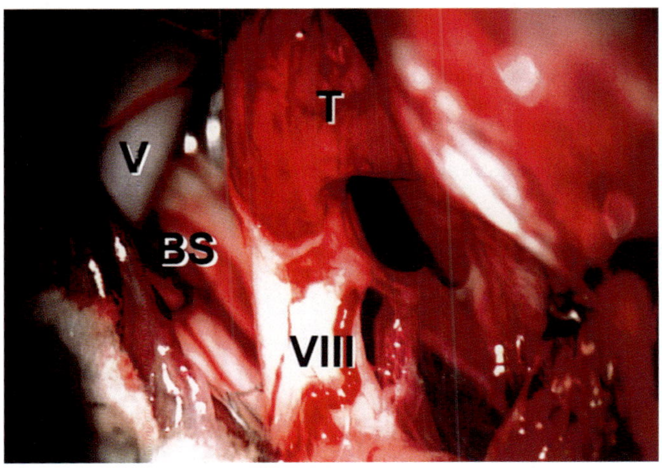


**FIGURE 11.4.** Microscopic view of a 1.2-cm acoustic neuroma in the right cerebellopontine angle. Notice the facial, vestibulocochlear *(VIII)*, and trigeminal *(V)* nerves in relation to the brainstem *(BS)* and tumor *(T)*. Posterior face of the temporal bone *(top right)* is seen.

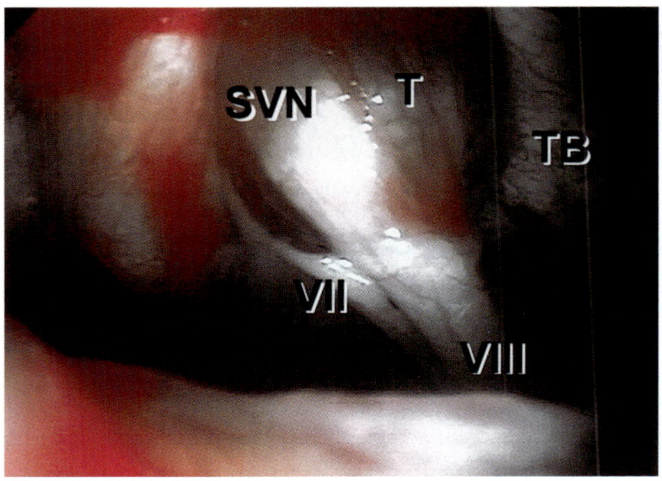


**FIGURE 11.6.** Endoscopic view of a 1.2-cm acoustic neuroma in the right cerebellopontine angle. A 30° endoscope shows the detailed relationship between the tumor *(T)*, the superior vestibular nerve *(SVN)*, the facial nerve *(VII)*, and the vestibulocochlear nerve *(VIII)*. With the 30° endoscope, it is possible to visualize the ventral aspect of the tumor before surgical exposure and manipulation of the internal auditory canal. *TB*, posterior face of the temporal bone.

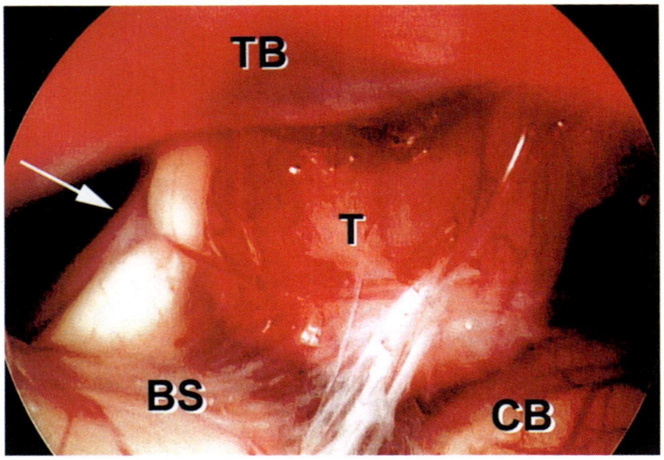


**FIGURE 11.7.** Endoscopic view illustrating the potential to visualize the neurovascular relationships within the cerebellopontine angle before retrosigmoid removal of a left 1.5-cm acoustic neuroma. The relation of the tumor *(T)* to the cerebellum *(CB)*, brainstem *(BS)*, and posterior face of the temporal bone *(TB)* is seen with a 0° endoscope. A small branch of the anterior inferior cerebellar artery *(arrow)* is tethered over the tumor and vestibulocochlear nerve, causing marked neural compression.

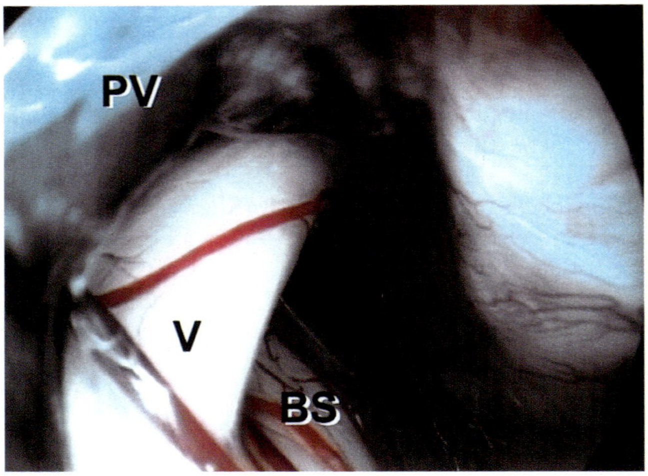


**FIGURE 11.9.** Endoscopic view illustrating the potential to visualize the neurovascular relationships within the cerebellopontine angle before the retrosigmoid removal of an acoustic neuroma. Cephalad (superior) to the tumor and facial-vestibulocochlear nerve complex, the trigeminal nerve *(V)*, brainstem *(BS)*, and petrosal vein *(PV)* (forming the superior petrosal sinus) can be seen.

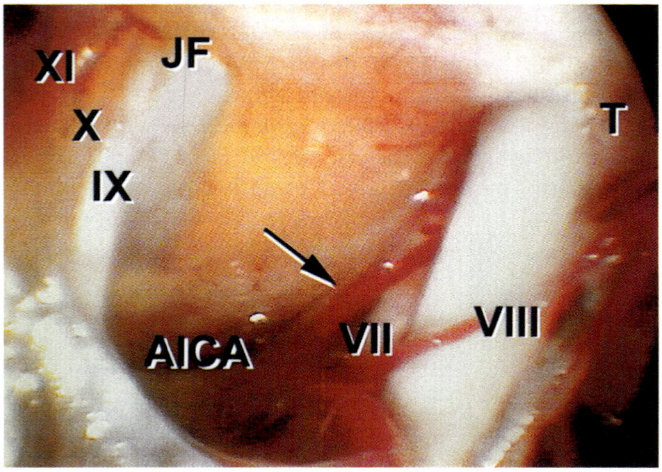


**FIGURE 11.8.** Endoscopic view illustrating the potential to visualize the neurovascular relationships within the cerebellopontine angle before the retrosigmoid removal of an acoustic neuroma. A 0° endoscope placed caudal (inferior) to a 0.5-cm acoustic neuroma *(T)* shows the anterior inferior cerebellar artery *(AICA)*, the labyrinthine artery *(arrow)*, facial nerve (*VII*), and vestibulocochlear nerve *(VIII)* in relation to the neural contents of the jugular foramen *(JF)*. *IX*, glossopharyngeal nerve; *X*, vagus nerve; *XI*, spinal accessory nerve.

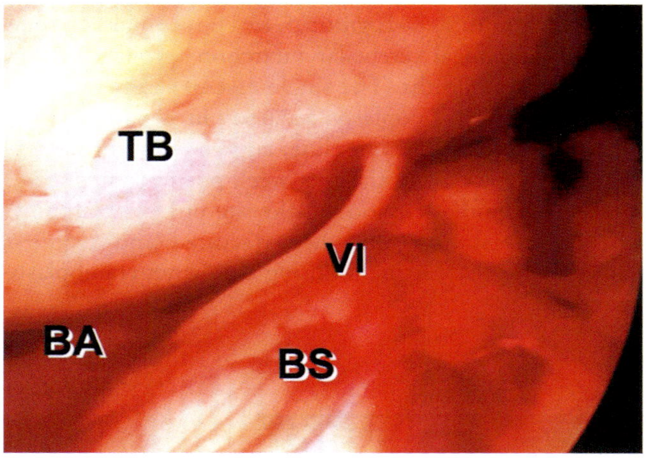


**FIGURE 11.10.** Endoscopic view illustrating the potential to visualize the neurovascular relationships within the cerebellopontine angle after the retrosigmoid removal of acoustic neuromas. Using a 0° endoscope, the abducens nerve *(VI)* can be seen entering Dorello's canal at the ventral petrous ridge of the temporal bone *(TB)*. The relationship between the brainstem *(BS)* and the basilar artery *(BA)* can be seen.

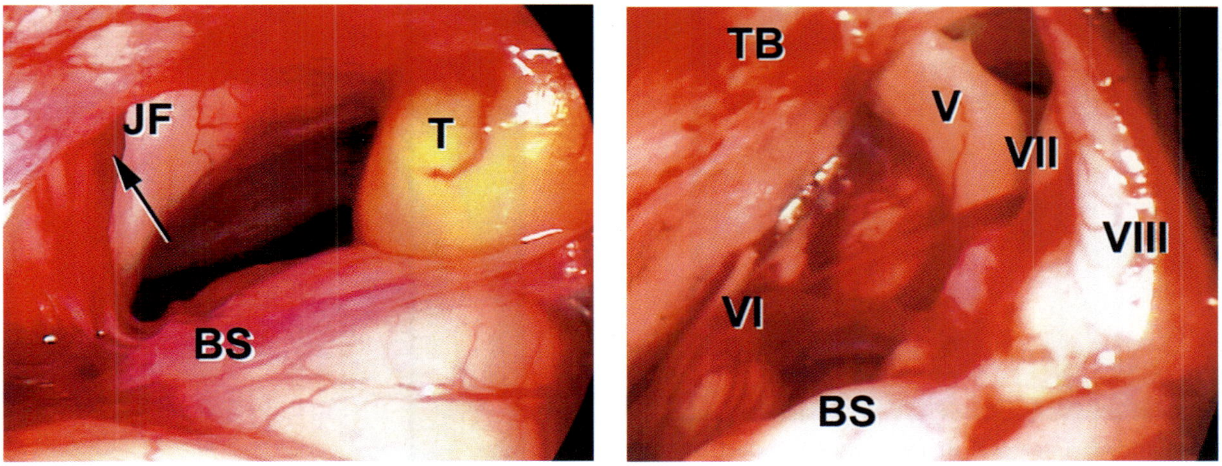


**FIGURE 11.11.** Endoscopic view illustrating the potential to visualize the neurovascular relationships within the cerebellopontine angle before and after retrosigmoid removal of a 1.7-cm left acoustic neuroma. **A:** Before removal, the tumor *(T)* can be seen in relation to the brainstem *(BS)* and jugular foramen *(JF)*. Cranial nerves IX, X, and XI *(arrow)* can be seen entering the jugular foramen. **B:** After retrosigmoid resection of the tumor, the vestibulocochlear *(VIII)*, facial *(VII)*, trigeminal *(V)*, and abducens *(VI)* nerves can be seen in relation to the brainstem *(BS)* and posterior face of the temporal bone *(TB)*.

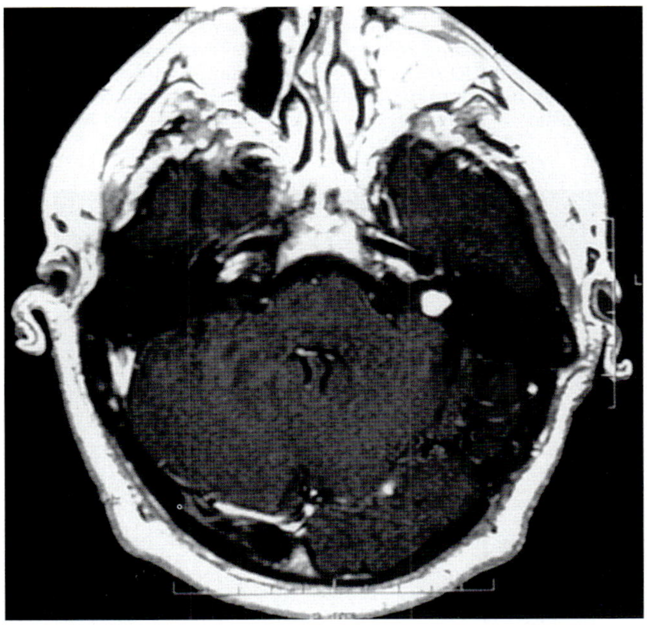

**FIGURE 11.12.** Preoperative axial T1-weighted magnetic resonance image with gadolinium enhancement shows an intracanalicular left acoustic neuroma resected using a retrosigmoid approach. Figures 11.13–11.15 show the corresponding endoscopic images of the cerebellopontine angle, tumor, and internal auditory canal.

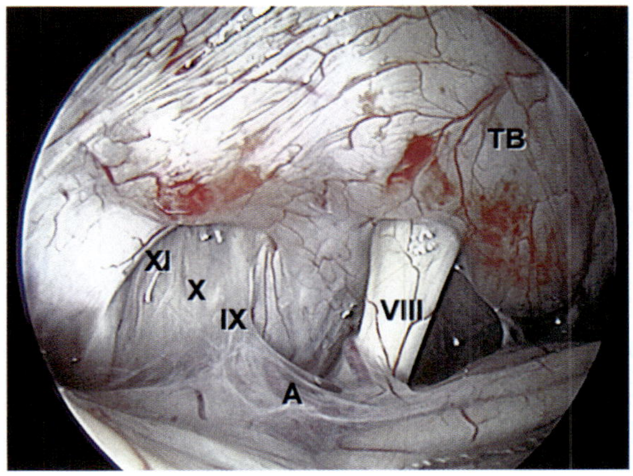


**FIGURE 11.13.** Panoramic view of cerebellopontine angle using a 4-mm, 0° endoscope before resection of left intracanalicular acoustic neuroma. The posterior face of the temporal bone *(TB)* is seen, as well as the porus acusticus and jugular foramen. *VIII,* vestibulocochlear nerve; *IX,* glossopharyngeal nerve; *X,* vagus nerve; *XI,* spinal accessory nerve; *A,* arachnoid.

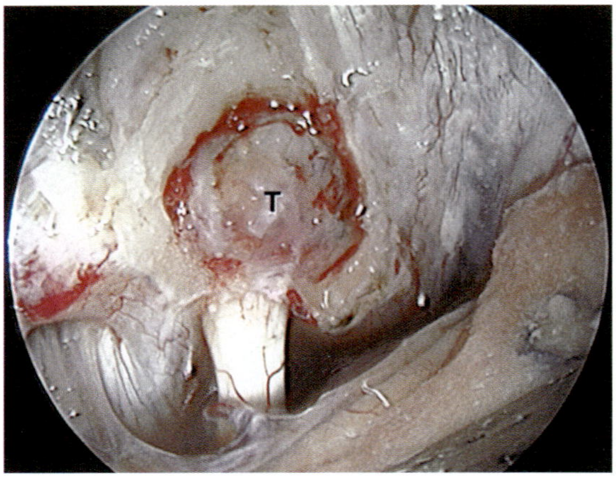


**FIGURE 11.14.** After removal of the posterior aspect of the internal auditory canal, the globular tumor *(T)* can be seen with a 4-mm, 0° endoscope.

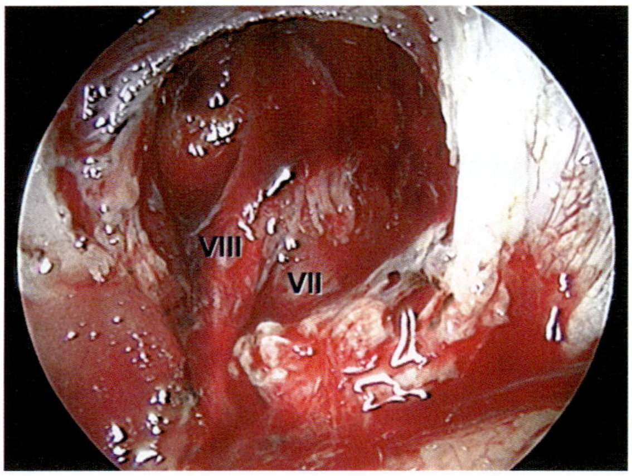


**FIGURE 11.15.** After removal of the tumor, a 4-mm, 30° endoscope shows no residual tumor in the fundus of the internal auditory canal. The intact facial *(VII)* and cochlear *(VIII)* nerves are shown.

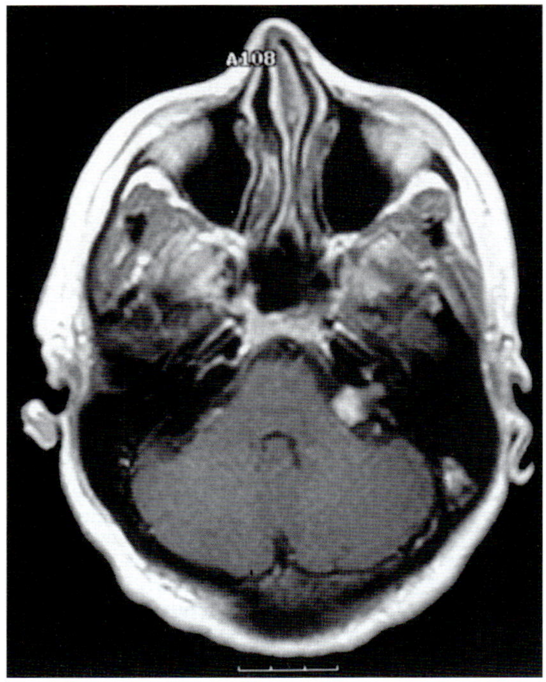


**FIGURE 11.16.** Preoperative axial T1-weighted magnetic resonance imaging with gadolinium enhancement shows a 1.0-cm, left acoustic neuroma resected using a retrosigmoid approach. Figures 11.17–11.19 show the corresponding endoscopic images of the cerebellopontine angle, tumor, and associated neural relationships to cranial nerves V, VI, VII, VIII, IX, X, and XI.

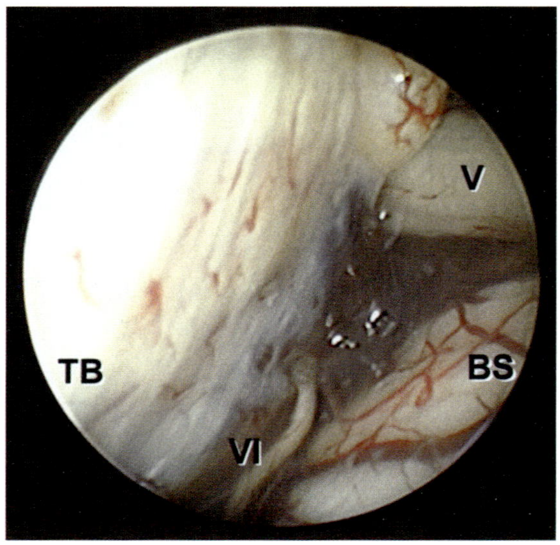


**FIGURE 11.17.** Before resection of the left, 1.0-cm acoustic neuroma, inspection of the posterior fossa with a 2.7-mm, 0° endoscope shows the posterior face of the temporal bone *(TB)*, brainstem *(BS)*, and trigeminal nerve *(V)*. The abducens nerve *(VI)* can be seen entering Dorello's canal at the petrous ridge.

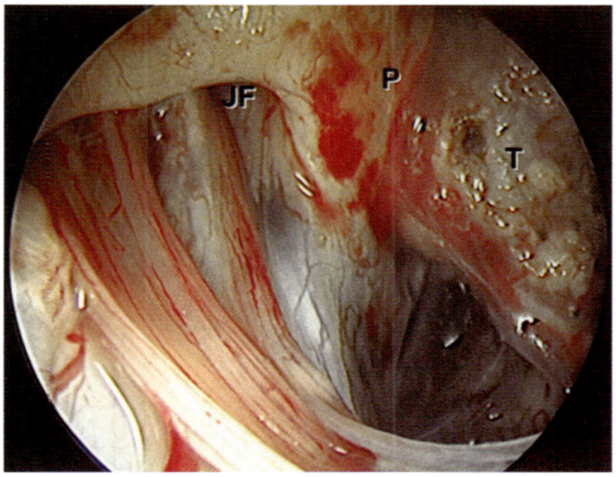


**FIGURE 11.18.** Examination of the posterior fossa using a 4-mm, 30° endoscope after beginning to debulk the extracanalicular tumor *(T)* shows the jugular foramen *(JF)* containing cranial nerves IX, X, and XI. Notice the relationship between the tumor and the porus acusticus *(P)*.

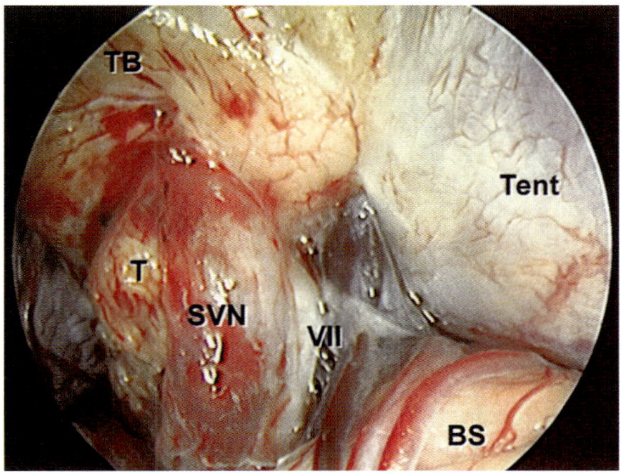


**FIGURE 11.19.** Placing the 4-mm, 30° endoscope cephalad (superior) and ventral (anterior) to the tumor *(T)* shows that the superior vestibular nerve *(SVN)* is splayed out over the tumor and demonstrates the position of the facial nerve *(VII)*. *BS,* brainstem; *TB,* temporal bone; *Tent,* tentorium.

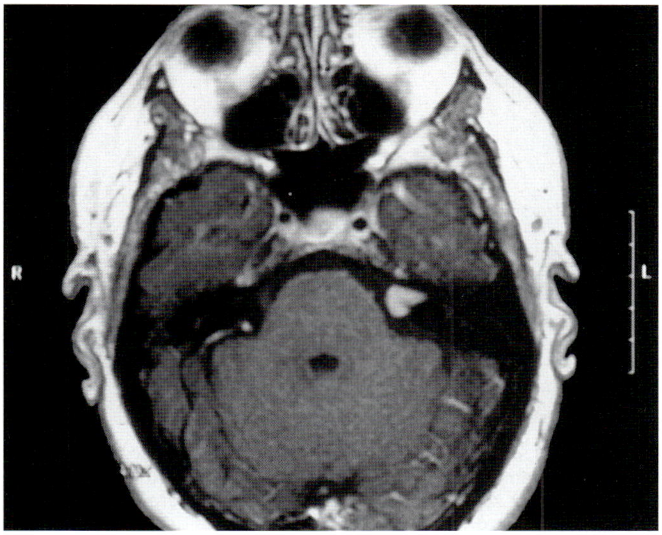


**FIGURE 11.20.** Preoperative axial T1-weighted magnetic resonance imaging with gadolinium enhancement shows a 1.2-cm, left acoustic neuroma resected using a translabyrinthine approach. Figures 11.21–11.23 show the corresponding endoscopic images of the cerebellopontine angle, tumor, brainstem, and root entry and exit zones for the vestibulocochlear and facial nerves.

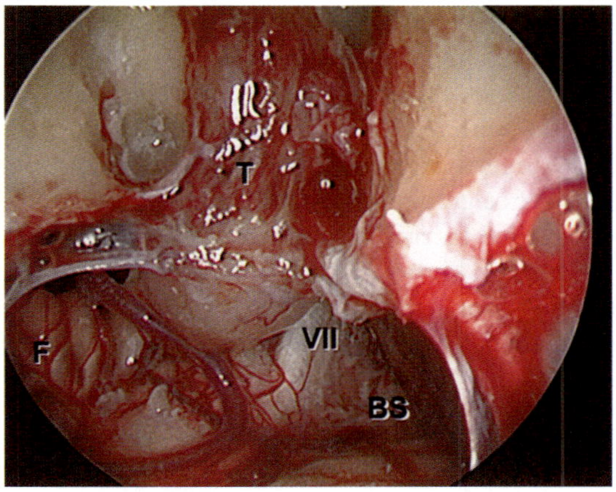


**FIGURE 11.21.** After completion of the translabyrinthine approach, a 4-mm, 45° endoscope shows the relation of the tumor *(T)* to the facial nerve *(VII)* and brainstem *(BS)*. Notice the root exit zone of VII. *F,* flocculus.

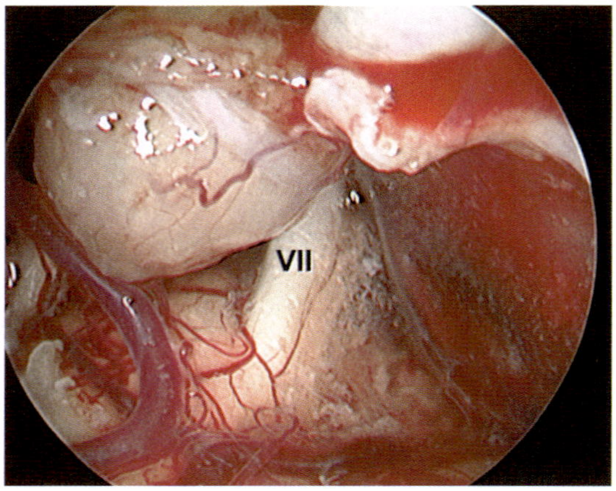


**FIGURE 11.22.** Placement of the 4-mm, 45° endoscope closer to the brainstem allows for better visualization of the facial nerve *(VII)* root exit zone and vascular supply of the brainstem in relation to the tumor.

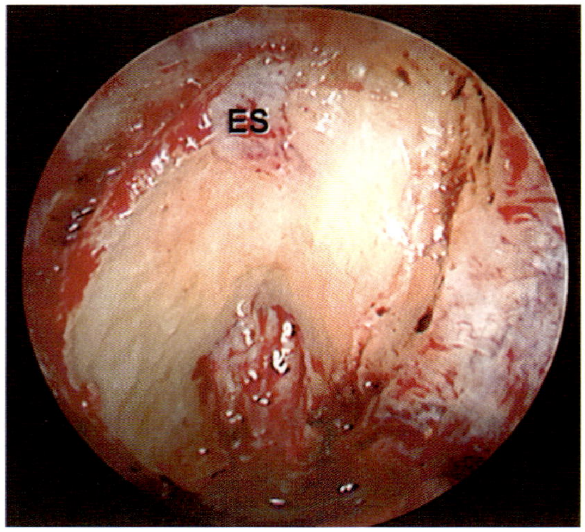


**FIGURE 11.24.** Inspection of the opened internal auditory canal using a 4-mm, 45° endoscope during the resection of a left, 1.7-cm acoustic neuroma using a retrosigmoid approach demonstrates the absence of open air cells in this patient. The intraosseous endolymphatic sac *(ES)* was exposed to determine the most lateral dissection of the internal auditory canal possible without violating the posterior semicircular canal. Notice the alternative perspective provided by the 45° endoscope when viewing the sheer wall created during the dissection between the posterior face of the temporal bone and the fundus of the internal auditory canal.

without opening the posterior semicircular canal. The surgical landmark used to determine this limit is the intraosseous endolymphatic sac (Fig. 11.24). An alternative method to accomplish this is performed with the addition of computer-guided stereotactic surgical instrumentation (see Chapter 3). One of the neuro-otologist–neurosurgeon teams (P.A.W. and G.A.M.) has been using the Stealth (Sofamor Danek, Memphis, TN) stereotactic system in conjunction with endoscopic techniques during acoustic neuroma surgery with laterally based tumors operated on using the retrosigmoid approach (Fig. 11.25). This method allows real-time determination of anatomic position during the surgery and shows the relationship between the IAC and the posterior semicircular canal. Samii and colleagues published their early experience with a microscope-based stereotactic navigational system used to accomplish the same purpose (14).

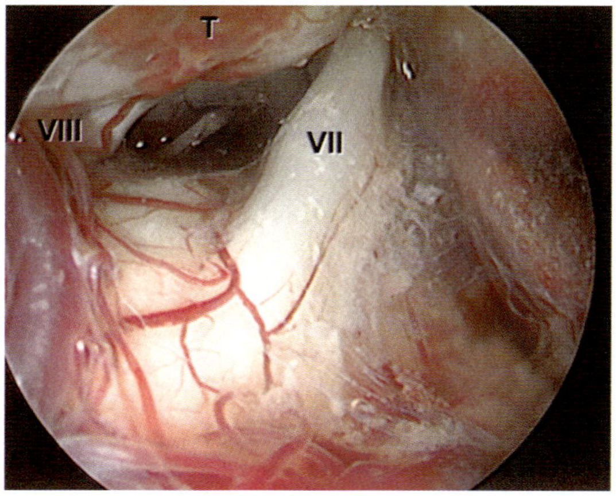


**FIGURE 11.23.** Deeper insertion of the 4-mm, 45° endoscope with the view angled in a caudal (inferior) direction shows the vestibulocochlear nerve *(VIII)* at the brainstem and the facial nerve *(VII)* in relation to the tumor *(T)*.

A complete tumor resection was achieved in 116 patients. In eight patients, near-total resection was completed. The tumor size for these eight patients ranged from 3 to 5 cm (mean, 3.5 cm). In all near-total resection cases, the tumor was extremely difficult to separate from the facial nerve because of attenuation of the nerve and adherence of the tumor. One of these patients was a 64-year-old woman with a 5-cm tumor that was extremely adherent to the brainstem, and a small amount of tumor was therefore left *in situ*. In four patients, subtotal resection was completed. The tumor size in group 1 ($n$=3) ranged from 2.5 to 4 cm (mean, 3.1 cm). The recidivistic tumor that was removed in a subtotal manner (group 2) was adherent to the facial nerve at the initial operation, and at the secondary surgery (P.A.W. and G.A.M.), only the component compressing the brainstem and trigeminal nerve was removed. In all four patients, the primary decision to perform a subtotal resection was based on facial nerve preservation and the preoperative wishes of each patient. After tumor removal, the endoscope was used to explore the fundus of the IAC. This clearly demonstrated the cranial nerves and bony landmarks. In 19 patients, residual tumor was identified endoscopically at the fundus of the IAC (Figs. 11.26 to 11.35) seven patients were operated by D.S.P. and his neurosurgical colleagues (group 1), and 12 patients were operated by

*(text continues on page 96)*

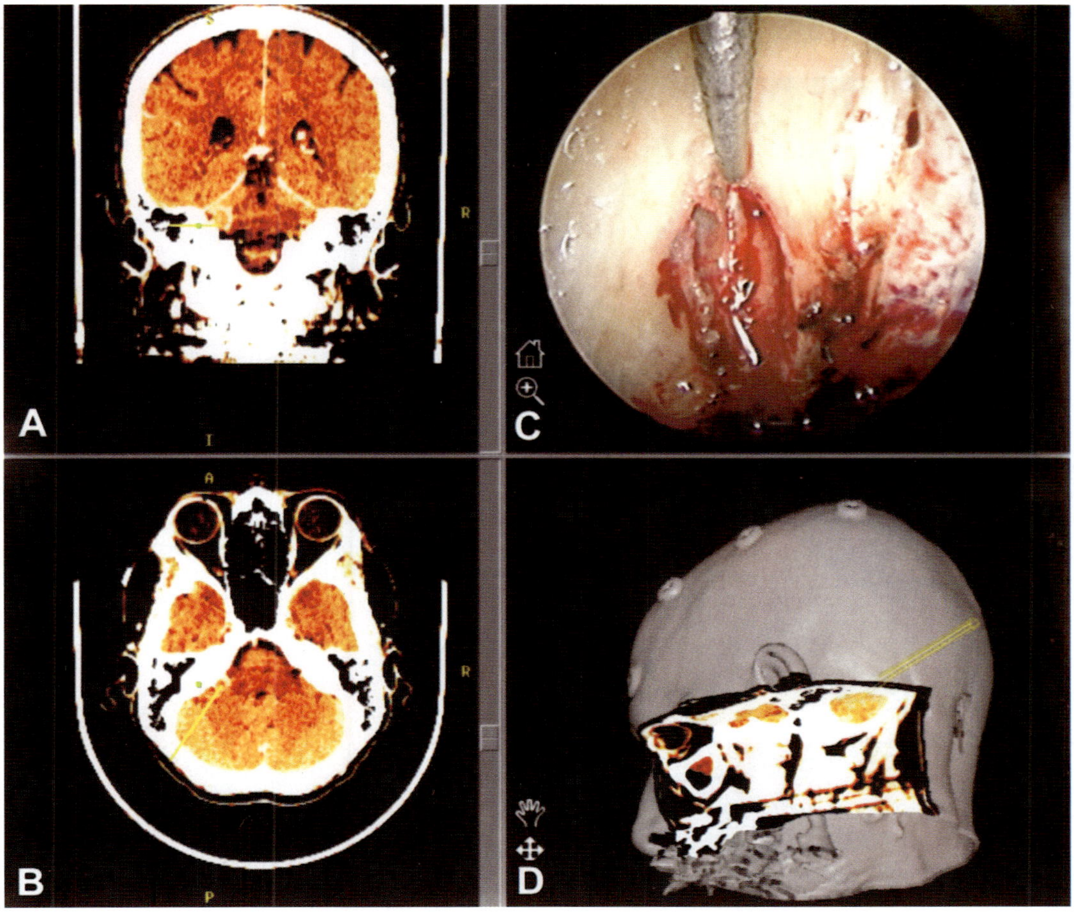


**FIGURE 11.25.** Computer-guided stereotactic endoscopic acoustic neuroma surgery with real-time viewing of the preoperative computed tomography (CT) data set after registration of fiducial markers. The computer workstation formats the CT data and can display the coronal **(A)** and axial **(B)** images containing the contact point of the blunt-tipped probe *(green dot).* Notice the left-right formatting convention. The window settings can be adjusted to emphasize bone when determining the lateral extent of internal auditory canal dissection relative to the posterior semicircular canal. A simultaneous operative image **(C)** using a 45° endoscope is also seen on the video monitor. Shown here is the blunt-tipped probe at the fundus of the opened internal auditory canal after a retrosigmoid resection of a left, 1.7-cm acoustic neuroma. A reconstructed image of the patient's head **(D)** demonstrates the adhesive fiducial markers on the head and the angle of surgical approach *(yellow pointer).*

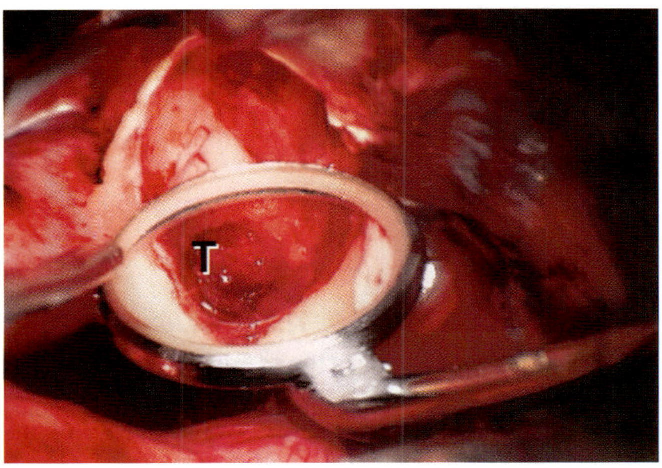


**FIGURE 11.26.** Microscopic view of the fundus of the internal auditory canal (IAC) and the residual tumor that can remain in the IAC after retrosigmoid transmeatal approach and resection of an acoustic neuroma. After resection of a 2.2-cm, left acoustic neuroma, residual tumor *(T)* can be seen at the fundus of the IAC using a small mirror and the operating microscope. As indicated at the top of this photograph, the residual tumor is not visible with the operating microscope alone.

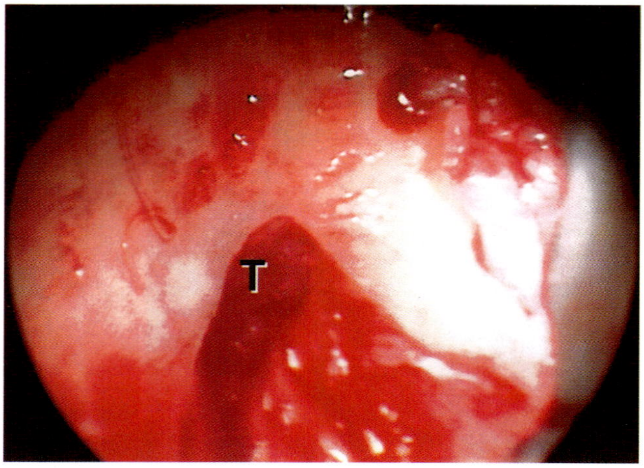


**FIGURE 11.27.** Endoscopic view of the fundus of the internal auditory canal (IAC) and the residual tumor that can remain in the IAC after retrosigmoid transmeatal approach and resection of an acoustic neuroma. A 30° endoscope shows residual tumor *(T)* at the fundus of the IAC after resection of a 1.5-cm, left acoustic neuroma using the retrosigmoid approach.

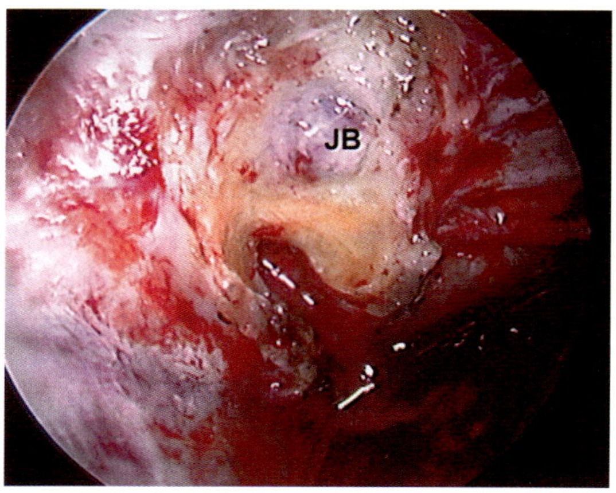


**FIGURE 11.28.** Endoscopic view of the fundus of the internal auditory canal (IAC) after retrosigmoid transmeatal approach and resection of a right, 3.0-cm acoustic neuroma. The tip of a 45° endoscope was held at a distance from the IAC and rotated so that the view is caudal (inferior) and lateral. A high-riding jugular bulb *(JB)* was uncovered to maximize exposure of the IAC. Notice that this view of the fundus is similar to that of the operating microscope. Figure 11.29 shows the view into the fundus and the residual tumor that was found.

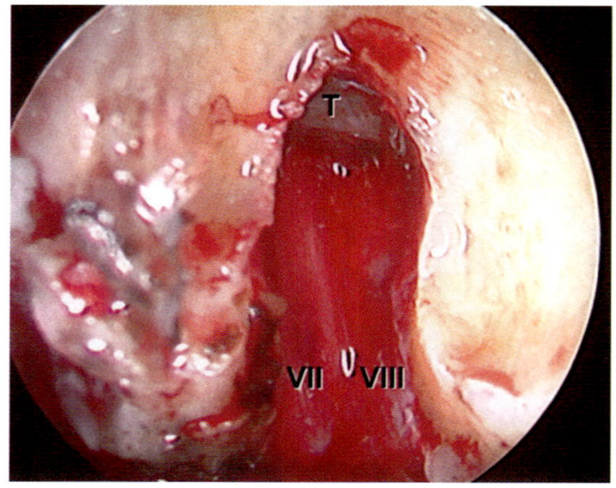


**FIGURE 11.29.** Endoscopic view of the fundus of the internal auditory canal using a 45° endoscope shows residual tumor *(T)* and the intact facial *(VII)* and cochlear *(VIII)* nerves.

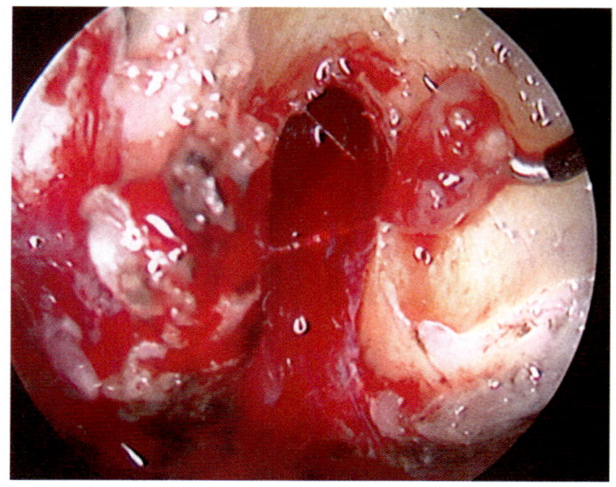

**FIGURE 11.30.** Using the 45° endoscope and a right-angled Kartush stimulus dissector (Xomed, Jacksonville, FL) the residual tumor is resected while preserving the facial and cochlear nerves.

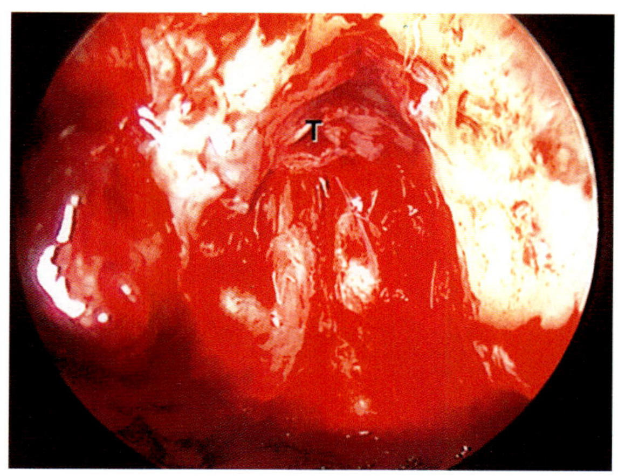


**FIGURE 11.31.** Examination of the internal auditory canal after resection of a right, 3.5-cm acoustic neuroma using a retrosigmoid approach with a 45° endoscope demonstrates residual tumor *(T)* at the fundus. This tumor was not visible with the operating microscope.

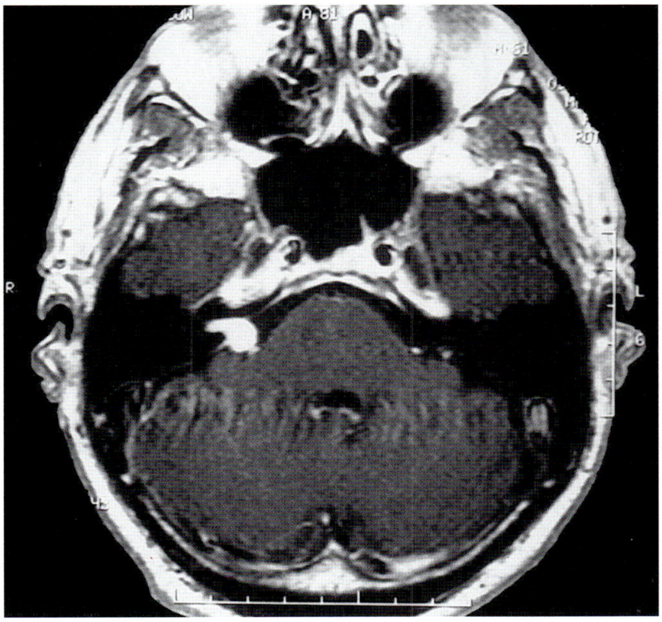

**FIGURE 11.32.** Preoperative axial T1-weighted magnetic resonance imaging with gadolinium enhancement shows a 1.2-cm, right acoustic neuroma resected using a retrosigmoid approach. Figures 11.33–11.35 show the corresponding endoscopic images of the internal auditory canal, residual tumor, and endoscopic removal of the residual tumor.

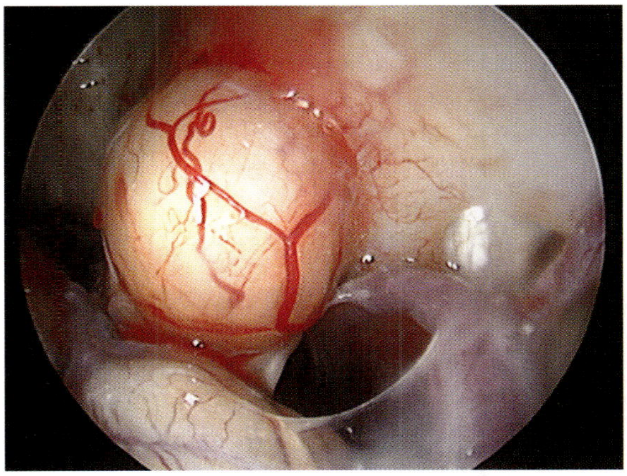

**FIGURE 11.33.** Initial inspection of the posterior fossa using a 4-mm, 0° endoscope shows the 1.2-cm extracanalicular portion of the tumor, the flocculus, and the neurovascular relationships around the tumor.

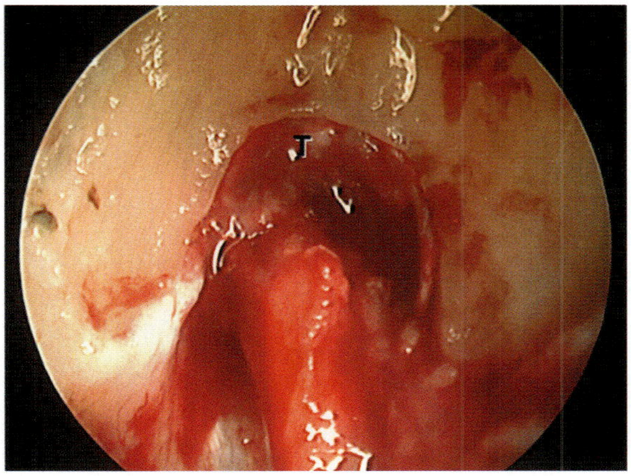

**FIGURE 11.34.** After resection of the tumor shown in Figures 11.32 and 11.33, residual tumor *(T)* was found at the fundus of the internal auditory canal using a 45° endoscope.

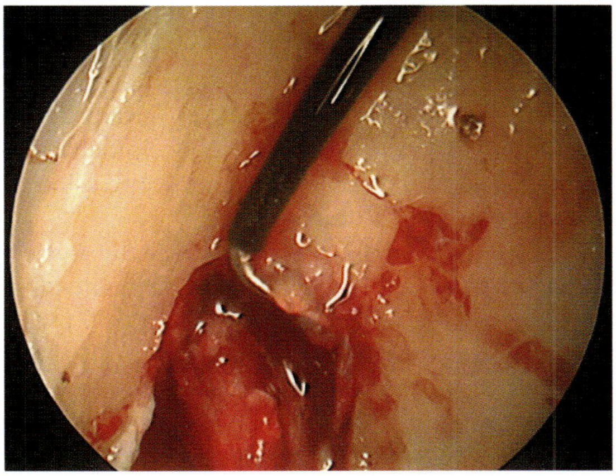

**FIGURE 11.35.** Using the 45° endoscope and a right-angled Kartush stimulus dissector (Xomed, Jacksonville, FL) the residual tumor is resected while preserving the facial and cochlear nerves.

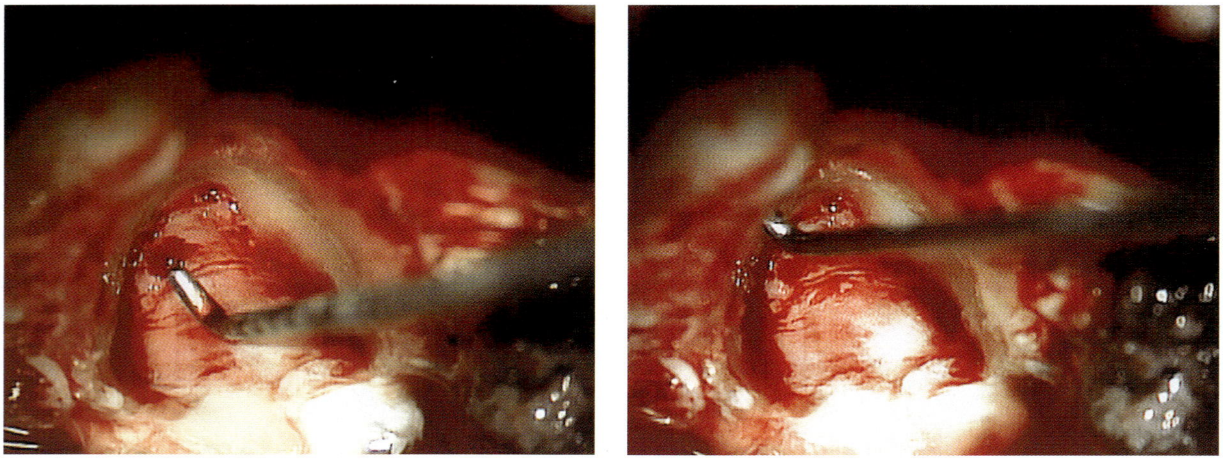

A B

**FIGURE 11.36.** Microscopic views of the fundus of the internal auditory canal (IAC) and the open air cells that can surround the IAC after retrosigmoid transmeatal approach to the IAC. **A:** A microscopic view of the IAC before opening the dura during resection of a 2.7-cm, right acoustic neuroma shows no open air cells, although a small, right-angled hook is posed to enter a large, opened air cell. **B:** The right-angled hook has been placed into the open air cell.

P.A.W. and his neurosurgical colleagues (group 2). All 19 patients underwent a retrosigmoid (suboccipital) approach, and with the use of the 30° or 45° endoscope, the residual tumor was removed in all cases.

Exposed air cells ($n$=51) not seen with the microscope during retrosigmoid approaches were identified endoscopically (group 1, $n$=43; group 2, $n$=8) (Figs. 11.36 to 11.38). In one of the translabyrinthine cases (group 3), the endoscope allowed identification of open air cells not visualized with the microscope. These were occluded individually using bone wax, and this was verified by the endoscope. Endoscopy provided additional anatomic information and documentation of nerve integrity (Figs. 11.39 to 11.44). In group 3, no displacement of the stapes footplate was identified.

One (0.9%) of the 111 patients undergoing a retrosigmoid or middle cranial fossa approach for tumor resection developed CSF rhinorrhea (group 1). This patient had resolution of the CSF rhinorrhea after 5 days of lumbar drainage of CSF and bed rest. Two patients undergoing a translabyrinthine approach for resection of their tumors (group 3) developed CSF rhinorrhea on postoperative day

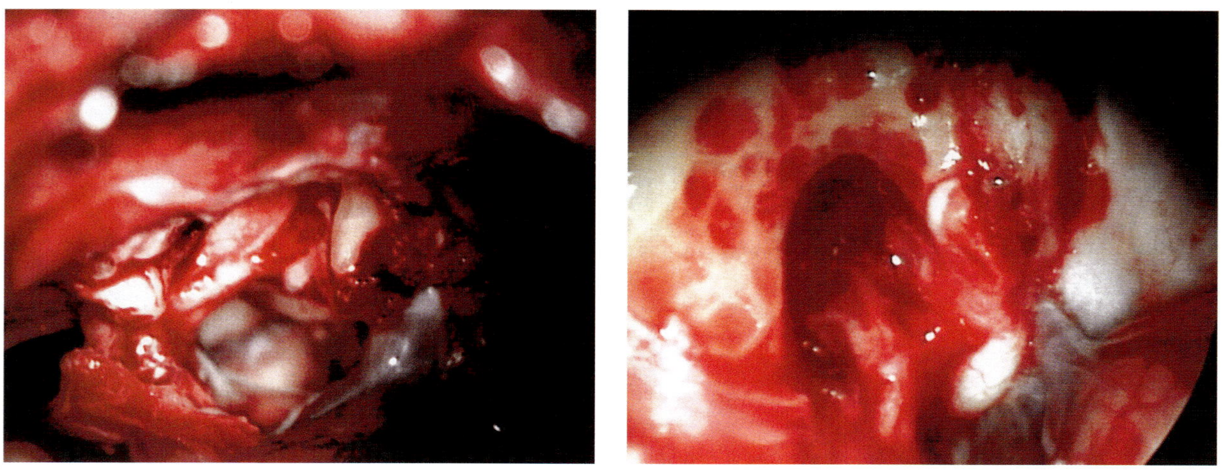

A B

**FIGURE 11.37.** Microscopic and endoscopic views of the fundus of the internal auditory canal (IAC) and the open air cells that can surround the IAC after retrosigmoid transmeatal approach to the IAC. **A:** The microscopic view after resection of a 1.5-cm, left acoustic neuroma using the retrosigmoid approach shows no open air cells. **B:** A 30° endoscope placed into the IAC shown in **A** demonstrates numerous open air cells that were not appreciated using the operating microscope.

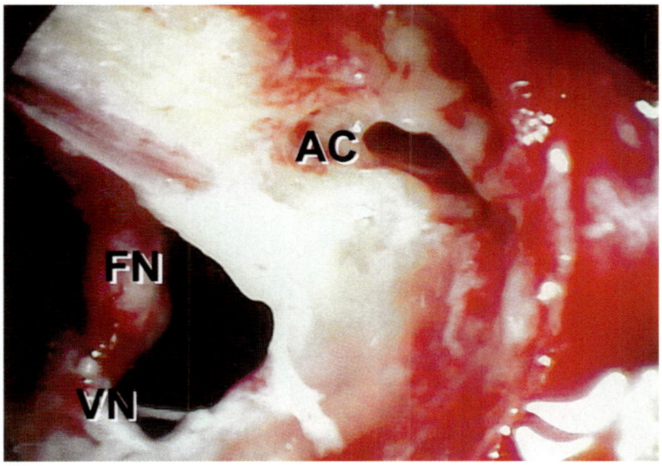


**FIGURE 11.38.** After resection of a left acoustic neuroma using the middle cranial fossa approach, the facial nerve *(FN)* and vestibular *(VN)* nerves can be seen using a 30° endoscope, as can a large, open air cell *(AC)* ventral (anterior) to the IAC.

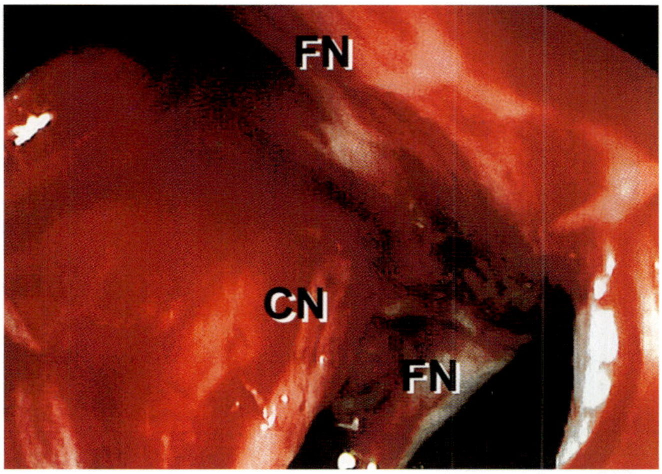


**FIGURE 11.39.** After middle cranial fossa approach and resection of an intracanalicular and 0.4-cm, extracanalicular, left acoustic neuroma, the course of the facial nerve *(FN)* and cochlear nerve *(CN)* can be seen with the 30° endoscope.

1. Although both cases resolved using lumbar drainage of CSF (8 to 10 mL/hour) for 4 to 5 days, one patient developed recurrent CSF rhinorrhea 14 months postoperatively and was found to have atrophy of her abdominal fat graft. Obliteration of her middle ear and eustachian tube resolved the CSF leakage. Of the 128 patients included in this series, only 3 (2.3%) experienced early postoperative CSF rhinorrhea. Two patients developed CSF leakage through the incision. In one patient (group 1), the incision was oversewn, which resolved the leak. In the second patient (group 3), a local wound infection was drained on postoperative day 5 by opening a small area of the scalp closure, thereby producing a CSF leak through the incision. Three days later, after intravenous antibiotics and local wound care, the scalp was oversewn, and the leak was stopped.

The adjunctive use of the endoscope did not significantly increase the operative time; only 15 to 30 additional minutes were required per case to set up, use, and digitally photograph the observed anatomic relationships.

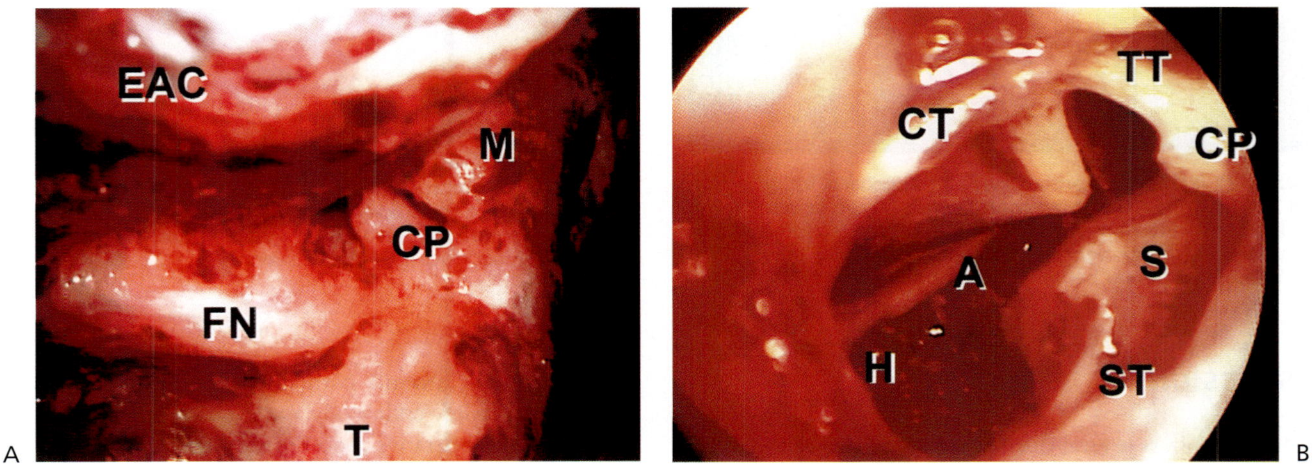


**FIGURE 11.40. A:** Microscopic view after translabyrinthine approach for resection of a 1-cm, left acoustic neuroma *(T)* shows the vertical segment of the facial nerve *(FN)*, cochleariform process *(CP)*, head of the malleus *(M)*, and the bony external auditory canal *(EAC)*. **B:** Placing a 0° endoscope at the facial recess shown in **A** allows visualization of the annular ligament *(A)*, stapes *(S)*, stapedial tendon *(ST)*, cochleariform process *(CP)*, tensor tympani tendon *(TT)*, chorda tympani nerve *(CT)*, and the hypotympanum *(H)*. The malleus and conical tympanic membrane are seen *(center)*.

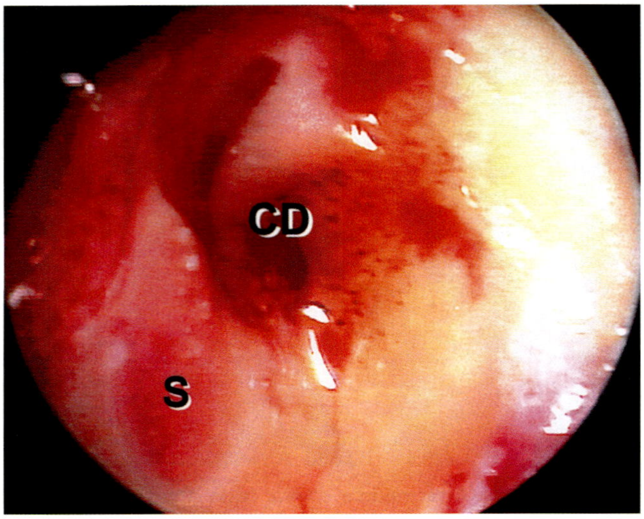


**FIGURE 11.41.** After a translabyrinthine approach for resection of a 1.5-cm, right acoustic neuroma, a 30° endoscope shows the undersurface of the stapes footplate *(S)* and oval window membrane surrounded by the annular ligament *(white rim)*. The entrance to the cochlear duct *(CD)* can be seen.

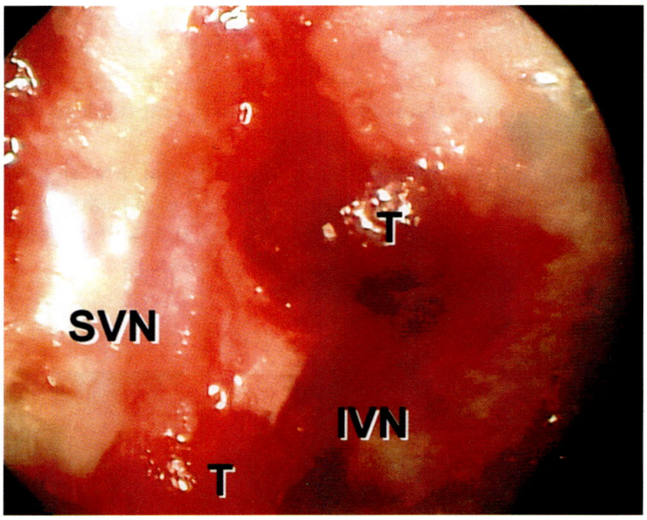


**FIGURE 11.42.** After translabyrinthine approach for resection of a 2.0-cm, right acoustic neuroma, tumor *(T)* can be seen at the fundus of the internal auditory canal *(bottom left)* and within the vestibule *(center right)*. The superior vestibular nerve *(SVN)* and inferior vestibular nerve *(IVN)* can be seen.

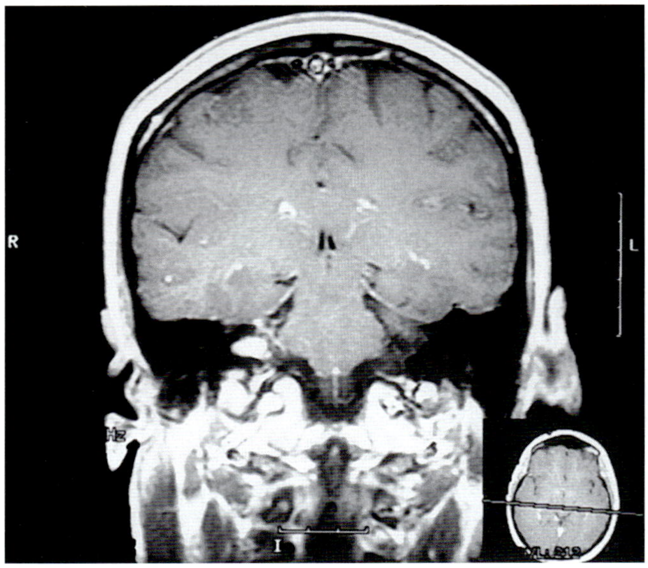


**FIGURE 11.43.** Preoperative coronal T1-weighted magnetic resonance imaging with gadolinium enhancement shows a 1.0-cm, right acoustic neuroma resected using a translabyrinthine approach. Figure 11.44 shows the corresponding endoscopic image of the stapes footplate, annular ring of the stapes, and entrance into the cochlea.

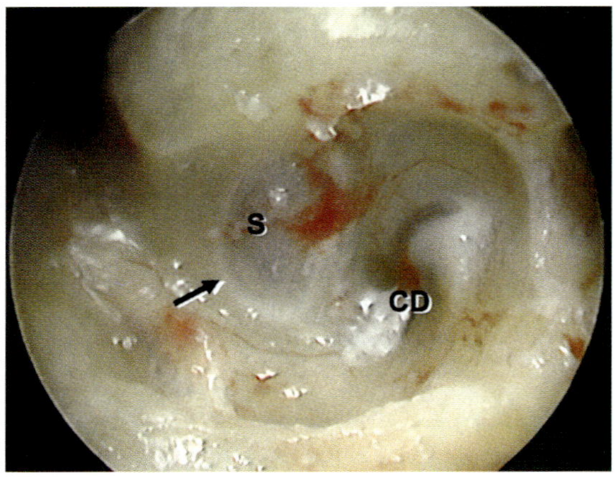


**FIGURE 11.44.** After a translabyrinthine approach for resection of a 1.0-cm, right acoustic neuroma, a 45° endoscope shows the undersurface of the stapes footplate *(S)* and oval window membrane surrounded by the annular ligament *(arrow)*. The entrance to the cochlear duct *(CD)* can be seen.

## DISCUSSION

Endoscopy offers several distinct advantages over the operating microscope that make it an excellent adjunctive tool during acoustic neuroma microsurgery. First, the high magnification gives excellent definition of perforating blood vessels, cranial nerves, and neural structures, which in many cases is superior to that achieved with the microscope. Second, the use of angled or flexible endoscopes allows the surgeon to "look around corners" and behind obstructing structures. Third, endoscopy has the theoretical advantage that a smaller operative procedure is required, which should reduce the operative morbidity.

There are also several notable disadvantages of endoscopy. These include the problems associated with blood soiling the tip of the endoscope, making visualization difficult or impossible; the lack of readily available instrumentation designed specifically for endoscopic neuro-otology;

and the poor overview of the operative field. The poor view is an important point, because the endoscope is placed adjacent to the lesion and does not allow the surgeon to look backward to prevent injury to structures next to the shaft of the telescope. The surgeon must be cognizant of potential thermal injury to structures caused by the heat generated by the light source. The image that the surgeon sees is two dimensional, which has certain unique problems when operating in a three-dimensional milieu, although the Xomed (Jacksonville, FL) and Sofamor Danek (Memphis, TN) companies have been approaching this problem with stereoscopic goggles and dual camera–endoscope systems. Because of the vast experience that most otolaryngologists have with endoscopic sinus surgery, the surgical techniques are familiar, and endoscopic dexterity has been mastered; however, maintaining three-dimensional orientation in the posterior fossa does require additional clinical experience. The primary challenge is that the surgeon must navigate around the lattice of nerves and arteries within the posterior fossa. Bimanual operating frequently is impossible because the endoscope sometimes must be held in one hand while the other is used to perform the surgery. This is not always the case, because it can be attached to a fixation device or held by the co-surgeon.

Endoscope-assisted craniotomy is an extension of the concept of "keyhole surgery," which suggests that a strategically placed small craniectomy, when combined with very high magnification and illumination, can offer excellent visual exposure of an intracranial lesion, sufficient to perform the necessary surgery. Our group has published our early experience with endoscopic vestibular neurectomy using a craniotomy measuring approximately 15 to 18 mm in diameter (10). One of the limitations of the operative microscope is that the angle of view is determined by the distance of the lens to the skull, retractor, or obstructing tissue, which is a function of the lens focal length; the longer the focal length, the narrower is the viewing angle. During most microsurgical procedures, the focal distance varies between 250 and 400 mm. If the operator looks through a door's keyhole at close range, nearly the entire room on the opposite side of the door can be seen, although nothing can be seen when the hole is viewed from a long distance. Endoscopes have focal lengths ranging from 5 mm to 20 mm, with the latter providing a much wider angle of view.

## Approaches to the Cerebellopontine Angle and Acoustic Neuroma Surgery

The endoscope seems well suited for dealing with lesions of the posterior fossa and CPA. Because the exposure is frequently narrow and the neurovascular relationships are tight, adequate illumination and exposure is not always possible. We have found that cranial nerves III through XII as well as the basilar artery and its branches can be easily identified (10,11,13). Other posterior fossa surgical indications have included microvascular decompression of the cranial nerves, vestibular neurectomy, and an assortment of intrinsic and extrinsic lesions involving the brainstem.

Incomplete tumor removal, especially within the IAC, does occur after retrosigmoid (suboccipital) resection (6) and rarely after translabyrinthine resection (7). The primary limitation in gaining lateral exposure of the IAC during the retrosigmoid approach is the restriction imposed by the need to maintain integrity of the posterior semicircular canal (14,15). Based on the morphometric analysis of 60 high-resolution temporal bone computed tomography (CT) scans, Blevins and Jackler found that an average of 3.0 mm (32% of the IAC length) must be left unexposed to avoid labyrinthine injury, with a range of 1.1 to 5.3 mm (9% to 58% of the IAC length) (16). Roberson and coworkers reported 35 patients with recurrent acoustic neuromas who all were operated originally using the retrosigmoid approach (6). During definitive revision surgery using the translabyrinthine approach, all 35 patients were found to have tumor extending all the way to the fundus. Based on the recurrence rate of five tumors in a series of 3,500 acoustic neuromas, the translabyrinthine approach appears to offer the lowest rate of tumor recurrence (7).

Tatagiba and colleagues presented their experience using glass lens and fiberoptic endoscopes for exploring the IAC after tumor excision (17). Although they identified no residual tumor at the fundus during endoscopic examination, this finding may reflect Samii's extensive experience with retrosigmoid surgery. In 19 (16.4%) of 116 patients who had total tumor removal, we found that tumor remnants were identified endoscopically that were not seen with the microscope (Figs. 11.26–11.35). In all of these patients (19 [19.8%] of 96), a retrosigmoid approach was used. Residual tumor was not visualized with any of the translabyrinthine or middle cranial fossa approaches. The use of the endoscope allows the anatomy of the fundus of the IAC and the cranial nerves within the IAC to be easily delineated, in contrast to the typical situation with microscopic visualization of the fundus of the canal, which can be impossible, and visualization of residual tumor using small mirrors may be difficult (Fig. 11.26).

CSF leaks may manifest through the incision, through the tympanic membrane as otorrhea, or through the eustachian tube and nasopharynx as rhinorrhea. The retrosigmoid, translabyrinthine, and middle cranial fossa approaches may expose pneumatized spaces of the temporal bone, allowing CSF to leak if not adequately sealed. During the past 15 years, detailed descriptions of the possible communications within temporal bones in cases of CSF rhinorrhea after posterior fossa surgery have been published by Harner and Laws (18). Communications may occur through the lateral end of the IAC, vestibule, and oval window into the middle ear; through the posterosuperior or posteromedial tracts (19–21); through air cells exposed during the retrosigmoid craniectomy; through the petrous apex and anterior air cell tract (3); and through the tubal openings of the peritubal cells directly into the osseous eustachian tube (4).

In an earlier report of comparing the rate of CSF rhinorrhea in 38 retrosigmoid acoustic neuroma cases without the use of the endoscope to the CSF rhinorrhea rate in 24 retrosigmoid acoustic neuroma cases with adjunctive endoscopy, we found that CSF rhinorrhea occurred in 18.4% of patients in the microsurgery group, whereas no patients in the endoscope-assisted group experienced this complication (5). Fifty-two (40.6%) of our 128 endoscope-assisted cases had air cells that were identified with the endoscope that were not seen with the microscope. An additional advantage with the use of the 30° endoscope in translabyrinthine approaches is that the undersurface of the stapes footplate (Figs. 11.41 and 11.44) can be identified, allowing assessment of stapes displacement as a route for CSF egress. One (0.9%) of our 111 patients who underwent a retrosigmoid or middle cranial fossa approach for resection of acoustic neuromas experienced transient CSF rhinorrhea that resolved by lumbar drainage of CSF. We think that the improved visualization and sealing the identified open air cells may be a critical factor in reducing the postoperative CSF rhinorrhea rate, certainly to levels well below the reported rate of 5% to 20% (1–5).

## CONCLUSIONS

Based on our expanded experience, we feel that endoscopes can be used safely during acoustic neuroma surgery and that, as an adjunct to the operative microscope, this modality does improve visualization of bony, neural, and vascular structures while minimizing retraction of these structures. Endoscopic exploration of the IAC after tumor removal using the 30° or 45° endoscope can reveal the presence of residual tumor and air cells that otherwise may result in recurrent tumor or CSF rhinorrhea, respectively, postoperatively.

## REFERENCES


1. Jackler RK. Acoustic neuroma (vestibular schwannoma). In: Jackler RK, Brackmann DE, eds. *Neurotology.* St. Louis: Mosby–Year Book, 1994:729–785.
2. Hoffman RA. Cerebrospinal fluid leak following acoustic neuroma removal. *Laryngoscope* 1994;104:40–58.
3. Millen SJ, Meyer G. Surgical management of CSF otorhinorrhea following retrosigmoid removal of cerebellopontine angle tumors. *Am J Otol* 1993;14:585–589.
4. Saim L, McKenna MJ, Nadol JB Jr. Tubal openings of the peritubal cells: implications for cerebrospinal fluid otorhinorrhea. *Am J Otol* 1996;17:335–339.
5. Valtonen HJ, Poe DS, Heilman CB, et al. Endoscopically assisted prevention of cerebrospinal fluid leak in suboccipital acoustic neuroma surgery. *Am J Otol* 1997;18:381–385.
6. Roberson JB Jr, Brackmann DE, Hitselberger WE. Acoustic neuroma recurrence after suboccipital resection: management with translabyrinthine resection. *Am J Otol* 1996;17:307–311.
7. Shelton C. Unilateral acoustic tumors: how often do they recur after translabyrinthine removal? *Laryngoscope* 1995;105:958–966.
8. King WA, Frazee JG, DeSalles AF, eds. *Endoscopic surgery of the central and peripheral nervous system.* New York: Thieme Medical Publishers, 1998.
9. Wackym PA, Rice DH, Schaefer SD, eds. *Minimally invasive surgery of the head, neck and cranial base.* Philadelphia: Lippincott Williams & Wilkins, 2001.
10. Wackym PA, King WA, Barker FG, Poe DS. Endoscope-assisted vestibular neurectomy. *Laryngoscope* 1998;108:1787–1793.
11. Friedland DR, Wackym PA. Evaluation of surgical approaches to endoscopic brainstem implantation. *Laryngoscope* 1999;109: 175–180.
12. King WA, Wackym PA. Endoscopically assisted surgery for acoustic neuromas (vestibular schwannomas): early experience using the rigid Hopkins telescope. *Neurosurgery* 1999;44: 1095–1102.
13. Wackym PA, King WA, Poe DS, et al. Adjunctive use of endoscopy during acoustic neuroma surgery. *Laryngoscope* 1999; 109:1193–1201.
14. Samii A, Brinker T, Kaminsky J, et al. Navigational-guided opening of the internal auditory canal via the retrosigmoid route for acoustic neuroma surgery: cadaveric, radiological, and preliminary clinical study. *Neurosurgery* 2000;47:382–388.
15. Roland PS, Meyerhoff WL, Wright CG, et al. Anatomic considerations in the posterior approach to the internal auditory canal. *Ann Otol Rhinol Laryngol* 1988;97:621–625.
16. Blevins NH, Jackler RK. Exposure of the lateral extremity of the internal auditory canal through the retrosigmoid approach: a radioanatomic study. *Otolaryngol Head Neck Surg* 1994;111: 81–90.
17. Tatagiba M, Matthies C, Samii M. Microendoscopy of the internal auditory canal in vestibular schwannoma surgery. *Neurosurgery* 1996;38:737–740.
18. Harner SG, Laws ER. Translabyrinthine repair for cerebrospinal fluid otorhinorrhea. *J Neurosurg* 1982;57:258–261.
19. Lang JL, Kerr AG. Pneumatization of the posteromedial air-cell tract. *Clin Otolaryngol* 1989;14:425–427.
20. Smith PG, Leonetti JP, Grubb RL. Management of cerebrospinal fluid otorhinorrhea complicating the retrosigmoid approach to the cerebellopontine angle. *Am J Otol* 1990;11:178–180.
21. Gordon DS, Kerr AG. Cerebrospinal fluid rhinorrhea following surgery for acoustic neurinoma—report of two cases. *J Neurosurg* 1986;64:676–678.

12

# ENDOSCOPE-ASSISTED SURGERY OF THE TRIGEMINAL, FACIAL, COCHLEAR, OR VESTIBULAR NERVE

PHILLIP A. WACKYM
WESLEY A. KING
GLENN A. MEYER
CHANDRANATH SEN
FRED G. BARKER
DENNIS S. POE

Endoscopic techniques have revolutionized the practice of surgery in a number of specialties. This is evident in looking at the impact of endoscopy in otolaryngology, neurosurgery (1), laparoscopy in abdominal surgery, arthroscopy in orthopedic surgery, and thoracoscopy in cardiothoracic surgery. In many situations, smaller incisions and exposures are possible, resulting in decreased postoperative pain, shorter recuperation, better cosmetic results, and shorter hospitalizations. Endoscopes have the ability to provide high magnification and illumination of the operative field, but in contrast to the operative microscope, the endoscopic view is not limited to the linear line of sight. With flexible and angled endoscopes, the surgeon can "look around corners," past obstructing tissue and structures. Initial reports of endoscope-assisted otologic and neuro-otologic surgery have been published, and the limits of these techniques are continuing to be explored (2–7). This chapter describes the use of endoscopes during surgery for neurectomy of the vestibular nerve or nervus intermedius and for cranial nerve microvascular decompression procedures.

The surgical position and operating room organization for all of these procedures is shown in Figure 12.1. In addition to the microsurgical instrumentation typically used for neuro-otologic cranial base surgery, 4- and 2.7-mm endoscopes (0°, 30°, 45°, and 70°) are available for use, together with a three-chip video camera (Stryker Endoscopy, Santa Clara, CA), video monitor (Sony Electronics, San Jose, CA), digital capture and storage system (Stryker Endoscopy), and S-VHS video recorder (Sony Electronics, San Jose, CA). Illumination was provided by a xenon light source (Stryker Endoscopy). An endoscope holder (Codman Endoscopy, Randolph, MA) attached to a Mayfield head frame (OMI Surgical Products, Cincinnati, OH) is necessary for bimanual operation if the co-surgeon is not holding the endoscope for the surgeon during the definitive portion of the procedure.

## VESTIBULAR NEURECTOMY

The rationale for unilateral deafferentation of a dysfunctional vestibular labyrinth is that the central nervous system is better able to compensate for a complete loss of vestibular function than a fluctuating partial loss. The single most common peripheral vestibular disorder requiring vestibular neurectomy is Ménière's disease, although most of these patients are successfully managed with medical therapy (8,9). Rarely, recurrent vestibular neuronitis or traumatic labyrinthitis requires unilateral ablation of vestibular function to achieve compensation. Vestibular neurectomy has the advantage of preserving hearing when patients have useful cochlear function. A survey of the American Otological Society and the American Neurotology Society performed nearly a decade ago revealed that almost 3,000 vestibular neurectomies had been performed in the United States since the introduction of the operating microscope (10).

Contraindications to vestibular neurectomy include bilateral peripheral vestibular disease, vertigo from an only hearing ear, indications of central nervous system pathology such as multiple sclerosis, physiologic old age, and poor medical condition. Additional clinical consideration should be given before ablative surgical procedures in elderly patients because they have more difficulty in compensating; however, destructive vestibular procedures remain an important treatment option for the elderly patient disabled by vertigo of peripheral origin. There are distinct advan-

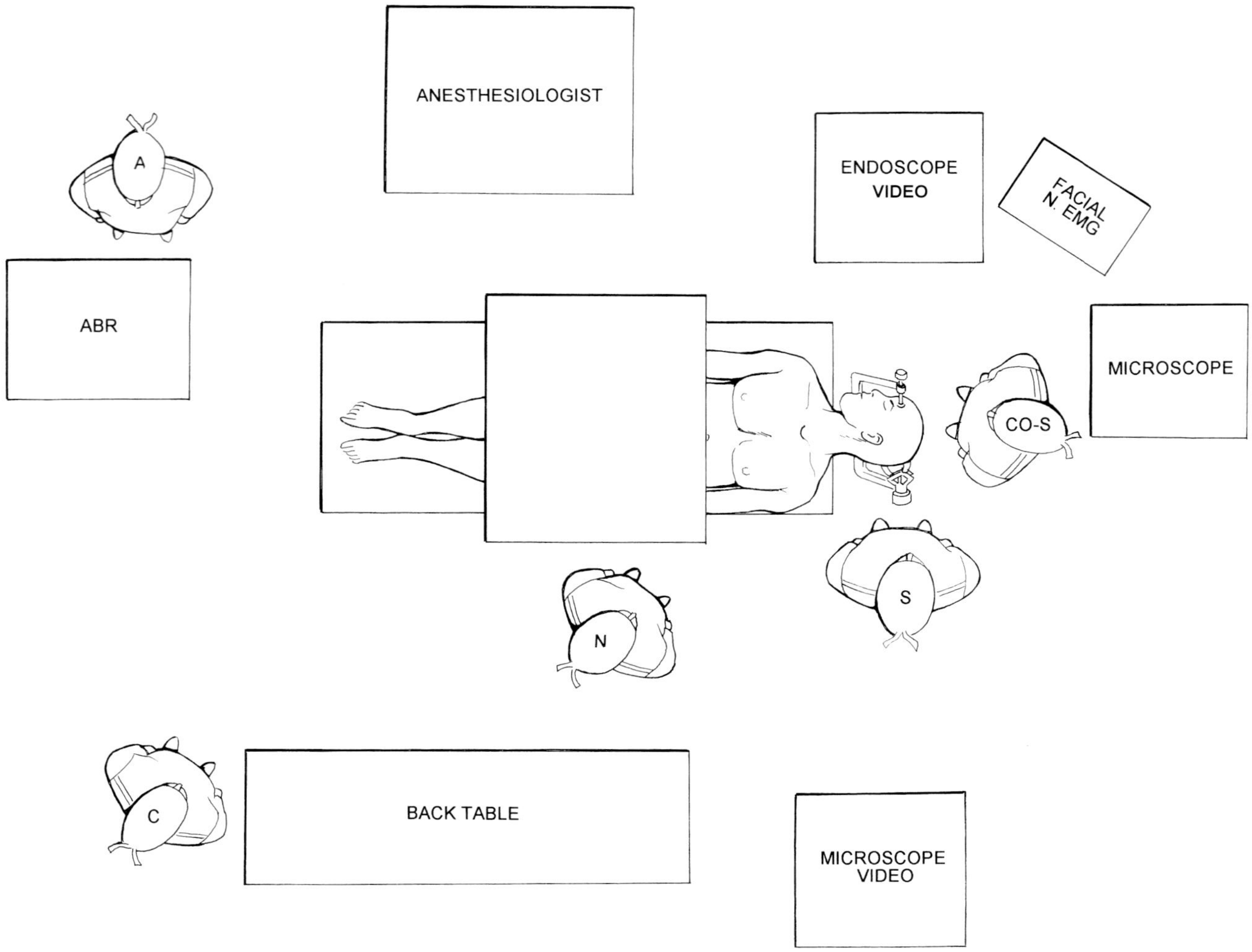


**FIGURE 12.1.** Patient position for endoscope-assisted surgery of the trigeminal nerve, facial nerve, cochlear nerve, or vestibular nerve. Notice the relationship between the video monitor and the surgeon. The surgical microscope is kept at hand and draped sterilely in case there is urgent need to use it instead of the endoscope. *A,* audiologist; *C,* circulator; *Facial n. emg,* facial nerve electromyography; *S,* surgeon; *CO-S,* co-surgeon; *N,* nurse; *ABR,* auditory brainstem evoked response monitor.

tages to each surgical approach, and these are briefly reviewed in the context of the application of endoscopic techniques to this procedure.

Charcot, who was a contemporary of Prosper Ménière and director of a famous neurologic clinic in Paris, has been credited with the first suggested intracranial division of the auditory nerve to eliminate the symptoms of Ménière's disease in 1874. This attribution was most consistently used by Walter Dandy (Fig. 12.2); however, Jackler, after translating the original French manuscript, suggested that this acknowledgment was inaccurate (11). It was not until October 6, 1908, in Philadelphia, that Frazier completed this procedure in a patient with persistent aural vertigo (12). A passage from the report of Frazier (12) summarizes the critical issue in the surgical management of patients with Ménière's disease: "Before this operation is undertaken in the future, one should determine by every means of precision whether the case falls in the category for which this form of treatment is especially applicable." It was Walter Dandy who first recognized that selective neurectomy of the vestibular nerve was possible (13): "In one of the patients . . . the vestibular and cochlear branches of the auditory nerve were separate and distinct. Such an anatomic variation would lend itself to division of the vestibular nerve without injuring the cochlear nerve and the hearing." In July 1932, McKenzie of Montreal was the first to selectively section the vestibular nerve while preserving hearing (14). Hugh Cairns of London performed a similar operation in February 1933, and Dandy performed this selective neurectomy in March 1933 (15,16). However, Dandy popularized the procedure, performing 607 neurectomies in 587 patients with Ménière's disease between 1924 and 1946

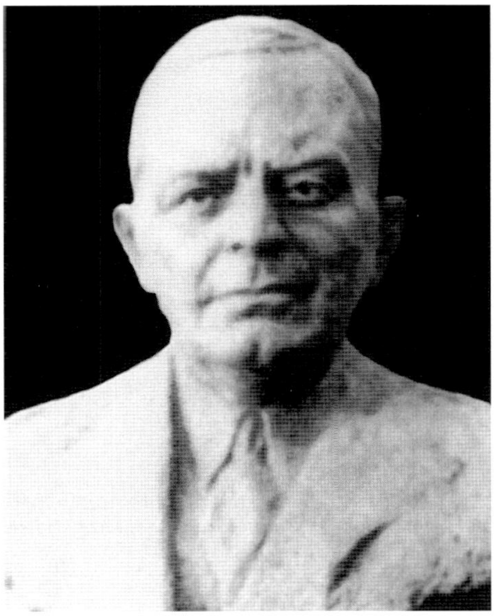

**FIGURE 12.2.** Emil Seletz sculpture of Walter Edward Dandy (1885–1946).

(16). The use of the middle cranial fossa approach to section the vestibular nerve was first reported in 1904 (17). There have been numerous advances in the surgical deafferentation of the peripheral vestibular system, which are described elsewhere (18). We initially reported 10 cases of endoscope-assisted vestibular neurectomy (2).

## Technique and Results

Fourteen patients with intractable unilateral Ménière's disease (Table 12.1) underwent a retrosigmoid craniotomy for neurectomy of the vestibular nerve or nervus intermedius, respectively. Endoscopy with a Hopkins telescope was used during each procedure to study posterior fossa anatomic relationships and to assist the neurectomy. Preoperative and postoperative audiometric evaluations were performed for all patients undergoing vestibular neurectomy. Thirteen of these patients had preoperative electronystagmography (ENG), and eight patients completed postoperative ENG. The 1995 American Academy of Otolaryngology–Head and Neck Surgery (AAO-HNS) Committee on Hearing and Equilibrium guidelines for the diagnosis and evaluation of therapy in Ménière's disease were used (19).

### *Operative Technique: Vestibular Neurectomy*

Each patient was positioned supine, with the head turned in the opposite direction of the affected ear. After 1 g/kg of mannitol and 10 mg of Decadron were administered intravenously, the patient was hyperventilated to achieve maximum cerebellar relaxation. A 4- to 6-cm linear skin incision was made approximately 10 to 15 mm posteromedial from the estimated position of the sigmoid sinus extending caudally for 6 cm, beginning just above the level of the transverse sinus (Fig. 12.3). After incising the nuchal muscles and elevating the periosteum, a single Adson cerebellar or articulated Weitlaner retractor was placed into the wound.

**TABLE 12.1. MÉNIÈRE'S DISEASE PATIENTS UNDERGOING VESTIBULAR NEURECTOMY: AAO-HNS 1995 REPORTING CRITERIA**

| | | | Electronystagmography (Canal Paresis)[b] | |
|---|---|---|---|---|
| Subject | Stage[a] | Age (yr)/Sex/Side | Preop (%) | Postop (%) |
| 1 | 4 | 49/F/AD | 44 | 100 |
| 2 | 1 | 56/F/AS | 82 | 100 |
| 3 | 2 | 62/F/AS | 73 | 100 |
| 4 | 1 | 43/F/AS | 26 | 100 |
| 5 | 1 | 34/F/AS | 29 | 100 |
| 6 | 2 | 16/F/AD | 28 | 100 |
| 7 | 3 | 62/F/AD | 78 | 100 |
| 8 | 3 | 60/F/AS | 84 | 100 |
| 9 | 3 | 34/F/AD | 29 | NA |
| 10 | 4 | 55/F/AS | 0 | NA |
| 11 | 3 | 34/F/AD | 0 | NA |
| 12 | 1 | 60/F/AS | 90 | NA |
| 13 | 3 | 36/F/AD | 38 | NA |
| 14 | 3 | 45/M/AS | NA | NA |

AD, auris dexter; AS, auris sinister; NA, not available.
[a]Staging is based on the four-tone average (pure-tone thresholds) at 0.5, 1, 2, and 3 kHz. Stage 1 (≤25 dB); Stage 2 (26–40 dB); Stage 3 (41–70 dB); Stage 4 (>70 dB).
[b]Canal paresis of affected ear, calculated after caloric irrigation.
From Committee on Hearing and Equilibrium guidelines for the diagnosis and evaluation of therapy in Ménière's disease. American Academy of Otolaryngology–Head and Neck Foundation, Inc. *Otolaryngol Head Neck Surg* 1995;113:181–185, with permission.

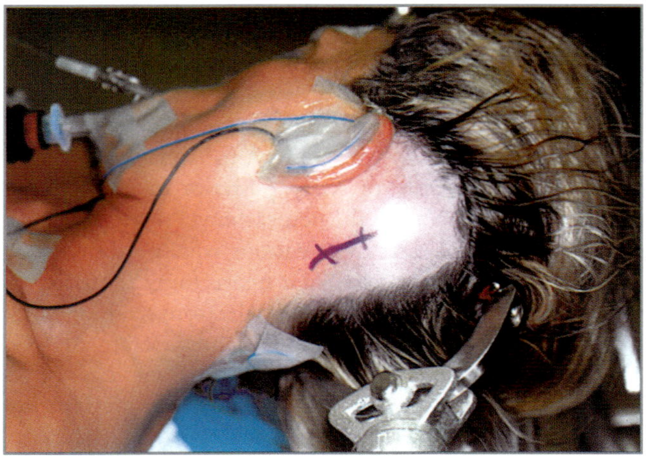

**FIGURE 12.3.** Endoscopic vestibular neurectomy for Ménière's disease. A 4-cm linear incision is designed that extends caudally from the transverse sinus. Notice the Mayfield head holder, which is used to attach the endoscope holder. Intraoperative auditory brainstem evoked response and facial nerve electromyography monitoring is performed during the vestibular neurectomy.

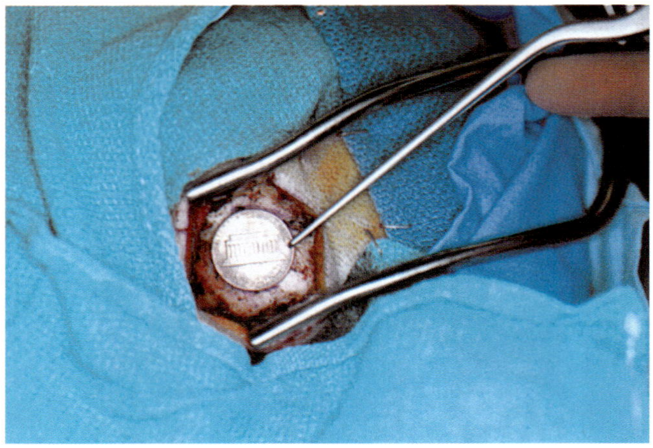

**FIGURE 12.5.** Endoscopic vestibular neurectomy for Ménière's disease. The retrosigmoid craniectomy is smaller than the diameter of this sterilized penny.

A retrosigmoid (suboccipital) approach was performed in all patients. The craniotomy was 18 to 25 mm in diameter (Figs. 12.4 and 12.5). After the craniotomy or craniectomy was performed, the dura was opened using a Y-shaped incision and was secured to the adjacent soft tissue. The cerebellum was gently elevated to expose the lateral medullary cistern, which on opening allowed release of cerebrospinal fluid. The lateral surface of the cerebellum was protected by placing moist Cottonoids before retracting it medially, exposing the cerebellopontine angle (CPA) and the vestibulocochlear nerve–facial nerve complex (Fig. 12.4). The cerebellum was maintained in this position by gravity or a small Greenberg or De Martel retractor blade.

In patients with useful preoperative hearing, intraoperative auditory brainstem evoked response (ABR) monitoring was performed, and in all subjects, unilateral needle electromyography of the orbicularis oris and oculi muscles was performed. A neuro-otologist and a neurosurgeon team (P.A.W. and W.A.K., P.A.W. and G.A.M., or D.S.P. and F.G.B.) performed each procedure. If adequate visualization of the vestibulocochlear nerve and facial nerve complex was possible, the remainder of the vestibular neurectomy was performed with one of the co-surgeons holding the endoscope while the other co-surgeon identified the vestibular nerve and completed the neurectomy. Alternatively, an articulated

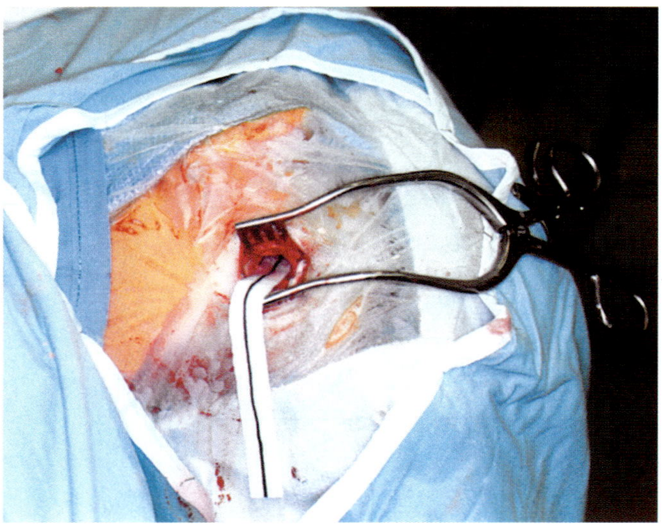

**FIGURE 12.4.** The craniectomy is shown with a Cottonoid (0.5 × 3 inches) in place over the cerebellum.

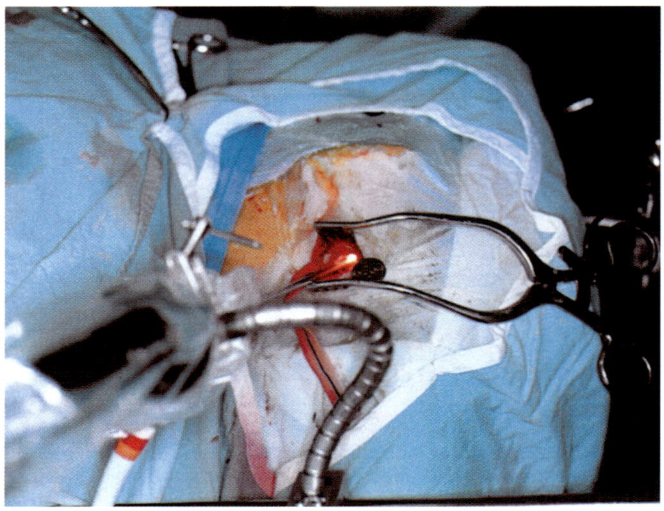

**FIGURE 12.6.** Endoscope shown entering the posterior fossa through the craniectomy and maintained in position using an endoscope holder. A sterilized dime is placed for scale.

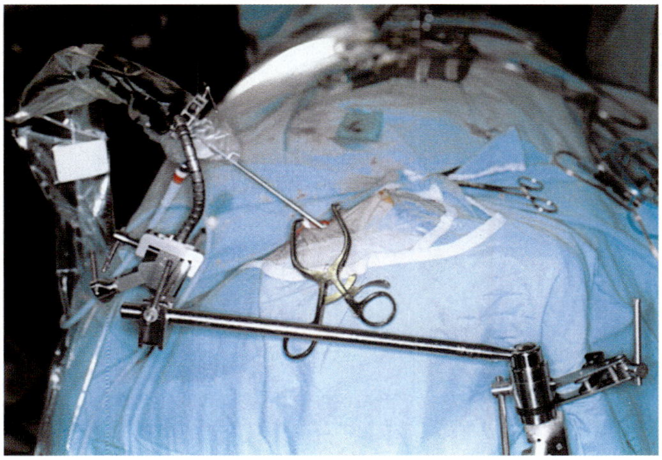

**FIGURE 12.7.** The articulated endoscope holder is shown attached to the Mayfield head frame and holder.

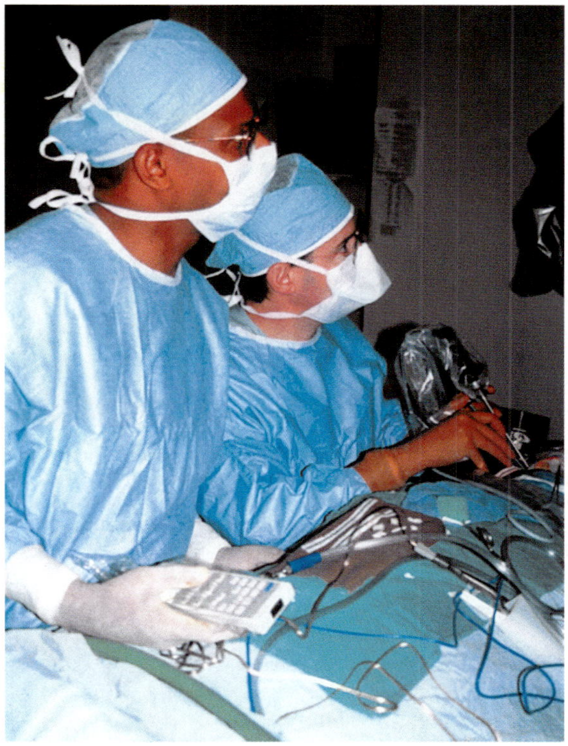

**FIGURE 12.9.** The surgeons visualize the operative field using the video monitor.

endoscope holder (Codman, Randolph, MA) was used while performing the neurectomy (Figs. 12.6–12.9).

All patients were examined with the rigid Hopkins rod endoscopes (4 mm, 0°; 4 or 2.7 mm, 30°) (Karl Storz, Culver City, CA; Smith & Nephew, Inc., Memphis, TN). Specific attention was paid to cranial nerves V through XI, the internal auditory canal (IAC), and the vascular anatomy (Fig. 12.10). Identification of the cleavage plane between the cochlear and vestibular nerves was sought, and in cases in which this division was not evident, 30°, 45°, or 70° endoscopes were used to identify this plane within the IAC. In no case was a transmeatal approach (i.e., opening the IAC) required.

The vestibular nerve was visually identified and the location of the facial nerve was confirmed by stimulating the nerve with 0.05-mA current and recording the electromyographic activity of the orbicularis oculi and oris muscles (Fig. 12.11). The vestibular nerve was then sharply sectioned (Fig. 12.12). While retracting the vestibular nerve using the microsuction in a lateral to medial direction, the vestibular nerve was again sectioned, completing the neurectomy (Fig. 12.13). A three-

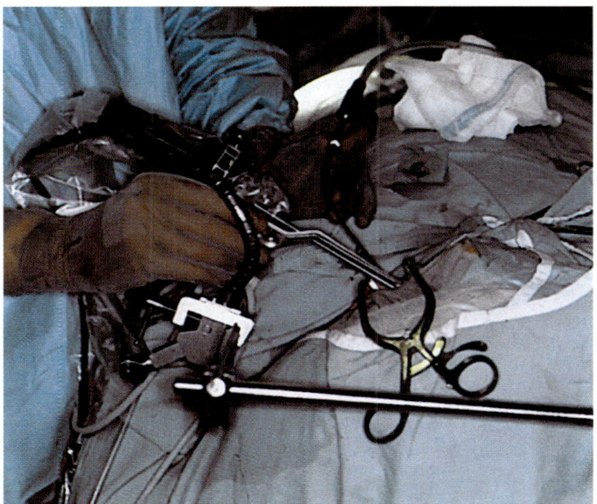

**FIGURE 12.8.** With the use of an articulated endoscope holder, the operating surgeon is free to use both hands in performing the neurectomy.

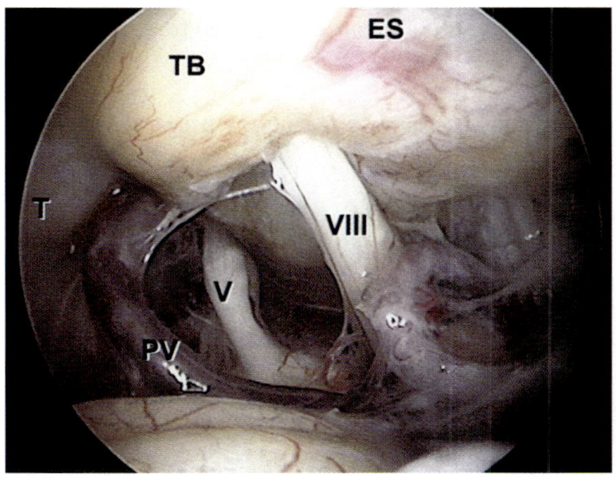


**FIGURE 12.10.** Endoscopic vestibular neurectomy for right Ménière's disease. An initial survey is performed with a 0° endoscope to gain orientation within the posterior fossa. *V,* trigeminal nerve; *VIII,* eighth nerve complex; *ES,* endolymphatic sac; *T,* tentorium; *TB,* posterior face of the temporal bone; *PV,* petrosal vein forming the superior petrosal sinus.

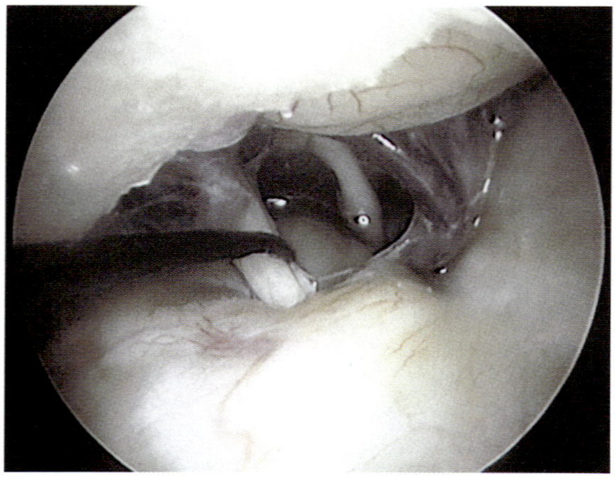

**FIGURE 12.11.** Confirmation of the facial nerve is accomplished using a stimulus-dissection instrument delivering 0.05-mA square wave current with a frequency of four times per second, each of 100 μs duration, and simultaneous electromyography recording from the orbicularis oculi and oris muscles.

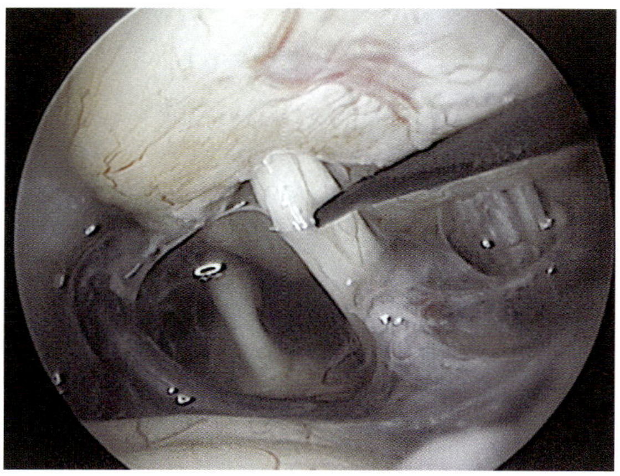

**FIGURE 12.12.** After identification of the cleavage plane between the vestibular and cochlear nerves, a stimulus-dissection instrument is used to isolate the vestibular nerve from the cochlear and facial nerves. The neurectomy is completed, and a segment of the vestibular nerve is resected to avoid the possibility of regeneration.

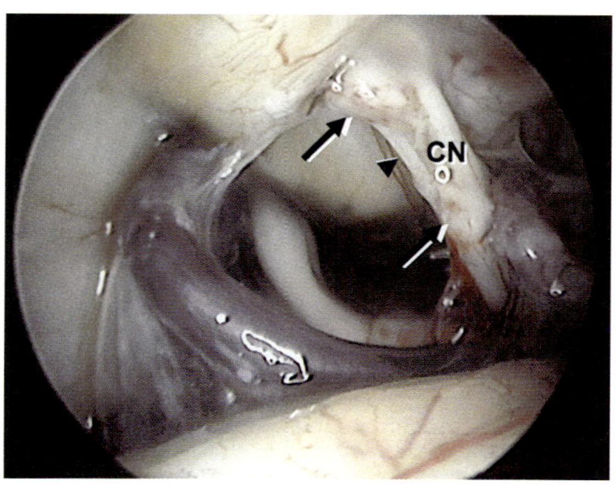


**FIGURE 12.13.** The cut ends of the right vestibular nerve *(arrows)* are seen with a 0° endoscope. *Arrowhead,* facial nerve; *CN,* cochlear nerve.

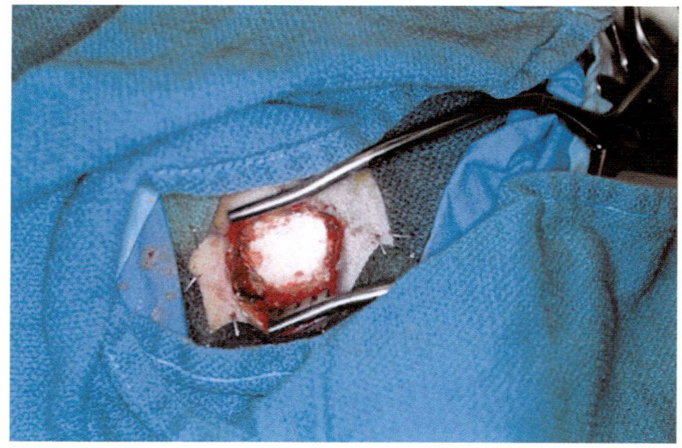

**FIGURE 12.14.** Titanium mesh is secured to the surrounding bone with screws (Synthes Maxillofacial, Paoli, PA), and a cranioplasty is completed using hydroxyapatite cement (BoneSource, Leibinger, Dallas, TX).

chip camera was attached to the lens of the endoscope, and the image was displayed on a 19-inch video monitor and captured on a S-VHS recorder or a digital dye-sublimation printer. After closure of the dura, hydroxyapatite cement cranioplasty (Leibinger, Dallas, TX) supported by a titanium mesh framework (Synthes Maxillofacial, Paoli, PA) (Fig. 12.14) was performed, and the wound was closed in layers.

## Results, Variations, and Complication

Complete neurectomy was achieved in all 14 patients. Endoscopy allowed improved identification of the nervus intermedius (Fig. 12.15) and of the facial, cochlear, and vestibular nerves and adjacent neurovascular relationships

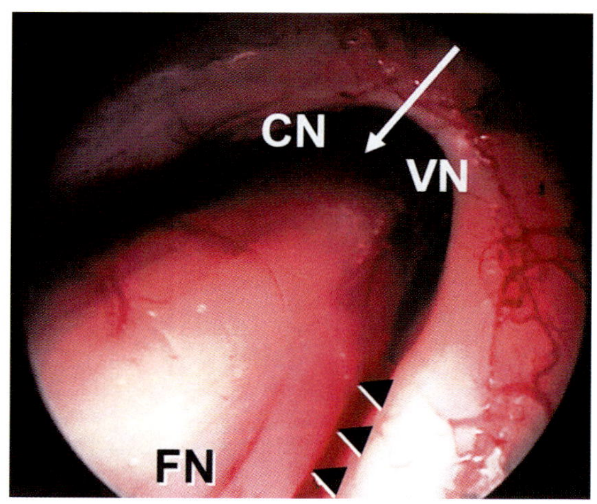


**FIGURE 12.15.** Variation on endoscopic vestibular neurectomy for left Ménière's disease. When a cleavage plane cannot be identified medial to the internal auditory canal (IAC), a 30° (45° or 70°) endoscope can be used to identify the cleavage plane *(arrow)* between the cochlear nerve *(CN)* and the vestibular nerve *(VN)* within the IAC. *Arrowheads,* nervus intermedius; *FN,* facial nerve.

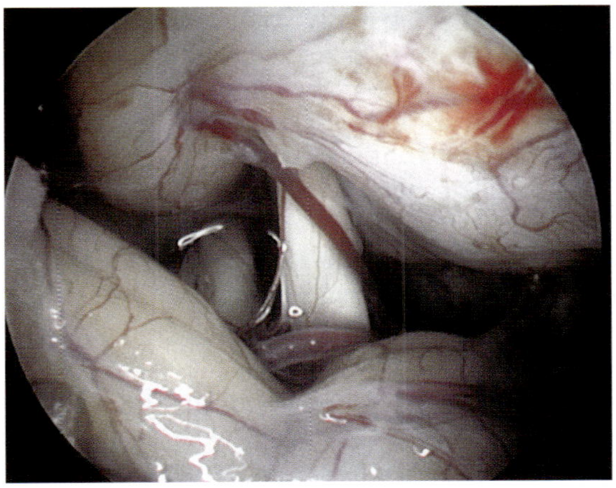

**FIGURE 12.16.** Variation on endoscopic vestibular neurectomy for right Ménière's disease. Several looping branches from the anterior inferior cerebellar artery (AICA) are seen around the vestibulocochlear nerve complex.

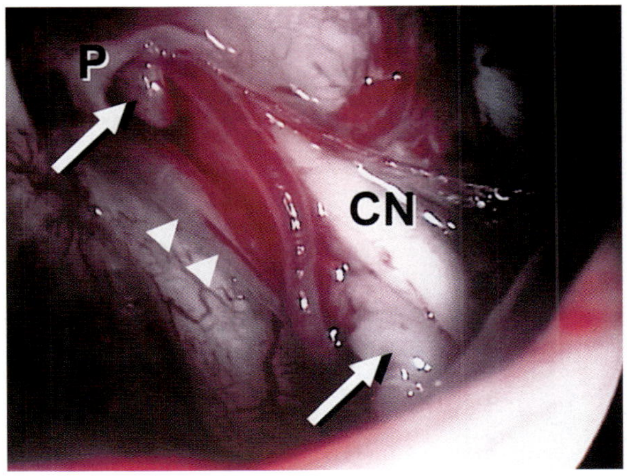


**FIGURE 12.18.** Variation on endoscopic vestibular neurectomy for right Ménière's disease. The cut ends of the vestibular nerve *(arrows)* are seen with a 30° endoscope beneath a large branch of the anterior inferior cerebellar artery (AICA) looping through the porus acusticus *(P)* into the IAC. *Arrowheads,* facial nerve; *CN,* cochlear nerve.

without the need for significant retraction of the cerebellum or brainstem (Figs. 12.10–12.13 and 12.15–12.20). Endoscopic identification of the cleavage plane between the cochlear and vestibular nerves medial to or within the IAC (*n*=3) was not seen with the microscope; however, they were identified using a 30°, 45° or 70° endoscope in all cases (Fig. 12.15). After identifying the cleavage plane between the cochlear and vestibular nerves within the IAC, it was developed medially before neurectomy. Vascular loops and branches of the anterior inferior cerebellar artery (AICA) passing into the IAC were also better appreciated (Figs. 12.16–12.20). In all patients with Ménière's disease, elimination of the recurrent episodes of vertigo (*n*=14) or otolithic crisis of Tumarkin (*n*=2) (two patients experienced attacks of true vertigo or otolithic crisis of Tumarkin) was achieved (Table 12.1); however, two patients later developed bilateral Ménière's disease. All patients who underwent postoperative ENG (*n*=8) were found to have complete vestibular deafferentation. None of the patients experienced postoperative cerebrospinal fluid (CSF) leakage, headache, or facial paresis or paralysis. One patient suffered complete hearing loss during retractor placement, probably caused by vascular insufficiency of the cochlea. Despite removal of the retractor when ABR changes were observed and placement of papaverine on the arteries feeding the vestibulocochlear complex, no measurable hearing returned. Complete vestibular deafferenta-

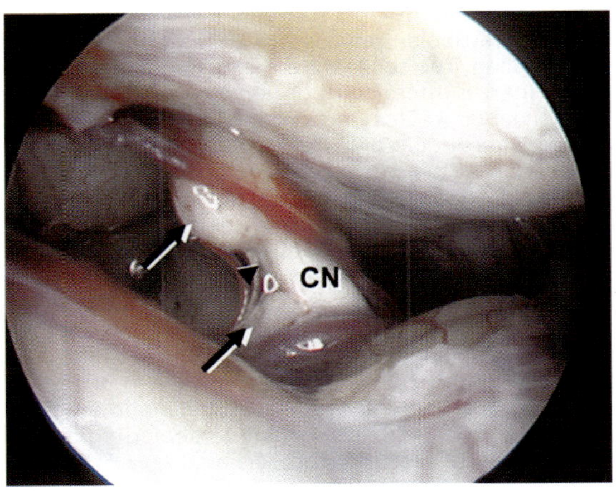


**FIGURE 12.17.** Variations on endoscopic vestibular neurectomy for right Ménière's disease. The same branches of the anterior inferior cerebellar artery (AICA) seen in Figure 12.16 are seen intact after completion of the vestibular neurectomy with a 0° endoscope. After neurectomy, an intact cochlear nerve *(CN)* and facial nerve *(arrowhead)* are seen adjacent to the cut ends of the vestibular nerve *(arrows)*.

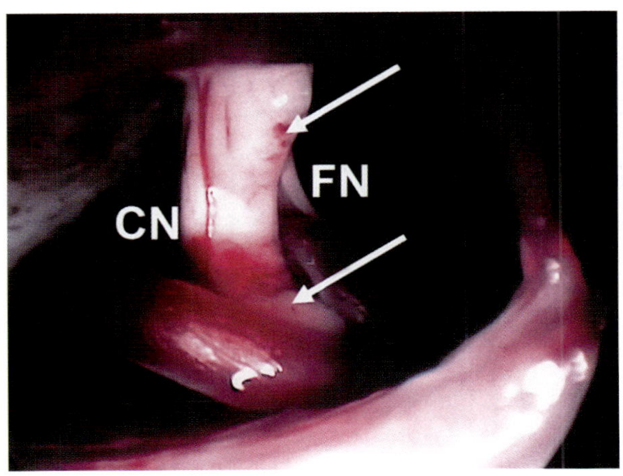


**FIGURE 12.19.** Variation on endoscopic vestibular neurectomy for left Ménière's disease. A 0° endoscopic view after vestibular neurectomy shows the cut ends of the vestibular nerve *(arrows)* and the cochlear nerve *(CN)*. Multiple looping branches from the anterior inferior cerebellar artery (AICA) are seen, one of which separates the CN and vestibular nerve from the facial nerve *(FN)*.

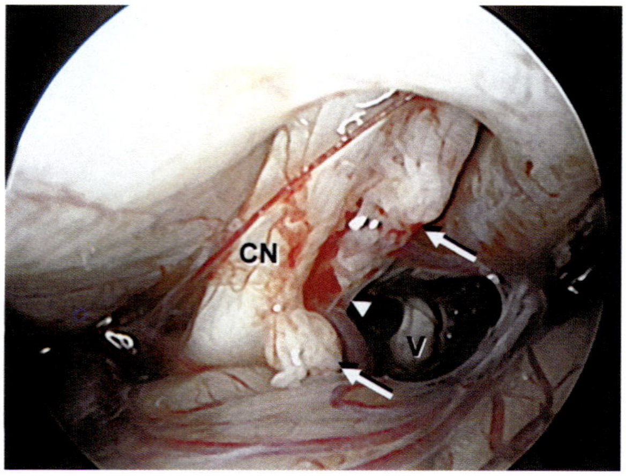


**FIGURE 12.20.** Complication of endoscopic vestibular neurectomy for left Ménière's disease. One patient from our series suffered irreversible, profound hearing loss during retractor placement. After neurectomy, an intact cochlear nerve *(CN)* and facial nerve *(arrowhead)* are seen adjacent to the cut ends of the vestibular nerve *(arrows)*. *V*, trigeminal nerve.

tion was achieved with anatomic preservation of the facial and cochlear nerves (Fig. 12.20).

## Discussion

The advantages and limitations of the various approaches to vestibular neurectomy have been reviewed (20). These approaches include the middle cranial fossa and the posterior fossa approaches, of which there are a number of variations, including the retrolabyrinthine approach; the retrosigmoid–internal auditory canal approach; and the combined retrolabyrinthine-retrosigmoid approach (10, 21). The middle cranial fossa approach provides the only exposure that allows resection of the primary afferent vestibular ganglia (Fig. 12.21). This accomplishes two goals: complete deafferentation of the vestibular periphery while preserving auditory function and elimination of the possibility of vestibular nerve regeneration. The significant advantages of posterior fossa over middle cranial fossa vestibular neurectomy are decreased risks of facial nerve injury and hearing loss. There are two principal disadvantages to posterior fossa vestibular neurectomy. First, the vestibular nerve fibers commingle with cochlear nerve fibers

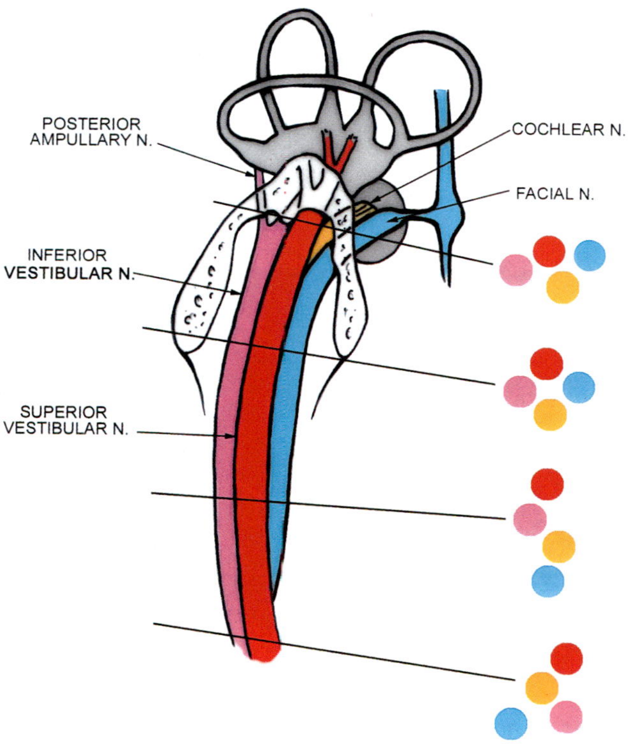


**FIGURE 12.21.** Anatomy of the seventh and eighth cranial nerves as seen from the surgical position during a left retrosigmoid–internal auditory canal approach. Notice the 90° rotation of the cochlear and vestibular nerves.

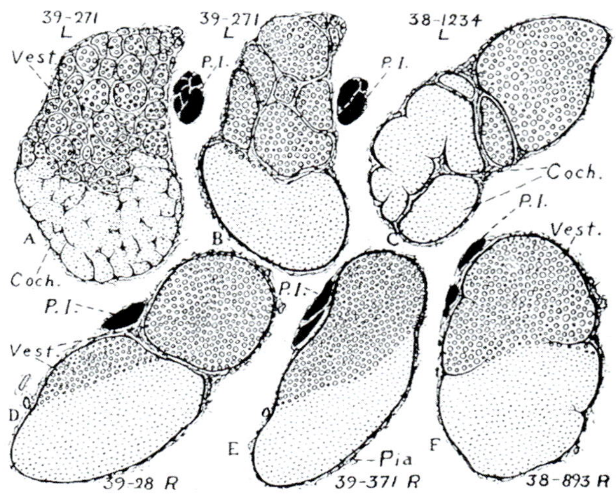


**FIGURE 12.22.** Diagrams show the cable-like patterns of the eighth cranial nerve, in cross sections, from human adults. The cochlear and vestibular regions are distinguished by different types of stippling. The solid white areas *(P.I.)* represents the pars intermedia (nervus intermedius or nerve of Wrisberg) of the seventh cranial nerve. **A:** Cross section slightly central to the vestibular ganglia. The cochlear and vestibular portions consist of many small bundles, with the cochlear beginning to fuse. **B:** A section of the same nerve as in **A** taken 2 mm further centrally, showing complete fusion of the cochlear and several vestibular fasciculi. The vestibular bundles ultimately fuse with each other and with the cochlear component until a single trunk is formed (similar to **E**). **C:** A case in which neither cochlear nor vestibular nerves are completely fused through most of the course in the internal auditory meatus and subarachnoid space. **D:** Example of the condition in which the eighth nerve is represented by two distinct trunks, one of which was apparently purely vestibular and the other was mostly cochlear, but with a prominent vestibular region amounting to about one fifth of the cross-sectional area of the cochlear trunk. **E:** Example of a common condition in which there is a single trunk, a little more than half of which (on microscopic examination) is found to be vestibular and the rest cochlear. **F:** A case in which incomplete glial septa roughly indicate the division between cochlear and vestibular trunks. Typically, there are at least a few vestibular fibers on the cochlear side of such septa. (From Rasmussen GL. Studies of the VIIIth cranial nerve of man. *Laryngoscope* 1940;50:67–83, with permission.)

proximal to Scarpa's ganglia, and it is possible to have an incomplete vestibular deafferentation or a partial hearing loss (22,23) (Fig. 12.22). Second, with sectioning the vestibular nerve, the potential for regeneration exists, whereas with the middle cranial fossa approach to vestibular neurectomy, resection of the primary afferent somata within Scarpa's ganglia eliminates any possibility of regeneration (24,25). We resect a segment of the vestibular nerve (Figs. 12.13 and 12.16–12.20) to avoid this possibility. In contrast to the 98% elimination of vertigo reported after the middle cranial fossa approach to vestibular neurectomy (26), 90% to 92% of patients undergoing posterior fossa vestibular neurectomy are relieved of vertigo (19,21). This difference may reflect imperfect patient selection or incomplete transection of the vestibular nerve.

The incidence of early CSF leakage in vestibular neurectomy is approximately 10% (10). The retrosigmoid–internal auditory canal approach has been associated with postoperative headache, described as severe in 75% of patients (27). The cause of the headache is unclear, although bone dust has been suspected (3,26). Both of these issues are related to opening the IAC, and with the procedure reported here, this transmeatal approach is not needed (28). However, we are reporting a modest series of patients, and it may be necessary to open the IAC in some cases if the cleavage plane between the cochlear and vestibular nerves is not seen using the 30°, 45°, or 70° endoscopes within the IAC. One of our patients suffered profound hearing loss during retractor placement. The microvascular decompression literature indicates that the incidence of ipsilateral hearing loss attributed to cerebellar retraction occurs in 2% to 8% of patients (29,30).

## NEURECTOMY OF THE NERVUS INTERMEDIUS

Endoscope-assisted surgery can be used to perform rhizotomy of other cranial nerves. An example of another application, neurectomy of the nervus intermedius for intractable geniculate neuralgia, is described subsequently.

*Case:* A 47-year-old woman with unilateral right otalgia for 4 months was initially treated for presumed otitis externa with ototopical agents and prednisone without relief. She was then referred to P.A.W. for further evaluation. An audiogram demonstrated normal thresholds and discrimination, and tympanometry findings were normal. Otologic, neuro-otologic, and complete head and neck examination findings were within normal limits. She then underwent a temporal bone computed tomography (CT) scan and magnetic resonance imaging (MRI) with gadolinium enhancement of the temporal bones, internal auditory canals, and skull base; the findings were unremarkable. An evaluation by an oral surgeon failed to reveal temporomandibular joint arthropathy. A trial of carbamazepine (Tegretol), followed by baclofen (Lioresal) and gabapentin (Neurontin) over a 12-month interval, was completed without change in her otalgia. Erythrocyte sedimentation rate, Lyme titers, and full laboratory evaluation results were normal. The patient underwent a retrosigmoid posterior fossa craniotomy with endoscope-assisted section of the nervus intermedius for a presumed geniculate neuralgia (Fig. 12.23). Three and one-half years after surgical intervention, the patient reports resolution of her otalgia with decreased, but not absent, sensation of the right posterior concha and no other neurologic deficits.

Geniculate neuralgia as the cause of primary otalgia is rare; however, anatomic and clinical studies have shown that there is a sensory component to the seventh cranial nerve that can be implicated in geniculate neuralgia (31) (Fig. 12.24). Sensory innervation to the cutaneous areas of the internal and external ear are complex, because the ear is the locus for cranial nerves V, IX, and X ; the nervus intermedius (Wrisberg's nerve) (32); and the upper cervical dorsal roots. Management of cases that are refractory to conservative therapy are managed surgically. The index case of primary otalgia treated with nervus intermedius section, reported by Clark and Taylor, established geniculate neuralgia as a definite clinical entity (31).

Before diagnosing a patient with geniculate neuralgia, an extensive differential diagnosis should be entertained. Otitis; temporomandibular joint disease; Eagle's syndrome; carcinoma of the nasopharynx, temporal bone, external auditory canal, or pinna; vascular lesions; and referred pain from cerebellopontine angle, laryngeal, and pharyngeal sites must be excluded. A complete neurologic, otologic, and dental evaluation is paramount.

Sensory ablation attempts have centered on section of the nervus intermedius, with or without section of other cranial nerves; section of the greater superficial petrosal nerve; and resection of the geniculate ganglion (33). Others have found vascular loops in relation to these cranial nerves and advocate decompression or nervus intermedius section combined with microvascular decompression of other cranial nerves (34). Major series report 72% to 90% success rate with sectioning of the nervus intermedius (33,34).

The facial nerve has two major components: the larger motor component supplying the facial musculature and a smaller component, the nervus intermedius, containing sensory and parasympathetic nerve fibers. The nervus intermedius, has distinct features and can be considered a separate cranial nerve. Its sensory portion is responsible for taste sensation on the anterior two thirds of the tongue, as well as sensation of the external auditory canal and concha. The parasympathetic portion of the nerve supplies secretomotor fibers to the lacrimal, submandibular, sublingual, nasal, and palatine glands.

The nervus intermedius, as described by Rhoton and colleagues (35), can be divided into three principal segments. The *proximal portion* is adherent to the eighth nerve just anterior to the superior vestibular nerve at the brain-

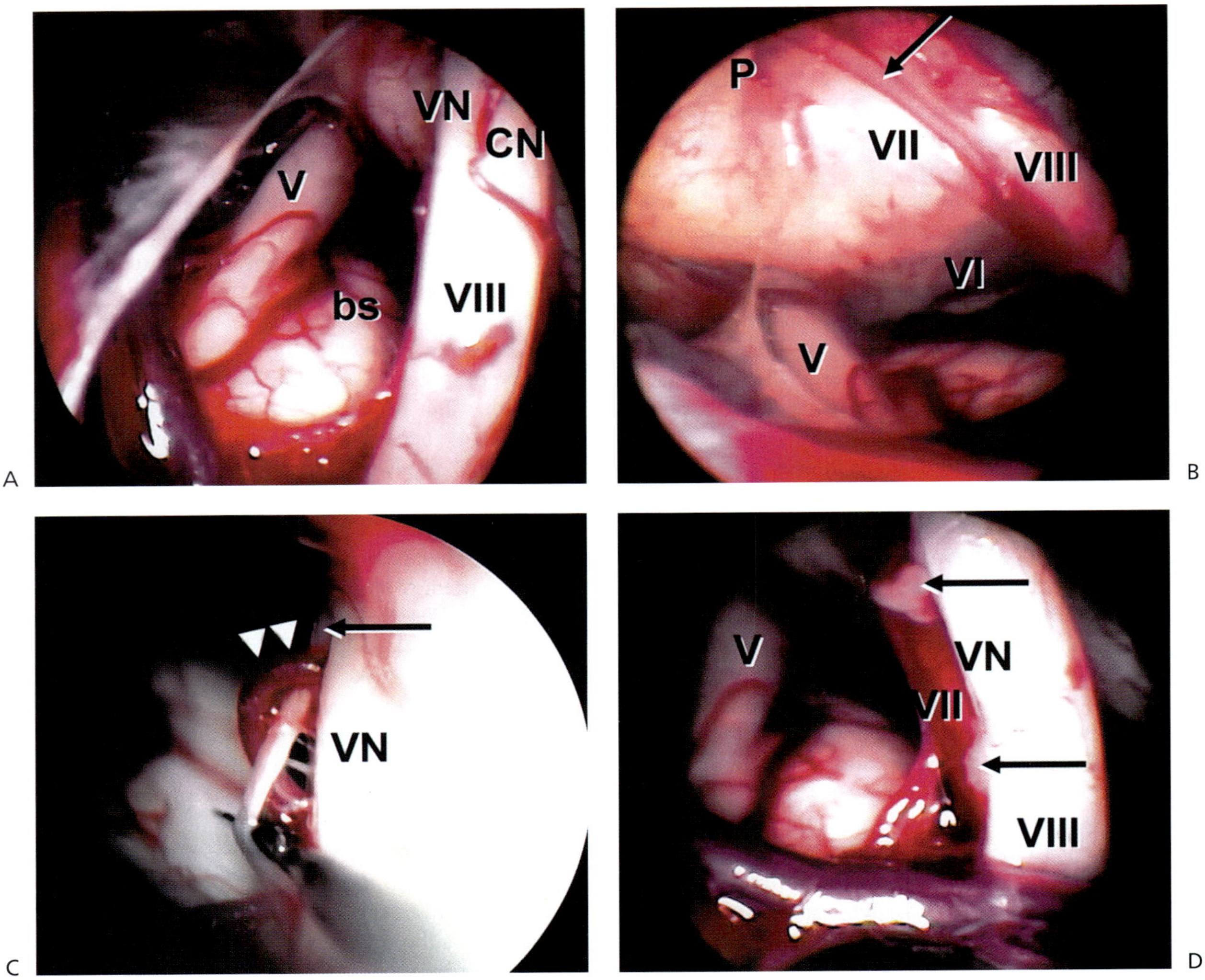


**FIGURE 12.23.** Endoscopic view of the right nervus intermedius within the posterior fossa in relation to the trigeminal *(V)*, abducens *(VI)*, facial *(VII)*, and cochleovestibular *(VIII)* nerves. **A:** Initial view into the posterior fossa and cerebellopontine angle. The cleavage plane between the vestibular nerve *(VN)* and cochlear nerve *(CN)* can be seen distal to the vestibulocochlear nerve *(VIII)*. *bs,* brainstem. **B:** Intermediate segment of the nervus intermedius *(arrow)* seen entering the porus acusticus *(P)*.**C:** The nervus intermedius *(arrow)* in this patient is seen to be separated from the VN by a looping branch of the anterior inferior cerebellar artery *(arrowheads)* before neurectomy. **D:** Cut ends of the nervus intermedius *(arrows)* are seen between cranial nerves VII and VIII. The anterior inferior cerebellar artery is seen in the foreground at the root entry zone of the vestibulocochlear nerve, and the trigeminal nerve *(V)* is seen in the background.

stem. The *intermediate segment* lies free between the seventh and eighth cranial nerves (Fig. 12.23). The *distal segment* becomes incorporated into the seventh nerve, usually within the porus acusticus (Fig. 12.15). In cadaveric studies by Rhoton and colleagues, most instances the nervus intermedius existed as a single nerve trunk, but in the remainder, it was composed of as many as four rootlets. In approximately 20% of cases, the nervus intermedius is adherent to the eighth nerve throughout the area between the brainstem and the porus acusticus. In these cases, the posterior lip of the internal auditory canal must be unroofed to allow access if the use of a 30°, 45°, or 70° endoscope fails to identify this plane. Arteries coursing to supply the brainstem dorsal to the eighth nerve may be found passing between the seventh and eighth nerves as far laterally as the internal auditory meatus. In 5 of 37 cases, a branch of the anterior inferior cerebellar artery was seen to enter the internal acoustic meatus with the seventh and eighth nerves, give rise to the labyrinthine artery, and then loop back to supply the brainstem.

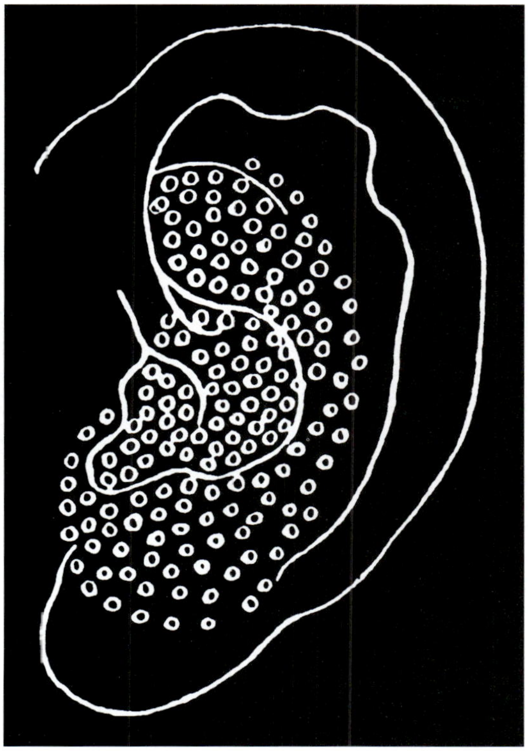

**FIGURE 12.24.** J. Ramsay Hunt described the distribution of the sensory component of the seventh nerve in his clinical studies of patients with herpes zoster oticus. This figure from his 1937 paper illustrates the sensory distribution of the nervus intermedius in the auricle. (Adapted from Hunt JR. Geniculate neuralgia (neuralgia of the nervus facialis). *Arch Neurol Psychiatry* 1937;37:253–283, with permission.)

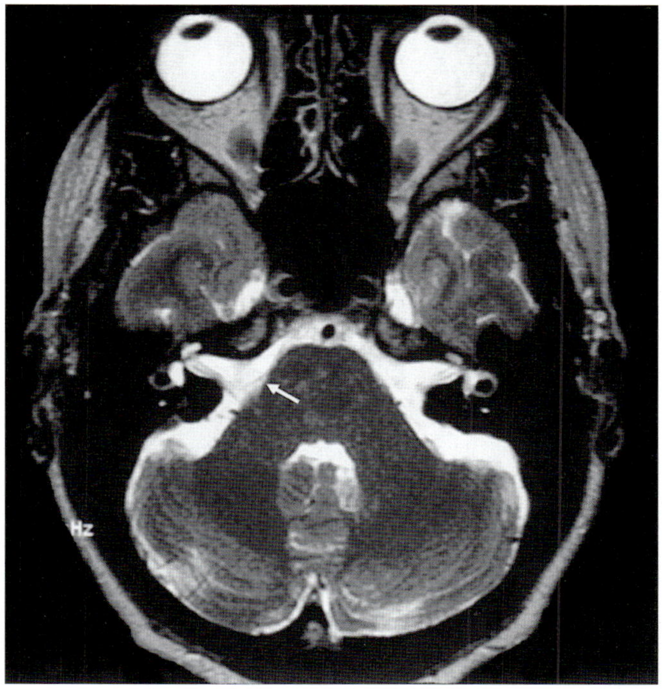


**FIGURE 12.25.** T2-weighted magnetic resonance imaging shows a vessel crossing the right root entry zone of the eighth nerve complex *(arrow)*. Normal cochlea, vestibular apparatus, and cochlear and inferior vestibular nerves are shown.

## MICROVASCULAR DECOMPRESSION

Microvascular compression syndromes have been described for the trigeminal, facial, cochlear, and vestibular nerves as a cause of trigeminal neuralgia (i.e., tic douloureux), hemifacial spasm, subjective tinnitus, and vestibular dysfunction, respectively (36). We have performed endoscope-assisted microvascular decompression for all of these entities, except vascular loop-induced vestibulopathy. Case examples are shown in Figures 12.25–12.34. In all cases, improvement or resolution of the symptoms was achieved.

### Microvascular Decompression for Tinnitus

A 54-year-old woman presented with intractable right unilateral tinnitus. She had been managed medically for several years and did not have an acoustic neuroma based on MRI studies. However, a large vessel crossing the root entry zone of the vestibulocochlear complex was identified on MRI (Fig. 12.25). She elected to undergo microvascular decompression using endoscopic techniques. Intraoperative ABR

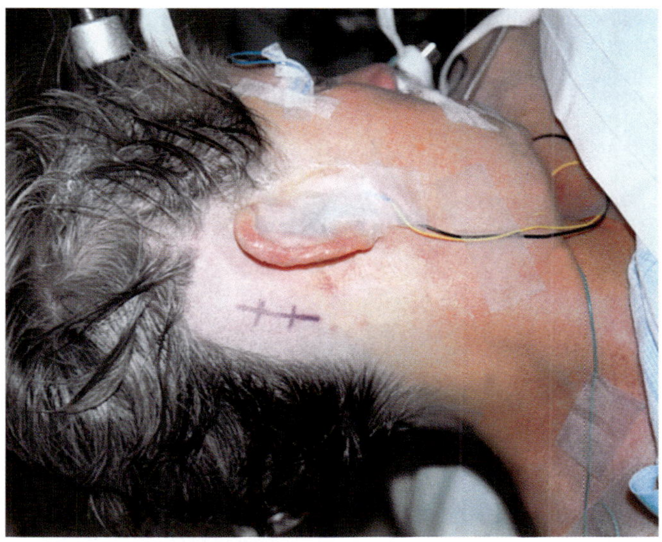

**FIGURE 12.26.** Endoscopic microvascular decompression for right intractable tinnitus. A 3- to 4-cm linear incision is designed that extends caudally from the transverse sinus. Notice the Mayfield head holder, which is used to attach the endoscope holder. Intraoperative auditory brainstem evoked response monitoring and facial nerve electromyography monitoring are performed during the microvascular decompression procedure.

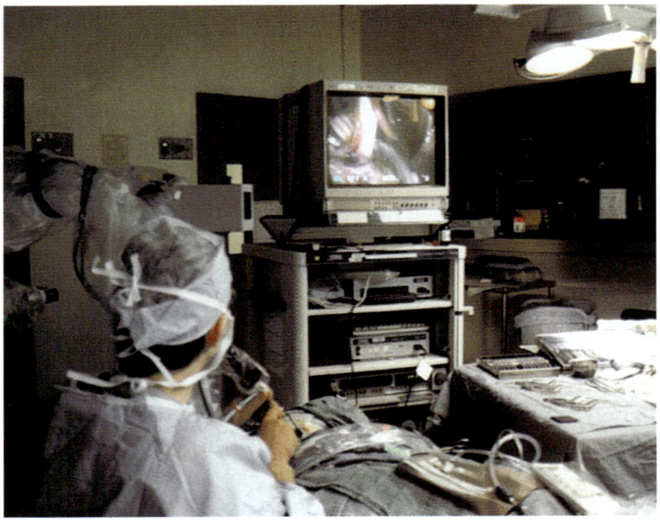

**FIGURE 12.27.** Intraoperative view of the patient, surgeon, and video monitor shows the microvascular decompression.

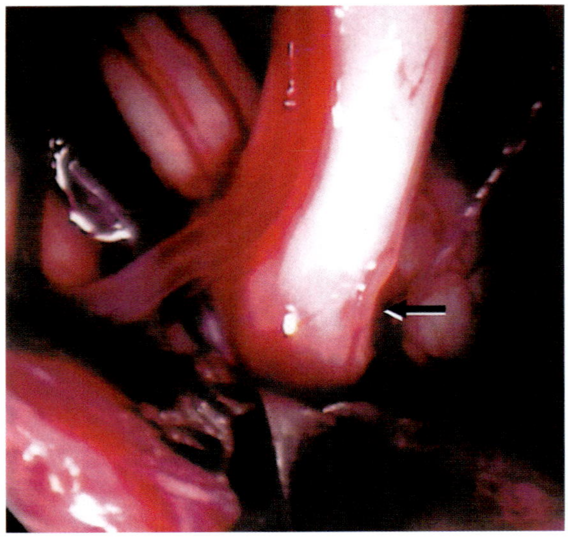

**FIGURE 12.29.** After mobilization of the vein crossing the root entry zone, indentation and demyelination of the cochlear nerve can be seen *(arrow)*.

and facial nerve monitoring was performed, and a small incision and craniotomy, as described in the vestibular neurectomy section of this chapter, was completed (Fig. 12.26). On inspection of the CPA, a vein was found to compress the root entry zone of the cochlear nerve, and numerous branches of the AICA were found surrounding the vestibulocochlear nerve (Figs. 12.27 and 12.28). After mobilization and elevation of the vein, the cochlear nerve was seen to be demyelinated and indented at the compression site (Fig. 12.29). Teflon felt was placed between the mobilized vessels and the vestibulocochlear nerve complex (Fig. 12.30). She experienced subjective improvement of her tinnitus, in that the character changed to a higher frequency that was of much lower intensity and only intermittent in nature. It is now 3 years after the decompression. During this interval, approximately 1 year after the surgery, she experienced a decrease in her pure tone average by 15 to 20 dB in the affected ear.

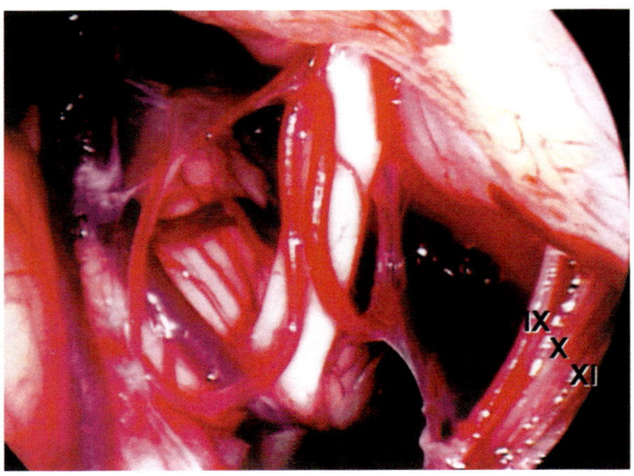


**FIGURE 12.28.** Initial endoscopic view of the eighth nerve complex *(center)* and cranial nerves *IX, X,* and *XI* entering the jugular foramen *(right)*. Numerous arterial branches from the anterior inferior cerebellar artery are seen over the vestibulocochlear nerve, as well as a single vein crossing the root entry zone of the cochlear nerve.

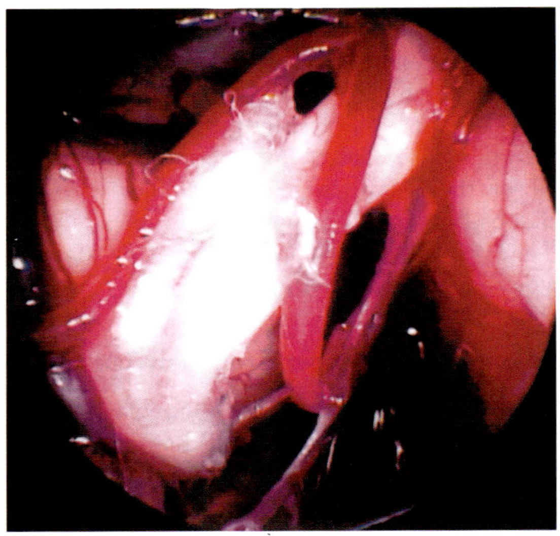

**FIGURE 12.30.** Teflon felt is placed between the vestibular and cochlear nerves and the branches from the anterior inferior cerebellar artery and the vein crossing the root entry zone of the vestibulocochlear nerve.

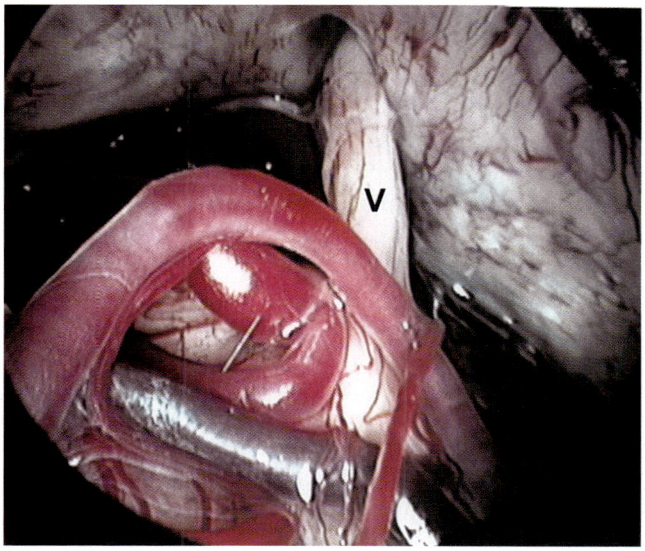


**FIGURE 12.31.** Microvascular decompression for right trigeminal neuralgia. Initial view on exposure of the right cerebellopontine angle using a 4-mm, 0° endoscope. Multiple arteries and veins are in contact with the trigeminal nerve *(V)* at the entry zone to the brainstem.

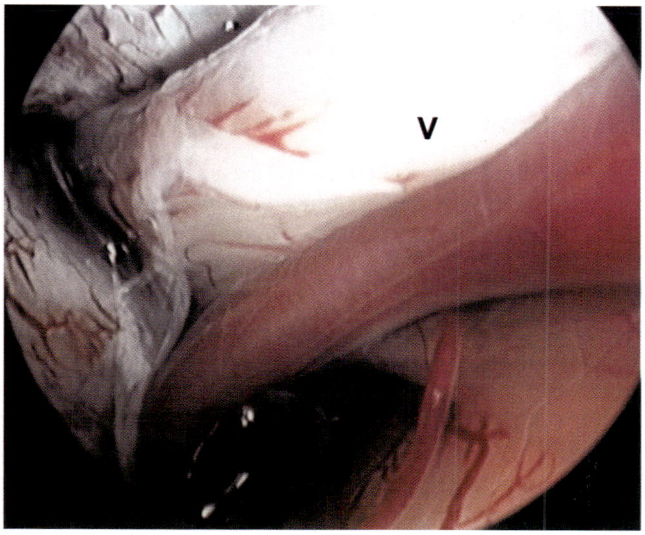


**FIGURE 12.33.** Microvascular decompression for right trigeminal neuralgia. After elevation of the large superior cerebellar artery compressing the trigeminal nerve *(V)*, the view of the nerve using a 30° endoscope demonstrates displacement from the nerve.

## Microvascular Decompression for Trigeminal Neuralgia or Hemifacial Spasm

Six patients with trigeminal neuralgia and two patients with hemifacial spasm who failed medical management underwent endoscope-assisted microvascular decompression by us. Anatomic compression of the nerve entry or exit zone was demonstrated in all eight patients. In each case, an arterial loop was felt to be responsible for the patient's clinical symptoms; the superior cerebellar artery was found to be the offending vessel in the patients with trigeminal neuralgia and the AICA in the patients with hemifacial spasm. Multiple arteries and veins were identified in several cases adjacent to the dysfunctional cranial nerve at the brainstem junction (Figs. 12.31–12.34). Using the microscope alone, it was difficult to determine the offending vessel. However,

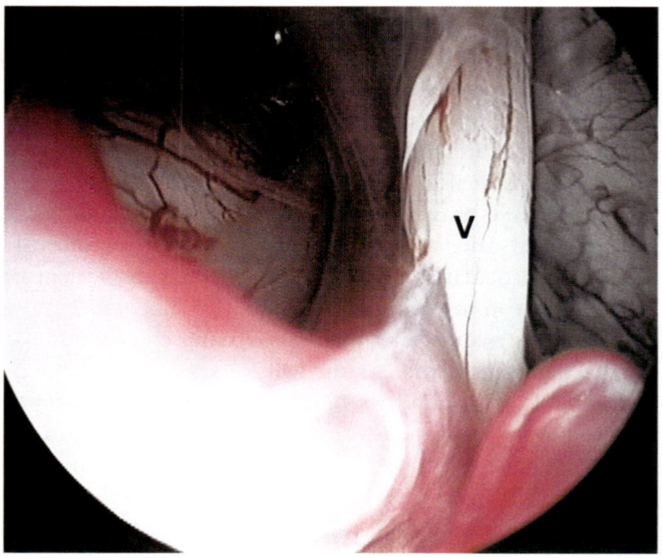


**FIGURE 12.32.** Microvascular decompression for right trigeminal neuralgia. Panoramic examination of the trigeminal nerve *(V)* using the 30° endoscope demonstrates compression by a large superior cerebellar artery.

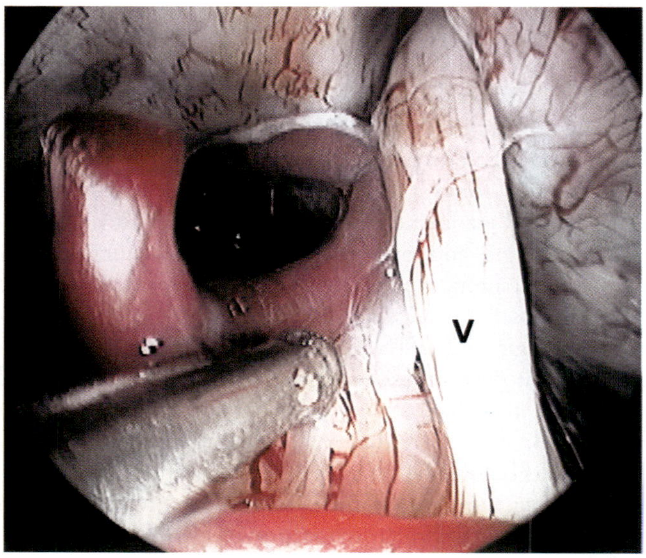


**FIGURE 12.34.** Microvascular decompression for right trigeminal neuralgia. Panoramic examination of the nerve used the 0° endoscope after decompression of the trigeminal nerve *(V)*.

in all cases, endoscopy clarified the exact site of the clinically significant compression.

## Discussion

Trigeminal neuralgia, hemifacial spasm, glossopharyngeal neuralgia, tinnitus, and disabling positional vertigo have all been associated with vascular compression (36). Microvascular decompression operations involve separating the compressive vessel from its point of contact with the cranial nerve root entry or exit zone and interposition of a prosthesis (usually Teflon felt) to prevent further nerve compression. Extensive experience has demonstrated that 62% to 64% of trigeminal neuralgia patients have a compressive artery, 12% to 24% have a compressive vein, 13% to 14% have an artery and a vein, and 8% have a tumor or vascular malformation pressing on the trigeminal nerve (37). The initial failure rate for microvascular decompression for trigeminal neuralgia is 2% to 7%, with a 3.5% per year incidence of a major recurrence (38–40). In the series of 1,185 patients who underwent microvascular decompression for trigeminal neuralgia reported by Barker and coworkers in 1996, there was a mean follow-up of 6.2 years and 30% of patients experienced a major recurrence, with 11% requiring a second microvascular decompression (41). The absence of a clear site of arterial compression has been associated with high recurrence rates (42). Patients found to have only venous compression and no arterial compression are more likely to suffer a recurrence (41). Kureshi and associates reported their surgical experience with 31 posterior fossa reexplorations for recurrent or persistent trigeminal neuralgia and hemifacial spasm (43). They discovered 3 (10%) cases in which there was new or previously unrealized arterial compression of neural structures. Similarly, for a series of microvascular compression syndrome patients reoperated after failure, the physicians reported identification of previously unseen arterial compression in 65.5% of the 116 patients (44). Liao and colleagues discovered persistent vascular compression in three of five patients undergoing repeat microvascular decompression (45).

Although some have doubted that microvascular compression of a cranial nerve can represent the cause of trigeminal neuralgia and other cranial nerve dysfunction syndromes, the literature indicates that the identification of an arterial vessel compressing the trigeminal nerve in trigeminal neuralgia and the facial nerve in hemifacial spasm and subsequent decompression results in higher cure rates and decreased recurrences than when a specific artery is not identified. We believe that some microvascular decompressions fail because the offending vessel has not been identified during the primary operation. Some of these failures occur because the microscope provides incomplete information about the anatomic relationship between the nerves and vessels. The 0° endoscope provides a panoramic view of the CPA, and angled endoscopes can "look around corners." Magnan and coworkers used an endoscope in 60 patients with hemifacial spasm and demonstrated that the operating microscope was able to visualize the offending vessel in 28% of cases, whereas the endoscope was effective in 93% of the same cases (46). We believe that the adjunctive use of the endoscope in microvascular decompression surgery can improve surgical outcomes.

## CONCLUSIONS

Endoscopy offers several distinct advantages over the operating microscope during surgery of the trigeminal, facial, cochlear, or vestibular nerves within the CPA that make it an excellent adjunctive tool to the microscope or independent modality during cranial base surgery. The high magnification gives excellent definition of perforating blood vessels, cranial nerves, and neural structures, which in many cases is superior to that achieved with the microscope. The use of angled or flexible endoscopes allows the surgeon to look around corners and behind anatomic structures blocking the view seen through a 0° microscope. Endoscopy also has the theoretical advantage that a smaller operative procedure is required, which should reduce the operative morbidity.

There are, however, several notable disadvantages of endoscopy. These include the problems associated with blood soiling the endoscope, making visualization difficult or impossible; the lack of readily available instrumentation designed specifically for endoscopic neuro-otology; and the poor overview of the operative field. This last point is an important one because the endoscope is placed adjacent to the lesion and does not allow the surgeon to look backward to prevent injury to structures next to the shaft of the telescope. The surgeon also must be cognizant of potential thermal injury to structures caused by the heat generated by the light source. Current endoscopic technology limits the image that the surgeon sees to two dimensions, which results in certain unique problems when operating in a three-dimensional milieu. Because of this, there is a steep learning curve to acquire endoscopic dexterity and three-dimensional orientation. Bimanual operating requires the use of an articulated endoscope holder or commitment of the co-surgeon to hold the endoscope.

There are additional limitations of endoscopic vestibular neurectomy. First, there is the lack of a significant true or expandable space through which the surgeon can manipulate multiple instruments. Second, it is necessary to navigate around the lattice of nerves and arteries within the CPA. Third, instruments are usually not passed through working channels of the endoscope or portals as they are during intraventricular neuroendoscopic surgery (1), but rather they must be passed along the side of the telescope. Because of these clinical problems, different endoscopic strategies and instruments must be used.

One of the limitations of the operative microscope is that the angle of view is determined by the distance of the lens to the skull, retractor, or obstructing tissue. This is a function of the lens focal length; the longer the focal length, the narrower is the viewing angle. During most microsurgical procedures, the focal distance varies between 200 and 400 mm. Using the previous analogy, if a person looks through a door's keyhole at close range, nearly the entire room on the opposite side of the door can be seen, although nothing can be seen when the hole is viewed from a long distance. This result is similar to what happens when using the endoscope with focal lengths ranging from 5 to 20 mm; a wider angle of view can be achieved.

Based on our experience, we believe that endoscopes can be used safely during retrosigmoid (suboccipital) surgery within the posterior fossa for vestibular neurectomy, neurectomy of the nervus intermedius, or microvascular decompression of cranial nerves. As an adjunct to or substitution for the operative microscope, this modality does improve visualization of bony, neural, and vascular structures while minimizing cerebellar retraction. Endoscopic exploration (with the 30°, 45°, or 70°endoscope) of the IAC when the cleavage plane between the cochlear and vestibular nerves cannot be identified medial to the IAC can demonstrate this cleavage plane, which can be developed medially before neurectomy, obviating a transmeatal approach and the increased risk of postoperative CSF leakage and headache.

## REFERENCES


1. King WA, Frazee JG, DeSalles AAF, eds. *Endoscopy of the central and peripheral nervous system.* New York: Thieme Medical Publishers, 1998:1–259.
2. Wackym PA, King WA, Barker FG, et al. Endoscope-assisted vestibular neurectomy. *Laryngoscope* 1998;108:1787–1793.
3. O'Donoghue GM, O'Flynn P. Endoscopic anatomy of the cerebellopontine angle. *Am J Otol* 1993;14:122–125.
4. McKennan KX. Endoscopy of the internal auditory canal during hearing conservation acoustic tumor surgery. *Am J Otol* 1993;14: 259–262.
5. Mangnan J, Chays A, Lepetre C, et al. Surgical perspectives of endoscopy of the cerebellopontine angle. *Am J Otol* 1994;15: 366–370.
6. Bottrill ID, Poe DS. Endoscopic-assisted ear surgery. *Am J Otol* 1995;16:158–163.
7. Rosenberg SI. Endoscopic otologic surgery. *Otolaryngol Clin North Am* 1996;29:291–300.
8. Glasscock ME III, Gulya AJ, Pensak ML, et al. Medical and surgical management of Ménière's disease. *Am J Otol* 1984;5: 536–542.
9. Santos PM, Hall RA, Snyder JM, et al. Diuretic and diet effect on Ménière's disease evaluated by the 1985 Committee on Hearing and Equilibrium guidelines. *Otolaryngol Head Neck Surg* 1993;109:680–689.
10. Silverstein H, Wanamaker H, Flanzer J, et al. Vestibular neurectomy in the United States—1990. *Am J Otol* 1992;13:23–30.
11. Jackler RK. Endoscope-assisted vestibular neurectomy [Letter, comment]. *Laryngoscope* 1999;109:1010–1011.
12. Frazier CH. Intracranial division of the auditory nerve for persistent aural vertigo. *Surg Gynecol Obstet* 1912;15:524–529.
13. Dandy WE. Ménière's disease: its diagnosis and a method of treatment. *Arch Surg* 1928;16:1127–1152.
14. McKenzie KG. Intracranial division of the vestibular portion of the auditory nerve for Ménière's disease. *Can Med Assoc J* 1936; 34:369–381.
15. Dandy WE. Treatment of Ménière's disease by section of only the vestibular portion of the acoustic nerve. *Bull Johns Hopkins Hosp* 1933;53:52–55.
16. Green RE. Surgical treatment of vertigo, with follow-up on Walter Dandy's cases: neurological aspects. *Clin Neurosurg* 1958;6: 141–151.
17. Parry RH. A case of tinnitus and vertigo treated by division of the auditory nerve. *J Laryngol Otol* 1904;19:402–407.
18. Silverstein H, Rosenberg S, Arruda J, et al. Surgical ablation of the vestibular system in the treatment of Ménière's disease. *Otolaryngol Clin North Am* 1997;30:1075–1095.
19. Committee on hearing and equilibrium guidelines for the diagnosis and evaluation of therapy in Ménière's disease. *Otolaryngol Head Neck Surg* 1995;113:181–185.
20. Wackym PA, Monsell EM. Revision vestibular surgery. In: Carrasco V, Pillsbury HC III, eds. *Revision otologic surgery.* New York: Thieme Medical Publishers, 1997:109–133.
21. Silverstein H, Norrel H, Rosenberg S. An evolution of approach in vestibular neurectomy. *Otolaryngol Head Neck Surg* 1990;102: 374–381.
22. Rasmussen GL. Studies of the VIIIth cranial nerve of man. *Laryngoscope* 1940;50:67–83.
23. Silverstein H. Cochlear and vestibular gross and histologic anatomy (as seen from the postauricular approach). *Otolaryngol Head Neck Surg* 1984;92:207–211.
24. Newman A, Honrubia V. Regeneration of the eighth cranial nerve in the bullfrog, *Rana catesbeiana. Exp Neurol* 1992;115: 115–120.
25. Monsell EM, Brackmann DE, Linthicum FH. Why do vestibular destructive procedures sometimes fail? *Otolaryngol Head Neck Surg* 1988;99:472–479.
26. Kronenberg J, Fisch U, Dillier N. Long-term evaluation of hearing after transtemporal supralabyrinthine vestibular neurectomy. In: Nadol JB, ed. *The Second International Symposium on Ménière's disease.* New York: Kugler & Ghedini Publications, 1989:481–488.
27. Silverstein H, Rosenberg SI. Retrolabyrinthine/retrosigmoid vestibular neurectomy. In: Brackmann DE, ed. *Otologic surgery.* Philadelphia: WB Saunders, 1994:490–500.
28. Saim L, McKenna MJ, Nadol JB Jr. Tubal and tympanic openings of the peritubal cells: implications for cerebrospinal fluid otorhinorrhea. *Am J Otol* 1996;17:335–339.
29. Bederson J, Wilson C. Evaluation of microvascular decompression and partial sensory rhizotomy in 252 cases of trigeminal neuralgia. *J Neurosurg* 1989;71:359–367.
30. Fritz W, Shafer J, Klein H. Hearing loss after microvascular decompression for trigeminal neuralgia. *J Neurosurg* 1988;69: 367–370.
31. Hunt JR. Geniculate neuralgia (neuralgia of the nervus facialis). *Arch Neurol Psychiatry* 1937;37:253–283.
32. Lustig LR, Jackler RK, Mandelcorn R. The history of otology through its eponyms I: anatomy. *Am J Otol* 1998;19:371–389.
33. Rupa V, Saunders RL, Weider DJ. Geniculate neuralgia: the surgical management of primary otalgia. *J Neurosurg* 1991;75: 505–511.
34. Lovely TJ, Janetta PJ. Surgical management of geniculate neuralgia. *Am J Otol* 1997;18:512–517.

35. Rhoton AL Jr, Kobayashi S, Hollinshead WH. Nervus intermedius. *J Neurosurg* 1968:29:609–618.
36. Schwaber MK. Vascular compression syndromes. In: Jackler RK, Brackmann DE, eds. *Neurotology.* St. Louis: Mosby–Year Book, 1994:881–903.
37. Rohrer D, Burchiel K. Trigeminal neuralgia and other trigeminal dysfunction syndromes. In: Barrow D, ed. *Surgery of the cranial nerves of the posterior fossa.* Park Ridge, IL: American Association of Neurological Surgeons, 1993:201–217.
38. Apfelbaum R. Surgery for tic douloureux. *Clin Neurosurg* 1984; 31:346–350.
39. Burchiel K, Clarke H, Haglund M. Long-term efficacy of microvascular decompression in trigeminal neuralgia. *J Neurosurg* 1988;69:35–38.
40. Sweet W. Trigeminal neuralgia: problems as to cause and consequent conclusions regarding treatment. In: Wilkins RH, Rengachary S, eds. *Neurosurgery update II.* New York: McGraw-Hill, 1991:366–372.
41. Barker FG, Jannetta PJ, Bissonette DJ, et al. The long-term outcome of microvascular decompression for trigeminal neuralgia. *N Engl J Med* 1996;334:1077–1083.
42. Mendoza N, Illingworth RD. Trigeminal neuralgia treated by microvascular decompression: a long-term follow-up study. *Br J Neurosurg* 1995;9:13–19.
43. Kureshi SA, Wilkins RH. Posterior fossa reexploration for persistent or recurrent trigeminal neuralgia or hemifacial spasm: surgical findings and therapeutic implications. *Neurosurgery* 1998;43: 1111–1117.
44. Wilkins RH. Cranial nerve dysfunction syndromes: evidence for microvascular compression. In: Barrow D, ed. *Surgery of the cranial nerves of the posterior fossa.* Park Ridge, IL: American Association of Neurological Surgeons, 1993:155–163.
45. Liao JJ, Cheng WC, Chang CN, et al. Reoperation for recurrent trigeminal neuralgia after microvascular decompression. *Surg Neurol* 1997;47:562–570.
46. Magnan J, Caces F, Locatelli P, et al. Hemifacial spasm: endoscopic vascular decompression. *Otolaryngol Head Neck Surg* 1997;117:308–314.

# 13

# ENDOSCOPIC SURGERY OF THE PITUITARY AND PARASELLAR REGION

HAREL DEUTSCH
WESLEY A. KING
PHILLIP A. WACKYM

## INDICATIONS

The development of endoscopic equipment and procedures has revolutionized the treatment of diseases in many surgical specialties. Endoscopic techniques enable smaller incisions and less tissue destruction, resulting in quicker postoperative recovery, increased patient satisfaction, and shorter hospital stays. Technologic advances in endoscopic equipment provide higher magnification and excellent illumination. Various angled endoscopes allow visualization of structures not previously accessible to surgeons. Techniques and indications for endoscopic surgery are being rapidly advanced in many surgical fields.

Schloffer and Hochenegg performed the first successful transsphenoidal surgery in 1908 in Vienna. Harvey Cushing perfected the transsphenoidal approach for sellar lesions in 1910 but abandoned the procedure in favor of open craniotomies because of the transsphenoidal approach's limited exposure. The incorporation of the operative microscope by Hardy and intraoperative fluoroscopy by Giout resulted in the transsphenoidal procedure's resurgence (Fig. 13.1).

Endoscopic transsphenoidal surgery may be performed for all the indications of the standard approach. Lesions accessible include microadenomas, macroadenomas, intrasellar cysts, and sellar metastasis. Patients with pituitary adenomas should be screened for hypopituitarism and for the oversecretion of pituitary hormones. Formal visual field testing is done to exclude compression of the optic chiasm. Patients with normal visual fields and normal hormone levels may be followed yearly with serial magnetic resonance imaging (MRI) scans. Surgery is indicated in patients with visual disturbances, hormone deficiencies, increasing tumor size, and uncertain diagnosis. Surgery is indicated for all patients with adenomas secreting adrenocorticotropic hormone (ACTH), thyroid-stimulating hormone (TSH), and growth hormone (GH). A significant reduction of morbidity can be achieved with surgical cure of ACTH, TSH, and GH oversecretion. Dopamine agonists are the preferred treatment for microprolactinomas and macroprolactinomas. Tumor shrinkage and normalization of hormone levels are achieved in most patients. Surgery is indicated for patients with prolactinomas not responsive to dopamine agonist therapy. Surgery is also indicated in patients who cannot tolerate dopamine agonist therapy.

## CONTRAINDICATIONS

Appropriate patient selection is essential for obtaining a good outcome. Endoscopic pituitary surgery contraindications are similar to contraindications for the standard transsphenoidal approach. Patients with sphenoid sinus infections should not undergo transsphenoidal surgery because of the risk of intracranial spread of infection and meningitis. The patient's anatomy can dictate the choice of operative procedure. Extremely small nares or multiseptated sphenoid sinuses may limit the surgeon's ability to maneuver the endoscope. Incomplete pneumatization of the sphenoid sinus may also contraindicate an endoscopic approach.

Tumor morphology may dictate the operative approach. Tumors with extensive suprasellar extension may require a craniotomy rather than a transsphenoidal approach. The tumor's consistency influences the surgical outcome. Most adenomas have a soft consistency and are easily and safely removed. Firm tumors can be difficult to remove using the transsphenoidal approach. Adequate preoperative radiologic evaluation is essential because of the wide range of pathologies found in the sella. For example, the misdiagnosis of an aneurysm as an adenoma can result in a potentially fatal complication. A vascular anomaly in the sella region may represent a contraindication for the transsphenoidal approach.

## PREOPERATIVE EVALUATION

Preoperative evaluation is essentially identical to the standard transsphenoidal procedure. The normal pituitary

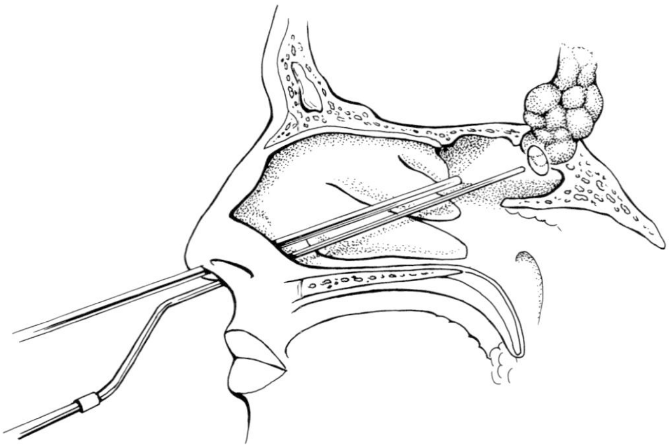

**FIGURE 13.1.** Illustration of the endoscopic transsphenoidal approach to the sella.

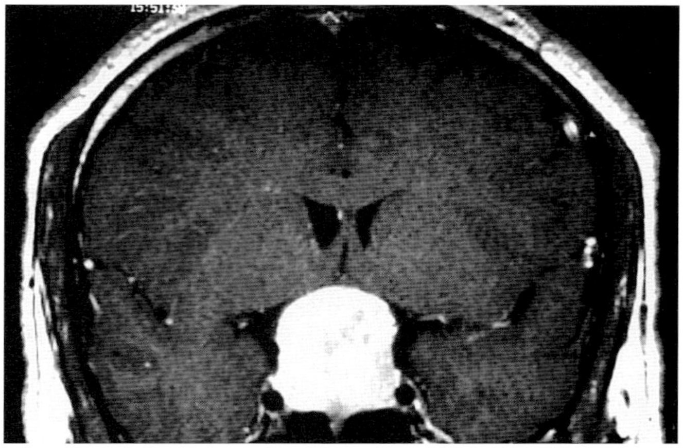

**FIGURE 13.2.** Coronal magnetic resonance imaging with gadolinium demonstrates a pituitary macroadenoma with compression of the optic chiasm.

gland is composed of an adenohypophysis and a neurohypophysis. The adenohypophysis originates as a diverticulum from the primitive foregut and contains the effector cells of the neuroendocrine system. The adenohypophysis is responsible for secreting eight hormones: GH, prolactin, follicle-stimulating hormone, luteinizing hormone, TSH, ACTH, melanocyte-stimulating hormone, and β-endorphin. Adenomas arising from endocrinologically active cells lead to hormone overproduction and associated syndromes. Large tumors place pressure on normal adenohypophysis cells and result in decreased hormone production. A detailed history and physical examination should be performed, and patients should be examined for any evidence of Cushing's disease, acromegaly, hyperthyroidism, or hypothyroidism. A full endocrine panel, including cortisol levels, TSH, thyroxine ($T_4$), testosterone, and prolactin levels should be assessed and appropriate replacement initiated before surgery. Formal visual field testing is important to establish whether a macroadenoma is exerting significant pressure on the optic chiasm.

A high-resolution MRI scan with and without intravenous gadolinium and special coronal and sagittal views of the pituitary are essential to delineate the sella anatomy. Some endoscopic surgeons also favor a high-resolution computed tomography (CT) scan of the sphenoid and sella to better assess the bony anatomy of the sphenoid (1).

## CASE EXAMPLE

A 52-year-old man presented with a chief complaint of headaches and blurry vision. His history was significant for approximately 9 months of diminished libido and worsening impotence. He also complained of generalized fatigue and decreased appetite. Physical examination findings were notable for a blood pressure of 110/60 mm Hg and bilateral gynecomastia. The patient demonstrated no cushingoid or acromegalic features.

Laboratory testing demonstrated a testosterone level of 123 ng/dL (normal range, 300 to 1,100 ng/dL), $T_4$ of 3 μg/dL (4 to 12 μg/dL), TSH of 12 mU/mL (0.5 to 5.0 mU/mL), and prolactin level of 58 ng/mL (<10 ng/mL). The somatomedin C level was normal. Visual field analysis demonstrated bitemporal hemianopsia. A brain MRI demonstrated a large sellar mass with suprasellar extension and compression of the optic chiasm (Fig. 13.2). The diagnosis of a clinically nonfunctioning pituitary adenoma was made.

The patient was scheduled for elective endoscopic transsphenoidal decompression. The patient tolerated the surgery and was discharged to his home on postoperative day 2. The patient noticed an immediate improvement in

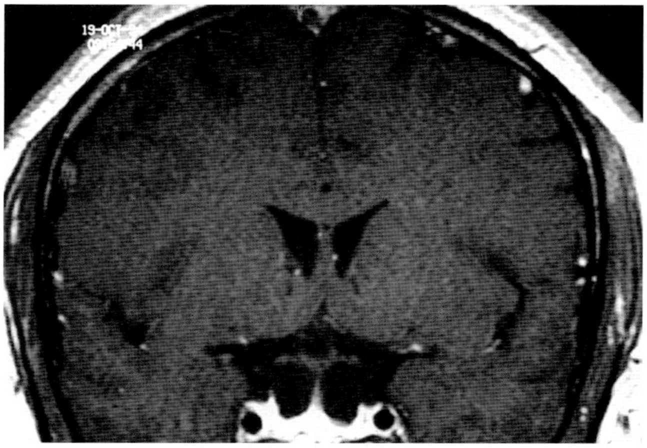

**FIGURE 13.3.** Postoperative coronal magnetic resonance imaging demonstrates complete tumor resection. The optic chiasm is well decompressed.

his vision. An MRI performed 3 months postoperatively demonstrated complete tumor resection (Fig. 13.3).

## INSTRUMENTATION

Several endoscopic approaches to the pituitary and parasellar region have been described, ranging from purely endoscopic to the standard transsphenoidal approaches with endoscope assistance. Instrumentation varies with the approach, and new instrumentation is being developed as endoscopic transnasal approaches gain popularity.

Most operations are performed using a 17-cm-long, 4-mm, 0° endoscope (Karl Storz, Culver City, CA). Additional 30° and 70° telescopes can provide oblique views into the sinuses and lateral walls of the sphenoid and sella, facilitating complete tumor resection. The 2.7-mm endoscopes can be used in children or patients with small nares, but optical resolution and illumination are reduced. Smaller scopes are also more fragile. Autoirrigation units can be used to keep the endoscopic lens free of blood. Self-retaining holders (Mediflex, Islandia, NY) are available to hold the endoscope in place and allow the surgeon to operate with both hands (Fig. 13.4).

The same instruments used in the standard microsurgical approach can be used for the endoscopic approach to the pituitary. Instruments employed in endoscopic sinus surgery systems are also useful in endoscopic approaches to the pituitary. Instruments designed specifically for endoscopic pituitary use are being developed (2). Standard equipment includes Frazier tip suctions in sizes of 3 to 9 French, forceps, Kerrison pituitary rongeurs, and curettes. Powered drills introduced endoscopically can be used to drill the floor of the sella.

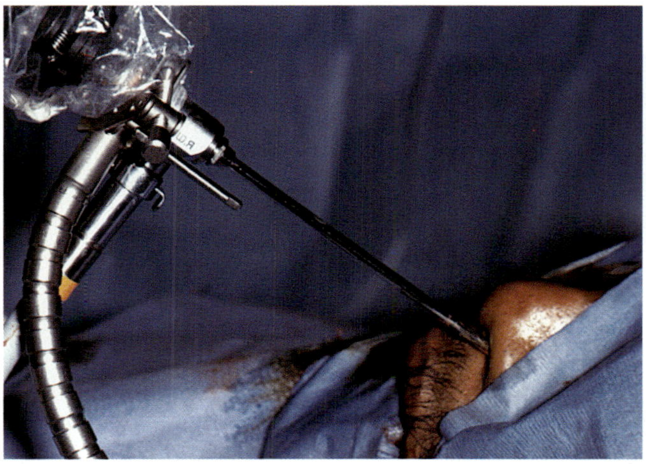

**FIGURE 13.4.** Self-retaining holders maintain the endoscope in place and allow the surgeon to operate with both hands. Alternatively, a surgical assistant may hold the endoscope.

## OPERATING ROOM LAYOUT

The patient is placed supine on an x-ray–compatible operating table under general anesthesia and endotracheal intubation (Fig. 13.5). The patient's head is placed in a three-point head-fixation system and tilted to the right with slight extension. The surgeon stands to the patient's right side, with an assistant to the surgeon's left. The scrub technician stands to the surgeon's right side and toward the foot of the table. The video monitor is positioned on the opposite side from the surgeon (i.e., on the patient's left side). The anesthesiologist and anesthesia equipment are positioned at the foot of the bed. A fluoroscopic C-arm is advanced to allow for lateral skull fluoroscopic images.

## ANESTHESIA

General endotracheal intubation with general anesthesia is used for endoscopic approaches to the pituitary and sella. Special armored tubing and positioning of the endotracheal tube in the right mouth corner is required to allow the surgeon complete access to the nose. The oropharyngeal cavity is packed with povidone-iodine–saturated gauze.

## OPERATIVE TECHNIQUE

The face and nares are prepared using a 5% povidone-iodine solution, and the abdomen is prepped for possible harvesting of a fat graft. Nasal mucosa vasoconstriction is achieved with topical Afrin and lidocaine with 1:100,000 epinephrine injected in the lateral wall of the nose, middle turbinate, uncinate process, and inferior turbinate. Blunt dissection is used to medialize the middle turbinate, allowing better visualization of the uncinate process (Fig. 13.6). The uncinate process is removed with rongeurs, exposing the bulla ethmoidalis. Sharp and blunt dissection is used to perform a complete ethmoidectomy (3). The posterior half of the middle turbinate is removed to increase the exposure. The sphenoid sinus generally lies behind the medioinferior quadrant of the posterior ethmoid wall. Probing with a suction or Freer elevator is used to identify the sphenoid sinus ostia. A small, oblique ridge of bone on the anterior wall of the sphenoid process lies laterally to the natural ostia of the sphenoid sinus (Fig. 13.7). Lateral fluoroscopy is used to confirm the correct location and trajectory (4) (Fig. 13.8).

The natural ostium is enlarged using pituitary Kerrison rongeurs or sphenoid punches. Most of the sphenoid anterior wall is removed to allow passage of the endoscope and instrumentation. The mucosa within the sinus is removed with rongeurs and blunt dissection, exposing the posterior sphenoid sinus wall and sella floor. The pituitary fossa is entered through the anteroinferior face. Opening too far forward results in entering the anterior cranial fossa. In

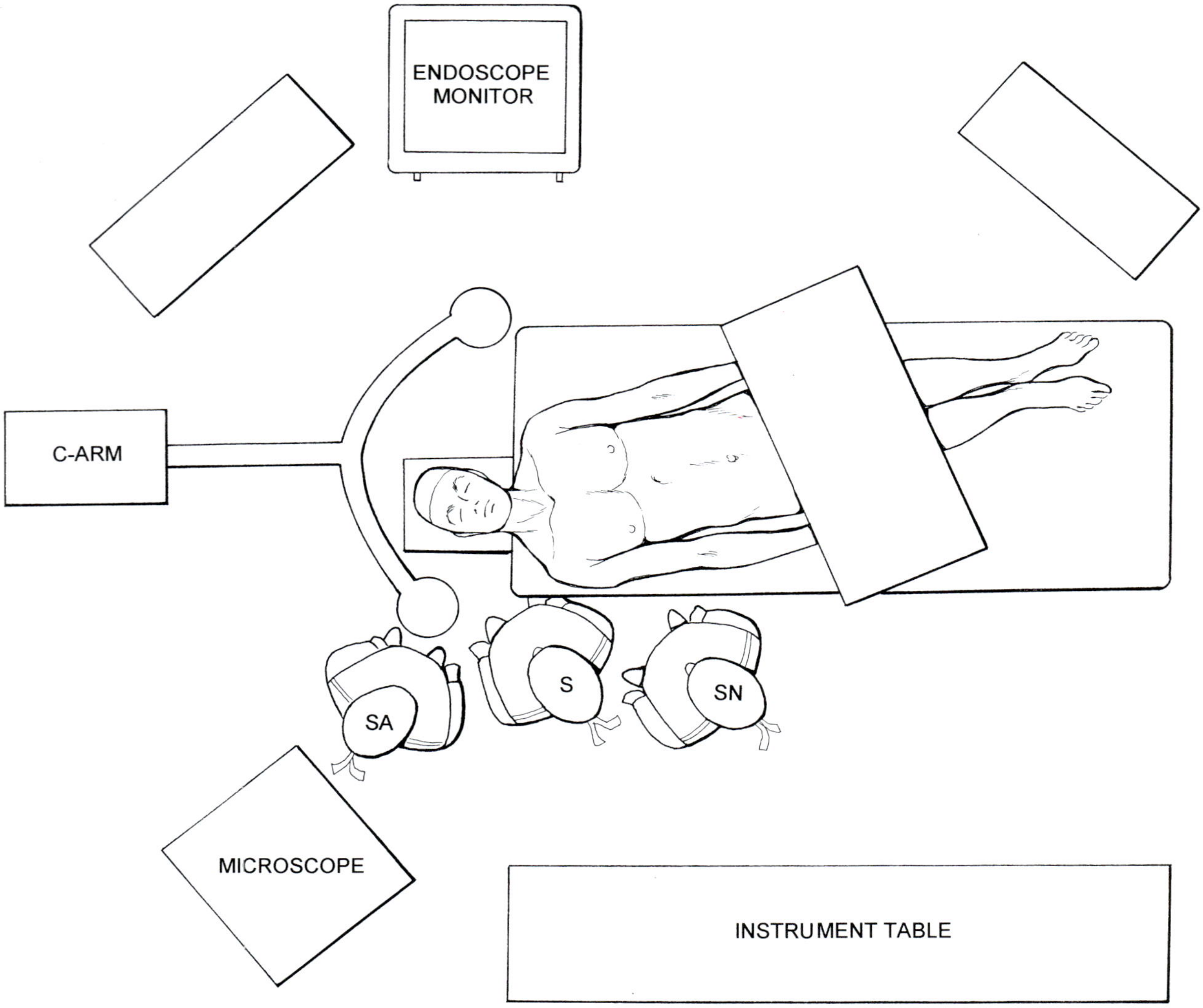


**FIGURE 13.5.** A typical operating room layout with the surgeon *(S)* at the patient's right side and with the surgical assistant *(SA)* positioned toward the head of the table and the scrub nurse *(SN)* positioned to the surgeon's right side. The fluoroscopic C-arm is positioned preoperatively to aid in intraoperative localization.

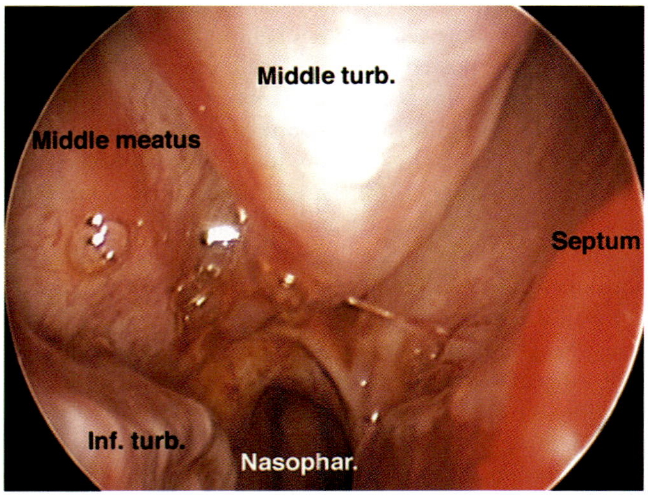


**FIGURE 13.6.** Initial introduction of the endoscope brings the middle turbinate, inferior turbinate, and septum into view.

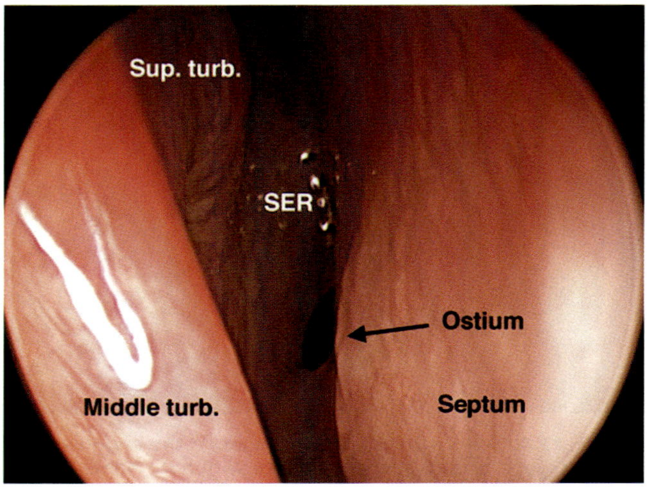


**FIGURE 13.7.** Displacing the middle turbinate laterally reveals the sphenoid ostium in the posterior sphenoethmoidal recess *(SER)* medial to the superior turbinate.

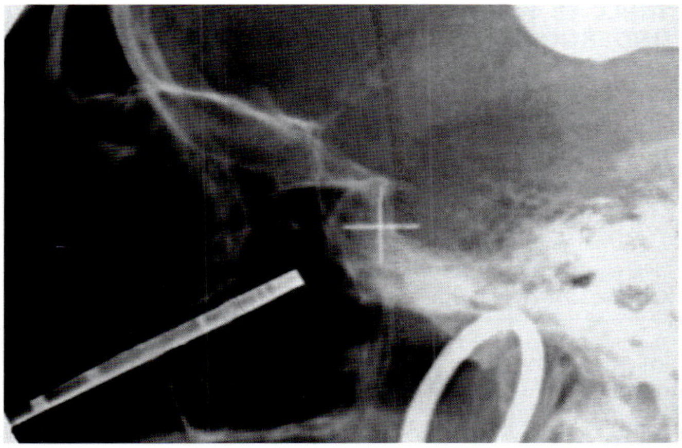

**FIGURE 13.8.** Intraoperative lateral fluoroscopic image confirms the endoscope's appropriate location near the sella *(cross).*

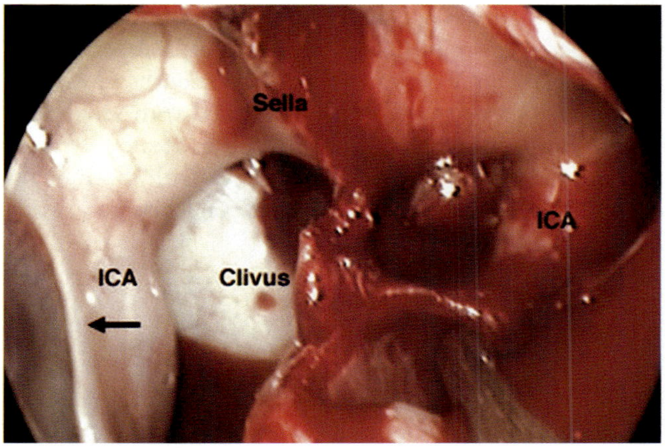


**FIGURE 13.10.** This intraoperative picture shows the carotid prominence of the carotid artery *(ICA)* in the lateral wall of the sphenoid sinus and the clivus posteriorly. An oblique septation *(arrow)* may be associated with the carotid canal.

cases of macroadenomas, the sella floor may be significantly thinned and can be opened simply with an osteotome or rongeur. Otherwise, small, high-speed drills with extended bits can be used.

At this point, the dura is coagulated with a bipolar cautery, and a cruciate incision is made using a scalpel. The tumor generally is removed using suction and various angled curettes (Fig. 13.9). As the tumor is removed, the endoscope is advanced into the empty pituitary fossa. Additional 30° and 70° angled telescopes are used to visualize the entire sella and ensure complete resection and avoidance of important structures such as the cavernous sinus and internal carotid arteries (Fig. 13.10). After tumor removal, hemostasis is secured. If cerebrospinal fluid (CSF) is seen during the operation, the sella is packed with a fat graft harvested from the abdomen. No nasal packing is required.

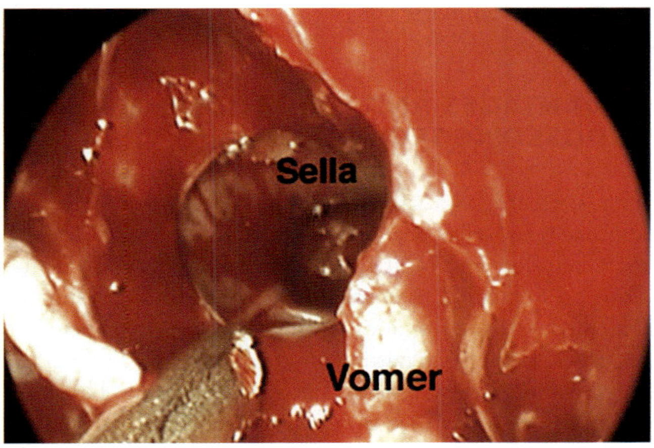


**FIGURE 13.9.** After enlargement of the sphenoid ostium the sphenoid sinus and the anterior wall of the sella are well visualized.

## SPECIAL POINTS

With practice, exposure of the sella can be achieved significantly faster than with standard microsurgical techniques. The decreased nasal dissection involved obviates the need for postoperative nasal packing and the associated postoperative patient discomfort. The angled endoscopes allow a full sella view, and surgery does not require blind dissection for tumor resection.

## POSTOPERATIVE CARE

Endoscopic transsphenoidal surgery is generally well tolerated by patients, who have few significant complications. Patients typically only remain in the hospital for 1 to 3 days. Most patients who do not demonstrate any evidence of diabetes insipidus (DI) are discharged home on postoperative day 1. All patients are placed on low replacement doses of steroids (1 mg of Decadron given twice daily) until endocrine evaluation demonstrates adequate serum cortisol levels. Patients are carefully instructed to be cognizant of the possibility of a CSF leak and its associated dangers.

Normalization of hormone levels while preserving normal pituitary function is the goal of therapy in endocrinologically active tumors. For prolactinomas, the goal of therapy is the normalization of prolactin levels to less than 25 ng/mL for at least 5 years. Galactorrhea should cease, and normal menstrual periods should resume. The purpose of surgery in Cushing's disease is to eliminate inappropriate secretion of ACTH and to preserve normal pituitary function. Satisfactory results in treating GH-secreting tumors include clinical improvements in the symptoms and signs of acromegaly and a fall in serum GH values to less than 2 ng/mL during a glucose tolerance test. Approximately 50%

to 70% of patients operated on for pituitary macroadenomas experience an improvement in vision postoperatively.

An MRI scan is typically obtained 3 months postoperatively. Residual adenoma can be followed with serial MRI scans, and recurrent tumor growth can be treated by reoperation or radiation therapy. Patients with hormonally active tumors undergo an endocrine evaluation to assess if further treatment is required.

## COMPLICATIONS

Endoscopic transsphenoidal surgery can be performed with extremely low mortality and low morbidity (5–8). Anesthetic complications in transsphenoidal surgery are rare. Patients with pituitary lesions are often deficient in one or more pituitary hormones. A comprehensive preoperative endocrine analysis is essential, and adequate stress doses of steroids should be given. Postoperatively, the patients' endocrine status should be followed carefully. Other medical complications are relatively rare and are commensurate with complications in other elective procedures.

Vascular injuries represent serious morbidities and can lead to death. Intraoperative mucosal bleeding and delayed postoperative bleeding can occur from the mucosal branch of the sphenopalatine artery. Damage to the carotid arteries, although rare, can occur in the sphenoid sinus or in the sella. Maintaining a midline trajectory during surgery is essential to avoiding carotid injury. Preoperative radiologic studies are essential in localizing the carotid artery. There are significant variations in the carotid's sellar course, and the distance between the two arteries can be only 4 mm or less. Heavy arterial bleeding signals intraoperative injury to the carotid artery, and the only treatment involves packing the operative field. Carotid artery injury can result in subarachnoid hemorrhage, vasospasm, false aneurysms, and carotid cavernous fistulas. A postoperative cerebral angiogram is essential to identify any of these complications. Approximately 25% of deaths occurring during standard transsphenoidal surgeries are attributable to vascular injuries (9).

Visual disturbances are also possible because of the close association of the chiasm, optic nerve, and the pituitary. Damage can occur through direct trauma, traction injury, or vascular compromise. Tumor bed hematomas can lead to postoperative visual loss. Injuries to the hypothalamus can also occur and may result in death. These patients are comatose and exhibit hyperthermia. Hypothalamic injury represents the most common cause of death in transsphenoidal surgeries.

In the postoperative period, several complications can be anticipated. Early recognition and appropriate treatment can circumvent catastrophic results. Patients should be closely monitored for DI with frequent serum sodium evaluations and careful accounting of patients' fluid intake and urine output. An elevated serum sodium level or excessive urine output may indicate DI, which results from manipulation of the pituitary stalk. Temporary postoperative DI occurs in 10% to 20% of standard microsurgical transsphenoidal cases. Permanent DI is much less common, occurring in 0.5% to 5% of patients. Delayed onset of the syndrome of inappropriate antidiuretic hormone can also occur about a week postoperatively, but it is unusual.

**TABLE 13.1. COMPLICATIONS IN 50 PATIENTS UNDERGOING ENDOSCOPIC TRANSSPHENOIDAL SURGERY**

| Complication | No. of Patients |
|---|---|
| Cerebrospinal fluid | 2 |
| Diabetes insipidus | |
| Temporary | 2 |
| Permanent | 1 |
| Decreased anterior pituitary function | 6 |
| Chronic sphenoidal sinusitis | 1 |

Jho HD, Carrau RL. Endoscopic endonasal transsphenoidal surgery: experience with 50 patients. *J Neurosurg* 1997;87:44–51, with permission.

Postoperative anterior pituitary insufficiency is one of the most commonly seen postoperative complications. Postoperative steroid therapy should be used in all postoperative patients until a thorough endocrine evaluation is complete. Adrenal insufficiency is a potentially serious complication if adequate steroid replacement therapy is not initiated (Table 13.1).

Cerebrospinal fluid rhinorrhea is another commonly encountered complication of the transsphenoidal approach. Patients developing CSF rhinorrhea are first treated using spinal drainage for several days. Failure to close the CSF fistulas using spinal drainage may indicate the need for reoperation with repair of the sella. Early recognition and treatment of CSF rhinorrhea is important because a CSF leak can lead to meningitis (10).

## ADVANTAGES AND LIMITATIONS OF THE ENDOSCOPIC TECHNIQUE

The standard transsphenoidal operation is an effective approach to sellar lesions and can be performed with extremely low morbidity. However, the approach's limitations are remedied to some extent by endoscopic surgery. The most serious limitation of the standard transsphenoidal approach is the very narrow surgical corridor. The narrow corridor limits the lateral and rostrocaudal view. This limitation can result in incomplete tumor resection or inadvertent injury to adjacent structures. The endoscope's short (5- to 15-mm) focal length enables a panoramic view of the sella with excellent magnification and illumination superior to the operative microscope. Angled scopes allow the surgeon to view the lateral parasellar and suprasellar compartments. Much of the dissection involved in standard transsphenoidal surgery is done blindly, and the most significant mortalities associated with the transsphenoidal surgery result from inadvertent injury to the hypothalamus or carotid arteries. The improved sellar visualization possible with the endoscope can reduce carotid and hypothalamus injury.

The standard transsphenoidal approach may employ a sublabial or nasal incision, which is occasionally associated with septal perforations, nasal deformities, or denervation or devascularization of the teeth. The approach can also be performed through the nostril, but the requirement of a nasal speculum further reduces the exposure and illumination. The endoscopic approach obviates the need for extensive intranasal dissection and therefore avoids the associated nasal and dental complications.

Although the endoscope offers many advantages to the transsphenoidal operation, it also has several disadvantages. The lack of a stereoscopic view with depth perception is a limitation of the endoscope. Stereoscopic scopes are being developed, but they potentially will be larger and may have lower resolution. Bleeding is more difficult to deal with using the endoscope. Excessive bleeding may necessitate conversion to a standard microsurgical transsphenoidal operation. The patient's anatomy can dictate the choice of operative procedure. Extremely small nares or multiseptated sphenoid sinuses may limit the surgeon's ability to maneuver the endoscope. Incomplete pneumatization of the sphenoid sinus makes an endoscopic approach very difficult. Another disadvantage relative to the standard approach is the learning curve involved in endoscopic transsphenoidal surgery.

## LITERATURE REVIEW

The standard microsurgical approach to the sella is a safe and effective surgical treatment for pituitary lesions. The transsphenoidal approach's narrow exposure has always posed a problem, leading to the use of the endoscope as an adjuvant to the standard microsurgical approach (11,12). Griffith and Veerapen reported the first endonasal approach to the sella in 1987 (13). The microscope was eventually eliminated and the endoscope was used in conjunction with a speculum. The approach was very similar to the standard transsphenoidal approach, and the nasal and dental complications were similar. Newer developments have led to the introduction of a purely endoscopic approach without the speculum introduction and the potential for a less destructive approach and improved tumor visualization and resection (2,6).

The endoscopic transnasal approach is making the transition from an experimental procedure to a more mature technique. Early studies demonstrated endoscopic transnasal operations could be performed safely and effectively, producing results similar to those for standard microsurgical techniques (5–8). Studies are attempting to refine the instrumentation and techniques, as well as report innovative approaches (14,15).

Only recent reports have compared results of endoscopic transnasal techniques with the traditional transsphenoidal microsurgical approach to determine whether the endoscopic approach has a useful role. Sheehan and colleagues retrospectively reviewed 26 patients undergoing endoscopic transnasal pituitary macroadenoma resection and 44 matched control patients (16). They concluded surgical resection, anterior pituitary function, visual fields, and complications were not significantly different between the two groups. The endoscopic group did have a significantly reduced operative time of 2.7 hours compared with 3.4 hours for patients undergoing a sublabial approach.

Koren retrospectively compared 20 patients undergoing an endoscopic approach to the sella with 20 patients undergoing a sublabial approach (17). The endoscopic approach was associated with a shorter operative time, shorter hospitalization time, absence of recurrent epistaxis snoring and denture problems, and lower incidence of septal perforation. The loss of nasal tip projection was found only in the group that had sublabial standard surgery. Endoscopically guided transseptal transsphenoidal surgery was time saving and resulted in fewer nasal and denture complications than the sublabial technique.

Although endoscopic transnasal surgery is still in its infancy, several studies have demonstrated that it holds great promise in minimizing several morbidities and increasing patient satisfaction. Refinement of the technique and more studies comparing results against patients undergoing the standard microsurgical approach are required.

## REFERENCES


1. Jho HD, Carrau RL. Endoscopic endonasal transsphenoidal surgery: experience with 50 patients. *J Neurosurg* 1997;87: 44–51.
2. Cappabianca P, Alfieri A, Thermes S, et al. Instruments for endoscopic endonasal transsphenoidal surgery. *Neurosurgery* 1999;45: 392–395; discussion 395–396.
3. Levine H, May M, Rontal M. *Complex anatomy of the lateral nasal wall: simplified for the endoscopic sinus surgeon.* New York: Thieme Publishers, 1993.
4. Kennedy D, Zinreich S, Rosenbaum A. Functional endoscopic sinus surgery: theory and diagnostic evaluation. *Arch Otolaryngol* 1985;111:576–582.
5. Jho HD, Carrau RL, Ko Y, et al. Endoscopic pituitary surgery: an early experience. *Surg Neurol* 1997;47:213–222; discussion 222–223.
6. Jho HD, Carrau RL. Endoscopy assisted transsphenoidal surgery for pituitary adenoma: technical note. *Acta Neurochir* 1996;138: 1416–1425.

7. Sethi DS, Pillay PK. Endoscopic management of lesions of the sella turcica. *J Laryngol Otol* 1995;109:956–962.
8. Heilman CB, Shucart WA, Rebeiz EE. Endoscopic sphenoidotomy approach to the sella. *Neurosurgery* 1997;41:602–607.
9. Black P, Zervas N, Candia G. Incidence and management of complications of transsphenoidal operation for pituitary adenomas. *Neurosurgery* 1987;20:920–924.
10. Teo C, Rahman S, Boop F. Complications of endoscopic neurosurgery. *Childs Nerv Syst* 1996;12:248–253.
11. Helal MZ. Combined micro-endoscopic trans-sphenoid excisions of pituitary macroadenomas. *Eur Arch Otorhinolaryngol* 1995;252:186–189.
12. Helal M. Combined micro-endoscopic transsphenoid excisions of pituitary macroadenomas. *Eur Arch Otorhinolaryngol* 1995; 252:186–189.
13. Griffith H, Veerapen R. A direct transnasal approach to the sphenoid sinus: technical note. *J Neurosurg* 1987;66:140–142.
14. Yaniv E, Rappaport ZH. Endoscopic transseptal transsphenoidal surgery for pituitary tumors. *Neurosurgery* 1997;40:944–946.
15. Rodziewicz GS, Kelley RT, Kellman RM, et al. Transnasal endoscopic surgery of the pituitary gland: technical note. *Neurosurgery* 1996;39:189–192; discussion 192–193.
16. Sheehan MT, Atkinson JL, Kasperbauer JL, et al. Preliminary comparison of the endoscopic transnasal vs the sublabial transseptal approach for clinically nonfunctioning pituitary macroadenomas. *Mayo Clin Proc* 1999;74:661–670.
17. Koren I, Hadar T, Rappaport ZH, et al. Endoscopic transnasal transsphenoidal microsurgery versus the sublabial approach for the treatment of pituitary tumors: endonasal complications. *Laryngoscope* 1999;109:1838–1840.

# 14

# ADJUNCTIVE USE OF ENDOSCOPY IN ANTERIOR CRANIAL BASE SURGERY

IBRAHIM SABIT
WILLIAM T. COULDWELL

## EVOLUTION OF MINIMALLY INVASIVE NEUROSURGICAL TECHNIQUES

### Historical Aspects

At the beginning of the twentieth century, large craniotomies were required to gain access to intracranial pathology and carried with them excessively high morbidity and mortality rates. This was largely unavoidable because of the limitations of poor preoperative diagnostic methods that failed to detect pathologic conditions until they had reached critical sizes. The poor intraoperative illumination and large surgical instruments that were tailored more for general surgery than neurosurgery required large craniotomies to allow adequate visualization of and access to the lesions. Despite the tremendous advances in neurosurgery during the past two decades, the fear of undergoing a "brain operation" is a direct result of these early practices of neurosurgery and the morbidity that was associated with them.

During the past century, surgery in general and neurosurgery in particular witnessed a dramatic increase in the emphasis on reducing preoperative and intraoperative traumatization of patients to decrease morbidity and mortality. This is evident in the introduction of the operating microscope with its superior illumination of the field, development of microneurosurgical techniques and instrumentation, neuronavigational systems, stereotactic neurosurgery, and intraoperative electrophysiologic monitoring, all of which have been of paramount importance in minimization of the trauma associated with brain surgery.

Concomitantly, advances in preoperative diagnostic methods such as computed tomography (CT), magnetic resonance imaging (MRI), use of contrast material in imaging, three-dimensional reconstruction images, and angiography have aided in determining with ever-increasing accuracy the size and location of intracranial lesions. Equally critical is the ability of these preoperative diagnostic tools to reduce intraoperative complications by providing meticulous details of the area involved and elucidating variations in normal anatomy. This preoperative knowledge of the details of the individual normal and pathologic anatomy of each patient has allowed the surgical approach to be conducted with minimal brain retraction and trauma, maximal access to the lesion, and avoidance of unnecessarily large craniotomies. In effect, this tailoring of the surgical approach to the individual patient was made possible by the improved diagnostic tools and better surgical equipment, and it has given rise to the frequently employed but not often understood concept of *keyhole microneurosurgery*.

### Keyhole Concept in Neurosurgery

Keyhole microsurgery is the realization par excellence of minimally invasive neurosurgery. Keyhole approaches refer to the ability to target a specific intracranial area with maximum efficacy while minimizing the size of the craniotomy required to achieve adequate exposure. A comparison is given between the sizes of atypical bone flap during a keyhole approach (usually 2 cm in diameter) and a standard craniotomy with an average flap of 7 to 8 cm in diameter. Using the rule of $A = \pi r^2$ for the area of a circle (r = radius of a circle), compare the area of 3.14 $cm^2$ obtained for the amount of exposure during a keyhole approach with the 38.46 $cm^2$ area for a standard craniotomy 7 cm in diameter—an area approximately 12.2 times greater is employed during the standard craniotomy!

The driving logic for the concept of keyhole microsurgery is that the size of the optic field is directly proportional to distance. A superficially lying meningioma would require a craniotomy that is at least as large as the lesion itself. By the same token, the size of a craniotomy required for a deep-seated basilar tip aneurysm could be smaller than the actual lesion itself. It is usually the size of the instrument that determines the extent of craniotomy, not the lesion itself, in keyhole microsurgery.

With the advances in preoperative diagnostic tools, the surgical team can be armed with the necessary information for targeting a specific intracranial location through the most size-effective anatomic window to reduce iatrogenic intraoperative trauma. A clear extrapolation of this concept is the absolute necessity of understanding the anatomy of the target region to safely take advantage of the existing anatomic corridors. Performed efficiently by the hands of an experienced team, keyhole approaches can significantly reduce the size of the craniotomy required, minimize brain and neural tissue retraction, and decrease the tension on important vascular structures.

## Technical Considerations in Endoscope-Assisted Microneurosurgery

Despite the clear advantages of using a keyhole approach in cranial base surgery, the technique still posseses significant disadvantages from an optical standpoint. By minimizing the size of the craniotomy, a marked narrowing of viewing angles and a decrease in the light intensity often hamper adequate visualization through the operating microscope. Consequently, important anatomic structures that lie in the penumbra of the light source are hidden from view (Fig. 14.1). This significant reduction of light-source intensity is particularly notable under high magnification because of the inverse optical relationship between magnification and brightness of field in the modern microscope. The adjunctive use of the endoscope has proved to be valuable in overcoming these shortcomings of keyhole approaches in neurosurgery. The operating endoscope effectively introduces increased light intensity to the operating field (250- to 350-W xenon light sources) and offers excellent visualization of the anatomic details through the advanced optics of the endoscope. Through the fish-eye effect of the endoscope, extended viewing angles allow the surgeon to "look around the corners" to examine vital structures hidden from the view of the microscope (Fig. 14.2). Rigid endoscopes are the most widely used in microneurosurgery because the quality of the optics in rigid endoscopes (lens scopes) are far superior to those employed in flexible endoscopes and because rigid endoscopes can be mounted on the headrest with retractor arms. The latter reason is particularly important because of the small cranial openings employed during keyhole approaches. By mounting the rigid microscope, a simultaneous view of the operating field can be obtained from the microscope and the endoscope while not interfering with the high degree of coaxial control of microinstrument manipulation required to safely perform the surgery. To this end, methods of image projection from the neuroscope can be tailored to suit the surgeon's needs.

Hopf and Perneczky devised terminology for the use of the endoscope in intracranial neurosurgery (1,2). The endoscope can be used alone or in conjunction with the operating microscope. In the latter method, images from the operating microscope and the endoscope can be alternated on a monitor and provide the most economic method to view both modalities. The route for surgical manipulation may be through the endoscope or outside the endoscope. Accordingly, they suggested categorizing the procedure as *endoscopic neurosurgery* (EN; endoscope used alone with surgical manipulation through the endoscope), *endoscope-assisted microneurosurgery* (EAM; endoscope used in con-

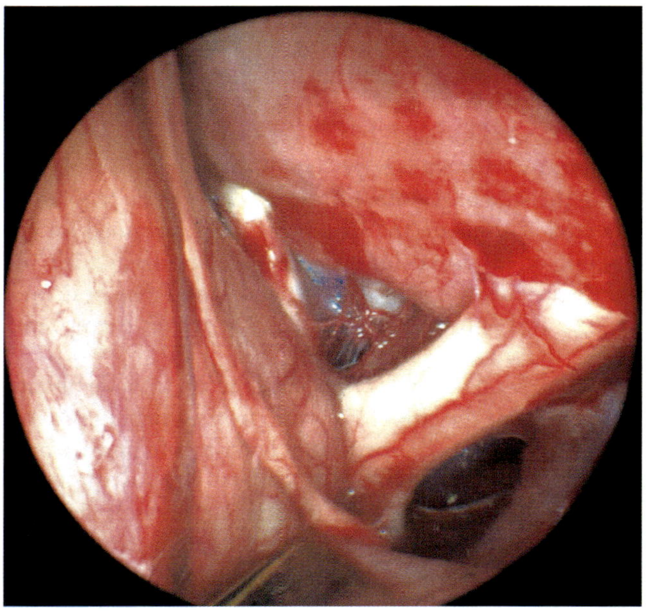

**FIGURE 14.1.** Standard surgeon's view through the binocular operating microscope, demonstrating the details of the suprasellar structures through an anterior keyhole approach. Notice the optic nerves, optic chiasm, and the pituitary stalk that is just visible to the left of the right optic nerve. The right internal carotid artery is adjacent and lateral to the right optic nerve.

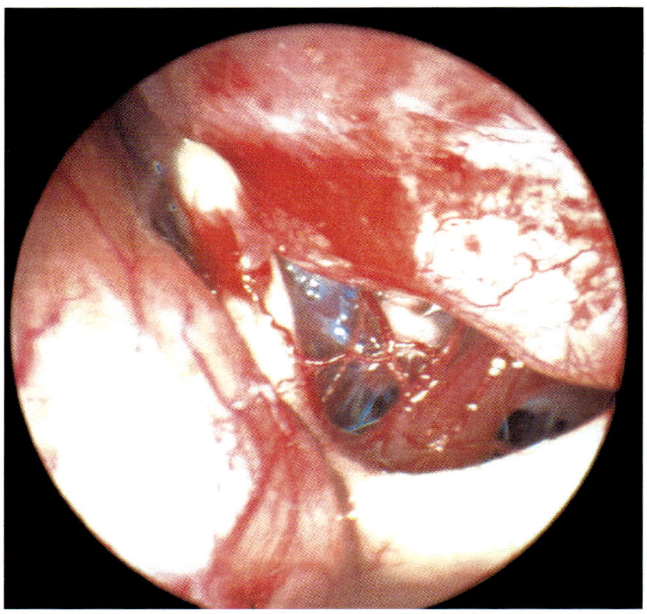

**FIGURE 14.2.** Similar view to that in Figure 14.1, but it is taken through the 0° endoscope. By advancing the endoscope, increased visualization of the pituitary stalk is possible.

junction with the operating microscope), and *endoscope-controlled microneurosurgery* (ECM; endoscope used alone but operating outside the endoscope). With new technology and the increased interest in endoscope-assisted neurosurgery, the simultaneous integration of imagery from the microscope and the endoscope on a single monitor is possible (Twin-Video System, Storz, Tuttlingen, Germany) and is advocated for intracranial keyhole approaches.

The advances in endoscopic instrumentation and increased experience with keyhole approaches have enabled the application of these techniques to skull base surgery, largely under the guidance of the otolaryngology members of the skull base team. The anterior skull base is an excellent anatomic region for application of endoscopy because of the relative lack of important vascular and arterial structures that traverse the skull base in this region. The proximity of the anterior skull base to the paranasal sinuses makes it a favorable region for endoscopic access (2–10). In this chapter, we discuss the application of endoscopy to the paranasal sinuses and its use during open craniotomy to facilitate exposure and access to various pathologic processes of the anterior skull base and adjacent regions.

## ANTERIOR SKULL BASE ENDOSCOPIC ANATOMY

The anterior cranial fossa provides support for the orbital frontal lobes and for the olfactory bulb and tracts (Figs. 14.3–14.6). Most of the bony floor of the anterior cranial fossa is composed of the orbital portion of the frontal bones. These bones, which cover the orbits bilaterally, are separated by the frontal crest, crista galli, cribriform plate of the ethmoid bone, and planum sphenoidale from anterior to posterior, respectively. The foramen cecum lies immediately behind the frontal bone in the midline; the ethmoid bone forms the posterior and lateral boundaries of this foramen. The posterior floor region, composed of the planum sphenoidale in the midline and the lesser wings of the sphenoid laterally, is an important area surgically because it is a location for posterior-extending olfactory groove and planum meningiomas, traumatic fractures, and a landmark for approaches to the suprasellar region and optic canals. From a surgical standpoint, it is important to recognize that the anterior cranial fossa is not flat; the cribriform region may extend inferiorly some distance between the orbits and is the lowest part of the anterior cranial fossa. The cribriform plate exhibits a variable number of foramina, which transmit the olfactory rootlets, covered by a sleeve of dura mater and arachnoid membranes, in addition to branches of the ethmoidal arteries that originate from the ophthalmic artery. The orbital roofs themselves are often irregular in contour, and this is the reason in part for the subfrontal region of the brain having a predilection for contusion from head trauma, produced by translational movement of the base of the brain across the rough bony surface.

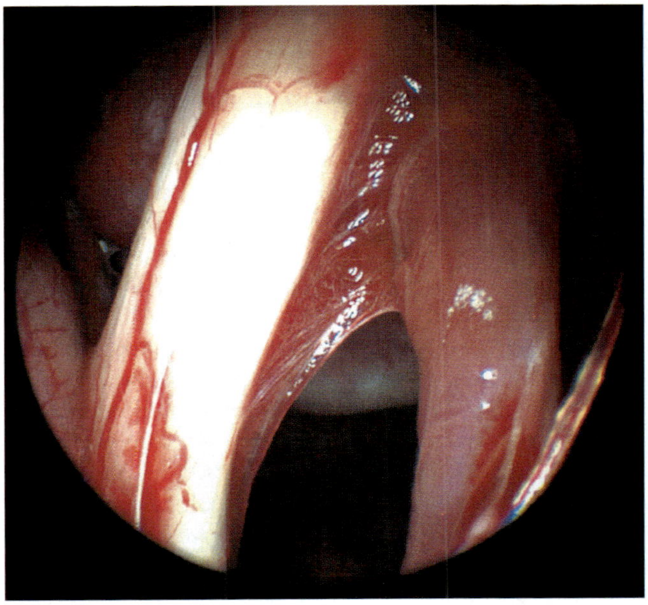

**FIGURE 14.3.** Endoscopic photograph taken of the opticocarotid cistern. The size of the endoscope permits placement of the surgeon's eye directly at the level of the cistern. Notice the right optic nerve and the carotid artery. The dorsum sellae is visualized posteriorly between these structures.

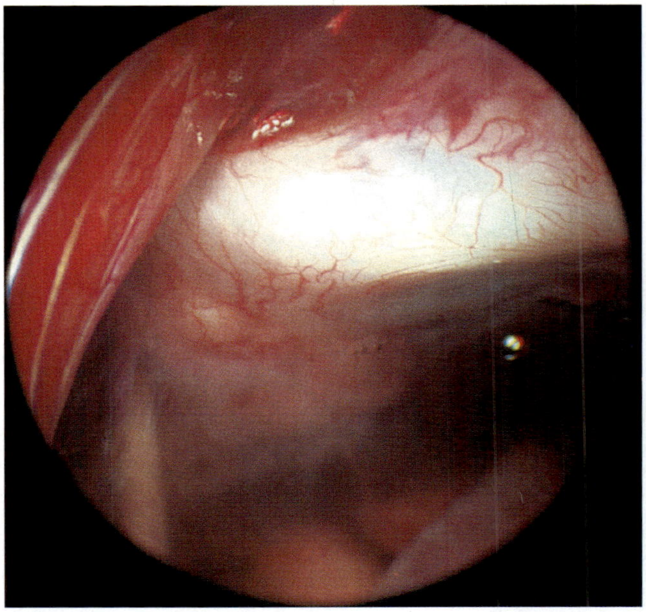

**FIGURE 14.4.** Endoscopic view through the opticocarotid cistern. The structure to the upper left is the pituitary stalk entering the diaphragma sellae. This particular view could not be obtained through a conventional microscope. Notice the contralateral oculomotor nerve at the 7 o'clock position and the basilar artery at the 5 o'clock position.

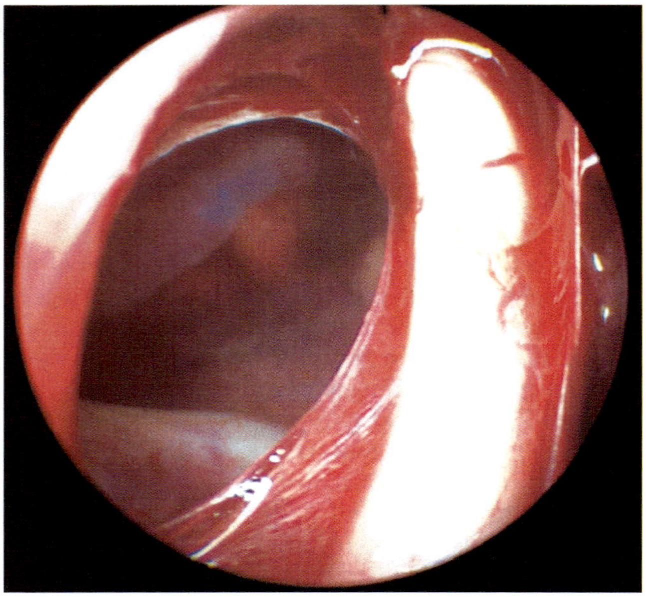

**FIGURE 14.5.** Endoscopic (0°) view of the ipsilateral third (oculomotor) nerve just lateral to the carotid artery. The surgeon may now see behind the carotid, a view not achievable with the standard operating microscope. The basilar artery is between the carotid and the third nerve in a deeper visual plane.

Direct access to the midline skull base may be obtained through the nasal cavity to the region of the cribriform plate and olfactory groove (11,12). More lateral exposure may be gained through the ethmoid sinuses and frontal sinuses. Posteriorly, endoscopy through the sphenoid sinus enables access to the anterior cranial fossa (through the planum sphenoidale) or the sella turcica. Laterally in the sphenoid, exposure is limited by the carotid arteries and their course in the lateral wall of the sphenoid sinus and the cavernous cranial nerves more superiorly at the level of the sella turcica and the cavernous sinus.

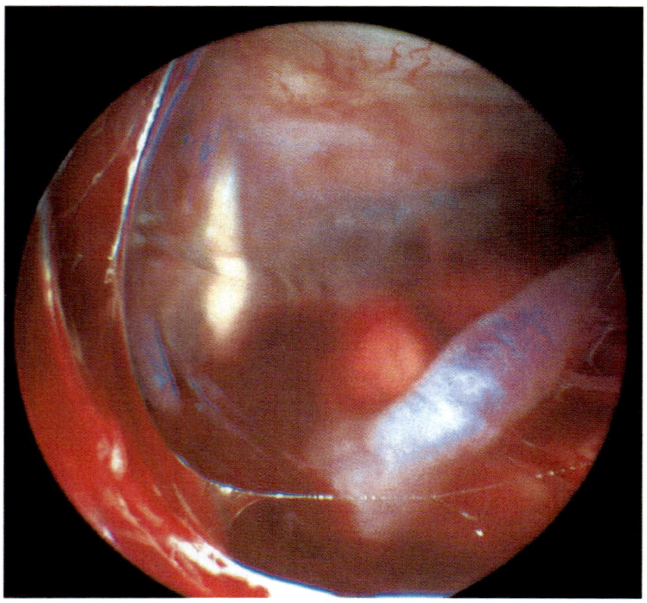

**FIGURE 14.6.** Endoscopic view beyond the optic nerves through the opticocarotid cistern. The basilar artery is clearly visualized in its upper and middle segments. The belly of the pons is seen beneath the basilar artery, and the contralateral oculomotor nerve is emerging from the interpeduncular cistern.

## APPLICATIONS OF ENDOSCOPY TO SURGERY OF THE ANTERIOR SKULL BASE

### Surgical Approaches to the Anterior Skull Base

To better illustrate the utility of the endoscope in surgery of the anterior skull base, a brief illustration of the procedures employed to gain access to this area of the cranial base is warranted. Traditionally, a standard bifrontal transbasal craniotomy has been the mainstay of the intracranial component of craniofacial resection. The patient is placed in a supine position with the head elevated 10° to 15°. Further elevation is contraindicated to avoid the risk of venous air embolism to the superior sagittal sinus in case it is violated or intentionally ligated during the course of the operation. The bone flap elevated depends on the exposure desired. For maximal exposure, a bifrontal flap is raised. The careful placement of bilateral burr holes at the keyhole region allows visualization of the anterior floor above the orbit. A low cut just above the floor provides maximum exposure of the floor with minimal bifrontal retraction (Fig. 14.2). For lesions with large posterior extensions for which access to the sphenoid sinus and clivus are desired, the extended transbasal approach provides excellent basal visualization. Supplementing the standard bifrontal approach with an orbitofrontal osteotomy to remove the orbital floor and supraorbital rims performs this. If only limited anterior skull base exposure is necessary, a unilateral variation of the bifrontal craniotomy, such as a unilateral frontotemporal flap, is performed. This is used to gain middle fossa exposure for extensive lesions involving the midline and unilateral middle fossa. Further anterior extension of this approach may be obtained by performing an orbitofrontal osteotomy.

A minimally invasive supraorbital keyhole approach was described by Cohen (13). The technique uses a small eyebrow incision, followed by a supraorbital craniotomy with a bone flap of only 2.5 cm × 1.5 cm, extending from the medial aspect of the supraorbital nerve to the frontal process of the zygomatic bone (Fig. 14.6). Several features of the supraorbital keyhole approach make it ideal for endoscopy-assisted neurosurgery. The anatomy of the suprasellar area offers clear advantages for an anterior keyhole approach. The area is bordered laterally by the temporal lobe and posteriorly by the mesencephalon. Any attempt to approach from those trajectories requires some degree of brain retraction. However, an anterior trajectory to the suprasellar region requires no brain retraction because of the presence of "anatomic corridors" between the carotid artery and the optic nerve, between the carotid and oculomotor nerve, and the existence of a subchiasmatic route. The endoscope is introduced through these windows to gain access to lesions in suprasellar and interpeduncular cisterns and to supratentorial aneurysms. Because the approach is not predefined anatomically, it has the broadest field of indications. Careful preoperative imaging enables the surgeon to tailor such an elegant "microapproach" for more medial (subfrontal) or more lateral (pterional) exposure. Like the extended transbasal approach, removal of the supraorbital rim may supplement the supraorbital craniotomy to afford more access to basal structures in more extreme cases. There is minimal or no brain retraction required, significantly decreasing intraoperative trauma. The benign skin incision, hidden in the eyebrow, together with the lack of bone defect from the craniotomy, provides excellent cosmetic results. The net effect is a shorter, less eventful hospital stay with an expedited return of the patient to employment.

## OPEN SURGICAL AND ENDOSCOPIC MANAGEMENT OF CEREBROSPINAL FLUID FISTULAS

Iatrogenic trauma is an important source of leaks, usually in the case of neurosurgical violation of the anterior skull base in the region of the cribriform plate, opening of the frontal sinus, or during transsphenoidal sellar approaches. Otolaryngologists are prone to encounter leaks through several intranasal or sinus procedures, such as during rasping of the nasofrontal duct or other frontal sinus, ethmoid, and mastoid operations. Because leakage of CSF may complicate any type of skull base procedure, meticulous attention must be paid to the reconstitution of a dural barrier to prevent the development of a fistula. Persistent CSF leakage may result in death from meningitis, other manifestations of infection such as encephalomyelitis or cerebral abscess, intracranial hemorrhage, pneumocephalus producing encephalopathy, and various cranial neuropathies, the most common of which is hearing loss.

The option to institute antimicrobial prophylaxis in the face of a CSF leak remains controversial. Although there is irrefutable evidence of a decrease in the rate of meningitis with their use, it must be tempered with the risk of selecting resistant organisms. The previously reported necessity of immediate surgical intervention in cases of traumatic or iatrogenic fistulas is probably not justified. A judicious period of expectant management should be attempted, with the time before surgical closure tailored to the offending pathology. The length of conservative trial is controversial, with opinions ranging from 1 to several weeks. In cases of nonpenetrating traumatic lesions *without radiographic evidence of a major traumatic bony disruption*, a substantial course of conservative trial is indicated. We routinely attempt such conservative therapy for a period of at least 1 week in the patient with an uncomplicated basilar skull fracture and CSF leak; in the patient with a compound skull fracture with cerebral violation or gross communication with paranasal sinuses, an earlier exploration with irrigation, débridement, and dural repair would be warranted.

In the event of decided surgical repair, the site of the leak should be meticulously localized radiographically. This is accomplished usually with the aid of MRI and CT scanning with bone windows (to localize any associated bony defect along the base) and possibly the addition of water-soluble contrast dye to visualize the leak. Dye accumulation in adjacent paranasal sinuses is an indication of the approximate site of the leak if a bony defect is not seen. Delayed scanning performed 3 to 12 hours later may be helpful if the leak is not visualized on the initial study. If this technique fails to disclose the site of the leak, intrathecal administration of fluorescein or radioactive tracers such as indium ($^{111}$In-DTPA) may be of help in detection.

The surgical options for exposure include a primary intracranial or extracranial approach. Extracranial approaches, performed with the skull base team, offer less morbidity than standard craniotomy and have instigated a trend in some centers toward these approaches as the initial surgical strategy in the repair of traumatic and some spontaneous anterior fossa leaks. One disadvantage is the increased difficulty in localizing the leak intraoperatively inherent to the limited exposure offered. However, the valuable assistance that modern imaging has offered in the precise localization of the fracture site in posttraumatic lesions has obviated much of the need for earlier exploratory intracranial procedures. We have found the use of intraoperative computer imaging guidance (Radionics, Burlington, MA) to be helpful in limiting the exposure and precisely targeting the region of the skull base. Other investigators and we advocate this as the method of choice for the repair of noncomminuted basal fractures. There have been claims of superior results to craniotomy using the extracranial approach when previous intracranial repair was unsuccessful. Excluding these excellent reports, the literature generally acknowledges a similar recurrence rate (20%) for the two approaches. Taken together, the extracranial approach is advocated if the leakage site can be visualized and is accessible; endoscopic extracranial exploration should be the procedure of choice in cases without extensive bony disruption. The technique used by our skull base team includes obliteration of the dural defect with a fascial graft, with direct placement of the fascial graft between the skull base and the surrounding dura, if possible, to facilitate a seal. Postoperative lumbar puncture or continuous spinal drainage is performed to reduce intracranial pressure and promote a graft seal.

Tutino and colleagues (10) documented the potential for complete extradural dissections of the anterior skull base dura performed endoscopically through trephine openings. This obviates the use of the bicoronal skin incision and bifrontal bone flap, which are the mainstay of a complete extradural anterior skull base exploration. The investigators defined the craniofacial anatomy by endoscope to determine the best approach for dissecting endocranial structures. With experience, this interesting approach also could be a method for addressing CSF leaks, which would enable closure of larger dural defects by direct extradural dissection and placement of fascial grafts.

## ENDOSCOPY AS AN ADJUVANT TO ANTERIOR SKULL BASE TUMOR RESECTION

There are specific circumstances in which the endoscope may be helpful in resection of tumors of the anterior skull base.

### Aid to Visualization of Important Neurovascular Structures

Decreased cerebral blood flow and elevated local tissue pressure in neurosurgical procedures have been directly attributed to brain retraction (14,15). The prolonged obstruction or severe tension on intraparenchymal or extraparenchymal vascular structures intraoperatively that results from this retraction is probably a cause of postoperative strokes. Tumor resection through standard open craniotomy may be facilitated by endoscopic visualization of important neurovascular structures and their relation to the tumor, which may not be directly visualized by the operating microscope. The improved optic control afforded by endoscope-assisted microneurosurgery diminishes the need for retraction of brain tissue and neurovascular structures. One common use is during resection of large subfrontal skull base meningiomas. The posterior aspect of the tumor may be intimately associated with the anterior cerebral artery or its major branches. Dissection of the tumor from these arteries may be difficult during a standard bifrontal approach that is often used (12). The use of a side-angle endoscope enables adequate visualization of the vascular structures from the capsule of the tumor. The optic nerves and chiasm may be visualized and their location verified before dissection of the posterior aspect of the tumor. Fries and coworkers treated 205 cranial tumors in a series of 380 cases using endoscope-assisted microsurgery (16). Despite the smaller cranial opening, better visualization of the operative field using the endoscope minimized the retraction required and decreased the intraoperative time. There was no increase in postoperative morbidity compared with the approaches traditionally used for those lesions.

In a similar manner, Hopf and Perneczky (1) suggested that intraventricular cysts and suprasellar arachnoid cysts should be approached through the endoscope (i.e., EN). They observed that arachnoid cysts in more locations with greater potential for vascular injury, such as posterior fossa or sylvian arachnoid cysts, should be fenestrated using a combined microneurosurgical technique (i.e., EAM or ECM).

### Aid to Visualization of the Paranasal Sinuses

In tumors that invade the anterior skull base, such as paranasal sinus malignancies, meningiomas, or esthesioneuroblastomas, the endoscope may be used to visualize paranasal extension into the sphenoid, ethmoid, and frontal sinuses (Fig. 14.7). The scope may serve as an adjunct to standard bifrontal or unifrontal craniotomy, and such use may avoid the use of facial incisions and transfacial exposure to address or guide tumor resection in these regions. We examined the extent of access to the paranasal sinuses by a bifrontal endoscope-assisted microneurosurgery approach alone, not compounded with external facial incisions as in a lateral rhinotomy. In this model, adequate access to the ethmoid or frontal sinuses and visualization of the nasopharynx can be easily achieved with a flexible endoscope. The inferomedial half of both maxillary sinuses can also be visualized by the microscope alone when viewed from above. The posterolateral halves and superior aspect of the maxillary sinuses are easily visualized with a flexible endoscope. Employment of the endoscope as a supplement to bifrontal craniotomy can alleviate the need for any additional and unnecessary facial incisions by allowing the surgeon to see areas hidden from the field of view of the microscope. The increased use of endoscopic guidance in this region has limited facial incisions for tumors of the anterior skull base with sinus extension.

## ENDOSCOPY AS AN ADJUVANT TO PITUITARY SURGERY

There has been considerable interest in the use of endoscopy as an adjuvant in resection of pituitary adenomas and other lesions in the region of the sella and suprasellar cistern. Work by our group (9) and others (3,4,17) has demonstrated that visualization of the sella and suprasellar cistern is greatly enhanced by the use of a rigid endoscope. The volume of exposure of the suprasellar region, superiorly and laterally, is enhanced by the endoscope by "placing the surgeon's eye" at the level of the sella. The variation in the anatomic architecture of the sphenoid sinus mandates a particular order of bone removal, particularly during the lateral sphenoidectomy, to avoid injury to the anterior loop of the carotid artery. The artery indents on the superior part of the posterolateral wall of the sinus, and in 66% of cases, the artery is covered by less than 1 mm of bone in the cadaveric specimen and only by the mucosa of the sphenoid sinus in 4% (18). The inferior medial wall of the optic canal protrudes into the superior lateral aspect of the sphenoid sinus. The osseous shielding of the optic nerve in this location may be very thin or lacking, leaving the nerve vulnerable to injury from surgical manipulation and thermal damage (18). The wide-angle view afforded by the endoscope during the infrasellar and sellar removal of bone and mucosa affords the surgeon better visualization of this often modestly illuminated area, enabling safer dissection. Large, superiorly extending pituitary tumors often require dissection above the level of the planum sphenoidale, and the safety of this maneuver is increased with the better visualization afforded by the endoscope. The use of the scope allows localization of the optic chiasm and cranial nerves, enabling a more aggressive resection of lesions with extension to the suprasellar cistern. However, laterally invasive lesions still pose significant limitations of this technique because of the lack of adequate surgical access to the many vital anatomic structures that lie in the cavernous sinus.

Most surgeons using endoscopic guidance for tumor resection in the region of the sella are using a rigid endoscope to avoid the necessity for nasal dissection, placement of the nasal speculum-type Hardy retractor, and the operating microscope. In most cases, the endoscope is used for visualization of the procedure through one nostril while microsurgical instruments are introduced through the contralateral nostril. Thereafter, dissection of the rostrum of the sphenoid sinus and floor of the sella proceeds in a fashion similar to that for standard microsurgical transsphenoidal adenomectomy. This limits the amount of nasal dissection performed and maintains the integrity of the nasal cartilage and the mucosa overlying the floor of the nasal cavity, vomer, and nasal cartilage. This technique has been used preferentially for smaller pituitary tumors and has been demonstrated to be safe and effective. It may reduce the nasal complications associated with standard transnasal dissection and has reduced the length of postoperative hospitalization (3,4,17).

The endoscope may be used to assist the intrasellar and suprasellar dissection of tumor during standard microsurgical transsphenoidal tumor resection. The endoscope may be inserted after removal of the sellar tumor and used to inspect the lateral cavernous sinus regions to ensure complete tumor removal. Similarly, the endoscope may be used to visualize the suprasellar region as described previously. Adoption of the endoscope as an adjuvant tool in pituitary surgery by both of these techniques is gaining widespread acceptance.

For pituitary lesions with marked lateral extension to the compartment of the cavernous sinus, efforts by our group have focused on developing a minimally invasive, endoscope-assisted, combined transmaxillary-transsphenoidal approach (19). The technique employs an extracranial corridor to the sellar and infrasellar region by following the course of the infraorbital nerve (i.e., terminal branch of the maxillary branch of the trigeminal nerve) to the foramen rotundum. The thick bone of the floor of the middle fossa medial to the foramen rotundum is then enlarged, and drilling is safely propagated medially toward the lateral sphenoid wall. After the anterior aspect of the lateral wall is removed and the sinus opened, the mucosa is stripped from the sphenoid sinus and the major septum extracted using pituitary forceps. With an endoscope, the extent of ipsilateral carotid artery and optic nerve protection are assessed, and more extensive bone drilling can safely be conducted to medially extend the osteotomy into the opened sphenoid sinus. The wide angles of viewing and excellent illumination afforded by the endoscope are again crucial to the safe propagation of the approach. The thin bone of the sellar floor covering the medial cavernous compartment is thinned with a 2-mm diamond burr and removed using microsurgical dissection to avoid injury to the dural sac covering the pituitary gland. With the sellar floor removed, access to the entire ipsilateral cavernous sinus and infrasellar fossa is gained, as well as proximal control of the con-

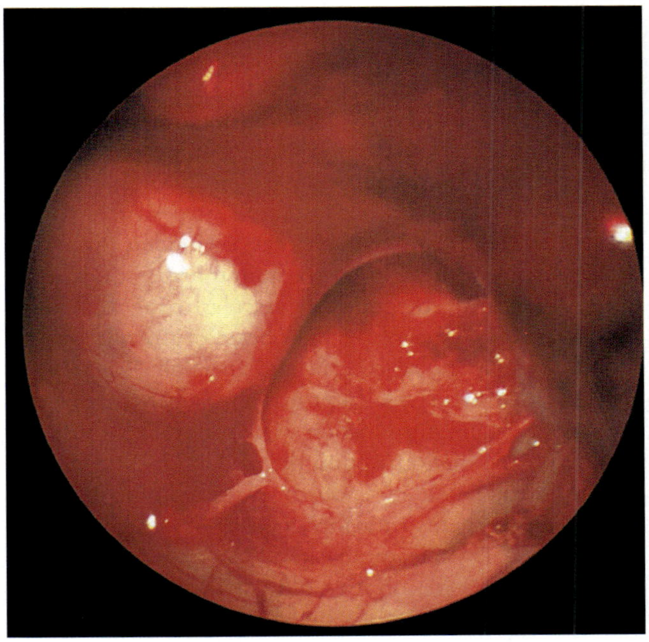

**FIGURE 14.7.** Endoscopic (30°) visualization of the sphenoid through a minimal window. This view was obtained between the second and third ($V_2$ and $V_3$) divisions of the trigeminal nerve during an anterior transcavernous approach to a spheno-orbital meningioma. The tumor grew into the sphenoid sinus from the adjacent posterior orbit and anterior cavernous sinus. At surgery, the skull base team removed the tumor in the sphenoid sinus using endoscopic guidance and exposure of the sphenoid adjacent to the optic nerve (through the planum sphenoidale) and between the superior orbital fissure and $V_2$ and between $V_2$ and $V_3$, respectively. Notice the sella turcica at the 10 o'clock position.

tralateral intracavernous carotid artery. By identifying the neural and vascular contents of the cavernous early, more medial exposure can be performed with decreased risk of iatrogenic injury to open the sphenoid sinus and expose the infrasellar region and contralateral carotid. Rhoton and associates reported that the distance between the intracavernous carotid arteries ranged from 4 to 18 mm (18). For large, invasive midline pathology of the cavernous sinus, approaching the lesions from the inferolateral orientation afforded by this procedure can be a safer alternative than aiming the direction of the approach directly at the medial cavernous compartment and the carotid arteries. Adequate proximal and distal control of the ipsilateral carotid artery is established, as well as endoscopic visualization of the medial aspect of the contralateral carotid artery. The approach can be a safe alternate route for exposing locally aggressive lesions as craniopharyngiomas and recurrent aggressive pituitary adenomas with significant lateral extension and involvement of the intracavernous carotid artery that would otherwise require a transsphenoidal and pterional approach.

## ENDOSCOPY AS AN ADJUVANT IN THE MANAGEMENT OF VASCULAR LESIONS

Because of their anatomic characteristics, aneurysms of the anterior cranial fossa are favorably situated for treatment by a keyhole microsurgical approach. Vascular lesions in the anterior cranial fossa permit a minimally invasive approach requiring little or no retraction of the brain or neurovascular structures. However, limitations of the keyhole approach include poor illumination of deeply seated structures and poor visualization of structures that are hidden from view by the shadow of the light source from the operating microscope. Microinstruments and vascular clips often fall directly along the axis of the light beam of the microscope, causing loss of optical control and increasing the risk of intraoperative aneurysmal rupture. This is particularly hazardous during the introduction of aneurysm clips into the field and manipulation around the neck of the aneurysm.

The introduction of endoscopy-assisted microvascular surgery has been instrumental in overcoming the optical limitations of keyhole approaches. Side-angle viewing may be used for direct visualization of the backside of the vascular lesion to help identify perforators or other relevant anatomy without any retraction of neurovascular structures. The endoscope then can be maintained in one anatomic corridor to safely guide the introduction of the clip to the neck of the aneurysm through another corridor. After placement of the aneurysm clip, an endoscope may be used to check accurate blade placement and preservation of all vessels. Without the benefit of the endoscope, adequate visualization and manipulation of the lesion cannot be achieved without significant tissue retraction, increasing the risk of rupture and postoperative vascular accident. This method is particularly useful in clip ligation of aneurysms of the anterior communicating complex because the vascular anatomy of these aneurysms may be complicated by the multitude of vessels in the region and the perforators emanating from the A1 segments.

The supraorbital approach described previously is an excellent keyhole approach for addressing vascular regions arising in the anterior cranial fossa, sellar region, and the anterior part of the circle of Willis (20,21). In addition to providing adequate visual control and dissection of the ipsilateral circle of Willis, the versatility of the approach affords good control of the contralateral arterial structures. The contralateral ophthalmic artery, medial loop of the internal carotid artery, M1 segment of the internal carotid artery, A1 segment of the anterior cerebral artery, and posterior communicating vessels can all be adequately controlled by this approach (2,16). Van Lindert and colleagues reported successful clipping of 139 supratentorial aneurysms through this technique (22). The versatility of head positioning (10° to 60°) and bone flap used in the approach also allows a contralateral (cross-court) approach, and this method was used by the Van Linder group for vascular lesions arising from the posterior cerebral artery and superior cerebellar artery. For aneurysms of the medial carotid-ophthalmic segment, the small opening limits adequate dissection of the aneurysm sac and proximal control before clipping. This can be overcome by endovascular placement of a balloon in the proximal carotid artery.

With a trajectory along the anterior skull base, endoscope-assisted microsurgical application of this approach has been a favorable technique to address lesions as far posterior as the interpeduncular fossa (7). Previously, this region was approached using a frontotemporal craniotomy with retraction of the carotid artery or its branches and oculomotor nerve for adequate visualization. The minimal supraorbital craniotomy with endoscopic aid offers a direct approach to visualization of the region without manipulation of these important structures. For adequate visualization and safe manipulation of aneurysm clips in this region, the endoscope was found to be of paramount importance.

## CONCLUSIONS

As experience with the endoscope by neurosurgeons and otolaryngologists increases and with further refinements in instrumentation, endoscopes will be used more often in the management of a variety of lesions. Endoscopy enables the surgeon to look and work behind structures that are hidden from microscopic view. Endoscopes help to minimize craniotomy exposure, because they offer increased visualization of anatomic regions when used alone or to complement the operating microscope. Facial dissections for the removal of craniofacial tumors have decreased, in part because of the greater visualization offered by the endoscope. This trend should continue as surgeons gain experience and become comfortable with the use of endoscopes.

## REFERENCES


1. Hopf NJ, Perneczky A. Endoscopic neurosurgery and microneurosurgery for the treatment of intracranial cysts. *Neurosurgery* 1998;43:1330–1336.
2. Perneczky A, Fries G. Endoscope-assisted brain surgery. Part I. Evolution, basic concept, and current technique. *Neurosurgery* 1998;42:219–225.
3. Jho HD, Carrau RL. Endoscopic endonasal transsphenoidal surgery: experience with 50 patients. *J Neurosurg* 1997;87: 44–51.
4. Jho HD, Carrau RL, Ko Y, et al. Endoscopic pituitary surgery: an early experience. *Surg Neurol* 1997;47:213–222.
5. Kumon Y, Zenke K, Ohta S, et al. Operative results in fourteen cases of paranasal sinus and anterior cranial fossa lesions surgically treated by an extended transbasal approach. *No Shinkei Geka* 1995;23:889–895.
6. Matula C, Tschabitscher M, Day JD, et al. Endoscopically assisted microsurgery. *Acta Neurochir (Wien)* 1995;134:190–195.
7. Menovsky T, Grotenhuis JA, de Vries J, et al. Endoscope-assisted supraorbital craniotomy for lesions of the interpeduncular fossa. *Neurosurgery* 1999;44:106–110.
8. Rodziewicz GS, Kelley RT, Kellman RM, et al. Transnasal endoscopic surgery of the pituitary gland: technical note. *Neurosurgery* 1996;39:189–192.
9. Spencer WR, Das K, Nwagu C, et al. Approaches to the sellar and parasellar region: anatomic comparison of the microscope vs. endoscope. *Laryngoscope* 1999;109:791–794.
10. Tutino M, Betti G, Seminara P. Extradural endoscopic dissection of the anterior skull base. *J Craniofac Surg* 1997;8:454–459.
11. Couldwell WT. Surgery of the anterior skull base. *Otolaryngol Clin North Am* 1993;26:673–693.
12. Couldwell WT, Weiss MH. Olfactory groove meningiomas. In: Kaye AH, Black PMcL, eds. *Operative neurosurgery*. London: Churchill Livingstone, 1999.
13. Cohen AR, Perneczky A, Rodziewicz GS, et al. Endoscopic-assisted craniotomy: approach to the rostral brainstem. *Neurosurgery* 1995;36:1128–1129.
14. Arbit E, Diresta GR, Bedford RF, et al. Intraoperative measurement of cerebral and tumoral blood flow with laser-Doppler flowmetry. *Neurosurgery* 1989;24:166–170.
15. Miller JD, Stanek AE, Langfitt TW. Cerebral blood flow regulation during experimental brain compression. *J Neurosurgery* 1973;39:186–196.
16. Fries G, Perneczky A. Endoscope-assisted brain surgery. Part 2. Analysis of 380 procedures. *Neurosurgery* 1998;42:226–232.
17. Jho HD, Carrau RL. Endoscopy assisted transsphenoidal surgery for pituitary adenoma: technical note. *Acta Neurochir (Wien)* 1996;138:1416–1425.
18. Renn WH, Rhoton AL Jr. Microsurgical anatomy of the sellar region. *J Neurosurg* 1975;43:288–298.
19. Sabit I, Schafer S, Couldwell WT. Extranasal extradural combined transmaxillary-transsphenoidal approach to the cavernous sinus: a minimally invasive microsurgical model. *Laryngoscope* 2000;110:286–291.
20. Delashaw JB Jr, Tedeschi H, Rhoton AL. Modified supraorbital craniotomy: technical note. *Neurosurgery* 1992;30:954–956.
21. Delfini R, Raco A, Artico M, et al. A two-step supraorbital approach to regions of the orbital apex: technical note. *J Neurosurg* 1992;77:959–961.
22. Van Lindert E, Perneczky A, Fries G, et al. The supraorbital keyhole approach to supratentorial aneurysms: concept and technique. *Surg Neurol* 1998;49:481–490.


## SUGGESTED READING


Briant TD, Bird R. Extracranial repair of cerebrospinal fluid fistulae. *J Otolaryngol* 1982;11:191–197.

Brisman R, Hughes JE, Mount LA. Cerebrospinal fluid rhinorrhea. *Arch Neurol* 1970;22:245–252.

Cairns H. Injuries of the frontal and ethmoidal sinuses with special reference to cerebrospinal rhinorrhea and aerocoeles. *J Laryngol Otol* 1937;52:589–623.

Calceterra TC. Extracranial surgical repair of cerebrospinal fluid rhinorrhea. *Ann Otol* 1980;89:108–116.

Gamea A, Fathi M, el-Guindy A. The use of the rigid endoscope in transsphenoidal pituitary surgery. *J Larngol Otol* 1994;108:19–22.

Gunkel AR, Freysinger W, Thumfart WF, Pototschig C. Complete sphenoethmoidectomy and computer-assisted surgery. *Acta Otorhinolaryngol Belg* 1995;49:257–261.

Halves E, Bushe KA. Transsphenoidal operation on craniopharyngiomas with extrasellar extensions: the advantage of the operating endoscope. *Acta Neurochir Suppl (Wien)* 1979;28:362.

Hazan A, Roux FX, Levy D, et al. Use of endoscopy in pituitary surgery. *Neurochirurgie* 1998;44:327–330.

Heilman CB, Shucart WA, Rebeiz EE. Endoscopic sphenoidotomy approach to the sella. *Neurosurgery* 1997;41:602–607.

Hirsch O. Successful closure of cerebrospinal rhinorrhea by endonasal surgery. *Arch Otolaryngol* 1952;56:1.

Hughes RG, Jones NS, Robertson IJ. The endoscopic treatment of cerebrospinal fluid rhinorrhea: the Nottingham experience. *J Laryngol Otol* 1997;111:125–128.

Sethi DS, Pillay PK. Endoscopic management of lesions of the sella turcica. *J Laryngol Otol* 1995;109:956–962.

Taniguchi M, Perneczky A. Subtemporal keyhole approach to the suprasellar and petroclival region: microanatomic considerations and clinical application. *Neurosurgery* 1997;41:592–601.

Vanaclocha V, Saiz-Sapena N. Surgical treatment of anterior skull base tumors. *Acta Neurochir (Wien)* 1997;139:857–868.

Van Alyea OE. Sphenoid sinus: anatomic study, with consideration of the clinical significance of the structural characteristics of the sphenoid sinus. *Arch Otolaryngol* 1941;34:225–253.

Yaniv E, Rappaport ZH. Endoscopic transseptal transsphenoidal surgery for pituitary tumors. *Neurosurgery* 1997;40:944–946.

# 15

# ADJUNCTIVE USE OF ENDOSCOPY IN LATERAL SKULL BASE SURGERY

**PHILLIP A. WACKYM**
**WESLEY A. KING**
**MICHELLE M. SMITH**
**GLENN A. MEYER**

The technical limits of neuro-otologic skull base surgery and neurosurgery have diminished to the point that virtually any tumor can be resected, and the morbidity and mortality of these types of surgical procedures have declined rapidly over the past two decades. Despite these advances, the application of endoscopes as adjunctive tools in lateral skull base surgery is relatively recent. Because many of the advantages, disadvantages, and instrumentation pertinent to lateral skull base surgery has been covered in several of the chapters included in Section II of this textbook, this chapter focuses on specific case examples, with an emphasis on anatomic regions and pathologies.

## PETROUS APEX

A wide variety of pathologies can involve the petrous apex (Table 15.1). The application of rigid endoscopes can be useful in the management of several of these diseases, and case examples are provided subsequently. The primary benefit of using endoscopes during surgery of the petrous apex is to allow visualization and resection of residual disease in the anterior petrous apex and surrounding the infratemporal internal carotid artery. Most of the diseases involving the petrous apex are slowly expanding lesions, and the most common signs and symptoms are eustachian tube dysfunction, often producing unilateral serous otitis media with effusion; headache, typically retro-orbital or radiating to the vertex (through dural traction); facial pain or numbness, with involvement of the trigeminal nerve in the area of Meckel's cave; diplopia, with involvement of the abducens nerve at Dorello's canal; hearing loss, tinnitus, vertigo, or facial paralysis, with involvement of the otic capsule or internal auditory canal; and cranial neuropathies. With anterior and superior extension of disease, dysfunction of cranial nerves III, IV, and VI can be produced, and with inferior extension, dysfunction of cranial nerves IX, X, XI, and XII can be produced.

### Chordoma

Chordomas are rare, slowly growing but aggressive neoplasms that originate from the primitive notochord (from the Greek *noton*, meaning back, and from *chorde*, meaning "cord"). These malignant tumors account for 1% to 4% of all malignant bone tumors and can be found along the cranioaxial skeleton. The three most common sites from which chordomas develop are the spheno-occipital base of the skull region (35%), the vertebral column (15%), and the sacrococcygeal area (50%) (1). Although rare, chordomas can also develop within the petrous apex (2). Based on biologic behavior and histopathologic features, chordomas can be divided into three types: conventional chordomas, chondroid chordomas, and dedifferentiated chordomas.

Conventional chordomas are the most common and lack the cartilaginous or additional mesenchymal components seen in chondroid or dedifferentiated chordomas (3). Both sexes are affected equally and usually present between the ages of 40 to 50 years; these tumors are uncommon in individuals younger than 20 years of age. The literature also contains reports of a greater male incidence, ranging from 2:1 to 3:2 (4). Patients with conventional chordomas of the skull base usually present with headache, diplopia, or ataxia, and any of the cranial nerves can be affected. The typical radiologic features are shown in Figures 15.1–15.5. A combination of surgery and radiation therapy provides the best opportunity to achieve a disease-free interval, although some authorities advocate reserving radiation therapy for recurrence of disease (5,6). The average survival is 4 to 8 years, and local recurrences are the rule rather than the exception (5). Metastases are uncommon, occurring in 2% to 10% of patients. The most common sites of metastases are the lungs, bones, lymph nodes, liver, and skin.

Figures 15.6–15.8 illustrate how the adjunctive use of rigid endoscopes can be applied to the microsurgical resec-

**TABLE 15.1. POTENTIAL APPLICATIONS OF ENDOSCOPE DURING SURGICAL MANAGEMENT OF PETROUS APEX DISEASES**

| |
|---|
| *Inflammatory Lesions* |
| Cholesterol granuloma |
| Epidermoid (cholesteatoma) |
| Mucocele |
| *Infectious Diseases* |
| Petrous apicitis |
| Skull base osteomyelitis |
| *Neoplasms* |
| Chordoma |
| Chondrosarcoma |
| Hemangiopericytoma |
| Langerhans cell histiocytosis (histiocytosis X) |
| Meningioma |
| Metastasis |
| Nasopharyngeal carcinoma |
| Paraganglioma (glomus tumor) |
| Schwannoma |

tion of chordomas. In this case example, after a postauricular Fisch type C infratemporal fossa approach to this tumor, endoscope-assisted surgery allowed identification of residual disease at the petrous apex (Fig. 15.7), and subsequent resection was accomplished endoscopically (Fig. 15.8). Similar applications of endoscopes with an angled view have been reported (7,8).

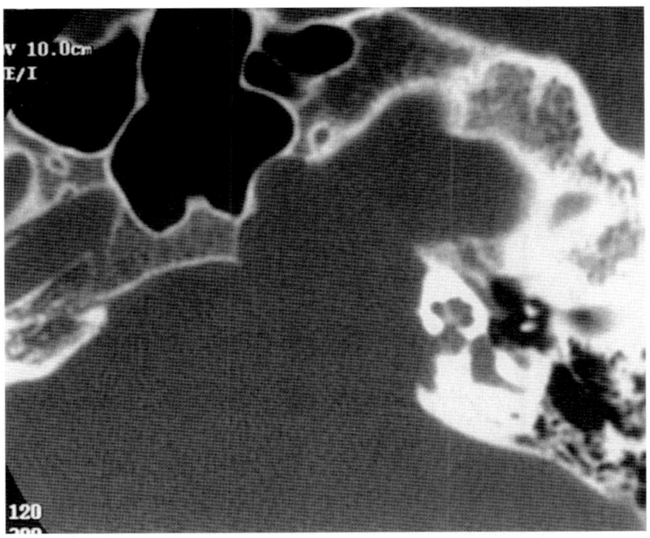


**FIGURE 15.1.** Axial computed tomography image of the left temporal bone filmed with the bone-window technique shows expansile soft tissue density mass within the left petrous apex adjacent to the petroclival fissure. The bone of the petrous apex appears expanded and remodeled. The lesion extends posteriorly into the porus acusticus.

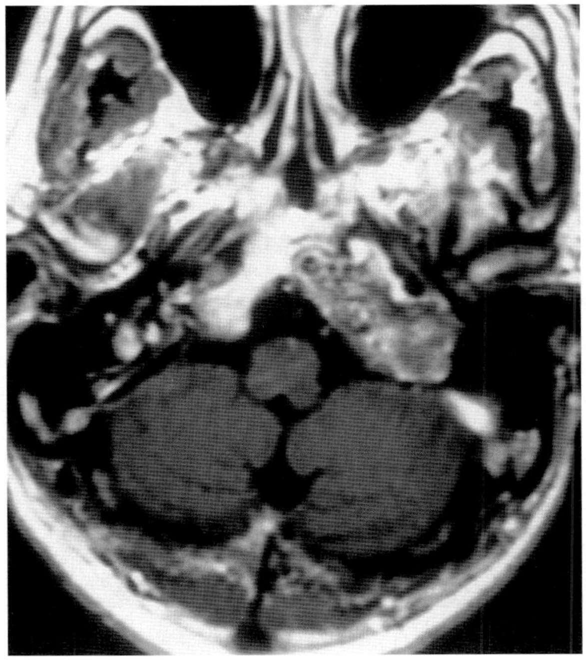

**FIGURE 15.2.** Axial, T1-weighted, postgadolinium magnetic resonance image shows the expansile lesion within the left petrous apex. The lesion enhances somewhat heterogeneously. The mass marginates the petrous segment of the left internal carotid artery posteriorly. Contrast enhancement is seen within the left sigmoid sinus posterior and lateral to the mass.

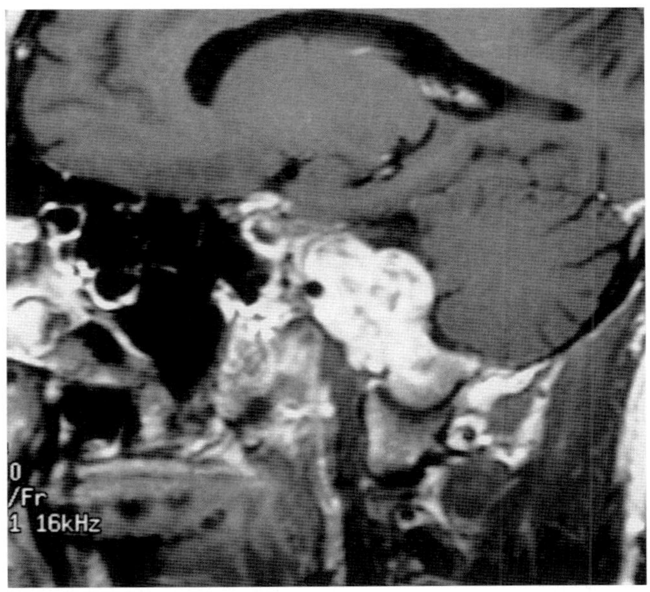


**FIGURE 15.3.** Sagittal, T1-weighted, postgadolinium magnetic resonance image shows a somewhat lobulated mass within the left skull base involving the petrous temporal bone. The mass enhances diffusely. At the anterior margin of the mass, the flow void of the petrous segment of the left internal carotid artery is appreciated. The lesion extends inferiorly into the left occipital condyle. No invasion of the adjacent cerebellum is observed.

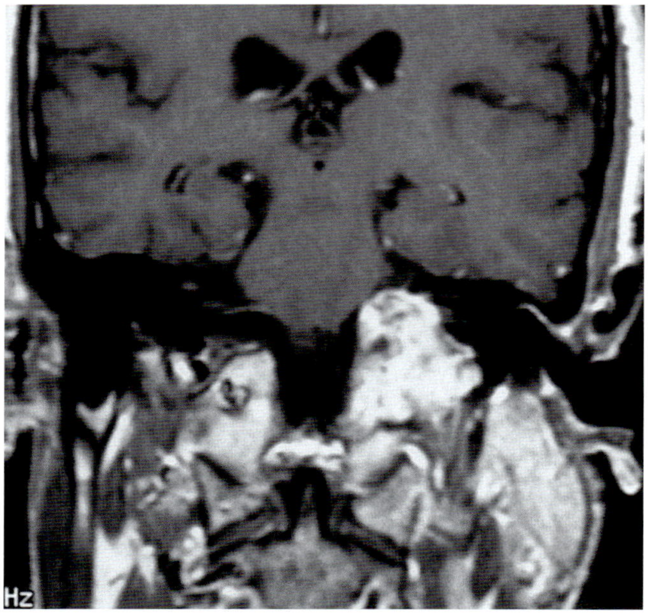


**FIGURE 15.4.** Coronal, T1-weighted, postgadolinium magnetic resonance image shows enhancing lesion within the left petrous apex and extending inferiorly into the occipital bone. The superior medial aspect of the lesion is adjacent to but does not compress the pons. No extension into the middle cranial fossa is observed on this image.

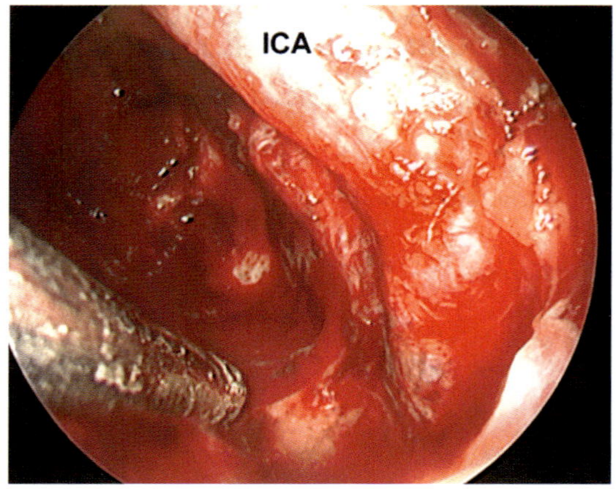


**FIGURE 15.6.** After a postauricular Fisch type C infratemporal fossa approach to the lateral and central skull base, this endoscopic view into the left petrous apex after resection of the tumor was seen. The infratemporal petrous internal carotid artery *(ICA)* was seen with a 4-mm, 0° endoscope. The petrous apex appears to be free of tumor.

Chondroid chordomas represent 25% to 35% of all cranial chordomas and are differentiated from conventional chordomas based on their inclusion of cartilaginous and chordomatous elements (5,6). The literature remains divided regarding the subclassification of these tumors as chordomas or chondrosarcomas (5). However, the biologic behavior, management, and prognosis remain the same as conventional chondromas (5,6).

Dedifferentiated chondromas are rare, constituting only 1% to 8% of all chordomas, and are differentiated from conventional chordomas based on their inclusion of malignant mesenchymal and chordomatous elements. These malignant mesenchymal elements can be fibrous histiocytoma, fibrosarcoma, or osteosarcoma. Dedifferentiated chordomas can arise as a primary tumor, within a recurrent conventional chordoma treated with surgery alone, or after radiation therapy for a conventional chordoma (5). In contrast to the conventional or chondroid chordomas, these are aggressive neoplasms that typically produce local recurrences and metastases. Most patients usually die of their disease within 6 to 12 months after diagnosis (5,6).

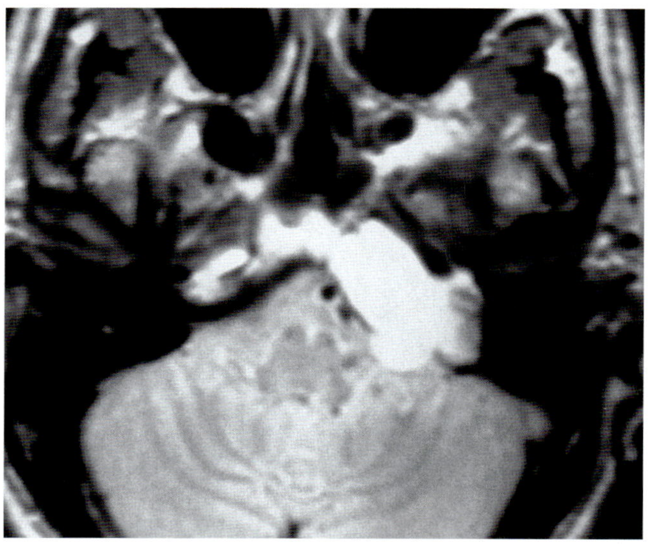

**FIGURE 15.5.** Axial, proton density–weighted magnetic resonance image shows well-circumscribed expansile petrous apex lesion on the left. On the T2-weighted sequence, the lesion is detected by the homogeneously high signal intensity. No flow voids are appreciated within the lesion. No edema within the adjacent left cerebellar hemisphere is observed. High signal intensity on long TR sequences is characteristic of chordomas and chondrosarcomas. The histopathologic diagnosis was chordoma.

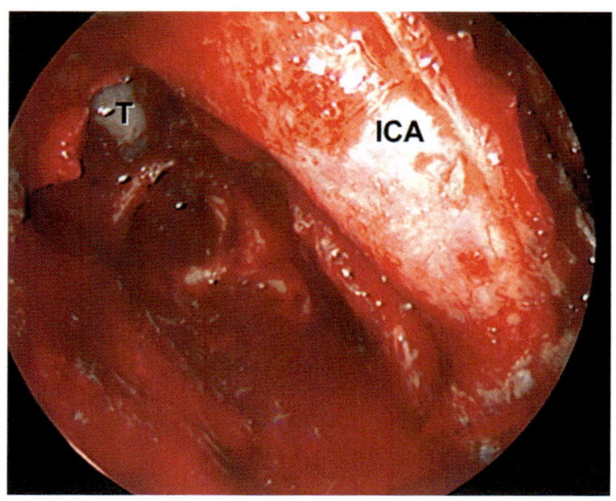


**FIGURE 15.7.** A 4-mm, 45° endoscope allows visualization of the anterior (ventral) portion of the petrous apex, and a small amount of residual tumor *(T)* is seen. All of the tumor has been removed from around the internal carotid artery *(ICA)*.

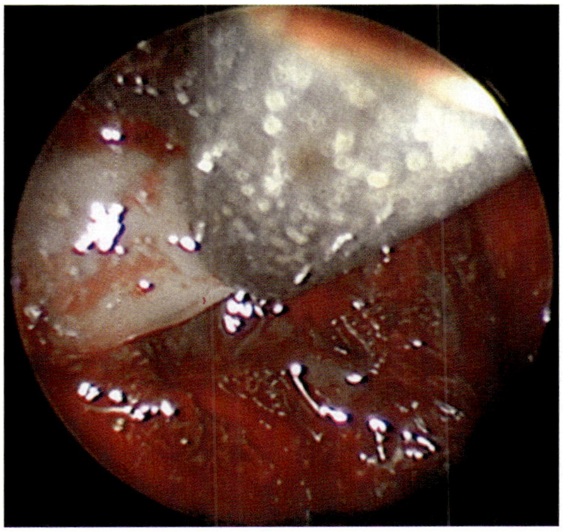

**FIGURE 15.8.** In this photograph, resection of the residual tumor can be seen. Visualization was provided by a 2.7-mm, 45° endoscope.

## Epidermoids

Epidermoids (i.e., congenital cholesteatomas, cholesteatomas, or pearly tumors) are unusual and represent 0.7% to 1.5% of all intracranial tumors (9,10). The cerebellopontine angle (40% to 60%) and petrous apex of the temporal bone are the most common skull base sites. They can be of intradural or intraosseous origin, and these tumors result from the growth of ectodermal inclusions trapped during embryogenesis. The computed tomography (CT) and magnetic resonance imaging (MRI) characteristics of a petrous apex epidermoid are shown in Figures 15.9–15.11. Histologically, they have a benign cyst wall lined with keratinizing squamous epithelium. Epidermoid cysts are filled with sterile, desquamated keratinaceous debris. Some cysts can have collections of cholesterol crystals or triglycerides and polyunsaturated fatty acids. At operation, they typically have a white, waxy appearance (Fig. 15.12), and it can be difficult to peel the epithelial matrix from neurovascular structures that the epidermoid has become adherent to. Angled endoscopes can be useful in the identification and removal of residual disease. Figure 15.12 shows the identification of residual epidermoid around the internal carotid artery in the

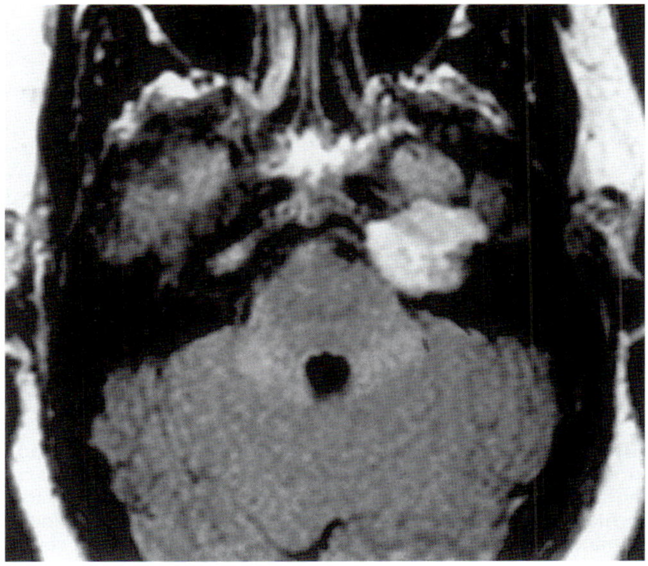

**FIGURE 15.10.** Axial, T1-weighted magnetic resonance image without gadolinium demonstrates a hyperintense expansile lesion of the left petrous apex. The lesion is anterior to the internal auditory canal. A normal-appearing left petrous internal carotid artery is appreciated.

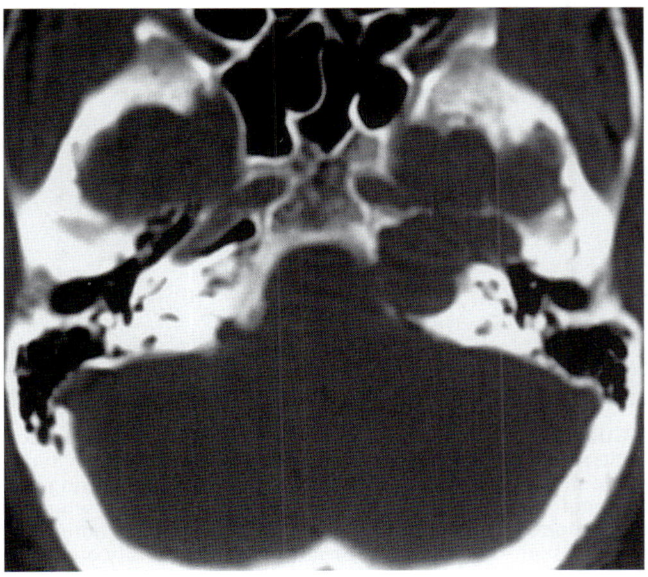

**FIGURE 15.9.** Axial computed tomographic examination of the head demonstrates well-circumscribed expansile lesion of the left petrous apex. There is bony remodeling but no aggressive bone erosion.

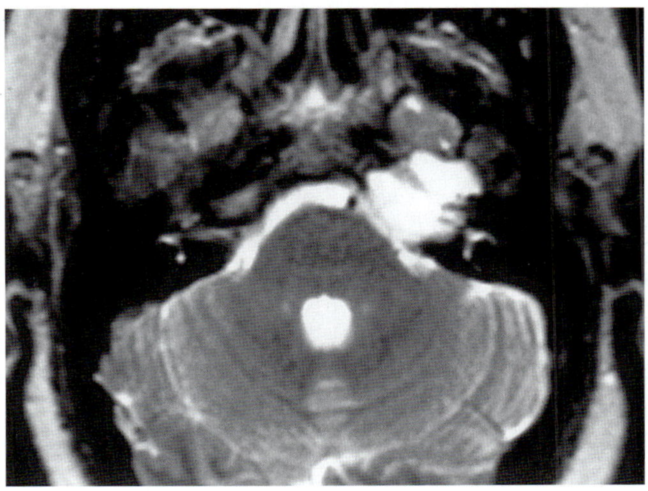

**FIGURE 15.11.** Axial, T2-weighted magnetic resonance image demonstrates that the lesion has homogeneously high signal intensity. The imaging features of the mass suggest an epidermoid tumor.

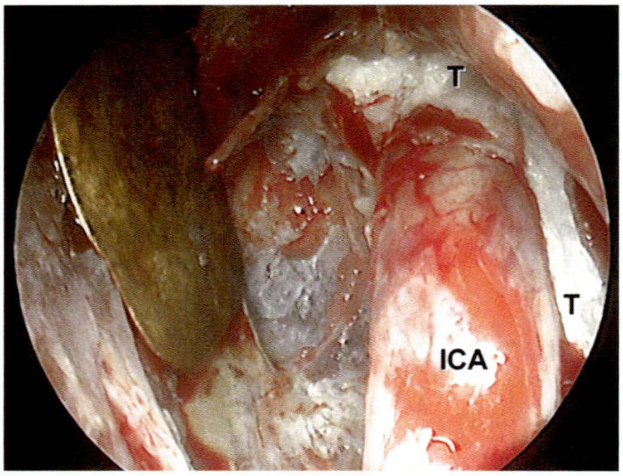


**FIGURE 15.12.** After a middle cranial fossa approach and exposure of the tumor, a 4-mm, 45° endoscope allows visualization of the petrous apex as viewed from the anterior limit of the cochlea. A malleable retractor *(left)* is seen retracting the middle cranial fossa and posterior fossa dura. A small amount of residual epidermoid tumor *(T)* is seen superior (cephalad) and lateral to the internal carotid artery *(ICA)*.

petrous apex, which was not visualized with the operating microscope. This residual disease was subsequently resected with endoscopic visualization. Endoscopes are similarly useful in removing epidermoids from the cerebellopontine angle, and their greatest utility is in removing the matrix from the lattice of cranial nerves within this anatomic region.

## CHOLESTEROL GRANULOMA

Cholesterol granulomas represent an inflammatory reaction including a foreign body–giant cell reaction to cholesterol, with associated fibrosis, vascular proliferation, hemosiderin-laden macrophages, and round cells. The pathogenesis begins with impaired ventilation of the middle ear and mastoid, which leads to a fluid accumulation with hemorrhage, cholesterol deposition, fibrous proliferation, and a foreign body granulomatous inflammatory reaction. Osteitis and bone erosion can occur. Predisposing factors include trauma; otitis media (i.e., serous otitis media or chronic otitis media, with or without cholesteatoma); previous otologic surgery; or barotrauma. The granulomas have various combinations of fluid and granulation tissue. The fluid can have the appearance of old motor oil or be bluish, brown, or yellow. They may occur in the middle ear, mastoid, or petrous apex (11,12). The CT and MRI features are useful in determining the preoperative diagnosis (12), and some of these features are illustrated in Figures 15.13 and 15.14. Surgical management of this entity requires drainage and permanent aeration of the petrous apex; however, total excision through a middle cranial fossa approach has been described (13). The case shown in Figures 15.13–15.15 was managed using the latter strategy. Figure 15.15 shows how an angled endoscope can be used to be certain that all of the

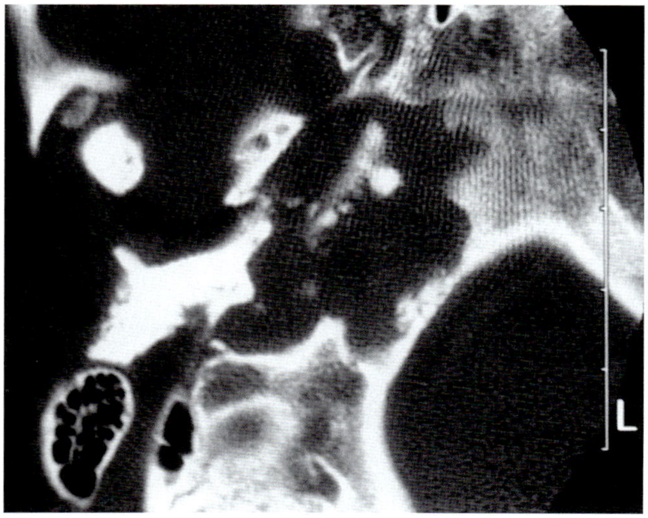


**FIGURE 15.13.** Axial computed tomographic examination of the right temporal bone demonstrates a slightly irregular mass within the right skull base with intact bony margins.

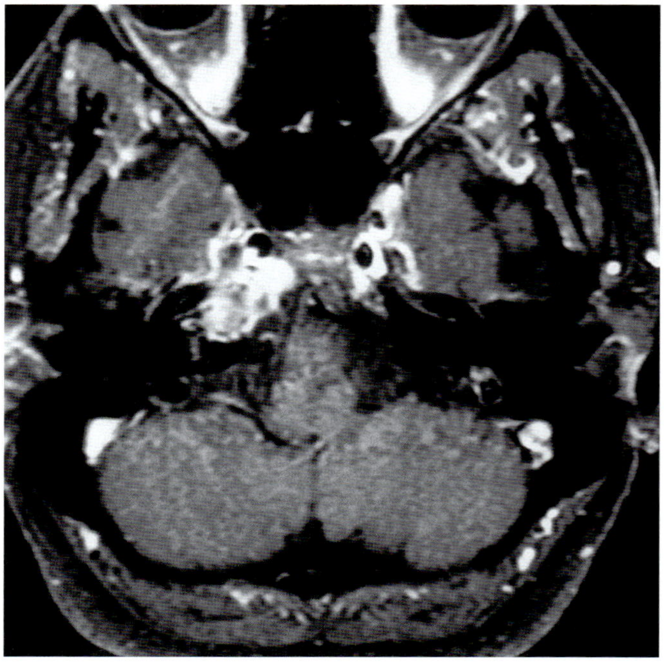

**FIGURE 15.14.** Axial, T1-weighted, gadolinium-enhanced magnetic resonance image obtained with the fat saturation technique shows high signal intensity within the lesion involving the right petrous apex. The flow void within the cavernous segment of the right internal carotid artery is displaced slightly anteriorly by the lesion. This lesion was of similar signal intensity on unenhanced T1-weighted images, and the signal intensity was high signal on T2-weighted sequences. It was proven to be a petrous cholesterol granuloma.

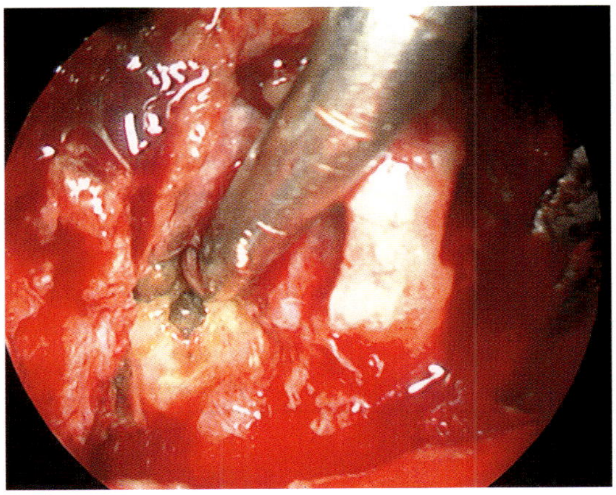

**FIGURE 15.15.** After a middle cranial fossa approach, a 4-mm, 45° endoscope was used to remove the cholesterol granuloma from the petrous apex. The endoscope was placed anterior to the petrous carotid artery, and the anterior view shows removal of the residual tumor from the petrous apex.

cholesterol granuloma has been excised from within the petrous apex.

## Langerhans Cell Histiocytosis

Histiocytosis (i.e., Langerhans cell histiocytosis or histiocytosis X) is a disorder of the reticuloendothelial system, and it is characterized by the proliferation of Langerhans cells. There have been descriptions of three clinical expressions of the disease, in decreasing degrees of severity: Letterer-Siwe disease, Hand-Schüller-Christian disease, and eosinophilic granuloma. In 1953, Lichtenstein (14) grouped all three diseases together based on the concept of their being one clinicopathologic entity, and coined the term *histiocytosis X*. The X reflected the unknown etiopathogenesis. In 1973, Nezelof and colleagues identified the Langerhans cell as the abnormally proliferating cell in histiocytosis (15). Subsequently, the term *Langerhans cell histiocytosis* replaced the term histiocytosis X. Although usually a disease of childhood, Langerhans cell histiocytosis can occur at any age, from birth to advanced age. The severity of the disease is usually related to the age of the affected individual, with the most severe and disseminated forms occurring in infants and young children. The incidence of Langerhans cell histiocytosis is 1 case per 200,000 to 350,000 people. The CT and MR characteristics are shown in Figures 15.16–15.18.

The spectrum of Langerhans cell histiocytosis ranges from a single bony site of involvement to disseminated disease of the viscera, bone marrow, lymphatic system, and skin. Diagnostic surveys are appropriate before treatment planning can be completed. Establishing a diagnosis based on histopathologic material is essential, and Figure 15.19 shows the endoscope-assisted biopsy of a 4-year-old boy with Langerhans cell histiocytosis isolated to the petrous apex. Table 15.2 shows the management strategies by stage of disease. Long-term prognosis depends on the stage of the disease: group 1 children have no functional impairment; group 2 children have a 65% to 100% survival rate; and group 3 children (infants) have a mortality rate of 65% to 95% (16).

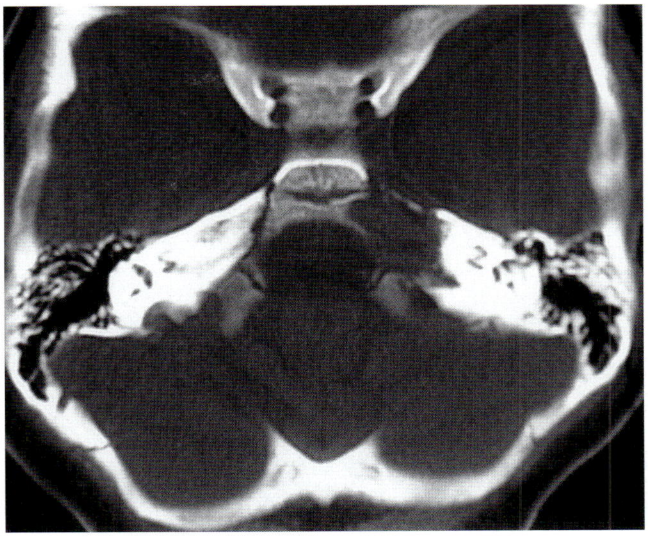

**FIGURE 15.16.** Axial computed tomography (CT) scan of the head of a 4-year-old boy at the level of the petrous apices demonstrates marrow-replacing lesion within the left petrous apex. The lesion has somewhat ill-defined margins and appears to cross the petroclival fissure into the lateral aspect of the clivus on the left. No internal calcifications are observed on the CT scan.

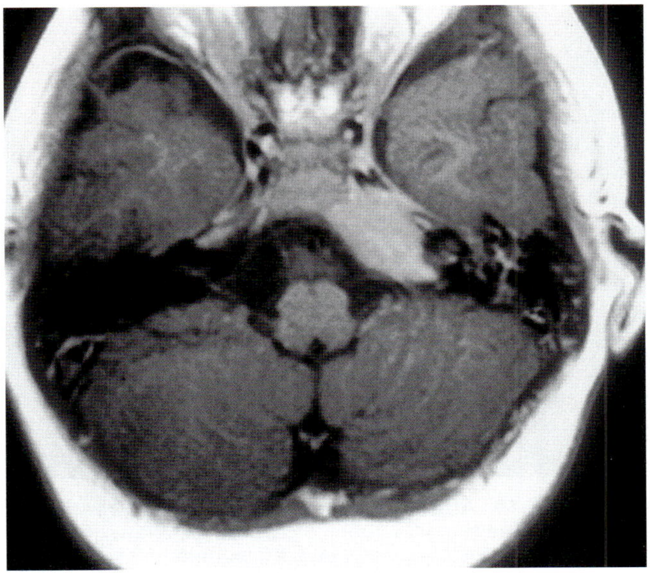

**FIGURE 15.17.** Axial, T1-weighted magnetic resonance image of the brain with gadolinium shows an enhancing mass within the left petrous apex. The lesion extends posteriorly into the porus acusticus and anteriorly into the region of Meckel's cave. No invasion of adjacent brain parenchyma is identified.

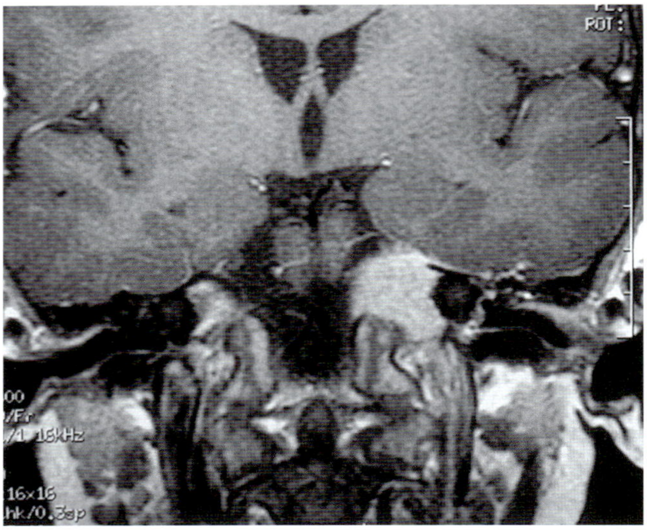

**FIGURE 15.18.** Coronal, T1-weighted, postgadolinium magnetic resonance image demonstrates the somewhat ill-defined enhancing lesion within the left petrous apex. On this image, the lesion extends superiorly into the left middle cranial fossa, and there is linear enhancement of the dura beneath the left temporal lobe suggesting dural invasion. Although this lesion was proven to be Langerhans cell histiocytosis (i.e., histiocytosis X), in the pediatric population, rhabdomyosarcoma can have a similar appearance.

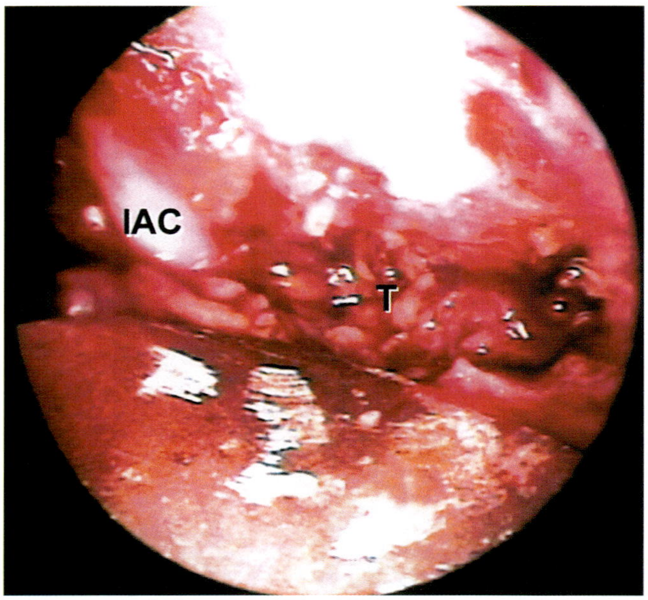


**FIGURE 15.19.** After a middle cranial fossa approach and exposure of the tumor, a 4-mm, 0° endoscope allows visualization of the petrous apex as viewed from middle cranial fossa toward the skull base (caudally). The Fisch middle cranial fossa retractor blade is seen at the petrous ridge *(bottom center)*. The dura remains intact over the contents of the internal auditory canal *(IAC)*. The tumor *(T)* fills the petrous apex. The biopsy result was consistent with Langerhans cell histiocytosis (i.e., histiocytosis X).

**TABLE 15.2. MANAGEMENT OF LANGERHANS CELL HISTIOCYTOSIS BY STAGE**

| Stage (Group) | Treatment |
|---|---|
| 1 (unifocal) | Biopsy and curettage<br>± Low-dose radiation therapy |
| 2 (multifocal) | Radiation therapy after biopsy<br>± Curettage<br>± Chemotherapy |
| 3 (disseminated) | Radiation therapy<br>Chemotherapy<br>± Thymic extracts |

## POSTERIOR FOSSA, TEMPORAL BONE, AND LATERAL SKULL BASE

### Posterior Fossa Arachnoid Cyst

Arachnoid cysts are rare, representing 1% of intracranial tumors (17–19). They are duplications of the arachnoid membrane, filled with cerebrospinal fluid (CSF), and usually manifest as space-occupying lesions. Arachnoid cysts can be primary or secondary. Primary arachnoid cysts result from an error in embryogenesis that leads to duplication of the outer secretory arachnoid membrane, with subsequent production and entrapment of CSF (17,18). A ball-valve mechanism with one-way flow of CSF into the cyst from the subarachnoid space has been proposed to explain the

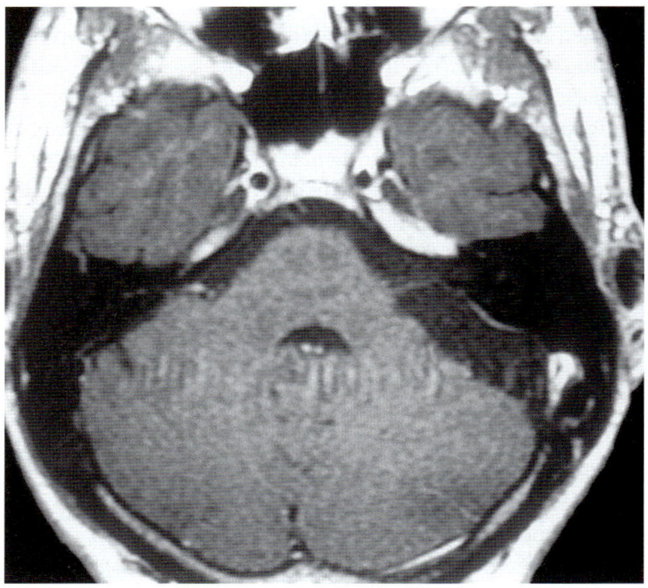

**FIGURE 15.20.** Axial, T1-weighted, postgadolinium magnetic resonance image demonstrates extraaxial collection within the left cerebellopontine angle that is isointense to cerebrospinal fluid. There is slight mass effect on the left middle cerebellar peduncle and left cerebellar hemisphere. The seventh and eighth cranial nerve complex can be seen anterior to the extraaxial collection.

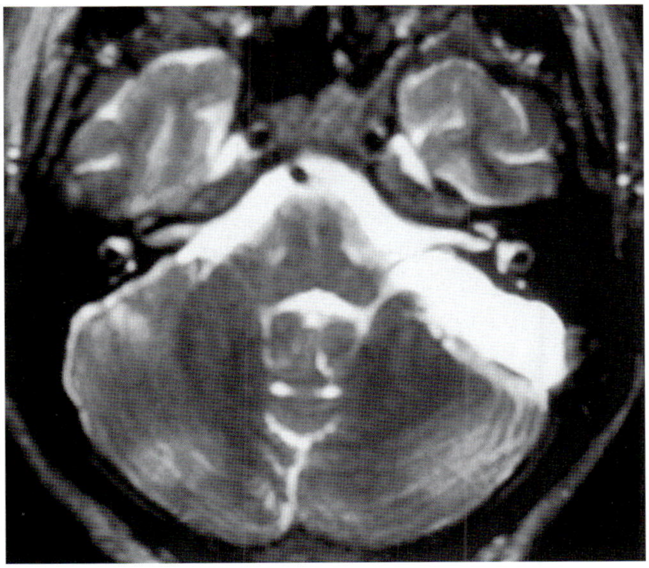

**FIGURE 15.21.** Axial, T2-weighted magnetic resonance image demonstrates high signal intensity within the lesion that is similar to cerebrospinal fluid. The lesion is well marginated and has characteristic features of an arachnoid cyst.

rapid change in symptoms occurring in some patients after experiencing increased intracranial pressure. Previous trauma, adhesive arachnoiditis, subarachnoid hemorrhage, or neoplasms cause secondary arachnoid cysts; however, it is possible that these arachnoid cysts are found incidentally during the imaging necessary to manage these putative predisposing diseases or conditions. Histologically, arachnoid cysts are CSF-filled spaces surrounded by a thin epithelial cell–lined membrane.

Arachnoid cysts of the posterior fossa can occur in three primary locations: laterocerebellar cysts (Figs. 15.20–15.23), which occur in the cerebellopontine angle; retrocerebellar cysts (Figs. 15.24 to 15.27), which occur on the dorsal aspect of the cerebellar hemisphere and compress the cerebellum; and clival cysts, which occur in front of the brainstem. The signs and symptoms observed in patients with a posterior fossa arachnoid cyst are quite variable and depend on the location of the cyst. Nonlocalized headaches are commonly experienced, as are generalized unsteadiness

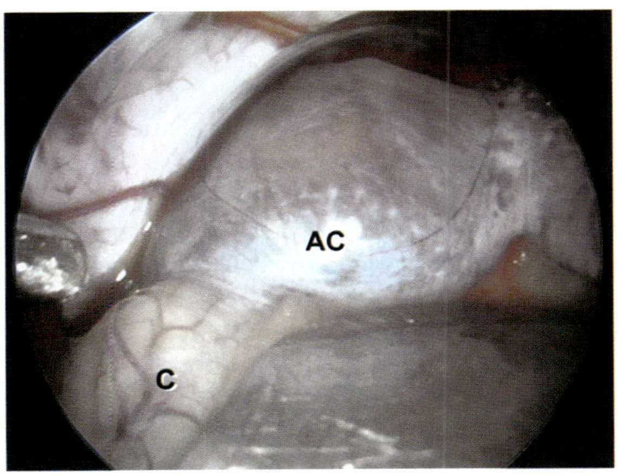


**FIGURE 15.22.** After a transtemporal (retrosigmoid) approach to the left posterior fossa, the arachnoid cyst *(AC)* can be seen within the cerebellopontine angle using a 4-mm, 0° endoscope. The cerebellum *(C)* was retracted to visualize the cyst. Notice the air-fluid level in the cerebrospinal fluid–filled arachnoid cyst.

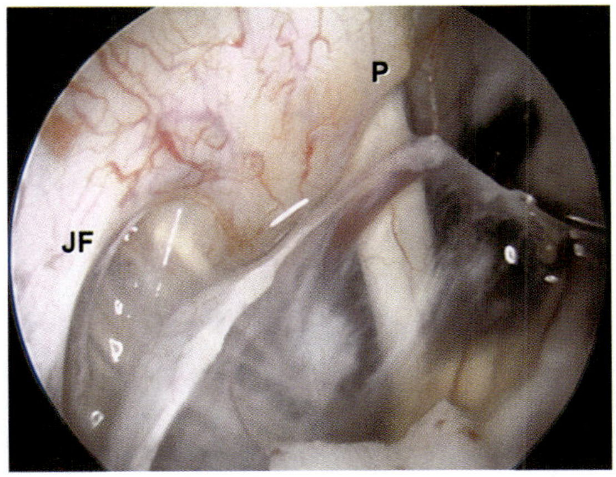


**FIGURE 15.23.** A 4-mm, 0° endoscope was used during the resection of the lateral and posterior walls of the arachnoid cyst. The medial cyst wall can be seen overlying the facial-vestibulocochlear nerve complex entering or exiting the porus acusticus *(P)* and the glossopharyngeal, vagus, and spinal accessory nerves exiting the skull base through the jugular foramen *(JF)*.

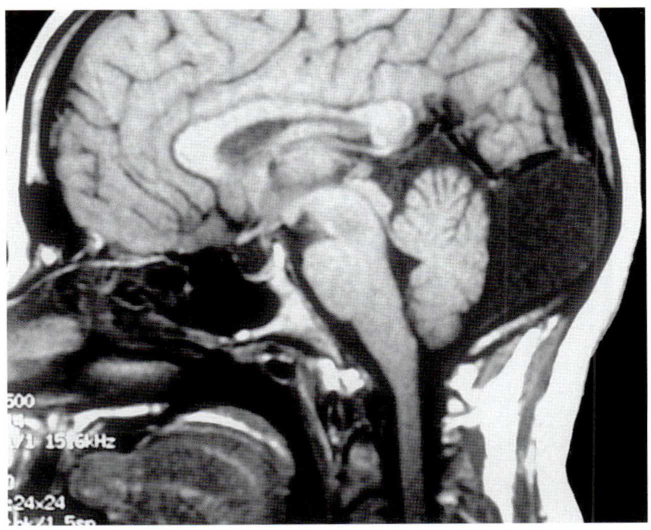

**FIGURE 15.24.** Sagittal, T1-weighted magnetic resonance image demonstrates a well-circumscribed extraaxial mass within the posterior fossa with T1-weighted signal similar to that of cerebrospinal fluid. The left cerebellar hemisphere is displaced anteriorly, and the flow void above the lesion within the straight sinus is displaced superiorly. Scalloping of the inner table of the calvarium suggests that the lesion has been present for some time.

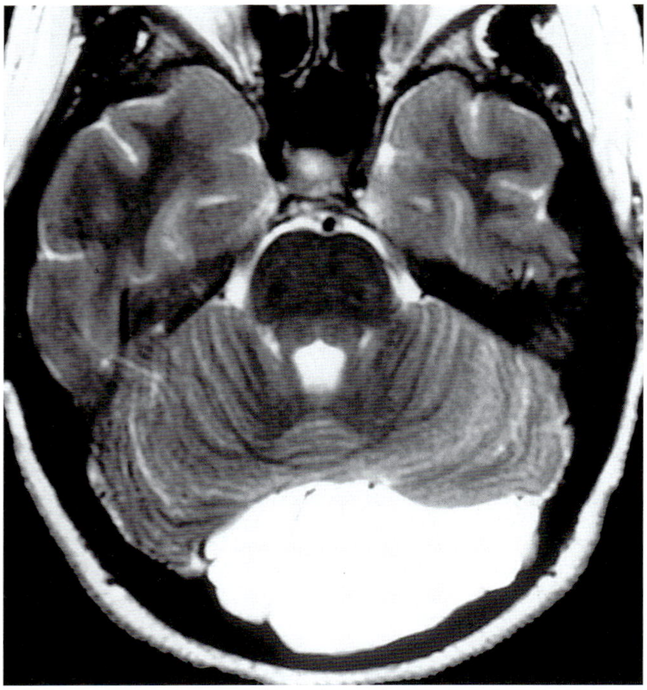

**FIGURE 15.25.** Axial, T2-weighted magnetic resonance image shows homogeneous signal throughout the extraaxial mass identical to that of cerebrospinal fluid. The mass effect on the falx cerebelli and cerebellum is observed, although there is no abnormal signal within the parenchyma to indicate edema or invasion. There is prominent scalloping of the inner calvarial margin on the left. The imaging features are characteristic of an arachnoid cyst.

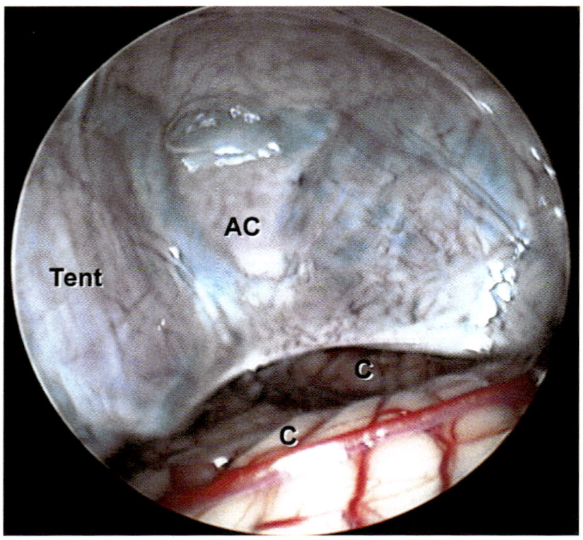


**FIGURE 15.26.** After a transtemporal (retrosigmoid) approach to the left posterior fossa, the cerebrospinal fluid–filled arachnoid cyst *(AC)* can be seen within the left and right posterior fossae using a 4-mm, 0° endoscope. The left *(foreground)* and right *(lower center)* cerebellar hemispheres *(C)* can be seen. Notice the cephalad (superior) extension of the arachnoid cyst to the tentorium *(Tent)*.

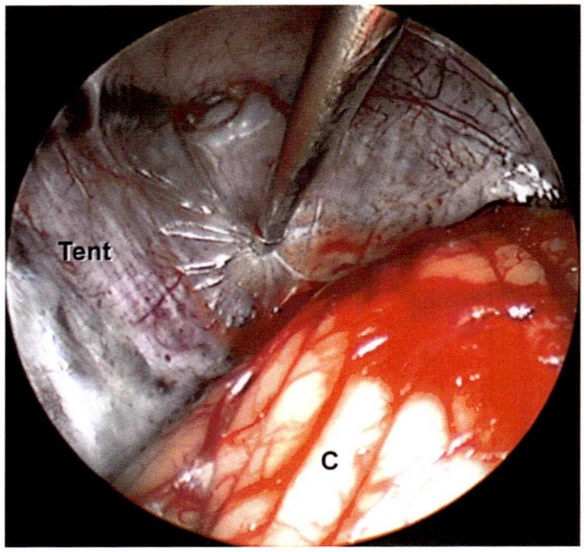


**FIGURE 15.27.** A 4-mm, 0° endoscope was used during the resection of the arachnoid cyst walls. Rhoton suction can be seen elevating the right lateral cyst wall from the right medial face of the occipital bone dura. The tentorium *(Tent)* is seen, as is the surface of the right cerebellum *(C)*.

and disequilibrium, and hearing loss, tinnitus, trigeminal nerve dysfunction, and facial nerve dysfunction have been described (17–19).

The patient presented in Figures 15.20–15.23 was struck by lightening and had vague symptoms suggesting left posttraumatic endolymphatic hydrops, including fluctuation of his hearing, left aural fullness, and disequilibrium. He initially responded to diuretics, but after his symptoms returned MRI demonstrated a left laterocerebellar arachnoid cyst (Figs. 15.20 and 15.21). He elected for surgical management through a left retrosigmoid approach and endoscopic resection of the cyst wall (Figs. 15.22 and 15.23). The endoscope allowed excellent visualization of the cyst wall, and his symptoms are markedly improved 2 years after resection.

Figures 15.24–15.27 illustrate a patient with large retrocerebellar arachnoid cyst. She was experiencing significant headaches and disequilibrium. All of her auditory and vestibular testing results were normal; however, MRI showed the cyst and cerebellar compression (Figs. 15.24 and 15.25). A small, left retrosigmoid craniotomy was performed, and the left and right retrocerebellar arachnoid cyst was resected with the use of a 4-mm, 0° endoscope (Figs. 15.26 and 15.27), obviating the need of a much larger craniotomy, a midline craniotomy, or bilateral craniotomies. Her symptoms resolved postoperatively. It remains controversial whether resection of most of the cyst wall with wide marsupialization or cyst-peritoneal shunting offers the best long-term outcome (17–19).

## Temporal Bone Meningocele

Encephaloceles represent the herniation of cranial contents beyond the normal confines of the skull. The term *encephalocele* includes several distinct entities: meningocele, a herniation of the meninges and CSF; encephalomeningocele, a herniation of the brain and meninges; and hydroencephalomeningocele, a herniation of cranial ventricles, brain, and meninges. Temporal bone encephaloceles are uncommon, with less than 150 reported cases. They can be classified by cause into five categories (20). Congenital encephaloceles result from disorders of ossification. Trauma-induced encephaloceles may occur after temporal bone trauma. Iatrogenic encephaloceles usually occur as a postoperative complication of mastoidectomy and were common in the preantibiotic era. Infection-induced encephaloceles occur in conjunction with chronic otitis media with and without cholesteatoma. Spontaneous encephaloceles are classified by exclusion, occurring in patients without prior history of trauma, surgery, or infection.

A large series and review of the literature by Lundy and colleagues (21) addressed the surgical management, which includes a transmastoid, middle cranial fossa, or combined approach. After repair, recurrence is rare.

Figures 15.28 and 15.29 demonstrate the MRI appearance of a temporal bone meningocele. This iatrogenic meningocele occurred through the posterior fossa into the mastoid and is shown in Figure 15.30. The application of endoscopic techniques in the repair of encephaloceles allows better visualization of the tissue to be reduced or amputated and provides the opportunity for repair to be accomplished through a smaller craniotomy.

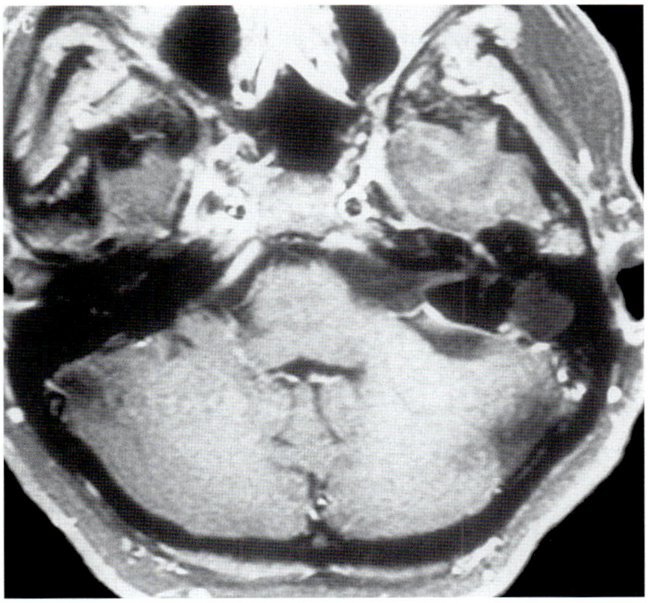

**FIGURE 15.28.** Axial, T1-weighted magnetic resonance image with gadolinium enhancement and fat saturation technique demonstrates a well-circumscribed lesion within the left mastoid with similar signal intensity to cerebrospinal fluid and no central enhancement. The left internal auditory canal, cochlea, and vestibule are unremarkable in appearance. A small amount of contrast enhancement can be seen within the left sigmoid sinus just posterior to the lesion.

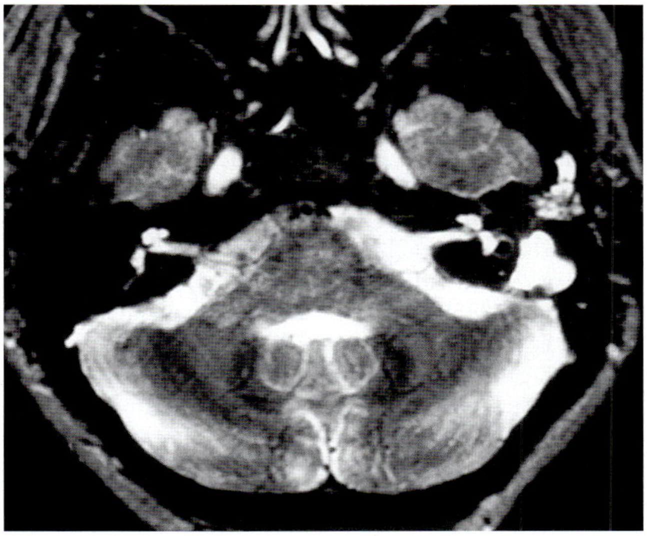

**FIGURE 15.29.** Axial, T2-weighted magnetic resonance image through the temporal bones demonstrates high signal intensity, which is similar to that of cerebrospinal fluid, within the left mastoid lesion. Additional high-signal-intensity fluid is seen within more anteriorly located left mastoid air cells in the squamous portion of the left temporal bone. The lesion was proven to be a meningocele extending into the mastoid (see Fig. 15.30).

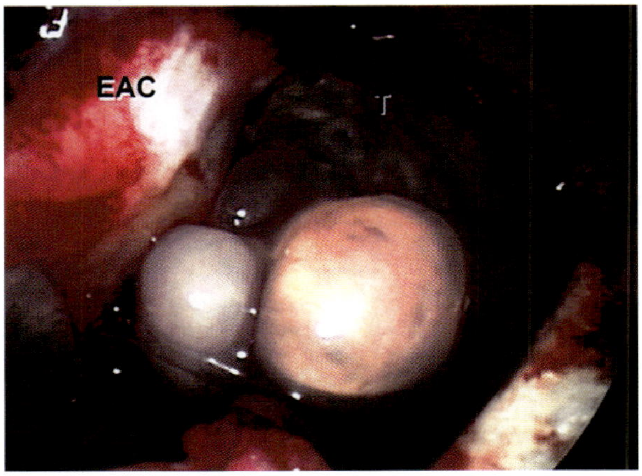


**FIGURE 15.30.** View into the left mastoid using a 4-mm, 0° endoscope. A multilobulated meningocele is filled with cerebrospinal fluid. Notice the external auditory canal *(EAC)* and the tegmen mastoideum *(T)*. This meningocele was resected, and the defect leading to the posterior fossa was closed with temporalis fascia and free bone grafts.

## Paragangliomas

Paragangliomas are a group of histologically similar neoplasms that arise from widely dispersed collections of specialized neural crest cells (i.e., chief cells), which are associated with segmental autonomic ganglia (i.e., paraganglia) throughout the body. They are derived from the neural crest and migrate in close association with the ganglia of the sympathetic nervous system (22). Paragangliomas can be divided into two main groups: adrenal and extraadrenal (Table 15.3). Adrenal paragangliomas are known as pheochromocytomas. Classification of head and neck paragangliomas is based on their anatomic location, and they include the carotid body, jugulotympanic, vagal, laryngeal, nasal, and orbital paragangliomas. Paragangliomas may be more common in Caucasians; however, there is not clear evidence to support this (23). They occur more frequently in women, and they typically manifest in the fourth or fifth decades of life (23). Paragangliomas have been described in patients as young as 6 months and as old as 88 years. Multiple or synchronous tumors occur in 3% to 10% of patients. A hereditary form of paraganglioma has been identified and is an autosomal dominant disorder linked to two loci: 11q13.1 and 11q22.3-q23 (24).

Jugulotympanic paragangliomas (i.e., glomus jugulare) grow in an insidious and slow pattern; however, they can be destructive, as was the case for the patient presented in Figures 15.31–15.34. Clinically, she had a vagal paresis and conductive hearing loss on the right side. The typical CT and MRI appearance of a glomus jugulare is shown in Figures 15.31–15.33. Based on her preoperative imaging studies, it was unclear whether she had extension into the posterior fossa (Fig. 15.33). During the surgical resection of this right glomus jugulare tumor by a Fisch type B infratemporal fossa approach and after completing the craniectomy anterior and posterior to the sigmoid sinus, a small dural incision was made, and a 4-mm, 0° endoscope was placed into the right posterior fossa. The endoscopic view provided no evidence that the tumor extended into the posterior fossa (Fig. 15.34). Postoperatively, she had recovery from the vagal paresis; however, because her external auditory canal was oversewn, she maintained her conductive hearing loss.

**TABLE 15.3. PARAGANGLIOMA CLASSIFICATION**

| Adrenal | Extraadrenal |
|---|---|
| Pheochromocytoma | Branchiomeric |
| | Aorticopulmonary |
| | Coronary |
| | Intercarotid |
| | Jugulotympanic |
| | Laryngeal |
| | Orbital |
| | Pulmonary |
| | Subclavian |
| | Intravagal |
| | Aorticosympathetic |
| | Visceroautonomic |

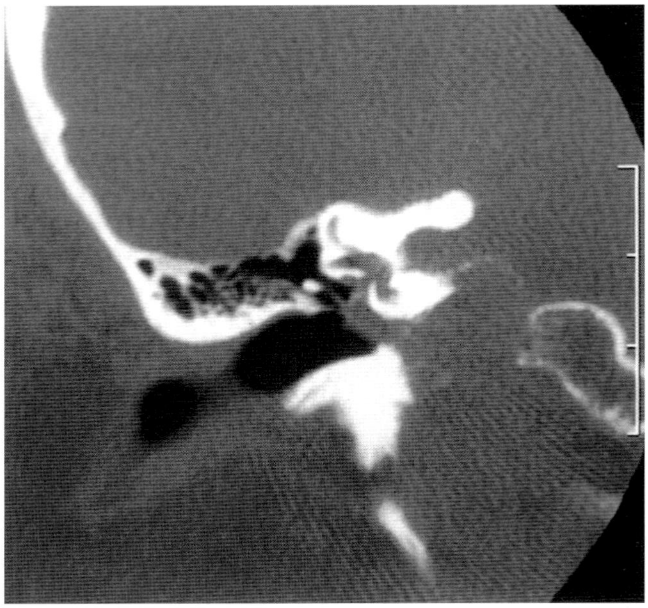

**FIGURE 15.31.** Coronal computed tomographic image of the right temporal bone filmed with the bone-window technique shows a mass involving the right jugular foramen with extension into the right middle ear cavity over the cochlear promontory. The lesion also extends into the medial aspect of the right internal auditory canal (IAC). There is a thin margin of bone between the IAC and the lesion.

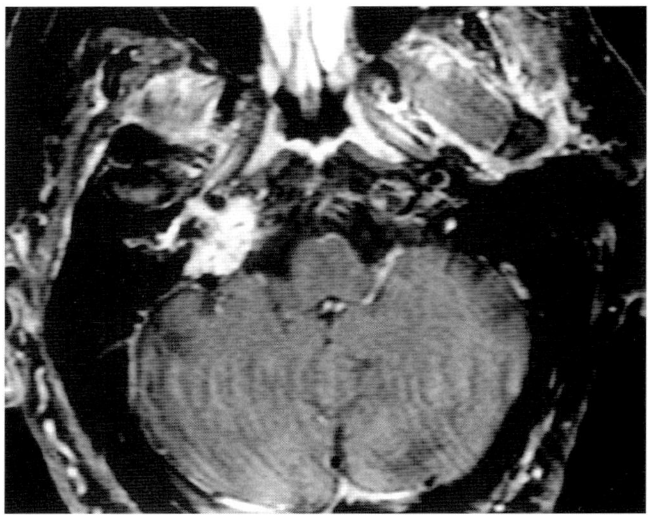

**FIGURE 15.32.** Axial, T1-weighted magnetic resonance image with gadolinium and fat saturation technique shows right skull base lesion at the level of the jugular foramen with ill-defined margins and diffuse enhancement. The lesion marginates the right internal carotid artery posteriorly. No invasion of the adjacent cerebellum is appreciated on this image.

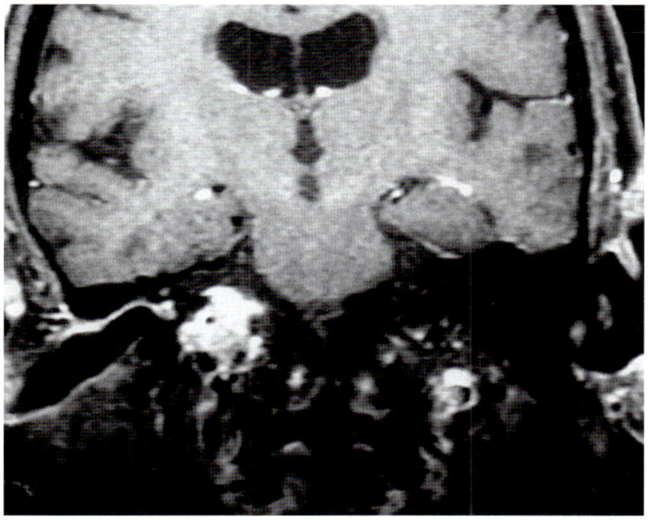

**FIGURE 15.33.** Coronal, T1-weighted magnetic resonance image with gadolinium and fat saturation technique shows ill-defined enhancing lesion involving the right jugular foramen. A punctate focus of signal void is seen within the lesion and is consistent with a flow void in this hypervascular glomus jugulare tumor. Possible extension of the tumor into the posterior fossa is seen.

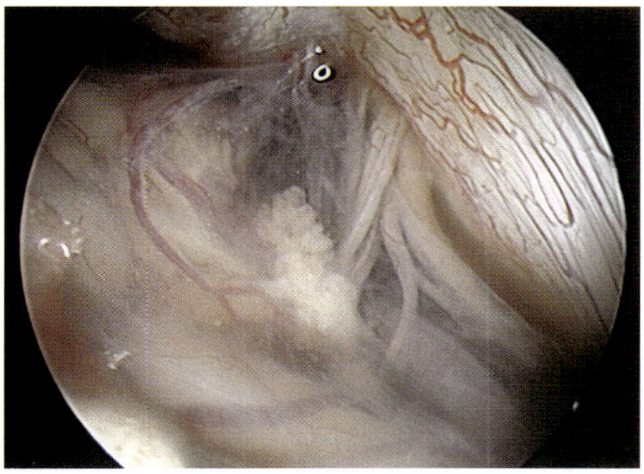

**FIGURE 15.34.** During the surgical resection of this right glomus jugulare tumor using a Fisch type B infratemporal fossa approach and after completing the craniectomy anterior and posterior to the sigmoid sinus, a small dural incision was made, and a 4-mm, 0° endoscope was placed into the right posterior fossa. This endoscopic view provided no evidence that the tumor extended into the posterior fossa. The glossopharyngeal, vagus, and spinal accessory nerves are seen entering the jugular foramen *(top center)*. Notice the choroid plexus *(center)*.

## MENINGIOMAS

Meningiomas are usually benign tumors that originate from the meningothelial arachnoid cells normally found in arachnoid villi adjacent to the dura (25). They tend to displace adjacent brain and nerves, and they characteristically invade dura, the venous sinuses, and underlying bone. Meningiomas account for 15% of all intracranial tumors, and their preferred sites are correlated with the location of arachnoid villi from which they arise. These include the parasagittal area along the dural sinuses, lateral cerebral convexities, sphenoid ridge, foramina of exit of the cranial nerves, and adjacent perineural sheaths of cranial nerves. They are generally well circumscribed, smooth or lobulated, and firm with a gray-white appearance. There are two characteristic macroscopic subtypes: en plaque or globular. En plaque tumors are flat and have a more marked tendency for invasion and to elicit hyperostosis.

The natural history of meningiomas is that they are slow-growing tumors in most cases; however, aggressively behaving tumors with metastatic potential have been reported. The size, symptom complex, rate of growth, and age and life expectancy must be taken into account when considering the management strategy. Preoperative angiography and embolization should be pursued when possible. The goal of surgery should be complete resection, including a dural margin and removal of any involved underlying bone.

### Petroclival Meningioma

Petroclival meningiomas present the greatest problems for achieving complete resection. The primary issues are surgical accessibility, avoidance of cranial nerve injury, and avoidance of vascular injury (26). Figures 15.35–15.40

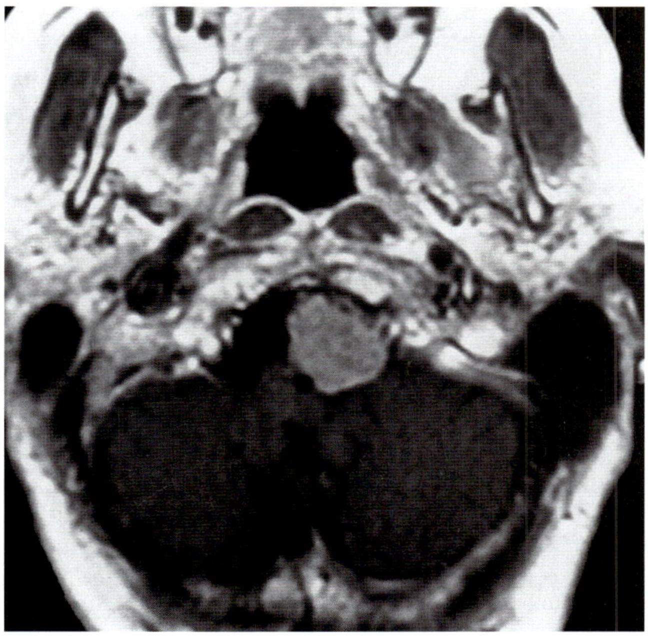

**FIGURE 15.35.** Axial, T1-weighted magnetic resonance image with gadolinium shows an extraaxial mass just above the foramen magnum displacing and compressing the medulla posteriorly and slightly toward the right. The lesion has well-circumscribed margins, abuts the dura, and enhances homogeneously.

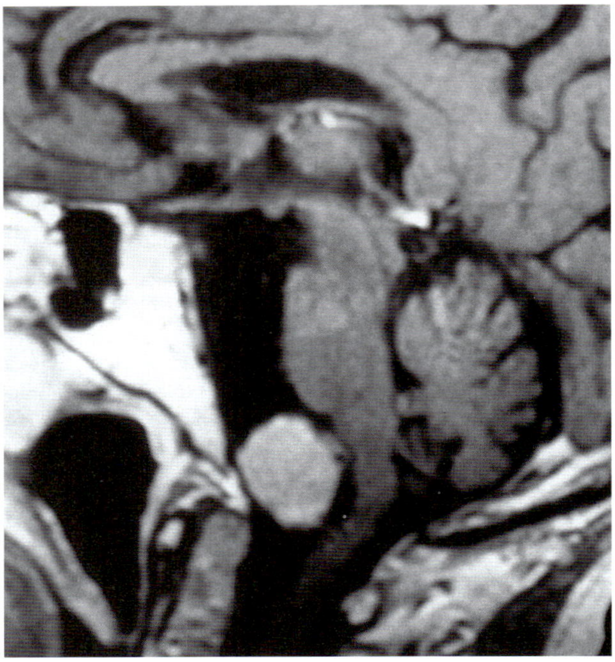

**FIGURE 15.36.** T1-weighted, sagittal magnetic resonance image after gadolinium administration shows the extraaxial mass at the anterior margin of the foramen magnum causing compression of the medulla posteriorly. Notice the normal marrow signal intensity within the clivus and the dens. The lesion does not invade the medulla. The imaging features are characteristic of a meningioma. Figures 15.37–15.40 show the endoscopic appearance before, during, and after resection of the tumor.

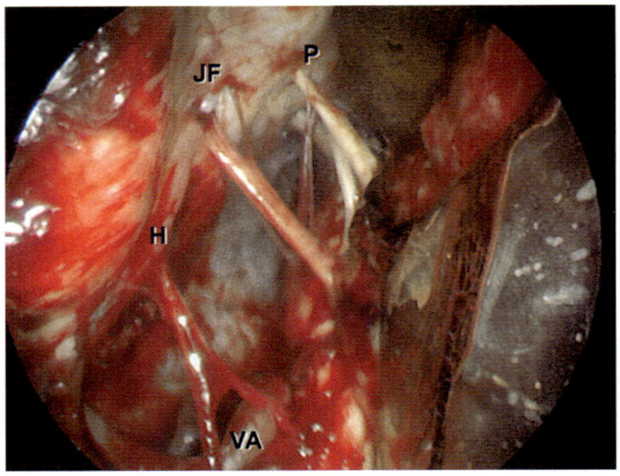


**FIGURE 15.38.** During resection of the meningioma, dissection between and beyond a lattice of cranial nerves was necessary. The vestibulocochlear nerves can be seen exiting the porus acusticus, and the facial nerve can be seen entering the porus acusticus *(P)*. The glossopharyngeal, vagus, and spinal accessory nerves are seen entering the jugular foramen *(JF)*. The hypoglossal nerve can be seen entering the hypoglossal canal *(H)*. Notice the right vertebral artery *(VA)*.

demonstrate such a challenging case. This petroclival meningioma was very low and produced significant brainstem compression (Figs. 15.35 and 15.36). As seen in Figures 15.37–15.40, rigid endoscopes were helpful in appreciating the neurovascular relationships surrounding the tumor.

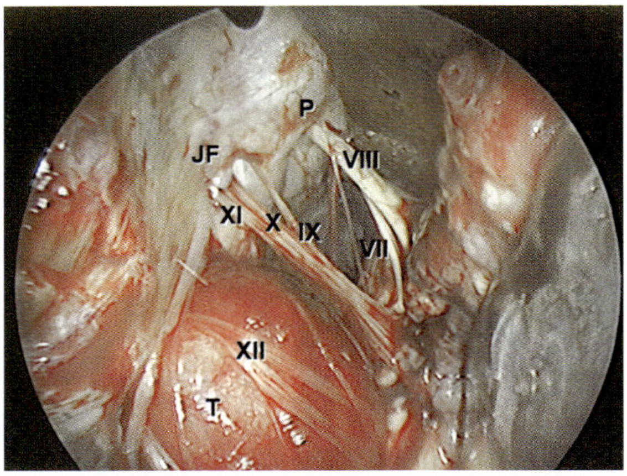


**FIGURE 15.37.** Intraoperative view of this caudally positioned left petroclival meningioma. The view with a 4-mm, 0° endoscope shows the petroclival junction *(left)* and ventral brainstem *(right)* in relation to the meningioma *(T)*. Cranial nerves *VII, VIII, IX, X, XI,* and *XII* are seen. Notice the porus acusticus *(P)* and jugular foramen *(JF)*.

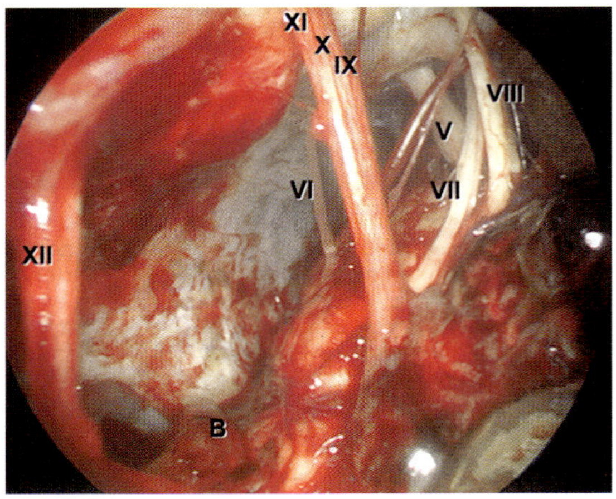


**FIGURE 15.39.** After tumor removal, advancement of the 4-mm, 0° endoscope shows the trigeminal *(V)*, abducens *(VI)*, facial *(VII)*, vestibulocochlear *(VIII)*, glossopharyngeal *(IX)*, vagus *(X)*, spinal accessory *(XI)*, and hypoglossal *(XII)* nerves. Notice the basilar artery *(B)*.

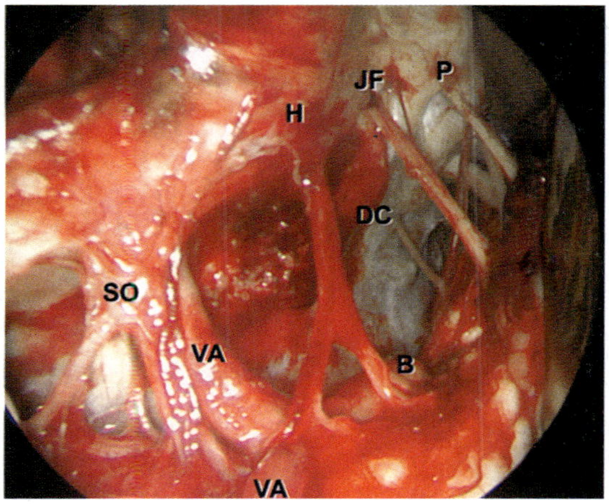


**FIGURE 15.40.** Panoramic view after tumor resection using a 4-mm, 0° endoscope shows the abducens nerve entering Dorello's canal *(DC)* at the anterior petrous apex; the vestibulocochlear and facial nerves at the porus acusticus *(P)*; the glossopharyngeal, vagus, and spinal accessory nerves entering the jugular foramen *(JF)*; the hypoglossal nerve entering the hypoglossal canal *(H)*; and the suboccipital nerve *(SO)*. Notice both vertebral arteries *(VA)* joining to form the basilar artery *(B)*.

## Orbital Apex Meningioma and Parasellar Meningioma

Figures 15.41–15.47 show two case examples of orbital apex and parasellar meningiomas. The typical CT and MRI findings are shown in Figures 15.41–15.43. The 4-mm, 0° and 30° endoscopes were helpful in defining the neurovascular relationships of the tumor, optic chiasm, internal carotid artery, and the optic and oculomotor nerves (Figs. 15.44–15.47).

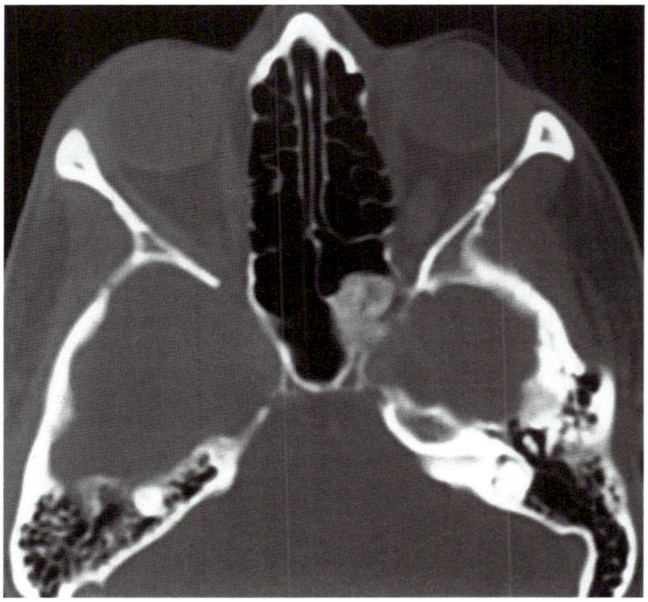

**FIGURE 15.41.** Axial computed tomographic examination of the head filmed with the bone-window technique demonstrates a calcified mass involving the left sphenoid sinus and medial wall of the left cavernous sinus. The lesion has a diffusely dense appearance and is well circumscribed. No extension into the left middle cranial fossa or orbital apex is appreciated, although there is some mass effect on the superior orbital fissure on the left. Histopathologic analysis demonstrated that this lesion was a meningioma.

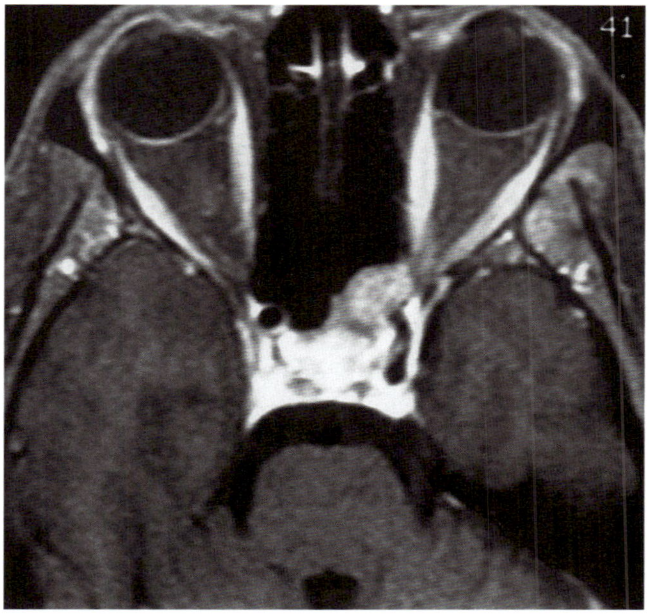


**FIGURE 15.42.** Axial, T1-weighted, postgadolinium magnetic resonance image with fat saturation technique demonstrates enhancement within the left sphenoid lesion. A normal-appearing flow void within the cavernous segment of the left internal carotid artery is appreciated.

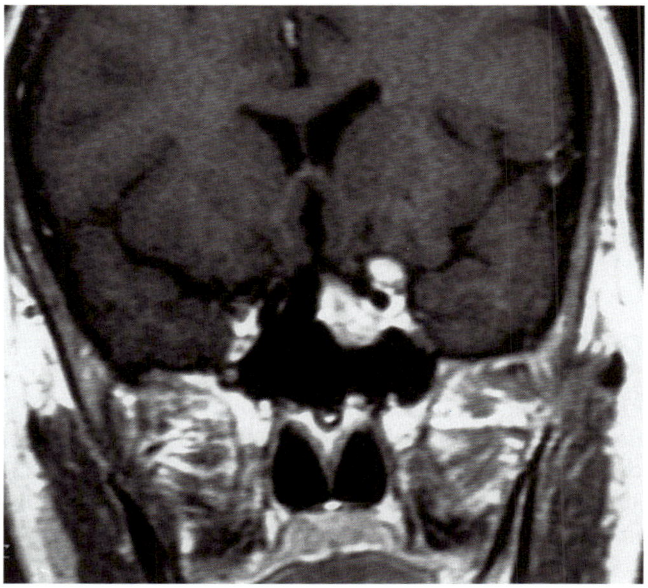

**FIGURE 15.43.** Coronal, T1-weighted, postgadolinium magnetic resonance image shows the well-defined left sphenoid lesion, which is diffusely enhancing. No compression of the cavernous carotid artery by this meningioma is seen, although it may be slightly elevated.

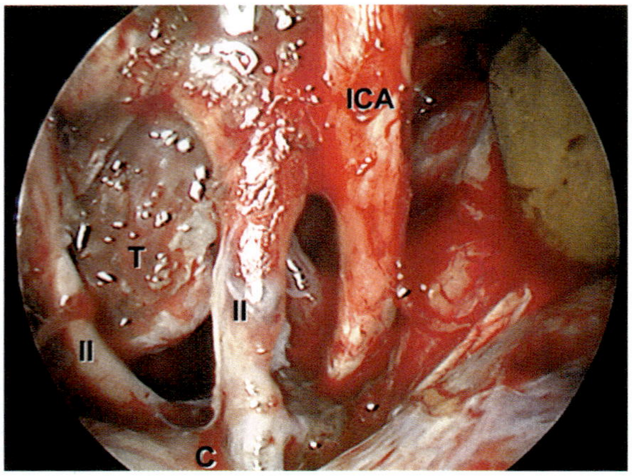


**FIGURE 15.44.** A 4-mm, 0° endoscope provides a panoramic view of the tumor *(T)* in relation to the left optic nerve *(II, center)*, the optic chiasm *(C)*, right optic nerve *(II, left)*, and left internal carotid artery *(ICA)*. This meningioma was resected, leaving this neurovascular lattice intact.

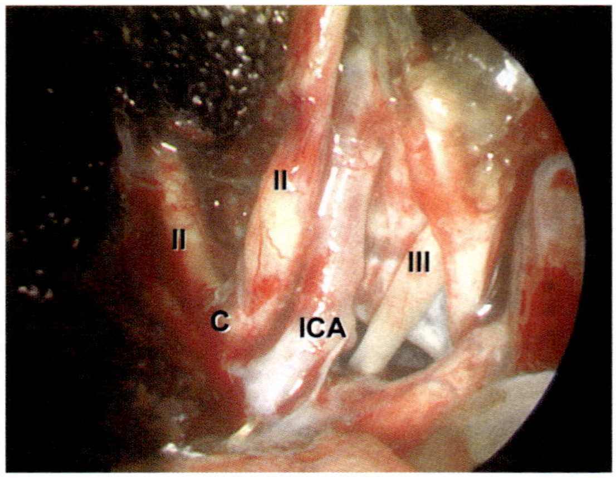


**FIGURE 15.46.** A 4-mm, 30° endoscope provides a slightly different perspective on this skull base anatomy. *II*, optic nerves; *III*, right oculomotor nerve; *C*, optic chiasm; *ICA*, internal carotid artery.

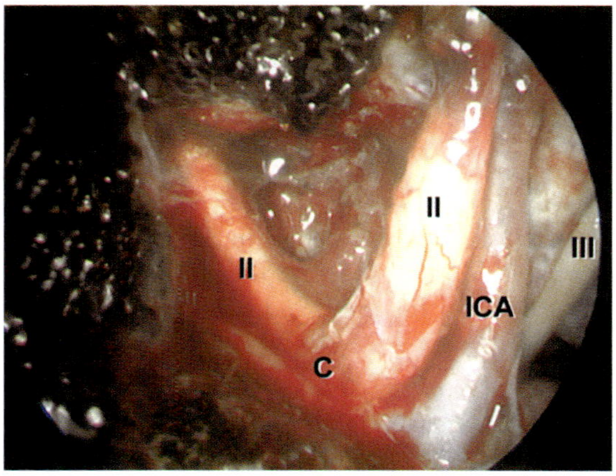


**FIGURE 15.45.** The endoscopic photographs shown in Figures 15.45–15.47 are examples of another skull base meningioma adjacent to the optic chiasm *(C)*. This tumor was approached from the right. This view with a 4-mm, 0° endoscope shows the right and left optic nerves *(II)*, as well as the right oculomotor nerve *(III)* and the internal carotid artery *(ICA)*.

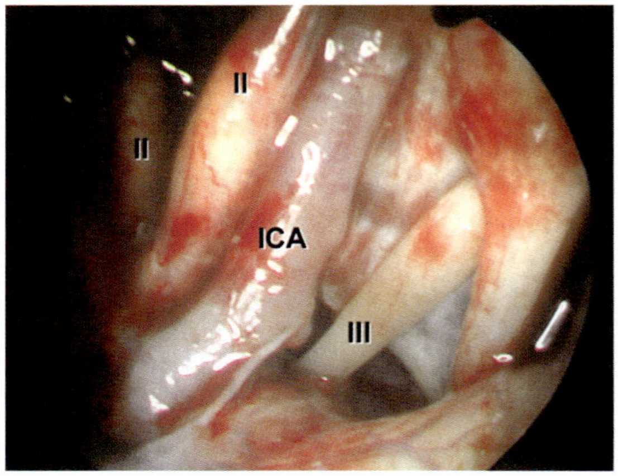


**FIGURE 15.47.** Comparison of this figure and Figure 15.46 shows how the position of the endoscope tip determines the degree of magnification. This photograph was taken with the tip of a 4-mm, 30° endoscope closer to the optic nerves *(II)*, the right internal carotid artery *(ICA)*, and the right oculomotor nerve *(III)*.

## CONCLUSIONS

Our experience indicates that endoscopes can be used safely during lateral skull base surgery and that, as an adjunct to the operative microscope, this modality does improve visualization of bony, neural, and vascular structures while minimizing retraction of these structures. The adjunctive use of endoscopes enhances our ability to surgically manage lateral skull base diseases.

## REFERENCES

1. Heffelfinger MJ, Dahlin DC, MacCarty CS, et al. Chordomas and cartilaginous tumors at the skull base. *Cancer* 1973;32:410–420.
2. Brown RV, Sage MR, Brophy BP. CT and MR findings in patients with chordomas of the petrous apex. *AJNR Am J Neuroradiol* 1990;11:121–124.
3. Barnes L, Peel RL, Verbin RS, et al. Diseases of the bones and joints. In: Barnes L, ed. *Surgical pathology of the head and neck.* New York: Marcel Dekker, 1985:883–1044.

4. Krespi YP, Levine TM, Oppenheimer R. Skull base chordomas. *Otolaryngol Clin North Am* 1986;19:797–804.
5. Barnes L, Kapadia SB, Nemzek WR, et al. Biology of selected skull base tumors. In: Janecka IP, Tiedemann K, eds. *Skull base surgery: anatomy, biology, and technology*. Philadelphia: Lippincott–Raven Publishers, 1997:263–289.
6. Gantz BJ, Perry BP. Skull base chordoma. In: Jackler RK, Driscoll CL, eds. *Tumors of the ear and temporal bone*. Philadelphia: Lippincott Williams & Wilkins, 2000:332–342.
7. Wackym PA, King WA, Poe DS, et al. Adjunctive use of endoscopy during acoustic neuroma surgery. *Laryngoscope* 1999; 109:1193–1201.
8. Wackym PA, King WA, Barker FG, et al. Endoscope-assisted vestibular neurectomy. *Laryngoscope* 1998;108:1787–1793.
9. Nager GT. Epidermoids involving the temporal bone: clinical, radiological and pathologic aspects. *Laryngoscope* 1975;85[Suppl 2]:1–22.
10. Samii M, Tatagiba M, Piquer J, et al. Surgical treatment of epidermoid cysts of the cerebellopontine angle. *J Neurosurg* 1996; 84:14–19.
11. Nager GT, Vanderveen TS. Cholesterol granuloma involving the temporal bone. *Ann Otol Rhinol Laryngol* 1976;85:204–209.
12. Smith PG, Leonetti JP, Klezker GR. Differential clinical and radiographic features of cholesterol granulomas and cholesteatomas of the petrous apex. *Ann Otol Rhinol Laryngol* 1988;97:599–604.
13. Gleason MJ, Fisch U, Makek M, et al. Mucosal cysts of the petrous apex. In: Fisch U, Valvanis A, Yasargil MG, eds. *Neurologic surgery of the ear and skull base*. Berkeley, CA: Kugler & Ghedini, 1989:3–10.
14. Lichtenstein L. Histiocytosis-X. *Arch Pathol* 1953;56:84–102.
15. Nezelof C, Basset F, Rousseau MF. Histiocytosis X: histiogenic arguments for a Langerhans' cell origin. *Biomedicine* 1973;18: 365–371.
16. Angeli SI, Alcalde J, Hoffman HT, et al. Langerhans' cell histiocytosis of the head and neck in children. *Ann Otol Rhinol Laryngol* 1995;104:173–180.
17. Daspit CP. Neurotologic aspects of posterior fossa arachnoid cysts. In: Jackler RK, Brackmann DE, eds. *Neurotology*. St. Louis: Mosby–Year Book, 1994:939–944.
18. Jallo GI, Woo HH, Meshki C, et al. Arachnoid cysts of the cerebellopontine angle: diagnosis and surgery. *Neurosurgery* 1997;40: 31–38.
19. Pappas DG, Brackmann DE. Arachnoid cysts of the posterior fossa. *Otolaryngol Head Neck Surg* 1981;89:328–332.
20. Wackym PA, Friedmann I. Unusual tumors of the middle ear and mastoid. In: Jackler RK, Driscoll CL, eds. *Tumors of the ear and temporal bone*. Philadelphia: Lippincott Williams & Wilkins, 2000:128–145.
21. Lundy LB, Graham MD, Kartush JM, et al. Temporal bone encephalocele and cerebrospinal fluid leaks. *Am J Otol* 1996;17: 461–469.
22. Kliewer KE, Cochran AJ. A review of the histology, ultrastructure, immunohistology, and molecular biology of extra-adrenal paragangliomas. *Arch Pathol Lab Med* 1989;113: 1209–1218.
23. Alford BR, Guilford FR. A comprehensive study of tumors of the glomus jugulare. *Laryngoscope* 1962;72:765–787.
24. Baysal BE, van Schothorst EM, Farr JE, et al. A high-resolution STS, EST, and gene-based physical map of the hereditary paraganglioma region on chromosome 11q23. *Genomics* 1997;44: 214–221.
25. Langford LA. Pathology of meningiomas. *J Neurooncol* 1996; 29:217–221.
26. Wackym PA, Blackwell KE. Abnormalities of the craniovertebral junction. In: Jackler RK, Brackmann DE, eds. *Neurotology*. St. Louis: Mosby–Year Book, 1994:1203–1231.

SECTION III

# PARANASAL SINUS SURGERY

# 16

# ANATOMY OF THE NASAL ACCESSORY SINUSES

**SAMUEL MÁRQUEZ**
**WILLIAM LAWSON**
**STEVEN D. SCHAEFER**
**JEFFREY T. LAITMAN**

## HISTORICAL PERSPECTIVE

The investigation of paranasal sinus anatomy may have begun with the great anatomist Galen in the second century ad, although his writings do not mention any of the sinuses by name (1). The depth and nature of descriptions of the sinuses have varied considerably through history, usually being mentioned within larger works. Notable in this regard were da Vinci's discussions of the maxillary sinus (2) and Berengario da Carpi's initial descriptions of the sphenoid sinus (3). It was not until the seventeenth and eighteenth centuries that studies began to focus on the sinuses themselves. Most of these works, however, were by individuals concerned not with precise anatomy but with more theoretical questions addressing functional explanations for the existence of these "hollow" spaces in the cranium (4,5). Anatomic observations by such individuals were not usually done for systematic assessment of structure but appear to have been used to buttress their particular functional theories (6).

In the late nineteenth century, the great Austrian anatomist Emil Zuckerkandl published the first detailed and systematic anatomic and pathologic description of the paranasal sinuses (7–9). His observations and illustrations were so precise and meticulous that they form the foundation for much current knowledge, and Zuckerkandl is regarded as the father of modern sinus anatomy (6,10).

During the preantibiotic era, in the early part of the twentieth century, anatomic studies focused on descriptions that could improve procedures for cannulation or drainage of pathologic sinuses (11–16). It became apparent that, after treatment, sinus infection often recurred in the same treated sinus and often spread and infected the other nontreated sinuses. These secondary infections were explained by the close and intimate relationships seen in the anatomy of the paranasal sinuses. At this time, the importance of understanding prenatal development as a vehicle to understand sinus surgery became more fully appreciated (17). Later, technologic advances led to the development of endoscopic and external sinus procedures. Having a knowledge of development, surgeons practicing endoscopic sinus surgery today primarily focus attention on the role of the ethmoid sinus in recurrent paranasal sinus infection (18). We are reminded that recurrent frontal or maxillary sinusitis was recognized earlier this century by Schaeffer (11), who stated that "the maxillary sinus is often a cesspool for infectious material from the sinus frontalis and certain of an anterior group of cellulae ethmoidales." This is an example of knowledge lost, only to be rediscovered when new interest in the sinuses arose after advances in imaging modalities, instrument technology, and the work of modern sinus surgeons (19,20).

A full description of the history, development, and anatomy of the paranasal sinuses would require a treatise in itself; this chapter focuses on the features of gross structure and development most relevant to surgical procedures. The chapter also addresses inconsistencies and vagaries in terminology, because they have often been a major source of confusion among those studying or operating on sinuses.

## PRINCIPLES OF DEVELOPMENT

A knowledge of paranasal sinus development provides an understanding of its complex anatomy, its intimate relationships, and the distinct drainage pathways associated with each sinus. Because detailed descriptions on the development of each sinus are found in the respective sections, the following text briefly discusses the principles and implications of paranasal sinus development.

All paranasal sinus development originates from the primordia of the cartilaginous nasal capsule, and completion begins with its budding into the bony elements of the cranium, establishing a communication network with the nasal cavity throughout life (21). The prenatal development of paranasal sinuses begins as an evagination of respiratory mucosal epithelium from the nasal capsule invading two bony elements of the splanchnocranium (i.e., maxillary and ethmoid bones). Although the initial development of all paranasal sinuses begins prenatally, the definitive frontal and sphenoidal sinuses are developmentally completed during their postnatal growth. Whether the early developmental stages serve as a prenatal template for postnatal formation and growth of the sinuses remains unclear.

The health and normal function of the paranasal sinuses depend on their having proper drainage and ventilation. During prenatal and postnatal developments, the communicating portals established between the sinuses and the nasal chamber are formed by the evaginations of respiratory mucosa, with each sinus having a distinct and patent pathway. The drainage pathways from all sinus ostia must navigate through intricate clefts or chambers and empty into a common space within the lateral wall of the nasal cavity (i.e., ethmoid infundibulum and superior meatus) before ultimately reaching the nasopharynx. The confluence of the sinus drainage pathways established in prenatal and postnatal development effectively links the sinuses together. The clinical implications of sinus development are evident by how rapidly infection can spread from one sinus to another. Knowledge of the development of paranasal sinus anatomy is essential in understanding the extension of sinus infection and in predicting the clinical course of patients.

## ETHMOID SINUS

### History, Development, and Anatomy

Galen was the first to describe the ethmoid bone as being sievelike in structure when referring to the cribriform plate (22). The honeycomb-like appearance of its air cells, combined with its intricate passageways and blind alleys, led investigators to refer to this bone as an ethmoid labyrinth (1). Van Alyea (23) stated that the very name "ethmoid labyrinth" implied structural intricacy. Descriptions regarding its shape have ranged from ethmoidal "bloc" (24) to pyramidal shape to trapezoidal "box" (25). Although Ritter (26) emphasized the ethmoid sinus as the principal support for the anterior cranial fossa, others saw it as a way to maximize the surface area of the mucosa and to absorb the energy of trauma, because its design permits the sinus to collapse to protect the eyes and the brain (25).

The ethmoid bone is considered the "keystone in the sinus system" (27) because each paranasal sinus drainage pathway is through or adjacent to its lateral wall. Along with the ethmoid, the maxilla, inferior conchae, and lacrimal and vertical plate of the palatine bones contribute to the intricate and irregular surface of the nasal cavity's lateral wall (28). The complex nature of these lateral wall structures can be best understood by reviewing the growth and development of the turbinates or conchae and of the ethmoid bone itself.

The extensive fetal developmental studies done by Schaeffer (17,29–31) showed no morphologic changes on the lateral wall until the thirty-eighth to fortieth day of prenatal growth, when two shallow grooves are observed above and below the region where the inferior nasal conchae or maxilloturbinal eventually develop (Fig. 16.1). Once mesenchymal differentiation in the area of the inferior nasal conchae ensues, it has the effect of producing a more prominent fold of the conchae and aids in accentuating the depth of these grooves or furrows. The developing folds are considered the primitive step for conchal formation, whereas these furrows constitute the future inferior and middle meatus. By the sixty-thrid to seventieth day of prenatal development, six major furrows develop along with their corresponding ridges or folds called the *ethmoturbinals* (i.e., turbinates arising from the ethmoid). Stammberger (32) divides these folds into two anatomic components: an anterior ascending portion (i.e., the ramus ascendens) and a posteroinferior descending more horizontal portion (i.e., ramus descendens). However, not all of these folds and furrows persist during the development of the fetus. For example, from the seventh month to term, the examiner could find three to five ethmoidal conchae with a corresponding number of intervening meatus, but after birth, because of fusion (21) or obliteration (29), only two or three ethmoidal conchae may persist [i.e., middle, superior, or supreme ethmoidal conchae (17)]. Although Santorini (33) was the first anatomist to describe all three ethmoidal conchae, the following commentary by Schaeffer (29) illustrates the confusion found in the literature regarding the "typical" number of conchae found present at birth: "Books generally describe and picture two ethmoidal conchae as the typical number, and apparently would have us think that three ethmoidal conchae are rather exceptional."

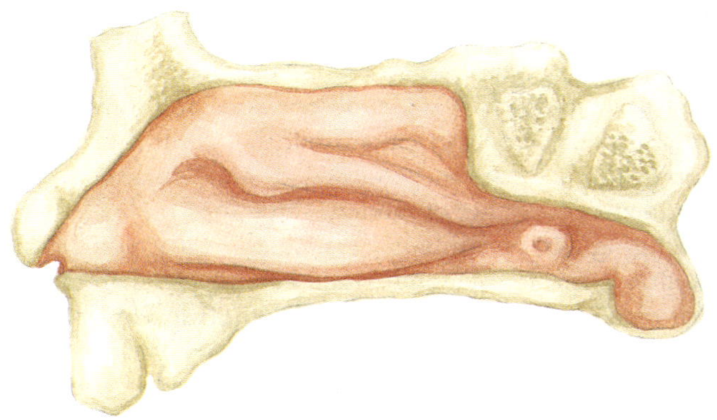

**FIGURE 16.1.** Parasagittal view shows the mucosal swellings and evaginations of the future concha of the lateral nasal cavity wall in a 190-day-old fetus. Notice the rudimentary nature of the superior nasal conchae. (Courtesy of Bridget Thomas McKnight, American Museum of Natural History, New York, NY.)

In a large series of cadaver material, Schaeffer (29) and van Alyea (23) showed that a supreme conchae was present in 62.5% and 67% of the subjects studied, and Zuckerkandl (34) recorded a supreme conchae in 80% of his 120 subjects. However, Lang and Sakals (35) reported only 17% of their subjects as having a supreme conchae, and Bingham and colleagues (36) found no supreme conchae in their samples. The issue regarding the typical number of ethmoidal conchae remains unclear.

The first primary furrow of the lateral nasal wall is located between the first and second ethmoturbinals, sometimes referred to as the first interturbinal furrow. The first ethmoturbinal (Fig. 16.2) is regarded by most investigators as the equivalent of the nasoturbinal found in higher mammals, including New World monkeys (e.g., howler monkey) and the lesser and great apes (e.g., gibbons, orangutans) (17,32,37–39). In humans, the nasoturbinal regresses during later development and never fully develops into a permanent turbinate. However, of anatomic and clinical interest, the ramus descendens of this "failed" first ethmoturbinal becomes the uncinate process, and the ramus ascendens becomes the agger nasi, both of which are important landmarks and are discussed later. The appearance of the first furrow is also an important developmental stage, because its descending anterior region becomes the ethmoid infundibulum and the superiorly ascending region becomes the frontal recess. The former is an important region where a number of the paranasal sinuses eventually drain into and through to the nasal cavity. The frontal recess undergoes further development, with additional furrows appearing or

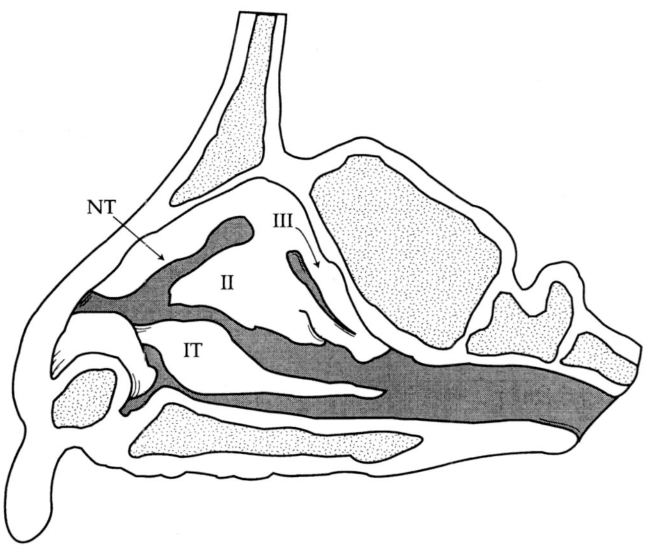


**FIGURE 16.2.** Parasagittal schematic drawing of the lateral nasal cavity wall of an Old World monkey shows the inferior turbinate *(IT)*, the nasoturbinal *(NT)*, middle turbinate *(II)*, and superior turbinate *(III)*. (Courtesy of Bridget Thomas McKnight, American Museum of Natural History, New York, NY.)

what Kasper (14) called "pits," which are outgrowths of epithelium that appear as spherical excavations in this region. Pneumatic invasion of the frontal bone originating from one of these pits in the frontal recess results in the development of the frontal sinus.

At birth, the ethmoid sinus consists of an anterior and posterior divisions. At that time, the fluid-filled ethmoids are difficult to recognize on routine radiography (40). Wolf and coworkers (41) reported the dimensions of the newborn's ethmoid sinus system to be 8 to 12 mm long (i.e., anteroposterior length), 1 to 5 mm high (i.e., superoinferior height), and 1 to 3 mm wide (i.e., medial-lateral width). They also found the anterior and posterior ethmoid air cells to be complete in number, although not in terms of adult size. Other studies have confirmed their findings (42). By 1 to 4 years of age, the ethmoids have rapidly expanded to 12 to 21 mm long, 8 to 16 mm high, and 5 to 11 mm wide. The ethmoid labyrinth may be visualized consistently by plain film radiography only after the first year postpartum and only if the air-filled divisions of the ethmoid sinus are well developed (43). At 4 to 8 years of age, the ethmoid sinus system is 18 to 24 mm long, 10 to 15 mm high, and 9 to 13 mm wide (41). By the twelfth year, the ethmoids have reached nearly adult size, with expansion during puberty primarily involving the bones outside the ethmoid capsule (44).

The designation of two divisions for the ethmoid sinus is best understood when reviewing the "architecture" of the ethmoid labyrinth (45). During development, the attachments of the various bony structures arising from the ethmoid (e.g., conchae, uncinate process) to the lateral wall are formed by one of several ground plates or *basal lamellae* (Figs. 16.3–16.9). Although the lateral attachments of these lamellae end abruptly, their medial aspects project beyond the labyrinth and form prominences, which extend into the nasal cavity. The most anterior of these lamellae is the lateral extension of the uncinate process. The *second lamella* is referred to as the plate of the bulla because its extension into the nasal cavity forms the bulla ethmoidales, and the third lamella serves as the attachment of the middle turbinate. The *third lamella* is an important anatomic structure, demarcating the division between the anterior ethmoid cells from the posterior cells and essentially dictating the drainage patterns of these air cells into the middle and superior meatus, respectively. It is also clinically significant because it is considered a natural boundary to the spread of infection into the posterior ethmoid, and it is the posterior landmark in anterior ethmoidectomy (46) (Fig. 16.10). As seen in Figures 16.3–16.9 and 16.11, this third lamella can be divided into three segments characterized by the anterior one third having a horizontal orientation and attaching superiorly, by the middle third considered the vertical portion and coursing posterior obliquely, and by the posterior

*(text continues on page 164)*

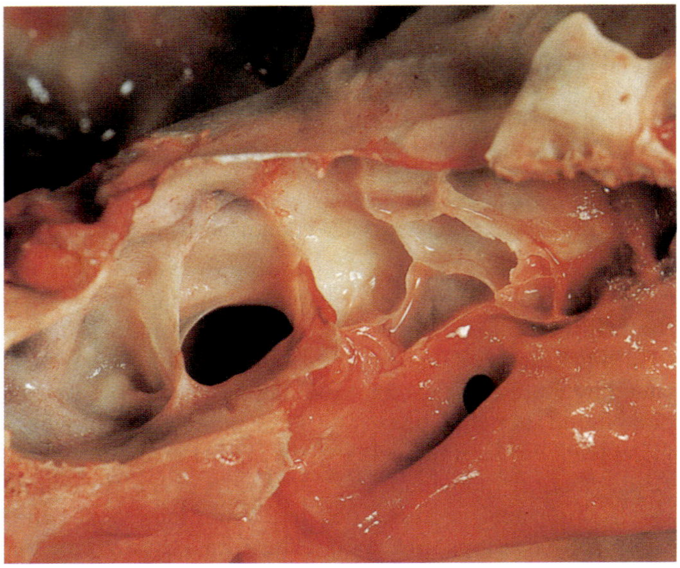

A

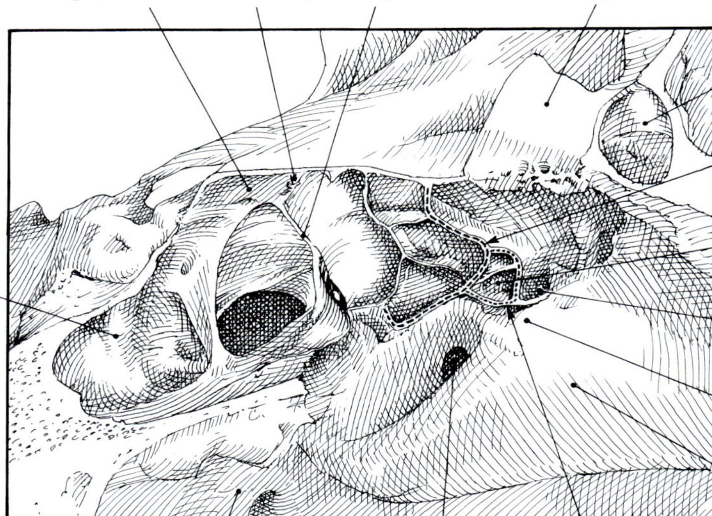


B

**FIGURE 16.3. A:** Extensively pneumatized sphenoid and ethmoid sinuses. **B:** Several basal lamellae are demonstrated along with the natural and accessory ostia of maxillary sinus.

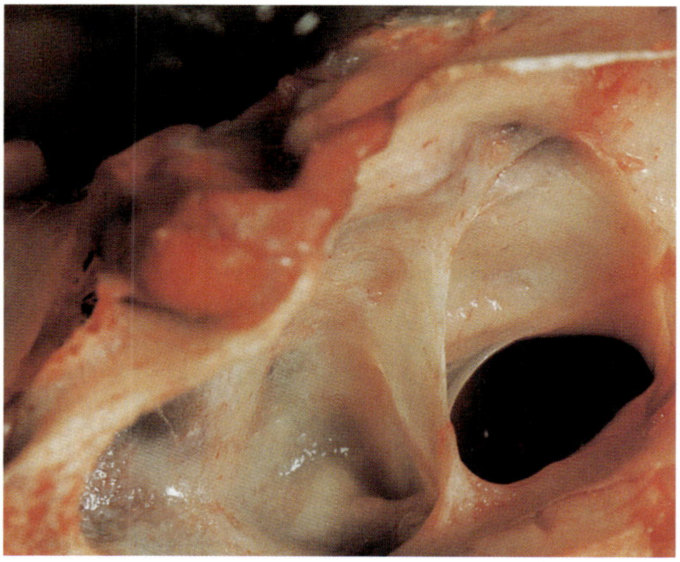

C

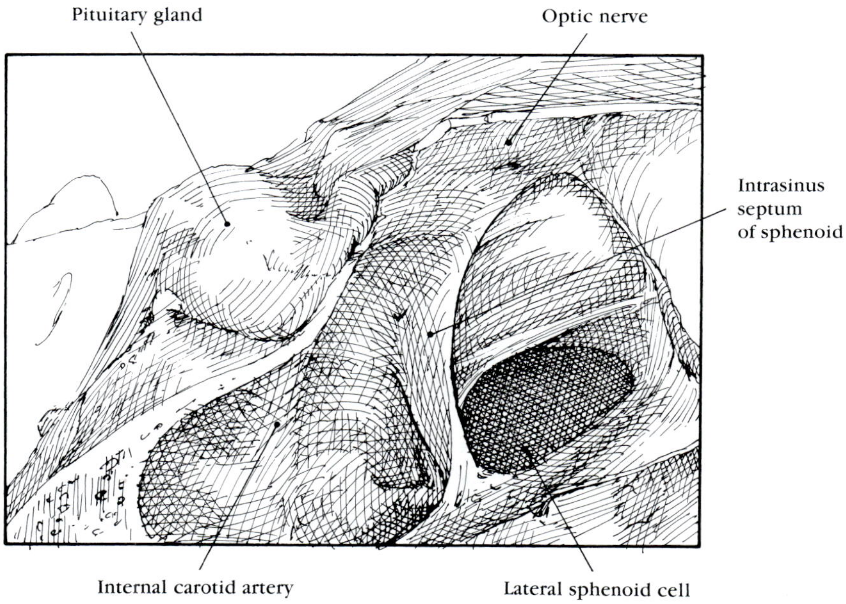


D

**FIGURE 16.3.** ***(continued)*** **C:** Enlargement of **A** shows the sphenoid and ethmoid sinuses. The medial aspect of optic nerve is exposed by ethmoid cells (similar to Onodi cells), and the internal carotid artery is traversing the lateral wall of the sinus. **D:** Extensive pneumatization of the ethmoid bone and extension of posterior ethmoid cells into the sphenoid bone are well demonstrated in this specimen. (From Rice DH, Schaefer SD, eds. *Endoscopic paranasal sinus surgery*, 2nd ed. New York: Raven Press, 1993, with permission.)

A

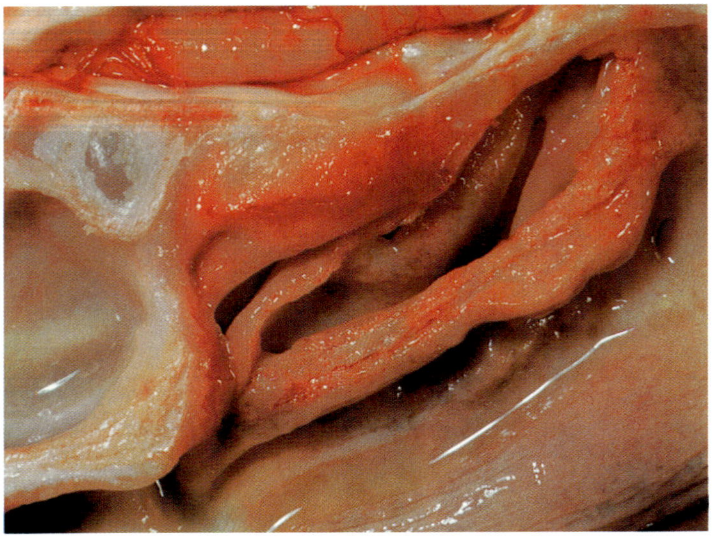

B

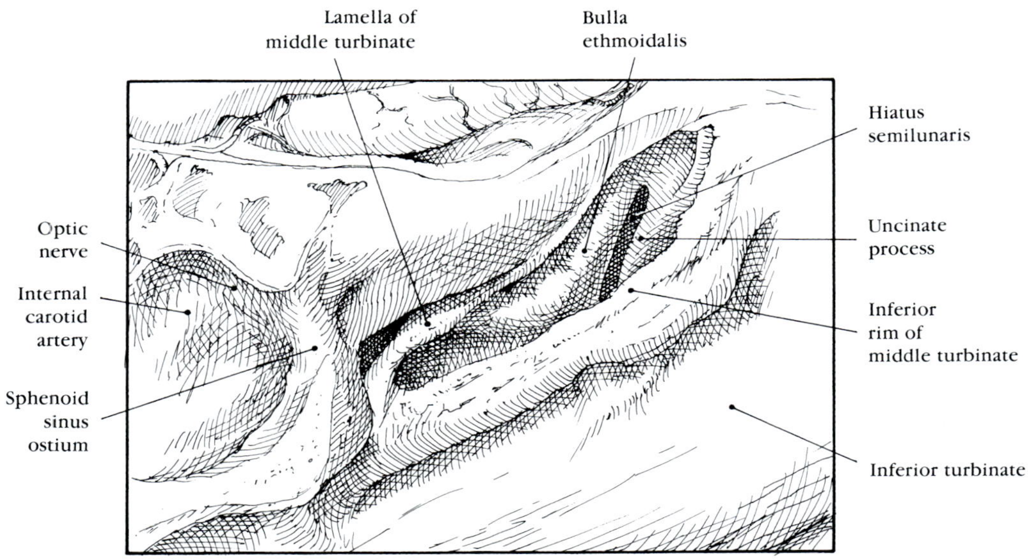


**FIGURE 16.4. A:** The body of the middle turbinate has been removed, leaving an intact rim of the middle turbinate. **B:** Diagram of **A** shows the course of the third lamella or basal lamella, which supports the middle turbinate. This lamella has three segments: a superior horizontal, an anterosuperior to posteroinferior oblique, and an inferior horizontal segment. (From Rice DH, Schaefer SD, eds. *Endoscopic paranasal sinus surgery*, 2nd ed. New York: Raven Press, 1993, with permission.)

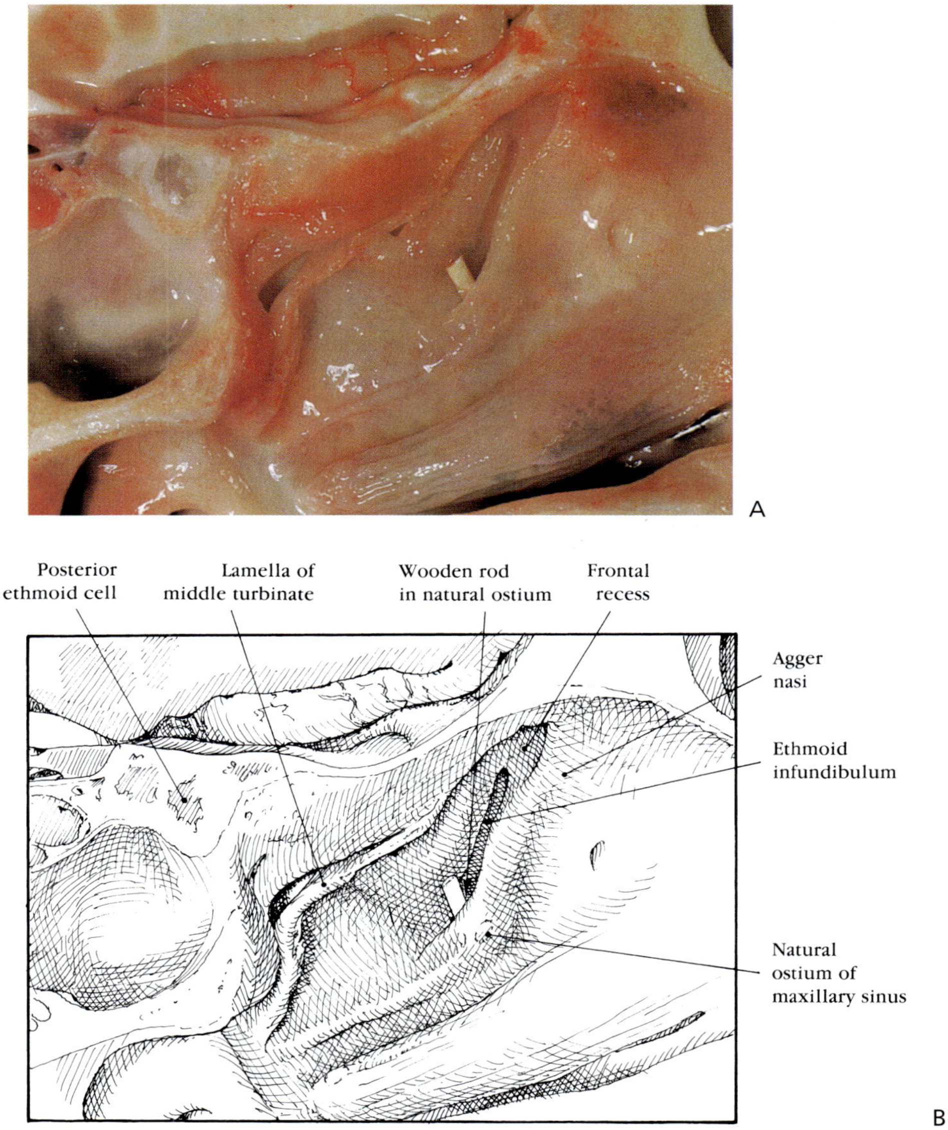


**FIGURE 16.5. A:** Dissection reveals the lateral nasal wall. The ostium of the maxillary sinus is cannulated by a wooden rod. **B:** Diagram of **A**. (From Rice DH, Schaefer SD, eds. *Endoscopic paranasal sinus surgery*, 2nd ed. New York: Raven Press, 1993, with permission.)

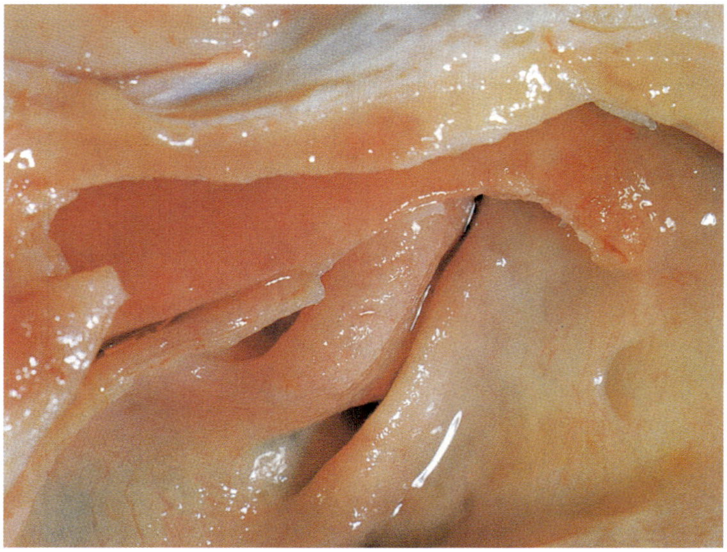

A

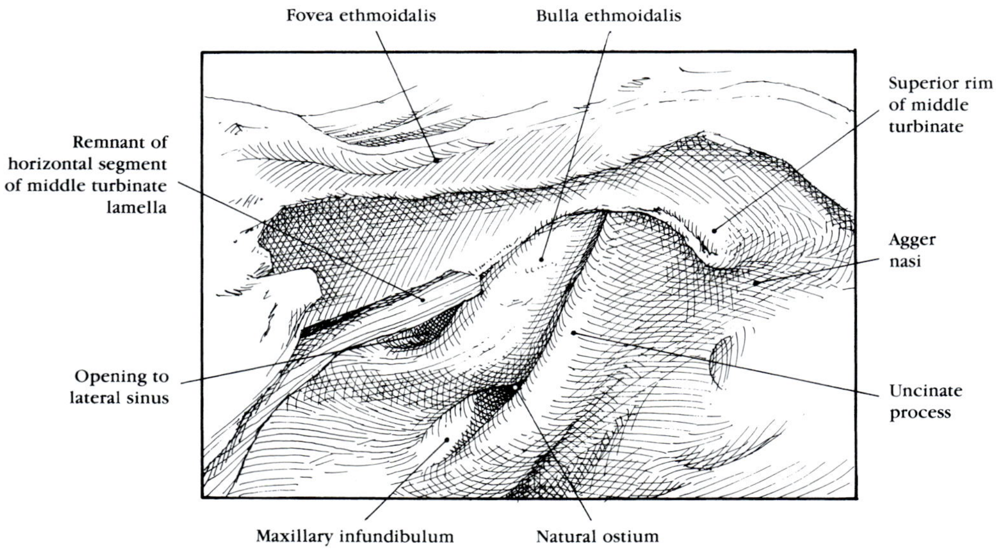


B

**FIGURE 16.6. A:** Enlargement of Figure 16.5A. **B:** The diagram illustrates a remnant of the posterior horizontal segment of basal lamella of the middle turbinate. The opening to the lateral sinus is located between the bullar and posterior ethmoid cells. (From Rice DH, Schaefer SD, eds. *Endoscopic paranasal sinus surgery*, 2nd ed. New York: Raven Press, 1993, with permission.).

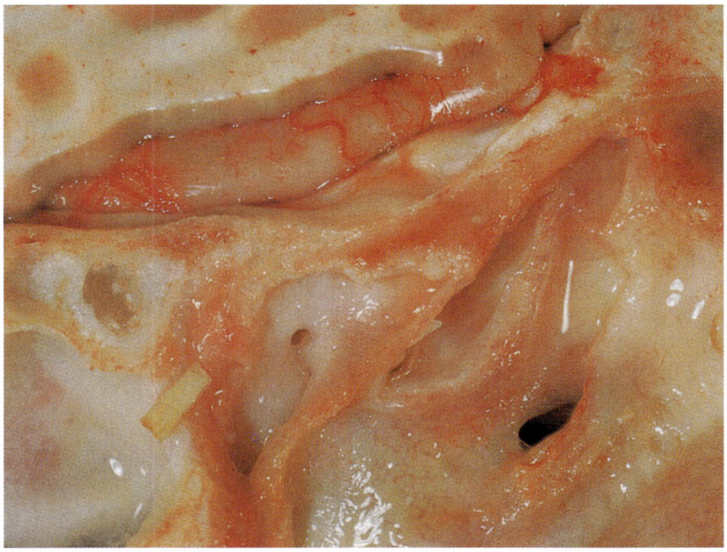

A

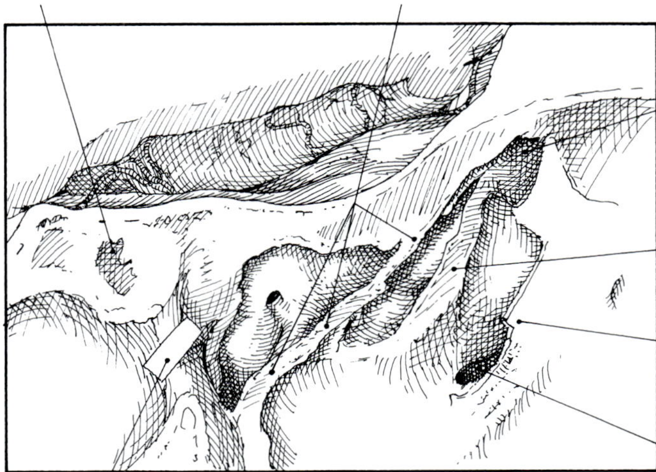


B

**FIGURE 16.7. A:** Medial aspect of bulla ethmoidalis and uncinate process have been removed to reveal lamella of middle turbinate and natural ostium of the maxillary sinus. **B:** Three of the lamellae or plates of bone from the lamina papyracea to the lateral nasal wall are illustrated. The most anterior lamella is from the uncinate process. The second lamella is the lateral extension of the anterior wall of the bulla. The third or basal (also known as grand) lamella provides the attachment of the middle turbinate to the lamina papyracea. (From Rice DH, Schaefer SD, eds. *Endoscopic paranasal sinus surgery*, 2nd ed. New York: Raven Press, 1993, with permission.)

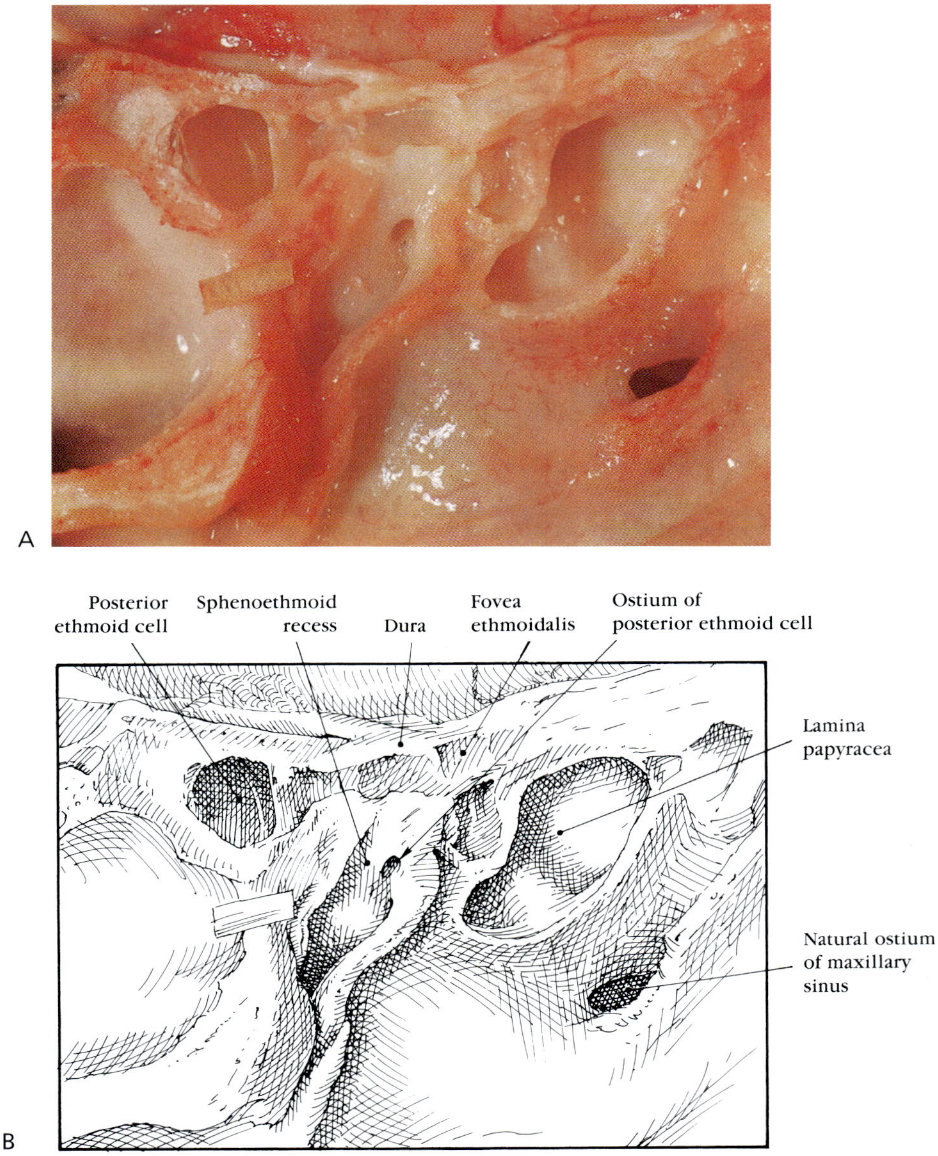


**FIGURE 16.8. A:** Further removal of the lateral nasal wall. **B:** Diagram of **A**. (From Rice DH, Schaefer SD, eds. *Endoscopic paranasal sinus surgery*, 2nd ed. New York: Raven Press, 1993, with permission.)

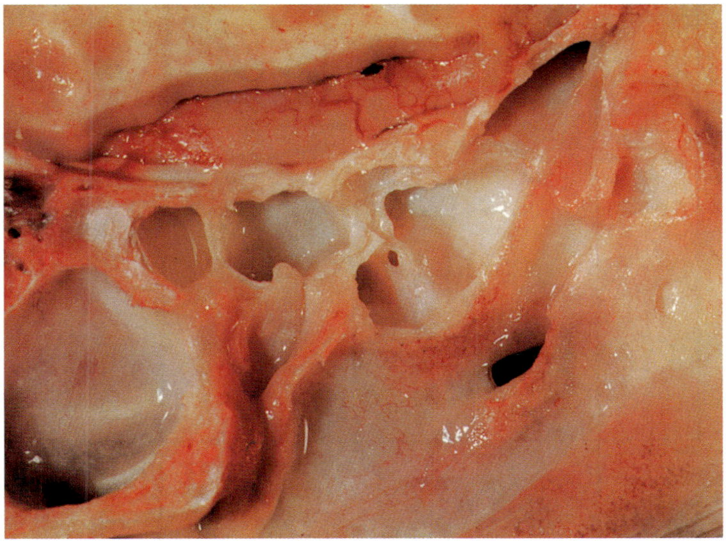

A

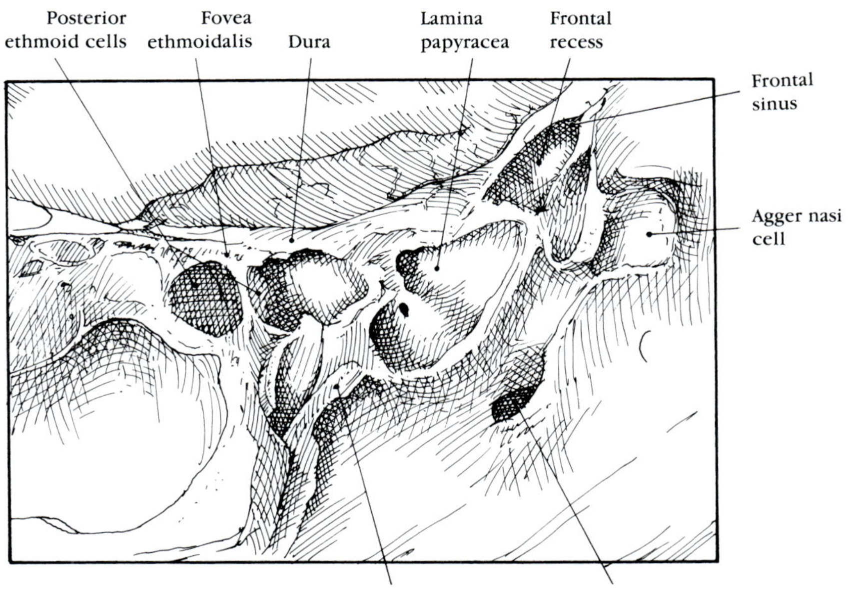


B

**FIGURE 16.9. A:** All ethmoid cells have been exposed to reveal their location within the ethmoid and adjacent bones. **B:** Notice the relation of the agger nasi (i.e., extramural infundibular cells) to the frontal sinus and the most posterior ethmoid cell to the sphenoid sinus. The latter is important because extramural ethmoid cells may be confused with the sphenoid sinus. (From Rice DH, Schaefer SD, eds. *Endoscopic paranasal sinus surgery*, 2nd ed. New York: Raven Press, 1993, with permission.)

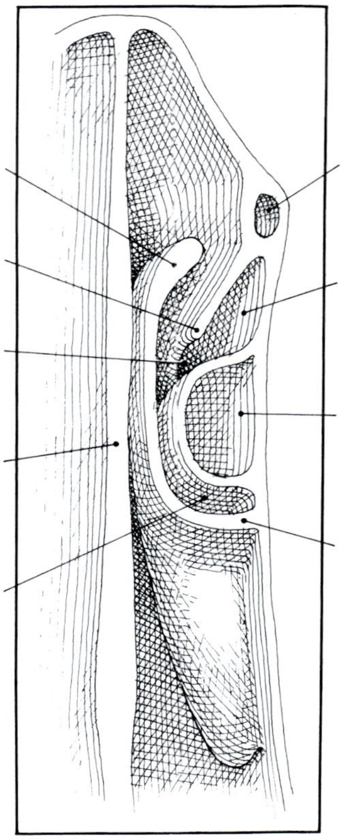


**FIGURE 16.10.** Diagram in the axial plane of the right lateral nasal wall. Notice the lateral sinus between posterior aspect of bulla ethmoidalis and third lamella or basal lamella of the middle turbinate. (From Rice DH, Schaefer SD, eds. *Endoscopic paranasal sinus surgery*, 2nd ed. New York: Raven Press, 1993, with permission.)

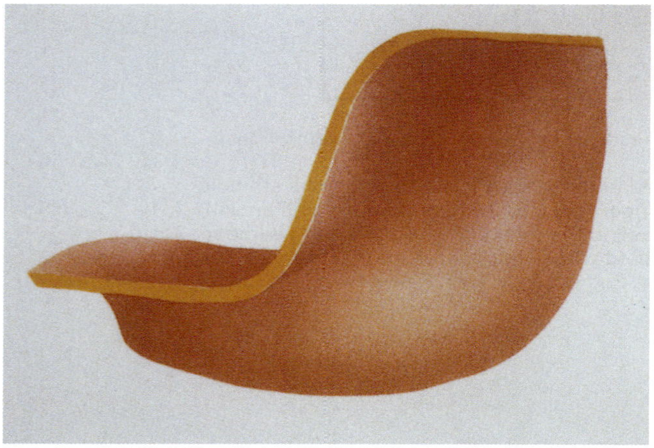

**FIGURE 16.11.** On the lateral surface of the middle turbinate, the yellow border signifies the areas of attachment of the lamella. Notice the anterior one third attaches superiorly, the middle third attaches to the lateral wall of nasal cavity in a somewhat vertical manner, and the posterior one third, although also attaching to the lateral wall, does so in a horizontal manner. (Adapted from Stammberger H. *Functional endoscopic sinus surgery*. Philadelphia: BC Decker, 1991, with permission.)

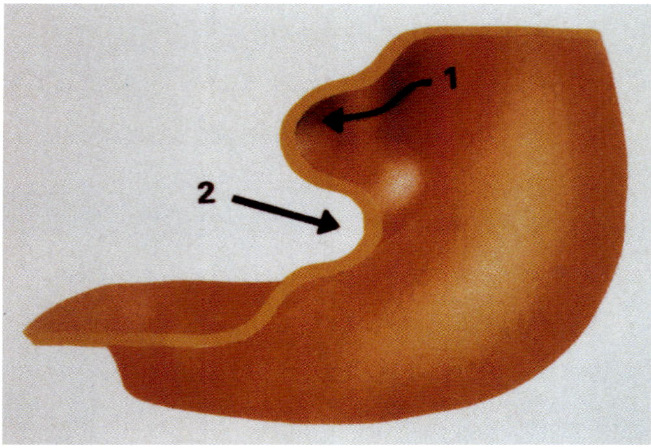


**FIGURE 16.12.** The basal lamella may become somewhat distorted because of the impinging ethmoid air cells, but the integrity of the barrier is nevertheless maintained. *1*, indentation by anterior ethmoid cells; *2,* indentation by posterior ethmoid cells. (Adapted from Stammberger H. *Functional endoscopic sinus surgery.* Philadelphia: BC Decker, 1991, with permission.)

one third assuming an inferior horizontal position and attaching laterally. The physical attachment of this basal lamella in three different planes (i.e., superior, vertical, and horizontal) provides much of the structural support of the middle turbinate (47). When this bony plate is removed during posterior ethmoidectomy, the turbinate loses its stability (18). This lamella is not always structurally fixed, and the ethmoid air cells during development have a tendency to expand to all available space, which Seydel (46) called "the struggle for space of the ethmoid." This results in air cells impinging and perhaps distorting the osseous barrier, but the lamella always remains intact and prevents intermingling of cells (23,32) (Fig. 16.12).

Another important variation in the ethmoid anatomy is the *lateral sinus*, which forms a space bounded laterally by the lamina papyracea, posteriorly by the lamella of the middle turbinate, anteriorly by the posterior aspect of the bulla ethmoidalis, and superiorly by the fovea ethmoidalis (Figs. 16.6 and 16.10). When the second lamella does not extend to the fovea ethmoidalis, the sinus lateralis continues anteriorly to the frontal recess. This gives rise, above the bulla, to a space is known as the *suprabullar furrow* or *suprabullar recess*, which communicates with the middle meatus. The *fourth lamella* is at the attachment of the superior turbinate, and when a supreme turbinate is also present, a *fifth lamella* arises lateral to this turbinate.

## Clinical Implications

In the adult, the ethmoid sinus viewed in a transverse section forms a pyramid, with the blunted apex located anteriorly and the wider base located posteriorly (Fig. 16.13). The entire sinus measures 4 to 5 cm anteroposteriorly, 2.5

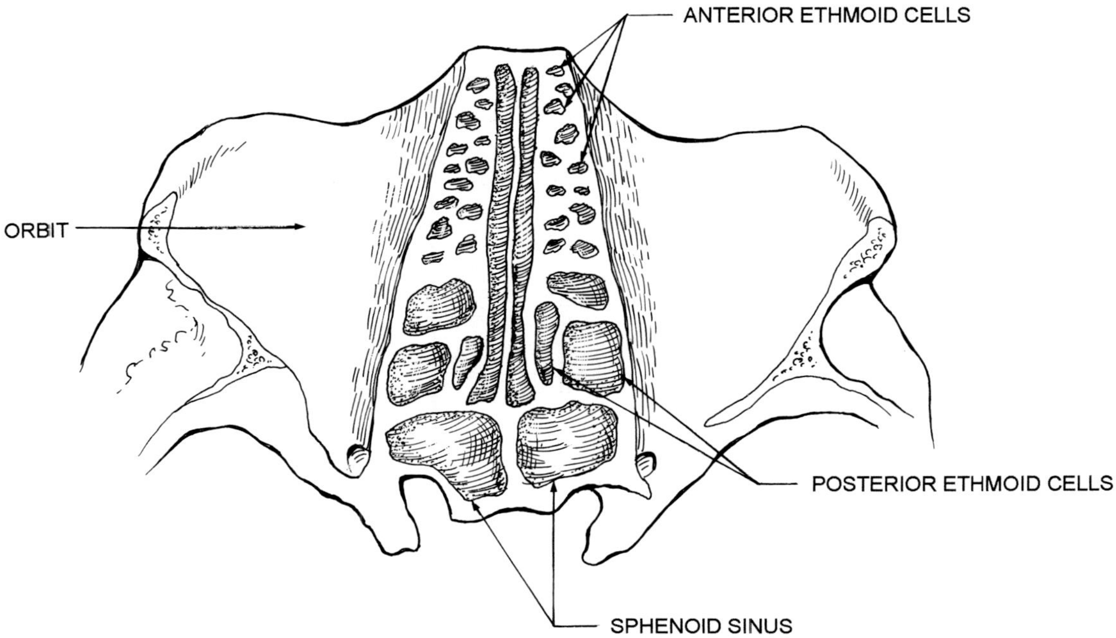


**FIGURE 16.13.** A transverse view of the ethmoid shows the width of the labyrinth increasing from anterior to posterior, whereas the number of cells decrease in the same direction.

cm inferosuperiorly, and 0.5 cm wide anteriorly and 1.5 cm posteriorly (48). Various descriptions of the ethmoid roof, such as fovea or foveolae ethmoidales, have caused considerable confusion over the years. Lateral to the cribriform plate and the insertion of the middle turbinate, numerous ethmoid air cells open superiorly and are closed by the frontal bone. Mosher (49) described this anatomy as follows: "[U]pon the whole length of the ethmoidal notch of the frontal bone there is a row of little half cells which is matched and completed by a similar row of cells on the upper surface of the lateral mass of the ethmoid bone."

Because the indentations, or foveolae,[1] of the frontal bone cover the corresponding clefts and cells of the ethmoid, the frontal bone is anatomically considered the roof of the ethmoid complex (50) (Fig. 16.14). Use of the term fovea to describe the entire ethmoid roof does not distinguish between the endonasal view and the endocranial perspective as viewed from the olfactory groove. These air cells are at or usually above the level of the cribriform plate. The term fovea or *foveola ethmoidalis* (fovea meaning "pit," rather than roof or tegmen), extends an average 2 to 3 mm above the more medial cribriform plate (Fig. 16.15). The plane of the fovea slopes inferomedial, with this bony plate

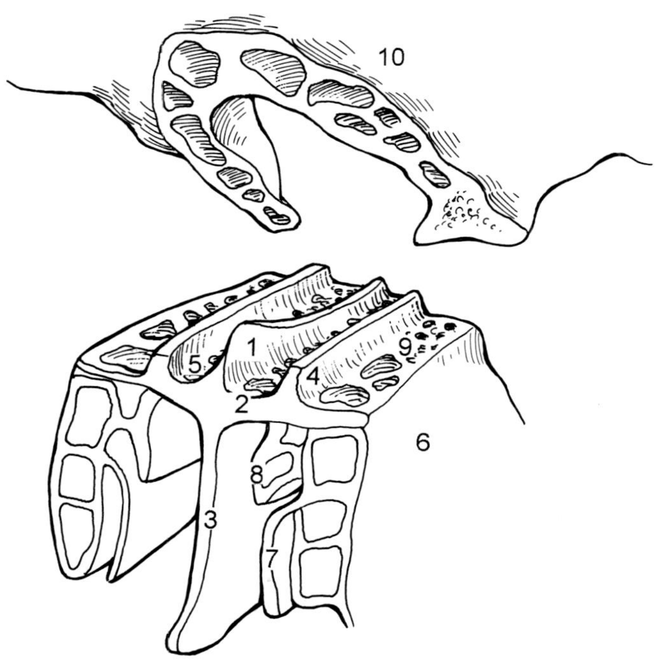


**FIGURE 16.14.** Schematic drawing shows the relationship between the ethmoid and frontal bones. Also illustrated are the crista galli *(1)*, lamina cribrosa *(2)*, septum *(3)*, lamina lateralis of lamina *(4)*, fossa olfactoria *(5)*, lamina papyracea *(6)*, middle concha *(7)*, superior concha *(8)*, ethmoidal clefts and cells open superiorly *(9)*, and os frontale with foveolae ethmoidales *(10)*.

[1]*Foveolae* from the Latin and *foveolae ethmoidales ossis frontalis*, meaning ethmoid pits of the frontal bone.

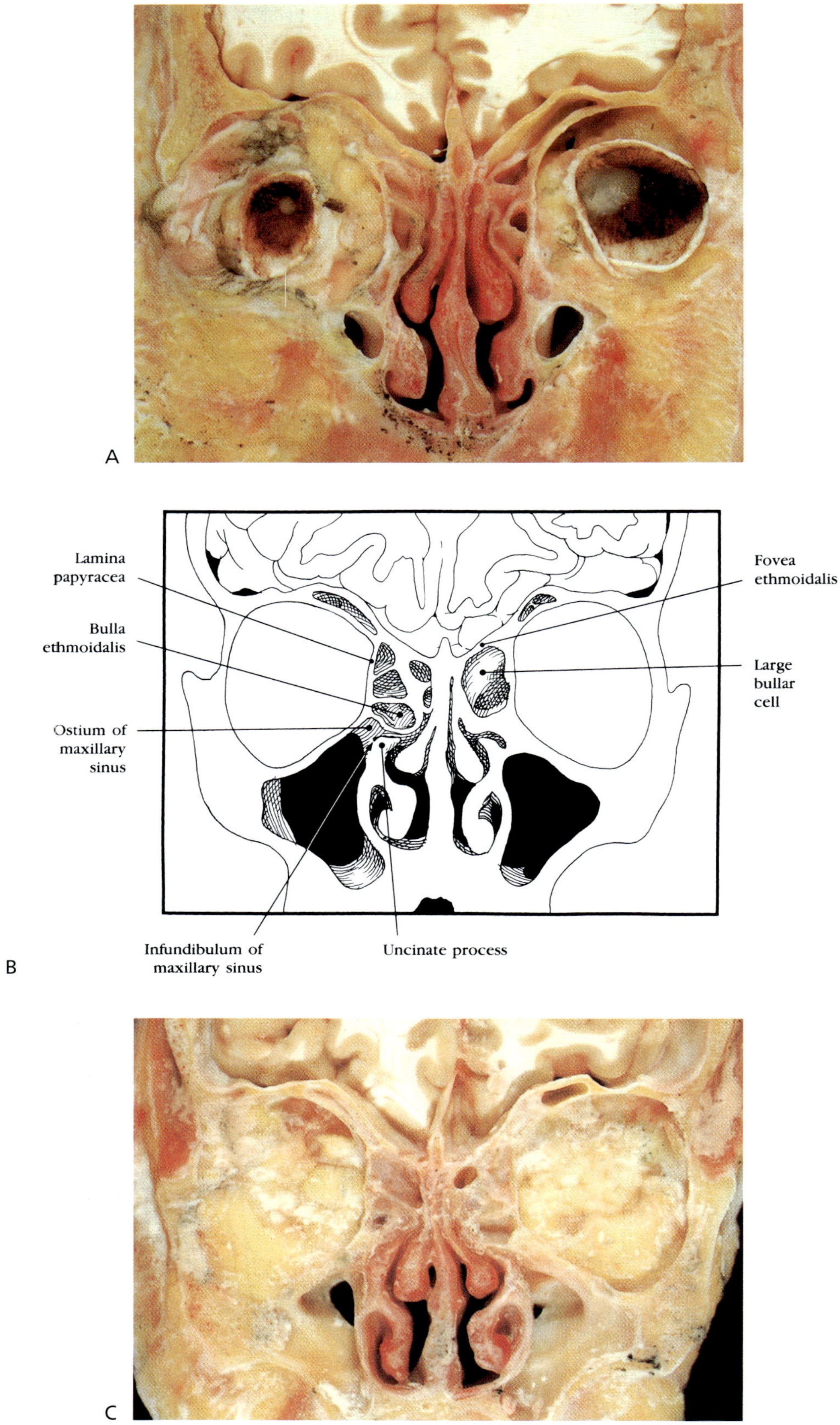


**FIGURE 16.15. A:** The anterior surface of the coronal section contiguous with Figure 16.20C is shown. It is at the level of the ventral aspect of the maxillary sinus. **B:** Notice the continuation of the infundibular cells. The most constant of these cells is the agger nasi, or pneumatization of the lacrimal bone. **C:** The posterior surface of the specimen in Figure 16.6A is shown. It includes the ventral portion of the maxillary sinus.

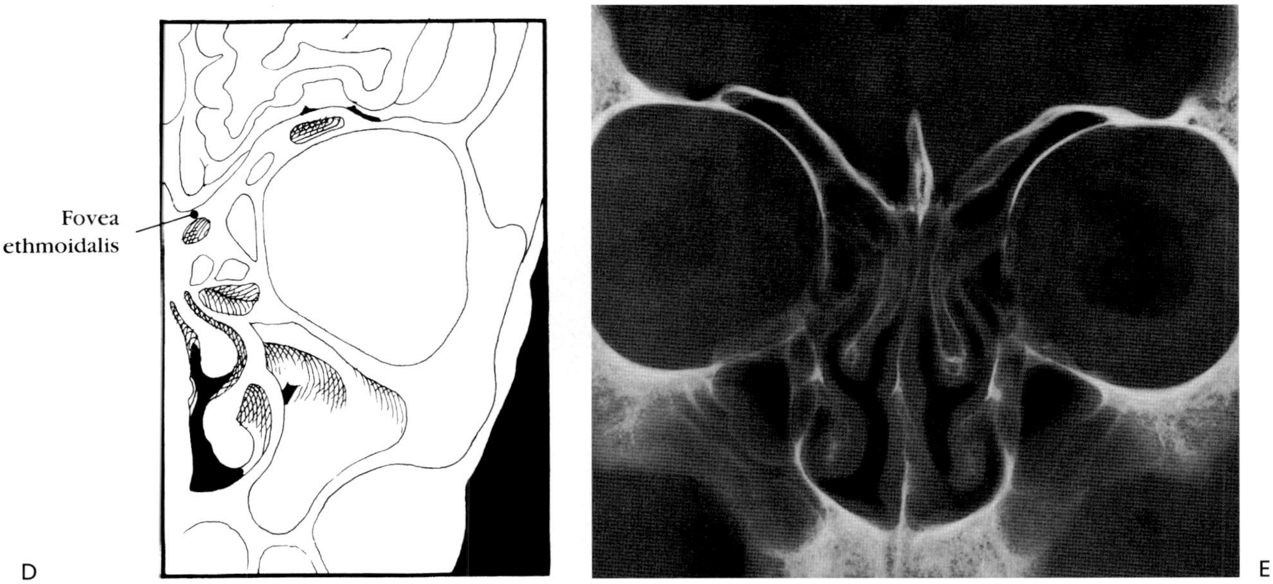


**FIGURE 16.15.** ***(continued)*** **D:** Residual infundibular and supraorbital cells are shown in this section. **E:** Plain radiograph of the specimen shown in **A** through **C**. (From Rice DH, Schaefer SD, eds. *Endoscopic paranasal sinus surgery*, 2nd ed. New York: Raven Press, 1993, with permission.)

sometimes at an acute angle to the cribriform plate. In such cases, the fovea is particularly vulnerable to penetration along the medial aspect. The lateral wall of the ethmoid bone is the *lamina papyracea* (i.e., orbital plate), which forms the most constant component (Figs. 16.15 and 16.16).

The actual size of the sinus and the number of cells present vary in each reported series. Van Alyea (23) examined 100 specimens, finding a range of 4 to 17 cells and averaging 9 cells per specimen. Schaeffer (51) found the most simple ethmoidal labyrinth to consist of only 3 cells and the most complex of 16 cells. When few cells occupy the ethmoid labyrinth, the cells are large, but when there are 12 to 16 cells "massed" together in the ethmoid region, each cell "struggles for space," resulting in the highly variable and irregularly formed ethmoidal air cells observed. The fact that the sinus is known as the "ethmoid labyrinth" attests to the intricacy of the structure and challenges our understanding of the anatomy.

For this discussion, cells are divided into those that are within the ethmoid region, or *intramural,* and those that are outside the ethmoid, or *extramural.* The intramural cells are further divided into the smaller but more numerous anterior cells and the larger posterior cells, with some authorities calling the ethmoid bulla the "middle cells" (Fig. 16.17). However, descriptions of a "middle ethmoid" or of "middle ethmoid cells" are considered incorrect because they are not based on developmental, anatomic, or functional grounds (50). The anterior ethmoid cells can be further subdivided based on their location or that of their ostia (23). However, cells of a given origin frequently invade the territory usually occupied by cells of another origin, and at least one investigator favors classification by the location of their ostia. Examples of several classifications are given in Table 16.1 (52).

Among the various classifications proposed, the Ritter nomenclature system conveys most clearly the origin and drainage of the ethmoid cells. Using Ritter's classification, the most anterior cells are the frontal recess cells (range, 0 to 4 cells), which arise from the anterosuperior growth of the ethmoid cells into the frontal bone (Figs. 16.4 and 16.11). These cells may come to rest within the frontal bone by forming the frontal sinus, giving rise to the *frontal bullae,* bulging into the frontal sinus floor, or forming the *supraorbital ethmoid cells* as they pneumatize the orbit (9,53). The inferior expansion of these cells can displace the nasofrontal duct, resulting in a tortuous or serpentine course of the duct.

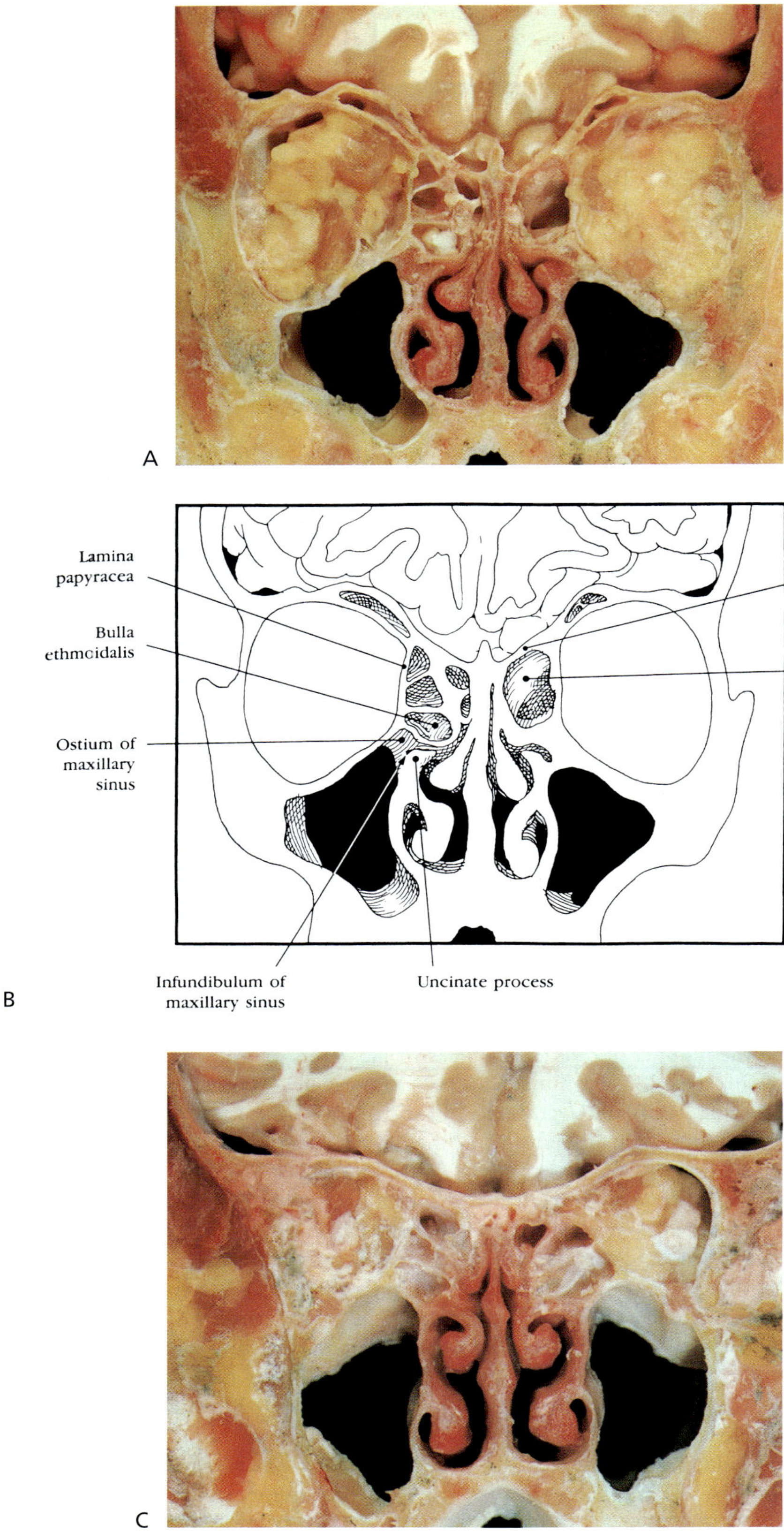


**FIGURE 16.16.** **A:** The anterior surface of the coronal section contiguous with specimen in Figure 16.15C is shown, which includes the midportion of the maxillary sinus. **B:** On the right of the specimen are several middle ethmoid cells, including bullar cells. On the left is a large bullar cell. **C:** The posterior surface of the specimen in **A** is shown, which exposes the middle ethmoid or bullar cells.

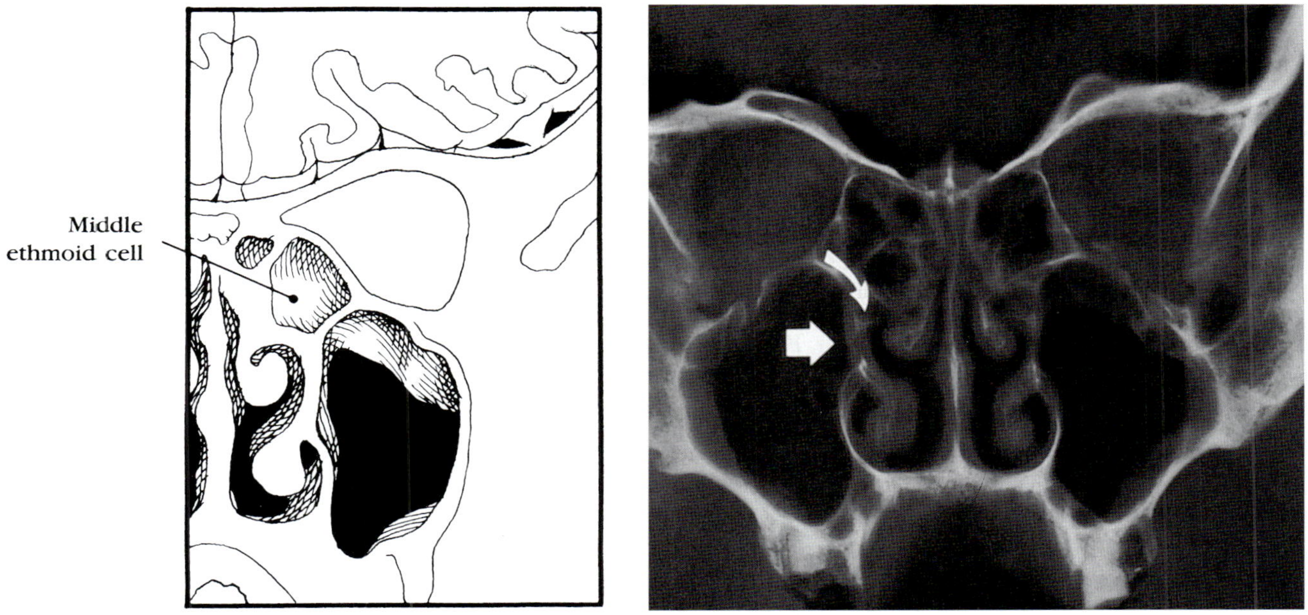


D

E

**FIGURE 16.16.** ***(continued)*** **D:** The illustration shows the middle ethmoid cells seen in **C**. **E:** Plain radiograph of the specimen in **A** through **C**. Notice the uncinate process projecting several millimeters superiorly *(curved arrow)*. The large arrow points to the membranous meatus. (From Rice DH, Schaefer SD, eds. *Endoscopic paranasal sinus surgery*, 2nd ed. New York: Raven Press, 1993, with permission.)

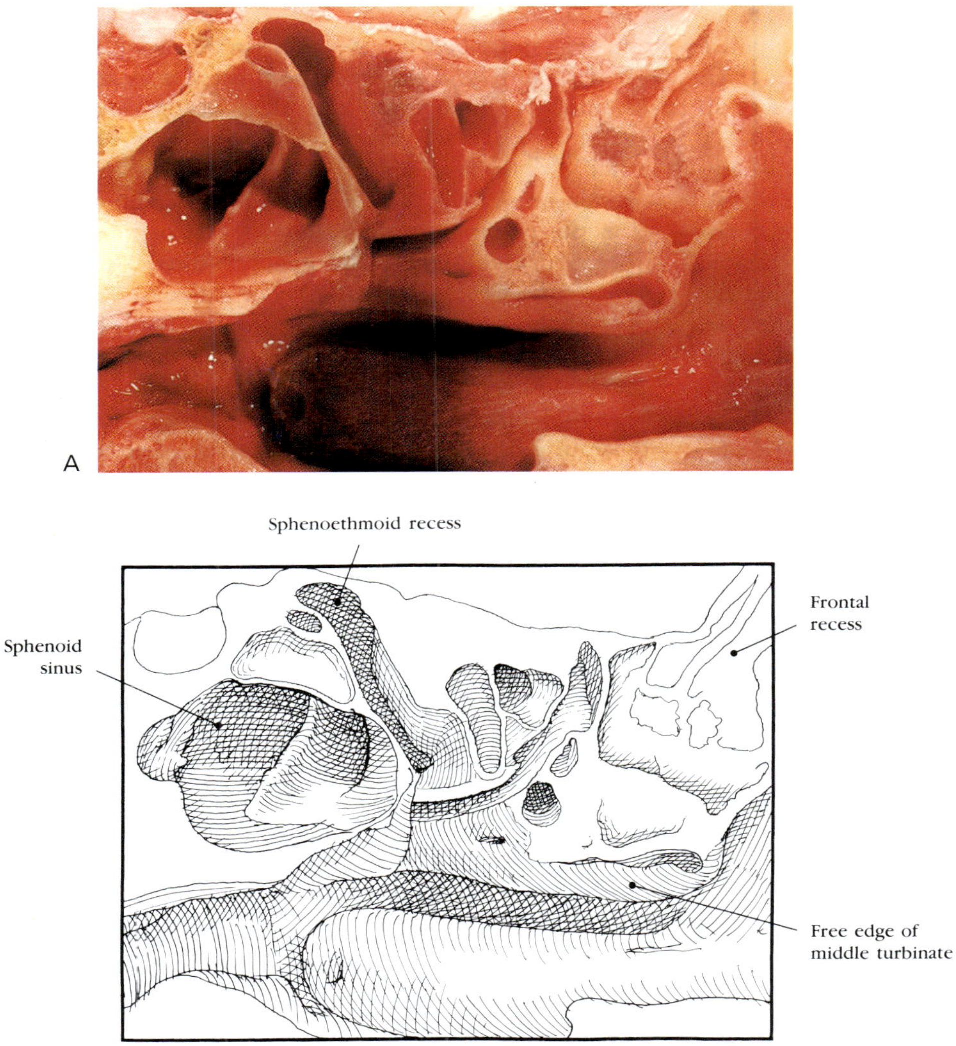


A

B

**FIGURE 16.17. A:** Parasagittal section through the middle turbinate is shown. **B:** Extensive pneumatization of the ethmoid bone is represented by the anterior and posterior ethmoid sinuses. (From Rice DH, Schaefer SD, eds. *Endoscopic paranasal sinus surgery*, 2nd ed. New York: Raven Press, 1993, with permission.)

**TABLE 16.1. CLASSIFICATION OF SINUS CELLS**

| | | |
|---|---|---|
| **Middle meatus cells** | **Anterior ethmoid cells** | **Anterior ethmoid** |
| Infundiular cells | Fontal recess | Fontal recess |
| Agger nasi | Infundibular | Infundibular |
| Terminal | Bullar | Bullar |
| Suprainfundibular | Conchal | Conchal |
| Inferior | Extramural (i.e., agger nasi) | Extramural |
| **Superior meatus cells** | **Posterior ethmoid cells** | **Posterior ethmoid** |
| Posterior cells | Intramural | Intramural |
| | Extramural (Ritter, 1978) | Extramural (Hollingshead, 1986) |
| **Supreme meatus** | | |
| Postreme cells (Van Alyea, 1939) | | |

The infundibular cells (range, 1 to 7 cells) are the second most anterior cells (Figs. 16.18–16.20). The most constant of these cells form the extramural cells, the *agger nasi*, through the pneumatization of the lacrimal bone (23). These cells are located on the lateral nasal wall immediately anterior to the middle turbinate and constitute an important landmark in intranasal procedures and external ethmoidectomy. They drain into the three-dimensional space of the *ethmoid infundibulum*, a pouch or trough that ends superiorly in the frontal recess (Figs. 16.3 and 16.5). In some individuals, the infundibular cells may be the origin of the frontal sinus (11) (Fig. 16.21). The ethmoid infundibulum lies anterior to the bulla ethmoidalis and is bounded medially by the middle turbinate (Fig. 16.5). The infundibulum is also the site of drainage for the frontal sinus and other anterior ethmoid cells involving the adjacent frontal, lacrimal, and nasal bones. Since Baron Alexis de Boyer first coined the term *infundibulum*, a Nomina Anatomica (NA) term, cells draining into this trough are also known as *Boyer's cells* (9).[2]

The bullar cells (range, 1 to 6 cells) are the most constant of the anterior ethmoid cells and together form a partial sphere lateral or beneath the middle turbinate, the *bulla ethmoidalis* (23) (Figs. 16.4–16.9, 16.16, 16.17, and 16.21). The term bulla ethmoidalis was first used by Zuckerkandl (9), although Grünwald (54) used the term lateral torus. Lang (55) gave its dimensions as 18 (9 to 28) mm long and 5.4 (2 to 13) mm high, whereas Zuckerkandl (9) reported lengths of 20 and 26 mm. By definition, this region of the ethmoid bone would not be called the bulla without pneumatization. A variable number of ethmoid air cells generally develop in the lamella of the bulla, producing the characteristic swelling described as the bulla ethmoidales (49). Even though the extent of pneumatization of the bulla is highly variable for individuals, a prominence is always detectable endoscopically and radiographically (10). The bullar cells drain into the middle meatus through crescentric ostia that lie superiorly, posteriorly, and parallel to the much larger semilunar cleft in the lateral nasal wall, the entrance of which Zuckerkandl described as the *hiatus semilunaris* (11,23). The hiatus semilunaris forms the curved groove between the bulla ethmoidalis that borders it posteriorly and the uncinate process, a ridge of bone formed by the ramus descendens of the first ethmoturbinal, that borders it anteriorly (48) (Figs. 16.10 and 16.21). The relationship of the hiatus to the middle turbinate is variable and is observed most commonly 11 to 20 mm posterior to the anterior aspect of the turbinate (12). Superiorly, the hiatus communicates with the *ethmoid infundibulum* (Fig. 16.5). The anteroinferior boundary of the hiatus semilunaris is the *uncinate process*, also a semilunar structure, which has an anterosuperior to posteroinferior sagittal orientation. It ranges from nearly flat to 4 mm high and 14 to 22 mm long, with its free margin occasionally projecting into the nasal cavity (12) (Figs. 16.4–16.9, 16.10, 16.21, and 16.22). The uncinate process, which is immediately posterior to the agger nasi bone, makes its visualization on the lateral nasal wall dependent on the anterior and inferior expansion of the middle turbinate.

The uncinate process is considered one of the most important surgical landmarks of the lateral nasal wall for endonasal sinus surgery. Its medial appendage is strategically located near the osteomeatal complex (OMC) (56).[3] The dynamics of this region are such that any abnormal

[2] According to Stammberger and colleagues (50), Boyer had named the cleft that Killian would later describe as the frontal recess.

[3] Naumann (56) coined the term *osteomeatal complex* to describe the region between the insertions of the inferior and middle conchae where the confluence of the frontal, ethmoid, and maxillary sinuses drains into before entering the nasal cavity.

A C B

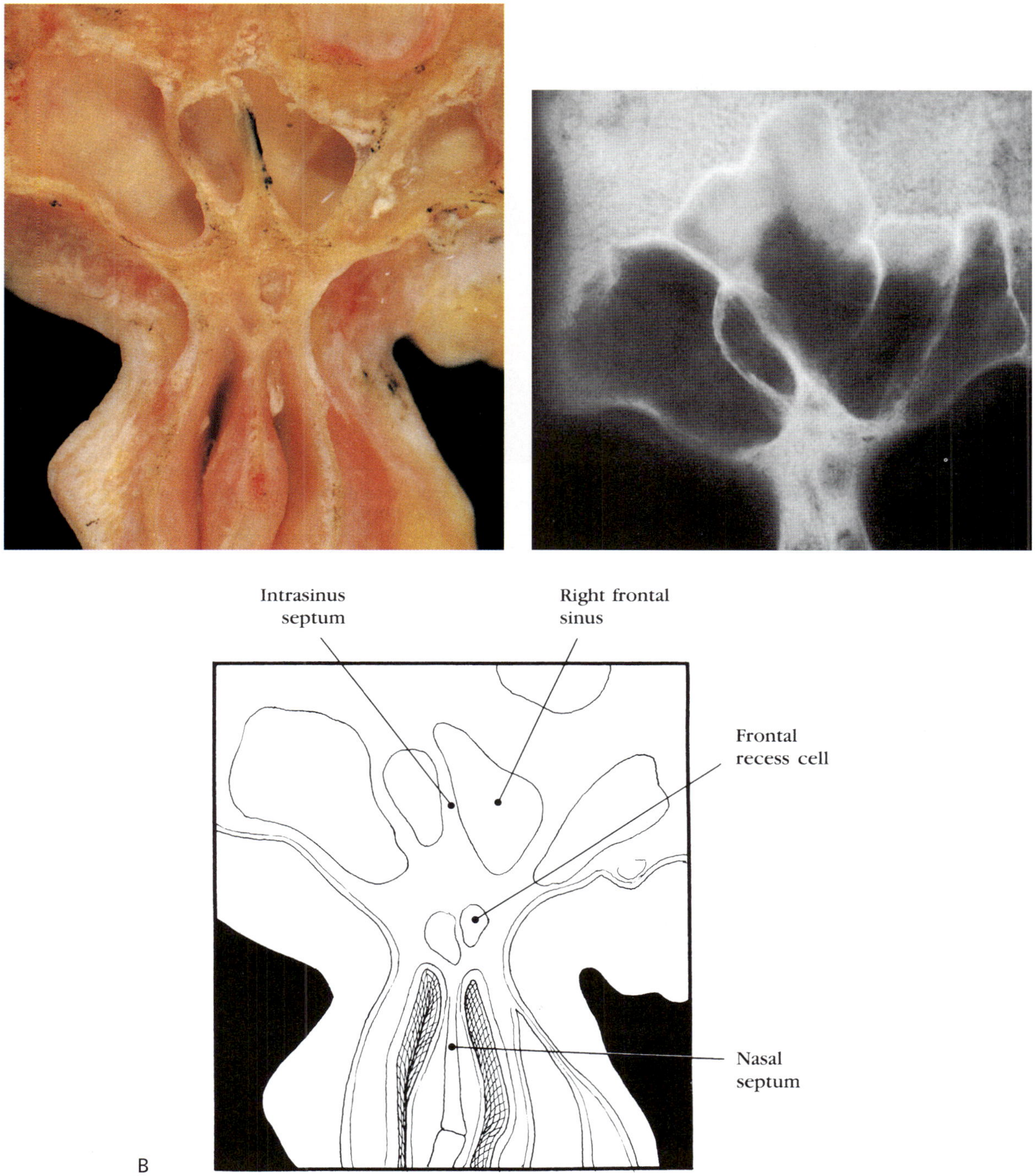


**FIGURE 16.18. A:** The posterior surface of the coronal section at the ventral aspect of the frontal sinus is shown. **B:** This section is sufficiently ventral to the body of the frontal sinus to include only a remnant of the frontal recess cells of the anterior ethmoid. **C:** Plain radiograph of the specimen shown in **A**. (From Rice DH, Schaefer SD, eds. *Endoscopic paranasal sinus surgery*, 2nd ed. New York: Raven Press, 1993, with permission.)

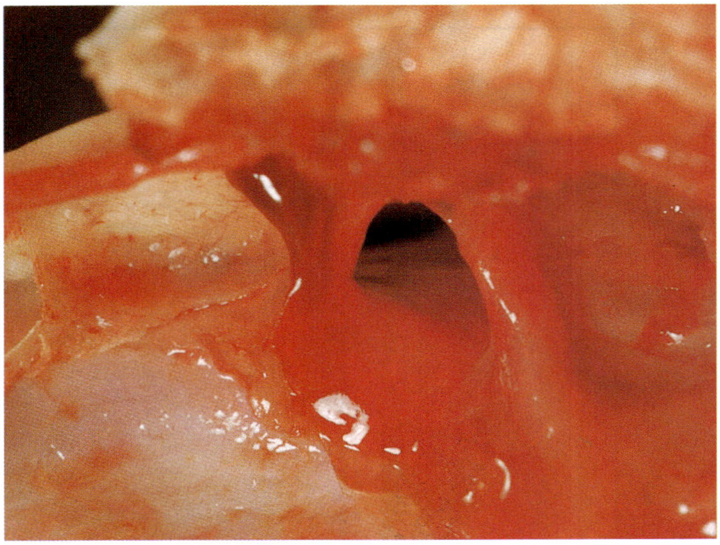

A

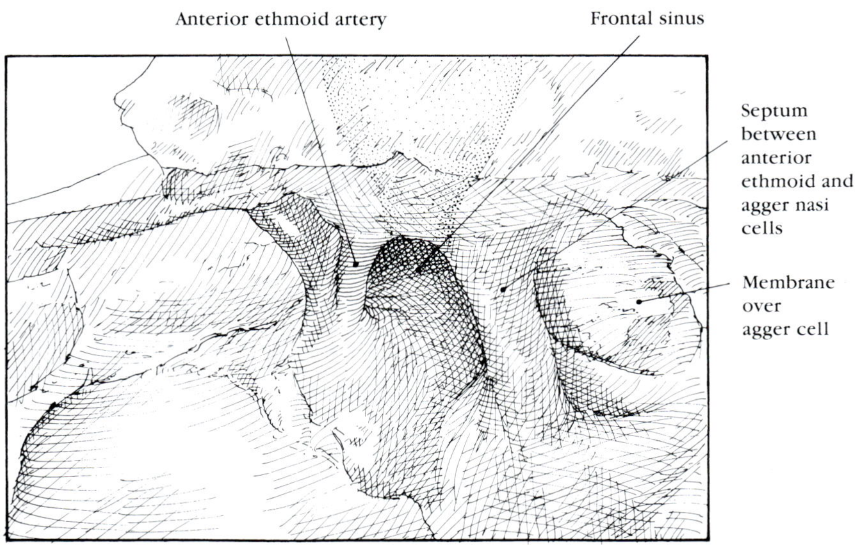


B

**FIGURE 16.19.** **A:** Frontal recess of the left ethmoid bone. **B:** Diagram of **A**. The relationship of the frontal sinus to the nose may be compared with an hourglass. The upper body of the glass is the frontal sinus, the neck is the ostium, and the lower body is the frontal recess. (From Rice DH, Schaefer SD, eds. *Endoscopic paranasal sinus surgery*, 2nd ed. New York: Raven Press, 1993, with permission.)

growth or excessive pneumatization of the uncinate process can potentially narrow and ultimately obstruct the outflow tract of multiple sinuses. Moreover, normal variations in the morphology of the uncinate process give rise to several patterns of drainage from the OMC (57) (Fig. 16.22). The first variation is an uncinate process coursing superolaterally to insert on the lamina papyracea (Fig. 16.22B). This variation leads to closure of the superior aspect of the infundibulum to form a blind pouch known as the *recess terminalis* and results in the communication of the frontal recess with the middle meatus medial to the ethmoid infundibulum. The frontal sinus drains into the nose medial to the ethmoid infundibulum and lateral to the middle turbinate. A second variation is an uncinate process extending superiorly to insert on or approximate to the fovea ethmoidalis, causing the frontal sinus to drain directly into the ethmoid infundibulum through the frontal recess (Fig. 16.22C). Another variation is extensive pneumatization of the uncinate process, which may obstruct drainage through the infundibulum (Fig. 16.22D).

The terminology regarding the anatomic boundaries of the hiatus semilunaris invites confusion. Some investigators

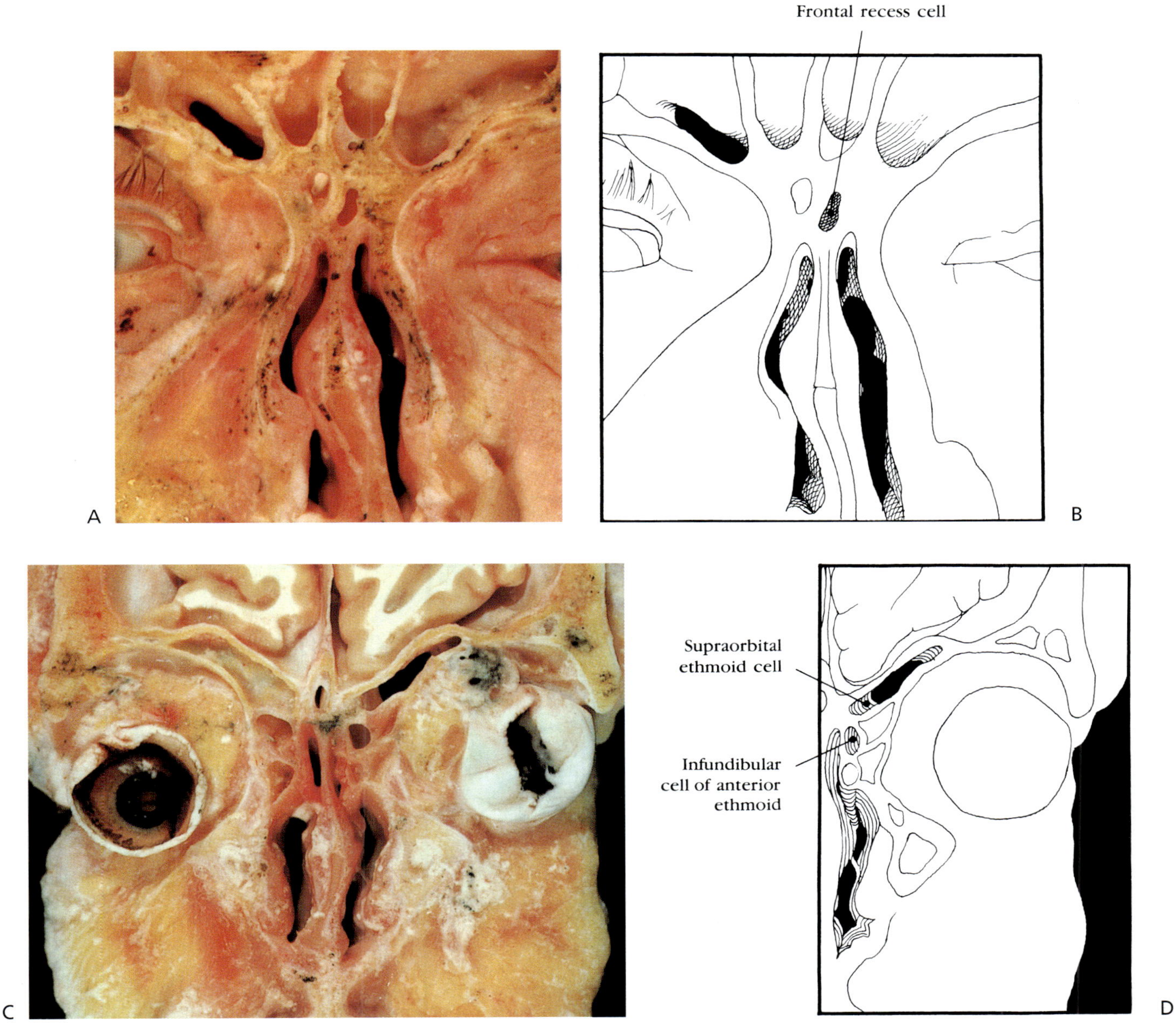


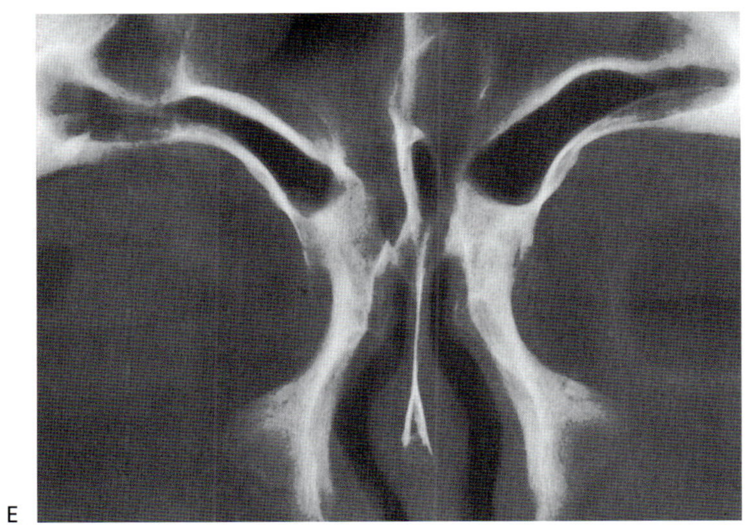


**FIGURE 16.20. A:** The anterior surface of coronal section through frontal sinus contiguous with the section in Figure 16.18A is shown. **B:** Notice the frontal recess cells seen in the coronal section in **A**. These cells are among the several possible origins of the frontal sinus. **C:** The posterior surface of the specimen in **A** is sectioned immediately dorsal to the principal cavity of the frontal sinus. **D:** The supraorbital ethmoid cells are shown immediately superior to infundibular cells of the anterior ethmoid. The lateral boundary of these cells is the lamina papyracea, which is the most constant structure in the ethmoid bone. **E:** Plain radiograph of the specimen shown in **A** through **C**. (From Rice DH, Schaefer SD, eds. *Endoscopic paranasal sinus surgery*, 2nd ed. New York: Raven Press, 1993, with permission.)

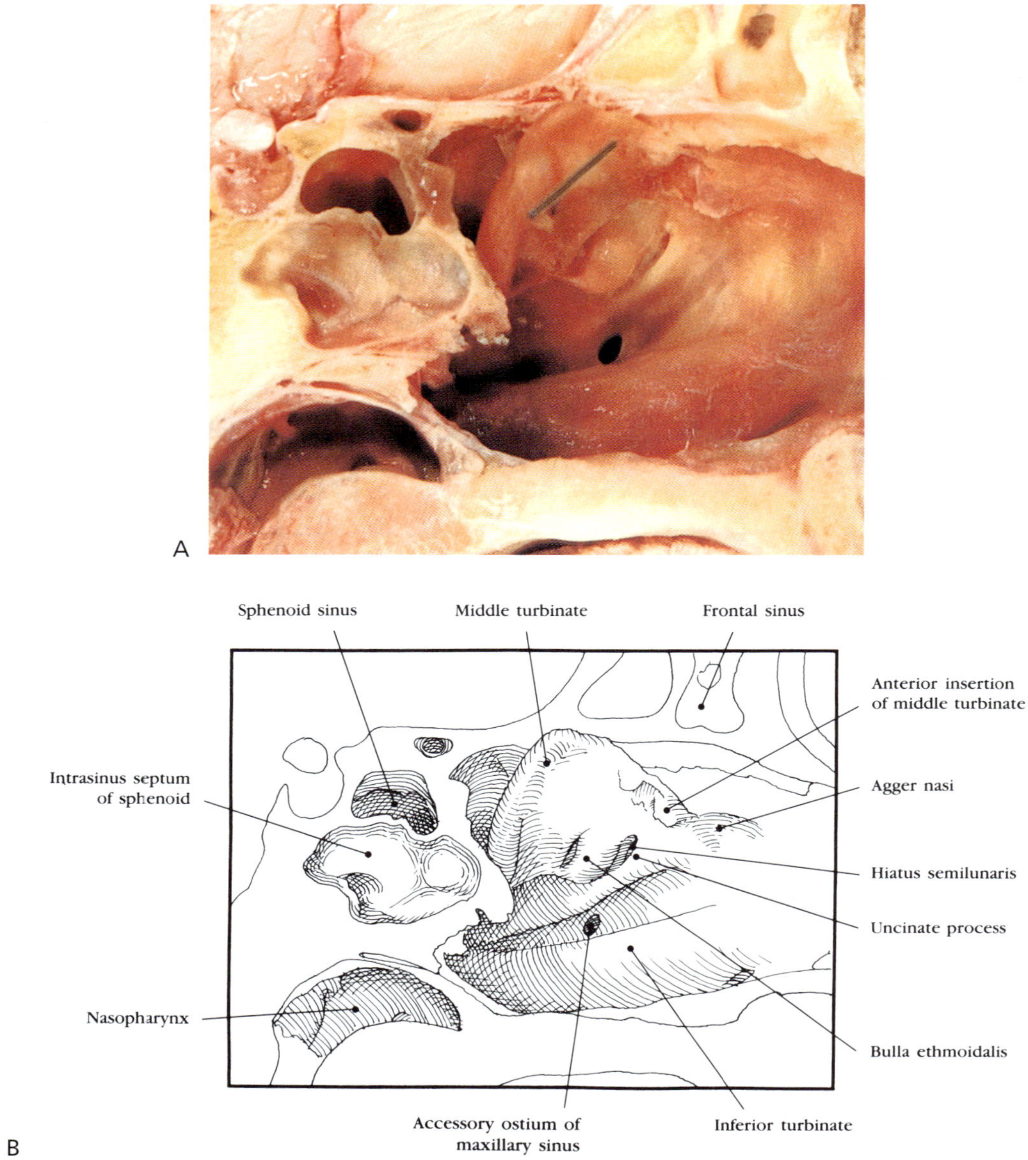


**FIGURE 16.21. A:** Midsagittal section shows the anatomy of the lateral nasal wall. The middle turbinate has been deflected superiorly to reveal the surface anatomy of the ethmoid sinus. **B:** The hiatus semilunaris appears as a depression between the bulla ethmoidalis and the uncinate process. Anterior to the uncinate ridge is the agger nasi, which is formed by pneumatization of the lacrimal bone by the infundibular cells of the ethmoid. The accessory ostium of maxillary sinus appears above the inferior turbinate. (From Rice DH, Schaefer SD, eds. *Endoscopic paranasal sinus surgery*, 2nd ed. New York: Raven Press, 1993, with permission.)

prefer to divide the hiatus semilunaris into anterior and posterior portions, but others tend to describe it as extending from the superior terminal of the frontal recess to the posterior aspect of the bulla, thereby substituting the anterosuperior portion of the hiatus for part of the ethmoid infundibulum. Others consider the infundibulum to be the bottom or most lateral region of the hiatus when describing the anterosuperior aspect as the ethmoid infundibulum (e.g., frontal recess to the bulla ethmoidalis), thereby designating that part of the infundibulum that communicates with the natural ostium of the maxillary sinus as the *maxillary infundibulum* (12,48) (Fig. 16.5). Various descriptions are given of the hiatus that include part of the infundibulum. The consensus is that the hiatus should be viewed as a two-dimensional structure, as Zuckerkandl (7) originally described, and should be regarded as the entrance into the infundibulum (50). Whatever terminology is used, these structures are important landmarks and constitute the route

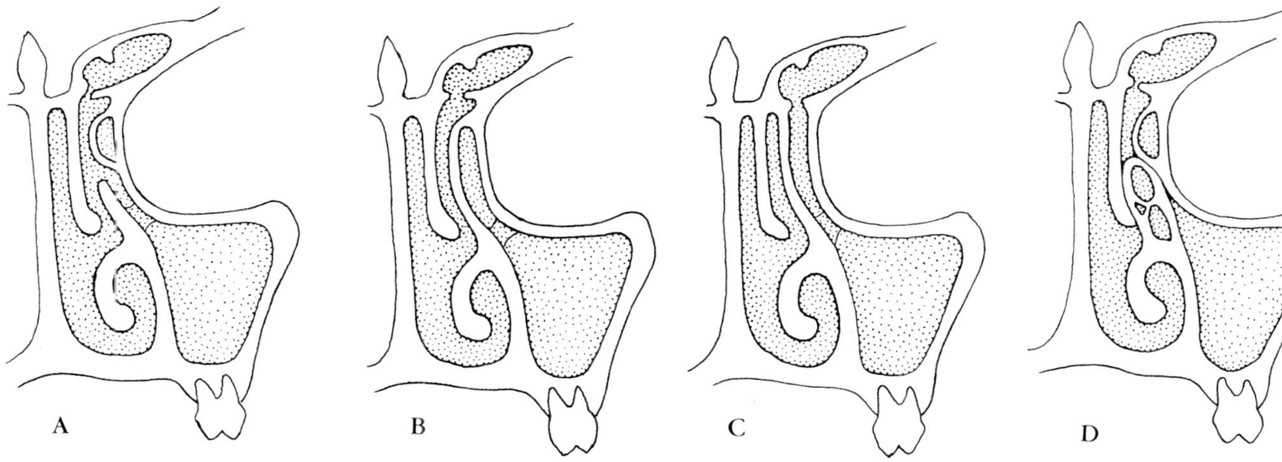


**FIGURE 16.22.** Variations in the uncinate process include the most common appearance of the uncinate process giving rise to this structure terminating in the nasal cavity **(A)**, the uncinate process inserting on the lamina papyracea to form a sinus terminalis **(B)**, the uncinate process fusing with the fovea ethmoidalis **(C)**, and an extensively pneumatized uncinate process partially obstructing outflow from the ethmoid and maxillary sinuses **(D)**. (From Rice DH, Schaefer SD, eds. *Endoscopic paranasal sinus surgery*, 2nd ed. New York: Raven Press, 1993, with permission.)

by which secretions can flow from the frontal and anterior ethmoid cells into the ostium of the maxillary sinus (11). Sometimes, a bony process develops from the attachment of the middle turbinate and projects laterally toward the orbit, but this is a rare event. Pneumatization of this process is called a *Haller cell* (Fig. 16.23). Because this cell is at the inferomedial aspect of the orbital rim, extensive pneumatization can impair outflow of the maxillary sinus, serve as a primary site of ethmoiditis, or increase the vulnerability of the eye to injury during endoscopic ethmoidectomy.

*Conchal cells* are ethmoid air cells that invade the middle conchae, and when these cells are located in the anterior aspect of the conchae, the condition is referred to as a *concha bullosa* (9,58) (Fig. 16.17). The bullosa cells are clini-

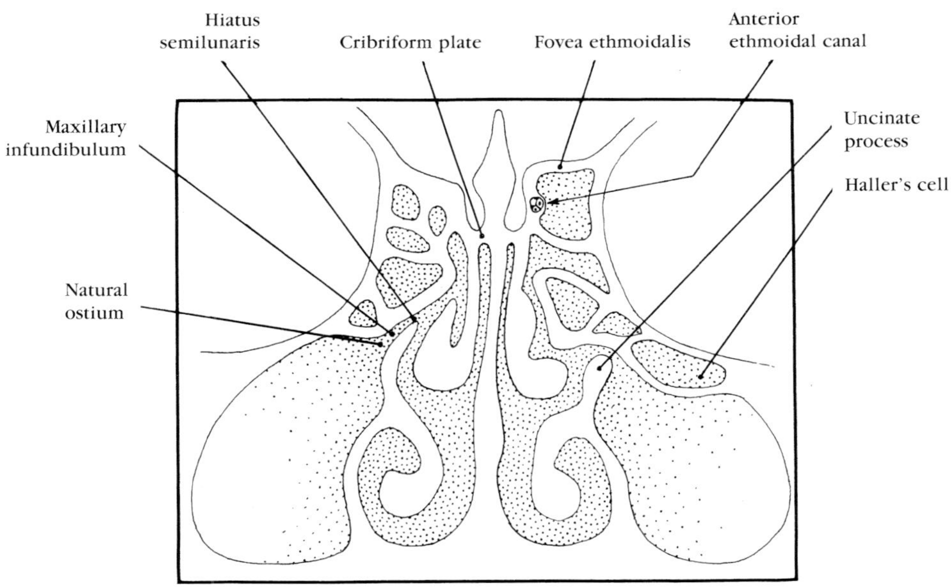


**FIGURE 16.23.** Schematic of the relationship of the paranasal sinuses to anterior cranial fossa and orbit. The anterior ethmoidal canal varies from 2 mm inferior to 4 mm superior to cribriform plate, and the posterior canal ranges from 0 to 3.1 mm superior to the cribriform. Pneumatization of the inferomedial orbit is known as a Haller cell. (From Rice DH, Schaefer SD, eds. *Endoscopic paranasal sinus surgery*, 2nd ed. New York: Raven Press, 1993, with permission.)

cally important because they can be an isolated source of recurrent ethmoiditis or may obstruct the middle meatus. The *middle turbinate*, being a medial appendage of the lateral nasal wall, overhangs the bulla ethmoidalis, the hiatus semilunaris, and the uncinate process (Fig. 16.14). Occasionally, the uncinate process and hiatus semilunaris are not covered by the downward expansion of this 3.5- to 4-cm-long important bony structure. Anteriorly, the middle turbinate is attached superiorly to the cribriform plate, with a 15° slope posteroinferiorly so that the posterior tip lies at or immediately inferior to the sphenopalatine foramen (53) (Fig. 16.24).

The *posterior ethmoid cells* (range, 1 to 7 cells), which invade the posterior ethmoid capsule, may also involve the middle turbinate, the sphenoid, the palatine, and the maxillary bones (Figs. 16.3, 16.5, 16.6, 16.16, and 16.17). An important form of the extramural extension of the posterior ethmoid cells is the migration of these cells to the medial aspect of the optic nerve within the sphenoid bone. Such cells located superiorly and inferiorly to the optic nerve are called *Onodi cells* (59). These cells are clinically important because the optic nerve may be covered by relatively thin bone and vulnerable to injury by dissection posterior to the anterior face of the sphenoid bone [anatomic relationships

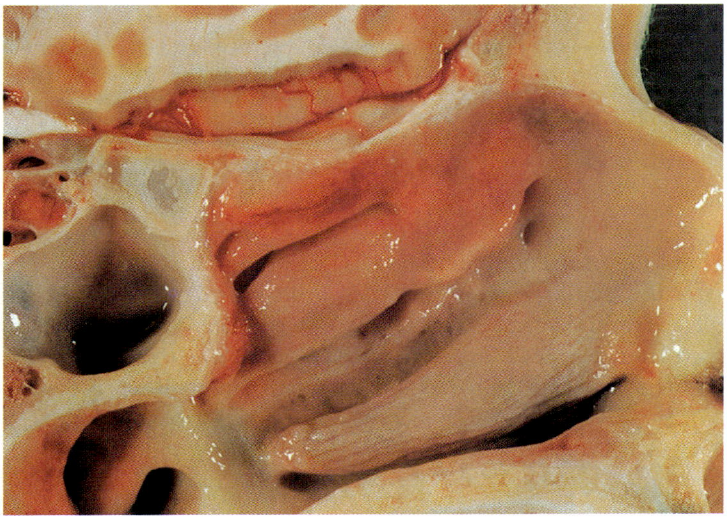

A

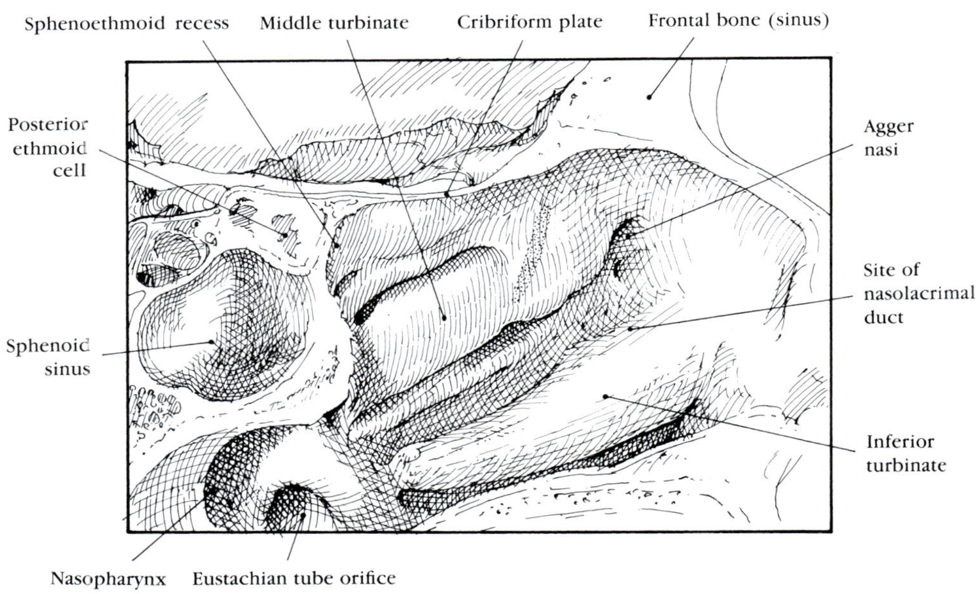


B

**FIGURE 16.24. A:** Most medial of a series of progressive dissections of the left lateral nasal wall. **B:** Diagram of **A** illustrates the surface anatomy. (From Rice DH, Schaefer SD, eds. *Endoscopic paranasal sinus surgery*, 2nd ed. New York: Raven Press, 1993, with permission.)

between optic nerve and paranasal sinuses are reviewed by Loeb (60) and in Fig. 16.3]. At the junction of the lamina papyracea and the frontal bone, the posterior ethmoidal artery enters the posterior ethmoids approximately 2 to 8 mm (average, 5 mm) anterior to the optic nerve. The *anterior ethmoidal canal* (Figs. 16.3 and 16.23) containing the artery (AEA) and the nerve of the same name runs between 1 mm inferior and 4 mm superior to the cribriform plate. The extraordinary course of the AEA originates from the orbital region and passes through the anterior ethmoid onto the anterior cranial fossa to finally enter the nasal cavity (61). A significant number of individuals have a natural dehiscence of this canal as it crosses the posterior aspect of the frontal recess at a region called *the dome of the ethmoid* (59,62). Injury to the AEA results in bleeding into the nasal cavity that can potentially cause the retraction of the vessel into the orbit, which leads to intraorbital bleeding and the danger of blindness. The *posterior ethmoidal canal* traverses the ethmoid bone at a plane approximately 1.5 mm above the cribriform plate, and it may also be partially dehiscent of bone.

## MAXILLARY SINUS

### History, Development, and Anatomy

The maxillary sinus has been referred to as the antrum of Highmore in honor of the English anatomist Nathanial Highmore, whose 1651 treatise, *Corporis Humani Disquisitio Anatomica,* described and illustrated this sinus (63). Clinical texts, however, continue to incorrectly credit Highmore as being the first to describe this sinus (64). Students of sinus anatomy history have noted other investigators who also described the maxillary sinus. Peter Paaw, for example, had already described it in his 1615 book, *Succenturiatus anatomicus* (65). Although Highmore's book primarily describes and illustrates the circulatory system of various systemic regions of the human body, undoubtedly because of his admiration and close association to Harvey,[4] the illustrated description of the maxillary sinus is what he is best remembered for (63) (Fig. 16.25). Nevertheless, recognition as the earliest known discoverer of the maxillary sinus would fall to Leonardo da Vinci, who illustrated and described this sinus in 1489 (6,66–69); Table 16.2 provides an overview of the earliest known investigators of the paranasal sinuses.

The maxillary sinus, lying within the body of the maxillary bone, is the largest and most constant of all four

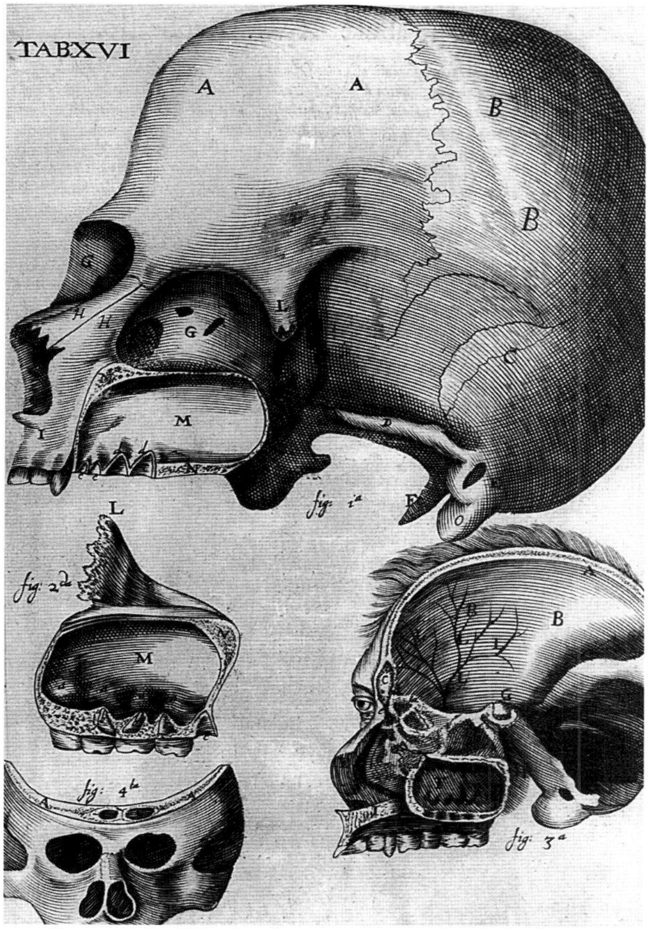


**FIGURE 16.25.** The original illustration of Highmore's description of the maxillary sinus as it appears on page 227 in his 1651 publication, *Discussion of the Human Body Anatomy and of the Blood Circulation.* (Courtesy of the New York Academy of Medicine Library, New York, NY.)

paranasal sinuses. Asymmetries of maxillary sinus size have been reported (70), but differences in the degree of asymmetry have not revealed any clear dominance of one particular side (71). An overall consensus is lacking regarding its shape, probably because of the great variability in its development (64). Cullen and Vidic (72) attempted to classify its prenatal morphology as elliptical, triangular, irregular, rectangular, and spherical. Anagnostopoulou and associates (73) classified 119 casts of adult maxillary sinuses from 60 dry skulls as semi-ellipsoid, paraboloid, hyperboloid, and conical. The maxillary sinus is generally described as being pyramidal (74), although Anon and colleagues (64) preferred the term tetrahedral to represent its morphology in three-dimensional space. Its anterior wall is the facial surface of the maxilla, where the facial vein and artery run, and the posterior wall is the infratemporal fossa, where the max-

[4] During 1642, while conducting studies on the embryonic development of the chick, Highmore and William Harvey became close colleagues. Highmore's 1651 treatise was the first anatomic textbook to accept Harvey's theory on the circulation of the blood.

**TABLE 16.2. PARANASAL SINUS ANATOMY HISTORY**

| Paranasal Sinus | Eponyms | First Described | Studies |
|---|---|---|---|
| Maxillary sinus | Antrum of Highmore | Leonardo da Vinci, 1489 | da Vinci, 1489 |
| Sphenoid sinus | | Giacomo Berengario da Carpi, 1521<br>Tillaux (1862)[a] | da Carpi, 1521 |
| Frontal sinus | | Volcher Coiter (1534–1576)<br>Basilius[b] | cited in Libersa et al, 1981<br>cited in Douglass, 1906 |
| Ethmoid sinus | | Galen (131–201) | Galen |

[a]Tillaux was the first to suggest that the sphenoidal sinus was part of the facial sinuses, although Johann Riolan (the younger) in 1649 was the first to recognize the paranasal sinuses as an entity (6).
[b]According to Douglass (69), Basilius was the first to describe the frontal sinus but offers no citation, as does Libersa and colleagues (1981), who cite Coiter as the first to describe this sinus.

illary artery[5] and vein are located. The medial wall constitutes the lateral wall of the nasal cavity, where a number of vascular structures are situated (i.e., branches of the sphenopalatine, the septal branch of the superior labial, and ethmoidal arteries). The superior wall or roof of this sinus is the floor of the orbit, and the floor of this sinus is the alveolar process of the maxilla. It becomes evident from its topographic relation to contiguous structures that infections and tumors of this sinus can spread in multiple directions, especially to the dentition (75,76).

Development of the maxillary sinus begins by the sixty-fifth day of gestation, making it the first sinus to develop *in utero* (77). Various researchers have reported different onsets of development. The initial onset of maxillary sinus development reported by Schaeffer (71) was the seventieth day; Kallius (78) timed the initial evagination during the middle of the third month; and Brandt and Roper-Hall (79) and Aubert (80) saw the fourteenth week as the beginning of maxillary sinus prenatal development. The initial stage of development of this sinus has been described primarily as a mucosal evagination (i.e., bud) into the lateral cartilaginous environment of the nasal capsule. However, Wang and coworkers (81) suggested that the mucosal evagination or outpouching of the nasal mucous membranes should be considered as a secondary event rather than the primary force. Although Schaeffer (71) described this pouch as a minute epithelial sac forming the anlage of the sinus, its presence precedes the appearance of the cartilage that later surrounds it. Wang and associates (81) showed that, during the nineteenth week *in utero*, the mucosa of the maxillary sinus makes direct contact with the maxillary bone only after the surrounding cartilaginous wall of the maxillary sinus begins to disappear through the degeneration and absorption of its cartilaginous cells. The exact location of this maxillary sinus outpouching stems from the primitive ethmoid infundibulum, also known as the uncibullous groove, which become the future uncinate and bulla ethmoidales structures. These structures demarcate the portal between the ethmoid infundibulum and nasal cavity (71). This developmental stage explains why any drainage from this sinus goes through the ethmoid infundibulum before reaching the middle meatus.

At birth, the sinus has an average volume of 6 to 8 mL but is fluid filled, making interpretation of plain film radiographs difficult (17,40). However, Weiglein and colleagues (82) reported that this sinus is of appreciable size at birth and can be identified on a Caldwell view. The maxillary sinus then undergoes two periods of rapid

[5] Based on the Nomina Anatomica (NA) adopted in Paris 1955. The maxillary artery, in the older Basle Nomina Anatomica (BNA), was referred to as the *internal maxillary artery* to distinguish it from the *external maxillary artery*, which is the *facial artery* in the NA.

**TABLE 16.3. EMBRYOLOGIC PATTERN OF DEVELOPMENT**

| Paranasal Sinus | Embryologic Appearance | Postnatal Appearance | Growth Spurt Interval |
|---|---|---|---|
| Ethmoid sinus | Development begins in third fetal month | Present at birth | First growth spurt between 1 and 4 years; second growth spurt between 4 and 8 years |
| Maxillary sinus | 65th day of gestation | Present at birth | First growth spurt between birth and 3 years; second between 7 and 12 years |
| Frontal sinus | Development begins in fourth fetal month | Detected at 7–12 years of age | Adult size completed by 20 years |
| Sphenoid sinus | Development begins in third fetal month | Detected at 3–4 years of age | By seventh year, sinus begins to extend posteriorly toward the sella turcica |

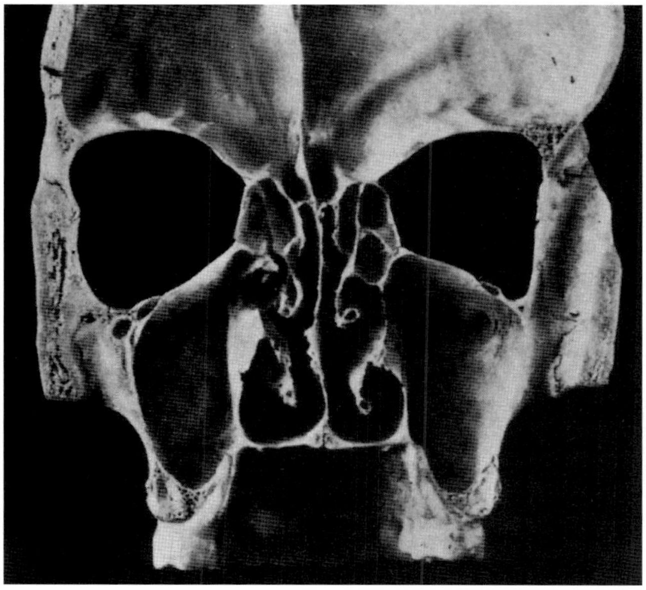

**FIGURE 16.26.** A coronal section of an adult human crania is shown in dorsal view to illustrate the descent of the maxillary sinus floor, falling below the level of the nasal cavity floor. (From Underwood AS. An inquiry into the anatomy and pathology of the maxillary sinus. *J Anat Physiol* 1920;44:354–369, with permission.)

growth: one between birth and 3 years and the other between 7 and 12 years (17,71). Between these two growth periods, at around 4 years of age, the sinus extends laterally past the infraorbital canal (83). After the second period of rapid growth (Table 16.3), subsequent expansion involves pneumatization of the alveolar process of the maxilla. Before growth is completed, there is a descent of the maxillary sinus from 4 mm above the floor of the nasal cavity at birth to the same level as the nasal floor at age 8 to 9 years and then a final drop of 4 to 5 mm below this level by adulthood (44) (Fig. 16.26; see Fig. 16.34). Because the descent of this sinus coincides with dental eruption, a long-held belief sees an intimate relationship between these two developmental events (84). Libersa and coworkers (85) and Márquez and associates (86), however, have demonstrated very poor and statistically insignificant relationships between molar eruption pattern and adult maxillary sinus form and between molar volume and adult sinus size, respectively.

## Clinical Implications

In the adult, the maxillary sinus can be roughly described as triangular, measuring 25 mm along the anterior limb of its base, 34 mm deep, and 33 mm high (17,44). The sinus can be partially compartmentalized by complete or incomplete septa. Knowledge of the incidence and morphology of maxillary sinus septa has clinical implications, especially in sinus lift operations performed preparatory to the placement of dental implants (87). In rare cases, separate cavities can exist in the posterior part of the sinus, which can be a source of persistent infection (88). The primary or *natural ostium* of this sinus is located in the superior aspect of the medial wall of the sinus and drains through its infundibulum into the hiatus semilunaris (Figs. 16.3 and 16.5 to 16.9). Despite a marked variation in position, most investigators see the ostia as being in the region of the posterior half of the infundibulum, or posterior to the midpoint of the bulla ethmoidalis (12,15,17). Lang and Papke (89) found that the ostium is located 1.3 to 11.5 mm (average, 4 mm) from the nasolacrimal duct (Fig. 16.27), and this proximity of the duct to the natural ostium makes it vulnerable to injury during middle meatus antrostomy. The pneumatization of the ethmoidal bulla and the height (e.g., medial and superior projection) of the uncinate process help to form a canal leading to the maxillary sinus, which was incorrectly called *maxillary infundibulum*.[6] This structure varies in depth (average, 5 mm) (71), orientation, and accessibility through the nose (12).

The *natural ostium* tends to be elliptical, measuring 1 to 20 mm long (71). *Accessory maxillary sinus ostia* were found in 15% to 40% of subjects examined by various investigators (12,15,71) (Figs. 16.3 and 16.21). These ostia may be located in the infundibulum or the membranous region of the medial sinus wall, with the latter being only a reduplication of the mucosa of the sinus and the lateral nasal wall. This membranous wall is known as the *membranous meatus* or *fontanelle*. This region is located inferior to the uncinate process and superior to the insertion of the inferior turbinate. Clinically, this site is particularly important because it may be used as an alternative to opening the natural ostium when the latter cannot be found during the performance of a middle meatus or supra-inferior turbinate antrostomy.

During the seventeenth century, antral trephination for suppuration was the most common maxillary sinus operation performed, followed by molar tooth extraction to create an oral-antral fistula for dependent drainage of an infected maxillary sinus (90). Historically, the next procedure for sinus drainage was an anterior wall approach above the canine fossa, which was maintained patent for irrigation procedures. Then came the Caldwell-Luc procedure, which combined the anterior wall approach with an intranasal antrostomy, and after removal of the infected mucosa, the intranasal incision was closed. Endoscopic sinus surgery is now performed primarily for treating infected maxillary sinuses (90).

[6] The maxillary infundibulum and frontal infundibulum are totally within their respected sinuses, appearing as funneling tunnels whose orientation is toward their natural ostia (50).

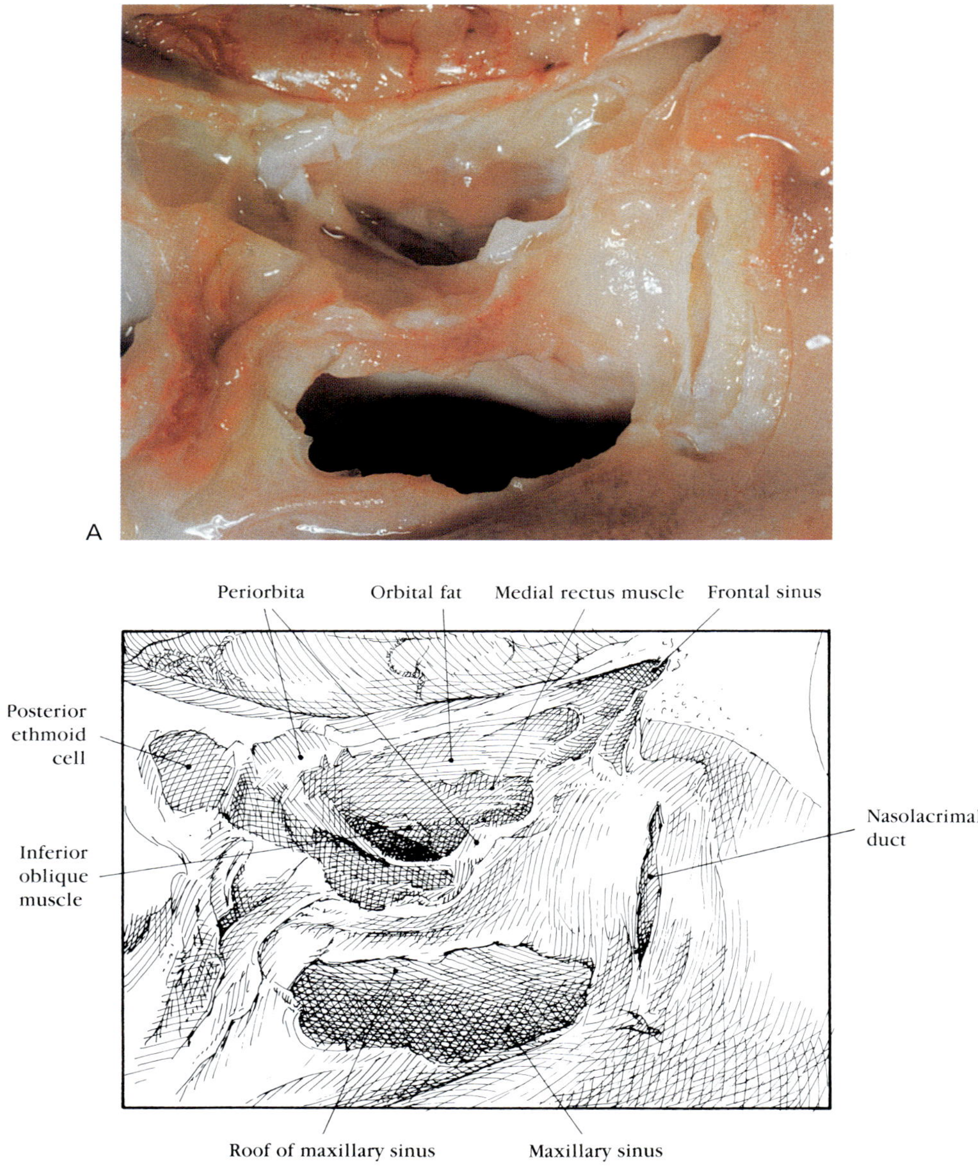


**FIGURE 16.27. A:** The lateral nasal wall has been exenterated to show the medial orbit, maxillary sinus, and nasolacrimal duct. **B:** The illustrated version of **A**. (From Rice DH, Schaefer SD, eds. *Endoscopic paranasal sinus surgery*, 2nd ed. New York: Raven Press, 1993, with permission.)

# FRONTAL SINUS

## History, Development, and Anatomy

Volcher Coiter of Holland, a pupil of Fallopius and Eustachius, is said to be the first to describe the frontal sinus (85). Berengario da Carpi (3) described the frontal bone region as having "two tables within which there is a notable vacuity so as to not weigh down the body." It was da Vinci, in 1489, who first recognized its existence and illustrated its morphology (2,91).

Development of the frontal sinus is initiated in the fourth fetal month, when the entire nasofrontal area is represented by the frontal recess (92), and it is the last paranasal sinus to develop (83). The usually paired frontal sinuses have several possible origins, each of which influences the relationship of this sinus to the lateral nasal wall and its drainage pattern within the middle meatus (93). In a study of 100 adult specimens and 15 late-term fetuses, Kasper (14) found the most common origin of the frontal sinus to be pits or furrows originating within the frontal recess that are considered rudimentary anterior ethmoid cells (described previously as frontal recess cells). These additional furrows are not to be confused with the previously described furrows that go on to become the meatus. Kasper (14) described these nasofrontal structures within the frontal recess as frontal pits because of their dimple-like appearance. What makes the anatomy of this region challenging is that there is neither a clear developmental pattern nor any constancy in the differentiation of these frontal pits. A person may have as many as four pits to a total absence of pit formation. When there is no pit formation, the frontal recess remains a simple blind outgrowth from the middle meatus without configuration of its lateral wall. The variability of which of these pits is present and which goes on to become the frontal sinus determines the specific pattern of sinus drainage. For example, the more remote or lateral the pits are from the ethmoid infundibulum, the more lateral the frontal sinus is and its communication with the nasal chamber, which is influenced by the impinging anterior ethmoid cells (14). Various developmental patterns are possible when all four pits are present, because each pit has the potential to become a frontal sinus (11). If the most anterior pit (i.e., pit 1) migrates in a ventral direction, it may pneumatize the agger nasi bone, becoming an agger nasi cell, and the second most anterior pit (i.e., pit 2) may migrate anterosuperiorly becoming the frontal sinus. The terms agger nasi (i.e., referring to the mound of bone) and agger nasi cell (i.e., referring to the pneumatization of the agger nasi bone) are not interchangeable, because each represents a distinct anatomic entity. Moreover, a markedly pneumatized agger nasi cell could have potential pathophysiologic consequences in frontal sinus drainage (94). Figure 16.28 demonstrates the relationship between the frontal sinus with its drainage tract and the agger nasi cell. Because the roof of the agger nasi cell is the floor of the frontal sinus and the posterior wall of the agger nasi cell is the anterior border of the frontal sinus drainage tract, a markedly inflated cell would theoretically interrupt its normal drainage and ventilation (94). Brunner and colleagues (95) have implicated the agger nasi cell in narrowing the frontal sinus outflow tract as a significant cause for the pathogenesis of frontoethmoid sinus pain and chronic frontal sinusitis. By the end of the second year of life, one of the anterior ethmoid cells migrates upward into the frontal bone to form the frontal sinus (96). Another means of frontal sinus formation results if no anterior ethmoid air cells develop in the frontal recess; ethmoid air cell extension from the ethmoid infundibulum can then create a frontal sinus (97).

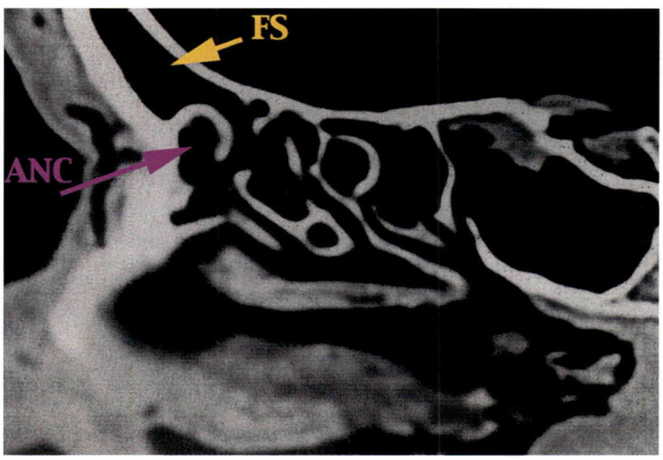


**FIGURE 16.28.** A two-dimensional computed tomographic reconstruction shows the topographic relationship of the frontal sinus *(FS)* and the agger nasi cell *(ANC)*. Notice that the roof of the ANC forms part of the floor of the FS.

The following text is a summary of the possible developmental patterns of the frontal sinus as a result of a direct outgrowth from the frontal recess region if no frontal pits are present; from one of the frontal pits within the frontal recess when present; and a direct outgrowth from the ventral portion of the ethmoid infundibulum by direct extension or from one of its cellular outgrowths (11). There also can be combinations of the possible patterns of development resulting in duplicate and even triplicate sinuses on one side alone (98).

At birth, the sinus has little clinical relevance, and it is often indistinguishable from the anterior ethmoid cells. Davis (99) tracked the frontal sinus postnatal development of 160 crania in persons ranging from birth to 16 years of age and recorded that an evagination into the vertical portion of the frontal bone occurred during the second year. At 3 years of age, the frontal sinus is observed 3.8 mm above nasion (i.e., a craniometric point defined as the junction between the nasal and frontal bones at the midline) and continues its vertical growth trajectory at an average annual rate of 1.5 mm until the fifteenth year. Final growth is completed before the twentieth year (44). Although as many as three sinuses have been reported in the literature (98) (Fig. 16.29), adult frontal sinuses consist generally of a pair which are asymmetric in nature (49). Tilley (100) illustrated the diversity of different frontal sinus morphologies, and he discredited using the prominences of the superciliary ridges as a guide in determining the presence and extent of the sinuses behind them. The potential of diverse initial growth patterns of the frontal sinus means that the adult sinus is highly variable such that each configuration is considered unique to each individual (101). Forensic identification of postmortem skeletal material based on the radiography of frontal sinus morphology has been used successfully in criminal investigations (102). Shapiro and Schorr (103) attempted to explain the vast differences observed in pneumatization patterns of the frontal bone and concluded that three factors may be ultimately responsible: craniofacial configuration, thickness of the frontal bone, and hormonal growth factors. Urken and coworkers (104) attempted to evaluate whether an overly "large"

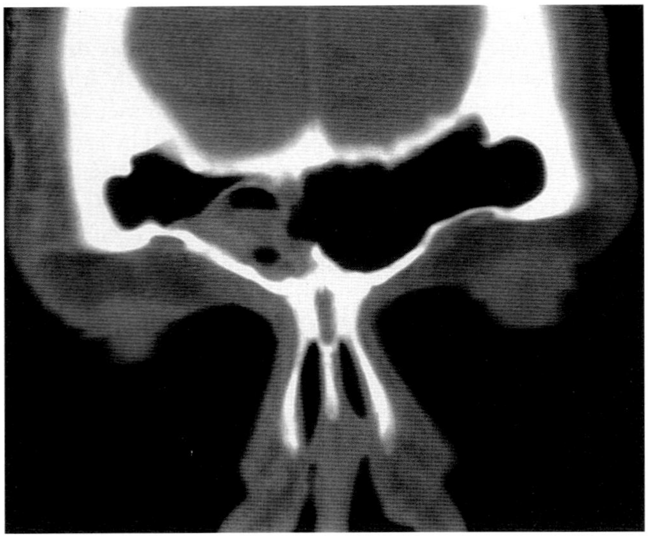

**FIGURE 16.29.** The frontal cell is visible within the right frontal sinus. There is an air-fluid level within the frontal cell. (Courtesy of Timothy L. Smith, M.D., M.P.H., Medical College of Wisconsin, Milwaukee, WI.)

frontal sinus might actually be abnormally inflated based on linear and derived area measurements as predictors of its "normal" variation. This led to a follow-up study in which Urken and associates (105) proposed three new categories to delineate the degree of excessive pneumatization based on aeration and bony changes of the sinus walls, which they called *hypersinus*, *pneumosinus dilatans*, and *pneumocele*.

## Clinical Implications

The adult frontal sinus, when viewed in a transverse section, has been classically described as pyramidal (49). The base or inferior floor of the pyramid is the orbital nasal portion of the splanchnocranium, the apex extends outward a variable distance over the orbit, the anterior wall is subcutaneous, and the posterior wall is cerebral. The adult frontal sinus has been measured as 28 mm high, 27 mm wide, and 17 mm long (106). This ideal sinus is a representative average, with the actual size and configuration reflecting the origin of the cavity and the superior development into the squama of the frontal bone (52). At the inferior aspect in the midsagittal plane, the anterior or outer table of the frontal sinus is approximately twice as thick as the posterior or inner table. The sinus is compartmentalized further by the intrasinus septa and marginated by irregular bone. The loss of definition of the scalloped border, or the intrasinus septa, on plain film radiographs indicates chronic infection (107).

In describing the anatomic relations of the frontal sinus and its connection to the nasal cavity, conflicting terms have caused confusion. For example, while some anatomists have concentrated on the frontal ostium (i.e., the "discharge" point), others have concerned themselves with the treatment of frontal sinus disease and the so-called nasofrontal duct (108). Historically, the communication of this sinus with the nasal cavity has been described as a distinct nasofrontal duct, although others prefer the term frontal recess. The term nasofrontal duct, which is used to describe the communication of the frontal sinus through the middle meatus and into the nasal cavity, is anatomically and developmentally incorrect. To confuse the issue even further, the terms frontal recess, frontal infundibulum, and nasofrontal duct have also been used interchangeable, when in reality they represent different anatomic structures (50). Conceptually, drainage of the frontal sinus has been likened to an hourglass, with the upper portion being the ostium (2 to 10 mm in diameter) and the frontal recess representing the lower portion beneath the neck. However, the term *frontal recess* introduced by Killian (109) is based on the prenatal observation of a space that is the continuation of the ascending branch of the first primary interturbinal furrow, with the descending branch becoming the ethmoid infundibulum.

The frontal sinus and the agger nasi cells are formed by pneumatization superiorly and anteriorly from the frontal recess region (32). Cells may develop in the frontal bone adjacent to the frontal sinus, a phenomena that Zuckerkandl (9) called the *bulla frontalis*. The frontal infundibulum was defined by Killian (109) as the superior opening of the frontal sinus drainage tract. The nasofrontal duct as defined by Lang (55) is any mucosal lined bony passage greater than 3 mm long. The developmental variability of the frontal sinus leads to the multiple observed drainage patterns, which can be further complicated by the highly variable pneumatization of the adjacent ethmoid air cells and by the position of the uncinate process. As an example, Lothrop (1898) reported a direct communication between the frontal sinus and ethmoid infundibulum in 47% of his 125 cadaver specimens, whereas Van Alyea (93) reported a 12.5% incidence in 112 cadavers. This prompted Stammberger (32) to conclude, "[I]t is senseless to name every recess or inlet that can be seen endoscopically, particularly when pathologic changes are present."

## Clinical Correlates

Serial computed tomography (CT) scans are necessary to demonstrate the sinus anatomy to gain access to the frontal sinus through the nasal cavity. In following air cells superiorly into the frontal sinus, it is important to dissect as far anterior as possible. The position of the AEA, by helping to identify the frontal recess and preventing an intracranial injury, forms an extremely important anatomic landmark in frontal sinus surgery. The vessel runs in a bony canal along the roof of the ethmoid labyrinth to form the posterior border of the frontal recess. Accordingly, surgery above the level of the canal must be anteriorly to enter the frontal sinus. Surgery posteriorly to it would violate the ethmoidal roof, resulting in a dural injury.

Accessing the frontal sinus through the nose may be hazardous because one of the visualized openings may not be the primary drainage of the frontal sinus and violating the floor of the anterior cranial fossa may lead to an intracranial injury. Moreover, scarring from previous surgery or pathologic conditions can make identification of the frontal recess impossible. This may require trephining the frontal sinus and transilluminating its floor by placement of a light source in the sinus or threading a probe through its ostium into the nasal cavity to guide further surgery. Intraoperative visualization has been aided by CT-guided visualization of the sinus and its outflow tract by electromagnetic and infrared navigational devices. Table 16.4 describes the clinical anatomic concerns.

**TABLE 16.4. IMPORTANT ANATOMIC RELATIONSHIPS AND THEIR SURGICAL IMPLICATIONS**

- Middle turbinate marks the junction of the roof of nasal cavity and ethmoidal labyrinth.
  - Surgery is performed laterally to avoid cribriform plate injury.
- Middle turbinate slopes downward along its posterior course.
  - To resect, scissors must be inclined downward; the posterior tip of middle turbinate and superior turbinate lie in the plane of the face of the sphenoid.
- Middle turbinate resection
  - Superior portion is maintained as a landmark; the posterior tip may be a source of bleeding and should be electrocauterized.
- The nasolacrimal duct runs downward at the anterior border of the attachment of the middle and inferior turbinates.
  - Inferior or middle meatus antrostomies must not be carried too far anteriorly to avoid duct injury.
- The nasofrontal duct drains into the infundibulum or frontal recess cells.
  - It cannot be safely enlarged, and the frontal sinus entered intranasally in every case.
- The natural ostium of the maxillary sinus is generally 1 to 2 cm beyond the anterior attachment of the middle turbinate.
  - Dissection anteriorly may injure the nasolacrimal duct; dissection superiorly penetrates the orbit.
- Fovea ethmoidalis is generally at a higher level than the cribrifrom plate
  - Thickness, yellow color, and sensitivity of bone are not reliable indicators; the higher the fovea, the weaker its medial wall and the more susceptible to fracture and perforation it is with intracranial entry.
- Posterior ethmoidal cells may extend behind the sphenoid face.
  - Dissection behind may produce optic nerve injury or cerebrospinal fluid (CSF) leak
- Posterior ethmoidal cells may be superior to the sphenoid sinus.
  - Dissection may produce CSF leak.
- Developmental abnormalities of anterior ethmoidal cells exist.
  - Hypoplasia of the uncinate process may lead to orbital injury on infundibulotomy; hyperplasia of agger nasi cells may block the frontal recess or impinge on the nasolacrimal duct, making it vulnerable to surgical injury.
- Ethmoidal labyrinth is placed superior and lateral to the middle turbinate in its posterior aspect.
  - Failure to follow cells upward may result in orbital injury.
- A narrow ethmoid variant may exist (the ethmoid may not widen posteriorly in a small number of cases).
  - Lateral dissection in a posterior cell my produce optic nerve injury.
- The lamina papyracea lies superiorly in the plane of the membranous middle meatus.
  - Middle meatus antrostomy must be made on the upper border of the inferior turbinate (supraturbinal) to prevent orbital injury.
- Sphenoid ostium lies about 7 cm and 30° from the nares.
  - Never blindly perforate into sinus; always cannulate transnasally or transseptally
- Sphenoid ostium is 8 mm below the cribriform plate.
  - Dissection superiorly carries the risk of intracranial injury; attempted entry should be made medially and inferiorly.
- Sphenoid ostium widening should be performed selectively.
  - Superior widening carries the danger of CSF leak; inferior widening carries the danger of sphenopalatine artery injury.
- Sphenoid sinus walls may be dehiscent laterally.
  - Instrumentation laterally may cause internal carotid artery injury.
- Sphenoid sinus may be partially encircled by medially displaced internal carotid arteries.
  - Dissection or fracture superiorly may cause arterial injury.

Adapted from Lawson W. The intranasal ethmoidectomy: evolution and an assessment of the procedure. *Laryngoscope* 1994;104(pt 2):1–49, with permission.

## SPHENOID SINUS

### History, Development, and Anatomy

In 1521, Giacomo Berengario da Carpi (3) was the first to describe the sphenoid sinuses, but it was Tillaux (110) who suggested that this sinus was part of the other paranasal sinus complex. According to Dixon (111), the sphenoid sinus is the most variable cuboidal sinus of all the paranasal sinuses. The average adult sinus has six surfaces: the anterior, posterior, superior, inferior, medial, and lateral walls. The sphenoid bone, where this sinus resides, is strategically located in one of the more complex regions in all of human anatomy. The endocranial surface of this bone serves as the seat for endocrine activity; as a conduit for cranial nerves responsible for vision, ocular movements, nasal mucosal gland stimulation, nasal sympathetic innervation; and as a major vascular supply for the nasal cavity.

Growth of the usually paired sphenoid sinus is initiated during the third month of intrauterine development (90,111). These two sinuses generally develop asymmetrically where usually one sinus encroaches on and limits the other's growth to a rudimentary size. The bony partition between the two sinuses has been incorrectly called *median septum*. Congdon (112) suggested the more appropriate term of *intersinus septum* because the partition is frequently found more lateral than medial, and this is the accepted term today. Complete or partial septation of the sinuses is a frequent occurrence because no clear pattern emerged from a number of studies (112). The variety of encroachment patterns, the pneumatization of contiguous structures, and the irregularities of its sinus septa are all considered to be within normal variation (92).

The sphenoid sinus begins development as an evagination of the nasal mucosa into the posterior portion of the cartilaginous nasal capsule. The inferoposterior expansion forms a pouchlike cavity in the cartilage, the wall of which is called the sphenoid conchae, or Bertini's ossicles (92). At birth, the pyramidal paired ossicles, whose spines are in contact with the medial pterygoid lamina and whose bases help to form the roof of the nasal cavity, begin to ossify. Around the time of birth, the sphenoid sinus is primarily an evagination of the sphenoethmoid recess, with essentially no growth until age 3 years. It is not until the third year of life that the sphenoid conchae becomes attached to the presphenoid and the cavity develops into the definitive sphenoid sinus (90). After this period, the sinus begins to pneumatize the sphenoid bone, and by the seventh year, the sinus extends posteriorly toward the sella turcica. Based on the prenatal development of the sphenoid bone (e.g., the anterior to posterior arrangement of its ossifications centers), Congdon (112) classified four types of sphenoid sinus pneumatization patterns: conchal, presphenoid, basisphenoid, and occipitosphenoid (i.e., the basilar part of the occipital bone). Based on a sample size of 181 specimens, Congdon (110) classified 5% as conchal, 4.5% between conchal and presphenoid types, 23.5% presphenoid, and the remaining 67% included basisphenoid and occipitosphenoidal types. Different incidences of these types of sphenoidal pneumatization have been reported over the years. For example, Hammer and Radberg (113) found conchal types in 2.5% of cases, presellar types (presphenoid) in 11%, postsellar types (basisphenoid) in 59%, and mixed types in 27%. In the most common developmental type, the postsellar, the sinus extends posteriorly toward the sella turcica by 7 years of age. Development may continue into adulthood, involving the basisphenoid and with arrest in pneumatization accounting for the tremendous variations in the sinus size. Such variations may produce recesses formed by the pneumatization of the sphenoid rostrum, the lesser wing of the sphenoid, and the orbital processes (114–116). Pneumatization of other bony structures have been reported for the pterygoid processes in 25% to 40% of adults and the anterior clinoid process in 13% (83). Donald (24) reported the occurrence of a septal recess, sometimes called a sphenovomerine bulla, which is pneumatization of the vomer. The tendency to pneumatize contiguous bony structures is not restricted to human development because it is also seen in our own CT-based investigations of the sinus anatomy of the African great ape (117) (Fig. 16.30).

The average adult sinus measures 20 mm high, 23 mm long, and 17 mm wide (44). The volume varies from 0.1 to 30 mL, with the average ranging from 5 to 7.5 mL (44,111). As the sinus expands, vessels and nerves in the lateral aspect of the body of the sphenoid bone come to lie as indentations in the wall of the sinus. Van Alyea (44) found a projection of the internal carotid artery into the lateral sinus wall in 65 specimens ($n$=100) and the projection being pronounced in 53 of them (16) (Figs. 16.31–16.34). Based on a study of 1,600 skulls, Dixon (111) found that the optic nerve was present as an indentation in the sinus wall in 8% of the specimens and the vidian nerve in 7% (Figs. 16.33–16.35). In this same study, Dixon reported that 22% of the skulls had an intrasinus septum, with dehiscence of the septum observed in only five specimens (Fig. 16.34). The primary septum was found in the midline in only one fourth of the subjects. More often than not, the septum grows asymmetrically, with most of the bony wall coursing to one side, and sometimes exhibits an S or C shape. Equally important is the thinning of the superior wall, which may separate the sinus from the dura by only 1 mm (53). Dehiscence of the sella floor is rare (9), and dehiscence of the lateral wall over the internal carotid artery is also uncommon, but the potential minimal bony covering of this vessel is a clinically important factor to consider.

*(text continues on page 191)*

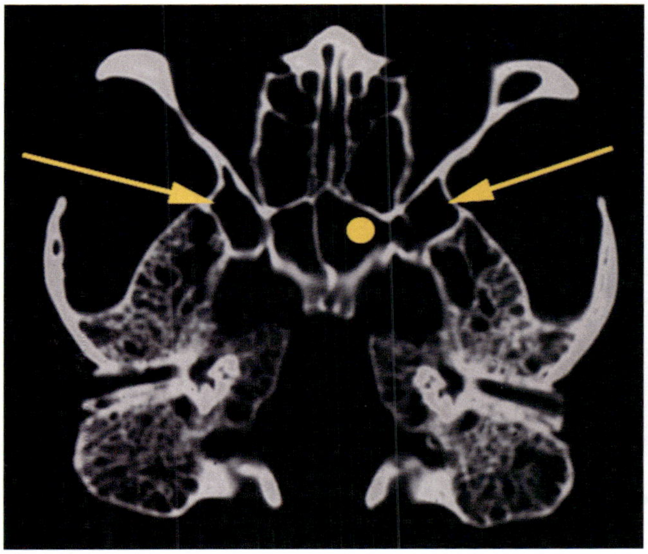

A

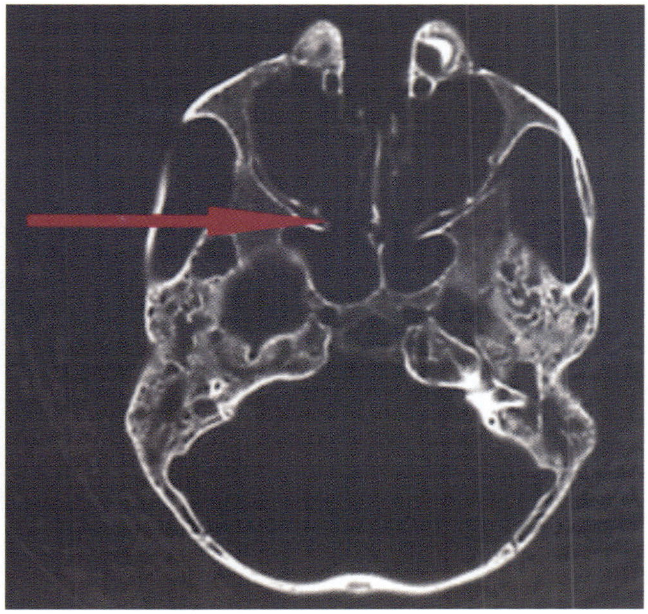

B

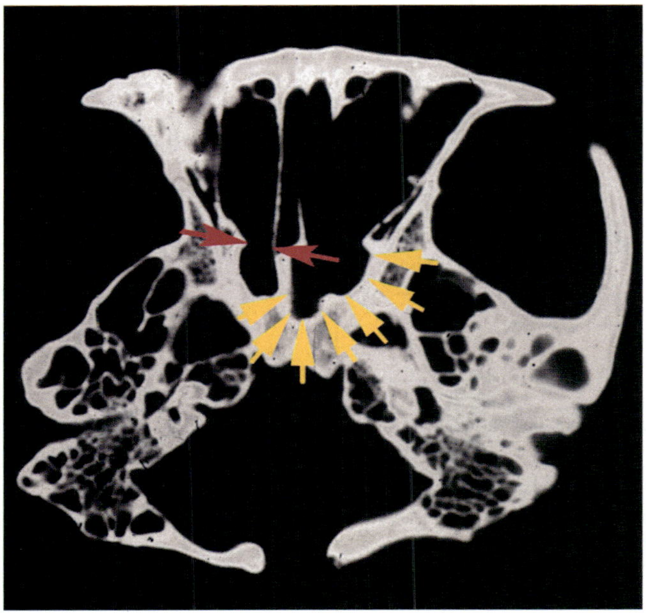

C

**FIGURE 16.30. A:** An axial scan of an adult gorilla shows the sphenoid sinus *(yellow dot)* invading and pneumatizing the pterygoid plates *(yellow arrows)*. **B:** An axial scan of a subadult orangutan shows what appears to be a sphenoid sinus but is actually the maxillary sinus invading the sphenoid bone. **C:** In an adult orangutan, the communication *(yellow)* between the left maxillary sinus and the evacuated sphenoid bone is clearly patent; the right maxillary sinus *(red arrow)* encroaches on the sphenoid bone.

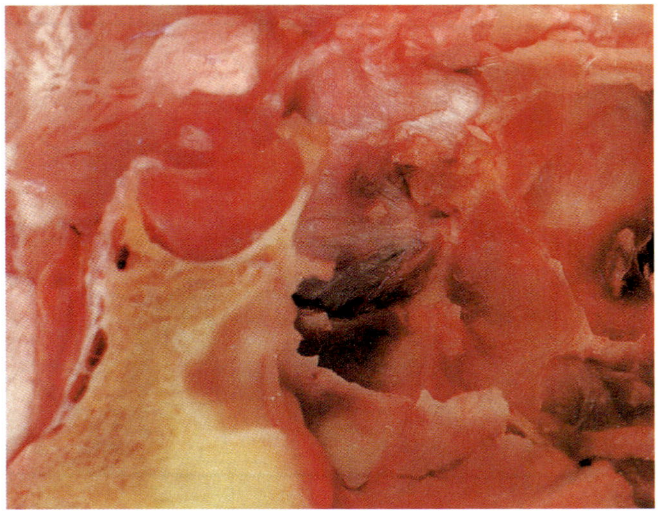

A

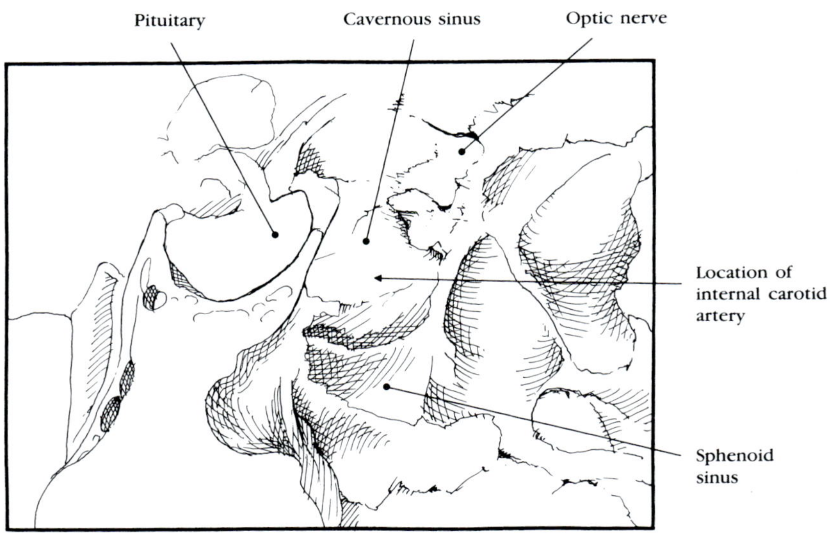


B

**FIGURE 16.31.** **A:** Parasagittal section through the sphenoid and posterior ethmoid sinuses. The lateral wall of these sinuses has been removed to expose the cavernous sinus and optic nerve. **B:** The proximity of the optic nerve and internal carotid artery to the lateral wall of the sphenoid and posterior ethmoid sinuses is illustrated. (From Rice DH, Schaefer SD, eds. *Endoscopic paranasal sinus surgery*, 2nd ed. New York: Raven Press, 1993, with permission.)

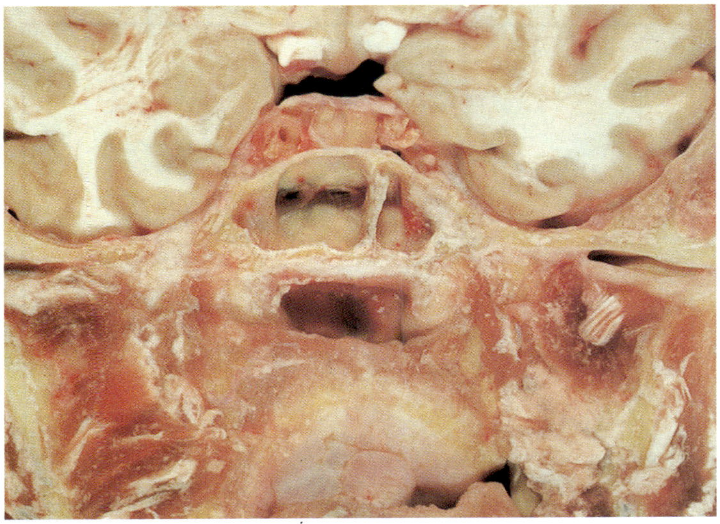

A

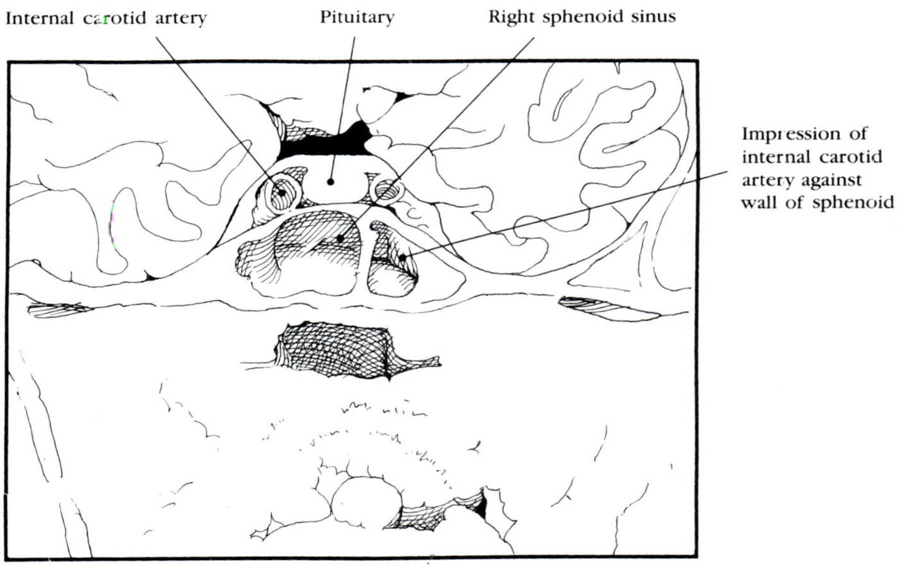


B

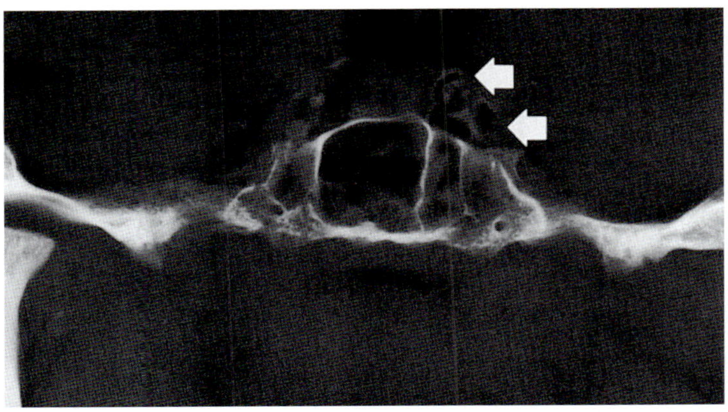

C

**FIGURE 16.32. A:** The anterior surface of the coronal section is contiguous with the section in Figure 16.35C at the level of the posterior sphenoid sinus. **B:** The drawing of **A** emphasizes the close relationship of the sphenoid sinus to important neurovascular structures. **C:** Plain radiograph of the specimen in **A**. The arrow points to the internal carotid. (From Rice DH, Schaefer SD, eds. *Endoscopic paranasal sinus surgery*, 2nd ed. New York: Raven Press, 1993, with permission.)

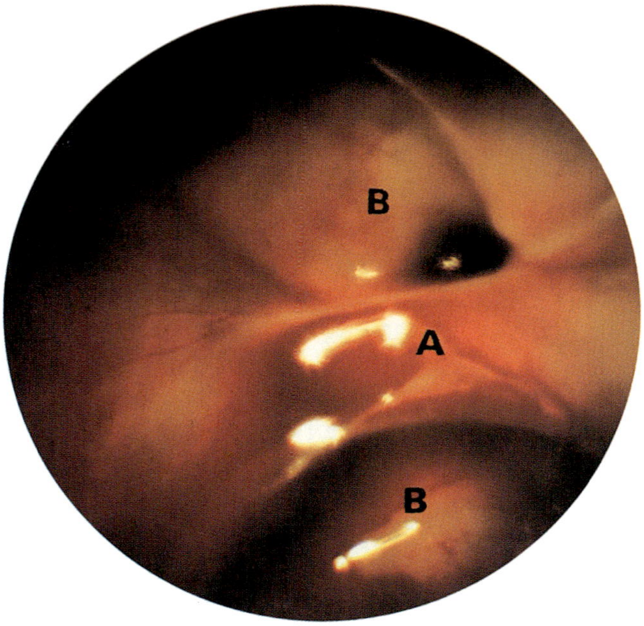


**FIGURE 16.33.** Lateral wall of left sphenoid sinus is visualized with a 25° endoscope. The optic nerve *(A)* horizontally crosses the internal carotid artery *(B)*. (From Rice DH, Schaefer SD, eds. *Endoscopic paranasal sinus surgery*, 2nd ed. New York: Raven Press, 1993, with permission.)

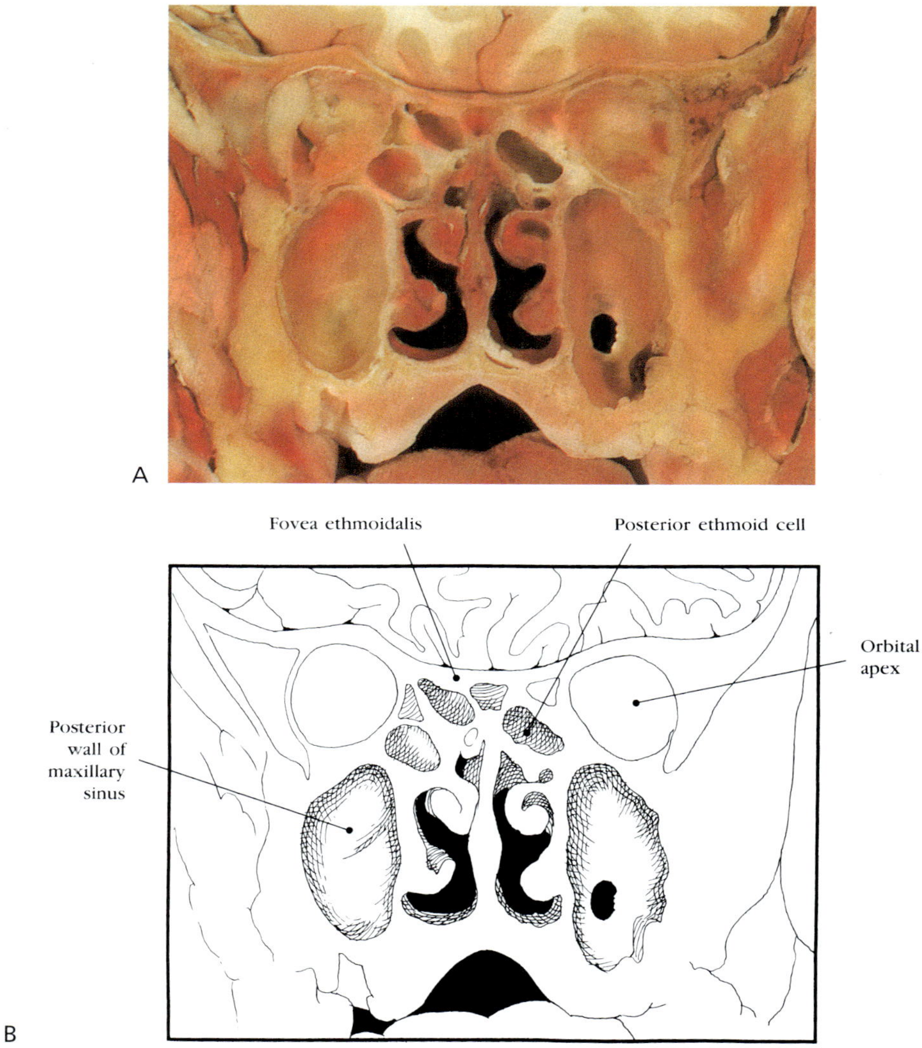


**FIGURE 16.34. A:** A coronal section exposes the posterior wall of the maxillary sinuses from an anterior perspective and is a reference for **C**. **B:** The residual maxillary cavity is shown along with the adjacent posterior ethmoid cells. Notice that the fovea ethmoidalis is properly identified.

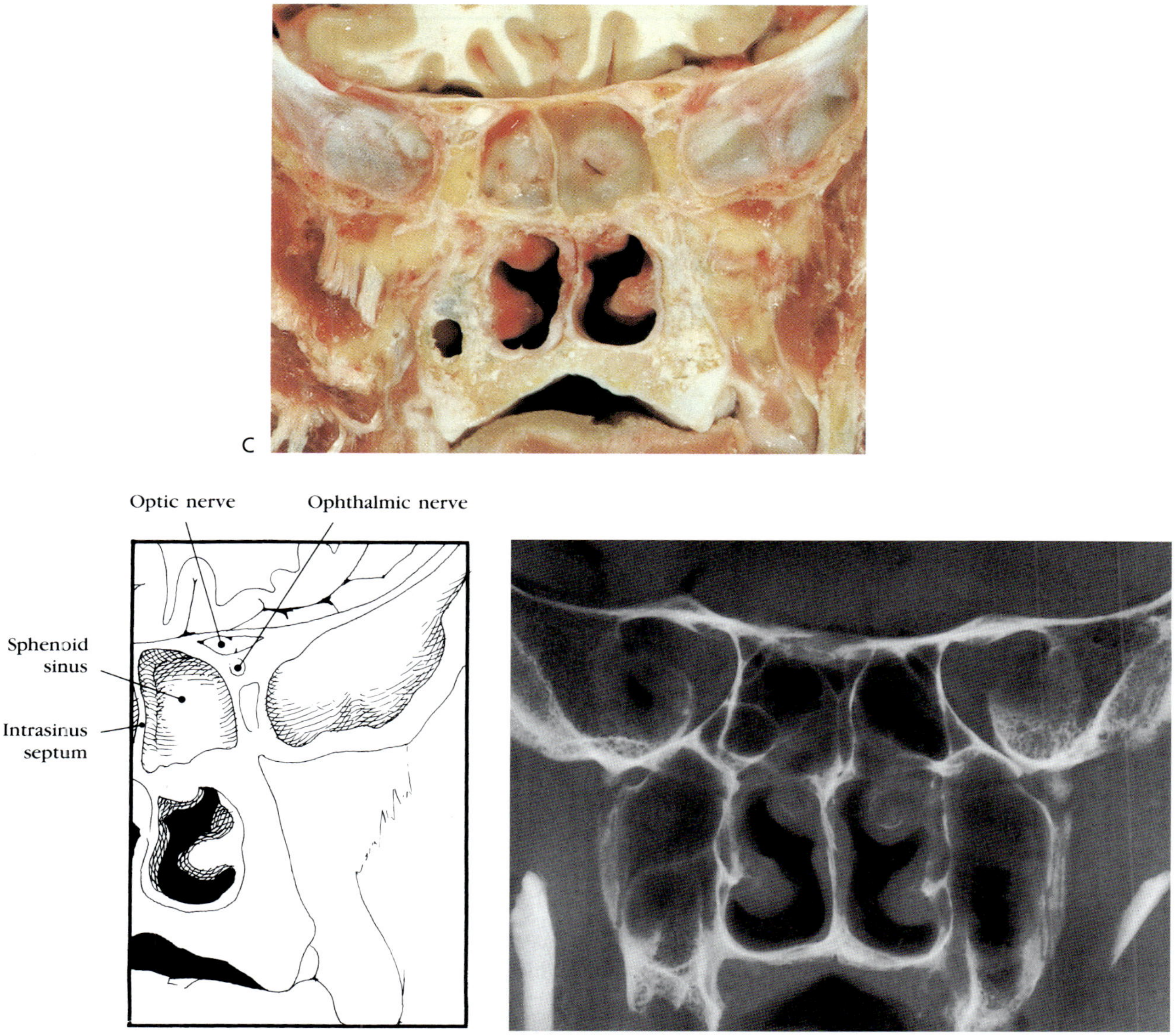


**FIGURE 16.34. *(continued)*** **C:** The posterior surface of the specimen in **A** is immediately dorsal to the maxillary sinus or at the plane of the pterygopalatine space. **D:** The dorsal surface of the anterior wall of the sphenoid sinus is visualized along with the nasopharynx. Notice the relationship of nerves to the sinus wall. **E:** Plain radiograph of the specimen in Figure 16.8 shows the remnant of the pterygoid plates and the convergence of the posterior ethmoids (Fig. 16.8A) and the sphenoid sinus (Fig. 16.8C). (From Rice DH, Schaefer SD, eds. *Endoscopic paranasal sinus surgery*, 2nd ed. New York: Raven Press, 1993, with permission.)

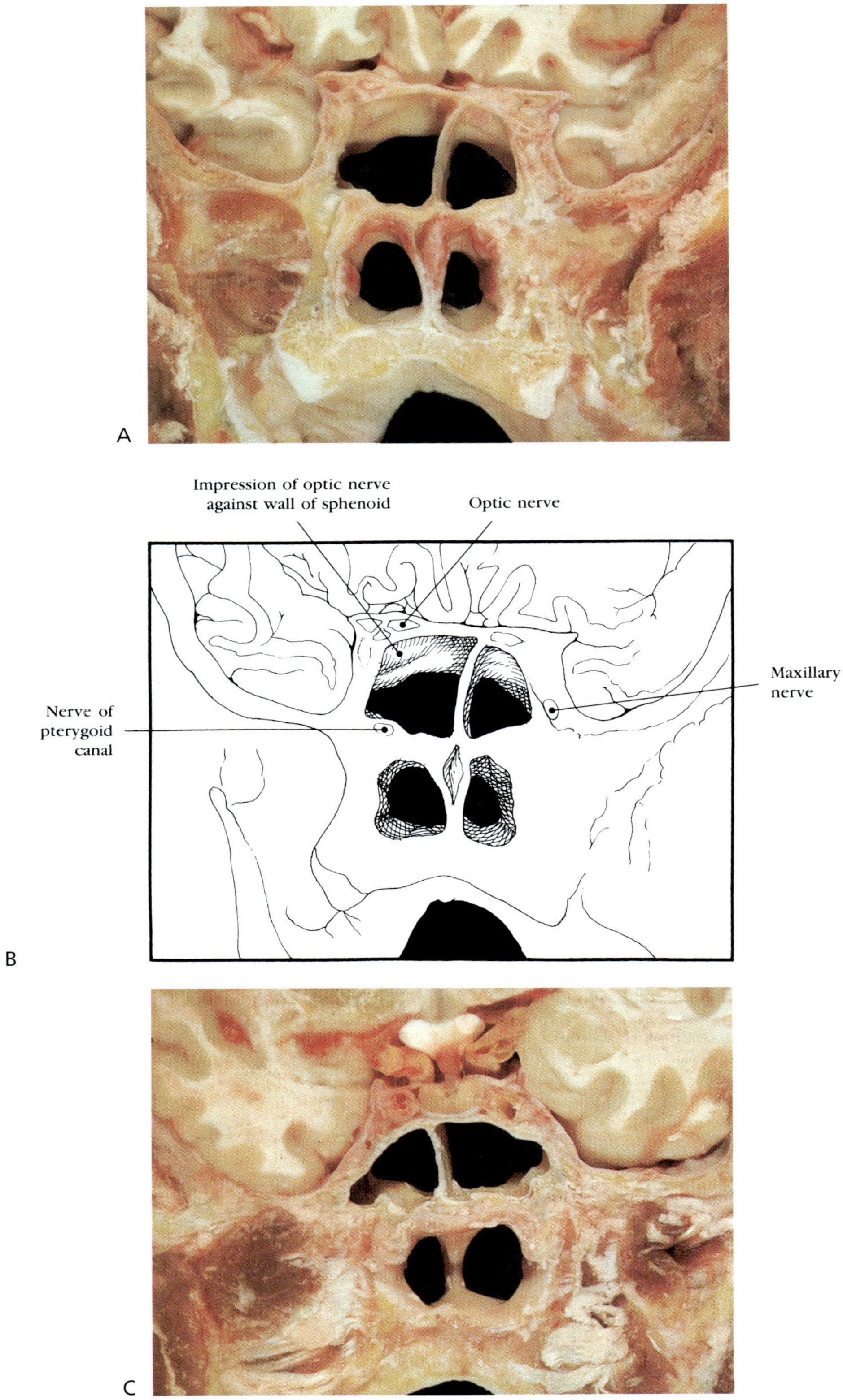


**FIGURE 16.35. A:** The anterior surface of the coronal section is contiguous with the specimen in Figure 16.34C or at a plane adjacent to the dorsal aspect of the anterior wall of the sphenoid sinus. **B:** The diagram of **A** shows the proximity of the optic nerve to the sphenoid sinus. Inferior to the sphenoid is the posterior choana. **C:** The posterior surface of the specimen in Figure 16.3A, which encompasses the principal cavity of the sphenoid sinus and the pituitary gland. (From Rice DH, Schaefer SD, eds. *Endoscopic paranasal sinus surgery*, 2nd ed. New York: Raven Press, 1993, with permission.)

### Clinical Implications

The sphenoid sinus drains by a single ostium into the sphenoethmoid recess. This ostium in the clinical setting is 2 to 3 mm in diameter and may be round or elliptical (44,111). The sinus depends on mucociliary flow for drainage because the ostium is typically 10 to 15 mm superior to the floor of the sinus, or 8 mm from the cribriform plate (range, 1 to 15 mm) and 5 mm lateral to the nasal septum (111). Our experience suggests that, in most cases, the ostium tends to be observed more inferior than superior to the average location and generally lies at a 30° angle from the floor of the nose. The pneumatization of the posterior aspect of the middle turbinate may make visualization of this ostium difficult. Because of the importance of such identification in surgery, various measurements have been reported (Figs. 16.21 and 16.24 and Table 16.5).

Of the many sinus surgical procedures done today, sphenoethmoidectomy is considered one of the more complex. Schaefer (18) reminds us of the comments offered by the surgeon Harris Mosher that, although referring to an ethmoidectomy procedure, could be applied here: "one of the easiest operations with which to kill a patient." To be performed safely and effectively, the sphenoethmoidectomy operation is based on the detailed anatomy of the paranasal sinuses. When surgical procedures were performed during the early twentieth century, they usually involved an external approach. Even though the intranasal sphenoethmoidectomy operation was first reported by Yankauer (118) at the Mount Sinai Hospital, the inherent danger of this procedure resulted in very little endonasal sinus surgery being performed until the 1986 introduction of the endoscope to the United States from Europe, where it had already been in use for more than a decade. With the advent of more sophisticated cross-sectional imaging techniques and refinements in instrumentation, the sphenoethmoidectomy operation is considered a valuable procedure for surgeons well grounded in the intricate anatomy of the nose and paranasal sinuses.

**TABLE 16.5. DISTANCES IN THE SPHENOID SINUS**

| Anatomic Site | Distance from Anterior Nasal Spine[a] | Distance from Anterior Nasal Rim[b] |
|---|---|---|
| Sphenoid ostium | 7 cm | — |
| Pituitory fossa | 8.5 cm | — |
| Inferior face of sphenoid | — | 5.7 cm |
| Posterior wall of sphenoid sinus | — | 7.6 cm |

[a]Dixon (1937) in living subjects.
[b]Mosher (1929) in cadavers.

## CONCLUSIONS

The appreciation of paranasal sinus anatomy by surgeons has had a long and rich history. From its earliest beginnings, clinicians have reported the most common treatment for sinus disease to be drainage. Initially, external procedures were employed because of difficulties in visualizing and conceptualizing the sinuses intranasally. With technologic advances in radiologic imaging and the development of innovative instrumentation, endonasal sinus surgery has been resurrected. For example, CT scanning and magnetic resonance imaging (MRI) have allowed the otolaryngologist to map and track precisely the extent of sinus disease. Moreover, cross-sectional imaging with CT or MRI allows unprecedented, rapid, and accurate assessment of inflammatory disease, and it may help distinguish it from a neoplastic process. Understanding of sinus morphology through anatomic dissections and radiologic imaging has brought endonasal sinus surgery from speculum rhinoscopy to endoscopic hypophysectomy. Although the benefits of these new technologies are many, the complexity of sinus anatomy and disease requires an array of approaches to be used. Even newer technologies will appear in our rapidly advancing technology-based world. The only aspect of sinus surgery that remains unchanged is our constant striving to better understand the intricate nature of these special spaces. Mastery of sinus anatomy continues to be *indispensable* for proper and safe sinus surgery.

## REFERENCES

1. Blanton PL, Biggs NL. Eighteen hundred years of controversy: the paranasal sinuses. *Am J Anat* 1969;124:135–148.
2. da Vinci L. Quaderni d'anatomia, I–VI. In: Fogli della Royal Library di Windsor, pubblicati da CL Vangensten, A Fonahn, H Hopstock. Christiania: F Dybwad, 1489:1911–1916.
3. Berengario da Carpi G. *Commentaria cum amplissimis additionibus super anatomia mundini una cum textu ejusdem in pristinum et verum nitorem redacto.* Bononiae, imp per H de Benedictis, 1521.
4. Bauhin C. *Theatrum anatomicum Caspari Bauhini,* 2. Basel: Auflage von J Th De Bry, 1621.
5. von Haller A. Elementa physiologiae corporis humani. Tumus Quintus: Sensus externi interni. Lausannae, 1769.
6. Stammberger H. History of rhinology: anatomy of the paranasal sinuses. *Rhinology* 1989;27:197–210.
7. Zuckerkandl E. *Normale und pathologische Anatomie der Nasenhöhle und ihrere pneumatischen Anhänge.* Vienna: Braumüller, 1882.
8. Zuckerkandl E. *Normale und pathologische Anatomie der Nasenhöhle und ihrere pneumatischen Anhänge. Anatomie der Nasenscheidewand,* Bd. II. Vienna: Braumüller, 1892.
9. Zuckerkandl E. *Normale und pathologische Anatomie der Nasenhöhle und ihrere pneumatischen Anhänge,* 2nd ed, Bd II. Vienna: Braumüller, 1893.
10. Lawson W. The intranasal ethmoidectomy: evolution and an assessment of the procedure. *Laryngoscope* 1994;104:1–49.
11. Schaeffer JP. The genesis, development, and adult anatomy of the nasofrontal region in man. *Am J Anat* 1916;20:125–143.

12. Myerson MC. The natural orifice of the maxillary sinus. I. Anatomic studies. *Arch Otolaryngol* 1931;15:80–91.
13. Simon E. Anatomy of the opening of the maxillary sinus. *Arch Otolaryngol* 1933;29:640–649.
14. Kasper KA. Nasofrontal connections: a study based on one hundred consecutive dissections. *Arch Otolaryngol* 1936;23: 322–343.
15. Van Alyea OE. The ostium maxillare: anatomic study of it surgical accessibility. *Arch Otolaryngol* 1936;24:553–569.
16. Rosenberger HC. The clinical availability of the ostium maxillae: a clinical and cadaver study. *Ann Otol Rhinol Laryngol* 1938; 47:177–182.
17. Schaeffer JP. *The nose, paranasal sinuses, nasolacrimal passageways, and olfactory organ in man.* Philadelphia: Blakiston, 1920.
18. Schaefer SD. An anatomic approach to endoscopic intranasal ethmoidectomy. *Laryngoscope* 1998;108:1628–1634.
19. Wigand ME, Steiner W, Jaumann MP. Endonasal sinus surgery with endoscopical control: from radical operation to rehabilitation of the mucosa. *Endoscopy* 1978;10:255–260.
20. Messerklinger W. Endosckopiche Diagnose und Chirugie der rezidivierenden Sinusitis. In: Krajina Z, ed. *Advances in nose and sinus surgery*. Zagreb, Yugoslavia: Zagreb University, 1985.
21. Negus V. *The comparative anatomy and physiology of the nose and paranasal sinuses.* London: E & S Livingstone, 1958.
22. Weir N. *Otolaryngology—an illustrated history*. Cambridge: Butterworth, 1990.
23. Van Alyea OE. Ethmoid labyrinth: anatomic study, with consideration of the clinical significance of its structural characteristics. *Arch Otolaryngol* 1939;29;881–902.
24. Donald PJ. Anatomy and histology. In: Donald PJ, Gluckman JL, Rice DH, eds. *The sinuses*. New York: Raven Press, 1995: 25–48.
25. Davis WE, Templer J. Parsons DS. Anatomy of the paranasal sinuses. *Otolaryngol Clin North Am* 1996;29:57–74.
26. Ritter FN. The middle turbinate and its relationship to the ethmoidal labyrinth and the orbit. *Laryngoscope* 1982;92:479–482.
27. Terrier G. *Rhinosinusal endoscopy: diagnosis and surgery*. Milan, Italy: Zambon, 1981.
28. Skillern RH. *The catarrhal and suppurative diseases of the accessory sinuses of the nose*. Philadelphia: JB Lippincott, 1923.
29. Schaeffer JP. The lateral wall of the cavum nasi in man, with especial reference to the various developmental changes. *J Morphol* 1910;21:613–707.
30. Schaeffer JP. The genesis and development of the nasolacrimal passages in man. *Am J Anat* 1912;13:1–24
31. Schaeffer JP. Types of ostia nasolacrimalis in man and their genetic significance. *Am J Anat* 1912;13:183–192
32. Stammberger H. *Functional endoscopic sinus surgery.* Philadelphia: BC Decker, 1991.
33. Santorini GD. *Observationes anatomicae*. Venetis: apud FB Recurti, 1724.
34. Zuckerkandl E. Die Siebbeinmuscheln des Menschen. *Anat Anz* 1892;7:13–25.
35. Lang J, Sakals E. Üer die höhle der Cavitas nasi, die Länge ihres Bodens und Maße sowie Anordnung der Conchae nasales und der Apertura sinus sphenoidalis. *Anat Anz* 1981;149:297–318.
36. Bingham B, Wang R-G, Hawke M, Kwok P. The embryonic development of the lateral nasal wall from 8 to 24 weeks. *Laryngoscope* 1991;101:992–997.
37. Paulli S. Über die pneumaticität des Schädels bei den Säugethieren. III. Über die morphologie des siebbeins und pneumaticität bei den Insectivoren, Hyracoideen, Chiropteren, Carnivoren, Pinipedien, Edentaten, Rodentiern, Prosimien und Primaten. *Morphol J* 1900;27:483–564.
38. Cave AJE, Haines RW. The paranasal sinuses of the anthropoid apes. *J Anat* 1940;74:493–523.
39. Moore WJ. *The mammalian skull*. Cambridge, UK: Cambridge University Press, 1981.
40. Wasson WW. Changes in nasal accessory sinuses after birth. *Arch Otolaryngol* 1933;17:197–211.
41. Wolf G, Anderhuber W, Kuhn F. Development of the paranasal sinuses in children: implications for paranasal sinus surgery. *Ann Otol Rhinol Laryngol* 1993;102:705–711.
42. Pransky SM, Low WS. Pediatric ethmoidectomy. *Otolaryngol Clin North Am* 1996;29:131–142.
43. Shapiro R, Jantzen AH. *The normal skull: a roentgen study*. New York: Paul Be Hoeber, 1960.
44. Van Alyea OE. *Nasal sinuses: an anatomic and clinical consideration*, 2nd ed. Baltimore: Williams & Wilkins, 1951.
45. Shambaugh GE. The construction of the ethmoid labyrinth. *Ann Otol Rhinol Laryngol* 1907;16:771–792.
46. Seydel O. Über die Nasenhöhle der höheren Säugetiere und des Menschen. *Gegenbaurs Morphol J* 1891;17:44–99.
47. Rice DH. Management of the middle turbinate in endoscopic surgery. *Operative techniques in otolaryngology–head and neck surgery.* 1995;6:144–148.
48. Mosher HP. The surgical anatomy of the ethmoidal labyrinth. *Ann Otol Rhinol Laryngol* 1929;38:869–901.
49. Mosher HP. The applied anatomy of the frontal sinuses. *Laryngoscope* 1904;14:830–855.
50. Stammberger HR, Bolger WE, Clement PAR, et al. Paranasal sinuses: anatomic terminology and nomenclature. *Ann Otol Rhinol Laryngol* 1995;104[Suppl 167]:7–16.
51. Schaeffer JP. The clinical anatomy of the ethmoidal labyrinth. *Laryngoscope* 1930;60:627–632.
52. Hollingshead WH. *Anatomy for surgeons: the head and neck.* New York: Harper & Row, 1968.
53. Ritter FN. *The paranasal sinuses: anatomy and surgical technique*, 2nd ed. St. Louis: CV Mosby, 1978.
54. Grünwald L. Deskriptive und topograhische Anatomie der Nase und ihrer Nebenhöhlen. In: Denker A, Kahler O, eds. *Die Krankheiten der Luftwege und der Mundhöhle*. Berlin: Springer-Bergman, 1925:1–95.
55. Lang J. *Clinical anatomy of the nose, nasal cavity and paranasal sinuses*. New York: Thieme Medical Publishers, 1989.
56. Naumann H. Pathologische Anatomie der chronischen Rhinitis und Sinusitis. In: *Proceedings of the VIII International Congress of Oto-rhino-laryngology*. Amsterdam: Excerpta Medica, 1965.
57. Isobe M, Murakami G, Kataura A. Variations of the uncinate process of the lateral nasal wall with clinical implications. *Clin Anat* 1998;11:295–303.
58. Schaeffer JP. On the genesis of air cells in the conchae nasales. *Anat Rec* 1910;4:167–180.
59. Lang J, Hass A. Über die Sagittalausdehnung des Sinus frontalis dessen Wanndicke, Abstande zur Lamina cribrosa, die Teife der sogenannten Olfactorious-Rinne und die Cannales ethmoidales. *Gegenbaurs Morphol J* 1988;134:459–469.
60. Loeb HW. A study of the anatomic relations of the optic nerve to the accessory cavities of the nose. *Ann Otol Rhinol Laryngol* 1909;9:243–276.
61. Kainz J, Stammberger H. The roof of the anterior ethmoid: a place of least resistance in the skull base. *Am J Rhinol* 1989;3:191–199.
62. Kennedy D. Functional endoscopic sinus surgery. *Arch Otolaryngol* 1985;111:643–649.
63. Highmore N. *Corporis humani disquisitio anatomica in qua sanguinis circulationem in quavis corporis particular plurimis typis novis, ac anygmatum medicorum succincta dilucidatione ornatum prosequutus est.* Hagae-Comitis: S Brown, 1651.
64. Anon JB, Rontal M, Zinreich SJ. *Anatomy of the paranasal sinuses.* New York: Thieme Medical Publishers, 1996.
65. Harle F. The history of maxillary sinus surgery—from Leonardo da Vinci until today. *Bull Hist Dent* 1992;40:79–84.

66. Sperber GH. Applied anatomy of the maxillary sinus. *J Can Dent Assoc* 1980;6:381–386.
67. Wendler D. Nathanael Highmore (1613–1685) und die Oberkieferhöhle. *Anat Anz* 1986;162:375–380.
68. Stoney P, MacKay A, Hawke M. The antrum of Highmore or of Da Vinci? *J Otolaryngol* 1991;20:456–458.
69. Douglass B. *Nasal sinus surgery with operations on nose and throat.* Philadelphia: FA Davis, 1906.
70. Hajnis K, Kustra T, Farkas LG, Feiglova B. Sinus maxillaris. *Z Morphol Anthropol* 1967;59:185–197.
71. Schaeffer JP. The sinus maxillaris and its relations in the embryo, child, and adult man. *Am J Anat* 1920;10:313–367.
72. Cullen RL, Vidic B. The dimensions and shape of the human maxillary sinus in the perinatal period. *Acta Anat* 1972;83:411–415.
73. Anagnostopoulou S, Venieratos D, Spyropoulous N. Classification of human maxillary sinuses according to their geometric features. *Anat Anz* 1991;173:121–130.
74. Alberti PW. Applied surgical anatomy of the maxillary sinus. *Otolaryngol Clin North Am* 1976;9:3–20.
75. Almagro AM, Marco JM, Galvis CG, Guiñon IB. Relaciones entre seno maxilar y apófisis alveolar maxilar superior: estudio anatomotopográfico. *Acta Otorrinolarygol Esp* 1995;46:409–415.
76. Boocock P, Roberts CA, Manchester K. Maxillary sinusitis in medieval Chichester, England. *Am J Phys Anthropol* 1995;98: 483–495.
77. Amedee RG. Sinus anatomy and function. In: Bailey BJ, ed. *Head and neck surgery–otolaryngology.* Philadelphia: JB Lippincott, 1993:342–349.
78. Kallius E. *Sinnesorgane-erst Abteilung-Geruchsorgan und Geschmacksorgan. Handbuch der Anatomie des Menschen.* Jena von Bardelebens, 1905.
79. Brandt W, Roper-Hall HT. Clinical aspects of the embryonic relations of paranasal sinuses to adjacent structures. *Med Presse* 1943:209:190–191.
80. Aubert F. Contribution à l'étude embryologique du sinus maxillaire chez l'homme. *CR Assoc Anat* 1929;20:571–573.
81. Wang R-G, Jiang S, Gu R. The cartilaginous nasal capsule and embryonic development of human paranasal sinuses. *J Otolaryngol* 1994;23:239–243.
82. Weiglein A, Anderhuber W, Wolf G. Radiologic anatomy of the paranasal sinuses in the child. *Surg Radiol Anat* 1992;14:335–339.
83. Scuderi AJ, Harnsberger HR, Boyer RS. Pneumatization of the paranasal sinuses: normal features of importance to the accurate interpretation of CT scans and MR Images. *AJR Am J Roentgenol* 1993;160:1101–1104.
84. Underwood AS An inquiry into the anatomy and pathology of the maxillary sinus. *J Anat Physiol* 1910;44:354–369.
85. Libersa C, Laude M, Libersa J-C. The pneumatization of the accessory cavities of the nasal fossae during growth. *Anat Clin* 1981;2:265–273.
86. Márquez S, Gannon PJ, Reidenberg JS, et al. The role of the primate maxillary sinus: respiratory reservoirs or evolutionary dead spaces? *Assoc Res Otolaryngol* 1998;21:178.
87. Krennmair G, Ulm C, Lugmayr H. Maxillary sinus septa: incidence, morphology and clinical implications. *J Craniomaxillofac Surg* 1997;25:261–265.
88. Som PM, Sacher M, Lanzier CF, et al. The hidden antral compartments. *Radiology* 1984;152:463–464.
89. Lang J, Papke J. Über die klinische Anatomie des Paries inferior orbitae und dessen Nachbarstrukturen. *Gengenbaurs Morphol J* 1984;130:1–47.
90. Tange RA. Some historical aspects of the surgical treatment of the infected maxillary sinus. *Rhinology* 1991;29:155–162.
91. Imperatori CJ. Leonardo da Vinci's contribution to laryngology, rhinology and phonetics. *Ann Otol Rhinol Otolaryngol* 1941;50: 979–994.
92. Van Alyea OE. Frontal cells. An anatomic study of these cells with consideration of their clinical significance. *Arch Otolaryngol* 1941;34:11–23.
93. Van Alyea OE. Frontal sinus drainage. *Ann Otol Rhinol Laryngol* 1946;55:267–277.
94. Talbot AR. Frontal sinus surgery in children. *Otolaryngol Clin North Am* 1996;29:143–158.
95. Brunner E, Jacobs JB, Lebowitz RA, et al. Role of the agger nasi cell in chronic sinusitis. *Ann Otol Rhinol Laryngol* 1996;105:694–700.
96. Shea JJ. Morphologic characteristics of the sinuses. *Arch Otolaryngol* 1936;23:484–487.
97. Brown MJ. Frontal sinusitis. *Ann Otol Rhinol Otolaryngol* 1941; 50:435–449.
98. Schaeffer JP. An unusual sinus frontalis. *Ann Surg* 1912;60: 396–400.
99. Davis WB. Anatomy of the nasal accessory sinuses in infancy and childhood. *Ann Otol Rhinol Otolaryngol* 1918;28:940–967.
100. Tilley H. An investigation of the frontal sinuses in 120 skulls from a surgical aspect, with cases illustrating methods of treatment of disease in this situation. *Lancet* 1896;2:866–870.
101. Schaeffer JP. Further observations on the anatomy of the sinus frontalis in man. *Ann Surg* 1916;64:665–671.
102. Ubelaker DH. Positive identification from the radiographic comparisons of frontal sinus patterns. In: Rathbun TA, Buikstra JE, eds. *Human identification: case studies in forensic anthropology.* Springfield, IL: Charles C Thomas, 1985:399–411.
103. Shapiro R, Schorr S. A consideration of the systemic factors that influence frontal sinus pneumatization. *Invest Radiol* 1980;15: 191–202.
104. Urken ML, Som PM, Lawson W, et al. The abnormally large frontal sinus. I. A practical method for its determination based upon an analysis of 100 normal patients. *Laryngoscope* 1987;97: 602–605.
105. Urken ML, Som PM, Lawson W, et al. Abnormally large frontal sinus. II. Nomenclature, pathology, and symptoms. *Laryngoscope* 1987;97:606–611.
106. Maresh MM. Paranasal sinuses from birth to late adolescence. *Am J Dis Child* 1940;60:55–78.
107. Wigh R. Mucoceles of the fronto-ethmoid sinuses. *Radiology* 1950;54:579–590.
108. Hartmann A. *Atlas der Anatomie der Stirnhöhle der vorderen Siebbeinzellen und des Ductus nasofrontalis mit erläuterndem Texte und Bemerkungen über die Behandlung der Stirnhöhleneiterung.* Weisbaden: Verlag von JF Bergmann, 1900.
109. Killian G. Anatomie der Nase menschilcher Embryonen. *Arch Laryngol Rhinol (Berl)* 1895;3:17–47.
110. Tillaux P. *Rôle des sinus de la face.* Paris: Thèse Méd., 1862.
111. Dixon FW. A comparative study of the sphenoid. *Ann Otol Rhinol Laryngol* 1937;46:687–698.
112. Congdon ED. The distribution and mode of origin of septa and walls of the sphenoid sinus. *Anat Rec* 1920;18:97–123.
113. Hammer G, Radberg C. Sphenoidal sinus: an anatomical and roentgenological study with reference to transsphenoid hypophysectomy. *Acta Radiol (Stockh)* 1961;56:401–422.
114. Sluder G. The anatomical and clinical relations of the sphenopalatine (Meckel's) ganglion to the nose and its accessory sinuses. *N Y Med J* 1909;90:293–298.
115. Cope VZ. The internal structure of the sphenoid sinus. *J Anat (Lond)* 1917;51:127–136.
116. Peele JC. Unusual anatomical variations in the sphenoid sinuses. *Laryngoscope* 1957;67:208–237.
117. Márquez S, Delson E, Silvers A, et al. The meaning of emptiness: pneumatization patterns of great ape paranasal sinuses via CT imaging. *Am Assoc Phys Anthropol* 1999;28:191.
118. Yankauer S. The complete spheno-ethmoid operation. *Laryngoscope* 1921;31:831–842.

# 17

# PATHOPHYSIOLOGY OF RHINOSINUSITIS

DANIEL I. BRANOVAN
STEVEN D. SCHAEFER

To attempt to summarize the pathophysiology of rhinosinusitis, one of the most common diseases of Western industrial society, is to embark on a work in progress. Although significant strides have been taken in elucidating some of the risk factors, environmental and pathogenic mediators, and molecular mechanisms leading to this chronic inflammatory condition, the full picture has yet to emerge. In the year 2000, when the scientific community celebrates one of sentinel achievements in science—deciphering the human gene—we are humbled by the gaps in knowledge of basic human pathophysiology. We hope the information presented in this chapter will ignite interest in future research and scientific investigation among the next generation of young scientists.

## EPIDEMIOLOGY

Although it may seem overly dramatic to place rhinosinusitis in the company of such common diseases of Western civilization as heart disease, cancer, and AIDS, the comparison is not overly exaggerated when the statistics are examined. Since the early 1990s, rhinosinusitis has held the distinction of the most frequent cause of physician visits in the United States. Up to 14% of the U.S. population report symptoms of rhinosinusitis lasting at least 3 months, and the incidence appears to be rising (1). More than $2.5 billion in direct medical costs is spent each year on treatment of the disease. If we were to factor in the proliferation of often necessary, but quite expensive surgical interventions, counterbalanced by just as pervasive a movement toward over-the-counter and alternative medical techniques in the treatment of rhinosinusitis, this disease would easily earn the dubious distinction of one of the most expensive illnesses suffered by the U.S. population (2).

## DEFINITIONS

Rhinosinusitis may be clinically defined as a condition manifested by an inflammatory response involving the mucous membranes of the nasal cavity and paranasal sinuses, fluids within these cavities, underlying bone, and olfactory neuroepithelium (3,4). This term is currently favored in the literature over the traditional "sinusitis" and appropriately so, given that it is far more descriptive of the disease process. The inflammatory process usually originates in the nasal cavity (i.e., rhinitis) and only thereafter proceeds to involve the paranasal sinuses (i.e., sinusitis). Because the respiratory mucosa of the nasal cavity and the paranasal sinuses is contiguous, it is readily apparent why "rhinitis" and "sinusitis" proceed in tandem most of the time (5,6). Symptoms associated with rhinosinusitis include nasal obstruction, nasal congestion, nasal discharge, nasal purulence, postnasal drip, facial pressure and pain, alteration in the sense of smell, cough, fever, halitosis, fatigue, dental pain, pharyngitis, otologic symptoms (i.e., ear fullness and popping), and headache (3).

Definitions of various stages of rhinosinusitis were standardized by a joined congress of the American Academy of Allergy, Asthma, and Immunology and the American Academy of Otolaryngology–Head and Neck Surgery in 1996. Rhinosinusitis may be stratified into four distinct stages: acute rhinosinusitis, subacute rhinosinusitis, chronic rhinosinusitis, and acute exacerbation of chronic rhinosinusitis (3). Pictorial description of the processes is helpful (Fig. 17.1), but brief definitions also are in order:

*Acute rhinosinusitis* denotes a bacterial infection and inflammatory process involving nasal mucosa and paranasal sinuses, lasting less than 12 weeks.

*Subacute rhinosinusitis* represents prolonged persistence of the inflammatory process, but without the severity of signs and symptoms of acute rhinosinusitis.

*Chronic rhinosinusitis* denotes persistence of acute symptoms beyond the 12-week course. An alternative approach relies on the radiologic findings of a computed tomography (CT) scan of the paranasal sinuses to define chronic rhinosinusitis as persistence of chronic inflamma-

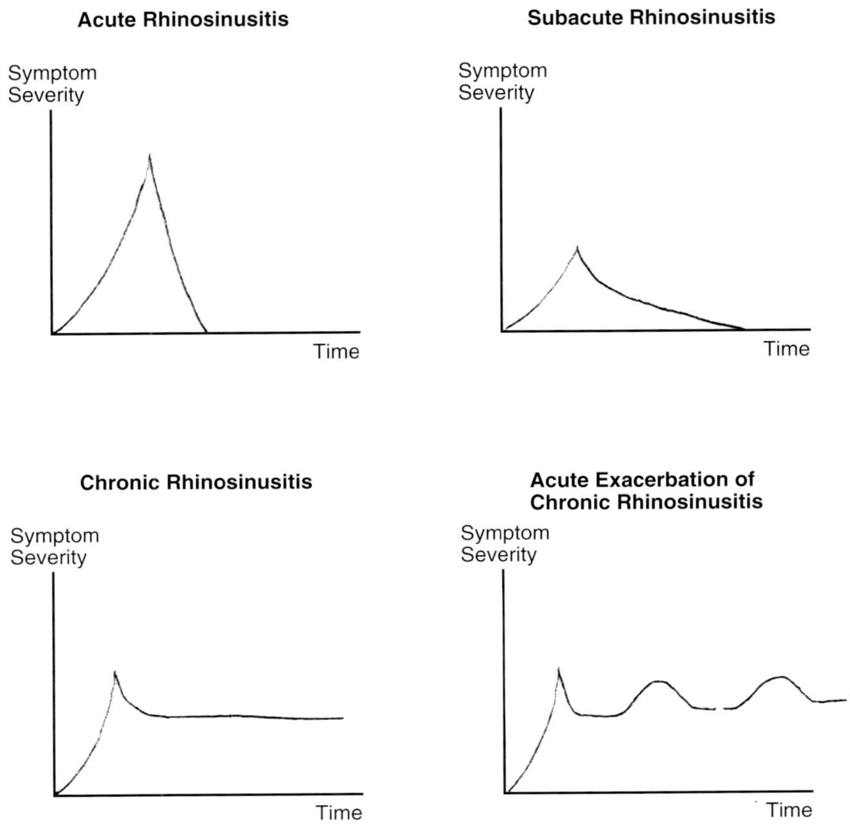


**FIGURE 17.1.** Stages of rhinosinusitis.

tory process in the paranasal sinuses after completion of 4- to 6-week course of appropriate antibiotic and steroid therapy.

*Acute exacerbation of chronic rhinosinusitis* represents a sudden worsening of symptoms and signs of chronic rhinosinusitis, representing increase in the inflammatory process, which never returns to the baseline healthy state with treatment.

Although the rigidity of these definitions is open to criticism, stratification of the disease process into at least the acute and chronic stages has proved beneficial from the standpoint of understanding the pathophysiology of the disease process and from the perspective of evaluating treatment protocols.

## THE VICIOUS CIRCLE OF RHINOSINUSITIS

How does a person develop acute rhinosinusitis, and how and why does it progress to chronic rhinosinusitis? To answer these and related questions, we must start at the very beginning of the inflammatory process. Most experts would agree that acute rhinosinusitis is a bacterial superinfection, which complicates routine viral upper respiratory infection (Fig. 17.2).

### Stage I: Viral Upper Respiratory Infection

A patient is exposed to an aerosolized secretory droplet, infected by a subtype of numerous species of upper respiratory viruses (most commonly rhinovirus, influenza virus, or parainfluenza virus). Anyone who has ever seen slow-motion photography of a human sneeze (7) may recall the dramatic sight of tens of thousands of tiny droplets infected with millions of viral particles spreading in the air in search of the next victim. Once such victim is found, exposure to the viral load results in contamination of the upper respiratory tract. Given the size of the aerosolized contaminate [100 to 2,000 Angstroms (8)] and normal breathing patterns of the patient, it is most likely that the viral load will be delivered primarily to the nasal mucosa. Virus particles waste no time in fulfilling their only mission in life: to be fruitful and multiply. They multiply within the confines of the nasal mucosa and the adjoining mucosa of the rest of the upper respiratory tract. The patient's immune response to viral infection responds by the release of inflammatory mediators, such as interleukin-8, which is chemotactic for neutrophils and T lymphocytes; RANTES, which targets eosinophils; and numerous other cytokines (9–12). An example of self-perpetuating inflammatory response is found in the recruitment to nasal mucosa of eosinophils from peripheral circulation.

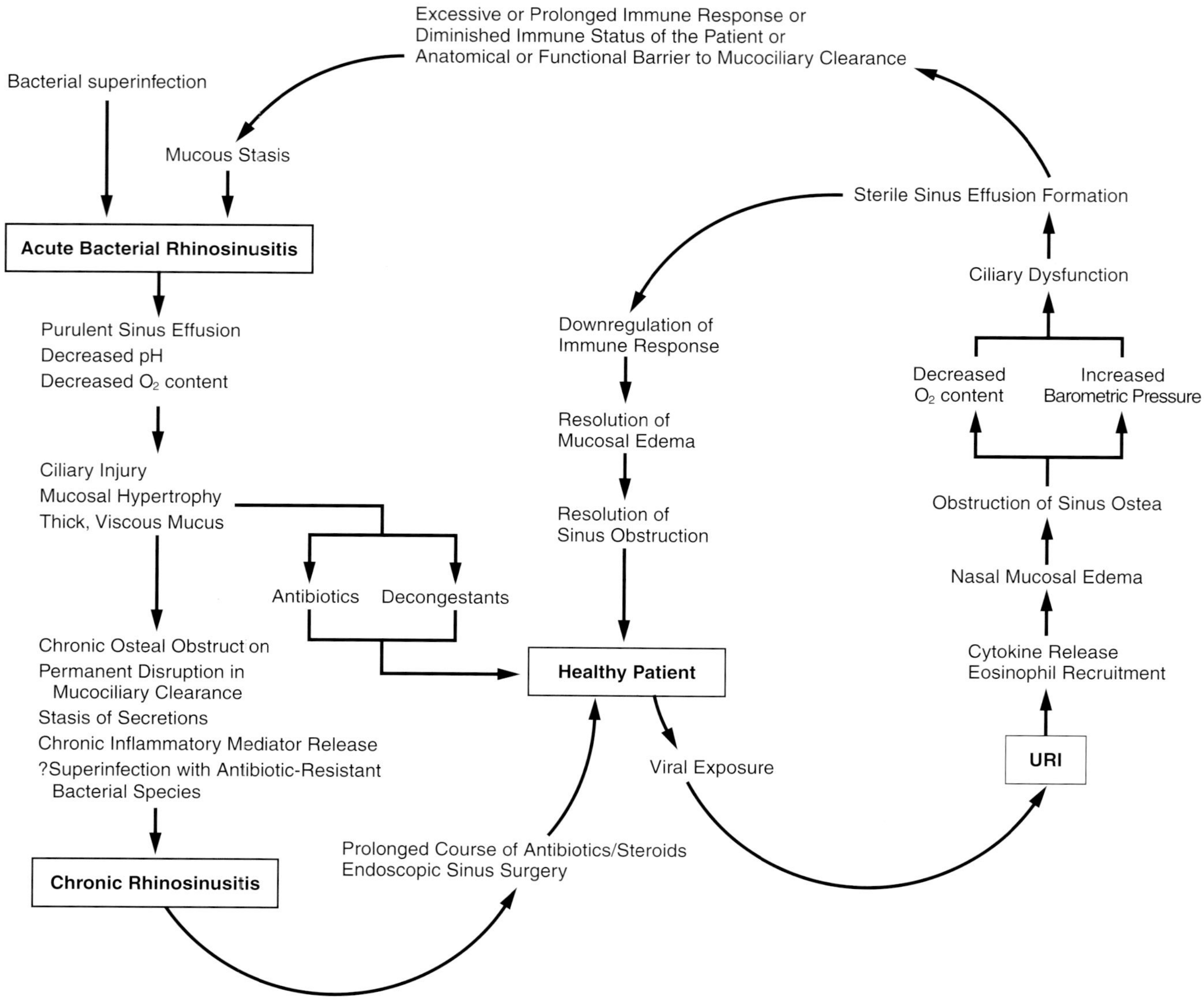


**FIGURE 17.2.** The vicious circle of rhinosinusitis.

Eosinophil survival within the mucosa is supported by increased production of granulocyte-macrophage colony-stimulating factor (GM-CSF) by the inflamed mucosal cells, which further primes mucosal cells for response to activating stimuli. Once activated, eosinophil products can alter epithelial ion transport processes and induce ciliostasis (2).

Maintained in this way, the inflammatory process persists and results in progression of edema of nasal mucosa, increase in cellular membrane permeability, increase in serous secretions within the mucosa of the nasal cavity and paranasal sinuses, and compromise of normal mucociliary clearance. Edema of the nasal mucosa may cause partial or near total obstruction of paranasal sinus ostia. The respiratory cycle then results in a relative decrease in barometric pressure within the affected sinuses (13). The latter may cause secretion of a transudate within the sinus cavity. When coupled with an increase in the secretory, exudative function of virally infected mucosal cells within the sinus, these processes often cause partial filling of the sinus cavities with serous or mucoid collection (14). Routine CT scans of paranasal sinuses of patients with a viral upper respiratory infection demonstrate fluid collection within paranasal sinuses in up to 95% of cases (15).

## Stage II: Delayed or Incomplete Resolution of Inflammatory Process

If this inflammatory process occurs in most viral upper respiratory infections, why does such a small percentage (5% to 10%) result in progression to acute bacterial rhinosinusitis? Unfortunately, a comprehensive answer to this most appropriate question must await further advances in our understanding of the intricacies of human immune system response. However, several mechanisms leading to the perpetuation of the inflammatory process may be postulated.

The first mechanism is an excessive or abnormally prolonged immune response. The virally induced inflammatory process may be more severe than normal because of high virulence of the viral agent, or it may progress for longer than the usual 7 to 10 days' duration. Although sinus secretions at this stage are relatively sterile as far as their bacterial counts are concerned, prolonged exposure to the neighboring highly contaminated environment of the upper respiratory tract and contamination of sinus contents with nasal secretions during snorting or nasal blowing maneuvers may seed the paranasal sinuses with sufficient bacterial counts to result in a bacterial superinfection of the sinus collection.

The second mechanism is a deficiency of the host immune response. A patient's relatively weakened immune system (e.g., chronic illness, diabetes, immune deficiencies) may reduce the period during which the patient may effectively fight off early bacterial superinfection of sinus contents.

The third mechanism is a deficiency in mucociliary clearance or a stasis of secretions. Normal mucociliary clearance mechanisms may be deficient from the outset or later become relatively impaired, contributing to stasis of secretions within the paranasal sinuses, eventually resulting in bacterial superinfection. The barrier to normal clearance of sinus secretions may take many forms: anatomic (e.g., obstruction of sinus ostia by marked nasal septal deviation or nasal polyps) or physiologic (i.e., impaired ciliary motility: congenital, as in Kartagener's syndrome, or acquired, such as exposure to toxins or cigarette smoke). Increased stasis of sinus secretions may result from altered viscosity of mucous envelope itself, as in cystic fibrosis, and other hyperviscidosis states.

## Stage III: Acute Rhinosinusitis

A combination of any or all of the predisposing factors result in progression from upper respiratory infection to full-blown bacterial superinfection of paranasal sinuses, or acute bacterial rhinosinusitis. The typical bacterial pathogens implicated in acute rhinosinusitis are the same as in other upper airway infections in Western society: *Streptococcus pneumoniae*, *Haemophilus influenzae*, and *Moraxella catarrhalis* (in the decreasing order of frequency) (Fig. 17.3) (16). The specific kinds of most common pathogens and rates and patterns of antibiotic sensitivity vary significantly by geographic locale (17).

In a typical patient, 7 to 10 days of generalized aches and pains coupled with abundant clear, watery rhinorrhea (i.e., symptoms typical of virally induced upper respiratory infection) may then be replaced by low-grade fever, facial pains, and purulent nasal discharge, which strongly suggest progression to acute bacterial rhinosinusitis. In the altered microenvironment of the paranasal sinus mucosa, the normally thin, almost translucent mucosal envelope is distorted to a thickened, edematous structure (Fig. 17.4). Purulent secretions become evident on the surface and may fill a large portion of the paranasal sinus volume. An electron microscopic view demonstrates that carefully ordered healthy cilia, normally beating in unison to propel the

**---- Stage I: URI ----**

**--- Stage II: Persistent Inflammatory --- Process**

**--- Stage III: Acute Bacterial -- Rhinosinusitis**

**--- Stage IV: Chronic Rhinosinusitis ---**

| Common Cold Viruses | Typical Upper Respiratory Infection Bacterial Species | Atypical Bacterial Species | Fungi |
|---|---|---|---|
| Rhinoviruses | S. pneumonia | S. aureus | |
| Influenza | H. influenza | P. aeruginosa | |
| Parainfluenza | M. catarrhalis | S. epidermididis | |
| | | Coagulase – staph | |
| | | Corynebacterium species | |
| | | Anaerobes | |

**FIGURE 17.3.** Spectrum of the infectious causes of rhinosinusitis.

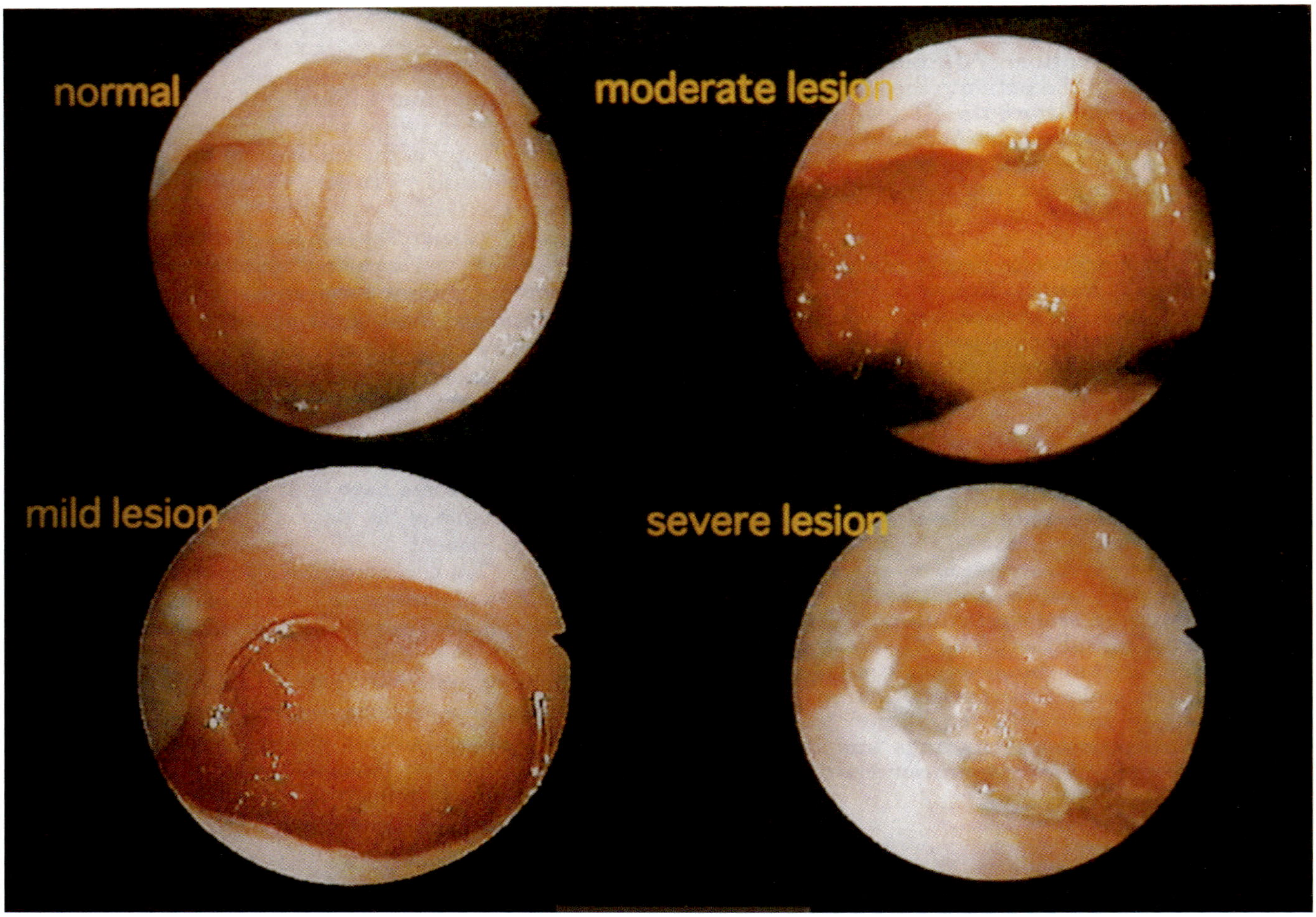


**FIGURE 17.4.** Endoscopic appearance of the maxillary sinus mucosa, showing progression from normal to acute inflammation to a chronic inflammatory state in response to infection. (From Asai K, Haruna S, Otori N, et al. Saccharin test of maxillary sinus mucociliary function after endoscopic sinus surgery. *Laryngoscope* 2000;110:117–122, with permission.)

A 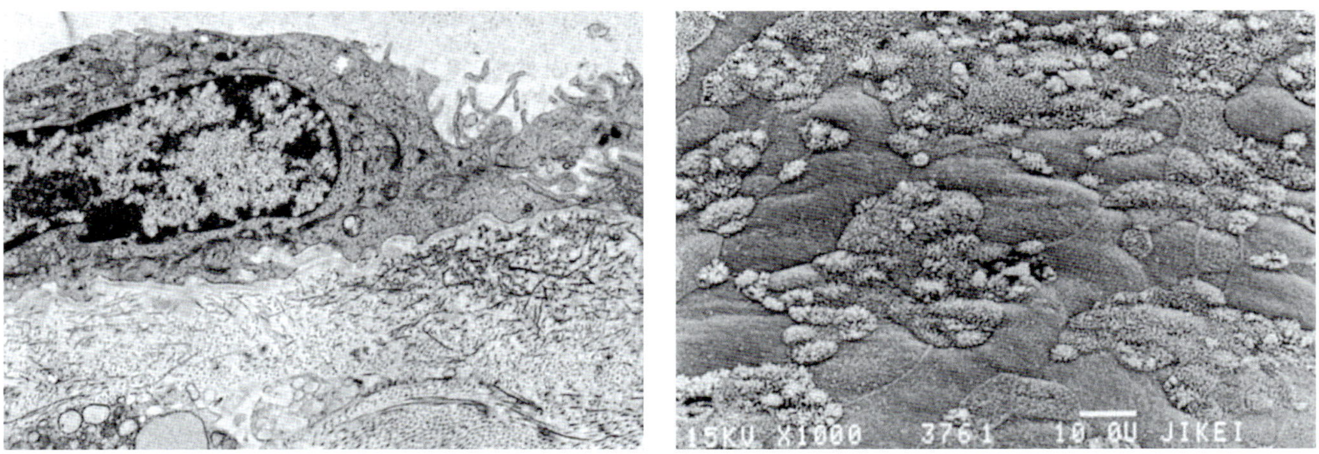 B

**FIGURE 17.5. A:** High-power microscopic view of inflamed sinus mucosa, demonstrating a decrease in the number of cilia and their disorder. (From Al-Rawi MM, Edelstein DR, Erlandson RA. Changes in nasal epithelium in patients with severe chronic sinusitis: a clinicopathologic and electron microscopic study. *Laryngoscope* 1998;108:1816–1823, with permission.) **B:** Scanning electron microscopic view of same process: the cilia are denuded on a large number of cells. (From Asai K, Haruna S, Otori N, et al. Saccharin test of maxillary sinus mucociliary function after endoscopic sinus surgery. *Laryngoscope* 2000;110:117–122, with permission.)

mucus toward sinus ostia, show evidence of structural damage, become denuded in some areas (Fig. 17.5), demonstrate decreased ciliary beat frequency, and to a great extent loose their coordinated contractile property (18–20). This damage results from a combination of several factors. Hypertrophic, edematous mucosa develops from the persistent inflammatory process, which is identified by the replacement of acute lymphocytic cellular infiltrate with monocytes and macrophages responsible for combating the bacterial threat. The diminished oxygen content and diminished pH within the sinus combine with the cytotoxic effects of bacterial exotoxins to inflict injury on the cilia (21). Stasis of mucous secretions creates a thick, viscous mucoid envelope, poorly amenable to mucociliary clearance (22).

Despite the severity of the apparent mucosal injury, experimental and epidemiologic evidence demonstrates that up to 50% of all bacterial sinus infections resolve spontaneously in healthy individuals without extraneous agents such as decongestants, topical steroids, and antibiotics (23,24). An investigation of sinus mucosa after such recovery demonstrates full resolution of the anatomic changes previously described, with restoration of mucosal integrity and ciliary function. Unfortunately, review of statistical data also demonstrates that, in up to 15% of cases (even among patients appropriately treated), the severity of mucosal injury in combination with anatomic obstruction of sinus ostia may produce long-standing changes in anatomy and physiology of paranasal sinus mucosa, leading to the development of chronic rhinosinusitis (25,26).

## Stage IV: Chronic Rhinosinusitis

To a great extent, the pathologic changes in anatomy and function of paranasal sinus mucosa in chronic rhinosinusitis reflect a continuum in the inflammatory process. However, the major distinction lies in the progressive severity and potentially irreversible nature of damage. Let us examine some of the underlying pathophysiologic changes identified within the sinus mucosa of chronic rhinosinusitis patients and appropriate experimental models.

### *Bacteriology of Chronic Rhinosinusitis*

Much controversy exists about the role of bacteria in chronic rhinosinusitis. Several studies have demonstrated three categories of bacterial infection in chronic rhinosinusitis (Fig. 17.3) (2,27–31). The first category includes microorganisms similar to those found in acute rhinosinusitis (*S. pneumoniae, H. influenzae*). Although recovered in high titers from sinus aspirates of chronic rhinosinusitis patients, their role in the inflammatory process as active agents remains to be defined. The second category includes microorganisms exclusive to chronic infections, and includes *Staphylococcus aureus* and *Pseudomonas aeruginosa*. These organisms have frequently been identified in patients who have resisted improvement after antibiotic treatment regimens and endoscopic sinus surgery. They likely play some role in the bacteriology of chronic rhinosinusitis in some patients, especially given selection of these frequently antibiotic-resistant organisms by multiple courses of broad-spectrum antibiotics during treatment of rhinosinusitis patients. The third category of microorganisms include *Staphylococcus epidermidis*, other coagulase-negative staphylococci, corynebacterium species, and anaerobes. Their titers have been traditionally low, and contamination of experimental cultures must be excluded. Despite the presence of high titers of multiple bacterial species in chronic rhinosinusitis patients, some studies have concluded that bacterial role in chronic rhinosinusitis is limited to opportunistic colonizers, not pathogenic agents (32).

### *Role of Inflammatory Mediators in Chronic Rhinosinusitis*

Given uncertainty regarding the role of bacterial agents in the pathophysiology of chronic rhinosinusitis, other agents responsible for mediating inflammatory response have been investigated. Chronic rhinosinusitis is characterized by inflammatory mucosal thickening and polyp formation with a predominantly eosinophilic infiltrate (33), which is believed to be mediated in part by the upregulation of Th2 cytokines, including interleukin-4, interleukin-5, and GM-CSF. Interleukin-4 is involved in IgE production and in eosinophil recruitment through upregulation of vascular cell adhesion molecule-1. Interleukin-5 and GM-CSF are involved in eosinophil growth and survival (34). Other studies support a role for Th2 cytokine receptors and other cytokine pathways in the mediation of inflammation in chronic rhinosinusitis (35,36).

The adherence of circulating leukocytes to the vascular endothelium is a critical step in the emigration of leukocytes through blood vessel walls to inflammatory lesions. Experimental evidence suggests that IL-1β in the paranasal secretion of chronic sinusitis induces the adherence of neutrophils to vascular endothelium and subsequent infiltration of neutrophils in the paranasal sinuses, contributing to the persistence of chronic rhinosinusitis (37). Neither cyclooxygenase enzymes (i.e., COX1 and COX2) appear to be upregulated in chronic sinusitis, suggesting that COX products do not have an important role as mediators of chronic upper airway inflammation (38). Nitric oxide (NO) serves an important function in a variety of physiologic and pathophysiologic processes in the body, including vasoregulation, hemostasis, neurotransmission, immunity, and respiration (39). Discovery of surprisingly high concentrations of NO in the nasal airway and paranasal sinuses has important implications for the understanding of airway physiology. Given its well-known bacteriostatic and antiviral properties, high NO levels in healthy nasal and paranasal airways may contribute to the first-line defense against microorganisms and to upregulation of ciliary activity (40). Studies of patients with chronic rhinosinusitis (as well as patients with primary ciliary dyskinesia and cystic fibrosis) have indicated decreased levels of NO in diseased paranasal sinuses (41). However, whether this represents decrease in sinus mucosal production of NO or a decrease of nasal NO entrance into sinuses secondary to osteal obstruction is not yet understood (2).

### Role of Altered Mucociliary Transport in Chronic Rhinosinusitis

The mucociliary transport system is an important defense mechanism by which the human body usually maintains its homeostasis by protecting the body against invading particles, including bacteria. This system includes two major functional mechanisms—ciliary transport and mucous secretory systems—each of which is usually complementary and cooperative (42). Mucociliary transport represents the first barrier of the nasal cavity and paranasal sinuses against various biologic and physical insults. Several studies have identified significantly delayed mucociliary transport at times in chronic rhinosinusitis patients. Findings indicate that this delay is determined by an increase in viscoelasticity of the mucus after the acute release of mediators of inflammation, together with a reduction in the periciliary stratum, which slows down the metachronous wave of mucociliary transport (43). Further work suggests that locally produced mucous glycoproteins may largely contribute to the high viscoelasticity of nasal mucus in chronic rhinosinusitis (44,45).

An increase in the viscocity of mucous secretions and decrease in mucociliary transport in chronic rhinosinusitis may also be related to increase in goblet cell secretory activity. The number of goblet cells in the normal mucosa in the paranasal sinuses is comparable to that in the nasal mucosa. There are relatively few mucosal glands in the healthy sinuses. In an animal model, after induced chronic infections, the number of goblet cells in paranasal sinuses increases. In pneumococcal sinusitis, the number reaches a peak after 3 weeks and then declines. In sinusitis induced by *S. aureus* and the anaerobic bacteria *Bacteroides fragilis*, the number increases over time and persists for 12 weeks. In patients with chronic sinusitis, the number of goblet cells is usually not affected, but the number of glands increases, and the glands usually have a pathologic shape. A decreased ciliary beating frequency correlates well with an increase in number of goblet cells (46).

Three hereditary disorders—primary ciliary dyskinesia (i.e., immotile-cilia syndrome or Kartagener's syndrome), cystic fibrosis, and Young's syndrome—are systemically associated with mucociliary transport failure, leading to male infertility and chronic sinopulmonary infections. Cystic fibrosis (CF) is the most commonly inherited disease in Caucasians and is caused by a mutation in the gene encoding a membrane transport protein (47,48). Cloning of the CF gene has offered new insights into electrolyte transport in respiratory epithelium. The CF transmembrane conductance regulator (CFTR) functions as a cAMP-activated chloride channel and as a regulator of chloride and sodium channels. Disruption of the gene results in marked increase in viscosity of sinus mucous secretions, mucous stasis, and consequent failure of the mucociliary transport system (2).

However, in most chronic rhinosinusitis patients, ciliary dyskinesias are primarily the result rather than the cause of chronic sinusitis. Patients with chronic sinusitis of uncertain origin exhibit a prominent loss of differentiated epithelial cell and ciliary defects, most of which probably result from the chronic disease process (49). Ciliary disorientation with consequent poor mucociliary effort has also been described in patients with chronic rhinosinusitis (50). All of these changes slow mucociliary clearance and lead to a vicious cycle producing chronicity. Patient studies and animal model work examining the relationship between anatomic abnormalities of ciliary ultrastructure resulting from chronic sinusitis and ciliary beat frequency before and after middle meatal antrostomy demonstrated reversibility of pathologic changes in ciliary ultrastructure and function on resolution of the osteal obstruction (51,52).

An increasing number of patients with human immunodeficiency virus (HIV) suffer from acute infectious sinusitis, and many suffer recurrent episodes at a higher rate than their non-HIV counterparts. Studies have demonstrated inherent delay of mucociliary clearance in HIV-infected patients, which is chronic, possibly irreversible, and in association with nasal obstruction, represents a major mechanism of the high acute and recurrent sinusitis rate in this population (53).

### Role of Osteomyelitis in Chronic Rhinosinusitis

Mucosal changes have been well described in chronic sinusitis, but little is known about the underlying bone, despite clinical and experimental evidence suggesting that bone may be involved in chronic sinusitis. Patients undergoing surgery for chronic sinusitis were found to have evidence of marked acceleration in bone physiology, with histologic changes including new bone formation, fibrosis, and the presence of inflammatory cells. These findings are consistent with osteomyelitis. This suggests that underlying bone may serve as a catalyst for chronic rhinosinusitis (54).

### Environmental Factors in Chronic Rhinosinusitis

Although no definitive studies linking environmental pollutants and chronic rhinosinusitis have been identified, there are a number of pollutants that are known to produce cellular damage in nasal mucosa: ozone, carbon dioxide, and nitric oxide. Resulting inflammatory response may result in exacerbation of existing disease or precipitate rhinosinusitis episode (2). More research in the field of toxic substance exposure and occupational safety needs to be done to reach more detailed conclusions.

## Associated Conditions

### Asthma

The association between asthma and sinusitis was recognized more than a century ago. Since 1980, several studies have documented that severe asthma improved after coexisting sinusitis was effectively treated medically or surgically (55–57). Because the mechanism relating sinusitis to asthma is unknown, several theories have been proposed: aspiration of infected sinus secretions into the lungs during sleep; triggering of pharyngobronchial reflex by seeding inflammatory process into the pharynx, resulting in hyper responsive airway; production in the infected sinus of cytokines and bronchoconstrictive mediators; enhanced vagal stimulation in the infected sinus producing direct bronchospasm; bronchospasm from excessive airway drying from mouth breathing; and production of bacterial toxins that induce partial beta blockade (58,59). There are data to support each of these hypotheses, although the three former ones have gained greater support. Studies have also revealed increased numbers of eosinophils and increased levels of CM-CSF, interleukin-3, and interleukin-5 in the tissues of chronic rhinosinusitis patients compared with those of control subjects. These findings suggest that sinusitis might induce asthma by stimulating eosinophil production and activation and thereby supplying peptidoleukotrienes ($LTC_4$ and $LTD_4$) and other asthmagenic eosinophil products (58). Given the incidence of chronic rhinosinusitis and asthma in the population, more work must be done in this field.

### Nasal Polyps

Nasal polyps represent the end process of chronic edematous swelling of the mucous membrane, which is probably a localized mediator-dependent reaction of the mucous membrane in the lamina propria (60). The most common site of origin is lateral nasal wall, although primary sinus mucosal changes may be observed. Significant structural alterations are observed in polypoid mucosa: an increase in inflammatory cells (especially eosinophils), predominance of cystic inspissated mucous glands, and dedifferentiation of epithelium. Persistent inflammatory process is though to be stimulated by cytokine upregulation, resulting in recruitment of eosinophils and basophils from circulation (2). During this process, eosinophil cationic protein is released from activated eosinophils. The number and ratio of activated and nonactivated eosinophils seem to be reliable indicators for the activity of chronic polyposis and chronic rhinosinusitis (60). The underlying cause of the initial inflammatory insult leading to polyp formation is, however, not well understood.

## Anatomic Obstruction of the Sinus Ostia in Chronic Rhinosinusitis

The main association between nasal polyps and chronic rhinosinusitis stems from the obstruction of sinus ostia by polypoid changes. Animal studies clearly demonstrate that osteal occlusion leads to development of negative pressure within the occluded sinus (13). Subsequent disruption in mucociliary transport system, mucous stasis, bacterial superinfection, and chronic inflammatory processes discussed elsewhere in the chapter then follow, leading to the perpetuation of chronic inflammatory state.

Several anatomic alterations in the anatomy of nasal cavity in the region of the osteomeatal complex (OMC) may predispose the patient to transient or persistent sinus osteal obstruction (Figs. 17.6 and 17.7). The most common

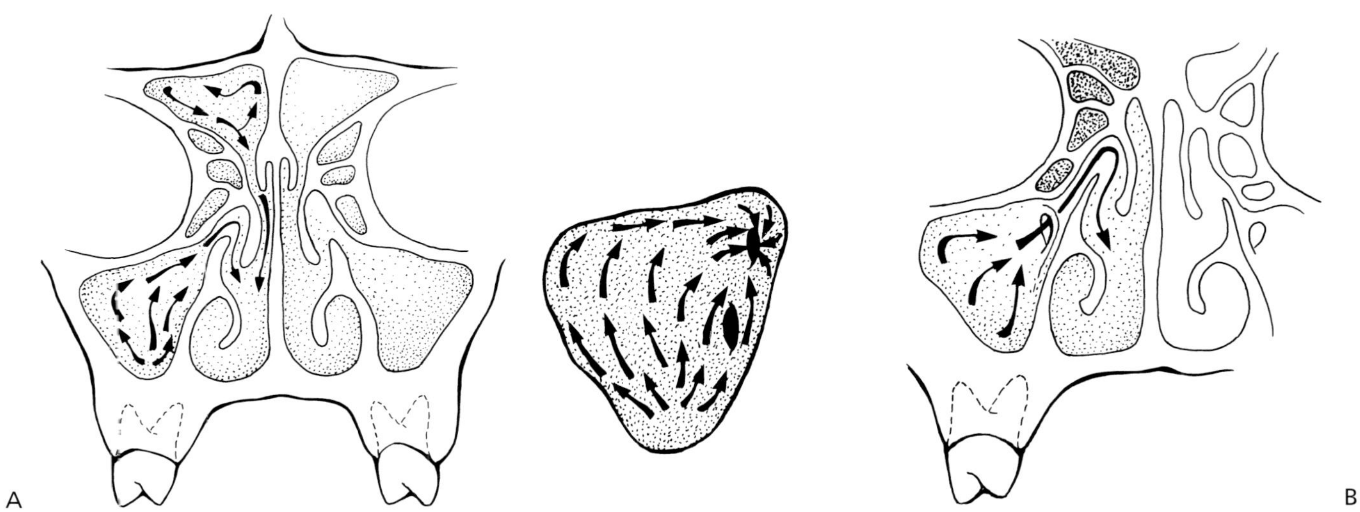

**FIGURE 17.6.** Normal patterns of mucociliary flow from the paranasal sinuses. **A:** Convergence of mucociliary flow from the ethmoid, maxillary and frontal sinuses. **B:** Details of mucociliary flow within the maxillary sinus. (Adapted from Donald PJ, Gluckman JL, Rice DH, eds. *The sinuses.* New York: Raven Press, 1995, with permission.)

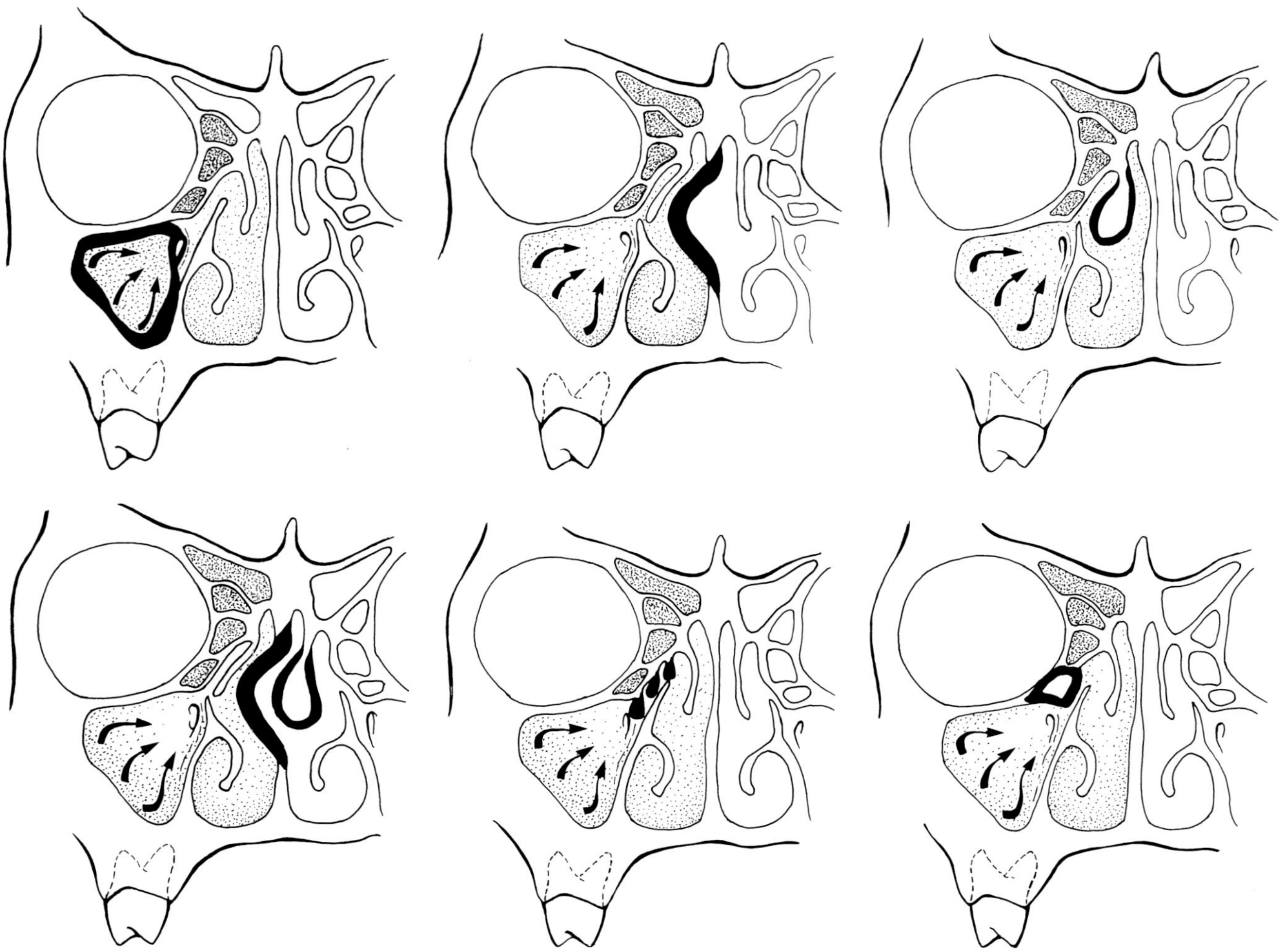


**FIGURE 17.7.** Anatomic obstruction of Maxillary sinus ostium **A:** Mucosal hypertrophy. **B:** Deviated nasal septum. **C:** Ipsilateral concha bullosa. **D:** Contralateral concha bullosa producing septal deviation. **E:** Extensive nasal polyps. **F:** Prominent Haller cell. (Adapted from Donald PJ, Gluckman JL, Rice DH, eds. *The sinuses.* New York: Raven Press, 1995, with permission.)

abnormalities include large nasal septal deflections, expansile concha bullosae, and atypical migration of ethmoid air cells during sinus development (i.e., agger nasi cells, Haller cells). Although the presence of any of these anatomic variants does not in itself correlate to the development of chronic rhinosinusitis, their compromise of the nasal cavity and OMC specifically is the main determinant of resultant sinus pathology.

Among the factors responsible for osteal compromise, the role of allergy in contributing to the development of chronic rhinosinusitis is important. Although there is some statistical correlation between allergic rhinitis and chronic rhinosinusitis in children (61) and between severe chronic rhinosinusitis and allergy in adults, there is no clear evidence that atopy in itself is implicated in the development of the chronic inflammatory process (2). Rather, the physical nature of OMC obstruction from the prolonged and extensive mucosal edema often seen in atopic patients is most significant. Although an association between allergic rhinitis and nasal polyposis offers another pathway to chronic rhinosinusitis, it is again through the mechanism of osteal compromise and obstruction.

### *Proposed Staging System for Chronic Rhinosinusitis*

Having completed the review of the pathophysiology of rhinosinusitis, it is tempting to venture into the clinical domains of diagnosis and treatment. Because these topics are best approached in a separate forum, we shall restrict our incursion to the proposal of a simple, clinically relevant model for staging of chronic rhinosinusitis (Table 17.1). There has been a proliferation of various staging classifications in the literature, with the Lund-Mackay system gain-

**TABLE 17.1. PROPOSED RHINOSINUSITIS STAGING SYSTEM**

| | |
|---|---|
| *For Pathology of the Nasal Cavity* | |
| S1 | Narrowing or partial obstruction of osteomeatal complex (e.g., polypoid changes, concha bullosa, septal spur) |
| S2 | Obstruction of osteomeatal complex (OMC) without significant nasal airway obstruction |
| S3 | Obstruction of OMC with significant nasal airway obstruction |
| S4 | Near complete or complete nasal airway and OMC compromise secondary to nasal polyps or inflammatory disease |
| *For Ethmoid Sinus Disease* | |
| S1 | Mucosal thickening in one or multiple cells |
| S2 | Partial opacification of anterior and/or posterior ethmoid cells |
| S3 | Complete or near-complete opacification of anterior OR posterior ethmoid cells |
| S4 | Complete or near-complete opacification of anterior AND posterior ethmoid cells |
| *For Maxillary, Frontal, and Sphenoid Sinus Disease* | |
| S1 | Mucosal thickening |
| S2 | Less than 50% of sinus opacified |
| S3 | Greater than 50% of sinus opacified |
| S4 | Complete sinus opacification |
| L1 | Anterior ethmoid cell involvement only |
| L2 | Anterior and posterior ethmoid cell involvement or posterior ethmoid cell involvement or maxillary sinus involvement alone or in conjunction with ethmoid sinus disease |
| L3 | Involvement of frontal or sphenoid sinus |
| L4 | Involvement of three or more sinuses on one side |
| R0 | No prior sinus surgery |
| R1 | Prior sinus surgery with residual uncinate process or antrostomy of inadequate size |
| R2 | Prior sinus surgery with complete removal of uncinate process and adequate size antrostomy |

*Staging*

| Stage 1 | Stage 2 | Stage 3 | Stage 4 |
|---|---|---|---|
| S1L1R0 | S2L1R0 | S3, L1–3, R0 | Any S, L4, R1 |
| S1L2R0 | S2L2R0 | S4, L1–3, R0 | Any S, Any L, R2 |
| | | Any S, L3, R0 | |
| | | Any S, L1–3, R1 | |

S, severity of the disease process; L, location, referring to site of sinus involvement; R, recurrence, referring to past surgical intervention history.
Each side should be staged separately.
When severity (S) grade varies within each anatomic subunit, the highest grade is accepted.
Bilateral involvement does not increase the actual stage number.
When unilateral disease is present, subscript "a" is added to the stage number.
When bilateral disease is present, highest stage of the two is reported, and subscript "b" is added.
When bilateral disease of similar stage is reported, subscript "c" is added.

ing acceptance by the Task Force on Rhinosinusitis of the American Academy of Otolaryngology–Head and Neck Surgery (AAO-HNS) (62). However, the main criticism levied against most of these remains their prohibitive complexity, reducing their implementation in clinical practice. To gain acceptance among the practicing otolaryngologists, the staging system must offer the following:

- Categories based on anatomy and pathophysiology of the disease
- Rapid, intuitive accounting system or staging criteria
- Results readily applicable in clinical situations and useful in communicating disease severity among physicians and to third parties

The classification given is based on radiologic criteria (i.e., findings on axial and coronal sections of noncontrast CT scan of paranasal sinuses). It is essential that CT findings correlate with the actual severity of chronic rhinosinusitis, not the acute inflammatory process during upper respiratory infection or acute rhinosinusitis stage. The classification given is to be employed only for patients who had undergone appropriate medical intervention (including 4 to 6 weeks of antibiotics in conjunction with oral or topical steroids) immediately before performing the staging CT scan. In the past, the main argument raised against systems relying on radiologic criteria had been their relatively poor correlation to patients' symptoms. However, we would argue that the true test of such classification system should be its ability to predict medical and surgical treatment outcomes. Patient symptoms and clinical history should be employed in conjunction with the staging system to determine the final treatment recommendation. Clinical outcome trials are under way to test the prognostic significance and efficacy of the proposed staging system.

## REFERENCES


1. Benson V, Marano MA. Current estimates from the 1993 National Health Interview Survey. National Center for Health Statistics. *Vital Health Stat* 1994;190:10.
2. Kaliner MA, Osguthorpe JD, Fireman P, et al. Sinusitis: bench to bedside. Current findings, future directions. *Otolaryngol Head Neck Surg* 1997;116:S1–20.
3. Lanza DC, Kennedy D. Adult rhinosinusitis defined. *Otolaryngol Head Neck Surg* 1997;117:S1–40.
4. Kern RC. Chronic sinusitis and anosmia: pathologic changes in the olfactory mucosa. *Laryngoscope* 2000;110:1071–1077.
5. May M, Levine HL, Schaitkin B, et al. Results of surgery. In: Levine H, May M, editors. *Rhinology and sinusology.* New York: Thieme Medical Publishers, 1993:176–192.
6. Gliklich R, Metson R. A comparison of sinus computer tomography (CT) staging system for outcome research. *Am J Rhinol* 1994;8:291–297.
7. *The sneeze.* (Motion picture sequences were filmed by Thomas Edison's assistant WKL Dickson in 1891. The Edison Kinetoscopic Record, the Library of Congress.)
8. Virus. In: *The Columbia Encyclopedia*, 6th ed. New York: Columbia University Press, 2001. [www.bartelby.com (online edition)].
9. Subauste MC, Jacoby DB, Richards SM, et al. Infection of a human respiratory epithelial cell line with rhinovirus: induction of cytokine release and modulation of susceptibility to infection by cytokine exposure. *J Clin Invest* 1995;96:549–557.
10. Noah TL, Becker S. Respiratory syncytial virus-induced cytokine production by a human bronchial epithelial cell line. *Am J Physiol* 1993;265[Pt 1]:L472–478.
11. Elias JA, Zheng T, Einarsson O, et al. Epithelial interleukin-11: regulation by cytokines, respiratory syncytial virus, and retinoic acid. *J Biol Chem* 1994;269:22261–22268.
12. Saji F, Nonaka M, Pawankar R. Expression of RANTES by IL-1 beta and TNF-alpha stimulated nasal polyp fibroblasts. *Auris Nasus Larynx* 2000;27:247–252.
13. Scharf KE, Lawson W, Shapiro JM, et al. Pressure measurements in the normal and occluded rabbit maxillary sinus. *Laryngoscope* 1995;105:570–574.
14. Facer GW, Kern EB. Sinusitis: current concepts and management. In: Bailey BJ, ed. *Head and neck surgery—otolaryngology.* Philadelphia: JB Lippincott, 1993:366–376.
15. Gwaltney JM Jr, Phyllis CD, Miller RD, et al. Computed tomographic study of the common cold. *N Engl J Med* 1994;330: 25–30.
16. Van Cauwenberge PB, Ingels KJ, Bachert C, et al. Microbiology of chronic sinusitis. *Acta Otorhinolaryngol Belg* 1997;51:239–246.
17. Penttila M, Savolainen S, Kiukaanniemi H, et al. Bacterial findings in acute maxillary sinusitis—European study. *Acta Otolaryngol Suppl* 1997;529:165–168.
18. Joki S, Toskala E, Saano V, et al. Correlation between ciliary beat frequency and the structure of ciliated epithelia in pathologic human nasal mucosa. *Laryngoscope* 1998;108:426–430.
19. Zakharova GP, Shabalin VV, Lantsov AA. Current methods for assessing mucociliary transport disorders in the diagnosis of chronic rhinosinusitis [in Russian]. *Vestn Otorinolaringol* 1998;4: 53–55.
20. Hinni ML, McCaffrey TV, Kasperbauer JL. Early mucosal changes in experimental sinusitis. *Otolaryngol Head Neck Surg* 1992;107:537–548.
21. Rohr AS, Spector SL. Paranasal sinus anatomy and pathophysiology. *Clin Rev Allergy* 1984;2:387–395.
22. Passali D, Ferri R, Becchini G, et al. Alterations of nasal mucociliary transport in patients with hypertrophy of the inferior turbinates, deviations of the nasal septum and chronic sinusitis. *Eur Arch Otorhinolaryngol* 1999;256:335–337.
23. Poole MD. A focus on acute sinusitis in adults: changes in disease management. *Am J Med* 1999;106[Suppl 5A]:38S–47S; discussion 48S–52S.
24. Fagnan LJ. Acute sinusitis: a cost-effective approach to diagnosis and treatment. *Am Fam Physician* 1998;58:1795–1802, 1805–1806.
25. Low DE, Desrosiers M, McSherry J, et al. A practical guide for the diagnosis and treatment of acute sinusitis. CMAJ 1997;156 [Suppl 6]:S1–S14.
26. Brook I. Microbiology and management of sinusitis. *J Otolaryngol* 1996;25:249–256.
27. Hsu J, Lanza DC, Kennedy DW. Antimicrobial resistance in bacterial chronic sinusitis. *Am J Rhinol* 1998;12:243–248.
28. Wald ER. Microbiology of acute and chronic sinusitis in children and adults. *Am J Med Sci* 1998;316:13–20.
29. Daele JJ. Chronic sinusitis in children. *Acta Otorhinolaryngol Belg* 1997;51:285–304.
30. Mortimore S, Wormald PJ, Oliver S. Antibiotic choice in acute and complicated sinusitis. *J Laryngol Otol* 1998;112:264–268.
31. Evans FO Jr, Sydnor JB, Moore WE, et al. Sinusitis of the maxillary antrum. *N Engl J Med* 1975;293:735–739.
32. Van Cauwenberge PB, Ingels KJ, Bachert C, et al. Microbiology of chronic sinusitis. *Acta Otorhinolaryngol Belg* 1997;51: 239–246.
33. Wright ED, Frenkiel S, Ghaffar O, et al. Monocyte chemotactic protein expression in allergy and non-allergy-associated chronic sinusitis. *J Otolaryngol* 1998;27:281–287.
34. Wright ED, Frenkiel S, Al-Ghamdi K, et al. Interleukin-4, interleukin-5, and granulocyte-macrophage colony-stimulating factor receptor expression in chronic sinusitis and response to topical steroids. *Otolaryngol Head Neck Surg* 1998;118:490-495.
35. Marney SR Jr. Pathophysiology of reactive airway disease and sinusitis. *Ann Otol Rhinol Laryngol* 1996;105:98–100.
36. Hamilos DL, Leung DYM, Wood R, et al. Chronic hyperplastic sinusitis: association of tissue eosinophilia with mRNA expression of granulocyte-macrophage colony-stimulating factor and interleukin-3. *J Allergy Clin Immunol* 1993;91[Pt 1]:39–48.
37. Itoh K, Katahira S, Matsuzaki T, et al. Retention fluids of chronic sinusitis induce neutrophil adherence to microvascular endothelial cells. *Acta Otolaryngol* 1992;112:882–889.
38. Demoly P, Crampette L, Lebel B, et al. Expression of cyclooxygenase 1 and 2 proteins in upper respiratory mucosa. *Clin Exp Allergy* 1998;28:278–283.
39. Djupesland PG, Chatkin JM, Qian W, et al. Nitric oxide in the nose and paranasal sinuses—respiratory tract physiology in a new perspective. *Tidsskr Nor Laegeforen* 1999;119:4070–4072.
40. Jain B, Rubenstein I, Robbins RA, et al. Modulation of airway epithelial cell ciliary beat frequency by nitric oxide. *Biochem Biophys Res Commun* 1993;191:83–88.
41. Lindberg S, Cervin A, Runer T. Nitric oxide (NO) production in the upper airways is decreased in chronic sinusitis. *Acta Otolaryngol* 1997;117:113–117.
42. Umeki S, Manabe T. Structure, function and pathophysiology of mucociliary transport system. *Nippon Rinsho* 1992;50:892–899.

43. Passali D, Ferri R, Becchini G, et al. Alterations of nasal mucociliary transport in patients with hypertrophy of the inferior turbinates, deviations of the nasal septum and chronic sinusitis. *Eur Arch Otorhinolaryngol* 1999;256:335–337.
44. Hattori M. Mucociliary function of chronic inflammation in upper and lower airways. *Auris Nasus Larynx* 1994;21:219–225.
45. Majima Y, Harada T, Shimizu T, et al. Effect of biochemical components on rheologic properties of nasal mucus in chronic sinusitis. *Am J Respir Crit Care Med* 1999;160:421–426.
46. Petruson B. Secretion from gland and goblet cells in infected sinuses. *Acta Otolaryngol Suppl* 1994;515:33–36, discussion 36–37.
47. Ruckes-Nilges C, Weber U, Popp C, et al. Ion transport in nasal and paranasal sinus mucosa in mucoviscidosis and chronic sinusitis. *HNO* 1999;47:157–166.
48. Coltrera MD, Mathison SM, Goodpaster TA, et al. Abnormal expression of the cystic fibrosis transmembrane regulator in chronic sinusitis in cystic fibrosis and non-cystic fibrosis patients. *Ann Otol Rhinol Laryngol* 1999;108:576–581.
49. Al-Rawi MM, Edelstein DR, Erlandson RA. Changes in nasal epithelium in patients with severe chronic sinusitis: a clinicopathologic and electron microscopic study. *Laryngoscope* 1998; 108:1816–1823.
50. Rayner CF, Rutman A, Dewar A, et al. Ciliary disorientation in patients with chronic upper respiratory tract inflammation.*Am J Respir Crit Care Med* 1995;151[Pt 1]:800–804.
51. Czaja JM, McCaffrey TV. The correlation between ciliary ultrastructure and ciliary beat frequency in experimental chronic sinusitis. *Am J Rhinol* 1998;12:317–323.
52. Elwany S, Hisham M, Gamaee R. The effect of endoscopic sinus surgery on mucociliary clearance in patients with chronic sinusitis. *Eur Arch Otorhinolaryngol* 1998;255:511–514.
53. Milgrim LM, Rubin JS, Small CB. Mucociliary clearance abnormalities in the HIV-infected patient: a precursor to acute sinusitis. *Laryngoscope* 1995;105:1202–1208.
54. Kennedy DW, Senior BA, Gannon FH, et al. Histology and histomorphometry of ethmoid bone in chronic rhinosinusitis. *Laryngoscope* 1998;108[Pt 1]:502–507.
55. Scadding G. The effect of medical treatment of sinusitis upon concomitant asthma. *Allergy* 1999;54[Suppl 57]:136–140.
56. Nakamura H, Kawasaki M, Higuchi Y, et al. Effects of sinus surgery on asthma in aspirin triad patients. *Acta Otolaryngol* 1999;119:592–598.
57. Ikeda K, Tanno N, Tamura G, et al. Endoscopic sinus surgery improves pulmonary function in patients with asthma associated with chronic sinusitis. *Ann Otol Rhinol Laryngol* 1999;108: 355–359.
58. Marney SR Jr. Pathophysiology of reactive airway disease and sinusitis. *Ann Otol Rhinol Laryngol* 1996;105:98–100.
59. Ozagar A, Dede F, Turoglu T, et al. Aspiration of nasal secretions into the lungs in patients with acute sinonasal infections. *Laryngoscope* 2000;110:107–110.
60. Appenroth E, Gunkel AR, Muller H, et al. Activated and nonactivated eosinophils in patients with chronic rhinosinusitis. *Acta Otolaryngol* 1998;118:240–242.
61. Rachelefsky GS, Goldberg M, Katz RM, et al. Sinus disease in children with respiratory allergy. *J Allergy Clin Immunol* 1978;61: 310–314.
62. Lund VJ, Kennedy DW. Staging for rhinosinusitis. *Otolaryngol Head Neck Surg* 1997;117:S35–40.

18

# OFFICE ENDOSCOPY

DALE H. RICE

Endoscopy forms the cornerstone of building a competent foundation for managing the patient with sinonasal disease in the office and the operating room. The novice sinus endoscopist's first step should be to gain familiarity with and then expertise in office examination of the nose with optical endoscopes. The experienced endoscopist should continue to use office endoscopy as the cornerstone of patient evaluation and management.

## ROUTINE EXAMINATION OF THE NOSE

The physician should develop a standard method for evaluating patients with sinus disease. Because such disease frequently is caused by obstruction of the ostia of the sinuses, each of these sites, along with the nasal septum, must be visualized. To accomplish this, the physician must have at least one standard 0° (and possibly one standard 30°) endoscope or one wide-angle 25° or 30° endoscope, a light cord, and a light source in the office. Such endoscopes are available in 4.0- and 2.7-mm diameters. The larger endoscopes offer a slightly better view of the nose, whereas the smaller ones are easier to use, particularly in children (Fig. 18.1). The smaller-diameter endoscopes are recommended for the solely pediatric practice. Flexible endoscopes can be used as an alternative to rigid endoscopes, but they are inherently optically inferior.

All endoscopists must realize the potential for confusion of landmarks and disorientation that may occur with the viewing limitations and magnification provided by optical endoscopes. Advancing the endoscope 30 to 10 mm from the object of interest produces an increase in magnification of 1.5-fold (Fig. 18.2) (1). Confusion of landmarks occurs with loss of perspective when the endoscope is held too close to the field of examination. The instrument is best used held at the maximum distance from the object of interest, which provides sufficient visualization, with closer advancement of the endoscope as needed to resolve details. The office examination should begin with the allocation of adequate time for vasoconstriction and, if needed, anesthesia to permit maximal visualization of the nasal cavity when septal deflections or a narrow airway compromise passage of an endoscope. Otherwise, the examination can proceed without either. Cottonoids saturated with 4% lidocaine or cocaine may be placed at the site of obstruction to provide further anesthesia. The nasal cavity can then be examined. One recommended routine is to initially advance the standard 0° or wide-angle 25° or 30° endoscope (usually the 2.7-mm-diameter endoscope) along the floor of the nose. In this way, the examiner can visualize the orifice of the nasolacrimal duct, inferolateral nasal wall, eustachian tube orifice, and nasopharynx (2). The second pass of the endoscope is immediately inferior to the middle turbinate and provides viewing of the sphenoethmoid recess, middle meatus, and sphenoid ostium. Each of these sites may be variably difficult to examine because of the presence of polyps, edematous mucous membrane, or pneumatization of the middle turbinate. The last pass of the endoscope should be directed toward the frontal recess, passing adjacent to the junction of the middle turbinate and the agger nasi cells.

## OFFICE SURGERY

### Requirements

Procedures such as biopsy, antral puncture, removal of several small or isolated large polyps, and control of epistaxis can be performed well in the office. All these procedures require the cooperation of the patient and are enhanced by the skill of the physician in administering topical and infiltrative anesthesia. In the more extensive procedures, regional blocks, such as anesthetizing the sphenopalatine nerve, may be particularly useful. In all procedures, the key to success is waiting 10 minutes or more after placement of the anesthetic agent to optimize its effect. The selection of further equipment to perform such procedures depends on the scope of the intended office surgery. As a minimum, we recommend purchas-

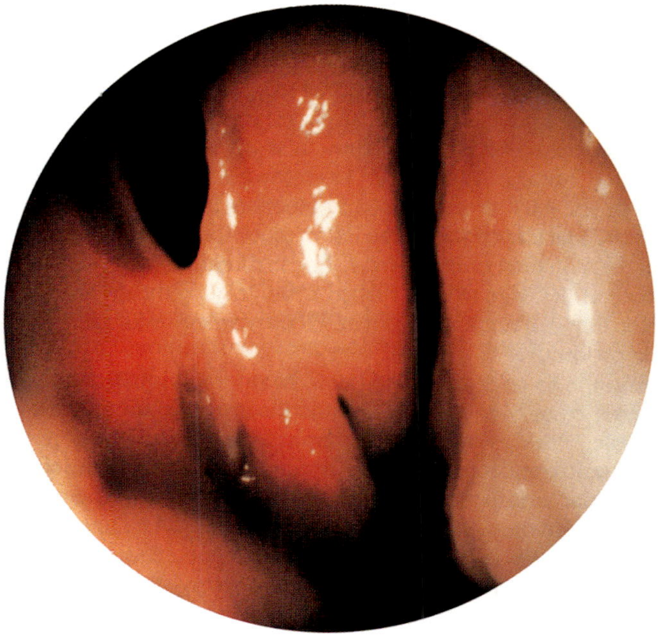

**FIGURE 18.1.** Photograph of synechia between middle turbinate and lateral nasal wall just superior to top of inferior turbinate. (From Rice DH, Schaefer SD, eds. *Endoscopic paranasal sinus surgery*, 2nd ed. New York: Raven Press, 1993, with permission.)

ing a 45° Weil-Blakesley forceps, curved suction canula, and if antral biopsies are to be performed, an antral trocar and forceps. Additional instruments, such as double-spoon forceps, can be added to the office set as they are needed.

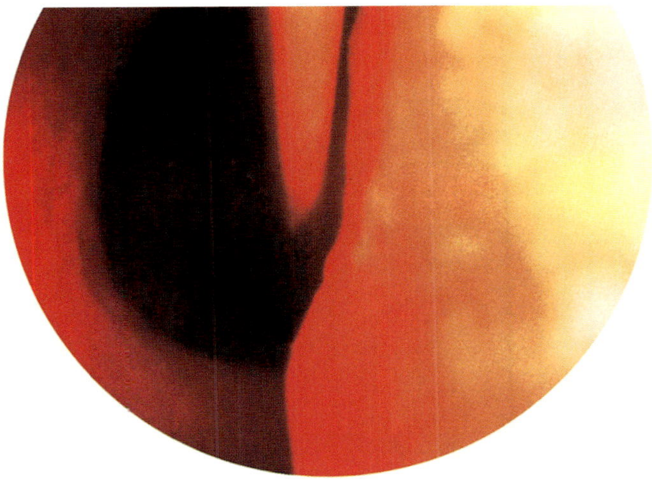

**FIGURE 18.2.** Photograph of well-healed postoperative middle meatus. Notice the thinness of the mucosa and of turbinate. (From Rice DH, Schaefer SD, eds. *Endoscopic paranasal sinus surgery*, 2nd ed. New York: Raven Press, 1993, with permission.)

## Antral Endoscopy

Endoscopic examination of the maxillary antrum is a simple procedure that can be performed well under local anesthesia and in an office setting. The antral puncture can be performed through the canine fossa or beneath the inferior turbinate. However, we recommend the former because visualization of the maxillary sinus is better and because the procedure is simpler and well tolerated by the patient. When puncturing the canine fossa, anesthesia should first be topical (4% cocaine or lidocaine on a cotton pledget), followed by infiltration of the appropriate agent. A 4-mm trocar is introduced under sterile conditions through the anterior wall of the maxilla using a rotating action that takes advantage of the design of the trocar and minimizes thrusting the instrument through the sinus. After the trocar is within the sinus, the stylet is removed, a 4-mm endoscope is passed into the sheath of the trocar, and the sinus is examined (Fig. 18.3). Biopsies can be taken by directing the trocar sheath under endoscopic control at the object of interest and then placing a forceps through the sheath or by using an optical forceps (i.e., endoscope with attached forceps) passed through the sheath of the trocar. Whatever method is used, antral endoscopy is a valuable alternative to Caldwell-Luc or conventional antrostomies as a means to inspect the maxillary antrum and to biopsy radiographically suspicious lesions.

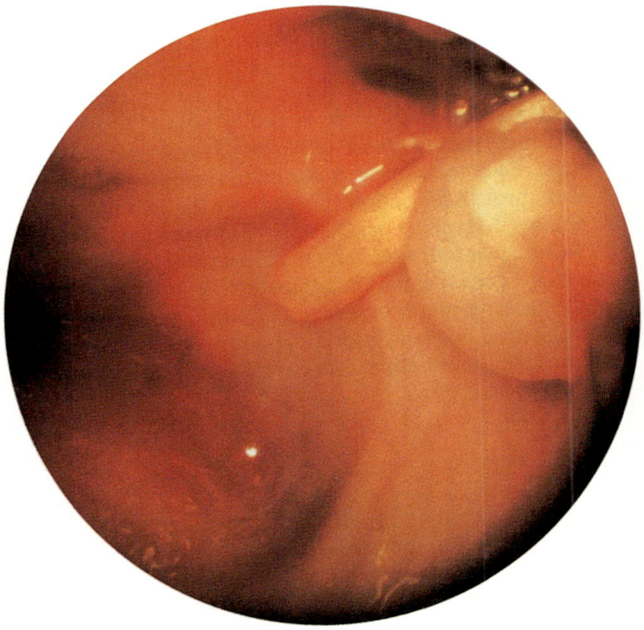

**FIGURE 18.3.** The right maxillary sinus is seen with a 25° endoscope inserted through a trocar through the canine fossa. A foreign body and polyp are seen on the right. (From Rice DH, Schaefer SD, eds. *Endoscopic paranasal sinus surgery*, 2nd ed. New York: Raven Press, 1993, with permission.)

## OPERATIVE EQUIPMENT SELECTION

The novice endoscopic surgeon is fortunate today to be able to choose among several excellent instrument manufacturers. The principal differences in the major optical companies reflect the philosophies of the surgeons who worked with these companies to develop equipment to best perform their particular surgical procedures. Many of these differences are more imagined than real. Those that are real concern the choice of endoscopes and the perceived value of suction irrigation, with the rest of the hardware being very similar.

### Optical Endoscopes

In selecting a sinus endoscope, one must consider the optical axis, degrees of vision, and the resolution at the visual periphery of the endoscope. The optical axis refers to the center of vision, and endoscopes are designated by their axis. The degree of vision is a measure of the actual size of the visual field of the instrument. For example, one endoscope may be a wide-angle 30° endoscope and the other a standard 45° endoscope, but the former instrument's field of vision eclipses the field of the latter. However, the former endoscope is only as useful as the skill of the optical manufacturer in minimizing distortion of the visual periphery, and all endoscopes are fabricated with relatively large angles of vision. To assist in evaluating these different types of optical endoscopes, we constructed a 4-inch-diameter sphere as a bench test. Each endoscope was placed in the center of the sphere, and a photograph was taken through the endoscope (Fig. 18.4 ). This helps illustrate that there are two basic choices that can be made: use two wide-angle endoscopes (25° or 30° and 70°) or four standard endoscopes (0°, 30°, 70°, and 90° or 120°). The 0° endoscope can be included with the former group of endoscopes, depending on the experience of the physician with a particular instrument. We tend to use the 0° endoscope if we are not using the 25°, wide-angle endoscope. The physician should evaluate these systems and decide which he or she prefers.

### Suction Irrigation

The suction-irrigation device consists of a endoscope sheath coupled to a handle. The purpose of suction irrigation is to prevent fogging of the endoscope by continuously drawing air past the lens and to remove blood on the lens through irrigation. If the suction irrigator does not do both of these tasks well, it is not worth purchasing. This instrument is not a prerequisite to performing endoscopic sinus surgery, and the sheath does slightly limit access to the operative field in the narrow nose. Fogging without the use of the irrigator can be minimized by periodic warming of the endoscope in hot water, using commercial defoggers (ELVIS or Endoscopic Laparoscopic Visual Improvement Sponge, Merocel Corp., Mystic, CT; FRED or Fog Reduction Elimination Device, Decide, Inc., Fort Worth, TX; Karl Storz, Los Angeles, CA) or by placing this instrument against the nasal mucous membrane. In most cases, the suction irrigator may not be worth the cost for the small amount of time that may be saved.

### Suction Forceps

The Weil-Blakesley forceps with a suction cannula welded to the inferior aspect of the shaft is a useful adjunct to the suction irrigator or an alternative to this device. This instrument provides a means to grasp soft tissue and thin bone and at the same time clear the operative field of blood. The

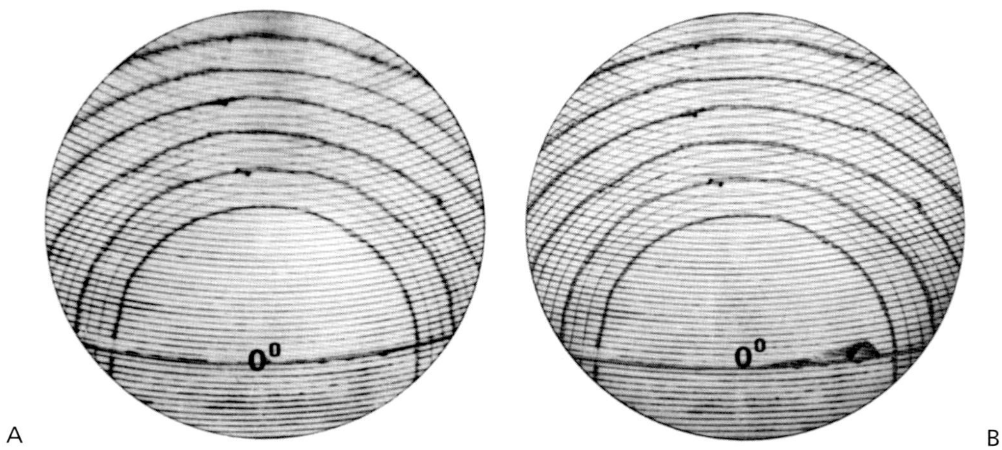


**FIGURE 18.4.** View of the 25° endoscope from one manufacturer **(A)** compared with a 30° endoscope from another **(B)**. (From Rice DH, Schaefer SD, eds. *Endoscopic paranasal sinus surgery*, 2nd ed. New York: Raven Press, 1993, with permission.)

disadvantage of the suction forceps is that the small diameter of the suction cannula results in frequent obstruction and need for cleaning, especially in patients with more severe disease. This instrument is available in straight and 45° configurations.

## Video Camera

The inclusion of a video camera in the surgical armamentarium is optional for most surgeons. Cameras are continuing to evolve in terms of smaller size and greater resolution. Such cameras do provide excellent visualization of the surgical procedure using a video monitor for the others in the operating room. Although cameras are available using couplings with or without a beam splitter, which provide the surgeon with visualization through the endoscope, we recommend the former. Using a camera without a beam splitter (i.e., operating from the video monitor) means that the surgeon is not aligning his or her eye in the same axis as the endoscope, and the dangers are greater in sinus surgery than in arthroscopy, which is performed without a beam splitter. In a teaching hospital, an endoscopic camera is practically a necessity and can be likened to a sidearm on the operating microscope. The ability to share the visualization of the operative field in a teaching institution may prove to be one of the most significant contributions of endoscopic sinus surgery given the inherent difficulty in training surgeons in sinus surgery.

## Additional Hardware

Of the various forceps manufactured, the 45° (or upturned) and 90° Weil-Blakesley (or Blakesley-Wilde) are the most useful. A retrograde antrum punch (sideward and backward cutting) forceps is helpful in enlarging the natural ostium of the maxillary sinus, and the double-spoon forceps is invaluable in removing tissue from the frontal and maxillary sinuses. A bent suction cannula provides a means of aspirating blood and secretions from the ethmoid, frontal, and maxillary sinuses. The rest of the sinus equipment armamentarium depends on the practice and the budget of the surgeon.

## REFERENCES

1. Wigand ME. *Endoscopic surgery of the paranasal sinuses and anterior skull base.* New York: Thieme Medical Publishers, 1990.
2. Kennedy DW, Zinreich J, Rosenbaum AE, Johns ME. Functional endoscopic sinus surgery. *Arch Otolaryngol* 1985;111:576–582.

# 19

# IMAGING OF THE PARANASAL SINUSES FOR FUNCTIONAL ENDOSCOPIC SINUS SURGERY

MICHELLE M. SMITH
TIMOTHY L. SMITH

Inflammatory disease of the paranasal sinuses is a common medical problem affecting an estimated 30 to 50 million people in the United States (1). Functional endoscopic sinus surgery has become standard surgical treatment for benign inflammatory disease of the paranasal sinuses that is refractory to medical therapy (2–4). High-resolution computed tomography (CT) is the imaging modality of choice for presurgical planning for endoscopic sinus surgery (5–7). CT evaluates the normal bony anatomy of the nasal cavity and paranasal sinuses, identifies any anatomic variants that may make a patient prone to recurrent inflammatory disease or at risk for injury during endoscopic surgery, and demonstrates disease present within the sinuses and occluding drainage pathways. CT and magnetic resonance (MR) imaging are also helpful in the evaluation of complications of endoscopic surgery.

## IMAGING TECHNIQUES

CT is the imaging modality of choice for evaluation of the sinonasal cavities before endoscopic surgery (5–7). CT defines the bony anatomy of the sinuses and osteomeatal complex (OMC) to better advantage than conventional radiography. In addition to evaluating the bony anatomy and air passages, CT demonstrates mucosal thickening, fluid, and calcifications within the sinuses. CT also provides visualization of the surrounding soft tissues of the orbits and anterior cranial fossa.

One of the major goals of CT imaging before endoscopic surgery is to identify irreversible disease within the sinonasal cavities. Patient preparation aimed at minimizing reversible disease is recommended before imaging. Therapy before imaging may include completion of a course of antibiotics to eliminate acute inflammatory disease, administration of antihistamines and decongestants to decrease mucosal congestion, and short course steroid therapy in cases of polyposis and allergy. Some physicians also recommend vigorous nose blowing and sympathomimetic nasal spray administration immediately before scanning (8).

Coronal sinus CT is performed with the patient in the prone position with the neck extended. Prone positioning allows mobile secretions to move away from the OMCs and to flow to the dependent portion of the maxillary antrum. Coronal imaging can also be performed in the supine position with the neck extended if the patient is unable to lie prone. The scan is angled approximately perpendicular to the hard palate (Fig. 19.1). The scan angle and field of view can be varied to avoid dental amalgam that can cause a streak artifact. Exposure settings of 125 kVp and 80 to 160 mA are recommended (9). Contiguous, 3-mm images are obtained from the anterior aspect of the frontal sinuses through the posterior aspect of the sphenoid sinuses. Images are printed at settings to optimize visualization of the air passages, bony anatomy, and soft tissues. In general, a window width of +2,000 Houndsfield units (HU) and a level of −200 HU are recommended.

In patients unable to undergo direct coronal imaging because of cervical spine disease or intubation, spiral (helical) scanning can be performed in the axial plane with the patient in the supine position. Images can then be reformatted in the coronal or sagittal planes. Axial scanning can be performed in addition to coronal images for patients undergoing surgery on the frontal, posterior ethmoid, and sphenoid sinuses. The axial plane is superior for evaluation of the posterior frontal sinus walls, for delineating the anatomic relationships between the posterior ethmoid and sphenoid sinuses, and for assessing the relationship of the optic nerves and internal carotid arteries to the sphenoid sinus. Scan exposure parameters for axial imaging are similar to those used for coronal imaging. The scan plane is oriented parallel to the palate. Three-millimeter-thick, contiguous images are obtained from the palate to the superior aspect of the frontal sinuses (Fig. 19.2).

MRI is superior to CT for evaluation of the soft tissues, but it is poor at defining bony anatomy, particularly at bone-air interfaces. Air and bone are both signal voids (i.e., no signal) on MRI and are therefore difficult to distinguish. MRI does not provide adequate detail of the bony anatomy and air passages required for presurgical planning for endoscopic sinus surgery. MRI does have a role in the evaluation of

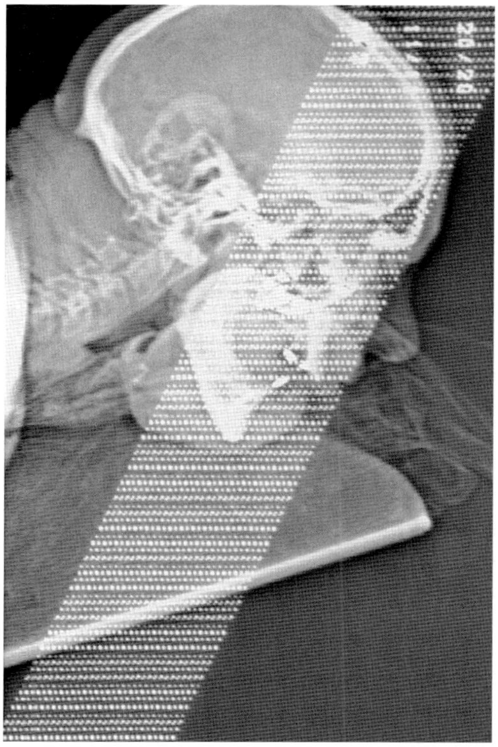

**FIGURE 19.1.** Lateral topogram image obtained before a coronal computed tomography scan. The patient is in the prone position, with the neck extended. The scanning plane is oriented perpendicular to the hard palate. Contiguous, 3-mm-thick images are obtained from the anterior wall of the frontal sinus to the posterior wall of the sphenoid sinus.

intracranial and orbital complications of endoscopic surgery and in the evaluation of sinonasal neoplastic disease.

## NORMAL ANATOMY

On sequential coronal CT images, the frontal sinuses are the most anterior structures to be encountered. The funnel-shaped frontal sinuses vary in the degree of pneumatization. The frontal sinuses are separated by a central septation, but additional septa may be present. Each frontal sinus drains by means of an ostium located in a depression at the medial and inferior aspect of the floor of the frontal sinus. The ostium is located at the superior aspect of the frontal recess (Fig. 19.3). The frontal recess forms the lower half of an hourglass, with the frontal sinus forming the upper half of the hourglass and the ostium forming the waist. Other structures seen on anterior images include the nasal fossae, cartilaginous nasal septum, the globes, and the floor of the anterior cranial fossa.

The superior, middle, and inferior turbinates are bulbous projections from the lateral nasal wall and divide the nasal cavity into three air passages: the superior, middle, and inferior meati. The posterior ethmoid air cells drain into the superior meatus, as do the sphenoid sinuses through the sphenoethmoidal recess. The middle meatus receives drainage from the frontal sinus through the frontal recess, the anterior ethmoid air cells through their ostia, and

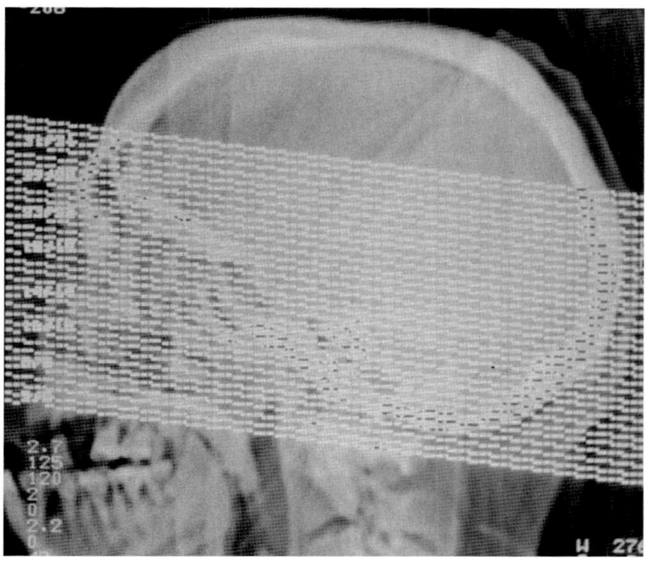

**FIGURE 19.2.** Lateral topogram image obtained before an axial computed tomography scan. The patient is supine, with the neck in neutral position. The scan plane is oriented parallel to the palate. Contiguous, 3-mm-thick images are obtained from the palate to the superior aspect of the frontal sinus.

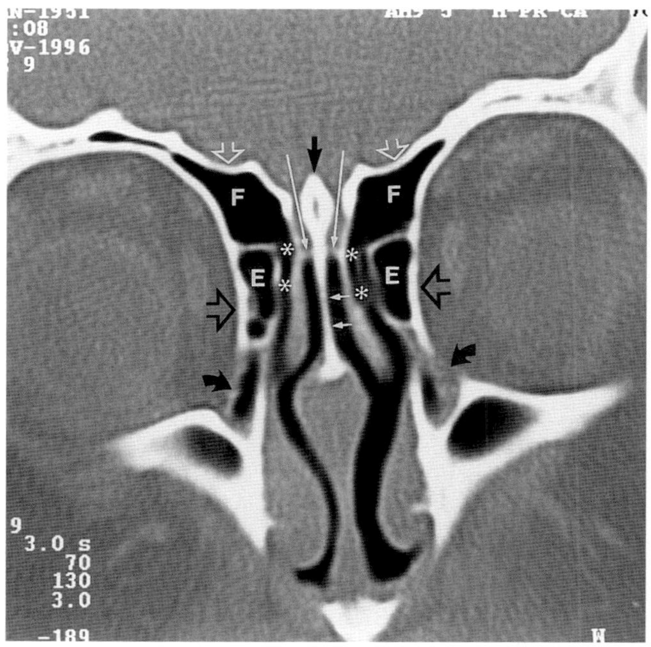


**FIGURE 19.3.** Coronal computed tomography through the posterior aspect of the frontal sinuses *(F)* shows patent frontal recesses *(asterisks)* bilaterally. Notice the anterior ethmoid air cells *(E)*, cribriform plates *(long white arrows)*, fovea ethmoidalis *(open white arrows)*, perpendicular plate of the ethmoid *(short white arrows)*, crista galli *(solid black arrow)*, lamina papyracea *(open black arrows)*, and nasolacrimal ducts *(curved arrows)*.

the maxillary sinuses through their ostia and the infundibulum. The nasolacrimal duct drains into the inferior meatus. The most anterior of the ethmoid air cells to be encountered are the agger nasi cells, which are located anterior to the nasolacrimal duct. On coronal CT images, the agger nasi cells are located anterior to the anterior aspect of the middle turbinates (Fig. 19.4). The anterior ethmoid cells are bordered anteriorly by the frontal process of the maxilla, superiorly by the frontal recess, inferomedially by the uncinate process, and inferolaterally by the lacrimal bone. The roof of the ethmoid labyrinth is the fovea ethmoidalis. It also functions as a portion of the floor of the anterior cranial fossa (Fig. 19.3). Medial to the fovea ethmoidalis is the cribriform plate, which comprises a medial lamella located medial to the vertical lamella of the middle turbinate (Fig. 19.3) and a very thin lateral lamella located lateral to the vertical lamella (Fig. 19.5).

The major structural elements comprising the OMC include the uncinate process, ethmoid infundibulum, hiatus semilunaris, middle meatus, ethmoid bulla, and middle turbinate. The uncinate process extends from the lateral nasal wall at the posteromedial aspect of the nasolacrimal duct to form the anteromedial border of the ethmoid infundibulum. The uncinate process has a "free" superoposterior edge. The uncinate process is bordered laterally by the infundibulum and medially by the middle meatus. The infundibulum is the air passage that connects the maxillary sinus ostium to the middle meatus at the hiatus semilunaris (Fig. 19.5). The hiatus semilunaris lies directly between the free margin of the uncinate process and the ethmoidal bulla (Fig. 19.5). The middle meatus is bordered laterally by the uncinate process and medially by the middle turbinate (Fig. 19.5). The ethmoid bulla is usually the largest anterior ethmoid air cell and is bounded anteriorly and inferiorly by the hiatus semilunaris, medially by the lamina papyracea, and superiorly by the anterior skull base (Fig. 19.5). If the bulla does not extend to the skull base, it is bounded superiorly by the suprabulbar recess. The middle turbinate is attached superiorly to the cribriform plate by the vertical lamella. Posteriorly, the middle turbinate is attached to the lamina papyracea by a second bony strut, the basal or ground lamella (Fig. 19.6). The basal lamella separates the anterior and posterior ethmoid air cells.

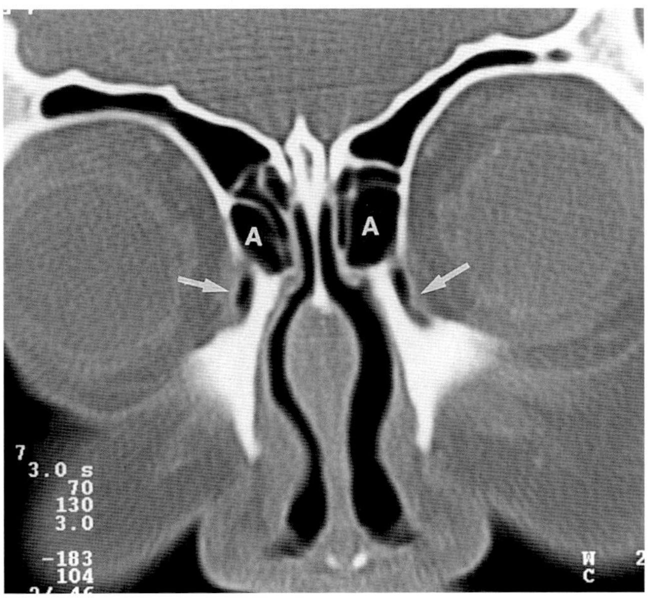


**FIGURE 19.4.** Anterior coronal image shows bilateral agger nasi air cells *(A)* located anterior to the superior aspect of the nasolacrimal ducts *(arrows)*. The frontal recesses course posterior to these air cells.

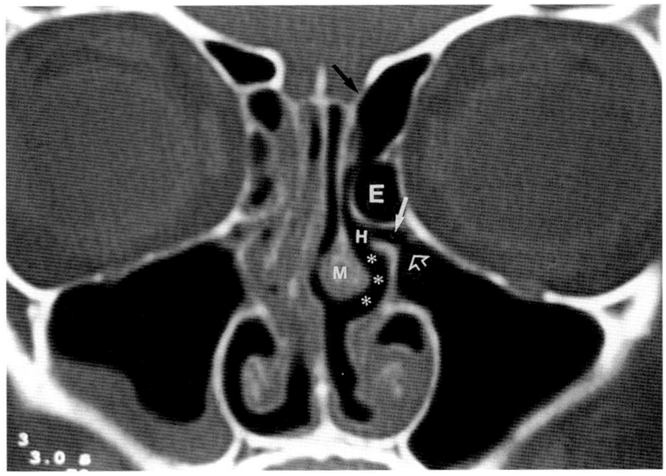


**FIGURE 19.5.** Coronal computed tomography at the level of the osteomeatal complex shows maxillary ostium *(open arrow)*, ethmoidal infundibulum *(solid white arrow)*, hiatus semilunaris *(H)*, middle meatus *(asterisks)*, ethmoidal bulla *(E)*, and middle turbinate *(M)*. Mucosal thickening occludes the right middle meatus and disease is seen within the ipsilateral maxillary and ethmoid sinuses. Notice the thin lateral lamella of the cribriform plate on the left *(black arrow)*.

The posterior ethmoid sinuses are located between the basal lamella of the middle turbinate and the sphenoid sinuses. The relationship of the posterior ethmoid cells to the sphenoid sinuses is seen to better advantage in the axial plane than the coronal plane. The number and size of the posterior ethmoid cells is highly variable. The sphenoid sinus is the most posterior in location and forms from pneumatization of the clivus and sphenoid bones. The sphenoid sinuses are most often separated by a dominant midline septum, but multiple septa may be present. The ostium of each sinus is located medially and superiorly along the anterior wall and drains into the sphenoethmoidal recess (Fig. 19.7). The sphenoethmoidal recesses are located just lateral to the posterior nasal septum. The sphenoid sinuses are bordered superoposteriorly by the sella turcica; superoanteriorly by the anterior cranial fossa and optic nerves; laterally by the orbital apices, cavernous sinuses, and foramen rotundum; and inferiorly by the posterior nasal cavity, vidian canals, and clivus (Fig. 19.8). Posteriorly, the

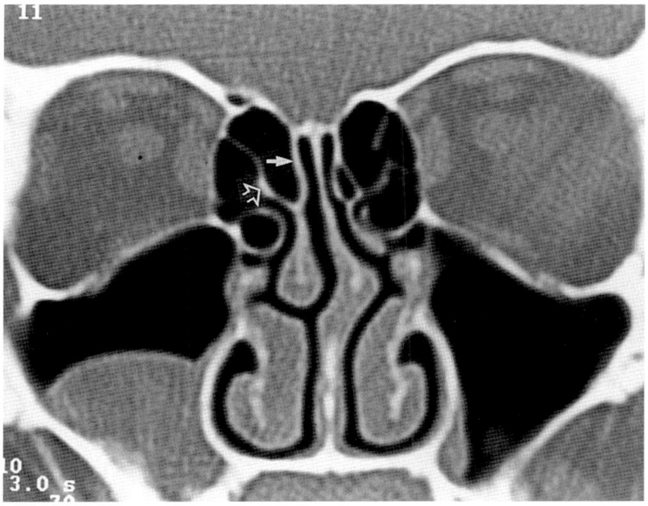

**FIGURE 19.6.** Coronal computed tomography at the level of the mid-maxillary antrum shows the two attachments of the middle turbinate the vertical lamella *(solid arrow)* and the basal lamella *(open arrow)*. A mucous retention cyst is seen within the alveolar recess of the right maxillary sinus, and a small amount of mucosal thickening is seen along the medial walls of both maxillary sinuses. There is leftward nasal septal deviation.

sphenoid sinuses are bordered by the internal carotid arteries and the clivus. The anatomy of the sphenoid sinuses and their relationship to surrounding structures of the central skull base are often best delineated in the axial plane (Fig. 19.9).

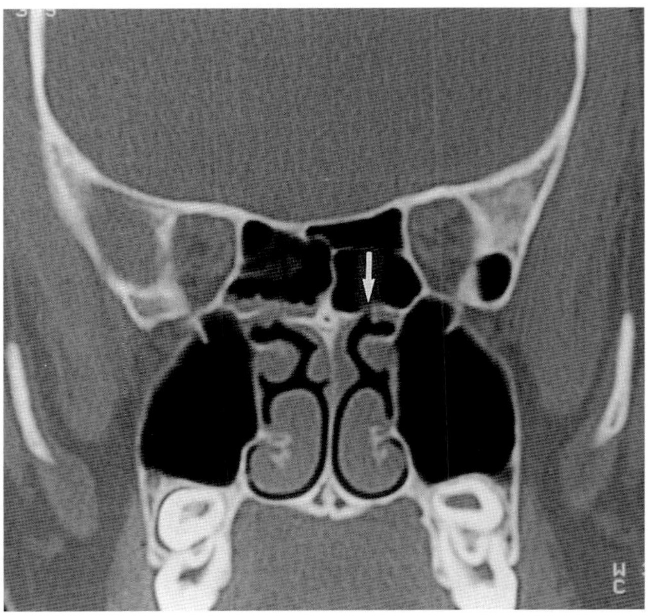

**FIGURE 19.7.** Coronal image through the posterior maxillary sinuses and anterior aspect of the sphenoid sinuses. The left sphenoid sinus ostium *(arrow)* is patent. The right sphenoid ostium is occluded by mucosal thickening. Fluid levels are seen within the right sphenoid sinus indicative of acute disease.

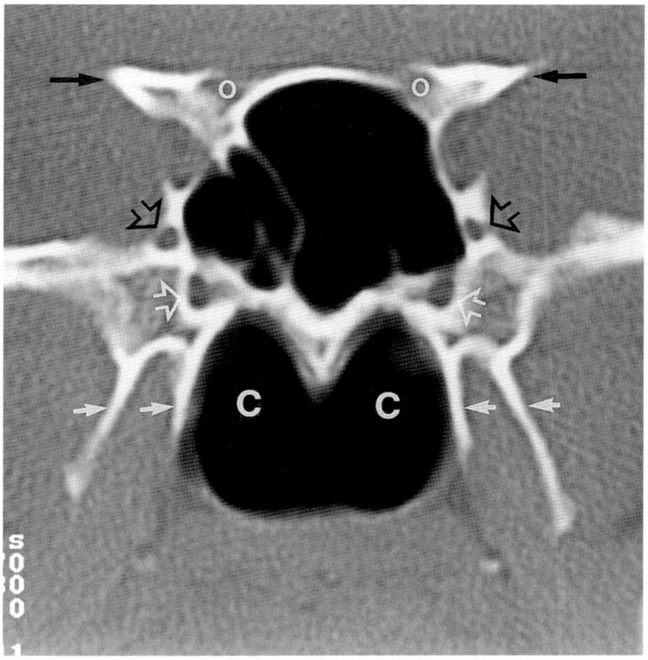


**FIGURE 19.8.** Coronal image through the posterior aspect of the sphenoid sinuses shows asymmetry in the volume of the sphenoid air cells. Anatomy surrounding the sphenoid sinuses includes optic nerves *(O)*, lesser wings of the sphenoid *(solid black arrows)*, foramen rotundum *(open black arrows)*, vidian (pterygoid) canals *(open white arrows)*, pterygoid plates *(solid white arrows)*, and choanae *(C)*.

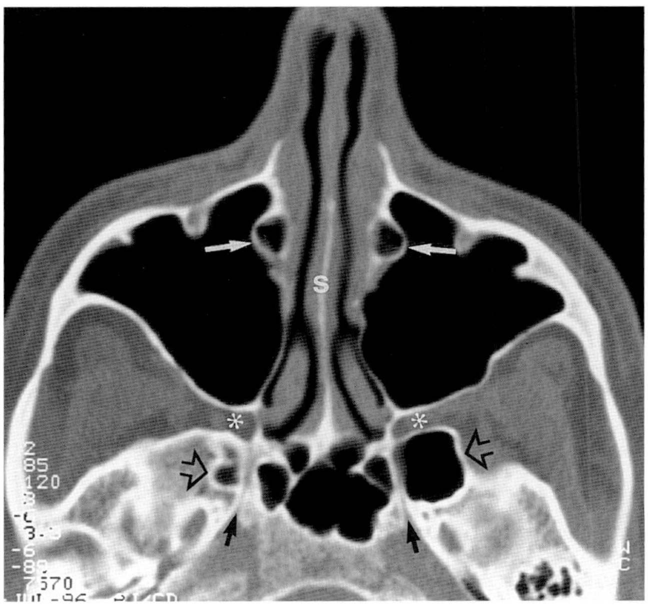


**FIGURE 19.9.** Axial computed tomography image through the mid-maxillary antrum shows nasolacrimal ducts *(white arrows)*, nasal septum *(S)*, pterygopalatine fossae *(asterisks)*, vidian canals *(solid black arrows)*, and pterygoid recesses of the sphenoid sinuses *(open black arrows)*.

## ANATOMIC VARIATIONS

### Nasal Septal Variants

#### *Septal Deviation*

Deviation of the nasal septum is a common anatomic variant seen in up to 44% of patients (10). Deviation from the midline may be diffuse and broad based, focal, or S shaped (i.e., double curvature). Associated anatomic variations of the turbinates, structures of the nasal wall, or palate may be present (Fig. 19.10). Septal deviation may be associated with narrowing of the middle meatus on the side to which the septum is deviated.

#### *Septal Spurs*

Septal spurs are frequently associated with deviation of the septum. They typically occur at the junction of the perpendicular plate of the ethmoid bone and the vomer. Spurs may be bony or cartilaginous. Septal spurs may impinge on the adjacent middle or inferior turbinate (Fig. 19.11).

#### *Septal Pneumatization*

The posterior superior aspect of the septum may be pneumatized. The air cell within the septum may be referred to

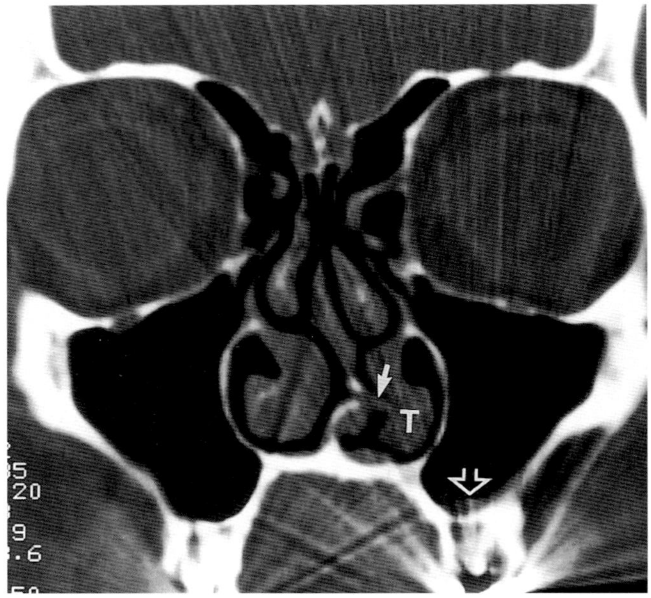


**FIGURE 19.11.** Coronal image shows leftward septal deviation with leftwardly directed cartilaginous spur *(solid arrow)* marginating the left inferior turbinate *(T)*. Mucosal thickening is seen within the alveolar recess of the left maxillary sinus *(open arrow)* although the osteomeatal complex is patent.

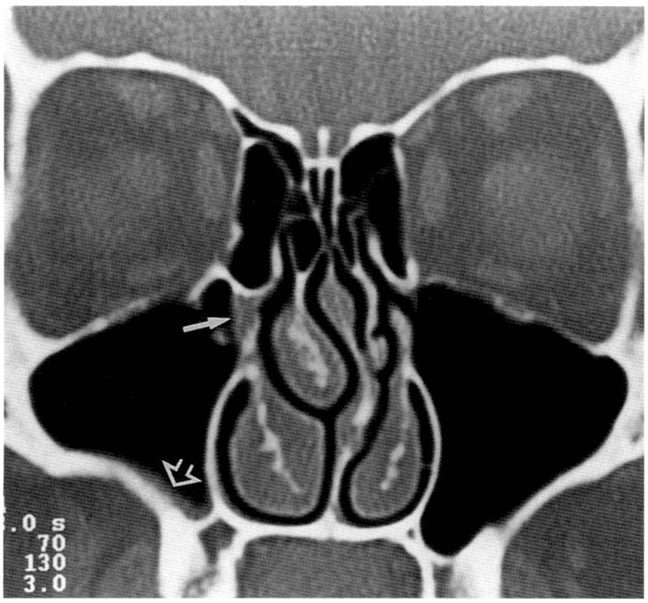


**FIGURE 19.10.** Coronal image shows leftward nasal septal deviation with associated hypoplasia of the left middle turbinate. Mucosal thickening occludes the right infundibulum *(solid arrow)*. Mucosal thickening is seen within the alveolar recess of the right maxillary sinus *(open arrow)*.

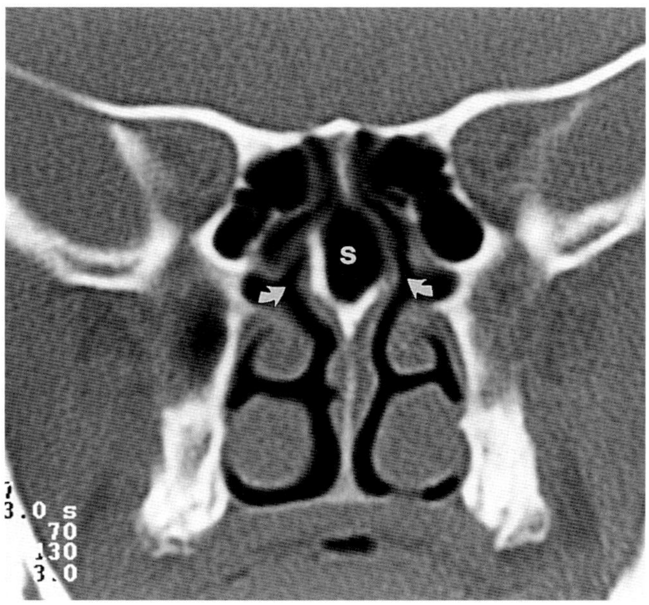


**FIGURE 19.12.** Coronal image through the posterior nasal cavity shows pneumatization of the posterior aspect of the nasal septum, or a "septal recess" *(S)*. The sphenoethmoidal recesses *(arrows)* are located just lateral to the septal recess.

as a *septal recess* (Fig. 19.12). The septal recess commonly drains into the sphenoid sinus. Disease within this type of cell may resemble a cephalocele. These entities can be easily differentiated with MRI.

## Ethmoidal Variants

### *Agger Nasi Cells*

Agger nasi cells are the most anterior of the ethmoid air cells and are extramural (i.e., not within the ethmoid bone). Because of variations in the anatomic descriptions of these air cells cited in the literature, the reported prevalence of these cells widely varies. For the purposes of coronal CT imaging, agger nasi cells are defined as those located anterior to the superior end of the nasolacrimal duct (Fig. 19.4). They may cause narrowing of the frontal recess and predispose to ipsilateral frontal sinus disease.

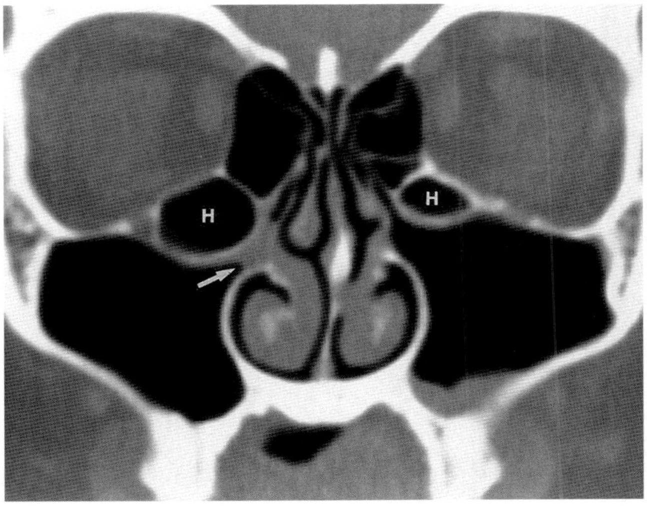


**FIGURE 19.13.** Coronal image at the level of the osteomeatal complex shows bilateral infraorbital ethmoid air cells, or Haller cells *(H)*. The right infraorbital ethmoid cell narrows the infundibulum that is occluded by mucosal thickening *(arrow)*. Although the left infundibulum is patent, there is disease within the left maxillary sinus.

### *Large Ethmoidal Bullae*

Large ethmoidal bullae may result in compromise of the OMC at the level of the infundibulum, hiatus semilunaris, or middle meatus.

### *Infraorbital Ethmoid Cells*

Infraorbital ethmoid cells (i.e., Haller cells) extend along the medial aspect of the orbital floor (i.e., medial roof of the maxillary sinus) (Fig. 19.13). They may be discrete air cells or drain into the infundibulum or maxillary sinus. Infraorbital cells may cause narrowing of the ethmoidal infundibulum, resulting in ipsilateral maxillary sinus disease (Fig. 19.14).

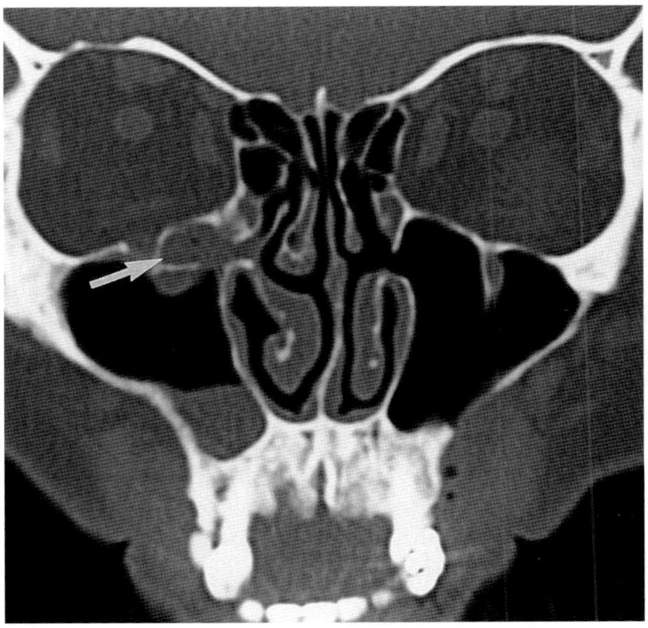

**FIGURE 19.14.** Coronal computed tomography at the level of the osteomeatal complex (OMC) shows a large right infraorbital ethmoid cell *(arrow)* with disease within the air cell and about its periphery. The right OMC is occluded, and there is mucosal disease within the ipsilateral maxillary sinus. There has been endoscopic surgery performed previously on the left with resection of the left uncinate process and partial ethmoidectomy.

### *Onodi Cells*

Onodi cells (i.e., sphenoethmoidal cells) are posterolateral extensions of posterior ethmoid air cells. They expand toward the orbital apex from the posterior ethmoid region and approximate the optic nerves. In this location, they predispose the optic nerve to injury during endoscopic surgery in the region. Onodi air cells are rare and are imaged to better advantage in the axial plane.

### *Low, Asymmetric Fovea Ethmoidalis*

An asymmetric, low-lying ethmoid roof is a potential risk factor for intracranial injury during endoscopic surgery of

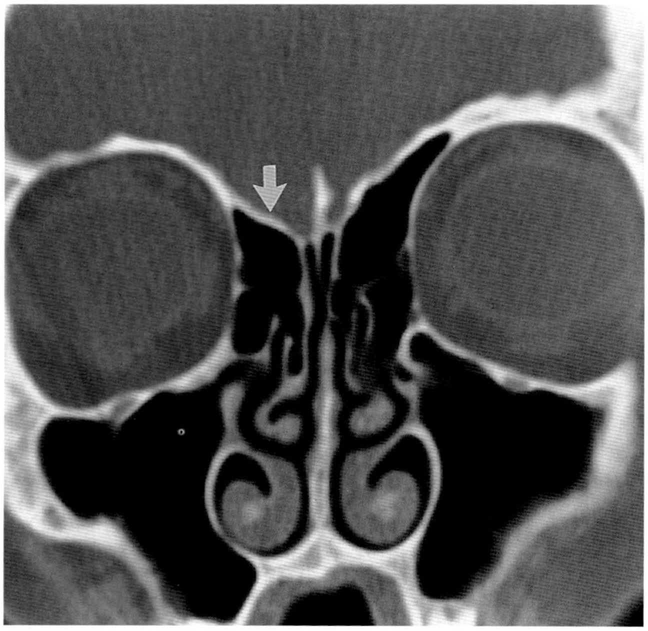

**FIGURE 19.15.** Coronal image shows asymmetry in the position of the fovea ethmoidalis with the right fovea *(arrow)* more inferior than the left. No dehiscence in the fovea is identified. Notice the paradoxical curvature of the middle turbinates.

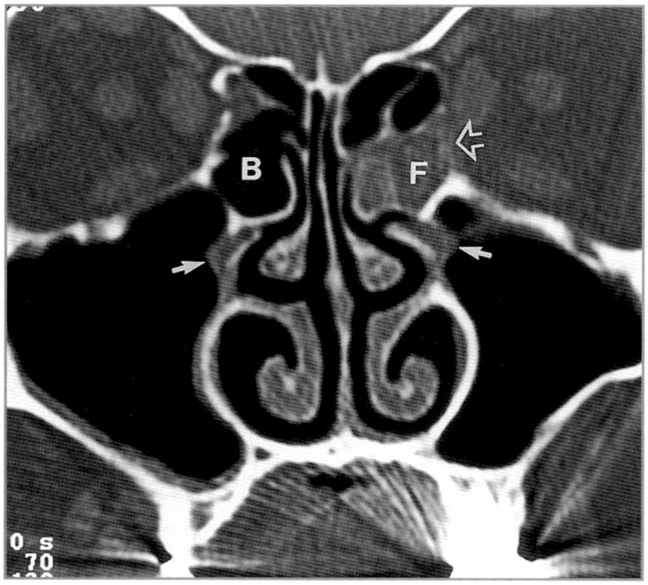


**FIGURE 19.16.** Coronal computed tomography through the mid-ethmoid labyrinths shows dehiscence of the left lamina papyracea *(open arrow)* with herniation of orbital fat *(F)* into the left ethmoidal bulla. Notice the well-aerated right bullar air cell *(B)*. There is mucosal thickening within the infundibula *(solid arrows)*.

the ethmoid air cells. Focal dehiscences of the fovea ethmoidalis or cribriform plate may be posttraumatic or congenital (Fig. 19.15).

### *Dehiscent or Medially Deviated Lamina Papyracea*

Similar to dehiscences within the fovea ethmoidalis and cribriform plate, dehiscences of the lamina papyracea may be posttraumatic or congenital. The dehiscence typically occurs at the point of attachment of the basal lamella. The bony defect predisposes the patient to orbital injury during endoscopic surgery because the deviated or dehiscent region may appear similar to the ethmoidal bulla endoscopically. The medial rectus muscle is prone to injury in patients with this variant (Figs. 19.16). Hypoplasia of the ethmoid labyrinth is a rare anatomic variant. The medial orbital wall is medially located in these patients, with orbital contents located in the expected position of the ethmoid air cells (Fig. 19.17).

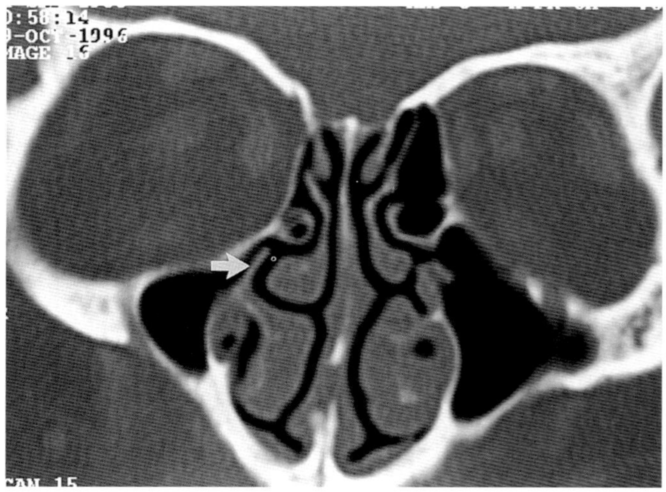

**FIGURE 19.17.** Coronal image shows hypoplasia of the right ethmoid labyrinth with a medial position of the right lamina papyracea. The medial aspect of the right orbit projects over the uncinate process *(arrow)* in the expected position of the ethmoidal bulla.

## Middle Turbinate Variants

### *Concha Bullosa*

Pneumatization of the middle turbinate is referred to as concha bullosa and may be unilateral or bilateral (Figs. 19.18 and 19.19). This variant is seen in up to 15% of the population. Concha bullosa may result in compromise of the middle meatus. A large concha may cause lateral displacement of the uncinate process and narrowing of the infundibulum. The air cavity in concha bullosa is lined by epithelium similar to that in the paranasal sinuses and is prone to similar inflammatory disease, including mucosal thickening, fluid, and mucocele formation (Fig. 19.20). Pneumatization of the inferior and superior turbinates is rare.

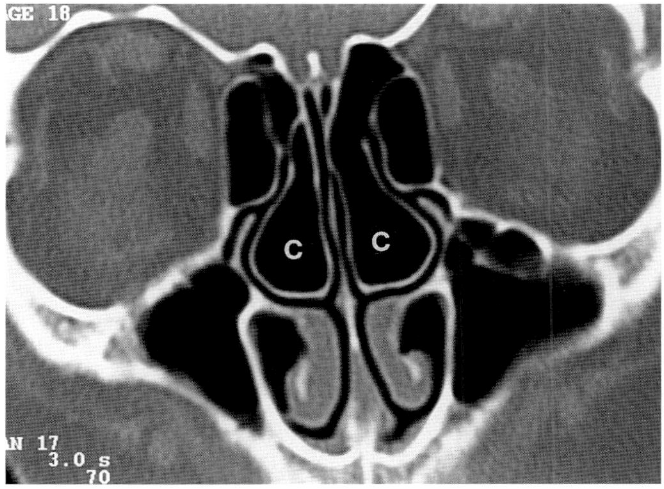


**FIGURE 19.19.** Coronal image shows large bilateral concha bullosa *(C)*. Despite the size of the middle turbinates, the osteomeatal complexes are patent.

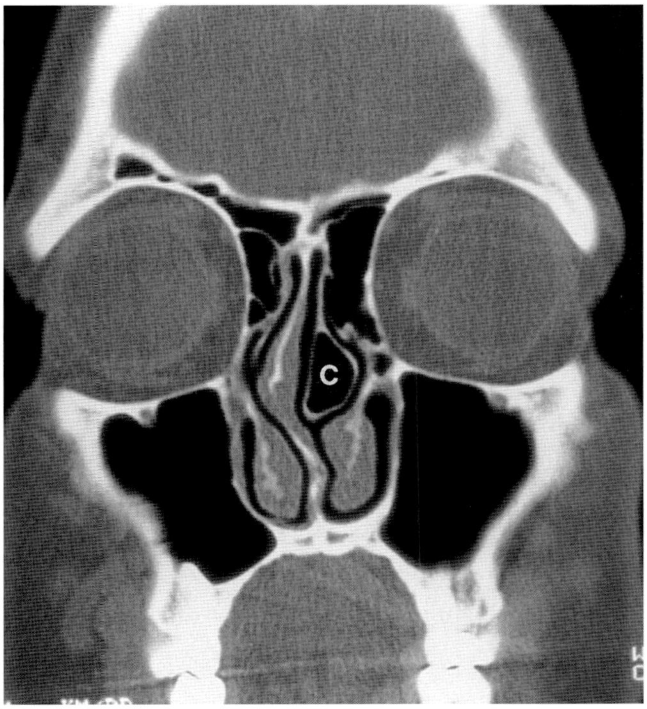


**FIGURE 19.18.** Coronal image shows pneumatization of the concha of the left middle turbinate or "concha bullosa" *(C)*. There is associated rightward deviation of the nasal septum.

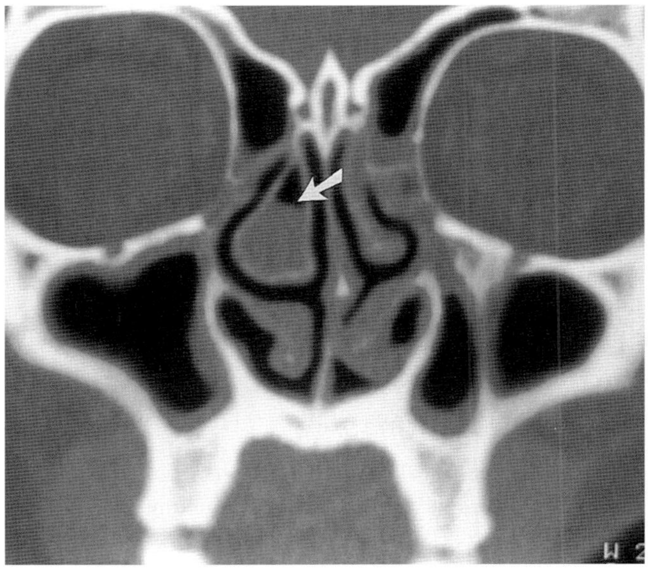

**FIGURE 19.20.** Coronal image shows large right concha bullosa with air-fluid level *(arrow)* indicative of acute inflammation. There is mucosal thickening within the maxillary, frontal, and left ethmoid sinuses. The osteomeatal complexes were occluded in this patient.

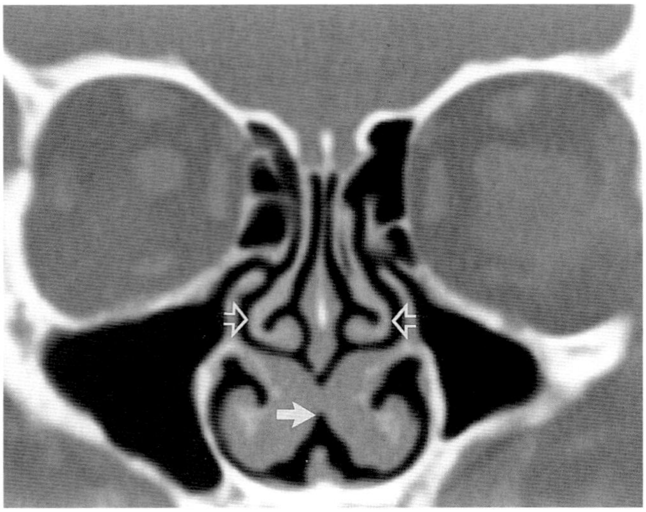

**FIGURE 19.21.** Coronal computed tomography image shows paradoxical curvature of the middle turbinates *(open arrows)* without compromise of the middle meatus on either side. Note large septal perforation *(solid arrow)* in this patient with a history of prolonged cocaine use.

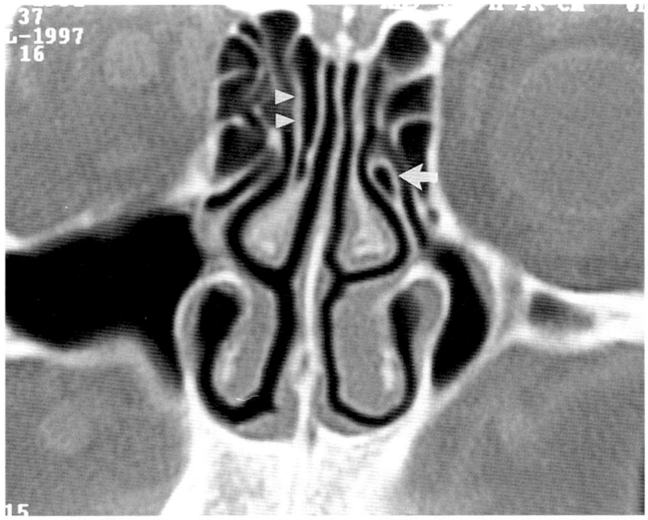

**FIGURE 19.22.** Coronal image shows pneumatization of the superior aspect of the left uncinate process *(arrow)*. No compromise of the middle meatus is appreciated. Also note pneumatization of the right vertical lamella *(arrowheads)*.

### *Paradoxical Curvature*

Paradoxical curvature of the middle turbinate occurs when the curvature of the concha is concave toward the nasal septum and convex toward the lateral nasal wall (Fig. 19.21). The curvature may involve the entire turbinate or be present focally. The configuration of the inferior aspect of the paradoxical middle turbinate is variable and may be pyramidal or club-shaped. Abnormalities of the vertical lamella and basal lamella are not usually associated with this variant. Paradoxical curvature may result in compromise of the middle meatus.

## Uncinate Process Variants

### *Pneumatized Uncinate*

The uncinate process can be considered to be a secondary turbinate. There may be extension of pneumatization into the uncinate process. Most often, pneumatization extends posteriorly from agger nasi cells into the uncinate. The anterior aspect of the uncinate is pneumatized more often than the posterior aspect, and pneumatization may be unilateral or bilateral. Uncinate process air cells may narrow the infundibulum or middle meatus. This anatomic variant is uncommon (Fig. 19.22).

### *Deviated Uncinate*

The position of the uncinate process is variable. The uncinate may be straight and vertically aligned or may be deviated medially or laterally. Laterally deviated uncinate processes may compromise the infundibulum, predisposing the patient to recurrent ipsilateral maxillary disease. The medially deviated uncinate may narrow the middle meatus or occlude it if fused to the vertical lamella of the middle turbinate (Fig. 19.23). In this case, the maxillary sinus drains into the middle meatus by an accessory ostium. The

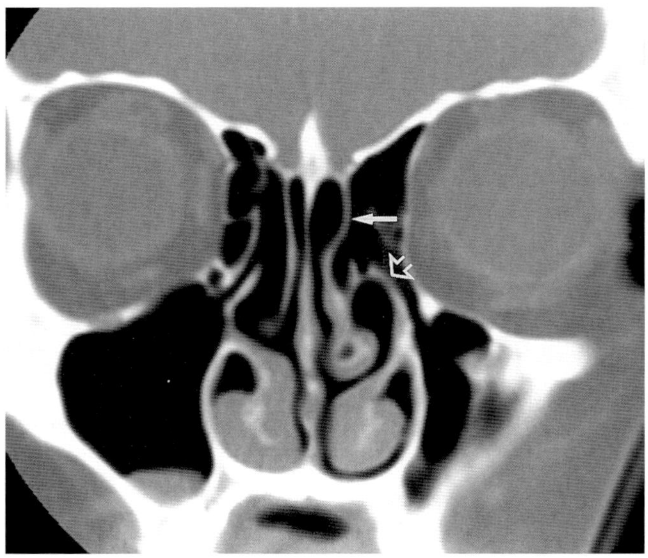

**FIGURE 19.23.** Coronal image shows medially deviated uncinate process *(open arrow)* that is fused to the vertical lamella of the middle turbinate *(solid arrow)*. This occludes the left middle meatus. The left maxillary sinus drains through an accessory ostium.

uncinate may also extend superiorly to the roof of the anterior ethmoid causing the infundibulum to end in a blind pouch referred to as the lamina terminalis. In these cases, the infundibulum drains into the posterior aspect of the middle meatus (9).

### *Atelectatic Uncinate*

The atelectatic uncinate process is lateral in position and may be fused to the medial orbital wall or lamina papyracea. This uncinate variation occludes the infundibulum. The ipsilateral maxillary sinus is often hypoplastic and at least partially opacified. The ipsilateral orbital floor is a low-lying structure. The position of the orbital floor and fusion to the uncinate predispose the patient to orbital injury during endoscopic resection of the uncinate.

## Sphenoidal Variants

### *Variable Pneumatization of the Sphenoid*

Pneumatization of the sphenoid sinus is highly variable. The sphenoid may be hypoplastic or extensively pneumatized with aeration of multiple recesses. Lateral extension of pneumatization may occur into the lesser wing of the sphenoid above the optic nerve or into the anterior clinoid processes inferior and lateral to the optic nerves. Pneumatization about the optic nerve may increase risk of injury during endoscopic surgery in the region. Extension of pneumatization into the greater wing may extend lateral to a line drawn between the pterygoid canal and foramen rotundum. These extensions excavate into the base of the pterygoid process and are referred to as pterygoid recesses (Fig. 19.24). Midline extensions may occur anteriorly into the nasal septum (i.e., septal recess) or posteriorly into the dorsum sella.

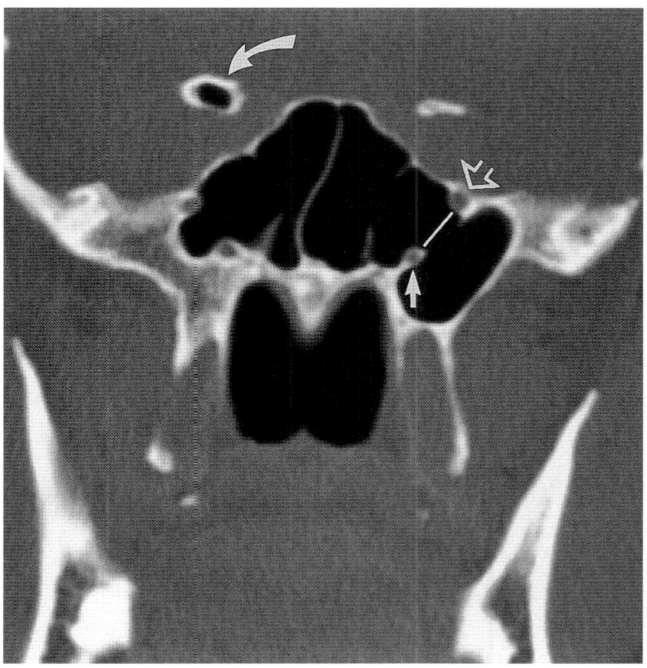

**FIGURE 19.24.** Coronal image through the sphenoid sinuses and choanae shows extension of pneumatization of the left sphenoid sinus lateral to a line drawn between the foramen rotundum *(open arrow)* and vidian canal *(closed arrow)*. Extension into the base of the pterygoid is called a pterygoid recess of the sphenoid sinus. There is pneumatization of the lesser wing of the sphenoid on the right *(curved arrow)*.

### *Medial or Dehiscent Internal Carotid Artery*

The internal carotid arteries may be medial in location and lie immediately behind the posterior wall of the sphenoid sinus. The bony covering over the artery may be extremely thin or absent, placing the vessel at risk during endoscopic sphenoid surgery (Fig. 19.25).

### *Sphenoid Septations*

Vertical septations within the sphenoid sinus may traverse the sinus obliquely and terminate posteriorly in the bony

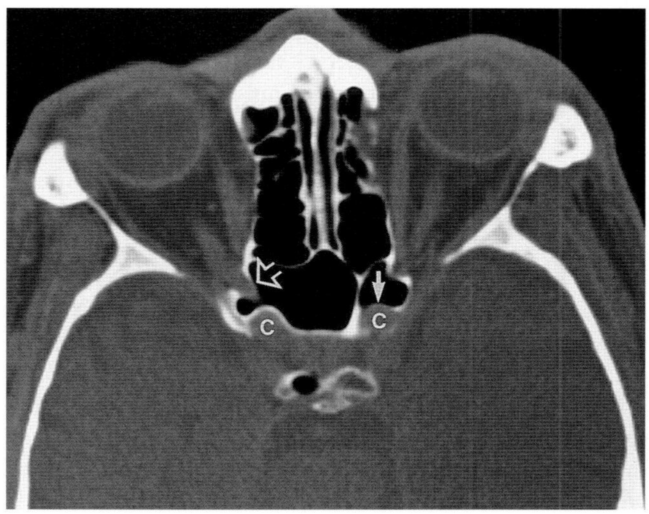


**FIGURE 19.25.** Axial computed tomography image shows both internal carotid arteries *(C)* bulging into the posterior aspect of the sphenoid sinuses. The bony covering over the left carotid canal is dehiscent *(solid arrow)*. Notice the pneumatization of the right sphenoid air cell around the right optic nerve laterally *(open arrow)* and into the dorsum sella posteriorly. There is a dehiscence of the left lamina papyracea from previous medial blow-out fracture.

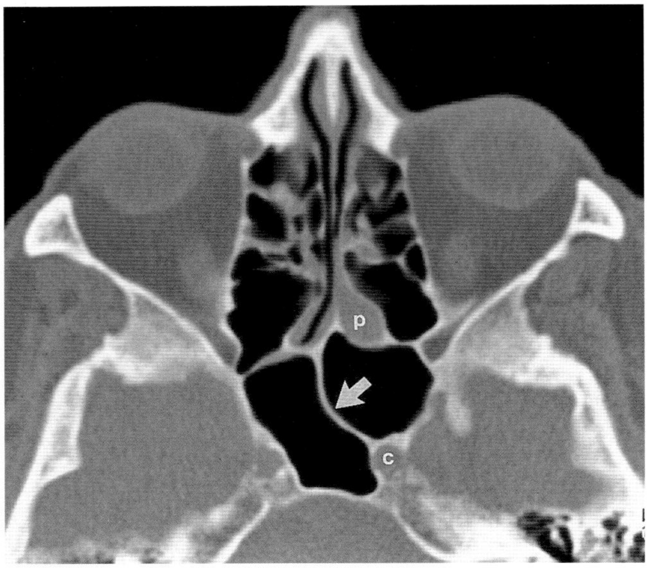


**FIGURE 19.26.** Axial image shows obliquely oriented septation *(arrow)* within the sphenoid fused posteriorly to the bony covering over the left internal carotid artery *(c)*. There is a polyp *(p)* within the left sphenoethmoidal recess. The mucosa is thickened within the ethmoid air cells bilaterally.

covering over the internal carotid artery, predisposing the vessel to injury (Fig. 19.26).

### *Optic Nerve Position*

The optic nerve may course along the roof of the sphenoid sinus or be surrounded by pneumatized portions of the sinus (Fig. 19.25). Optic nerves that bulge into the sphenoid sinus or posterior ethmoid sinuses are at risk for blunt trauma or transection at surgery.

## Miscellaneous Variants

### *Variable Pneumatization of the Frontal Sinus*

Similar to the sphenoid sinus, pneumatization of the frontal sinuses is highly variable. Pneumatization is typically asymmetric. Aplasia and hypoplasia of the frontal sinus is seen in up to 5% of the population. Extensive pneumatization of the frontal sinuses is not uncommon (Fig. 19.27). Extensions into the orbital plate of the frontal bone and into the anterior ethmoids may occur. Extension into the anterior ethmoids may be associated with absence of the ethmoidal bulla.

### *Pneumatization of the Crista Galli*

The crista galli may be aerated, and its ostium drains into the frontal sinus (Fig. 19.28). Obstruction of the ostium may result in mucosal thickening, fluid accumulation, or mucocele formation within this structure (Fig. 19.29). Recognition of this uncommon variant is important to avoid unnecessary extension into the anterior cranial fossa during surgery.

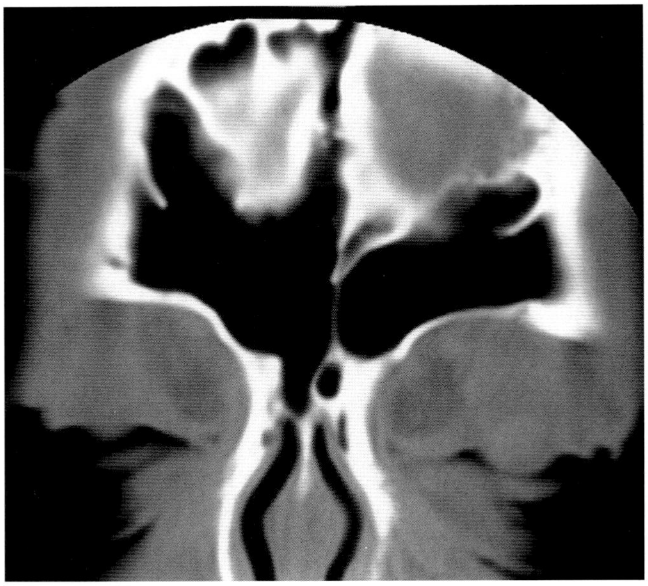

**FIGURE 19.27.** Coronal computed tomography image shows extensive pneumatization of the frontal sinuses with lateral extension over the orbits.

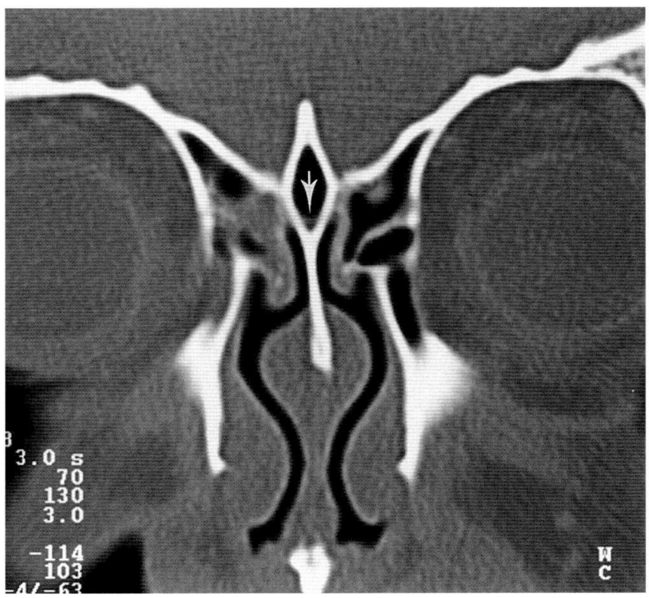


**FIGURE 19.28.** Coronal image shows pneumatization of the crista galli. There is a small amount of mucosal thickening within the inferior aspect of this air cell *(arrow)*. The crista galli drained into the right frontal sinus, which also showed mucosal thickening on more anterior images.

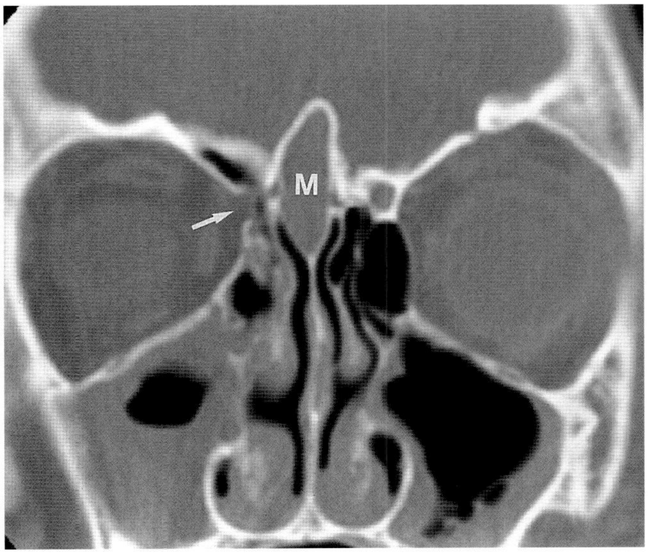


**FIGURE 19.29.** Coronal image shows opacification of a pneumatized crista galli with marked expansion consistent with mucocele formation *(M)*. Mucosal thickening and fluid is seen within the maxillary sinuses and the right ethmoids. There is a small dehiscence of the right lamina papyracea *(arrow)*.

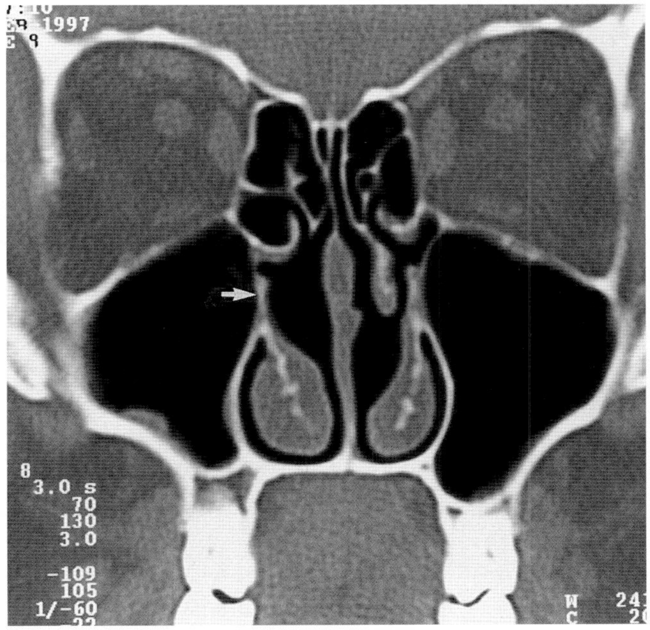


**FIGURE 19.30.** Coronal image at the level of the osteomeatal complexes in a patient after submucosal resection of the septum and right middle turbinectomy. The right uncinate process *(arrow)* was not resected. There is mucosal thickening within the right maxillary sinus.

### *Variable Pneumatization of the Maxillary Sinus*

Four recesses of the maxillary sinuses may be present. Palatine recesses extend medially into the hard palate from the inferior aspect of the maxillary antra. These recesses are bilateral and symmetric. Alveolar recesses are formed by extension of pneumatization into the superior alveolus. These are seen more frequently in edentulous patents. Alveolar recesses are close to the roots of the premolar and molar teeth. Infraorbital recesses result from pneumatization along the roof of the maxillary sinus medial to the groove for the infraorbital nerve. These extensions may be confused with infraorbital ethmoid (Haller) air cells. Extension of pneumatization into the malar bone results in formation of zygomatic recesses.

## POSTOPERATIVE EVALUATION

Postoperative CT evaluation can demonstrate the extent of surgery performed and help in the evaluation of residual or recurrent disease. Imaging studies can also be helpful in the management of surgical complications. Postoperative CT is best performed in the coronal plane. Optimally, the type and extent of surgery is known before scan interpretation so that focus can be placed on the appropriate areas. Specific items to assess after surgery include frontal recess patency; OMC patency; the extent of resection of the uncinate process, ethmoid bulla, and middle turbinate (Figs. 19.30 and 19.31); lamina papyracea contiguity; fovea ethmoidalis

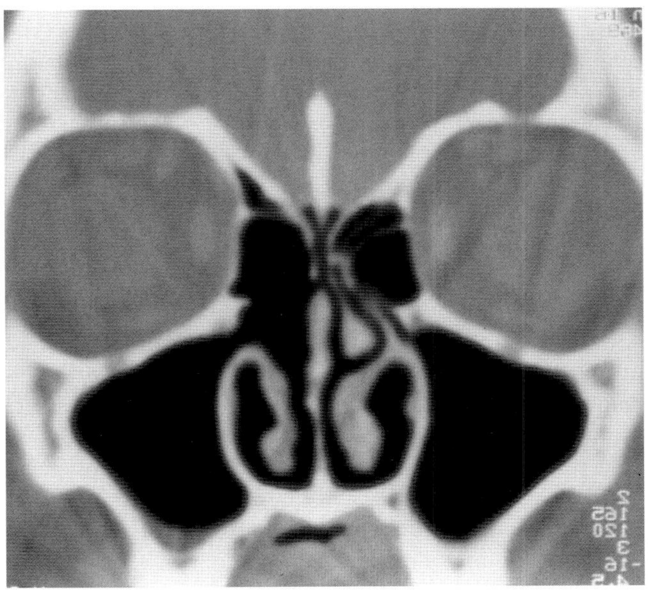

**FIGURE 19.31.** Computed tomography image after endoscopic surgery about the right osteomeatal complex shows a right ethmoidectomy, middle turbinectomy, and uncinectomy. The maxillary ostium is patent. There is minimal mucosal thickening in the alveolar recess of the right maxillary sinus. The lamina papyracea and fovea ethmoidalis are intact.

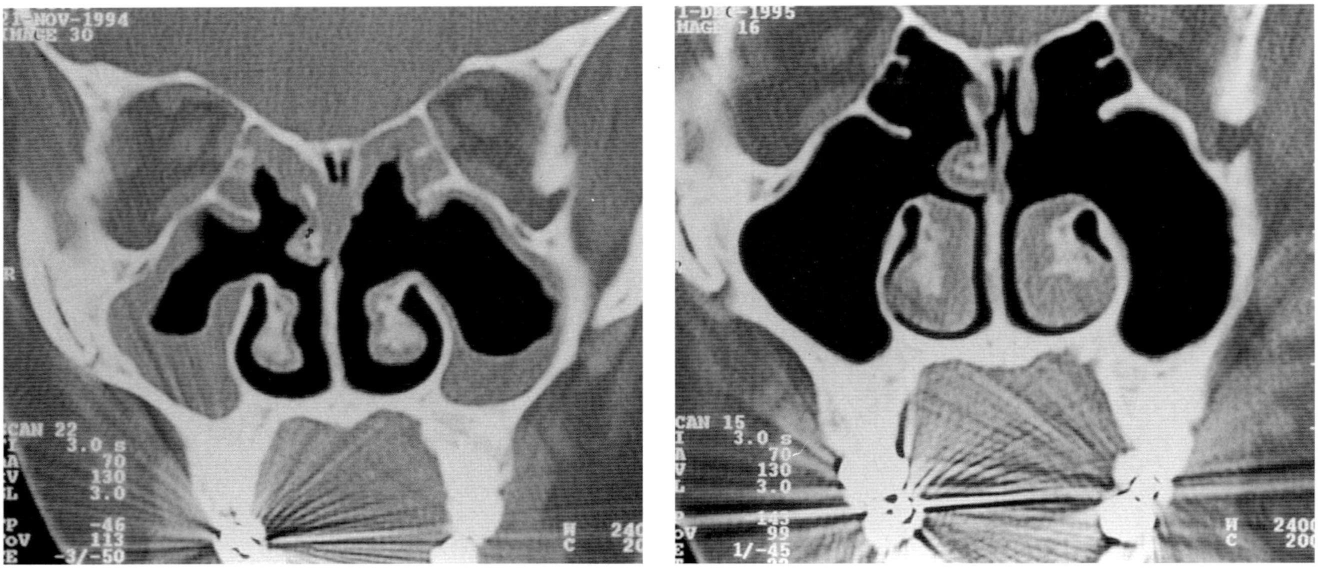

A B

**FIGURE 19.32. A:** Coronal image 1 week after bilateral uncinectomy, ethmoidectomy, and left middle turbinectomy shows circumferential mucosal thickening about the maxillary sinuses and ethmoidectomy cavities. These findings may reflect residual or recurrent disease or indicate postoperative changes this soon after surgery. **B:** Follow-up scan obtained 5 weeks after **A** shows resolution of those postoperative soft tissue changes.

integrity; and sphenoid sinus region for bony contiguity and integrity of adjacent structures such as the carotid arteries and optic nerves.

In the immediate postoperative period, it may be difficult to differentiate between residual or recurrent mucosal disease and expected postoperative soft tissue changes (Fig. 19.32). Imaging evaluation for recurrent disease is therefore best delayed until 6 to 8 weeks after the surgical procedure. Recurrent disease is reported in up to 18% of patients after endoscopic sinus surgery (Fig. 19.33). In addition to defining recurrent and residual disease, CT may demonstrate the formation of synechiae or adhesions between the middle turbinate and lateral nasal wall that can compromise the middle meatus.

Minor complications, including nasal synechiae, mild epistaxis, mild periorbital edema and hematoma, mild orbital or subcutaneous emphysema, and facial or tooth pain, generally do not require imaging evaluation. These minor complications typically resolve without intervention (11). CT or MRI may be indicated in cases of suspected injury to the orbit, brain, and internal carotid artery. MRI is the study of choice for evaluation of most intracranial complications of endoscopic surgery.

Orbital complications can include orbital emphysema, nasolacrimal duct injury, hematoma, abscess, breach of the lamina papyracea, medial rectus contusion or transection, and optic nerve injury. Injury to the lamina papyracea often occurs as the site of attachment of the basal lamella. Focal swelling or increased density within the belly of the medial rectus belly suggests injury to the muscle when associated with a defect in the medial orbital wall. Orbital hematomas may result from venous bleeding or arterial bleeding from injury to the anterior ethmoidal artery during ethmoidectomy. Hematomas appear as slightly hyperdense collections relative to other soft tissues on CT (Fig. 19.34).

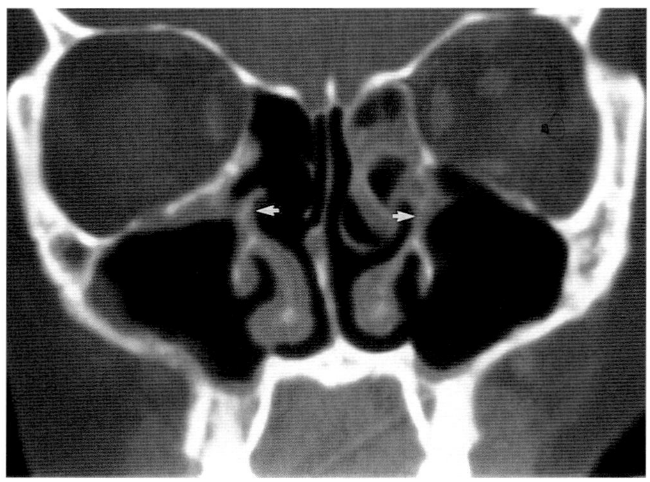

**FIGURE 19.33.** Postoperative coronal computed tomography image shows bilateral inferior antrostomies, right ethmoidectomy, and right middle turbinectomy. The uncinate processes *(arrows)* were not removed. The osteomeatal complexes are occluded by mucosal thickening bilaterally, and there is mucosal thickening within the maxillary sinuses and left ethmoids.

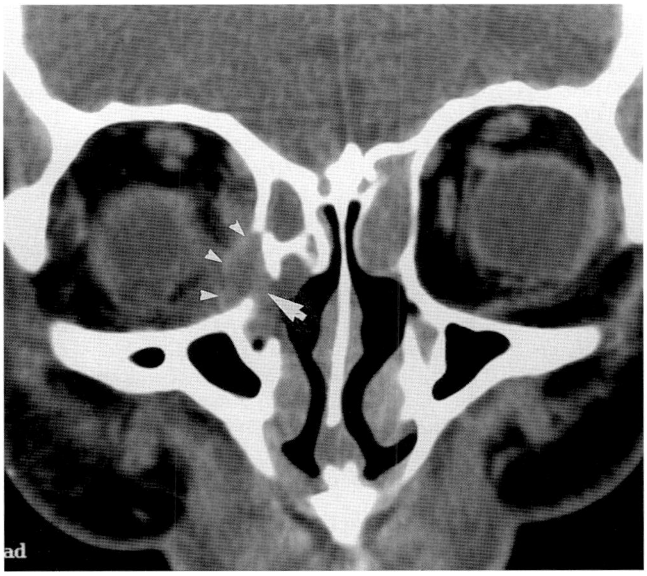


**FIGURE 19.34.** Coronal image with soft tissue windowing shows breach of the right lamina papyracea *(arrow)* that occurred during endoscopic surgery. There is an extraconal soft tissue mass *(arrowheads)* lateral to the bony defect consistent with hematoma.

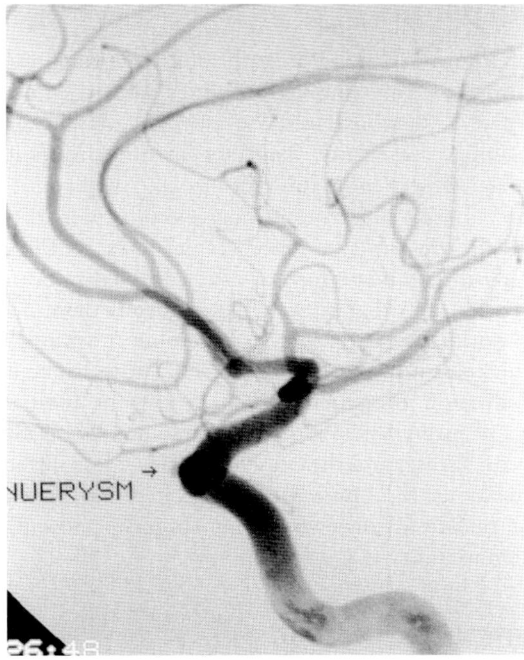


**FIGURE 19.35.** Digital subtraction angiographic image obtained in a patient with severe epistaxis after endoscopic sphenoid surgery. Left internal carotid artery injection shows small pseudoaneurysm projecting anteromedially from the internal carotid at the site of surgical injury. The vessel was subsequently sacrificed, with coils placed endovascularly.

Arterial injuries resulting in severe epistaxis may be caused by injury to the anterior ethmoidal artery or the internal carotid artery. Anterior ethmoidal artery injury is typically recognized immediately and treated surgically. Conventional angiography may be performed to determine the presence of and exact site of vessel injury. Internal carotid artery pseudoaneurysms appear as focal outpouchings from the vessel (Fig. 19.35). Pseudoaneurysms resulting from surgical trauma may be treated endovascularly with coiling of the pseudoaneurysm or internal carotid artery sacrifice, or they may be surgically clipped.

Fortunately, intracranial complications from endoscopic sinus surgery are unusual. Intracranial complications result from breach of the cribriform plate, fovea ethmoidalis, or sphenoid roof. The thin lateral lamella of the cribriform plate is the most common location for surgical injury. Complications may include postoperative cerebrospinal fluid (CSF) leak, pneumocephalus, subarachnoid hemorrhage, parenchymal hematoma, meningitis, cerebritis, brain abscess, and meningoencephalocele formation (Fig. 19.36). CSF leak can initially be evaluated with thin-section (1- to 2-mm) coronal CT. If a bony dehiscence within the cribriform plate, fovea ethmoidalis, or sphenoid roof is not demonstrated, cisternography can be performed with intrathecal contrast administration followed by CT. Unenhanced CT of the head is the initial study of choice for the evaluation of subarachnoid or parenchymal hemorrhage and pneumocephalus. MRI is the preferred modality for evaluation of intracranial infection and identification of meningoencephaloceles.

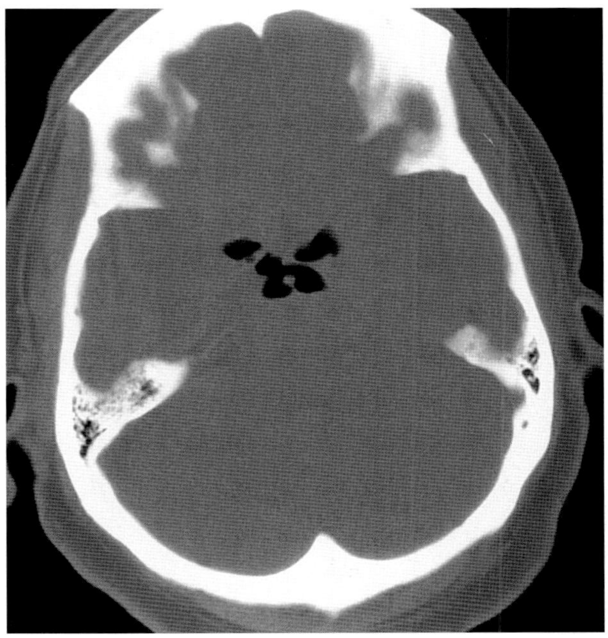

**FIGURE 19.36.** Axial computed tomography of the head with bone window technique in a patient with cerebrospinal fluid leak after endoscopic ethmoidectomy shows pneumocephalus within the suprasellar cistern.

## CONCLUSIONS

High-resolution CT is the study of choice for presurgical evaluation of the sinonasal cavities before endoscopic surgery. CT demonstrates the normal anatomy of the sinuses and nasal cavity, identifies anatomic variants that may make surgery more difficult or make the patient prone to injury during surgery, and may show incidental pathology within the orbits, anterior cranial fossa, or skull base. Scanning should be performed after completion of medical interventions, so that irreversible disease is demonstrated. CT is optimally performed in the prone position with a slice thickness no larger than 3 mm. CT can also be used in the evaluation of patients after surgery to evaluate the extent of surgical resection, the presence of residual or recurrent disease, and the presence of orbital or intracranial complications. MRI may also be indicated in the evaluation of complications of endoscopic surgery, particularly if intracranial injury is suspected.

## REFERENCES

1. Moss A, Parsons V. Current estimates from the National Health Interview Survey, United States, 1985. Hyattsville, MD: National Center for Health Statistics, 1986.
2. Kennedy DW, Zinreich SJ, Rosenbaum AE, et al. Functional endoscopic sinus surgery. Theory and diagnostic evaluation. *Arch Otolaryngol* 1985;111:576–582.
3. Rice DH. Endoscopic sinus surgery: results at 2-year followup. *Otolaryngol Head Neck Surg* 1989;101:476–479.
4. Schaefer SD, Manning S, Close LG. Endoscopic paranasal sinus surgery: indications and considerations. *Laryngoscope* 1989;99: 1–5.
5. Zinreich SJ, Kennedy DW, Rosenbaum AE, et al. Paranasal sinuses: CT imaging requirements for endoscopic surgery. *Radiology* 1987;163:769–775.
6. Laine FJ, Smoker WRK. The ostiomeatal unit and endoscopic surgery: anatomy, variations, and imaging findings in inflammatory diseases. *AJR Am J Roentgenol* 1992;159:849–857.
7. Mafee MF, Chow JM, Meyers R. Functional endoscopic sinus surgery: anatomy, CT screening, indications, and complications. *AJR Am J Roentgenol* 1993;160:735–744.
8. Babbel R, Harnsberger HR, Nelson B, et al. Optimization of techniques in screening CT of the sinuses. *AJNR Am J Neuroradiol* 1991;12:849–854.
9. Zinreich SJ, Benson ML, Oliverio PJ. Sinonasal cavities: CT normal anatomy, imaging of the osteomeatal complex, and functional endoscopic surgery. In: Som PM, Curtin HD, eds. *Head and neck imaging*, 3rd ed. Chicago: Mosby, 1996:97–125.
10. Earwaker J. Anatomic variants in sinonasal CT. *Radiographics* 1993;13:381–415.
11. Hudgins PA, Browning DG, Gallups J, et al. Endoscopic paranasal sinus surgery: radiologic evaluation of severe complications. *AJNR Am J Neuroradiol* 1992;13:1161–1167.

# 20

# ENDOSCOPIC PARANASAL SINUS SURGERY

DALE H. RICE

## ENDOSCOPIC PARANASAL SINUS SURGERY: ANTERIOR-TO-POSTERIOR APPROACH

### Indications

Endoscopic sinus surgery is based on two principles. First, obstruction in the anterior ethmoid may block the maxillary, frontal, and posterior ethmoid sinuses and, occasionally, the sphenoid sinus and eustachian tube. Stated another way, persistent disease in one of these sinuses most likely results from undiagnosed, untreated anterior ethmoid disease (1). Second, relief of obstruction in the anterior ethmoids may allow the other sinuses to drain and return to normal. The maxillary sinus ostium in particular lies in a gutter the infundibulum, where the purulent drainage from the ethmoids pours across it. It is implied in this concept that the mucosal disease is reversible with adequate drainage (2,3).

This technique is indicated whenever adequate medical management has failed in bacterial sinusitis. It is the first intervention of choice, and the technique often gives good results with minimum morbidity and rapid recovery.

### Contraindications

There are probably no absolute contraindications to this technique other than complicated frontal sinusitis, when more traditional techniques should be used. This approach would be inadequate for frontal sinusitis with an epidural or subdural abscess. A relative contraindication, particularly in inexperienced hands, would be ethmoiditis with an orbital complication. Extensive recurrent or chronic disease is probably better managed by a total sphenoethmoidectomy.

### Case Example

A 42-year-old woman had a 5-year history of recurrent right maxillary sinusitis. She had undergone numerous courses of antibiotics. With each course, the facial pain and mucopurulent rhinorrhea eventually stopped, only to recur within a few weeks. Two separate antral windows with irrigations failed.

Rhinoscopy revealed mucopurulent rhinorrhea coming from the middle meatus. The remainder of the physical examination findings were normal. A computed tomography (CT) scan (Fig. 20.1) revealed a completely opacified right maxillary sinus with obvious obstruction at the osteomeatal unit.

The patient underwent right endoscopic sinus surgery with removal of the uncinate process and bulla ethmoidalis. On completion of this operation, the opening to the maxillary sinus could be seen easily and was of adequate size, not needing to be enlarged. The patient did well postoperatively, and a CT scan (Fig. 20.2) showed complete clearing of the right maxillary sinus and an open osteomeatal unit (Fig. 20.3).

### Instrumentation

Richards, Karl Storz, and Richard Wolf make instruments that serve admirably for this operative technique (Fig. 20.4). The endoscopes come in different diameters and different optical axes. Most of the work in this technique can be performed with the 0°, 30°, and 70° or the wide-angle 25° or 30° and 70° endoscopes in 4-mm diameters. Much of the dissection can be performed with the 45° Weil-Blakesley forceps. The straight-biting, 90°, and reverse-biting forceps are frequently useful. A through-cut design is generally preferable, because this removes mucosa and bone more cleanly with less tearing of mucosa and with less denuded bone left behind.

### Anesthesia

Endoscopic sinus surgery can be performed under local or general anesthesia, depending on the preferences of

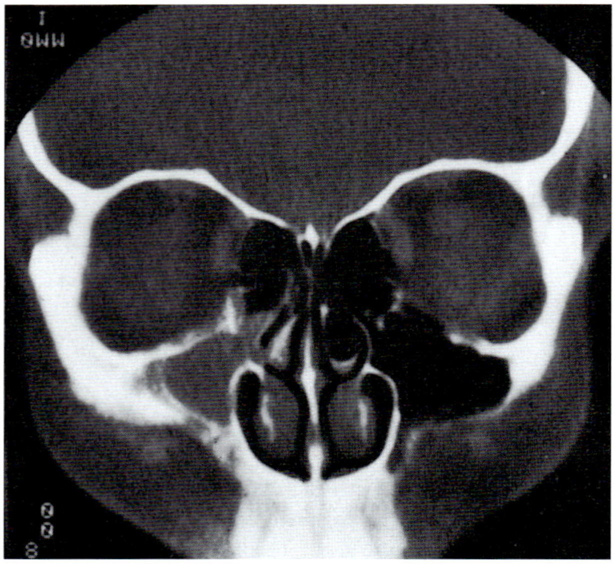

**FIGURE 20.1.** Axial computed tomography shows the opacified right maxillary sinus and obstructed osteomeatal complex. (From Rice DH, Schaefer SD, eds. *Endoscopic paranasal sinus surgery,* 2nd ed. New York: Raven Press, 1993, with permission.)

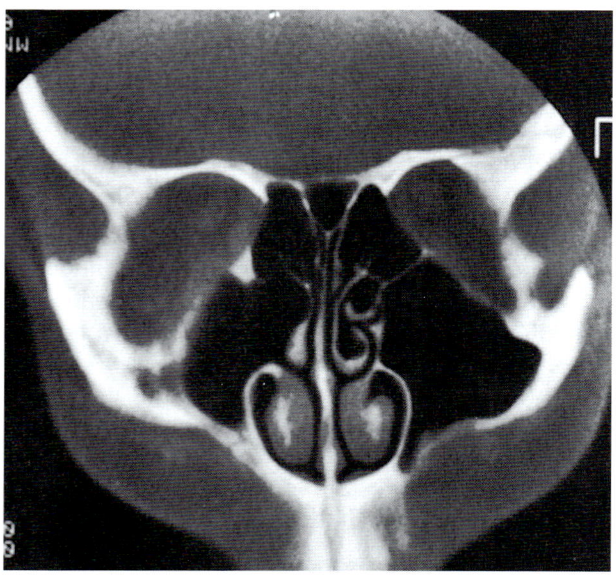

**FIGURE 20.2.** Postoperative computed tomography scan of the patient in Figure 20.1, showing complete clearing. (From Rice DH, Schaefer SD, eds. *Endoscopic paranasal sinus surgery,* 2nd ed. New York: Raven Press, 1993, with permission.)

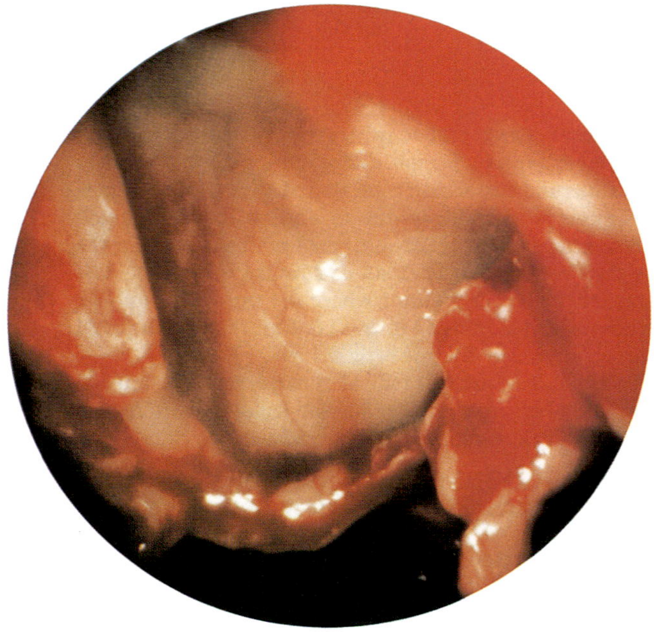

**FIGURE 20.3.** Endoscopic view of a middle meatal antrostomy. (From Rice DH, Schaefer SD, eds. *Endoscopic paranasal sinus surgery,* 2nd ed. New York: Raven Press, 1993, with permission.)

the surgeon and the patient. In either case, thorough vasoconstriction is imperative. This may be started in the preanesthetic holding area with Afrin or some other vasoconstrictive spray. In the operating room, the nasal cavity should be packed with Cottonoids, soaked (but wrung out) in 1% lidocaine with 1:100,000 epinephrine. After 5 minutes, the cotton pledgets should be removed, and the middle turbinate and lateral nasal wall is injected with 1% lidocaine with 1:100,000 epinephrine. It is frequently helpful also to inject the adjacent nasal septum if the mucosa is edematous. After the injections, another Cottonoid soaked in 1% lidocaine with 1:100,000 epinephrine should be inserted directly into the middle meatus. Another 5 minutes should be allowed to pass. For this technique, no more than 3 to 5 mL are needed per side. If there are significant polyps, they may be removed at this time in the traditional fashion with a headlight and forceps or with a microdebrider.

In 20% to 30% of patients, a septoplasty is indicated to correct nasal obstruction independent of the sinus disease or to remove a septal deflection at the level of the middle turbinate preventing adequate access for the instruments to perform the procedure or to perform adequate postoperative care. If indicated, the septoplasty should be performed first or second (i.e., after surgery on the open side but preceding surgery on the narrow side if necessary). Theoretically, elective septoplasty should be postponed to avoid exposing the septal cartilage to infection. In practice, this does not seem to pose a significant risk.

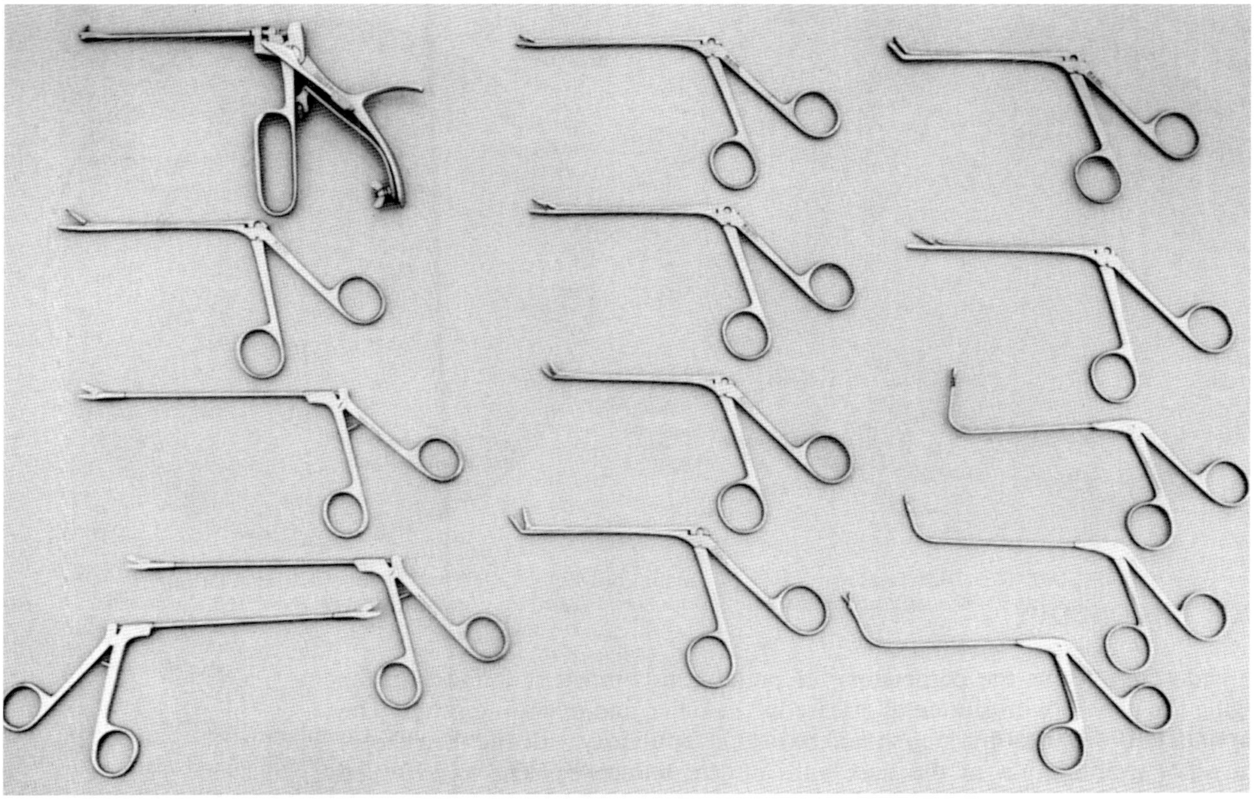

A

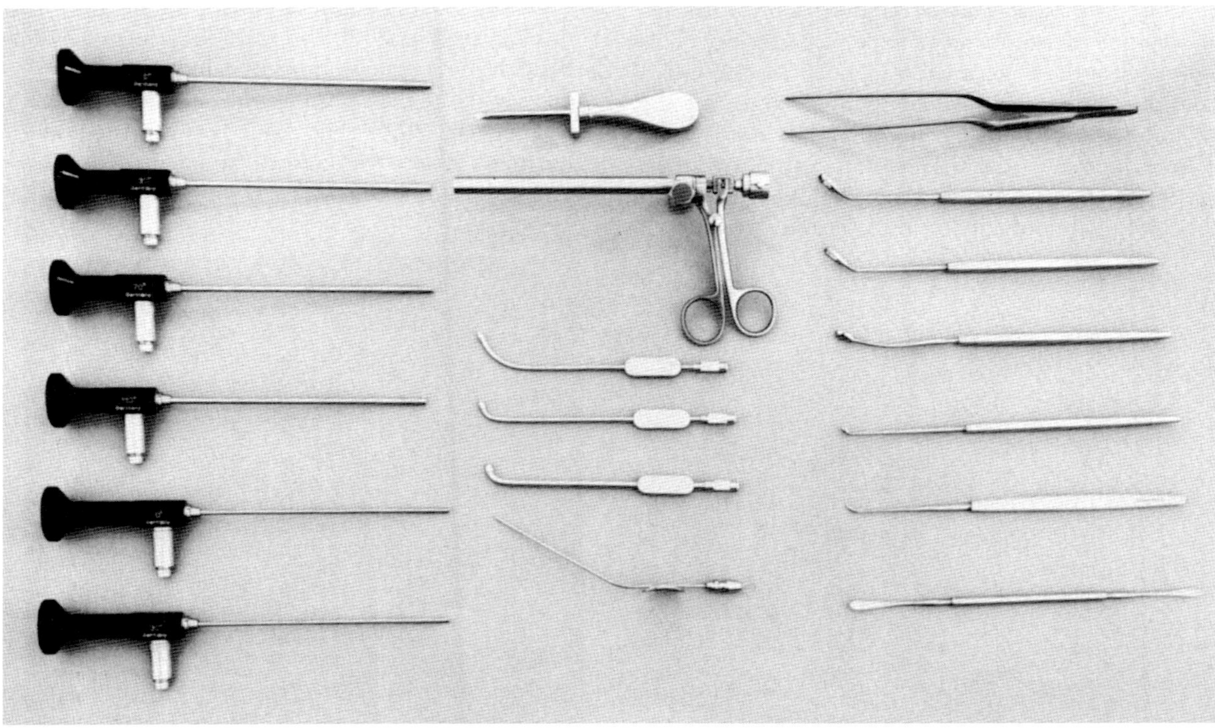

B

**FIGURE 20.4. A,B:** Examples of instruments and endoscopes available. (From Rice DH, Schaefer SD, eds. *Endoscopic paranasal sinus surgery,* 2nd ed. New York: Raven Press, 1993, with permission.)

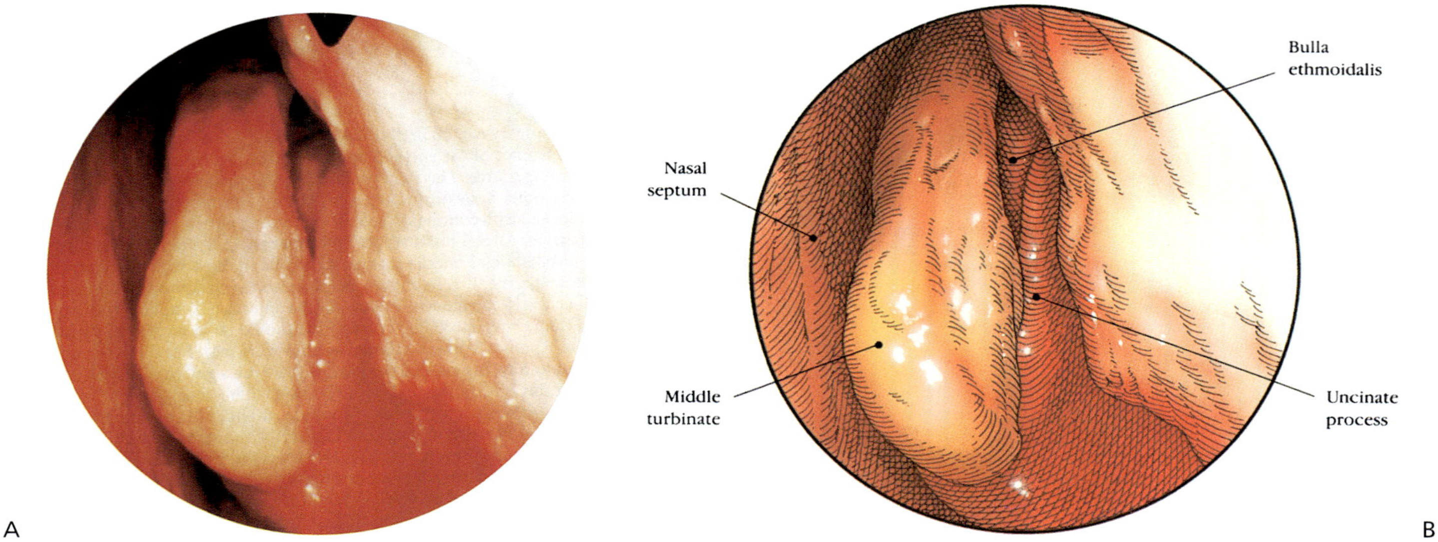


**FIGURE 20.5. A,B:** Endoscopic view and artist's drawing of a left middle meatus. (From Rice DH, Schaefer SD, eds. *Endoscopic paranasal sinus surgery,* 2nd ed. New York: Raven Press, 1993, with permission.)

## Operative Technique

### *Principal Maneuvers*

*Step 1:* Once the nasal mucosa is thoroughly vasoconstricted, a complete examination should be performed. This is best done with the 0° or a wide-angle 25° or 30° endoscope and should be performed gently to avoid tearing the mucosa and causing annoying bleeding. The nasal cavity should be examined systematically, with particular attention paid to the middle meatus (Figs. 20.5 and 20.6) and any other area of abnormality on the CT scan.

*Step 2:* The initial maneuver is to remove the uncinate process, which usually is immediately lateral to the anterior middle turbinate. This can be performed most elegantly by making an incision with the sickle knife or Cottle elevator (Fig. 20.7) and spreading the mucosa medially. Blakesley or Takahashi forceps can then be inserted so that one jaw is in the incision and one jaw is in the middle meatus (Fig. 20.8). The tissue between the jaws (i.e., the uncinate process) is grasped and removed. This should

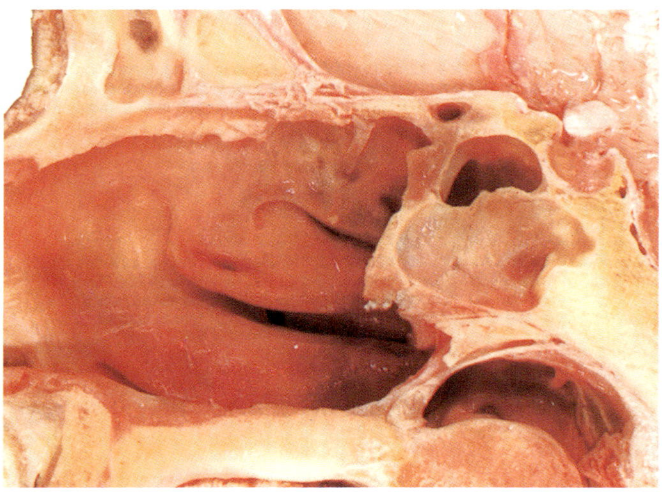

**FIGURE 20.6.** Parasagittal section shows the lateral nasal wall. (From Rice DH, Schaefer SD, eds. *Endoscopic paranasal sinus surgery,* 2nd ed. New York: Raven Press, 1993, with permission.)

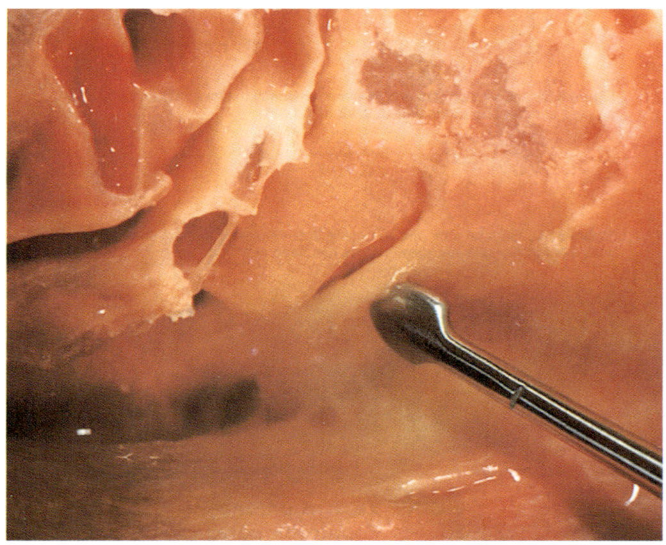

**FIGURE 20.7.** Photograph of the lateral nasal wall with the middle turbinate removed. The Cottle elevator is poised for uncinectomy incision. (From Rice DH, Schaefer SD, eds. *Endoscopic paranasal sinus surgery,* 2nd ed. New York: Raven Press, 1993, with permission.)

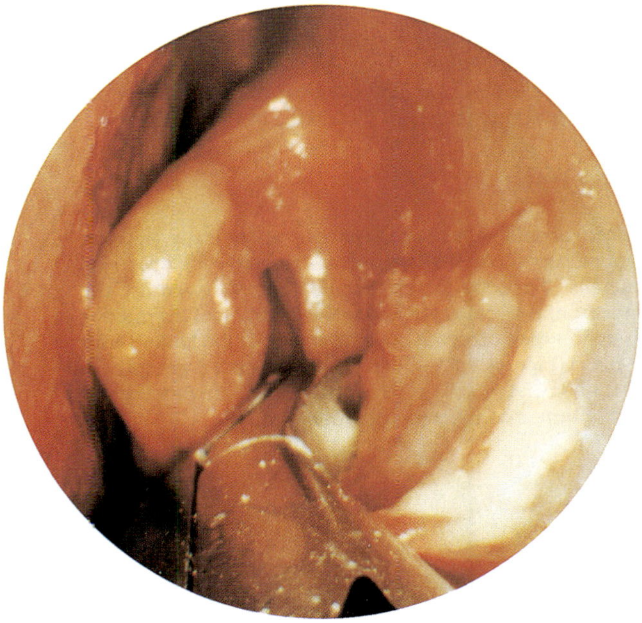

**FIGURE 20.8.** Endoscopic view of forceps removing an uncinate process. (From Rice DH, Schaefer SD, eds. *Endoscopic paranasal sinus surgery,* 2nd ed. New York: Raven Press, 1993, with permission.)

establish the initial correct plane of dissection. Bear in mind that the ethmoids are approximately 0.5 cm wide in this region.

*Step 3:* From this point on, the forceps should be held so the jaws open vertically, opening and closing parallel to the lamina papyracea. It is imprudent to turn the forceps so the pointed tips are directed laterally, unless the location of the lamina is precisely known. In general, the lamina lies in the same parasagittal plane as the maxillary ostium. Next, the forceps should be used to remove the remainder of the uncinate, if any, from the frontal recess superiorly to the insertion of the inferior turbinate inferiorly. The dissection then proceeds posteriorly across the hiatus semilunaris into the bulla ethmoidalis (Fig. 20.9). The bulla is treated similarly to the uncinate (Figs. 20.10 and 20.11). By removing the uncinate process and bulla ethmoidalis, the infundibulum is completely decompressed. In classic osteomeatal disease, the bulla eth-

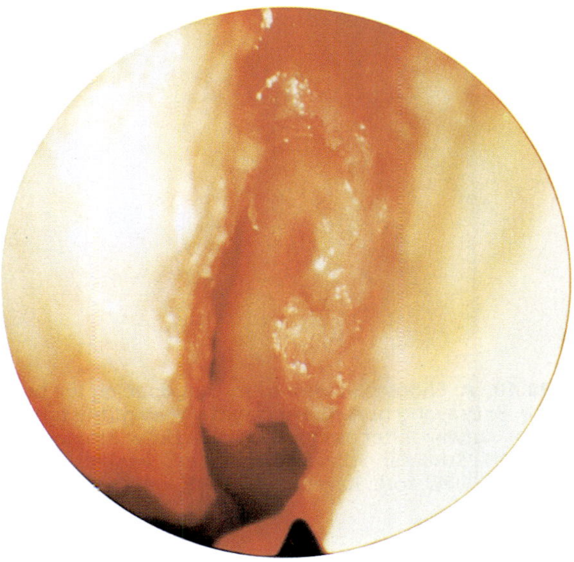

A

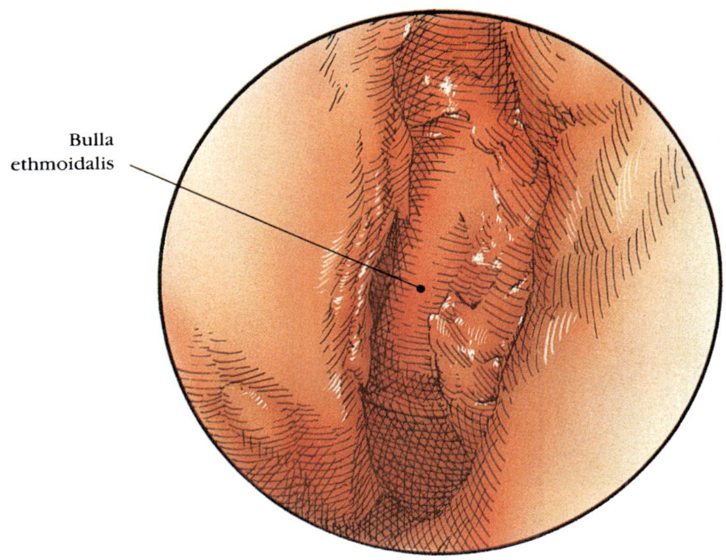


B

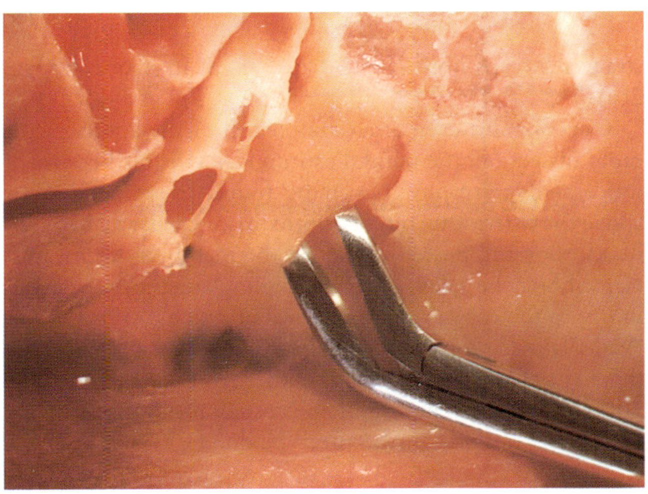

C

**FIGURE 20.9. A:** Endoscopic view with the uncinate removed. **B:** Drawing of **A**. **C:** Parasagittal view of forceps poised to open bulla ethmoidalis. (From Rice DH, Schaefer SD, eds. *Endoscopic paranasal sinus surgery,* 2nd ed. New York: Raven Press, 1993, with permission.)

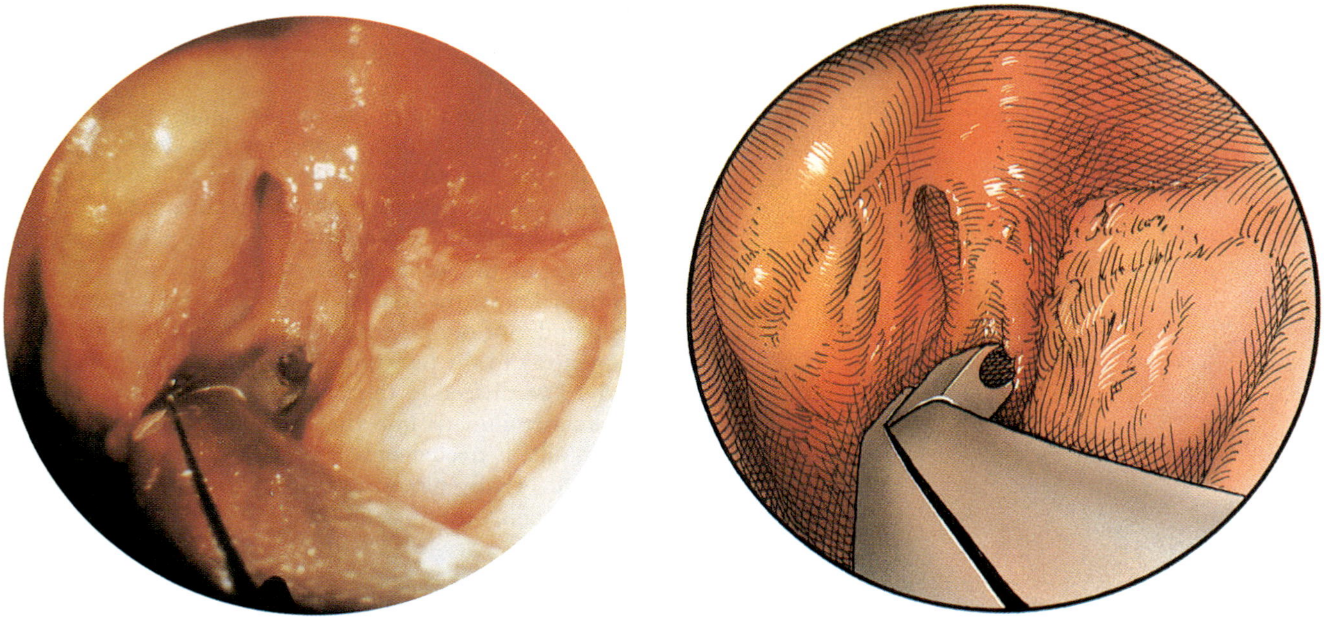

A

B

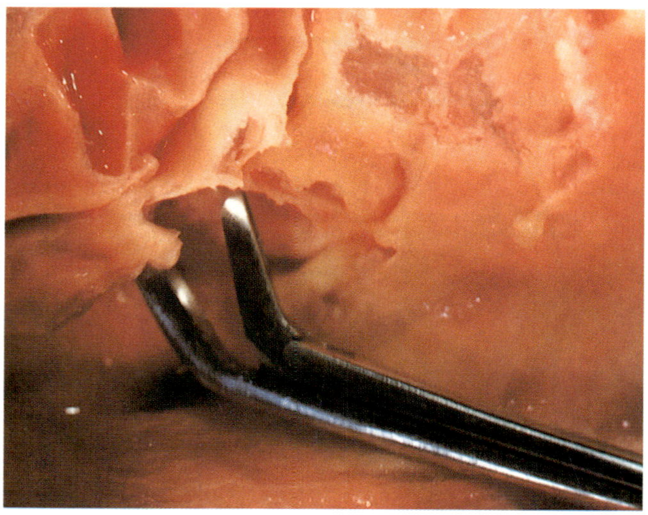

C

**FIGURE 20.10. A:** Endoscopic view of forceps opening the bulla ethmoidalis. **B:** Drawing of **A. C:** Parasagittal view of the forceps at the basal lamella after removal of the bulla ethmoidalis. (From Rice DH, Schaefer SD, eds. *Endoscopic paranasal sinus surgery,* 2nd ed. New York: Raven Press, 1993, with permission.)

moidalis may only need to be opened medially. A complete removal is probably unnecessary.

*Step 4:* At this point, the operation would be completed if there were no sinus disease other than the anterior ethmoids (Fig. 20.12). Usually, however, this is not the case. Most commonly, there is also maxillary sinus disease, and in that situation, the next step is to identify the natural ostium. Usually, this cannot be identified earlier in the procedure but often becomes visible as the inferior aspect of the uncinate and bulla are widely opened. If the natural ostium seems patent at this point, nothing further need be done. If it is not or if it is in question, it should be enlarged anteriorly using the reverse biting forceps or posteriorly with the straight forceps until it is 1.5 to 2.0 cm in diameter (Fig. 20.13).

Occasionally, even after completion of the anterior ethmoid dissection, the natural ostium is not visible because of mucosal hypertrophy. It can be found by palpating just above the inferior turbinate approximately halfway between its anterior and posterior ends in the membranous meatus. Care should be taken to avoid angling superiorly to avoid injury to the orbit. Gentle removal of mucosa with the 45° Weil-Blakesley forceps in this location will usually uncover the natural ostium, which should then be enlarged (Fig. 20.14). If the patient's problem is osteomeatal complex disease alone, nothing further need be done.

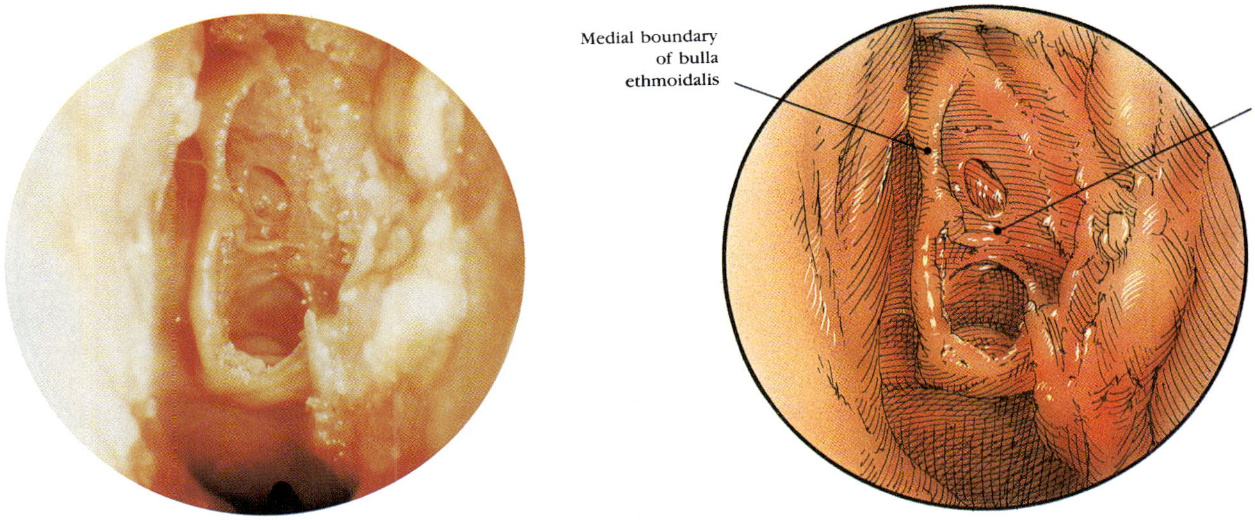


A

B

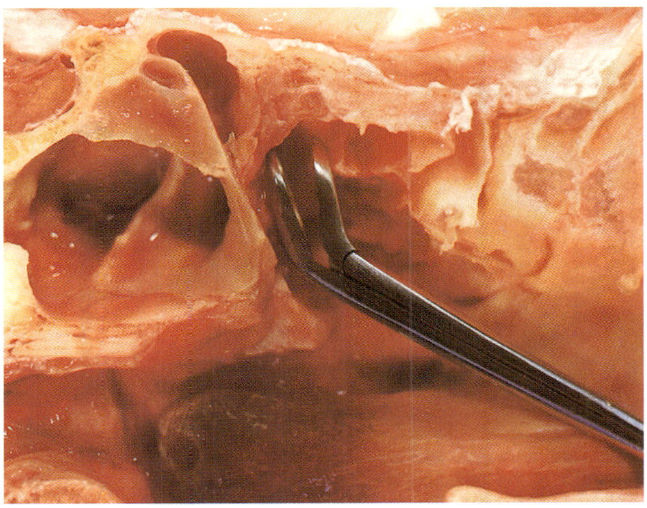

C

**FIGURE 20.11. A:**Endoscopic view of basal lamella after removal of uncinate and bulla. **B:** Drawing of **A. C:** Parasagittal view of forceps within posterior ethmoid air cells. (From Rice DH, Schaefer SD, eds. *Endoscopic paranasal sinus surgery,* 2nd ed. New York: Raven Press, 1993, with permission.)

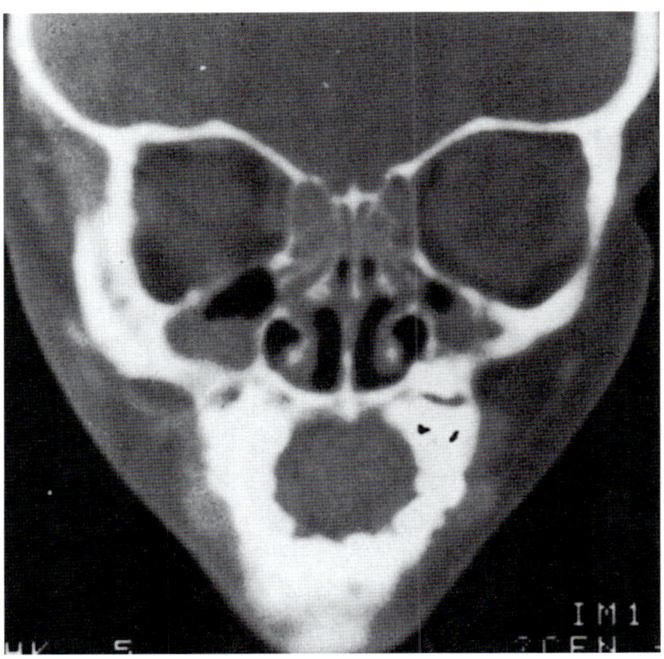

**FIGURE 20.12.** Coronal computed tomography scan shows typical anterior ethmoid and maxillary sinus disease. (From Rice DH, Schaefer SD, eds. *Endoscopic paranasal sinus surgery,* 2nd ed. New York: Raven Press, 1993, with permission.)

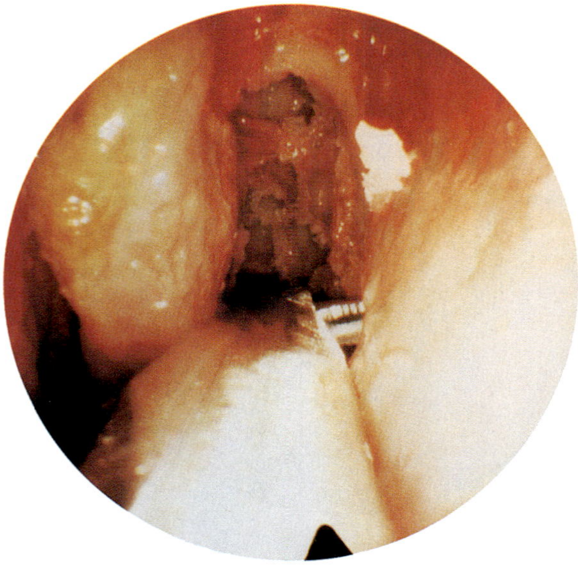

A

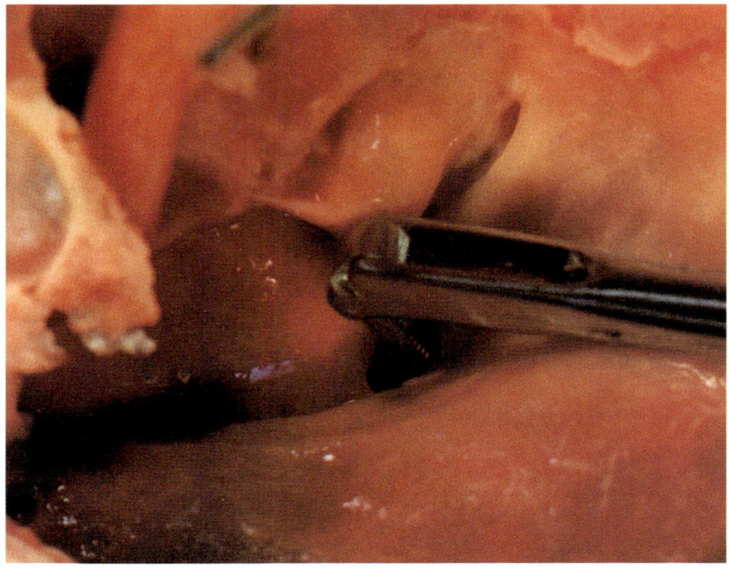

B

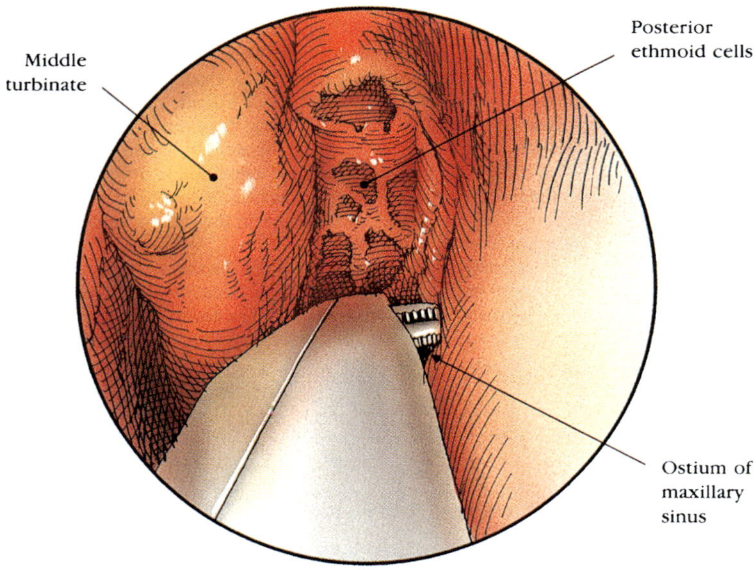


C

**FIGURE 20.13. A:** Endoscopic view of retrograde forceps enlarging maxillary ostium. **B:** Parasagittal view of the same subject. **C:** Drawing of **A**. (From Rice DH, Schaefer SD, eds. *Endoscopic paranasal sinus surgery,* 2nd ed. New York: Raven Press, 1993, with permission.)

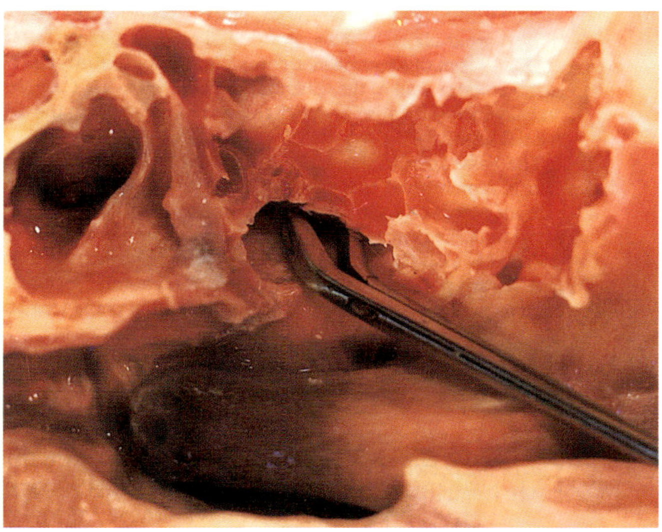

**FIGURE 20.14.** Forceps enlarging the maxillary ostium. (From Rice DH, Schaefer SD, eds. *Endoscopic paranasal sinus surgery,* 2nd ed. New York: Raven Press, 1993, with permission.)

### *Additional Maneuvers*

*Step 5:* If the patient also has *posterior ethmoid disease*, further dissection is indicated. At the completion of the preceding steps, the posterior limit of the operative field should be the basal (ground) lamella (Fig. 20.11A). This bony partition extends from the middle turbinate to the lamina papyracea and separates the anterior from the posterior ethmoid air cells. This partition should be penetrated in its vertical portion and the posterior cells entered. From this approach, a complete ethmoidectomy can be performed, stopping at the anterior wall of the sphenoid (Fig. 20.15). Care should be taken both laterally and superiorly because of the changing relationships to the orbit and to the anterior cranial fossa.

The basal lamella should be penetrated medially and inferiorly. It must be constantly remembered that the floor of the anterior cranial fossa slopes inferiorly as it extends posteriorly. The surgeon should think of entering the posterior ethmoids as a rotation downward of the instruments as much as an advancement of them. Progress should continue posteriorly along the lateral edge of the middle turbinate until the sphenoid is identified. The sphenoid ostium can usually be identified just posterior to the inferior edge of the superior turbinate. At this point, a complete ethmoidectomy can be performed with constant reference to the sphenoid posteriorly, the lamina papyracea laterally, and the skull base superiorly.

*Step 6:* If there is also *sphenoid disease*, the sphenoid can be entered after completion of the posterior ethmoidectomy (Fig. 20.16). The natural ostium usually can be identified just inferior and posterior to the inferior tip of the superior turbinate and can be enlarged in an inferior and medial direction. It is probably not wise to enlarge the ostium superiorly or laterally unless certain of the proximity of the superior and lateral walls. If the natural ostium cannot be

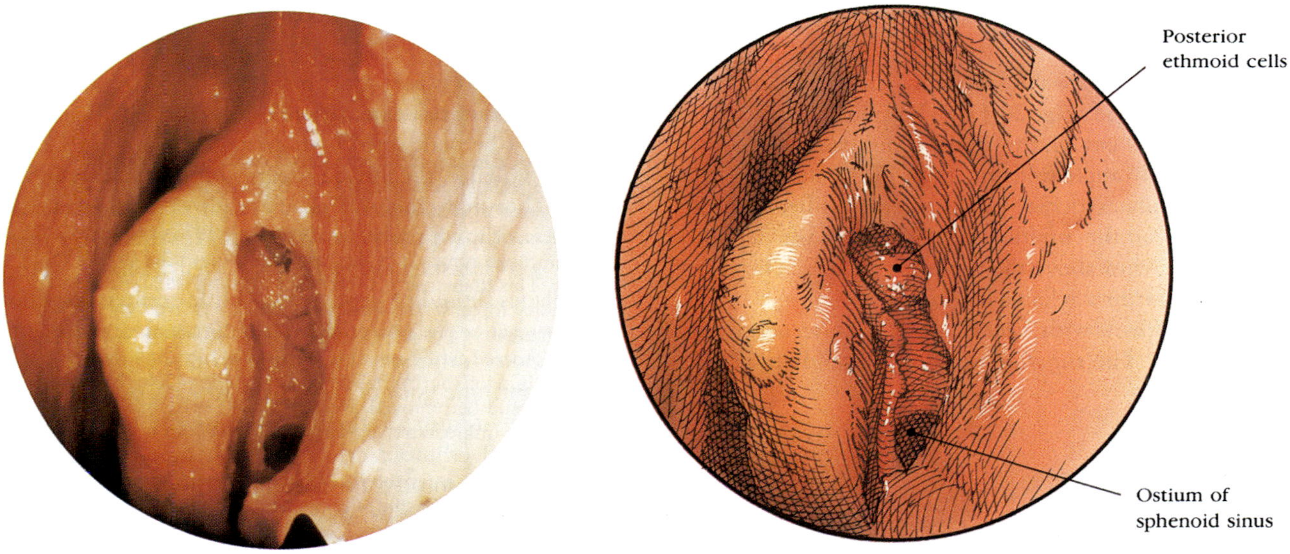


A

B

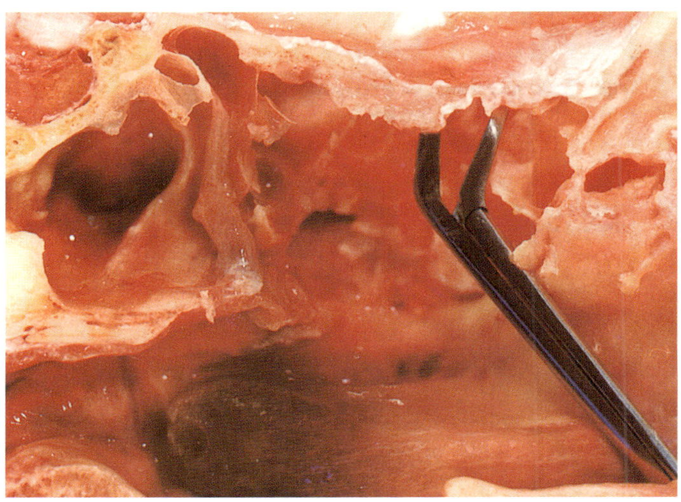

C

**FIGURE 20.15. A:** Endoscopic view after exenteration of the posterior ethmoid air cells. **B:**Illustration of **A. C:** Parasagittal view of angled forceps clearing air cells from the skull base. (From Rice DH, Schaefer SD, eds. *Endoscopic paranasal sinus surgery,* 2nd ed. New York: Raven Press, 1993, with permission.)

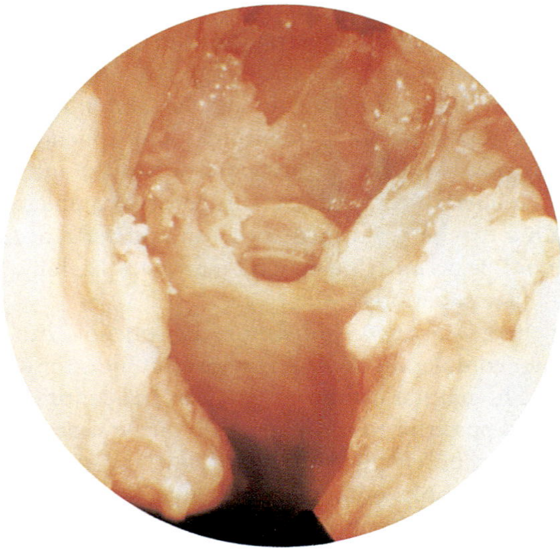

A

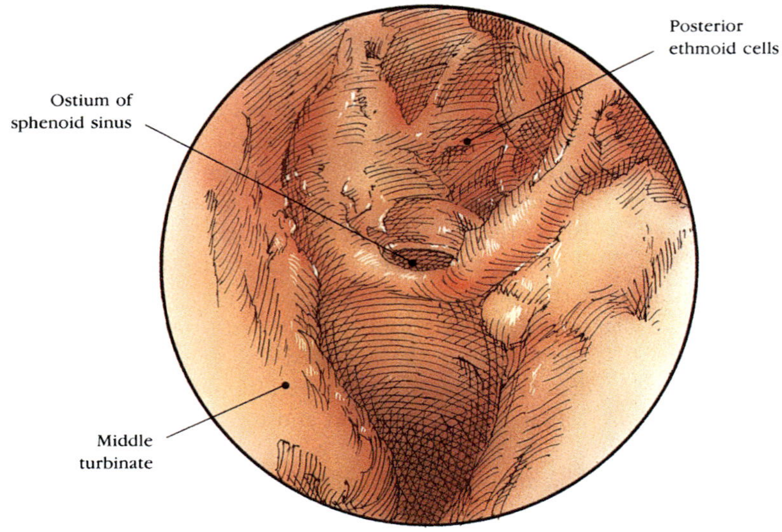


B

**FIGURE 20.16. A:** Endoscopic view of the posterior ethmoids with the sphenoid sinus ostium in view. **B:** Illustration of **A**. (From Rice DH, Schaefer SD, eds. *Endoscopic paranasal sinus surgery,* 2nd ed. New York: Raven Press, 1993, with permission.)

identified, the anterior wall of the sinus may be entered and the opening enlarged (Fig. 20.17). The sphenoid should be entered within 1 cm of the middle turbinate and never higher than a 30° angle from the floor of the nose. If there is doubt, the sphenoid may safely be entered between the posterior end of the middle turbinate and the septum, about 10 to 12 mm above the posterior choana. The superior turbinate forms a reliable landmark.

*Step 7:* In patients with *frontal sinus disease*, an additional step is required. The superior-anterior ethmoid air cells in

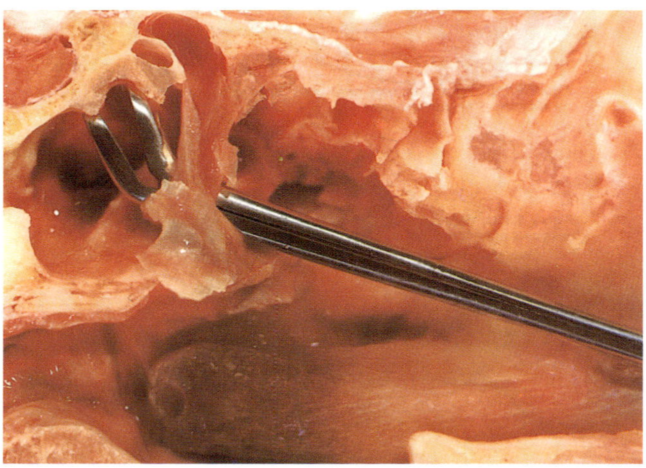

**FIGURE 20.17.** Parasagittal view of forceps within the sphenoid sinus. (From Rice DH, Schaefer SD, eds. *Endoscopic paranasal sinus surgery,* 2nd ed. New York: Raven Press, 1993, with permission.)

the frontal recess area must be opened, and the nasofrontal duct or ostium must be cleared of obstruction (Fig. 20.18). This must be performed with an angled endoscope to adequately visualize the area to ensure complete clearing of the duct. Thorough removal of these air cells is essential to ensure continued adequate drainage. This maneuver is most easily accomplished using the 45° Weil-Blakesley forceps. The blades should be kept vertical while exenterating the air cells immediately posterior to the anterior attachment of the middle turbinate. The surgeon should proceed cautiously until the floor of the frontal sinus is reached. At this point, the ostium of the frontal sinus is usually visible. Mucosa and ethmoid cells around it should be removed. The ostium is located posteriorly in the frontal sinus, and immediately posterior to the ostium is the fovea ethmoidalis. Mucosa usually should not be stripped from the ostium itself.

Occasionally, it may be necessary to enter the frontal sinus. Specially curved forceps are available for this purpose. The duct can be enlarged all the way into the sinus, but this step is rarely necessary (Fig. 20.19).

*Step 8:* In cases of *concha bullosa* disease, an air cell within the middle turbinate must be opened if it is diseased or if it has expanded the turbinate so that the lateral aspect encroaches on the middle meatus. This is best managed by entering the air cell at the anterior end of the middle turbinate with a sickle knife or the biting forceps (Fig. 20.20). After this, the lateral wall is removed sufficiently to establish adequate drainage and adequately enlarge the middle meatus (Fig. 20.21). When this is necessary, great care must be taken postoperatively to prevent adhesions between

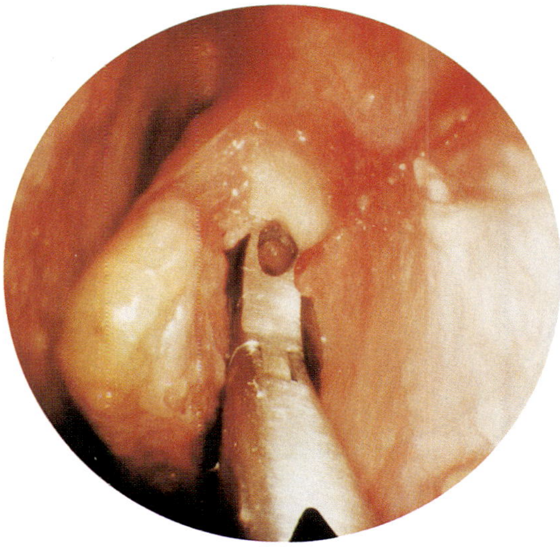

A

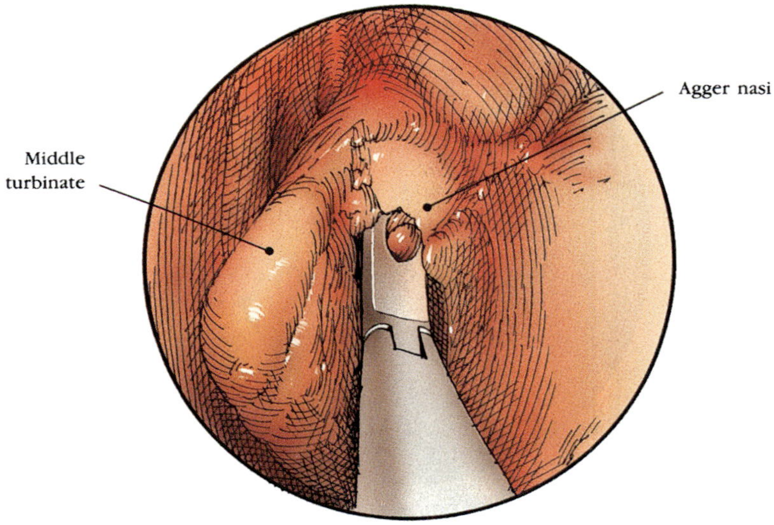


B

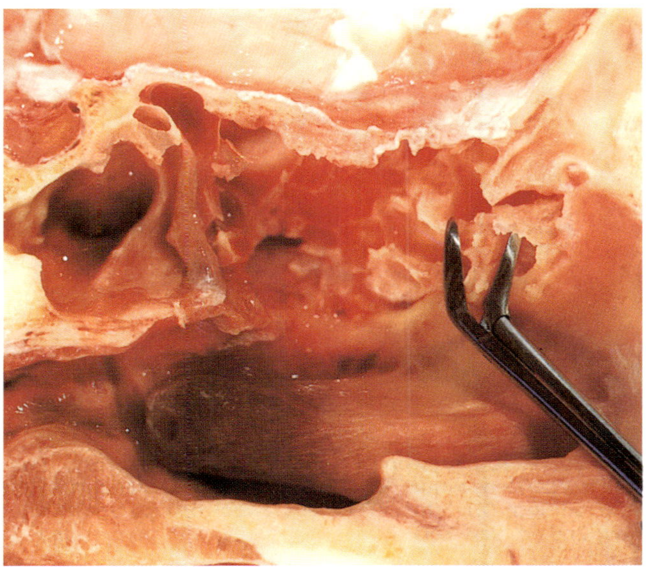

C

**FIGURE 20.18.** **A:** Endoscopic view of angled forceps opening the frontal recess. **B:** Illustration of **A.** **C:** Parasagittal view of **A**. (From Rice DH, Schaefer SD, eds. *Endoscopic paranasal sinus surgery,* 2nd ed. New York: Raven Press, 1993, with permission.)

the middle turbinate and the lateral nasal wall, because there is an opposing ring of denuded mucosa on the lateral surface of the middle turbinate. An alternative technique is to completely resect this lower portion of the concha bullosa—enough to uncover the anterior ethmoids and the maxillary sinus.

*Step 9:* If the *disease in the maxillary sinus* consists of edematous mucosa, polyps, and retention cysts, establishing adequate drainage through the natural ostium usually allows the mucosa to return to normal over time. Occasionally, there is disease that requires direct manipulation (e.g., pyocele, lesion that needs to be biopsied, allergic fungal mucus). Depending on location, this can be done in one of two ways. If routine endoscopic sinus surgery also has been required, the goal probably can be accomplished transnasally. Once the natural ostium has been enlarged, a nasoantral window can be created through the inferior meatus. The maxillary sinus can be observed with the endoscope through one opening while the forceps or curette is inserted through the other. With increased experience, all maneuvers can be performed through a generous middle meatal antrostomy.

If only the maxillary sinus is the problem, such as a lesion that must be biopsied, a canine fossa puncture can be performed with the trocar. The lesion can be identified by inserting the endoscope through the trocar sheath. The sheath is then pointed directly at the lesion, the endoscope is removed, the forceps are inserted, and the tissue removed.

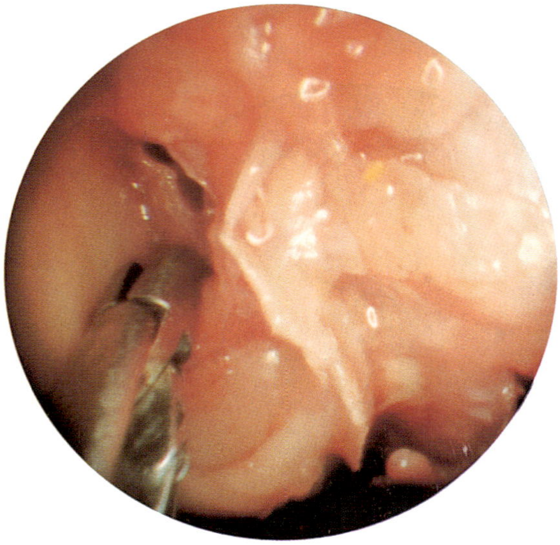

A

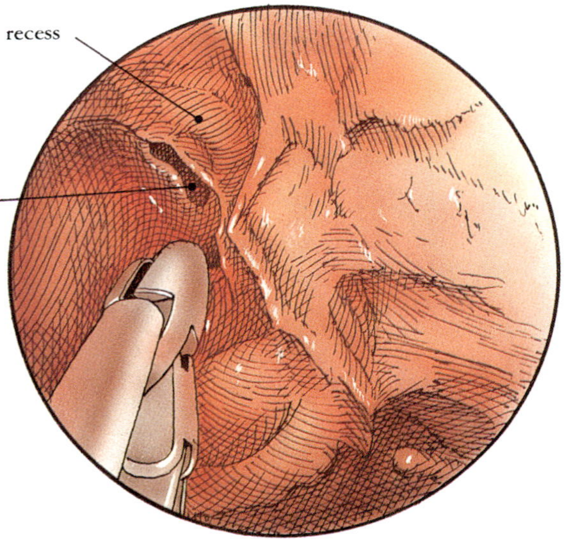


B

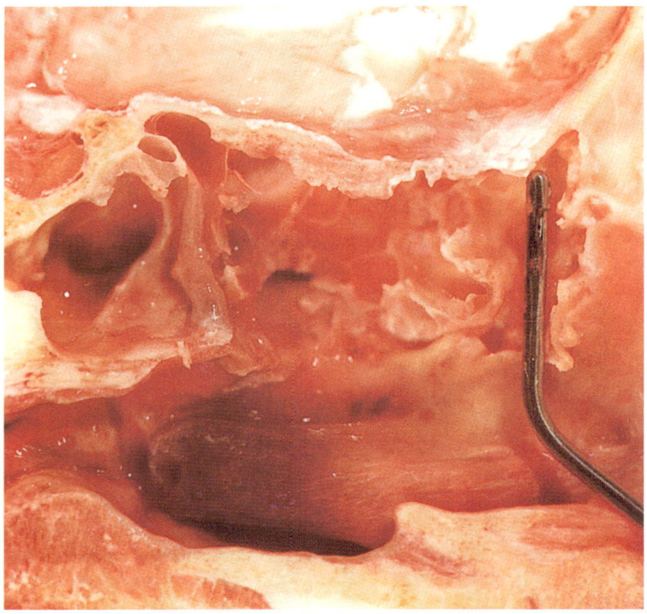

C

**FIGURE 20.19. A:** Endoscopic view of double-spoon forceps clearing the frontal sinus ostium. **B:** Illustration of **A. C:** Parasagittal view of **A**. (From Rice DH, Schaefer SD, eds. *Endoscopic paranasal sinus surgery,* 2nd ed. New York: Raven Press, 1993, with permission.)

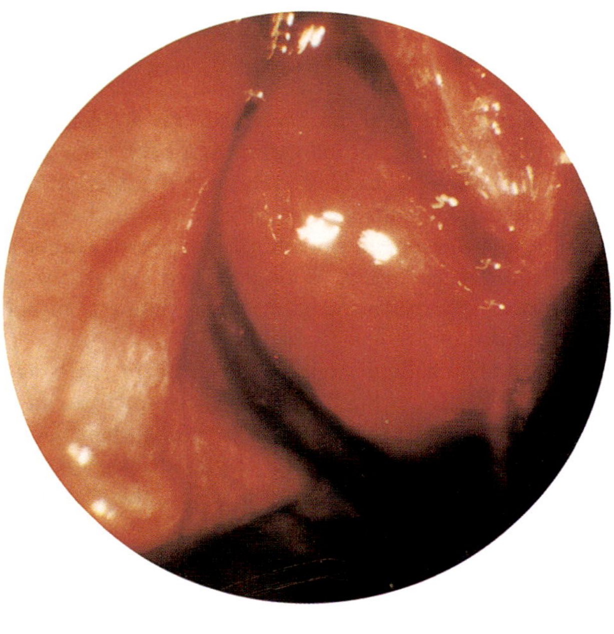

**FIGURE 20.20.** Endoscopic view of the concha bullosa. (From Rice DH, Schaefer SD, eds. *Endoscopic paranasal sinus surgery,* 2nd ed. New York: Raven Press, 1993, with permission.)

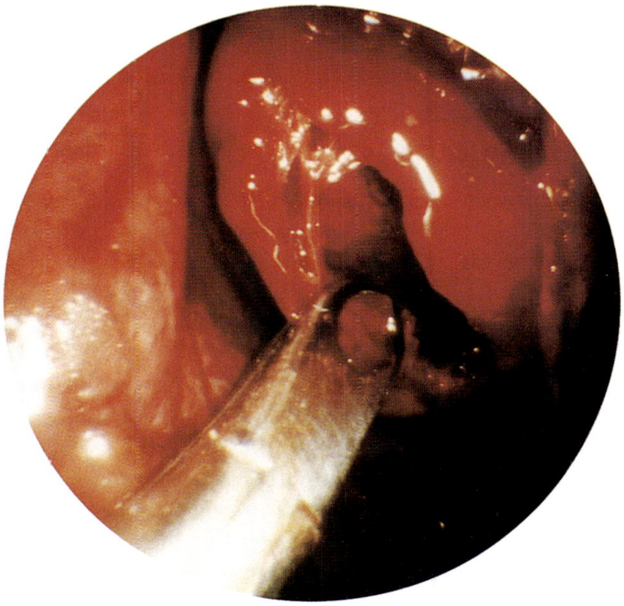

**FIGURE 20.21.** Endoscopic view showing the concha bullosa transected vertically and the lateral lamella being resected. (From Rice DH, Schaefer SD, eds. *Endoscopic paranasal sinus surgery,* 2nd ed. New York: Raven Press, 1993, with permission.)

If necessary, the optical forceps can be used through the sheath. With increasing experience, the canine fossa puncture becomes less necessary.

## Highlights

1. This procedure is most useful in the patient with chronic recurrent or refractory sinusitis when the anterior ethmoids are involved.
2. For most patients, it is probably the logical first invasive procedure.
3. This technique does not alter the nasal response to allergies in those patients who have them.
4. Care should be taken to avoid denuding the middle turbinate.
5. Opening agger nasi cells aids in postoperative cleaning and evaluation.
6. In patients with a narrow middle meatus but no concha bullosa, it may be advisable to resect part of the anterior-inferior, hanging end of the middle turbinate.

## Postoperative Care

Success in endoscopic sinus surgery requires more than performing the procedure correctly. Proper postoperative care is essential, and inadequate attention to detail can lead to failure. The objective is to keep the sinuses open and draining and to prevent scarring, which might subsequently occlude the ostia.

At the conclusion of the procedure, something should be done to minimize bleeding and crusting. Traditional gauze packing or Telfa gauze coated with an antibiotic ointment can be used. A third choice is to fill the operative site with an antibiotic ointment. Many other agents have been used, including Gelfilm, Gelfoam, fibrin glue, and various premade packs.

In the early postoperative period, the cavity should be inspected, and any clots or crusts should be removed. The patient should then begin nasal irrigations to keep the operative site clear. Considerable drainage should be expected and may continue several weeks. Irrigations should be performed as often as necessary to keep the site free of clots and crusts. This may be done effectively with a Grossan nasal irrigator attached to a Water Pik or a bulb syringe and continued until healing is complete. Some also use frequent vaporizer-like inhalations. Postirrigation application of a steroid nasal spray appears to aid healing, as does a 5- to 7-day course of antibiotics. For patients with nasal allergies, long-term results seem better with indefinite continuation of twice-daily saline irrigations coupled with steroid or cromolyn sodium nasal sprays. The ultimate objective is a wide open, mucosally covered middle meatus.

## Complications

In the standard, unmodified anterior-to-posterior technique, complications should be few and usually minor. Dissection too superiorly can lead to a cerebrospinal fluid leak. If this is recognized intraoperatively, it should be repaired endoscopically with fascia and fibrin or superglue, using a mucosal flap if possible. If it is recognized postoperatively, conservative treatment should be instituted unless it is clearly too large to seal spontaneously. If closure does not occur within 4 to 6 weeks, operative closure should be performed. Depending on the location and size, this may be done endoscopically or externally.

Dissection too laterally may lead to a breech of the lamina papyracea. The CT scan should be studied carefully preoperatively. Approximately 10% of people have an incomplete lamina papyracea. If previous ethmoid procedures have been performed, the lamina may have suffered an asymptomatic injury. If orbital fat is encountered, dissection should stop immediately in that area. Packing should not be used. If the injury is minimal, the patient can be expected to have some ecchymosis of the medial canthal area and lower eyelid, which will resolve in several days. Additional breech demands an immediate ophthalmologic evaluation.

Dissection in the posterior ethmoids and sphenoid is more dangerous and is discussed in Chapter 29. Dissection too anteriorly can lead to damage to the nasolacrimal apparatus. The bone around the lacrimal sac and the nasolacrimal duct is usually more dense, and this serves as a warning. However, even if either structure were injured, it would probably heal spontaneously. If epiphora persists, an intranasal endoscopic dacryocystorhinostomy can be performed (4).

It is possible also to damage the medial wall or floor of the orbit when exploring or enlarging the natural ostium of the maxillary sinus. Careful study of the preoperative CT scan shows the proximity of the orbit to the area of the natural ostium. In general, the orbit is closer anteriorly than posteriorly, and the search for the ostium should begin more posteriorly when it cannot be seen readily. In this situation, careful palpation usually identifies the ostium. The instrument should always be advanced in an inferolateral direction and never superiorly.

## ENDOSCOPIC TOTAL SPHENOETHMOIDECTOMY: POSTERIOR-TO-ANTERIOR APPROACH

### Indications

Total sphenoethmoidectomy is reserved for the patient with sinusitis or polyps extensively involving (i.e., a minimum of the ethmoid, sphenoid, and maxillary sinuses) the ipsilateral or bilateral paranasal sinuses. This is a particularly useful procedure in the patient with significant disease who no longer has conventional landmarks (e.g., middle turbinate) as a result of previous surgery. The technique is specifically intended to permit the surgeon to progress anteriorly from the sphenoid sinus, a landmark whose location cannot be altered, to exenterate the ethmoid sinus using the fovea ethmoidalis as the superior boundary of the dissection (5,6).

### Contraindications

There are no contraindications to this procedure in the otherwise healthy patient, as long as the disease process is confined to the paranasal sinuses.

### Case Example

A 32-year-old woman was referred with a 10-year history of repeated episodes of facial pain, mucopurulent rhinorrhea, nasal airway obstruction, and polyps. Previous medical management included immunotherapy, nasal steroids, and numerous courses of antibiotics during episodes of acute sinusitis. Previous surgical management included bilateral Caldwell-Luc procedures and intranasal ethmoidectomies 4 years earlier.

Physical examination revealed total obstruction of both nasal cavities with polyps, which precluded endoscopic visualization of the lateral nasal wall. CT scanning showed extensive disease of the paranasal sinuses (Fig. 20.22).

Operative management consisted of bilateral endoscopic intranasal sphenoethmoidectomies, frontal sinusotomies, and middle meatal antrostomies. At surgery, the sinuses were filled with both polyps and dense, inspissated secre-

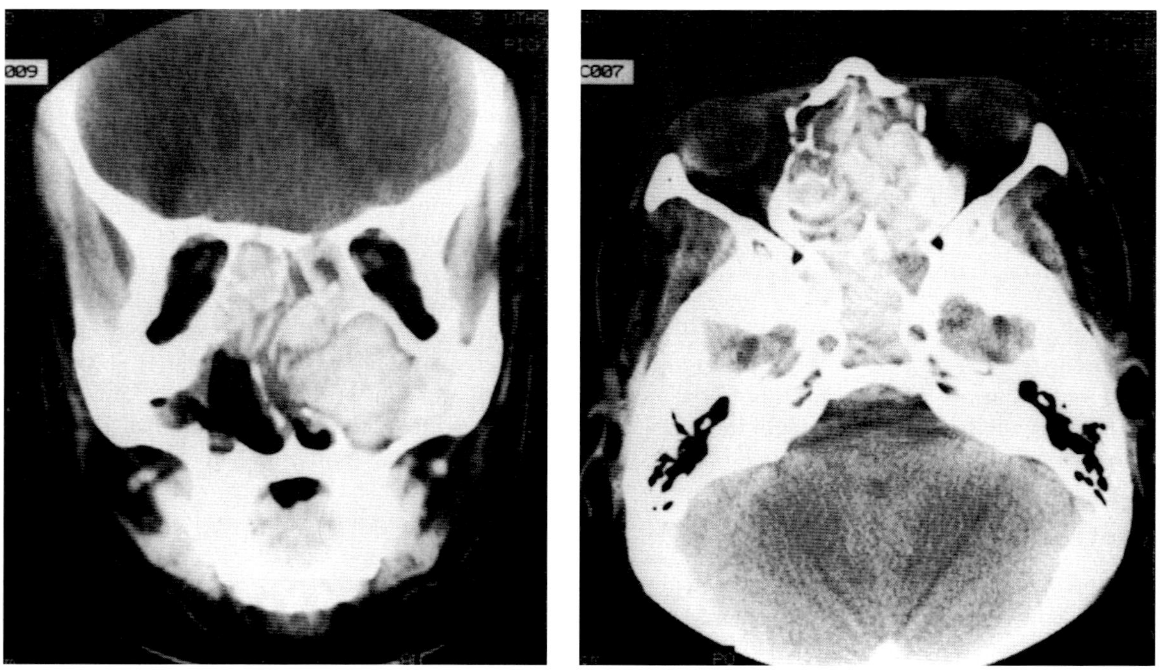


A B

**FIGURE 20.22. A:** Coronal computed tomography scan. **B:** Axial computed tomography scan of the same patient. (From Rice DH, Schaefer SD, eds. *Endoscopic paranasal sinus surgery,* 2nd ed. New York: Raven Press, 1993, with permission.)

tions. Results of the pathologic examination of the surgical specimen were consistent with allergic fungal (*Bipolaris*) sinusitis (7). The postoperative course was unremarkable, and the patient returned to work within a week of surgery. Follow-up care included nasal steroids and frequent endoscopic examination of the sinuses to observe for regrowth of polyps and fungus, which has not occurred.

## Instrumentation

A variety of available endoscopes may be used to perform a total sphenoethmoidectomy. Figure 20.4 shows equipment manufactured by three companies. Several instruments are particularly useful for this technique. First, a suction-irrigation system may be beneficial in dealing with increased bleeding that can occur in this more extensive procedure. Saline is decanted on the endoscope to clean the lens of blood. Second, forceps (i.e., double-spoon forceps manufactured at various angles) have been developed specifically to permit the removal of tissue within the recesses of the maxillary and frontal sinuses. Third, suction forceps have proved a useful alternative to suction irrigation in some cases. These instruments are available in straight and angled designs. Fourth, sinus punch forceps are useful for sphenoidotomy and frontal sinusotomy. In some cases, similar instruments can be found that serve the same function, such as the use of the universal handle and its various accompanying forceps.

## Anesthesia

The posterior-to-anterior approach for total sphenoethmoidectomy can be performed under local or general anesthesia. I prefer general anesthesia because of the extensive nature of the procedure and to avoid aspiration from posterior nasal bleeding. However, in selected patients, the combination of infiltrative anesthesia and a sphenopalatine block by means of the greater palatine foramen is an acceptable alternative to a general anesthetic. In all cases, before prepping and draping the patient, the lateral wall of the nose, middle turbinate, and face of the sphenoid are injected with 1% lidocaine with 1:100,000 epinephrine. Before this, the nose is sprayed with Afrin or an equivalent vasoconstrictive agent and packed with gauze saturated with a similar solution. If a septoplasty is indicated for airway obstruction or accessibility to the posterior paranasal sinuses, the septum also is injected at this time. On average, 20 to 25 mL of 1% lidocaine with 1:100,000 epinephrine is used for bilateral procedures and septoplasty. In our initial experience, approximately 32% of patients required a septoplasty for either airway obstruction or visualization of the posterior nasal cavity (8). Currently, less than 20% of our general sinus patients undergo septoplasty. After completing the injection of the nose, the vasoconstrictive agent–saturated packing is replaced in the nasal cavity. The patient is then prepped and draped for surgery so that the sterile field includes the brow superiorly and the upper lip inferiorly. When general endotracheal anesthesia is used, a sterile plastic drape may be placed over the upper lip and chin to permit visualization of the endotracheal tube for monitoring the airway.

## Surgical Procedure

*Step 1:* When indicated, a septoplasty is performed before beginning endoscopic sinus surgery. The nose is examined with an appropriate 25° or 30°, wide-angle endoscope or standard 0° and 30° endoscopes (Fig. 20.23). Care should be taken to clearly delineate the middle turbinate, the osteomeatal complex, the anterior wall of the sphenoid sinus, and the lateral wall of the nasal cavity.

*Step 2:* The inferior aspect of the middle turbinate is transected with two incisions using turbinate scissors. The first incision is parallel to the inferior free margin of the turbinate and removes approximately the inferior one third of this structure. The second incision begins at the midportion of the turbinate in an anterior-to-posterior direction and is directed superoposteriorly toward the upper aspect of the anterior wall of the sphenoid sinus, ending near the superior turbinate. This second incision results in a partial opening into the posterior ethmoid cells (Fig. 20.24). This step can be modified to include only the posterior incision and thereby preserve the entire anterior segment of the middle turbinate (Fig. 20.25).

*Step 3:* Depending on the extent of the disease, the sphenoid sinus may be identified as lying at approximately the same level as the posterior insertion of the middle turbinate near the superior turbinate, or it may be necessary to

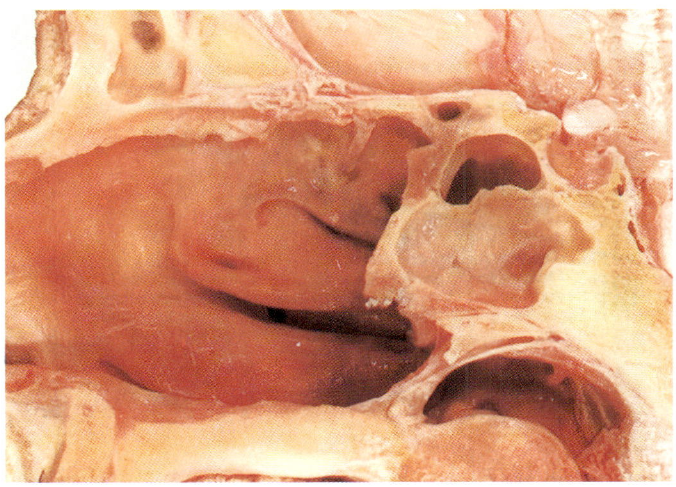

**FIGURE 20.23.** Endoscopic view of the normal left side of the nasal cavity. (From Rice DH, Schaefer SD, eds. *Endoscopic paranasal sinus surgery,* 2nd ed. New York: Raven Press, 1993, with permission.)

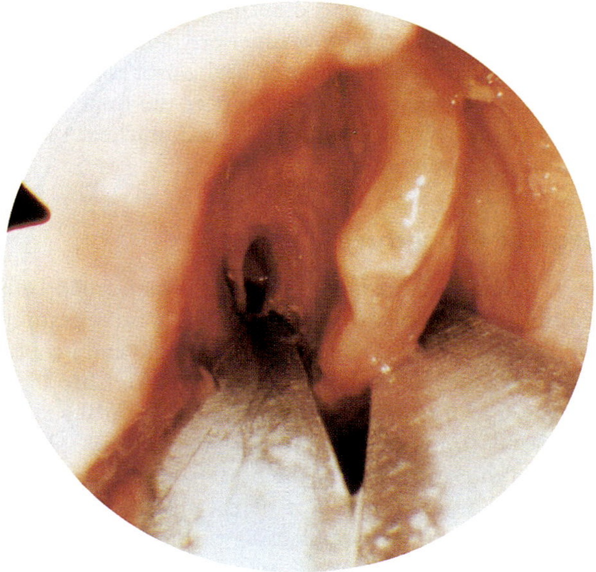

**FIGURE 20.24.** Endoscopic view of turbinate scissors about to resect the inferior aspect of the middle turbinate. (From Rice DH, Schaefer SD, eds. *Endoscopic paranasal sinus surgery,* 2nd ed. New York: Raven Press, 1993, with permission.)

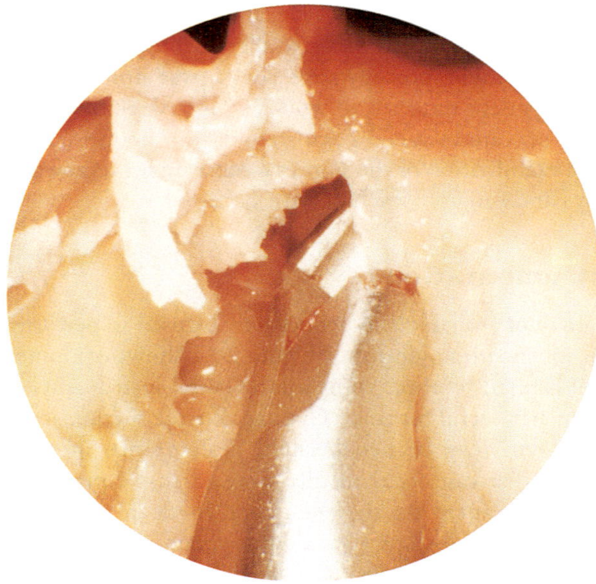

**FIGURE 20.26.** Endoscopic view of exposure of the sphenoid by partial resection of the posterior middle turbinate. (From Rice DH, Schaefer SD, eds. *Endoscopic paranasal sinus surgery,* 2nd ed. New York: Raven Press, 1993, with permission.)

remove additional posterior ethmoid cells (Fig. 20.26). In the latter case, 45° Weil-Blakesley ethmoid forceps are used for this purpose (Fig. 20.27). The endoscope should be positioned so as to permit full visualization of every aspect of the entire surgical procedure. In locating the sphenoid ostium, the physician should recall that this structure is approximately 7 cm from the maxillary spine at an angle of 30° from the nasal floor. This ostium may be confirmed by using a calibrated probe, such as a Cottle elevator, or rigid suction. Punch forceps are used to remove the anterior wall of the sphenoid sinus inferior to the ostium of this cavity (Fig. 20.28). The sinus is then examined endoscopically, and biopsies are taken as necessary. The convexity formed by the internal carotid artery can be visualized in the lateral wall of the sphenoid sinus, as can in some cases the optic nerve in the superior lateral aspect of the sphenoid sinus

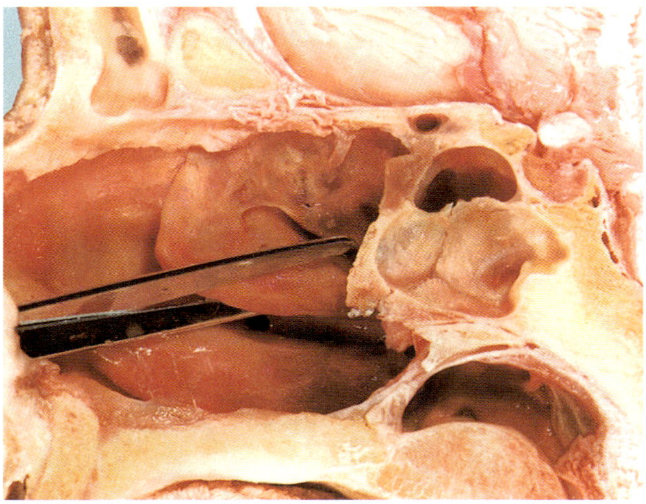

**FIGURE 20.25.** Parasagittal view of turbinate scissors placed to resect the middle turbinate to gain access to the posterior ethmoids. (From Rice DH, Schaefer SD, eds. *Endoscopic paranasal sinus surgery,* 2nd ed. New York: Raven Press, 1993, with permission.)

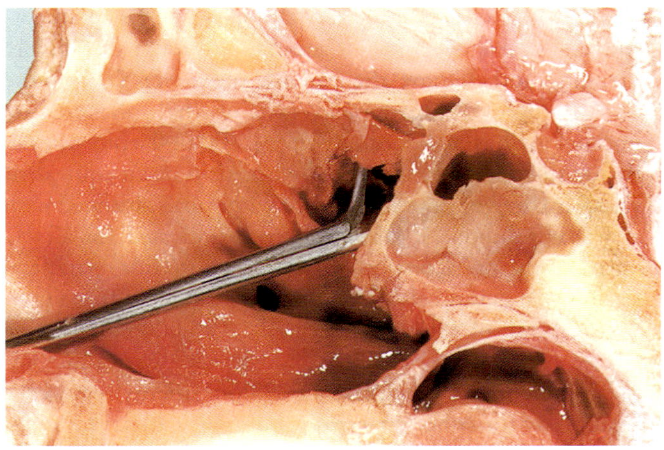

**FIGURE 20.27.** Parasagittal view of forceps clearing the posterior ethmoid air cells to obtain access to the sphenoid. (From Rice DH, Schaefer SD, eds. *Endoscopic paranasal sinus surgery,* 2nd ed. New York: Raven Press, 1993, with permission.)

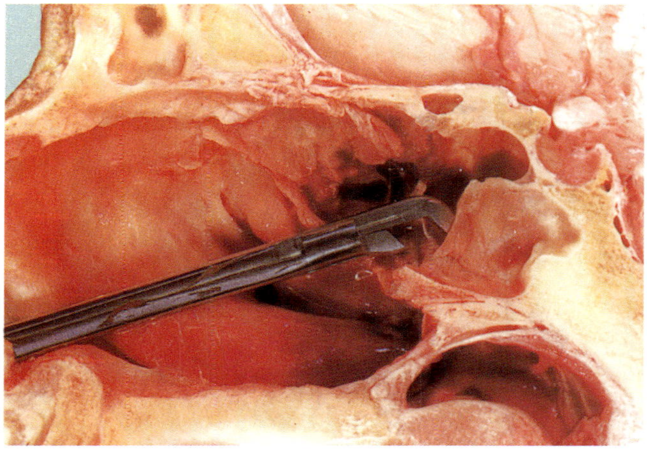

**FIGURE 20.28.** Parasagittal view of punch forceps enlarging the sphenoid ostium. (From Rice DH, Schaefer SD, eds. *Endoscopic paranasal sinus surgery,* 2nd ed. New York: Raven Press, 1993, with permission.)

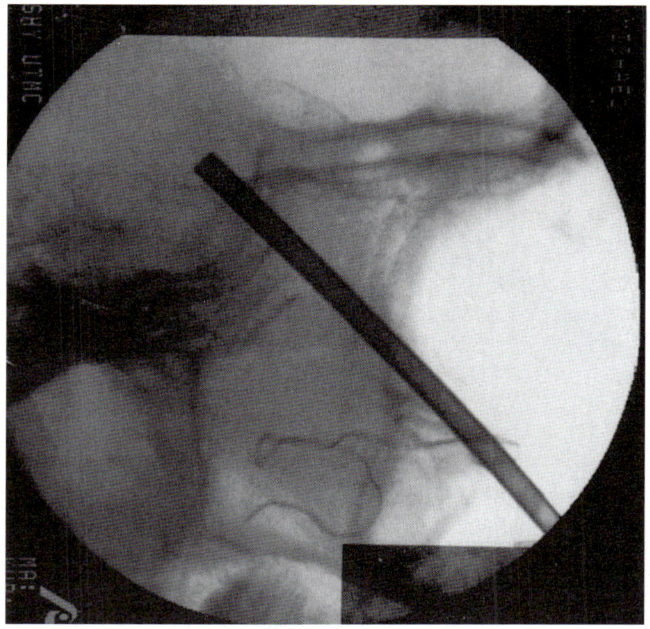

**FIGURE 20.30.** Intraoperative lateral radiograph shows the location of the endoscope within the sphenoid sinus. (From Rice DH, Schaefer SD, eds. *Endoscopic paranasal sinus surgery,* 2nd ed. New York: Raven Press, 1993, with permission.)

(Fig. 20.29). In some patients, the boundaries of the sphenoid sinus may have been altered by expansile processes eroding the skull base. When the boundaries or location of the sphenoid sinus is in question, radiography using an image intensifier in the lateral position is useful (Fig. 20.30), or an image guidance system should be used.

*Step 4:* After completion of the sphenoidotomy, the posterior ethmoid cells are reentered and exenterated, using the combination of the 45° and 90° Weil-Blakesley ethmoid forceps (Fig. 20.31). Care is taken to identify the fovea ethmoidalis, which serves as the superior boundary of the dissection (Fig. 20.32). This landmark should be identified throughout the rest of the procedure. While visualizing the fovea ethmoidalis, the anterior ethmoid cells are exenterated. The anterior limit of this procedure

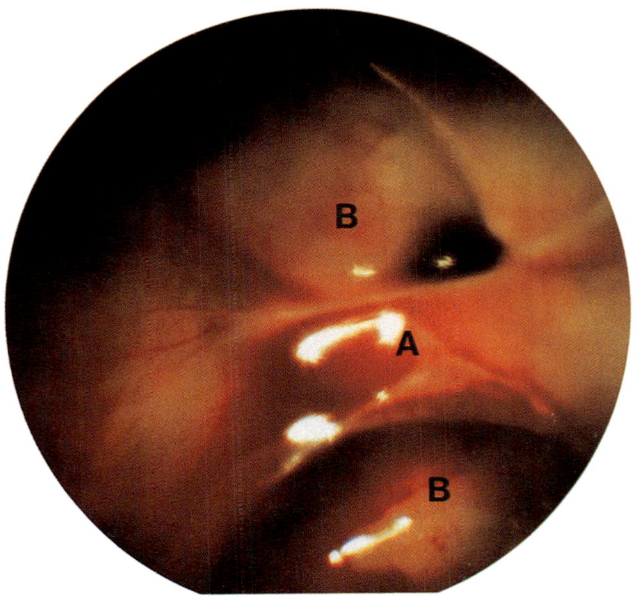


**FIGURE 20.29.** Endoscopic view of the anterior sphenoid sinus, showing the optic nerve (*A*) and carotid artery (*B*) impressions in the lateral wall. (From Rice DH, Schaefer SD, eds. *Endoscopic paranasal sinus surgery,* 2nd ed. New York: Raven Press, 1993, with permission.)

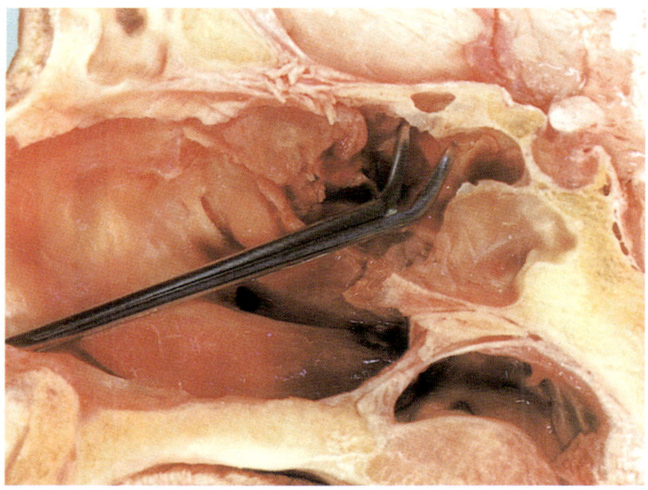

**FIGURE 20.31.** Parasagittal view of angled forceps exenterating the posterior ethmoid air cells. (From Rice DH, Schaefer SD, eds. *Endoscopic paranasal sinus surgery,* 2nd ed. New York: Raven Press, 1993, with permission.)

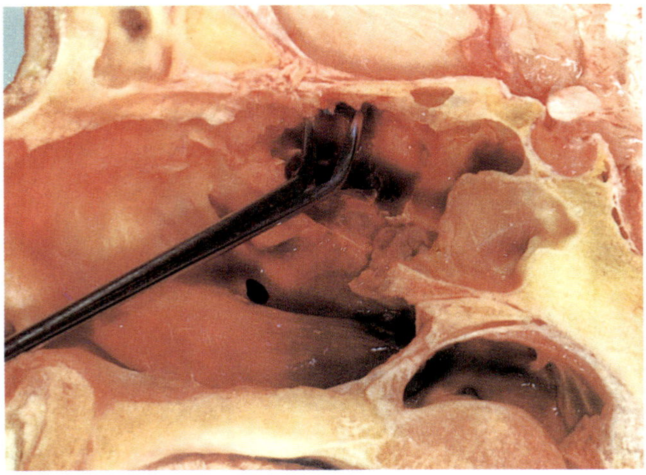

**FIGURE 20.32.** Parasagittal view of forceps resting on the roof of the ethmoid (i.e., skull base). (From Rice DH, Schaefer SD, eds. *Endoscopic paranasal sinus surgery,* 2nd ed. New York: Raven Press, 1993, with permission.)

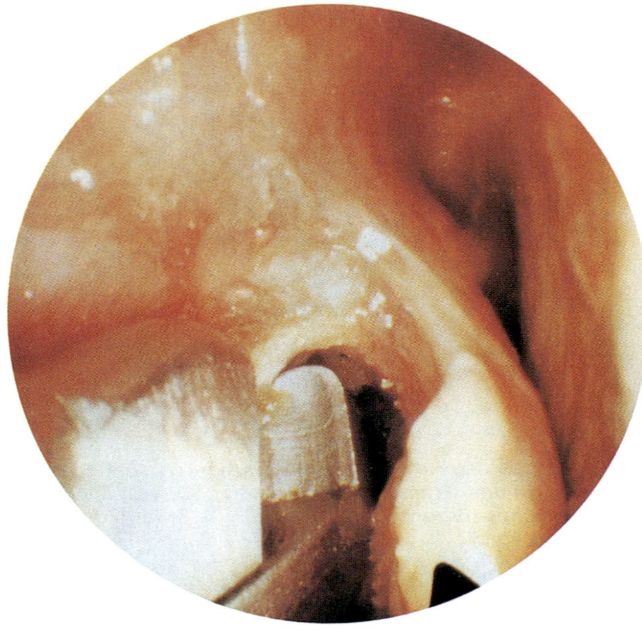

**FIGURE 20.33.** Endoscopic view of the frontal recess being exenterated. (From Rice DH, Schaefer SD, eds. *Endoscopic paranasal sinus surgery,* 2nd ed. New York: Raven Press, 1993, with permission.)

is reached when the frontal recess cells of the ethmoid are removed and the nasofrontal ostium or duct is identified (Fig. 20.33).

*Step 5:* The ostium or duct of the frontal sinus is inspected for patency (Fig. 20.34). All frontal recess cells are carefully exenterated to preclude the postoperative obstruction of the outflow of the frontal sinus. The ostium or duct of this sinus is not entered unless there is radiographic evidence of frontal sinusitis. In many individuals, the removal of the frontal recess cells may be sufficient to resolve recurrent frontal sinusitis. This passage may be cannulated with a curved suction canula and inspissated secretions removed. If the outflow of the frontal sinus is obstructed or tissue must be removed from this sinus, the anterior wall of the ostium or duct can be removed partially using a curette or diamond burr. Using the appropriate endoscope (i.e., wide-

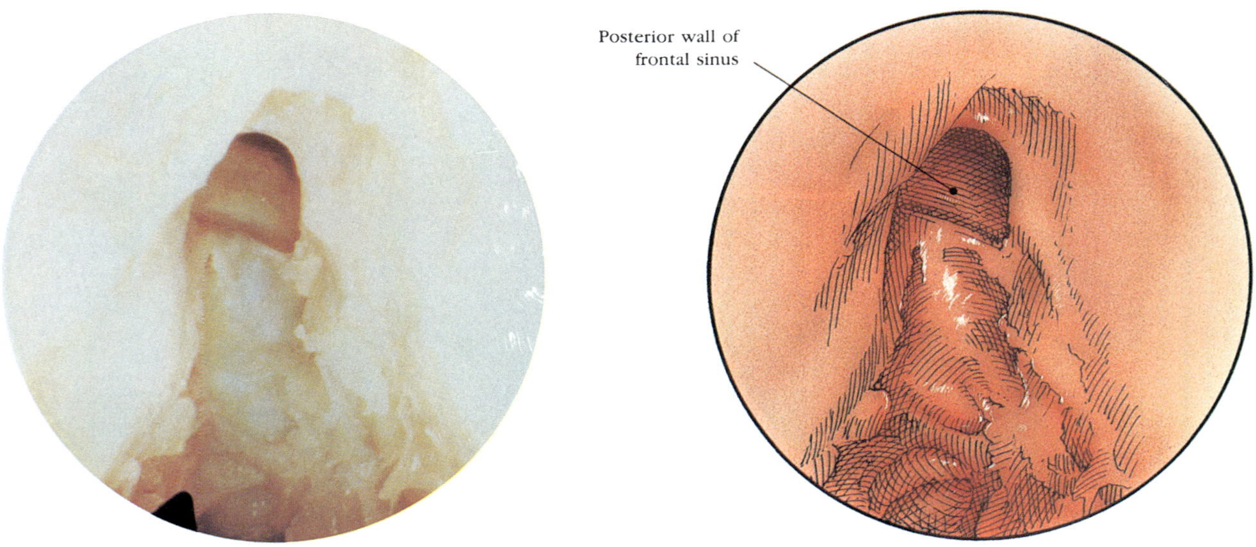


A B

**FIGURE 20.34. A:** Endoscopic view of the frontal ostium. **B:** Illustration of **A**. (From Rice DH, Schaefer SD, eds. *Endoscopic paranasal sinus surgery,* 2nd ed. New York: Raven Press, 1993, with permission.)

angle 70° endoscope or standard 90° endoscope), the frontal sinus can be examined. The various angled double-spoon forceps are useful for removing lesions within the frontal sinus (Fig. 20.35). By resecting the agger nasi cells, the frontal recess cells and ostium or duct of the frontal sinus are better visualized. When a 4-mm suction probe can easily be passed into the frontal sinus, good healing of this passage can be expected.

*Step 6:* The placement of a middle meatal antrostomy can be performed at the beginning or at the end of this procedure. Usually, it is beneficial to perform this at the beginning if the ostium of the maxillary sinus can clearly be identified by visualization or palpation. The retrograde forceps are then used to enlarge this ostium. In many patients, this is not the case, and the antrostomy is performed at the end of the procedure. This step is begun by using a 45° or 90° Weil-Blakesley forceps, small curved suction, or ostium probe placed immediately above the superior surface of the inferior turbinate and directed in a strictly inferolateral direction. In many patients, this aspect of the lateral wall of the nose is membranous and can be distinguished from the adjacent bone by palpation. After the forceps have entered the maxillary sinus, they may be opened and then withdrawn to force the mucous membrane of the medial aspect of the antrum into the nose to permit its removal. The Weil-Blakesley forceps and retrograde forceps are useful to enlarge the antrostomy to approximately 1.5 cm. This entire maneuver must be performed with great care to avoid injury to the adjacent orbit. The maxillary sinus is inspected with the more acutely angled endoscopes (i.e., wide-angle 70° endoscope or standard 70° and 120° endoscopes), and tissue may be removed using the double-spoon forceps.

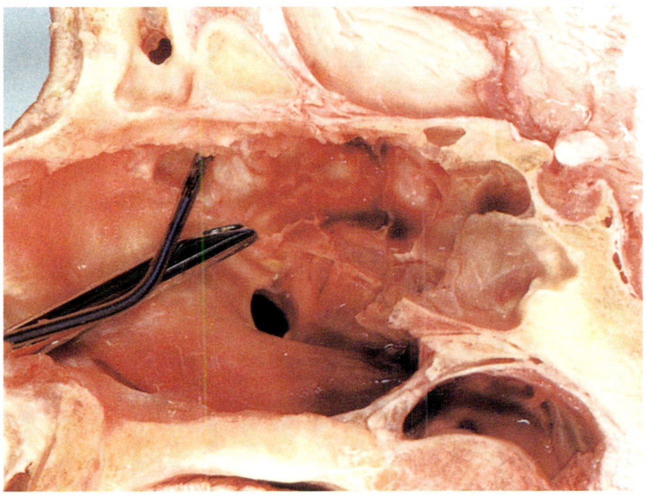

**FIGURE 20.35.** Parasagittal view of double-spoon forceps at the frontal ostium. (From Rice DH, Schaefer SD, eds. *Endoscopic paranasal sinus surgery,* 2nd ed. New York: Raven Press, 1993, with permission.)

*Step 7:* The last step is inspection of the entire operative field for residual fragments of bone and mucous membrane. It is important to remove these, because they may obstruct the outflow of the sinus or form a later nidus for infection. The nasal cavity may then be irrigated with normal saline. If a septoplasty has been performed, the application of septal splints between the septum and middle turbinate is recommended. Packing should be kept to a minimum and may consist of instilling water-soluble antibiotic ointment under endoscopic visualization within the actual sinus cavities. Most often no form of packing is employed.

## Highlights

1. Total sphenoethmoidectomy is designed to eliminate the need for other more invasive procedures, such as Caldwell-Luc, transantral or external ethmoidectomy, and osteoplastic flap with fat obliteration, in most patients with extensive paranasal sinus disease.
2. As in all endoscopic paranasal sinus surgery, the eyes must be included in the sterile field and monitored closely.
3. Partial resection of the agger nasi cells is useful in permitting inspection of the ostium or duct of the frontal sinus.
4. Gross polyps can be removed using a headlight or with a microdebrider before injection of local anesthetic to permit accurate placement of the anesthetic agent.

## Postoperative Care

The patient is given an instruction sheet before surgery that outlines the activities to be performed and avoided. The most important of these is irrigation of the nose with normal saline on the second postoperative day. This is best accomplished using a nasal irrigation attachment for the Water Pik. Saline can be purchased by the liter or made by having the patient use 2 cups of boiled water for every teaspoon of salt. The patient is instructed to irrigate a minimum of 2 cups of saline (or until the effluent from the nose is clear) three times each day for the first 4 weeks. The patient is encouraged thereafter to irrigate the nose indefinitely at least once each day.

Postoperative visits begin on the fourth through sixth days. The nose is carefully cleaned of dried secretions and blood approximately once each week for the first 3 weeks. After the operative field has been covered by mucous membrane, the office visits are less frequent. However, patients are encouraged to maintain periodic visits in the hope of recognizing and correcting early recurrent disease. Some patients recover slowly and tend to have low-grade sinusitis. These patients benefit from weekly irrigation of the involved sinus by the physician with one part hydrogen peroxide to four parts saline.

Nasal steroids are begun by the end of the first postoperative week, and antibiotics are discontinued by the fifth postoperative day. In the nonallergic patient without polyps and without other contraindications such as pregnancy, these medications are used for approximately 6 months. In the allergic or polyp patient, nasal steroids form an important long-term adjuvant to the medical and surgical management.

## Complications

The two major potential complications of endoscopic total sphenoethmoidectomy are the same as those with conventional approaches to the sinuses: injury to the eye and brain.

### *Ophthalmologic Injuries*

During performance of the ethmoidectomy or the antrostomy, the lamina papyracea can be perforated and the orbital tissues injured. The most common of these injuries is disruption of the orbital fat and hemorrhage. In a minor compromise of these structures, the outcome is only ecchymosis in the medial canthal region. Orbital hematoma may occur and may require immediate surgical intervention by lateral canthotomy and drainage. Orbital hematoma may be vision threatening. Less common is partial or complete transection of the medial rectus or superior oblique muscles. The least common injury is direct trauma to the optic nerve. In the normal patient, the optic nerve is surrounded by dense bone, and if the surgeon follows the rule of avoiding the removal of such bone, injury is unlikely. In the rare patient, the optic canal may be partially dehiscent, exposing the nerve in the sphenoid or posterior ethmoids. Such unusual events point out the need to always visualize well any area within the sinuses before removing tissue. Occasionally, this may be anticipated on the preoperative CT scan.

### *Neurologic Injuries*

The most common neurologic complication of sinus surgery is cerebrospinal fluid fistula. This tends to result from avulsion of the olfactory filia, penetration of the fovea ethmoidalis, or fracture of this bony plate. The first problem can be avoided by remaining lateral to the middle turbinate during surgery. The second cause of cerebrospinal fluid fistula is best prevented by painstaking visualization of the fovea. The last cause of this complication is inadvertent torquing of the fovea during the removal of the ethmoid labyrinthine bone.

Whatever the cause, minor injuries can be repaired intraoperatively using fibrin glue or cyanoacrylic and fascial or muscle grafts applied under endoscopic control. In such cases, a lumbar drain may be useful in controlling the fistula.

Another major but uncommon neurologic complication is laceration of the internal carotid artery. This vessel is most vulnerable in the sphenoid, because it impinges on the lateral wall of the sinus, and like the optic nerve, the bony covering of the artery may be dehiscent. Careful visualization of the lateral wall of the sphenoid sinus is necessary. Other complications include subarachnoid hemorrhage, pneumocephalus, frontal lobe injury, and various central nervous system infections.

## REFERENCES


1. Messerklinger W. Endoskopische diagnose und chirurgic der rezidivierenden sinusitis. In: Krajina Z, ed. *Advances in nose and sinus surgery*. Zagreb, Yugoslavia: Zagreb University, 1895.
2. Stammberger H. Endoscopic endonasal surgery-concepts in treatment of recurring rhinosinusitis. Part 11. Surgical technique. *Otolaryngol Head Neck Surg* 1986;94:147–156.
3. Stammberger H. Endoscopic surgery for mycotic and chronic recurring sinusitis. *Ann Otol Rhinol Laryngol* 1985; 119[Suppl I]:111.
4. Rice DH. Endoscopic intranasal dacryocystorhinostomy. *Am J Rhinol* 1988;2:127–128.
5. Wigand ME. Transnasal ethmoidectomy under endoscopic control. *Rhinology* 1981;19:7–12.
6. Wigand ME, Steiner W, Jaurnann MP. Endonasal sinus surgery with endoscopical control: from radical operation to rehabilitation of the mucosa. *Endoscopy* 1978;10:255–260.
7. Manning S, Schaefer SD, Close LG, et al. Culture-positive allergic fungal sinusitis. *Arch Otolaryngol Head Neck Surg* 1991;117: 174–178.
8. Schaefer SD, Manning S, Close LG. Endoscopic paranasal sinus surgery: indications and considerations. *Laryngoscope* 1989;99: 1–5.

# 21

# ENDOSCOPIC MANAGEMENT OF FRONTAL SINUS DISEASE

FREDERICK A. KUHN
AMIN R. JAVER

## INDICATIONS

Historically, frontal sinus disease was treated surgically using the external approach and obliterative procedures (1–3). It was later thought that preservation of the frontal sinus and maintenance of the patency of the nasofrontal recess and internal frontal ostium resulted in a better overall outcome. This idea led to the development of external procedures designed to remove disease from the frontal sinus and reestablish the frontal sinus pathways (4). Lynch described a procedure to remove part of the sinus floor, the entire sino-orbital wall, and as much of the sinus mucosa as possible. He advocated placement of a rubber tube into the newly created nasofrontal connection to maintain its patency (5). Because of a significant failure rate (approximately 30%) several modifications to the original procedure were introduced, including the use of stents of various materials ranging from gold to Silastic sheeting (6–8). This later evolved into the use of mucosal free grafts (9) and split-thickness skin grafts (10) with limited success. Mucoperiosteal flaps as described by Sewall and later modified by McNaught and Boyden resulted in better outcomes (11). Several modifications and outcomes of these procedures have been reported since the original description. Dedo and colleagues described their 25-year experience with the external frontoethmoidectomy and Sewall-Boyden reconstruction. They reported a 97% patency rate for the nasofrontal pathway (12). Overall, these modifications resulted in long-term failure rates between 15% and 20% (13).

Over the past decade, functional endoscopic sinus surgery (FESS) has been accepted as the procedure of choice for the surgical management of chronic sinusitis (14–16). Because of the complex anatomy of the frontal recess, endoscopic intranasal approaches to this region continue to be an area of controversy (17–19). Several investigators have devoted much energy to renewing interest in the Lothrop procedure (18,19). We are highly selective in its use. Maintenance of mucous membrane in the frontal sinus drainage pathway is the key to a successful functional outcome. We do not advocate the use of powered instrumentation in the frontal recess except for the occasional use of a curved débriding blade to remove curetted debris from the frontal recess region (20). FESS advocates removal only of tissue necessary to relieve obstruction, thereby restoring natural sinus drainage and ventilation. The ideal method in dealing with the frontal drainage pathway would be to carry out a careful and delicate dissection from below using the appropriate instrumentation and causing the minimum amount of damage to the mucosa of the internal frontal ostium. Using the correct technique and with increasing experience, the success rates of the endoscopic intranasal frontal sinusotomy have surpassed those of the external approach in centers specializing in sinus diseases (15,20). It has less morbidity than nonendoscopic sinus procedures, can be done on an outpatient basis, has a shorter convalescent period, and leaves no external scarring on facial skin (14–16,21). Preservation of normal frontal sinus anatomy has the advantage that future radiologic or endoscopic evaluation is not distorted (17).

The frontal sinus is the most challenging of the four paranasal sinuses to treat endoscopically. Its anterosuperior location and complex relatively narrow frontal recess anatomy makes visualization difficult and predisposes it to stenosis. Significantly serious complications are possible because of the proximity of the frontal recess to the anterior ethmoid artery, orbit and anterior cranial fossa. However, with full knowledge of the anatomy and potential pitfalls and a thorough preoperative evaluation, the FESS surgeon can successfully restore normal frontal sinus physiology (22).

Indications for endoscopic frontal sinusotomy are derived from assessment of the patient's history, diagnostic endoscopy, and the computed tomography (CT) scan. Endoscopic intranasal frontal sinusotomy can be used successfully in most primary cases of chronic frontal sinusitis and in revision frontal sinus surgery. It can also be used in place of trephine to treat acute frontal sinusitis, but bleeding may be a problem because of the inflammation. Other applications are to the treatment of frontal sinus mucoceles (16) and frontal recess inverting papillomas (23,24).

Frontal sinus allergic fungal sinusitis, mucoceles with erosion of the posterior table or superior orbital wall, inverting papilloma of the frontal sinus, and extensively pneumatized frontal sinuses are contraindications to obliteration. These conditions are best managed with an intranasal endoscopic approach or a combined osteoplastic flap and intranasal approach, after which the frontal recess and internal frontal ostium can be followed postoperatively in the office.

## CONTRAINDICATIONS

Endoscopic frontal sinusotomy is contraindicated for frontal sinus tumor, inverting papilloma of the frontal sinus, broadly based osteomas, frontal recess stenosis, and laterally based mucoceles.

Invasive malignancies involving the frontal sinus and extending into the orbit or cranium should not be dealt with endoscopically (25). Inverting papillomas only rarely involve the frontal sinuses. Most involvement of the frontal sinuses is limited to the frontal recess region, but occasionally, part or all of the sinus can be involved. Published series list an incidence of between 1% and 16% (26). Inverting papilloma involving the frontal sinus proper should not be dealt with using a conservative endoscopic procedure by itself. It is better dealt with using an osteoplastic flap without obliteration together with an endoscopic approach from below in the same operation. This may be one indication for the intranasal modified Lothrop procedure. Broadly based osteomas are also not adequately dealt with using the endoscopic technique by itself (27,28).

Significant stenosis of the frontal recess from previously performed endoscopic surgery or a superiorly pneumatized agger nasi cell may require an extension of the endoscopic approach by using the above and below approach (22) or a frontal sinus rescue procedure (29). A 4-mm burr hole in the anterior wall of the frontal sinus can allow simultaneous visualization and instrumentation of the stenotic area from above and below (22).

In acute frontal sinusitis, the slightest indication of an incipient central complication (e.g., meningitis, abscess, cavernous sinus thrombosis), osteomyelitis of the frontal bone with sequestration, or acute visual or visual field loss or blindness leads us to use one of the external anterior approaches. Mucoceles can generally be treated using the intranasal endoscopic approach unless one is located so far laterally that it cannot be reached endoscopically over the frontal recess.

## PREOPERATIVE EVALUATION

A thorough evaluation, including a complete history and review of previous surgical records, is important. An outcome measure, such as RSOM-31 or SNOT-20 (30), including postnasal drainage, intermittent fever, frontal pressure, and headache, is helpful for documentation and follow-up. The nature of the headache should be reviewed in detail to exclude a nonsinus cause. Contingent medical disorders, such as allergies, asthma, congenital illnesses, or immune deficiencies are important to document.

Endoscopic description of abnormalities such as polyps, purulence, concha bullosa, persistent uncinate process, frontal recess scarring, presence or absence of partially resected turbinates (31), and the absence of landmarks should be documented. Computer-assisted photography is an excellent means of documentation (Fig. 21.1). In a patient with previous endoscopic surgery, direct examination of the frontal recess may be possible using the 30° or 70° telescopes. Any purulence or allergic mucin should be obtained endoscopically and cultured for bacteria and fungi to accurately select treatment (Fig. 21.1).

All patients with chronic frontal sinusitis should be given a substantial trial of medical therapy. A 3- to 6-week trial of culture-directed antibiotics used with combinations of

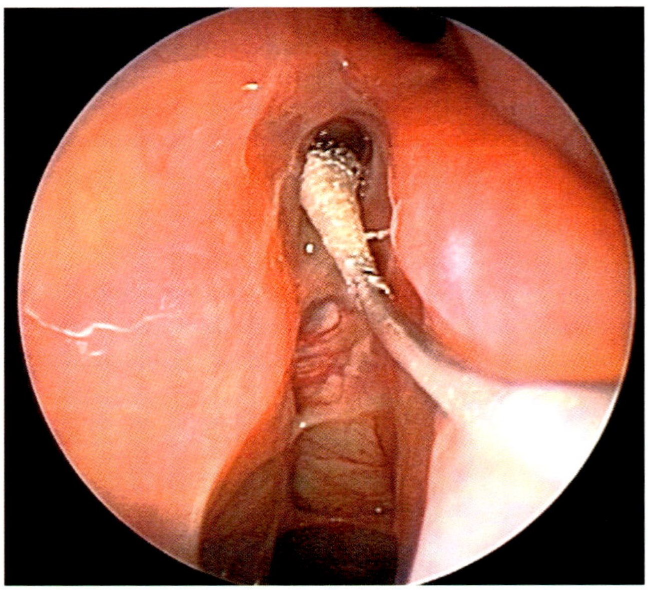

**FIGURE 21.1.** The 70° endoscopic view shows a culture sample being taken from the frontal sinus with a 90° angled suction tip.

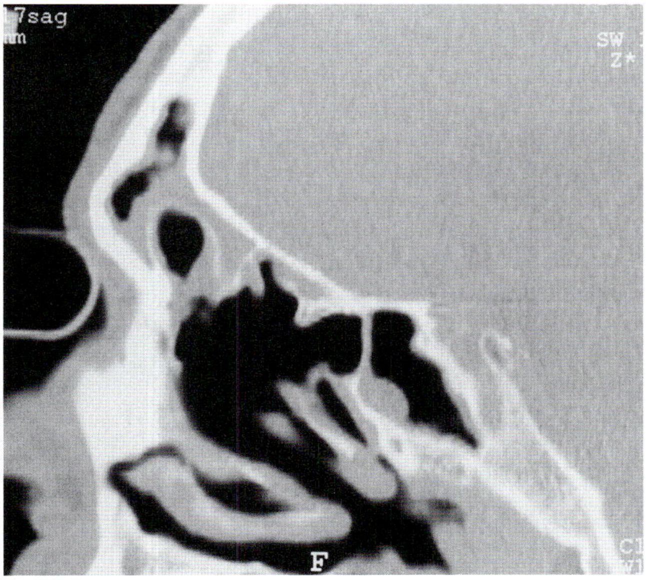


**FIGURE 21.2.** Case 1: Preoperative computed tomography scan shows an obstruction of the frontal sinus.

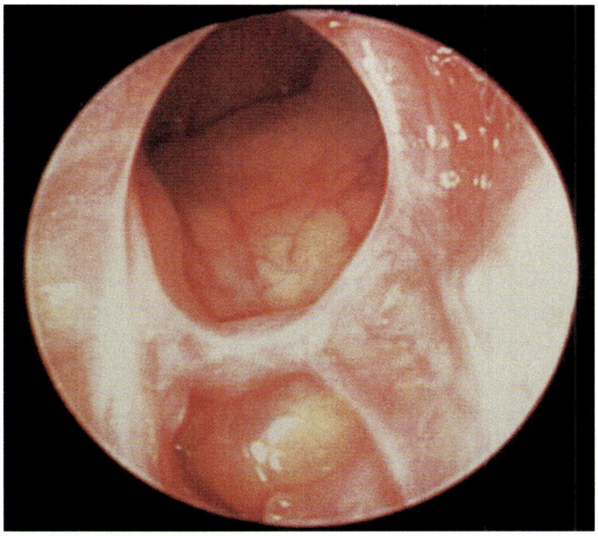

**FIGURE 21.3.** Case 1: One-year postoperative frontal recess view with a 70° endoscope.

decongestants, mucolytics, topical or oral steroids, or antihistamines may be indicated. Immunotherapy should be considered for patients with an allergic component to their sinusitis. Failure of extensive, individualized medical therapy to alleviate symptoms within 6 to 8 weeks warrants a CT scan to exclude an anatomic obstruction. If frontal sinus or recess disease is identified radiographically or endoscopically, the patient is counseled about the potential risks and benefits of FESS.

The standard coronal CT scan of the sinuses provides much information, but it is inadequate to understand three-dimensional frontal recess anatomy. Sagittal reconstructions provide the most information for evaluating the anterior-posterior dimension (Fig. 21.2). Thin axial sections (1 mm) and helical scans provide safe corneal radiation levels, excellent sagittal and coronal reconstructions, and clearly show frontal sinus anatomy and the various cells that obstruct the frontal sinus (32). The benefit of the thin axial sections extends to the use of frameless stereotactic surgical navigation devices (33).

## CASE EXAMPLES

### Case 1

A 53-year-old, white man presented with a history of sinus surgery 2.5 years previously. He had suffered from sinus infections since surgery, and for the previous 6 months, he had chronic purulent drainage and fullness in the midface and forehead despite maximum medical management. His initial RSOM-31 score was 11 for six of the nasal symptoms. CT showed bilateral residual agger nasi cells and frontal cells with bilateral frontal recess obstruction (Fig. 21.2). Endoscopically guided cultures were positive for *Staphylococcus aureus*. Bilateral revision ethmoidectomies and frontal sinusotomies were performed. One year after surgery, his sinus symptoms have cleared, and both frontal sinuses remain widely patent and easily visualized on follow-up examinations (Fig. 21.3). His 1-year follow-up RSOM-31 score was 0 for the same set of nasal symptoms.

### Case 2

A 39-year-old man presented with a 7-year history of chronic sinusitis, aspirin-sensitive asthma, and nasal polyposis. All his symptoms and asthma started in 1991, after he returned from the Gulf War, where he was exposed to vehicle exhaust and smoke from burning human waste. His preoperative RSOM-31 test revealed extensive nasal symptoms, with a University of Pennsylvania smell test indicating complete anosmia. He had a history of one previous endoscopic sinus surgery in September 1994. Nasal endoscopy revealed polyposis from floor to roof in the region of the middle turbinate, with loss of landmarks secondary to previous middle and superior turbinate resections. Cultures revealed *Serratia marcescens* and heavy growth of fungi *Paecilomyces*. His serum IgE level was 355 (normal range, 0 to 150). A review of his CT scans revealed complete bilateral opacification with evidence of

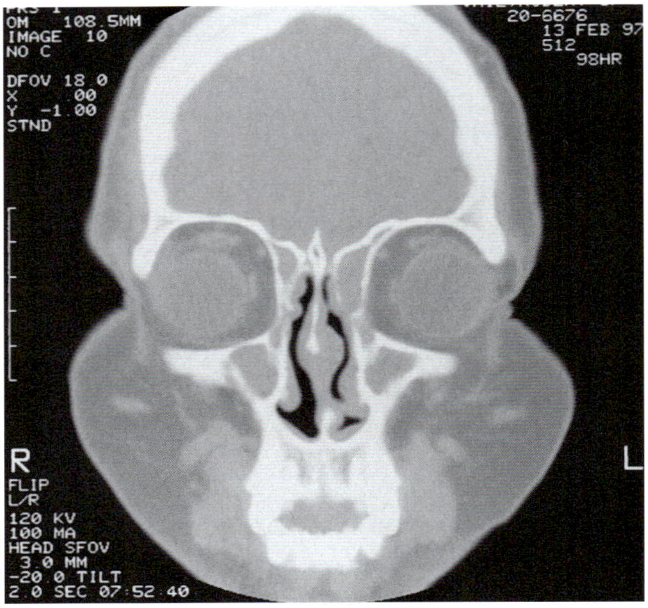


**FIGURE 21.4.** Case 2: Preoperative computed tomography shows complete frontal sinus opacification and suggests allergic fungal sinusitis and medial orbital wall dehiscence.

typical allergic fungal sinusitis from his previous and current scans (Fig. 21.4). He also had evidence of dehiscence of the left lamina papyracea. He had extensive bilateral revision FESS using stereotactic computer-assisted navigation (SCAN) or image-guided surgery (Fig. 21.5). A large amount of allergic mucin was retrieved from his frontal sinuses. Intranasal endoscopic frontal sinusotomies were performed with mucous membrane preservation despite extensive scarring and lateralized middle turbinate remnants bilaterally. Postoperative follow-up revealed well-healed frontal ostia with normally functional frontal sinuses. He has been placed on a treatment protocol for allergic fungal sinusitis (34).

## INSTRUMENTATION

The location of the frontal recess requires specialized instruments for this surgery. Frontal recess suction and nonsuction, 45° and 90° curettes, forceps, and seekers have been developed over the past decade and continue to evolve to

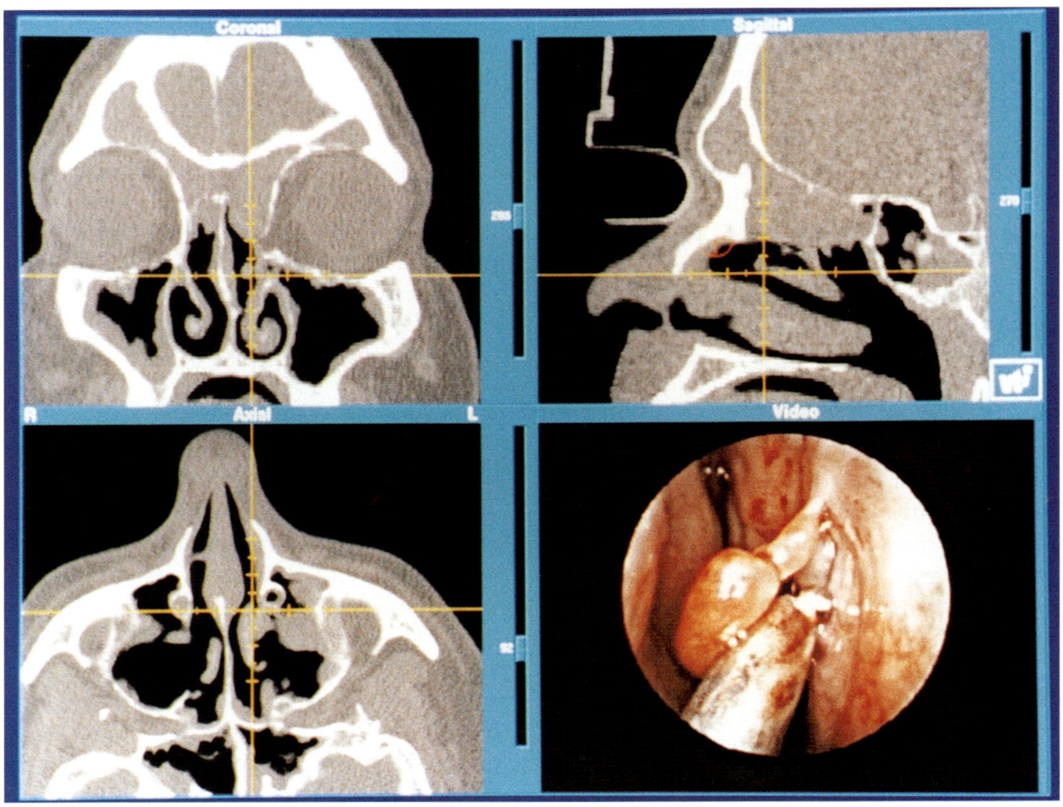


**FIGURE 21.5.** Case 2: Intraoperative view using the InstaTrak (Visualization Technologies, Inc., Boston, MA) navigational device.

solve this problem (Fig. 21.6). The 90° hook on the frontal sinus ostium seeker helps palpate, identify, and remove bony debris from the frontal ostium and the frontal recess. Additional necessary instruments include giraffe forceps; the forceps must be available in side-to-side and front-to-back biting orientations. The curettes are extremely useful for dissecting soft tissue and bony cell walls out of the frontal recess to a position where they may be grasped and removed. An instrument that has proven extremely valuable in this region is the frontal sinus mushroom punch and the through-cutting Heuweisser (Karl Storz), which aids in the removal of horizontal shelves created by bone or scar obstructing the frontal recess. Although most FESS carried out for the other paranasal sinuses uses the 0° endoscope, the frontal recess requires visualization with the 30° and 70° telescopes. The 8- and 9-French malleable suctions (Karl Storz) angled at 45°, 90°, and 110° are necessary to aspirate in this area. The angled instruments are generally intended for use below the telescope, reaching around its anterior end (Fig. 21.7). Consequently, the 45° instruments work well with the 30° scope, and 90° instruments complement the 70° endoscope. Powered instrumentation should not play a significant role in endoscopic frontal sinus surgery in most cases.

Revision endoscopic frontal sinus surgery is even more challenging in the presence of significant frontal recess scar tissue and lateralized middle or uniturbinates (31). A uniturbinate refers to scarring from previous surgery between a partially resected middle turbinate and the superior turbinate, resulting in the formation of a single, more posteriorly based turbinate. Surgery in this situation can be greatly enhanced with the use of an intraoperative image guidance system that can allow precise dissection in the region of the frontal recess (Fig. 21.5). Development of specifically angled tips to reach the frontal recess and internal frontal ostium has made image-guided surgery even more useful in this region (31) (Fig. 21.8).

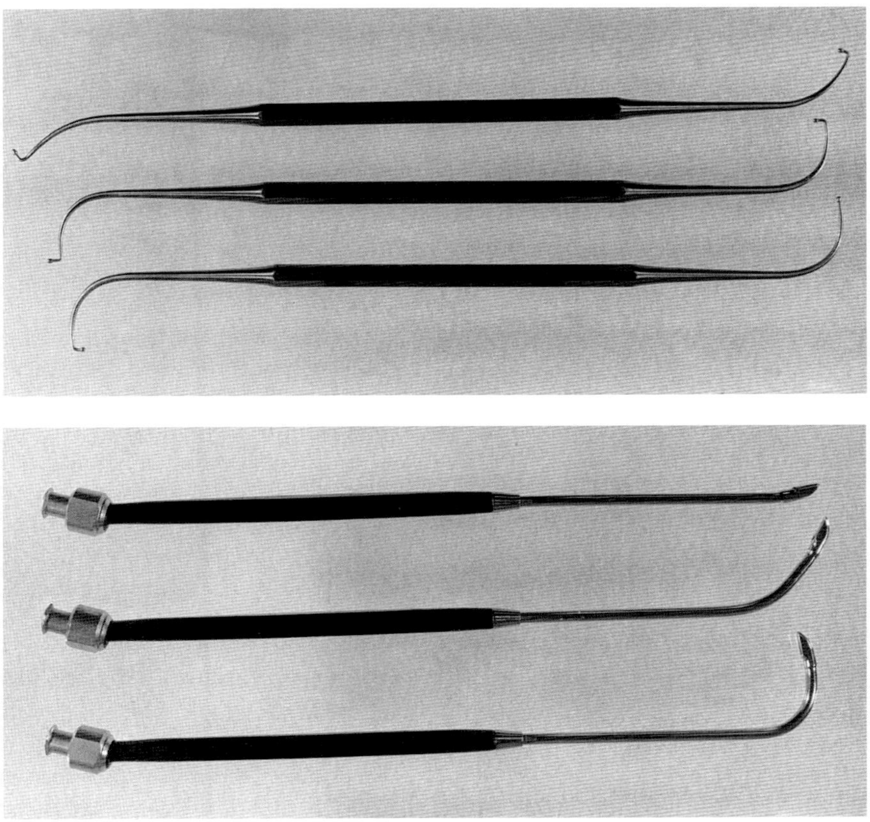

A

B

**FIGURE 21.6. A:** Latest addition of Kuhn frontal sinus seekers by Karl Storz (Tuttlingen, Germany). **B:** Suction Kuhn frontal sinus curettes developed by Med Trek (Germany).

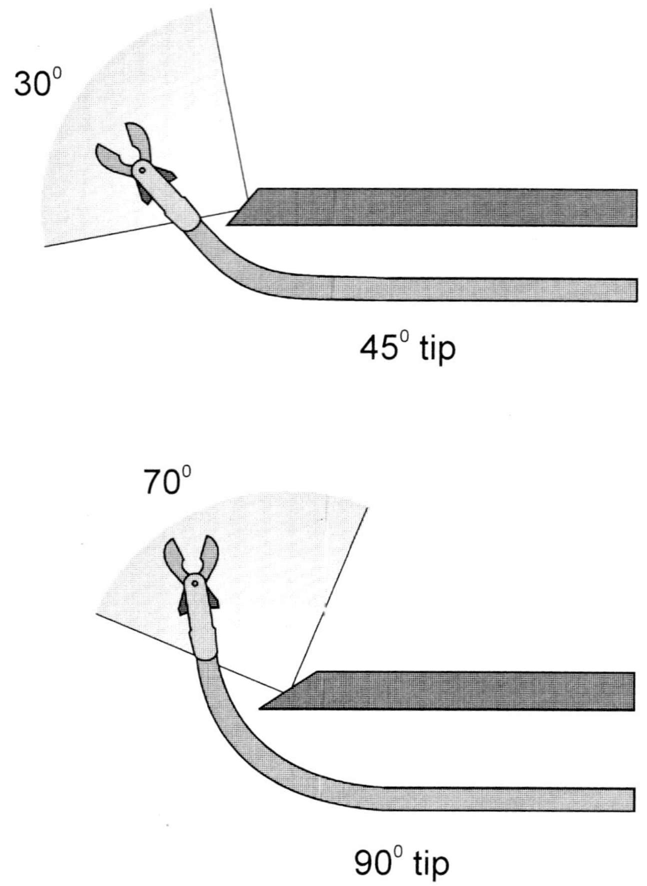


**FIGURE 21.7.** Correct use of 45° and 90° instruments with 30° and 70° telescopes.

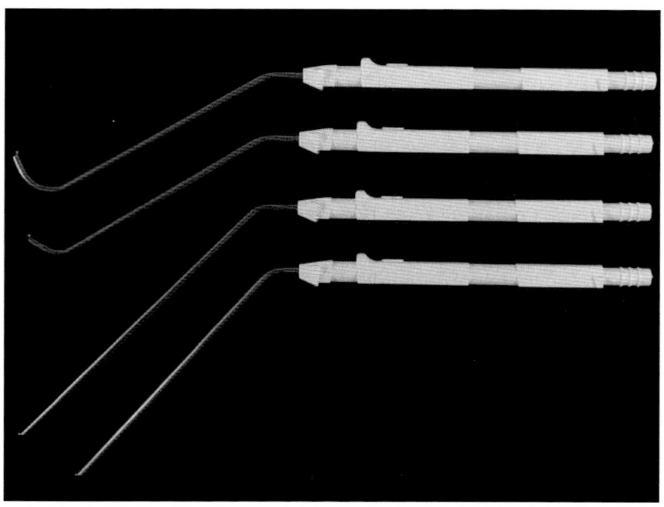

**FIGURE 21.8.** Curved suction tips available for the InstaTrak (Visualization Technologies, Inc., Boston, MA) image-guided system.

## OPERATING ROOM LAYOUT

The operating room layout for endoscopic frontal sinusotomy does not differ from the basic layout for all FESS cases. We operate from a 20-inch monitor placed directly in front of the operating surgeon. We sit on comfortable operating chairs for all our endoscopic procedures (Fig. 21.9).

## ANESTHESIA

In properly selected patients, local anesthesia with sedation has several advantages over general anesthesia. A significant decrease in blood loss has been demonstrated in endoscopic cases carried out under local anesthesia (35). An awake patient's feedback may alert the surgeon if the dissection approaches orbital periosteum or dura. However, in predictably prolonged cases, general anesthesia may prove to be much more comfortable for the patient and the surgeon.

An oxymetazoline (Afrin)–soaked length of cotton gauze is placed in the middle meatus while the patient is being prepped and draped. This is then removed, and an injection using 1% Xylocaine with 1:100,000 epinephrine is carried out with an effort to infiltrate the most superior and anterior aspect of the middle meatus and the anterior buttress of the middle turbinate, as well as the anteroinferior aspect of the uncinate. While awaiting vasoconstriction, complete nasal endoscopy is carried out, correlating endoscopic and CT findings.

## OPERATIVE TECHNIQUE

### Anatomy

Any discussion of frontal sinus surgery must begin with an anatomic review of the cells, which may potentially obstruct the frontal recess. These include agger nasi cells, supraorbital ethmoid cells, frontal cells type I through IV, frontal bulla cells, suprabullar cells, and interfrontal sinus septal cells. The first three types are the more common anterior ethmoid cells, which pneumatize the frontal recess and cause frontal sinus obstruction or confuse the operating surgeon about whether the frontal sinus has been opened. Further details and discussion of these cells can be found elsewhere (17,29,36–39).

A successful surgical outcome requires thorough clinical and radiologic frontal recess evaluation. This includes thin axial-section CT with sagittal reconstruction to determine the cell types that may be involved in its obstruction. If disease in the frontal recess does not resolve after prolonged medical treatment, the obstruction must be removed before drainage from the frontal sinus can be effected.

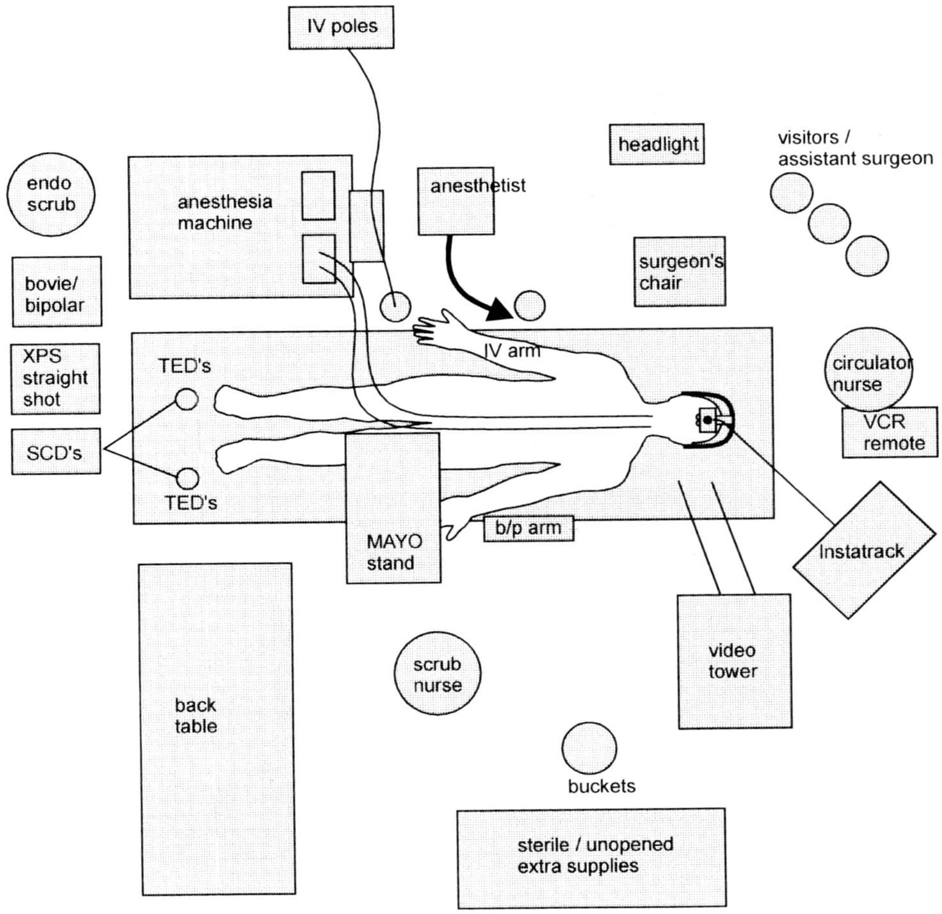


**FIGURE 21.9.** Operating room layout. Two pads on bed; eggcrate foam under head and heels; 3 suctions; call family every 20–30 minutes. *SCD*, sequential compression device; *TED*, compression hose; *XPS*, tissue debrider/powered dissector.

## Operative Method

### *Principal Methods*

It is imperative that the frontal recess mucous membrane be preserved using a delicate surgical technique. Removal of the mucous membrane leads to osteoneogenesis, scarring, and frontal sinus stenosis (36). In a previously unoperated patient, the procedure is carried out in the following manner:

*Step 1:* The uncinate process is removed and the natural maxillary ostium identified using the technique previously described by Owen and Kuhn (40). The maxillary sinus outflow tract is left undisturbed.

*Step 2:* The ethmoid bulla and posterior ethmoids are then removed if there is evidence of disease extending into this region. If a complete ethmoidectomy is being done, the surgeon should go through the basal lamella to the face of the sphenoid. The face of the sphenoid is followed superiorly to the skull base. The skull base is then followed anteriorly from posteriorly, removing all lamella with through-cutting instruments. The posterior and anterior ethmoids should be cleaned out first. As the anterior ethmoid artery is approached, the skull base begins sloping sharply upward. This is the posterior entrance to the frontal recess (Fig. 21.10). The surgeon's movements should be from posterior to anterior, with very limited side-to-side action, protecting the orbit and anterior cranial fossa. Great care is taken to avoid injuring the lamina papyracea laterally and the lateral lamella of the cribriform plate medially. The weakest point of the entire anterior skull base is at the roof of the ethmoid where it is penetrated by the anterior ethmoid artery (28). This corresponds to the lateral lamella of the cribriform plate. The bone may only be 0.1 to 0.2 mm thick at this point. This area is even more susceptible to injury in a Keros type III anatomic variation, in which the olfactory groove is deep

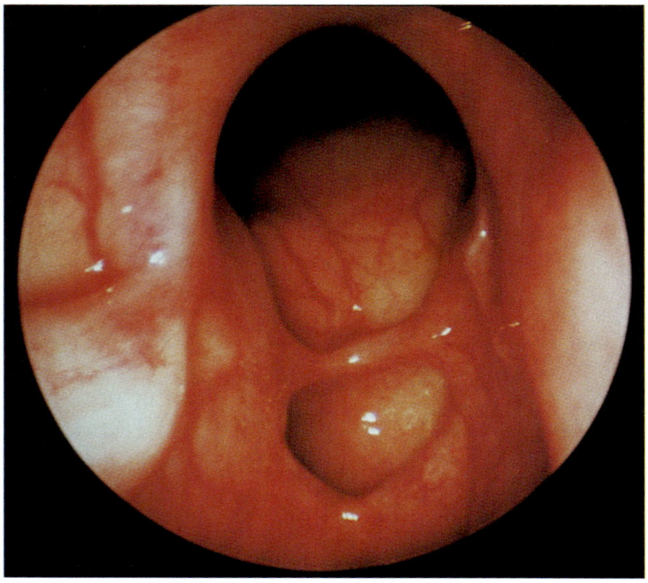

**FIGURE 21.10.** The 70° endoscopic view of the frontal recess and sloping skull base, showing the anterior ethmoid artery.

creating a taller lateral lamella of the cribriform plate (36) (Fig. 21.11).

*Step 3:* The angled frontal recess curettes can then be slipped up the posterior frontal recess wall behind any bony cellular elements which occupy the frontal recess (Fig. 21.12A). The curette and cell walls can then be pulled down and forward. The bony fragments are then removed with giraffe forceps (Fig. 21.12B). This step is repeated carefully until the internal frontal ostium is visualized and its obstruction removed.

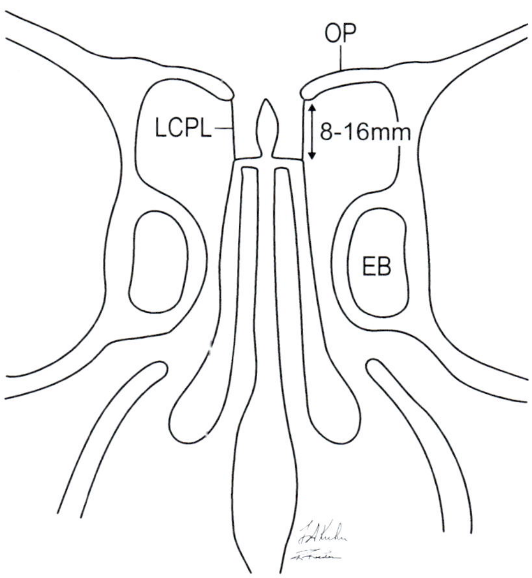


**FIGURE 21.11.** Keros type III configuration with a deep olfactory groove. *EB*, ethmoid bulla; *LCPL*, lateral cribriform plate lamellae; *OP*, orbital plate.

## Methods for Special Situations

*Step 4a:* If the patient has an agger nasi cell, the posterior wall and dome of the agger nasi cell must be removed. The superior aspect of the dome can sometimes be removed most easily with a frontal sinus mushroom punch after breaking down the posterior and medial walls with the 90° curettes.

*Step 4b:* If the patient has a supraorbital ethmoid cell, the common wall between the frontal sinus and the supraorbital ethmoid cell should be removed as high into the frontal recess as possible (Fig. 21.13). If these walls are not adequately removed, they may become chronically edematous because of mucociliary mucous clearance disruption, resulting in frontal sinus obstruction. Disruption of mucociliary flow patterns in partially removed cells leads to mucus recirculation and edema, which may close off the drainage pathways.

*Step 4c:* Interfrontal sinus septal cells can be challenging to deal with. One of the major problems is the difficulty translating the CT appearance into the endoscopic view (Fig. 21.14). Interfrontal sinus septal cells generally empty into the frontal recess medial and anterior to the internal frontal ostium. It may be difficult distinguishing between these two ostia (Fig. 21.15).

*Step 4d:* If the patient has had the anterior aspect of the middle turbinate resected with lateralization of the remnant stump obstructing the frontal recess, a *frontal sinus rescue* procedure can be carried out (41). This involves removal of the anterior middle turbinate stump together with the mucous membrane on its medial aspect. The mucous membrane on its lateral aspect is carefully maintained and draped medially over the denuded area where the previous stump with its mucous membrane had laid. This results in a large, mucosalized opening into the previously obstructed frontal sinus (Fig. 21.16).

If only anterior ethmoidectomy is necessary, the basal lamella may be followed upward to the skull base and frontal recess, as described by Loury (42), or in the case of isolated frontal sinus disease, the ethmoid bulla may be left intact, as described by Sethi (unpublished data, Vienna, Austria, 1998). The only pitfall with this technique is not removing the bulla lamella completely and leaving a supraorbital ethmoid cell undetected behind it. It is much better to follow the middle turbinate basal lamella to the skull base instead and then work forward.

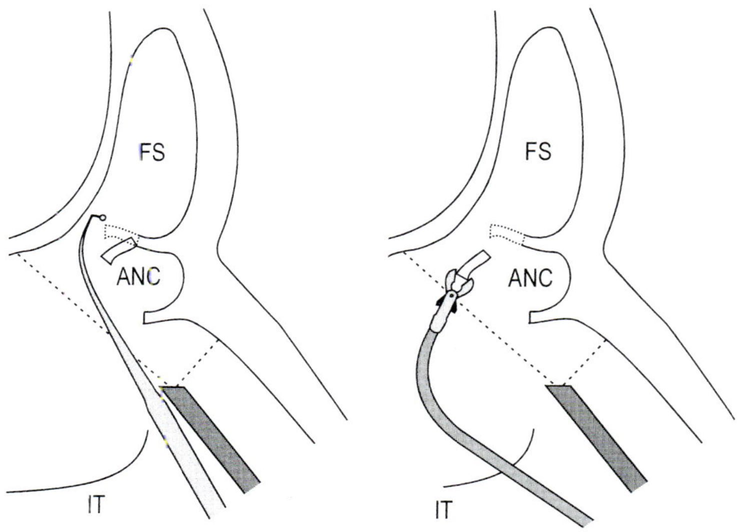


**FIGURE 21.12.** Frontal endoscopic sinusotomy technique using a 70° endoscope and 90° instrumentation to remove bone and a mucous membrane obstruction.

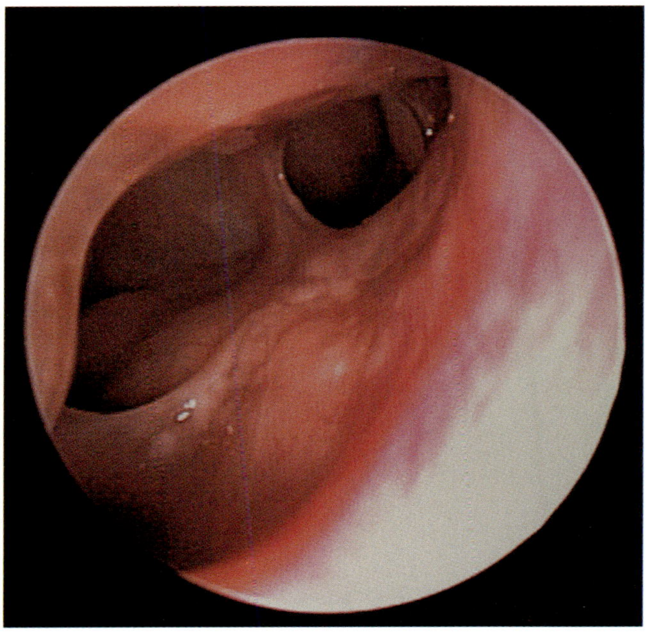

**FIGURE 21.13.** The 70° endoscopic postoperative view shows the partition between a supraorbital ethmoid cell and the frontal sinus.

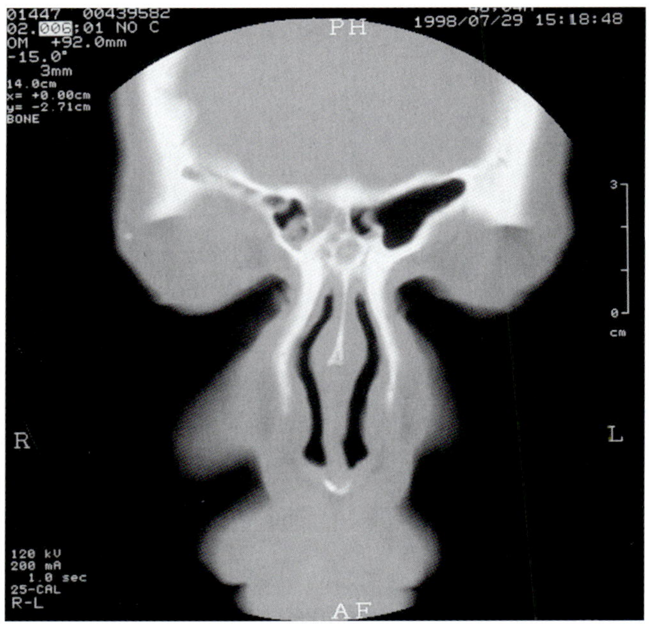


**FIGURE 21.14.** Coronal computed tomography shows an opacified intersinus septal cell.

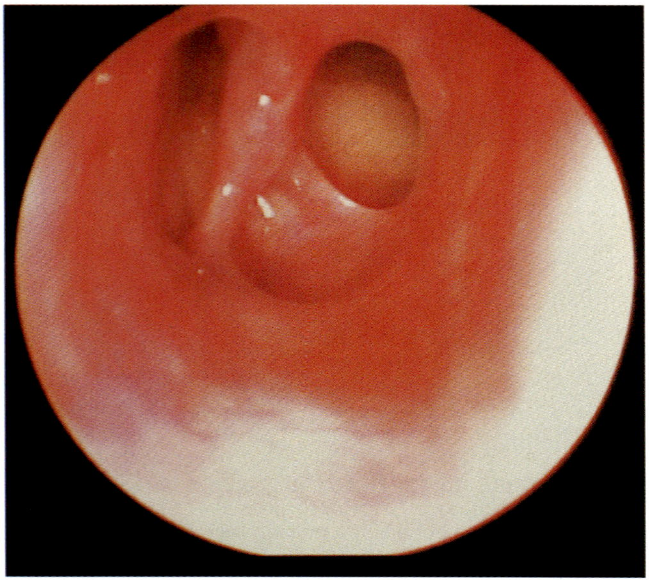

**FIGURE 21.15.** The 70° endoscopic view of the drainage pathway of a left sided intersinus septal cell (*left*) and internal frontal ostium (*right*).

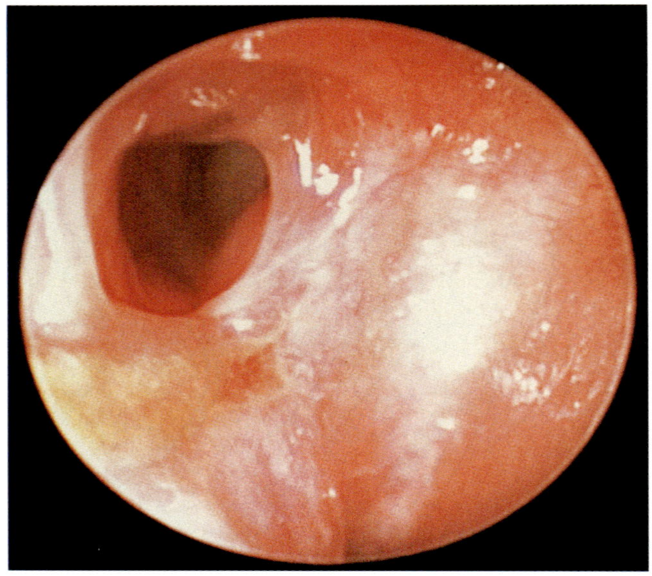

**FIGURE 21.16.** The 70° endoscopic view of a healed frontal sinus opening after a frontal sinus rescue procedure.

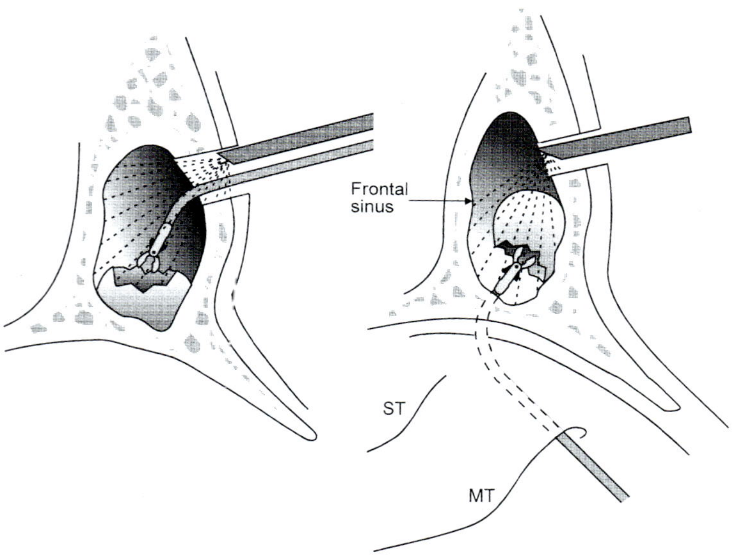


**FIGURE 21.17.** The "above and below" approach using an anterior table trephine.

### Additional Methods

In some cases, the intranasal endoscopic technique by itself is insufficient. Revision cases may be complicated by dense bone and frontal recess scarring. Frontal cells or superiorly pneumatized agger nasi cells may be unreachable endoscopically. In such special situations, an external frontal sinus trephination can be made to work on the frontal recess simultaneously from above and below.

*Step 1:* As completely as possible, an endoscopic intranasal frontal sinusotomy is first carried out as described previously.

*Step 2:* A 2-cm incision is made in the medial aspect of the eyebrow, angling the incision through the skin to match the angulation of the hair shafts. Once through the skin, blunt dissection is used down to the periosteum.

*Step 3:* Staying supraperiosteal, the tissue is slid superiorly and medially well above the supraorbital ridge. An incision is then made in the periosteum, and using a 4-mm burr, a hole is made into the anterior frontal sinus table.

*Step 4:* A 30° or 70° endoscope can then be inserted through the burr hole to inspect the frontal sinus, and cultures can be taken directly from the sinus.

*Step 5:* An angled scope is then parked at the upper outer entrance of the burr hole, and curettes or other instruments can be inserted into the sinus to break down bony shelves or scar tissue so that it can be removed with giraffe forceps from below (Fig. 21.17). When wider exposure is necessary, as after failed fat obliteration of the frontal sinus, an osteoplastic flap may be necessary rather than a trephine to "unobliterate" the frontal sinus. In many instances, these "above and below" approaches may provide the only opportunity to restore normal sinus ventilation and drainage (21).

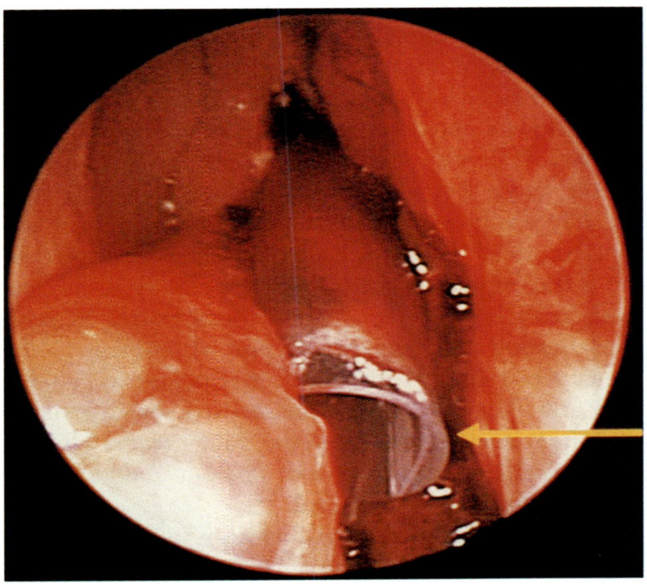

**FIGURE 21.18.** Endoscopic view of a rolled silostic sheet placed in the left frontal sinus.

If the dissected frontal recess is too narrow, stenting may be carried out to maintain patency. Soft rather than rigid stents have yielded the best results (8). Thin Silastic rolled into a stent provides soft support of the surgically manipulated frontal recess (Fig. 21.18). An 8- or 10-French pediatric biliary T-tube can also be cut to create a T-shaped stent that fits loosely into the internal frontal ostium. There has been some concern regarding the formation of a biofilm on the stents that can result in multiple antibiotic–resistant bacteria (43). The development of medically coated stents is in progress at our center to counter this problem.

## Highlights

1. The preservation of peripheral mucous membrane in the frontal recess and internal ostium is crucial for success of this procedure.
2. The surgeon must always be aware of the presence of supraorbital ethmoid cells that may masquerade as part of the frontal sinus if the CT scan is not critically evaluated.
3. In most instances, the intranasal endoscopic approach can be accomplished successfully without the need for an external procedure.
4. In revision cases with extensive scarring or extremely superiorly pneumatized frontal or agger nasi cells, the surgeon may need to resort to an external trephine, allowing an "above and below" approach.
5. The dissection should always be carried out in a posterior-to-anterior direction, and meticulous technique should be used to remove all free bone particles and debris from the frontal recess to prevent future scarring and osteitis.
6. Postoperative endoscopic care is integral to the success of endoscopic frontal sinusotomy. The availability of proper office equipment to perform postoperative care is critical, and if it is not available, the procedure should not be done.

## Postoperative Care

Proper immediate and long-term postoperative care begins in the operating room and has a pivotal role in achieving a good functional result (44). Good postoperative care requires proper office instrumentation, a schedule of postoperative visits, intranasal endoscopic débridement, patient counseling, and postoperative medical management.

The most important factors in achieving good functional results are scar prevention and avoiding middle meatus collapse. Mucous membrane preservation and postoperative fibrin clot débridement are extremely important aspects of scar prevention. Because fibrin clot can progress to granulation tissue and then scar, it is important to perform postoperative endoscopic débridement in the office. This removes as much clot as possible before it becomes organized. However, the clinician should not cause bleeding in the aggressive pursuit of fibrin clot removal, because this starts the process over again. Removal of mucous membrane in a difficult area such as the frontal recess, especially if the bone is curetted, rasped, or drilled, stimulates osteoneogenesis, with potential bony closure of ostia and recesses.

Middle meatal collapse can result in disaster. It can prevent inspection of the frontal recess and may end up obstructing the frontal and other sinus cavities. If there is any doubt of middle turbinate stability at the end of the procedure, it is wise to "Bolgerize" it (44). To reduce fibrin clot accumulation in the middle meatus, a middle meatal spacer is placed intraoperatively and removed on the fourth postoperative day (44).

To accomplish adequate postoperative débridement in the frontal recess, the surgeon must have the proper equipment. Office instrumentation should include 30° and 70° endoscopes, malleable suctions curved to 45° and 90°, 45° and 90° frontal sinus curettes, and a frontal ostium seeker. The 45° and 90° frontal recess giraffe forceps opening front-to-back and side-to-side are also required if proper postoperative office débridement in the frontal recess region is desired. The 45° instruments are used in conjunction with the 30° telescope, and the 90° instruments are used in conjunction with the 70° endoscopes (Fig. 21.7).

On the first postoperative day, the nose may be cleaned back to the middle meatus to remove some of the crusting, and the patient is told to begin saline irrigations. The need for postoperative antibiotics and steroids is assessed, depending on findings at surgery. On day 4, the patient returns for middle meatal spacer removal and endoscopic cleaning, with the clinician paying particular attention to the ethmoid roof and frontal recess. The patient is then reinstructed in the use of saline irrigations and encouraged to perform them more vigorously (Table 21.1). The third visit is 1 week later. Nasal endoscopic débridement is again performed, removing fibrin clot and polyps with débridement of any devitalized bone. The patient is continued on saline irrigations. The need for postoperative antibiotics and steroids is reassessed at each visit. The fourth postoperative visit is 2 weeks later if the frontal recess looks good at the third visit. Nasal endoscopy is performed, evaluating the need for additional cleaning and the progress of healing. Revision procedures may be performed as necessary in the office: breaking down synechiae, removing polyps, and placing spacers if the middle turbinate starts to lateralize. If the patient is doing well at this visit (21 to 25 days postoperatively), the next visit is scheduled approximately 3 weeks later.

**TABLE 21.1. RECIPE AND PATIENT INSTRUCTIONS FOR POSTOPERATIVE SALINE NASAL IRRIGATIONS**

| | |
|---|---|
| Hypertonic Saline | 3 heaping teaspoons of canning or pickling salt<br>2 heaping teaspoons of baking soda<br>1 quart of water |
| Instructions | Irrigate each nostril with 1 to 2 measuring cups of the saline mixture three or four times daily. This is designed to help clean the crusts, dried blood and clots out of the nose and to reduce the required cleaning in the office on your postoperative visits. |

Antibiotics and steroids are used when needed, but are not part of the routine. If the patient does not have an infection at the time of surgery, antibiotics are generally not prescribed. Endoscopically guided cultures are obtained by aspirating the sinus contents into a Luekens trap with a curved suction or a Xomed (Jacksonville, FL) Sinus Secretion Collector as a matter of routine when purulence is noticed (Fig. 21.2). Hypertonic saline irrigation is an important part of the healing process. We prefer non-iodized, pickling or sea salt rather than table salt to minimize the amount of irritants contacting the nasal mucous membrane during the healing process. We do not favor the use of powered dental irrigation devices for fear that the device may become colonized with bacteria such as *Pseudomonas.* Instead, disposable 60-mL irrigating syringes are used which can be washed and dried or thrown away and replaced as necessary.

## Complications

Potential intraoperative complications include penetration of the intracranial cavity posteriorly and medially and of the orbit laterally. Bleeding, cerebrospinal fluid leak, and a floppy middle turbinate are other possible early complications. The posterior frontal recess wall is composed of the skull base and anterior cranial fossa. Medially, just below the internal frontal ostium, lies the lateral cribriform plate lamella, which is extremely thin. Both are easily penetrable. Laterally, the frontal recess is bounded by the medial and superior orbital walls, which are relatively more dense than the lateral cribriform plate lamella. Anteriorly is only the hard, dense bone of the anterior frontal ostium buttress. Consequently, the primary direction of working in the frontal recess should be from posterior to anterior, pulling away from the thin skull base. Alternatively, the surgeon can work from medial to lateral in the frontal recess. The two directions that are unsafe to work are from anterior to posterior and from lateral to medial.

The anterior ethmoid artery, which is in the vicinity of the dissection, can also be penetrated, resulting in potentially severe bleeding or retro-orbital hematoma. Periorbital ecchymosis is probably the most common early complication but has an incidence of less than 1%.

Synechia between the middle turbinate and the lateral nasal wall is one of the most common late complications; this can be reduced by minimizing trauma to the lateral middle turbinate surface during insertion of the endoscopes and instruments. A study at our institution showed that previous partial resections of the middle turbinate resulted in a greater chance of frontal recess obstruction (31). Encephalocele formation due to a defect in the anterior skull base is a late complication. All patients are advised of the risk of recurrent or persistent sinusitis and the possible need for additional surgery.

## ADVANTAGES AND LIMITATIONS OF THE ENDOSCOPIC TECHNIQUE

The endoscopic intranasal approach to the frontal recess and sinus allows the surgeon to relieve obstruction, reestablish the physiologic mucociliary pathway, and provide aeration of the sinus using a less morbid, more easily tolerated procedure than the previously used external procedures. In most instances, the patient can be discharged home the morning after surgery. In the rare event that an external approach is required, it only involves an anterior wall trephine that allows simultaneous endoscopically directed dissection of the frontal recess from above and below. A major prerequisite of performing the procedure is an adequate amount of experience and patience on the part of the surgeon to ensure minimal trauma to the circumference of the frontal recess mucosa while achieving adequate removal of obstructing bone and scar tissue.

Endoscopic surgery of the frontal recess is not favored in the treatment of invading malignancies involving the frontal sinus, for intracranial or intraorbital complications arising from acute sinusitis, and for extreme laterally based mucoceles. In most other instances, a carefully performed endoscopic frontal sinusotomy can result in a ventilated, physiologically normal frontal sinus.

## REFERENCES


1. Reidel BM. In: Denker A, Kahler O, eds. *Handbuch der Hals-Nasen-Ohren Heilkunde*, vol 2. Berlin: Springer-Verlag, 1926; 806–808.
2. Brieger. *Arch Ohren Nasen Kelkopfheilk* 1895;39:213.
3. Killian G. De Killian'sche radicaloperation chronischer Stirnhohleneiterungen; II. Weiteres Kasuistisched Material und Zusammenfassung. *Arch Laryngol Rhinol* 1903;13:59-88.
4. Nguyen QA, Leopold DA. Current concepts in the surgical management of chronic frontal sinusitis. *Otolaryngol Clin North Am* 1997;30:355–370.
5. Lynch RC. Techniques of a radical frontal sinus operation, which has given me the best results. *Laryngoscope* 1921:31:1–5.
6. Anthony DH. *South Med J* 1940;33:949.
7. Ingals EF. Intranasal drainage of the frontal sinus. *Ann Otol Rhinol Laryngol* 1917;26:656–668.
8. Neel HB III, Whicker JH, Lake CF. Thin rubber sheeting in frontal sinus surgery: animal and clinical studies. *Laryngoscope* 1976;86:524–536.
9. Mihoefer W. *Arch Otolaryngol* 1928;7:133.
10. Negus VE. *BMJ* 1947;1:135.
11. Baron SH, Dedo HH, Henry CR. The mucoperiosteal flap in frontal sinus surgery (the Sewall-Boyden-McNaught operation). *Laryngoscope* 1973;80:1266–1280.
12. Dedo HH, Broberg TG, Murr AH. Frontoethmoidectomy with Sewall-Boyden reconstruction: alive and well, a 25-year experience. *Am J Rhinol* 1998;12:3:191–198.
13. Porto DP, Duvall AJ. Long-term results with nasofrontal duct reconstruction. *Laryngoscope* 1986;96:858–862.
14. Metson R. Endoscopic treatment of frontal sinusitis. *Laryngoscope* 1992;102:712–716.
15. Schaefer SD, Close LG. Endoscopic management of frontal sinus disease. *Laryngoscope* 1990;100:155–160.
16. Kennedy DW, Josephson JS, Zeinreich SJ, et al. Endoscopic sinus surgery for mucoceles: a viable alternative. *Laryngoscope* 1989;99:885–895.
17. Kuhn FA, Bolger WE, Tisdale RG. The agger nasi cell in frontal recess obstruction: an anatomic, radiologic and clinical correlation. *Oper Tech Otolaryngol Head Neck Surg* 1991;2:226–231.
18. Close LG, Lee NK, Leach JL, et al. Endoscopic resection of the intranasal frontal sinus floor. *Ann Otol Rhinol Laryngol* 1994; 103:952–958.
19. Becker DG, Moore D, Lindsey WH, et al. Modified transnasal endoscopic Lothrop procedure: further considerations. *Laryngoscope* 1995;105:1161–1166.
20. Kuhn FA. The endoscopic frontal recess approach to chronic frontal sinusitis. Presented at the 20th Advanced Functional Endoscopic Sinus Surgery Course, Savannah, GA, October 1998.
21. Bent JP, Spears R, Kuhn FA. An alternative to frontal sinus obliteration. Presented at the Southern Section of the Triologic Society, Marco Island, FL, January 14, 1994.
22. Bent JP, Kuhn FA. In: Stankiewics, ed. *Advanced endoscopic sinus surgery.* St. Louis: Mosby, 1995:13–23.
23. Waitz G, Wigand ME. Results of endoscopic sinus surgery for the treatment of inverted papillomas. *Laryngoscope* 1992;102: 917–922.
24. McCary WS, Gross CW, Reibel JF, et al. Preliminary report: endoscopic versus external surgery in the management of inverting papilloma. *Laryngoscope* 1994;104:415–419.
25. Har-El G, Lucente FE. Endoscopic intranasal frontal sinusotomy. *Laryngoscope* 1995;105:440–443.
26. Shohet JA, Duncavage JA. Management of the frontal sinus with inverted papilloma. *Otolaryngol Head Neck Surg* 1996;114: 649–652.
27. May M, Levine HL, Mester SJ, et al. In: May M, Levine HC, eds. *Endoscopic sinus surgery.* New York: Thieme Medical, 1943; 105–175.
28. Stammberger H, ed. *Functional endoscopic sinus surgery.* Philadelphia: BC Decker, 1991.
29. Owen RG, Kuhn FA. The supra orbital ethmoid cell. *Otolaryngol Head Neck Surg* 1997;116:254–261.
30. Leopold D, Ferguson BJ, Piccirillo JF. In: Anon JB, ed. Outcomes assessment. Report of the Rhinosinusitis Task Force Committee meeting. *Otolaryngol Head Neck Surg Suppl* 1997: 558–568.
31. Javer AR, Kuhn FA. The uniturbinate. In: Stammberger H, Wolf G, eds. *Proceedings ERS & ISIAN meeting.* Bologna, Italy: Monduzzi Editore, 1998:3–7.
32. Sillers MJ, Kuhn FA, Vickery CL. Radiation exposure in paranasal sinus imaging. *Otolaryngol Head Neck Surg* 1995;112: 248–251.

33. Metson R, Gliklich RE, Cosenza M. A comparison of image guidance systems for sinus surgery. *Laryngoscope* 1998;108: 1164–1170.
34. Kuhn FA, Javer AR. Allergic fungal rhinosinusitis: our experience. *Arch Otolaryngol Head Neck Surg* 1998;124:1179–80.
35. Stankiewicz JA. Complications in endoscopic intranasal ethmoidectomy: an update. *Laryngoscope* 1989;99:686–690.
36. Kuhn FA. Operative techniques in chronic frontal sinusitis: the endoscopic frontal recess approach. *Oper Tech Otolaryngol Head Neck Surg* 1996;7:222–229.
37. Kuhn FA. In: Gluckman JL, ed. *Renewal of certification study guide in otolaryngology—head and neck surgery.* Iowa: Kendall/ Hunt Publishing, 1998:171–181.
38. Bent J, Kuhn FA, Cuilty C. The frontal cell in frontal recess obstruction. *Am J Rhinol* 1994;8:185–191.
39. Merritt R, Kuhn FA. The interfrontal sinus septal cell. *Am J Rhinol* 1996;10.
40. Owen RG Jr., Kuhn FA. Demystifying the maxillary sinus ostium. *Am J Rhinol* 1995;9:313–320.
41. Citardi MJ, Javer AR, Kuhn FA. Revision endoscopic frontal sinusotomy with mucoperiosteal flap advancement: the frontal sinus rescue procedure. *Otolaryngol Clin North Am* 2001;34: 123–132.
42. Loury MC. Endoscopic frontal recess and frontal sinus ostium dissection. *Laryngoscope* 1993;103:455–458.
43. Reid G. Bacterial colonization of prosthetic devices and measures to prevent infection. *New Horizon* 1998;6:558–563.
44. Kuhn FA, Citardi MJ. Advances in postoperative care following functional endoscopic sinus surge. *Otolaryngol Clin North Am* 1997;30:470–490.

# 22

# SUBTLETIES IN ENDOSCOPIC SURGERY OF THE SPHENOID SINUS

TIMOTHY L. SMITH
ROBERT J. TOOHILL
TODD A. LOEHRL

## INDICATIONS AND HISTORICAL PERSPECTIVE

Endoscopic sphenoid surgery is most commonly indicated for chronic sphenoid sinusitis, but the endoscopic approach may also be used to manage fungal sinusitis, cerebrospinal fluid (CSF) leaks, mucoceles, and various benign growths and neoplasms (1).

Before the availability of endoscopes, isolated sphenoid sinus disease was approached transnasally using calibrated cannulas, angles, measurements, and the "experienced rhinologist's sensation of having slipped into a cavity" (2). Roentgenograms on lateral view were taken with probes and cannulas to verify appropriate placement. Van Alyea described the average distance from the inferior nasal spine to the sphenoid ostium as 58 mm using an angle of 23.5° with the cannula 1 cm above the nasal floor at the nares. The average distance from the anterior part of the nares to the ostium was 68 mm. Review of the literature demonstrates a fairly consistent 5-mm difference between male and female specimens. For the most part, there is agreement that the sphenoid ostium in adults is between 65 and 75 mm from the anterior nares (2–4) (Fig. 22.1).

Many approaches have been used to access sphenoid sinus disease. The transseptal approach has been used in cases of bilateral disease and requires submucous resection to the rostrum of the sphenoid with removal of the anterior face and a portion of the intersinus septum. The transantral approach was often used in cases of pansinusitis and required extensive enlargement of the maxillary sinus ostium posteriorly to allow visualization of the posterior ethmoids and sphenoid sinus. The external fronto-ethmo-sphenoidal operation was reserved for radical resection of sinus disease, including the sphenoid sinus. The transpalatal approach has generally been reserved for access to tumors involving the sphenoid sinus with extension into the nasopharynx. Before the availability of endoscopes, the operating microscope was frequently used with these approaches.

Modern management of sphenoid sinus disease almost always includes the use of endoscopes because of the excellent visualization afforded by them and the instrumentation designed to complement them (5). As experience with endoscopic sinus surgery has increased, the use of endoscopes has expanded to complement and sometimes replace traditional skull base approaches. In the era of endoscopic surgery, visualization by the surgeon has never been better and the morbidity suffered by the patient never less.

## PREOPERATIVE EVALUATION

Preoperative evaluation includes a complete history and physical examination. Headache is a common complaint in sphenoid disease and is often described as retro-orbital, occipital, or vertex in location. Visual symptoms, including blurring of vision, diplopia, transient loss of vision, and isolated oculomotor palsy, must be elucidated and require consultation with ophthalmology (6–8).

Nasal endoscopy using 0° and 30° endoscopes allows identification of sphenoethmoid recess polyps and other obstructions (1,9). It also permits endoscopically guided cultures to maximize medical therapy. Although preoperative sinus CT scanning usually is performed in the coronal plane, axial-plane scanning can be very helpful in imaging the sphenoid ostia, sphenoid septa configurations, sphenoethmoid (Onodi) cells, and carotid artery and optic nerve relationships with the lateral sphenoid wall. Bone erosion of the sphenoid walls requires further evaluation with magnetic resonance imaging (MRI) because encephaloceles and carotid artery aneurysms, along with other structures unsafe to biopsy, have been reported (9a). Imaging of the sphenoid sinus is further discussed in Chapter 19.

Medical therapy is maximized in patients with chronic sinus disease. Isolated sphenoid sinusitis raises the clinical suspicion of gastroesophageal reflux disease, and antireflux medications are considered. Ulualp and colleagues demon-

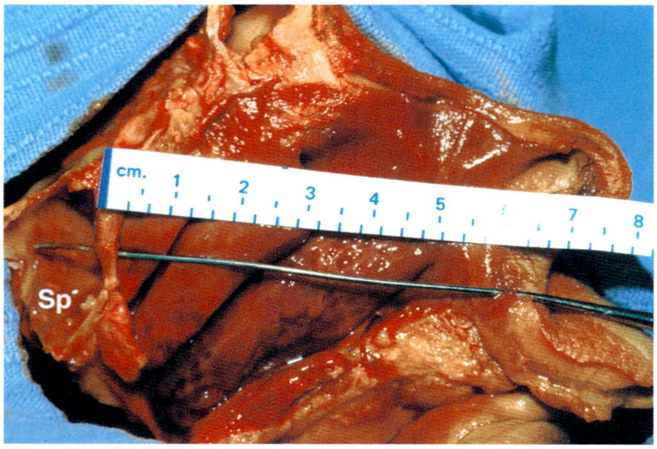


**FIGURE 22.1.** In adults, the sphenoid ostium is 65 to 75 mm from the anterior nares. *Sp,* sphenoid.

strated a higher occurrence of pharyngeal reflux of gastric acid by 24-hour three-site pH monitoring in patients with chronic sinusitis compared with normal controls (10). These patients frequently have no preceding chronic nasal or sinus symptoms. A high degree of suspicion is warranted for selected patients when no other obvious cause is found.

Preoperatively, culture-directed antibiotics are continued to the day of surgery. In patients with significant mucosal inflammation, systemic steroids are initiated at least 1 week preoperatively. Patients are educated regarding the surgeon's desire to medically reduce mucosal inflammation for the day of surgery.

## CASE EXAMPLES

### Case 1

A 67-year-old man presented with chronic vertex headaches for several months that were associated with recurrent purulent sinusitis. His symptoms improved after long courses of antibiotics, only to return within days after cessation of the antibiotics. CT scan of the sinuses revealed significant ethmoid mucosal thickening and opacification. The left sphenoid sinus contained a soft tissue density consistent with a cyst or polyp (Fig. 22.2).

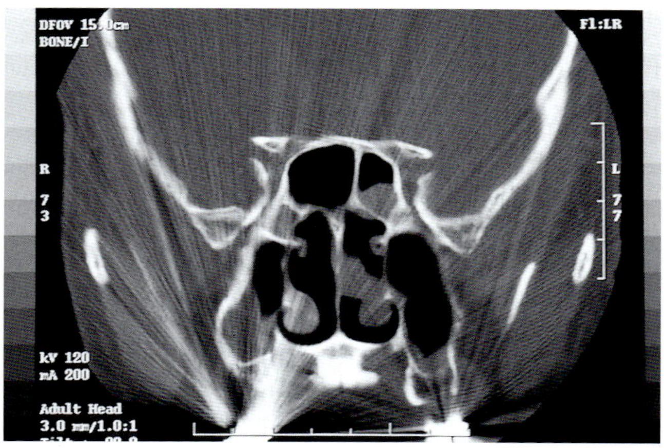


**FIGURE 22.2.** Computed tomography demonstrates a left sphenoid sinus soft tissue density "cyst."

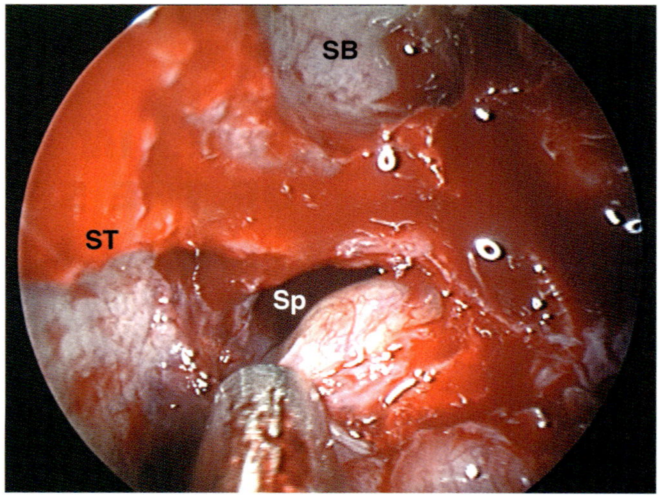


**FIGURE 22.3.** Cyst excised from the left sphenoid sinus. *ST,* superior turbinate; *SB,* skull base; *Sp,* sphenoid sinus.

The patient underwent endoscopic ethmoidectomy and transethmoidal sphenoidotomy. Gentle suctioning of the anterior inferior aspect of the sphenoid sinus demonstrated a cyst attached and the anterior inferior aspect of the sphenoidostomy (Fig. 22.3). Instrumentation of the cyst revealed purulent debris (Fig. 22.4). The cyst was gently excised. The patient's symptoms improved postoperatively, with resolution of chronic daily headaches.

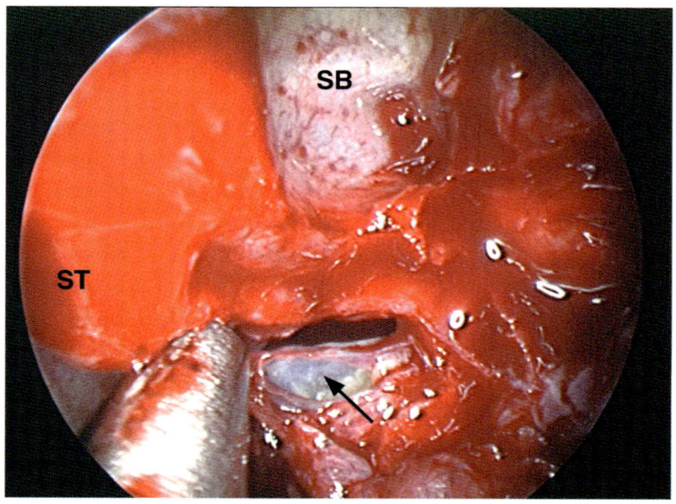


**FIGURE 22.4.** Purulent material within the sphenoid cyst. *ST,* superior turbinate; *SB,* skull base; *Sp,* sphenoid sinus; *arrow,* interior of the cyst.

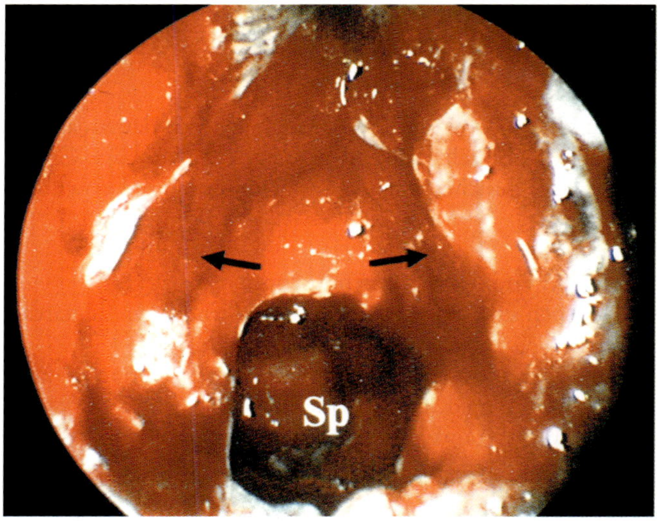


**FIGURE 22.5.** Transseptal approach to the sphenoid. The mucoperiosteal flaps are reflected away from the face of the sphenoid *(arrows)*. *Sp,* large sphenoidotomy.

## Case 2

A 60-year-old woman previously underwent sublabial, transseptal, transsphenoidal hypophysectomy for a pituitary adenoma. She had right CSF rhinorrhea 1 week postoperatively and was transferred to our institution for management. Endoscopic examination revealed clear fluid emanating from the right sphenoethmoidal recess. The CSF leak failed to respond to conservative management, including bed rest and lumbar drain placement for 5 days, and the patient underwent transseptal approach to the sphenoid sinus for repair of CSF leak (Fig. 22.5). At operation, the sphenoid sinus was filled with muscle, with CSF flowing around it. Removal of this muscle allowed endoscopic visualization of the large, surgically created defect in the floor of the sella turcica (Fig. 22.6). Endoscopic evaluation with a 45° endoscope revealed a defect in the diaphragma sellae with clear spinal fluid flowing through the defect.

CSF was drained through the lumbar drain to reduce the CSF pressure, and abdominal fat was harvested to fill the sella but allow space for reconstruction of the floor of the sella with bone cement. Lumbar drainage was discontinued after postoperative day 3, and the patient was discharged home and has had no recurrence of CSF leak with follow-up to 1 year.

## Case 3

A 45-year-old woman had previously undergone right sphenoethmoidectomy and right partial middle turbinate resection for allergic fungal sinusitis. Six months postoperatively, she noticed the onset of right-sided headaches and nasal congestion. Endoscopic evaluation revealed a mucosa-lined mass within the right sphenoethmoid recess (Fig. 22.7). The sphenoid ostium could not be visualized. CT revealed a heterogeneous mass filling the right sphenoid sinus and protruding into the sphenoethmoidal recess, which was consistent with recurrent allergic fungal disease. No bone erosion was observed.

A transnasal endoscopic approach to the sphenoethmoidal recess and sphenoid sinus was used. Marsupialization of the mucosa in the sphenoethmoidal recess revealed fungal material filling the cyst and sphenoid sinus

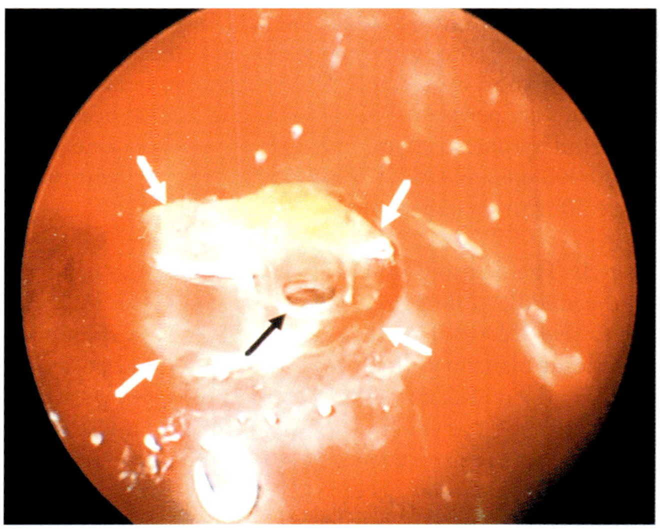

**FIGURE 22.6.** Endoscopic view of a large defect in the floor of the sella *(white arrows)* and a defect in diaphragma sellae *(black arrow)*.

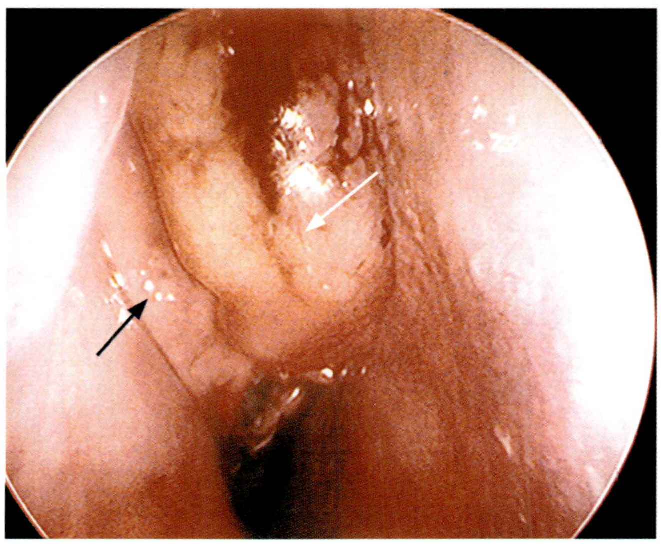

**FIGURE 22.7.** Mucosa-lined mass protrudes from the right sphenoethmoid recess *(white arrow)*. The superior turbinate *(black arrow)* and the septum *(S)* are shown.

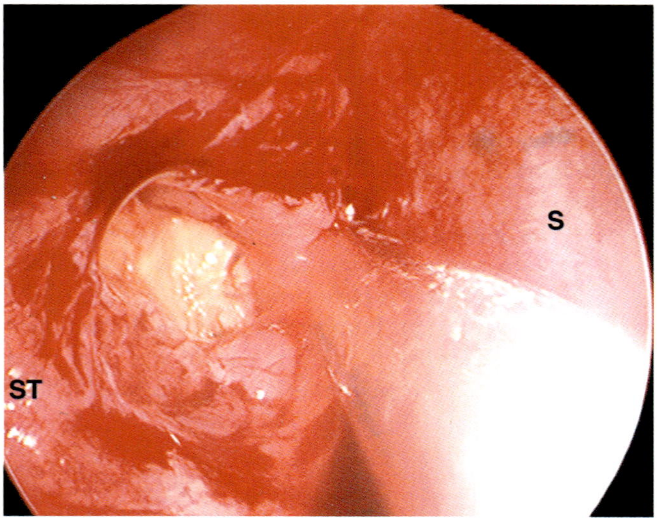


**FIGURE 22.8.** Removal of the anterior lining of the mass demonstrates fungal debris filling the sphenoid sinus. *S*, septum; *ST*, superior turbinate.

(Fig. 22.8). Endoscopic enlargement of the sphenoidotomy allowed complete removal of the fungal debris from the sphenoid sinus (Fig. 22.9).

Postoperatively, a 6-week tapering dose of systemic steroids, topical steroid spray, and weekly débridement of the sphenoid allowed complete resolution of disease with a patent sphenoidotomy.

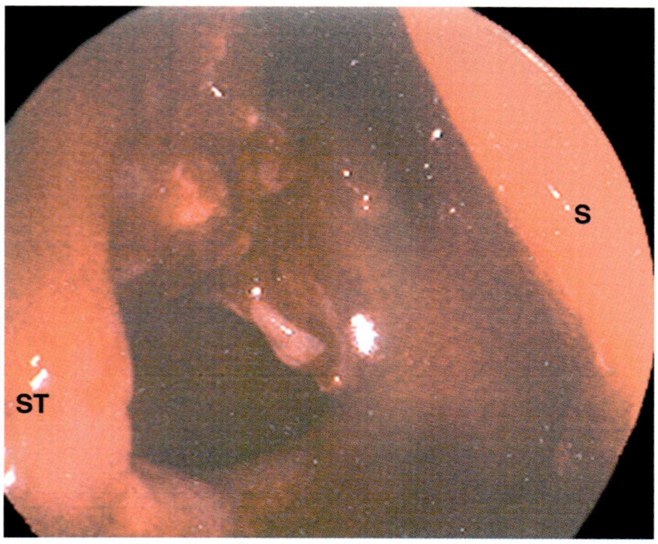


**FIGURE 22.9.** Large right sphenoidotomy after complete removal of fungal debris. *S*, septum; *ST*, superior turbinate.

## INSTRUMENTATION

The following instruments are required:

- Beaded probe with 5-cm, 7-cm, and 9-cm demarcations
- Sphenoid punch (Storz Instruments, Culver City, CA)
- Kerrison punches, 2 and 3 mm, upbiting and downbiting
- J curette
- 0°, 30°, and 45° 4-mm endoscopes
- 9-French Frazier suction with 5-, 7-, and 9-cm demarcations
- 3.5- and 4.0-mm power microdebrider; straight and Rad-40 (Xomed, Jacksonville, FL)
- Straight, 45° and 90° Blakesley-Wilde forceps, standard and through-cutting

## ANESTHESIA

General or local anesthesia can be used for endoscopic sphenoid surgery and depends on surgeon and patient preference. There are some diseases processes for which more extensive manipulation of the sinus is necessary, and general anesthesia may be preferential in these cases. Regardless of local or general anesthesia, topical vasoconstrictive agents are used and injections with 1% lidocaine with 1:100,000 epinephrine are used in all cases. Our technique is as follows:

***Step 1:*** Oxymetazoline spray (0.05%) is applied in the holding area. This begins the decongestion process and decreases systemic absorption of topical cocaine to be used subsequently.

***Step 2:*** Cottonoids saturated with oxymetazoline (0.051 %) solution are placed intranasally. It is critical that atraumatic technique is used. An attempt is made to place one pledget in the middle meatus. Pledgets are left undisturbed for 10 minutes while the surgeons scrub and the endoscopic instrumentation is prepared. The pledgets are removed and injections are performed using a 25-gauge spinal needle on a control syringe containing 8 mL of 1% lidocaine with 1:100,000 epinephrine. The tip of the needle is bent to an angle 30° from parallel.

***Step 3:*** The first injection is near the posterior attachment of the middle turbinate at the site of the sphenopalatine artery (Fig. 22.10). Slow, gentle infusion of 3 mL produces significant blanching of the lateral nasal wall and posterior aspect of the middle turbinate. Alternatively, if the posterior attachment of the middle turbinate cannot be visualized (e.g., polyps, extensive edema), injection of the greater palatine foramen may be necessary. This is performed transorally with an angled, 22-gauge spinal needle. The foramen is most often located medial to the second maxillary molar

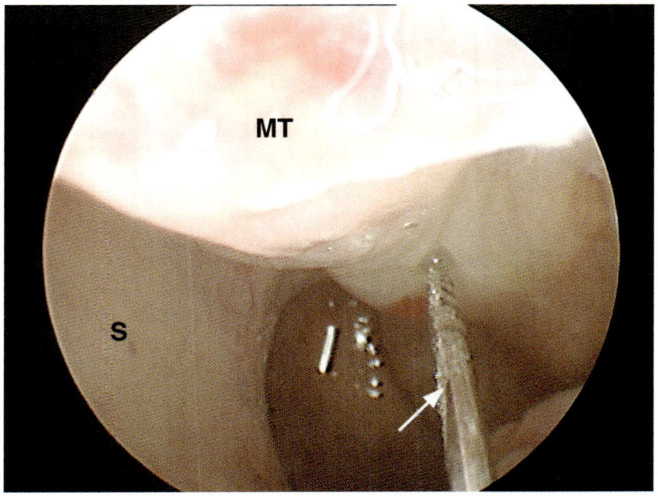


**FIGURE 22.10.** Injection at the posterior attachment of the left middle turbinate. *S,* septum; *MT,* middle turbinate; *arrow,* 25-gauge spiral needle.

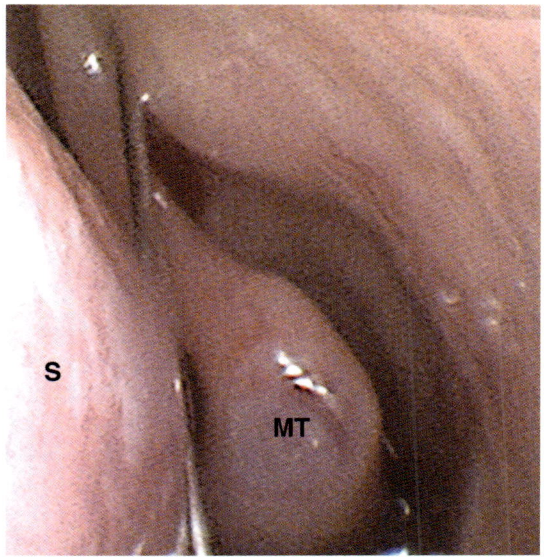


**FIGURE 22.12.** Injection of the anterior-superior attachment of the left middle turbinate *(MT)*. *S,* septum.

and may often be palpated with the finger as a depression in the palatal mucosa. Aspiration is required to avoid intraarterial injection. While this technique is proven and safe, temporary blindness has been reported.

***Step 4:*** The second injection is to the inferior aspect of the middle turbinate approximately 1.5 cm posterior to the head of the middle turbinate (Fig. 22.11). An attempt is made to direct the needle slightly laterally so that the lateral mucosa of the turbinate receives the agent. Approximately 1.5 to 2 mL are administered.

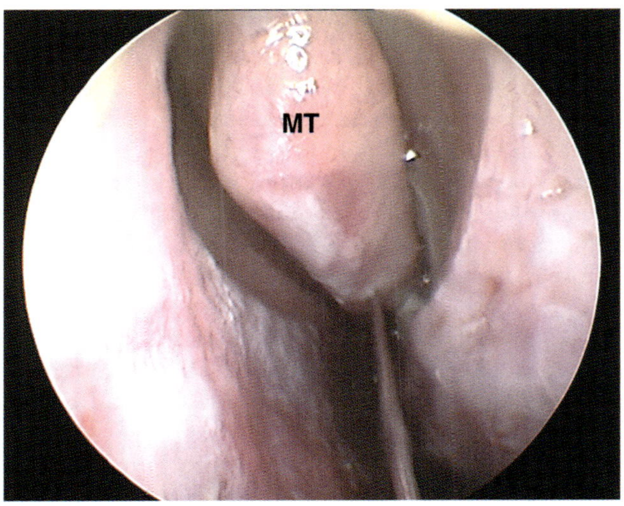


**FIGURE 22.11.** Injection in middle aspect of the left middle turbinate *(MT)*.

***Step 5:*** The final injection is to the anterior-superior attachment of the middle turbinate. Slow infusion results in blanching of the anterior aspect of the middle turbinate and the uncinate process (Fig. 22.12).

## OPERATIVE TECHNIQUE

Gentle diagnostic nasal endoscopy allows the surgeon examination of the middle meatus, sphenoethmoidal recess, and nasopharynx. The sphenoid sinus is generally approached using the transethmoidal route but, depending on the extent of disease and surgeon preference, may also be approached transnasally medial to the middle turbinate through the sphenoethmoidal recess. This transnasal route usually requires lateral retraction of the middle turbinate and risks destabilization of the middle turbinate and subsequent lateralization. The anatomically spacious nose may allow this direct transnasal approach without the risk of turbinate destabilization (4).

### Endoscopic Transethmoidal Sphenoidotomy

***Step 1:*** Resection of the uncinate process reveals the maxillary ostium and provides room within the middle meatus. The ethmoid bulla is resected, allowing early identification of the lamina papyracea and revealing the lateral extent of dissection.

***Step 2:*** The basal lamella is identified and penetrated inferior and medially, approximately 1.5 cm above its posterior extent at the level of the maxillary roof (11,12). Care must be taken to preserve the middle turbinate attachment to the lateral nasal wall, or the destabilized middle turbinate will almost certainly lateralize in the postoperative period. The posterior ethmoids are identified, but further posterior dissection is avoided before identification of the sphenoid, because further dissection risks breach of the skull base and creates bleeding, making identification of the sphenoid more difficult.

***Step 3:*** The basal lamella is examined, and a small area of the inferior and medial aspect is resected to reveal the superior meatus (Fig. 22.13). This, in essence, fenestrates the middle turbinate, providing excellent visualization of the superior meatus. The inferior aspect of the superior turbinate should be visualized. The inability to identify this critical landmark generally requires further inferior and medial dissection. However, only that portion of the inferior basal lamella that is necessary to visualize the superior turbinate should be resected. If there is any question regarding location, the J curette can be placed medial to the middle turbinate while the surgeon visualizes what is thought to be the superior meatus through the ethmoid.

***Step 4:*** Dissection of the lateral aspect of the basal lamella is performed to identify the lamina papyracea and enlarge the access to the posterior ethmoids.

***Step 5:*** Attention is directed back to the superior turbinate, which is gently manipulated so that the natural ostium of the sphenoid sinus can be identified. Identification of the natural ostium may require minimal resection (2 to 3 mm) of the inferior aspect of the superior turbinate (Fig. 22.14). In cases of severe disease, the ostium may not be visible with

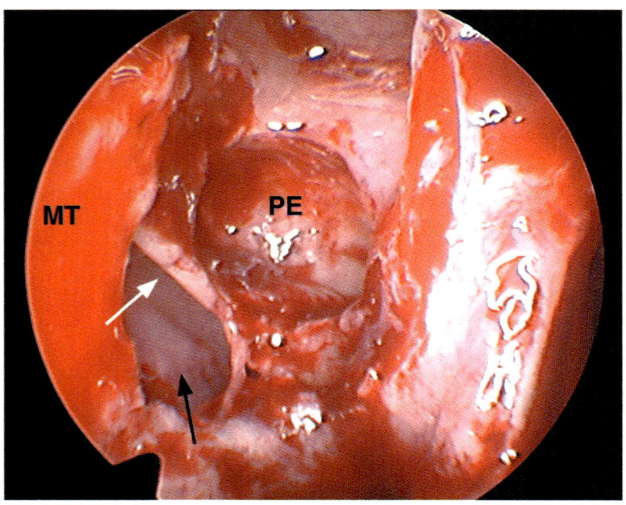


**FIGURE 22.13.** Transethmoidal approach to the left sphenoid. The basal lamella has been penetrated, and the superior turbinate *(white arrow)* is identified. The sphenoethmoid recess *(black arrow)* is indicated. *MT,* middle turbinate; *PE,* posterior ethmoid.

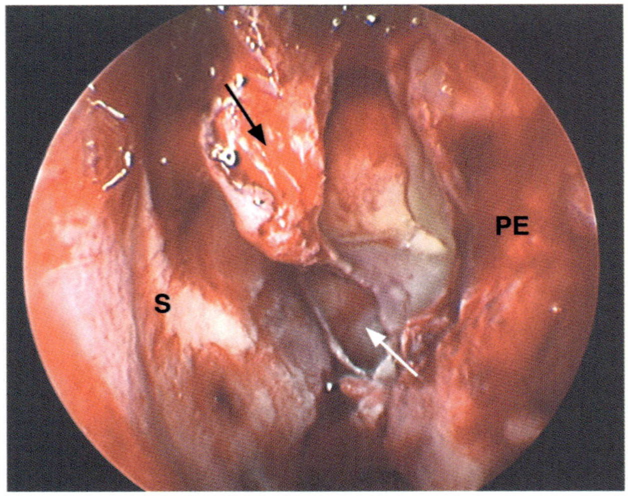


**FIGURE 22.14.** The natural ostium of the sphenoid sinus *(white arrow)* is identified in the transethmoidal approach. *S,* septum; *PE,* posterior ethmoid cell; *black arrow,* superior turbinate.

these maneuvers. Starting low, gentle probing with a blunt instrument with dilation of the natural ostium allows certain identification of the sphenoid sinus. The ostium is then enlarged inferiorly under direct visualization. Passing the endoscope into the sphenoid allows visualization of the lateral wall and roof and reveals the remaining sphenoid face. A J-curette can often be placed within the sinus directed laterally and seen through the translucent anterior wall. This "shelf" of bone may then be safely removed. During this portion of the resection, the surgeon must keep in mind the critical parasphenoidal structures.

## Additional Techniques

### *Transnasal Endoscopic Approach*

***Step 1:*** The endoscope is passed medial to the middle turbinate, with visualization of the superior turbinate and sphenoethmoidal recess. The natural ostium is visualized or probed with appropriate measurements confirmed. The distance from the superior rim of the choana is noted and is generally between 1.5 and 2 cm. It is sometimes necessary to remove the posterior portion of the middle turbinate for adequate visualization. This is performed with endoscopic scissors as described by Stankiewicz (13).

***Step 2:*** The natural ostium is dilated with a blunt instrument, or alternatively, closed, small, straight forceps are placed within the ostium and opened to dilate the ostium.

***Step 3:*** The sphenoid ostium is enlarged with 2-mm Kerrison forceps or a sphenoid punch. Some surgeons prefer to fracture the anterior wall posteriorly with a Frazier suction or other instrument, but great care should be taken with any "plunging" maneuver.

### Sublabial Transseptal Approach

***Step 1:*** After injection of the gingivobuccal sulcus with 1% lidocaine with 1:100,000 epinephrine solution, an incision is made from the premolar on one side to the premolar on the opposite side. Care is taken to allow an appropriate gingival cuff of mucosa for closure. The anterior nasal spine and inferior aspect of the piriform aperture are identified.

***Step 2:*** The nasal spine is followed to the caudal aspect of the cartilaginous septum, and a mucoperichondrial flap is elevated on the preferred side. Bilateral inferior nasal mucosal tunnels are elevated while leaving the mucoperichondrial flap attached to the cartilaginous septum on one side. This allows disarticulation of the septal cartilage from the maxillary crest. The cartilaginous septum is also separated from the posterior perpendicular plate of the ethmoid bone.

***Step 3:*** With the cartilaginous septum with attached flap retracted, the mucoperiosteal flaps are elevated from the ethmoid bone until the sphenoid rostrum is identified. Resection of the ethmoid bone is performed with cutting instruments so that the cribriform plate is not exposed to torquing forces.

***Step 4:*** Elevation of the mucosa from the rostrum of the sphenoid generally allows identification of the natural sphenoid ostia. Endoscopes can be quite helpful in identification. The Hardy retractor is placed so that the mucosa is retracted, allowing visualization of the sphenoid ostia. The sphenoid punch or Kerrison punch can be used to resect the anterior wall, allowing unparalleled access to the entire sphenoid sinus. The midline bone can be quite thick and require a 4-mm osteotome and mallet for complete resection. Endoscopes and microscopes may be used to aid visualization and thorough removal of disease (14).

## SPECIAL POINTS

There is an anatomic blend of the roof of the sphenoid superiorly and laterally with the roof of the ethmoid and of the lateral wall of the sphenoid to the posterior aspect of the lamina papyracea. When severe ethmoid disease is present, identifying the sphenoid and following these structures enables safer removal of ethmoid disease.

The sphenoethmoid recess is the space between the superior turbinate laterally, the olfactory fossa superiorly, and the nasal septum medially (15). Septal deviation, middle and superior turbinate hypertrophy, and severe inflammatory mucosal edema can compromise the sphenoethmoid recess.

Revision endoscopic sphenoidotomy can be very hazardous because of the lack of anatomic landmarks, scar tissue, and osteoneogenesis, which may occur at the anterior sphenoid face. Fortunately, the superior turbinate is a nearly constant and reliable landmark for revision cases.

Unless the natural ostium of the sphenoid sinus is directly visualized, opening of the anterior wall of the sphenoid sinus should always be preceded by measurement with a beaded probe or other instrument to confirm appropriate measurements.

Enlarging the natural ostium of the sphenoid can potentially be done, to some degree, circumferentially. However, there are limitations in every direction. In Van Alyea's dissection of 100 cadaver specimens, the sphenoid ostium demonstrated variable location in relation to the sinus (2). In 52%, the ostium was nearer the sphenoid roof than the floor of the sinus. In 34%, the ostium was equidistant from the roof and floor of the sinus, and in 14%, it was nearer the floor. For the entire group of specimens, the average distance from the ostium to the sphenoid roof was 7.7 mm, and from the ostium to the floor of the sinus was 10.7 mm. Medially, the sphenoid rostrum and septum limit enlargement almost immediately because of the fairly thick bone in this region despite the fact that the ostium averages 5.2 mm from the midline (16). Inferiorly, injury to the nasoseptal division of the sphenopalatine artery may result in vigorous hemorrhage. Superiorly, opening the cleft between the ethmoid and sphenoid bones may result in CSF fistula. Laterally, the sphenoid can be opened flush with the lateral aspect of the sinus cavity, keeping in mind the parasphenoidal structures.

Disease and soft tissue within the sphenoid sinus can be instrumented and removed after a wide sphenoidostomy is created. However, many feel that polypoid disease that is adherent to the superior, lateral, and posterior walls is better left rather than risking carotid injury.

Vital structures such as the carotid artery and optic nerve tend to be more exposed in a well-pneumatized sphenoid (17) (Fig. 22.15). In a cadaver study of 30 specimens, the carotid produced an identifiable bulge in the lateral wall in 93% (18). The optic nerve protruded into the superolateral aspect of the sphenoid in 100%. In 3% to 5% of specimens, there was no bony covering of these critical structures. Although the rate of true dehiscence varies in a number of studies, the findings of a "very thin bony covering" and true dehiscence occur in a significant proportion of patients.

The sphenoid sinus may pneumatize to the extent that structures outside of the sphenoid body are pneumatized, leading to the development of recesses. Potential recesses of the sphenoid sinus include (in decreasing frequency) the infraoptic or opticocarotid recess, inferolateral recess, pterygoid recess, and posterior clinoid recess (16).

Bony septa may deviate and insert into the bony covering of the carotid artery (13% to 40%) or into the bony covering of the optic nerve (3% to 7%). Accessory septa may occur in 30% to 69% of specimens (16).

Ethmoid cells can pneumatize lateral and to some extent superior to the sphenoid sinus. In these cases, these poste-

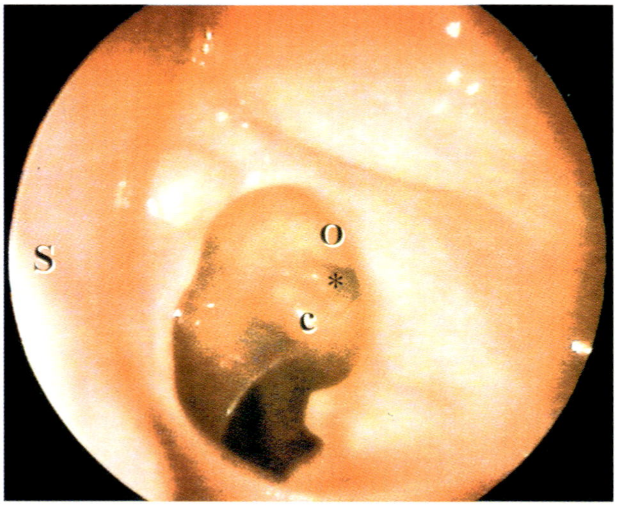


**FIGURE 22.15.** Postoperative appearance of sphenoidotomy. *S*, septum; *O*, prominence of the optic nerve; *c*, prominence of the carotid artery; *asterisk*, opticocarotid recess.

rior ethmoid cells are known as sphenoethmoid cells or Onodi cells (16). The optic nerve and carotid artery are often exposed in these cells, and attempts to locate the sphenoid sinus posterior to these cells can place these critical structures in harm's way. The optic nerve may be prominent within the lateral wall of other posterior ethmoid cells as well. Many experienced endoscopic surgeons feel that the optic nerve is at greater risk during ethmoid surgery than sphenoid surgery.

## POSTOPERATIVE CARE

At the conclusion of the operation, all bone fragments are removed, and devitalized bone and mucosa are resected. No packing, sponge, or absorbable materials are required in most cases. Nasal saline sprays are recommended several times per day, and we routinely reinstitute nasal steroid sprays on the first postoperative day. Antibiotics are directed by culture results from the preoperative period and are adjusted accordingly when microbiology reports from the operation are available. Steroid tapers, initiated at least 1 week before surgery, are continued as dictated by observations of mucosal disease at the time of surgery.

The postoperative follow-up for the endoscopic sinus surgery patient is very labor intensive. The routine patient is seen on postoperative days 6 and 13 for endoscopic débridement in the office. Crusting, devitalized mucosa, and bone are resected and any synechiae lysed. Patients demonstrating any sign of adverse scarring, extreme crusting, or ostial stenosis are seen more frequently. Patients generally require weekly follow-up for the first 6 to 8 weeks and then every 1 to 2 months for the first year.

## COMPLICATIONS

### Hemorrhage

In the context of endoscopic sphenoid surgery, hemorrhage generally occurs in one of three forms: bothersome mucosal oozing, significant hemorrhage from a named vessel, and life-threatening hemorrhage from the carotid artery.

The most common bleeding seen is the bothersome mucosal oozing that may limit visualization and increase operative time occasionally requiring termination of the procedure (4). Prevention and planning are critical to avoiding hemorrhage. Patients should be maximally medically treated preoperatively, including topical and systemic steroids and antibiotics when indicated to help reduce mucosal inflammation. We educate the patient regarding the risks of bleeding and the implications of bleeding in the context of endoscopic sinus surgery. This helps to improve compliance with preoperative medications that many patients would rather avoid. It also reminds patients of the reasons to avoid aspirin and aspirin-containing products 2 weeks before surgery. On the day of surgery, maximum mucosal decongestion is obtained before injections as outlined in the procedures section.

During endoscopic surgery, the surgeon remembers that blood drains along the mucosa from superior to inferior and from anterior to posterior. Atraumatic technique with every endoscopic maneuver and mucosal preservation are paramount.

Significant hemorrhage may occur in sphenoid surgery because of bleeding from the sphenopalatine artery, posterior ethmoid artery, or branches thereof. Careful penetration of the basal lamella at the appropriate level generally avoids injury to the sphenopalatine artery. If the surgeon's approach is too inferior and lateral, the branching sphenopalatine artery may be encountered. Pressure and topical vasoconstrictors followed by judicious use of suction electrosurgery may be sufficient to stop the hemorrhage. Endoscopic ligation of the sphenopalatine artery is effective in recalcitrant cases but is rarely necessary (19,20). Other sites where bleeding may be encountered are where the posterior ethmoid artery traverses the skull base and in the mucosa inferior to the sphenoid ostium, where the nasoseptal division of the sphenopalatine artery is located (3). Avoidance is the rule. Suction electrosurgery should not be used to control ethmoid artery bleeding because of the risk of CSF fistula.

Carotid artery injury is devastating and often not survivable. The endoscopic surgeon should approach the sphenoid sinus with the assumption that the carotid artery is dehiscent and that any tissue or disease within the sphenoid sinus is attached to it. In the case of carotid artery injury, the "carotid drill" should be used as a guideline for management (21).

### Cerebrospinal Fluid Fistula

CSF leak generally results from attempted entry superior to the sinus, aggressive superior enlargement of the sphenoidostomy, or avulsion of the superior turbinate with resultant skull base injury. Intraoperative recognition of the classic CSF washout of blood in the region of dural injury allows immediate repair without the need for lumbar drainage in most cases. We prefer a free mucosal graft from the contralateral septum bolstered with Surgicel and Gelfoam packing. CT of the head is performed postoperatively to identify intracranial complications, and the patient is placed on bed rest for 48 hours with the head elevated 30°. Antibiotics are not prescribed. Intrasphenoid CSF leaks may be treated with fibrin glue, with or without mucosal or adipose tissue grafts (22).

## Ostium Closure

Sphenoid ostium closure may result from "hard" scar tissue formation and osteoneogenesis or "soft" mucosal edema and polyp recurrence. The former requires revision surgery, and the latter may be amenable to medical therapy. The importance of maximum medical management and postoperative care cannot be overemphasized (23). Early recognition of ostial stenosis during postoperative endoscopic débridement may prevent closure.

## Turbinate Destabilization and Lateralization

The anatomic attachments of the middle turbinate must be well understood to avoid destabilization and subsequent lateralization. Careful penetration of the basal lamella with preservation of the middle turbinate's lateral attachment can prevent destabilization in most cases. Despite this, at the conclusion of the case, the surgeon should verify turbinate stability. For an unstable turbinate, one of two options should be used: placement of a temporary spacer within the middle meatus (i.e., the medial mucosa of the turbinate and opposing septal mucosa are scored to allow synechiae formation in some cases) or partial resection of the middle turbinate (24).

## Optic Nerve Injury

Although the optic nerve is more likely injured in the posterior ethmoid region, surgical trauma may also occur when the lateral sphenoid wall is instrumented. An immediate ophthalmology consultation is critical, and optic nerve decompression may be necessary (25).

## Orbital Hemorrhage

Orbital hemorrhage generally occurs in one of two forms: slow venous and rapid arterial. Slow venous hemorrhage may take several hours to fully develop and generally responds to medical management, including an ophthalmology consultation, removal of any packing, orbital massage, intravenous mannitol (1 to 2 g/kg over 30 to 60 minutes) and acetazolamide (500 mg) (26).

Rapid arterial bleeding results in rapid proptosis and orbital tension. Immediate action is required to prevent permanent sequelae. An immediate ophthalmology consultation is initiated along with medical therapy described for slow venous hemorrhage. Surgical management may be necessary if excessive orbital pressures continue and include lateral canthotomy and orbital decompression along with incision of the periorbita by approach most comfortable to the surgeon.

## Temporary Blindness from Injection

Injection of the greater palatine foramen rarely has resulted in temporary visual deficits. While frightening for the patient and surgeon, all episodes have reversed within 2 hours after surgery. It is critical to distinguish this self-limiting blindness from blindness due to direct optic nerve injury or orbital hematoma. As with all orbital complications, it is desirable to have a good working relationship with ophthalmology colleagues before performing difficult endoscopic cases.

## Circular Flow

The sphenoid sinus is considered to be more resistant to the circular flow phenomenon than the maxillary sinus. However, circular flow has resulted in persistent sphenoid sinusitis. If the sphenoidotomy is created inferior to the natural ostium, mucopurulence may flow from the natural ostium down the face of the sphenoid and back into the sphenoid sinus (27) (Figs. 22.16 and 22.17). When medical manage-

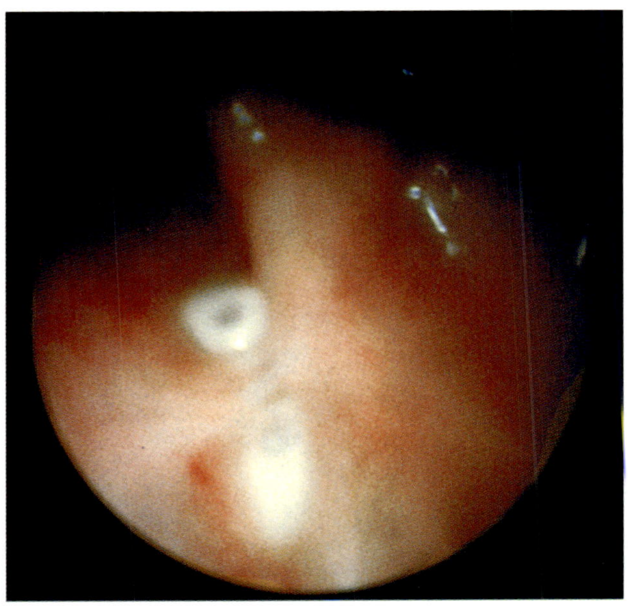

**FIGURE 22.16.** Postoperative appearance of the anterior face of the sphenoid with purulent material.

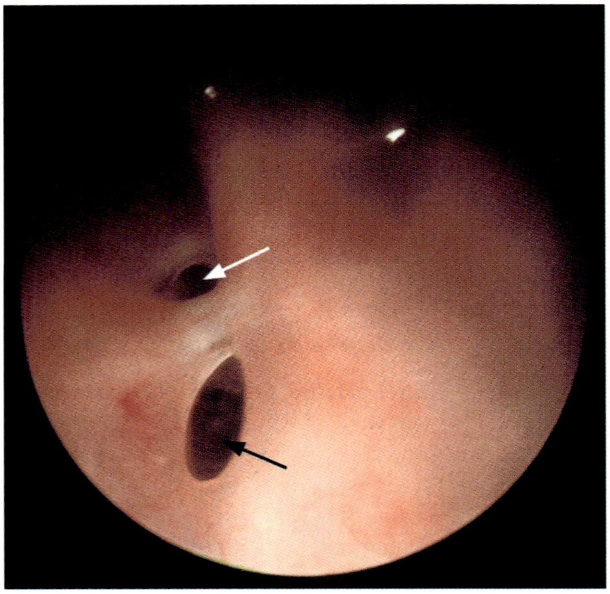

**FIGURE 22.17.** After purulent material is suctioned away, the natural sphenoid ostium *(white arrow)* and surgically created ostium *(black arrow)* are seen.

ment fails to cure the patient, revision sphenoidotomy connecting the two ostia should allow resolution of disease. We attempt to connect the natural ostium to the surgical sphenoidotomy at the time of initial surgery (Fig. 22.18).

## Olfactory Impairment

Olfactory impairment may result from overresection of the superior turbinate or avulsion of olfactory neuroepithelium from the olfactory cleft. If superior turbinate resection is required, the resection should be minimized, and through-cutting instruments should be used to prevent stripping of olfactory neuroepithelium (11,12).

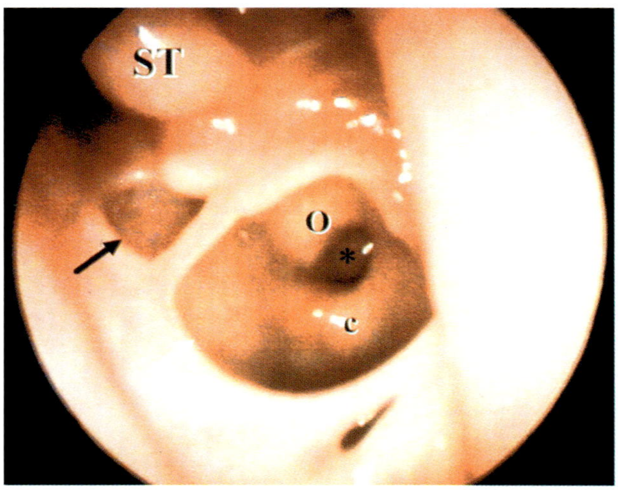


**FIGURE 22.18.** Postoperative appearance of left sphenoidotomy. The natural *(black arrow)* and surgically created *(white arrow)* ostia are separate. *ST,* superior turbinate; *O,* prominence of the optic nerve; *c,* prominence of the carotid artery; *asterisk,* opticocarotid recess.

## REFERENCES


1. Sethi DS. Isolated sphenoid lesions: diagnosis and management. *Otolaryngol Head Neck Surg* 1999;120:730–736.
2. Van Alyea OE. *Nasal sinuses: an anatomic and clinical consideration.* Baltimore: Waverly Press, 1951.
3. Lang J. *Clinical anatomy of the nose, nasal cavity, and paranasal sinuses.* New York: Thieme Medical Publishers, 1989.
4. Stankiewicz JA. *Advanced endoscopic sinus surgery.* St. Louis: Mosby–Year Book, 1995.
5. Lin WS, Hung HY. Transnasal endoscopic surgery of sphenoid sinus aspergillosis. *J Laryngol Otol* 1993;107:837–839.
6. Muneer A, Jones NS. Unilateral abducens nerve palsy: a presenting sign of sphenoid sinus mucoceles. *J Laryngol Otol* 1997;111: 644–646.
7. Sellars SL, De Villiers JC. The sphenoid sinus mucocele. *J Laryngol Otol* 1981;95:493–502.
8. Moriyama H, Nakajima T, Honda Y. Studies on mucoceles of the ethmoid and sphenoid sinuses: analysis of 47 cases. *J Laryngol Otol* 1992;106:23–27.
9. Sethi DS, Lau DPC, Chee LWJ, et al. Isolated sphenoethmoid recess polyps. *J Laryngol Otol* 1998;112:660–663.

9a. Deasy NP, Jarosz JM, Al Sarraj S, et al. Intrasphenoid cephalocele: MRI in two cases. *Neuroradiology* 1999;41:497–500.

10. Ulualp SO, Toohill RJ, Hoffmann R, et al. Possible relationship of gastroesophagopharyngeal acid reflux with pathogenesis of chronic sinusitis. *Am J Rhinol* 1999;13:197–202.
11. Bolger WE, Keyes AS, Lanza DC. Use of the superior meatus and superior turbinate in the endoscopic approach to the sphenoid sinus. *Otolaryngol Head Neck Surg* 1999;120:308–313.
12. Orlandi RR, Lanza DC, Bolger WE, et al. The forgotten turbinate: the role of the superior turbinate in endoscopic sinus surgery. *Am J Rhinol* 1999;13:251–259.
13. Stankiewicz JA. Sphenoid sinus mucocele. *Otolaryngol Head Neck Surg* 1989;115:735–740.
14. Moses RL, Keane WM, Andrews DW, et al. Endoscopic transseptal transsphenoidal hypophysectomy with three-dimensional intraoperative localization technology. *Laryngoscope* 1999; 109:509–512.
15. Stammberger HR, Kennedy DW. Paranasal sinuses: anatomic terminology and nomenclature. The Anatomic Terminology Group. *Ann Otol Rhinol Laryngol Suppl* 1995;167:7–16.
16. Elwany S, Elsaeid I, Thabet H. Endoscopic anatomy of the sphenoid sinus. *J Laryngol Otol* 1999;113:122–126.
17. Cheung DK, Attia EL, Kirkpatrick DA, et al. An anatomic and CT scan study of the lateral wall of the sphenoid sinus as related to the transnasal transethmoid endoscopic approach. *J Otolaryngol* 1993;22:63–68.
18. Sethi DS, Stanley RE, Pillay PK. Endoscopic anatomy of the sphenoid sinus and sella turcica. *J Laryngol Otol* 1995;109:951–955.
19. Snyderman CH, Goldman SA, Carrau RL, et al. Endoscopic sphenopalatine artery ligation is an effective method of treatment for posterior epistaxis. *Am J Rhinol* 1999;13:137–140.
20. Bolger WE, Borgie RC, Melder P. The role of the crista ethmoidalis in endoscopic sphenopalatine artery ligation. *Am J Rhinol* 1999;13:81–86.
21. Sofferman R. Complications: prevention and management—carotid artery and optic nerve injury. Presented at the First Inter-

national Symposium on Contemporary Sinus Surgery, Pittsburgh, PA, November 4–6, 1990.
22. Stankiewicz J. Cerebrospinal fluid fistula and endoscopic sinus surgery. *Laryngoscope* 1991;101:250–256.
23. Moriyama H, Yanagi K, Ohtori N, et al. Healing process of sinus mucosa after endoscopic sinus surgery. *Am J Rhinol* 1996;10:61–66.
24. Fortune DS, Duncavage JA. Incidence of frontal sinusitis following partial middle turbinectomy. *Ann Otol Rhinol Laryngol* 1998; 107:447–453.
25. Luxenberger W, Stammberger H, Jebeles JA, et al. Endoscopic optic nerve decompression: the Graz experience. *Laryngoscope* 1998;108:873–882.
26. Jones KR. In: Weissler MC, Pillsbury HC, eds. *Complications of endoscopic sinus surgery*. New York: Thieme Medical Publishers, 1995:90–93.
27. Yanagisawa E, Weaver EM. Endoscopic view of the recirculation phenomenon of sphenoid sinus drainage. *Ear Nose Throat J* 1996;75:69–70.

# 23

# ENDONASAL MICRO–ENDOSCOPIC MANAGEMENT OF FRONTAL SINUS DISEASE

WOLFGANG DRAF
RAINER WEBER

## INDICATIONS AND CONTRAINDICATIONS

Endonasal opening of the frontal sinus has a long tradition. Operations through the medial floor of the frontal sinus were carried out by Schaeffer as early as 1890 (1), and reports were published in 1899 by Spiess (2), 1905 by Ingals (3), 1906 by Halle (4), and 1907 and 1908 by Good (5,6). A wide variety of special instruments were developed early on: frontal sinus rasps designed by Good, Schaefer or Wigand; frontal sinus curettes designed by Schaefer, Wagener, and Kuhn-Bolger; frontal sinus drills designed by Halle, Ingals, Spiess, and Watson-Williams; and spacers designed by Good or Ingals. The most important instruments in this operation are special burrs (7), which make it possible with a relatively low risk (at that time without a microscope) to fashion a wide communication between the frontal sinus and nose. Newer developments include the frontal sinus punch (Smith & Nephew, Memphis, TN), designed by Bachert, or the frontal sinus stent (Smith & Nephew), designed by Rains.

For many years, the endonasal approach was abandoned because of severe complications. With the introduction of optical aids, such as the microscope (8), microscope plus endoscope (9–11), and endoscope (2–14), and the development of new instruments, a renaissance of endonasal sinus surgery took place. Endonasal frontal sinus surgery was established as a routine procedure for treating inflammatory disease and for other special indications (15–38). Draf (10) developed a classification system for endonasal frontal sinus drainage procedures that was somewhat extended by May and Schaitkin (26) (Table 23.1).

The indications for different methods of frontal sinus drainage are shown in Table 23.2. Contraindications to endonasal micro–endoscopic frontal sinus surgery include situations in which the pathologic process cannot be reached or in which stable drainage cannot be maintained despite type III drainage or insertion of a stent for 6 months (36):

- Recurrent sinusitis or mucocele after a Lynch operation extended far laterally (Fig. 23.1)
- Infection after reconstruction the frontal sinus wall with foreign material, which must be removed and a reconstruction performed with autogenic bone
- Large tumors or tumors in the lateral or cranial area
- Mucopyoceles in the lateral area
- Major bony defect of the anterior or posterior wall [reconstruction with calvarial bone indicated (see Case 4)]
- Endocranial complications with epidural abscess, subdural empyema, or frontal lobe abscess

**TABLE 23.1. ENDONASAL FRONTAL SINUS DRAINAGE: DRAF TYPES I–III AND NASOFRONTAL APPROACH TYPES I–IV**

| Draf Classification[a] | NFA Classification[b] | Extent of Surgery |
|---|---|---|
| Type I | NFA I | Anterior ethmoidectomy with drainage of the frontal recess without touching the frontal sinus outflow tract |
| Type II | NFA II | Removal of the frontal sinus floor between the middle turbinate medially and the lamina papyracea laterally |
| | NFA III | Removal of the frontal sinus floor between the nasal septum medially and the lamina papyracea laterally |
| Type III | NFA IV | Type II drainage on both sides and removal of the upper part of the nasal septum and the lower part of the frontal sinus septum |

[a] Classification according to Draf (10,16,34).
[b] Nasofrontal approach according to May and Schaitkin (26).
NFA, nasofrontal approach.

**TABLE 23.2. INDICATIONS FOR DIFFERENT DRAINAGE METHODS FOR THE FRONTAL SINUS**

| Type I (Frontal Recess) | Type II (Enlarged Drainage) | Type III (Median Drainage) |
|---|---|---|
| Chronic sinusitis without opacification of FS or opacified *without* risk factors (aspirin intolerance, bronchial asthma, sinusitis triad) or opacified in primary surgery | Large anterior-posterior diameter (>1 cm)<br>Hypoplastic internal nasal spine<br>Larger drainage necessary<br>No severe polyposis | Small anterior-posterior diameter (<1 cm)<br>Hyperplastic internal nasal spine<br>Opacified FS in chronic polypoid pansinusitis *with* risk factors (aspirin intolerance, bronchial asthma, sinusitis triad) |
| | Endocranial or orbital complication in acute sinusitis<br>Osteomas in the infundibulum and other benign tumors<br>CSF leak in the inferior and medial part<br>Recurrent barotrauma | Endocranial or orbital complication in acute or chronic sinusitis<br>Osteomas in the infundibulum and other benign tumors<br>CSF leak in the inferior and medial part<br>Revision surgery in chronic pansinusitis and after type II drainage<br>Special underlying disease (e.g.,muco-viscidosis, Kartagener syndrome, immotile cilia syndrome) |

CSF, cerebrospinal fluid; FS, frontal sinus.

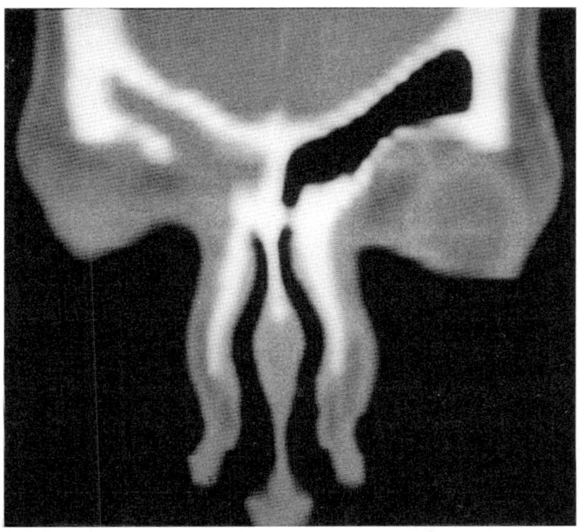

A

**FIGURE 23.1. A:** Preoperative computed tomography (CT) scan shows complete opacification of the right frontal sinus with a bony defect of the frontal sinus floor after a Lynch operation. **B:** Coronal *(left)* and axial *(right)* CT scans after a Lynch operation show stenosis of the frontal sinus outflow tract over a long distance *(asterisk)* compared with the wide-open drainage of the other side.

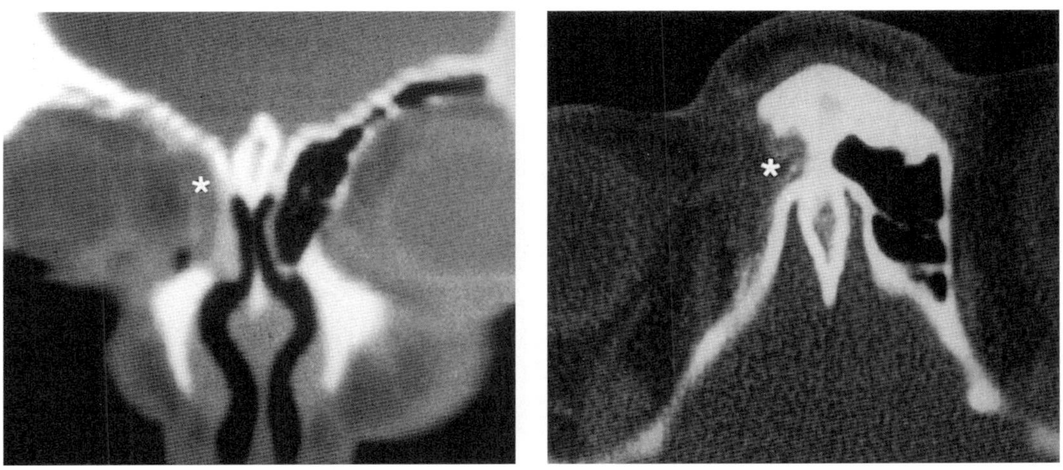

B

An osteoplastic flap procedure with or without fat obliteration is indicated in most of these cases (39–42).

## PREOPERATIVE EVALUATION

The preoperative evaluation should include the patient's history, seeking the following information:

- Symptoms, such as headache, olfaction disorder, runny nose, postnasal drip, and stuffy nose
- Accompanying diseases, such as bronchial asthma, analgetic hypersensitivity, immunologic disorder, and immotile cilia syndrome
- Previous surgery or trauma

The preoperative workup may also include nasal endoscopy (43,44), computed tomography (CT), an olfaction test, and acoustic rhinometry or rhinomanometry. Magnetic resonance imaging (MRI) may be needed in cases of orbital or endocranial complications. The need for surgery is determined by findings of the history, endoscopy, and CT (11).

### Case Examples

***Case 1:*** A 53-year-old woman developed swelling and redness in the right periorbital region (Fig. 23.2A) along with severe pain and double vision. She had no history of trauma or previous surgery. The CT examination revealed a mucocele of the anterior superior ethmoid medially with an subperiosteal abscess in the right orbit (Fig. 23.2B,C), but the other sinuses were normal. The ocular bulb was dislocated laterocaudally, producing exophthalmus. Because of a sufficiently wide anterior-posterior diameter and hypoplastic spina nasalis interna, an endonasal approach was used to achieve type II drainage of the frontal sinus. The lamina papyracea was partially removed, and the subperiosteal abscess was drained using a silicone tube for 3 days. After this procedure 6 years ago, the frontal sinus has remained open, and disease has not recurred (Fig. 23.2D).

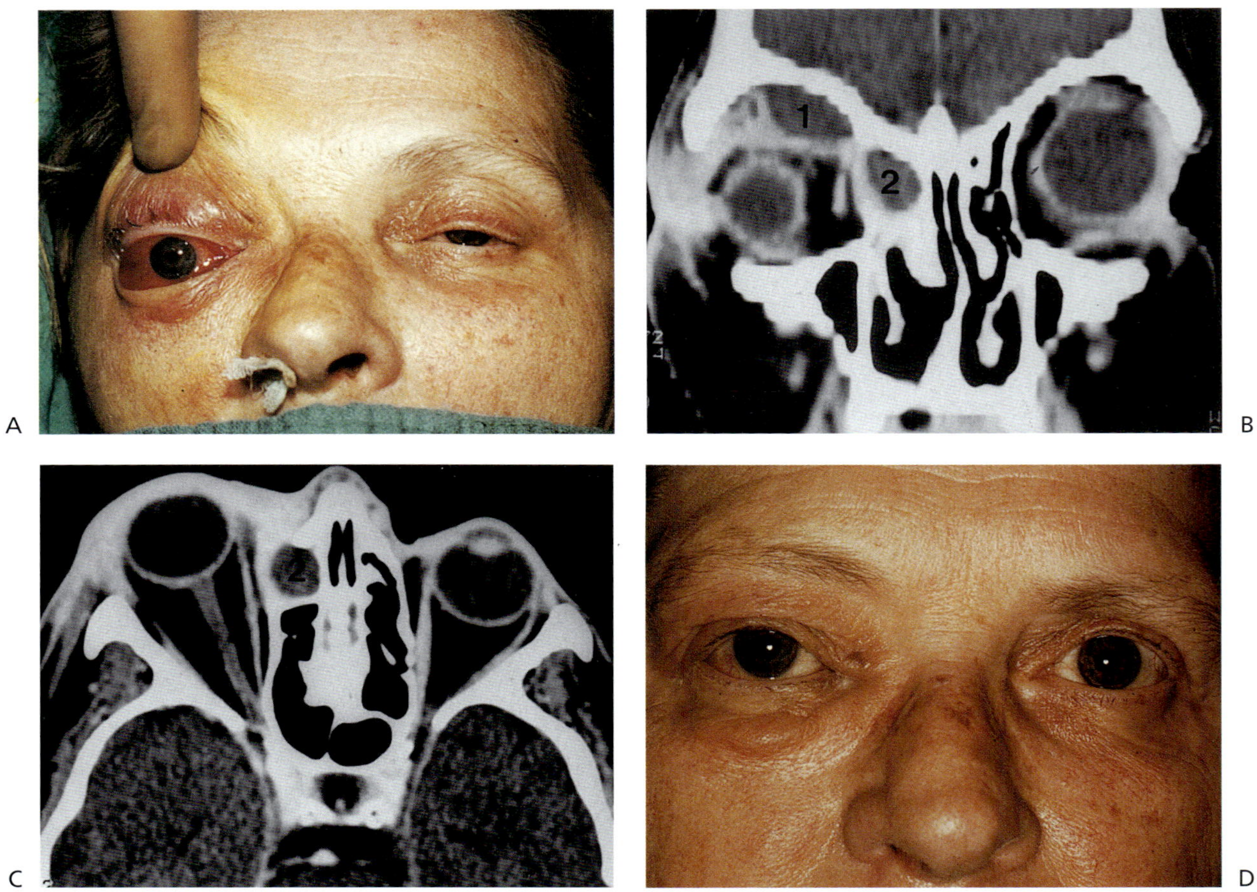


**FIGURE 23.2.** Mucocele of the anterior superior ethmoid occurs medially, with an subperiostal abscess in the right orbit. **A:** Patient before surgery. **B:** Preoperative coronal computed tomography (CT) scan. **C:** Preoperative axial CT scan. **D:** Patient 3 months after surgery. *1,* subperiostal abscess, *2,* mucocele.

***Case 2:*** A 51-year-old woman had undergone bilateral Caldwell-Luc operations many years previously, and 10 years ago she had a Lynch operation on the left side. After the procedure, she complained of double vision, severe pain in the orbital region, and swelling and redness of the periorbital region on the left side. For 6 months, swelling was evident above the medial canthus. CT examination revealed a mucocele of the medial aspect of the left frontal sinus with erosion of the lamina papyracea (Fig. 23.3A,B), but the other sinuses were normal. Because of a sufficiently wide anterior-posterior diameter and hypoplastic spina nasalis interna, an endonasal approach was indicated. To prevent recurrent stenosis of the frontal sinus outflow tract after collapse of its weak lateral wall, type III drainage was performed. Five years postoperatively, the frontal sinus is open and normal (Fig. 23.3C).

***Case 3:*** A 43-year-old woman had undergone bilateral Caldwell-Luc procedures 17 years ago and endonasal type I frontal sinus drainage 1 year ago because of chronic polypoid sinusitis. She developed persistent frontal pain. CT examination revealed complete opacification of both frontal sinuses, but the other sinuses were normal (Fig. 23.4A,B). Because of a small anterior-posterior diameter, endonasal type III frontal sinus drainage was indicated. Despite significant shrinkage of the opening postoperatively, sufficient drainage has been maintained for 8 years (Fig. 23.4C).

***Case 4:*** A 55-year-old man developed bilateral periorbital swelling and redness and a reddish frontal bulging of the forehead within 2 days (Fig. 23.5A). CT examination revealed almost complete opacification of the ethmoid cells on both sides and an osteoma of the left ethmoid (Fig. 23.5B). The frontal sinus outflow tract was completely obstructed by bone formation (Fig. 23.5C). The left frontal sinus was completely opacified, with major destruction of the anterior frontal sinus wall (Fig. 23.5D). An endonasal approach was contraindicated because of total bony obstruction of frontal sinus drainage and the major defect of the anterior wall. An osteoplastic procedure was performed using a coronal incision with fat obliteration and reconstruction of the anterior wall with calvarial split bone. An endonasal pansinus operation was also performed to remove the osteoma.

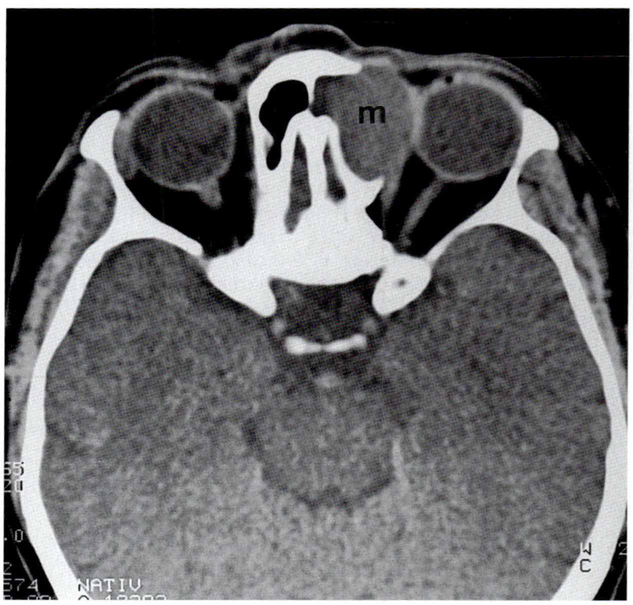


A

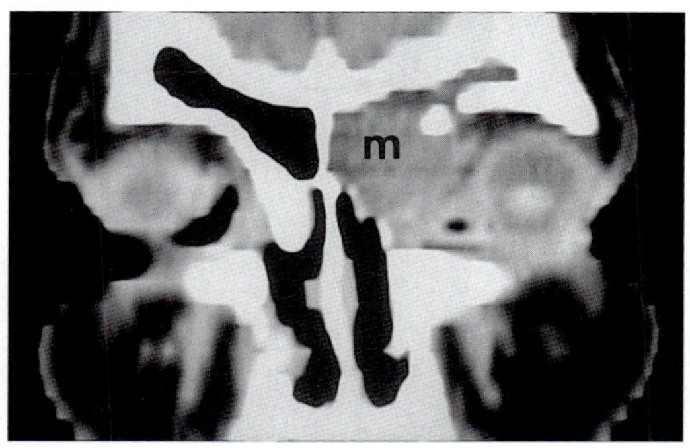


B

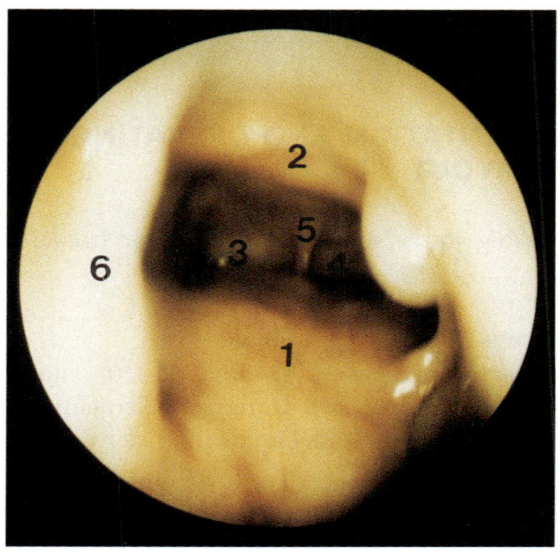


C

**FIGURE 23.3.** Medial mucocele of the left frontal sinus with erosion of the lamina papyracea. **A:** Preoperative axial computed tomography (CT) scan. **B:** Preoperative coronal CT scan. **C:** Endoscopic view 4 months after endonasal type III drainage. *m,* mucocele; *1,* posterior wall of frontal sinus; *2,* anterior wall; *3,* right frontal sinus; *4,* left frontal sinus; *5,* remnant of the interfrontal sinus septum; *6,* nasal septum.

A

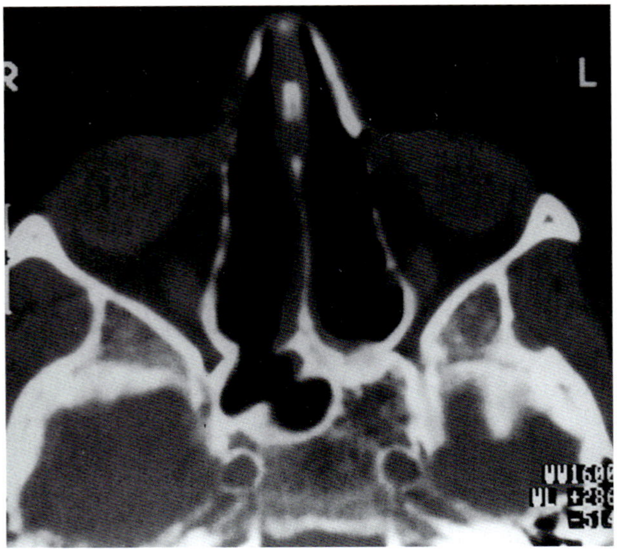


B

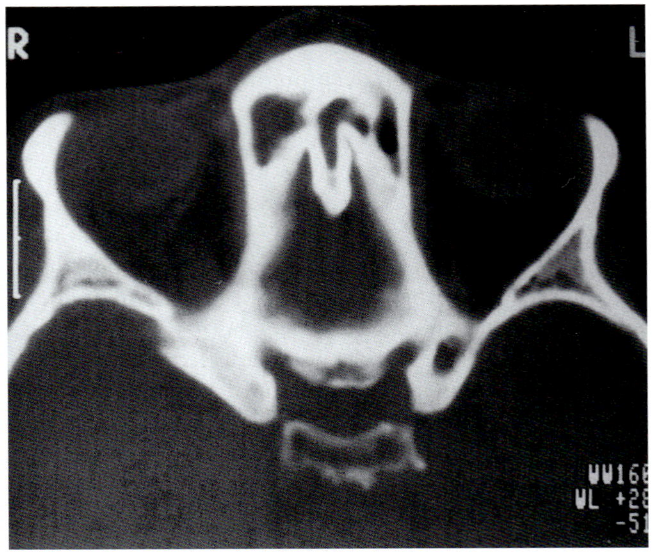


C

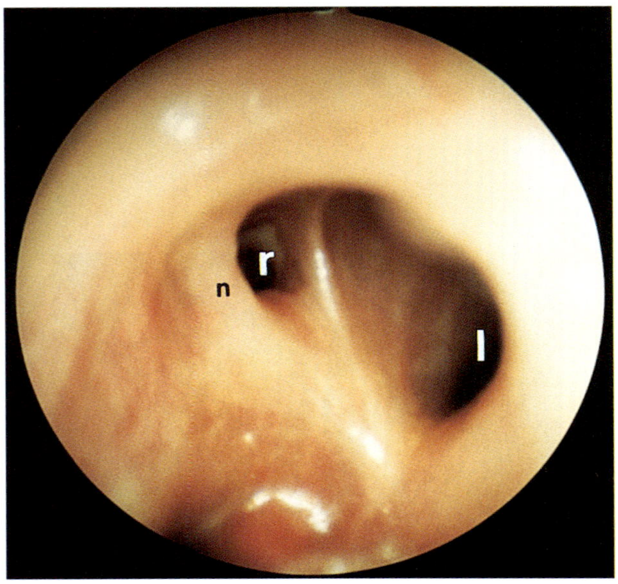


**FIGURE 23.4.** Persistent frontal sinusitis after type I drainage. **A:** Preoperative axial computed tomography (CT) scan shows a normal ethmoid sinus. **B:** Preoperative axial CT scan shows complete opacification of both frontal sinuses and their small anterior-posterior diameters. **C:** Endoscopic view 3 years after surgery with a sufficiently wide opening of both frontal sinuses from the left side. *r,* right frontal sinus; *l,* left frontal sinus; *n,* scarring at the upper margin of the reduced nasal septum.

## INSTRUMENTATION AND OPERATING ROOM LAYOUT

The following instruments are required for frontal sinus drainage:

- Microscope (250- or 300-mm objective)
- Suction-irrigation device, handle, and 30° endoscope with video monitor (Storz, Tuttlingen, Germany)
- Shaver: microresector XPS (Xomed, Jacksonville, FL)
- Cholewa self-retaining speculum (Storz, Tuttlingen, Germany)
- Nasal forceps of various sizes and angles (0°, 45°, 90°)
- Cutting forceps, straight and upward cutting, in various sizes and angulations (Stuemed, Würzburg, Germany and Storz, Tuttlingen, Germany)
- Snare (sharp)
- Nasal scissors
- Suction device (straight, angled 90°)
- Diamond burr (extra-long handpiece)

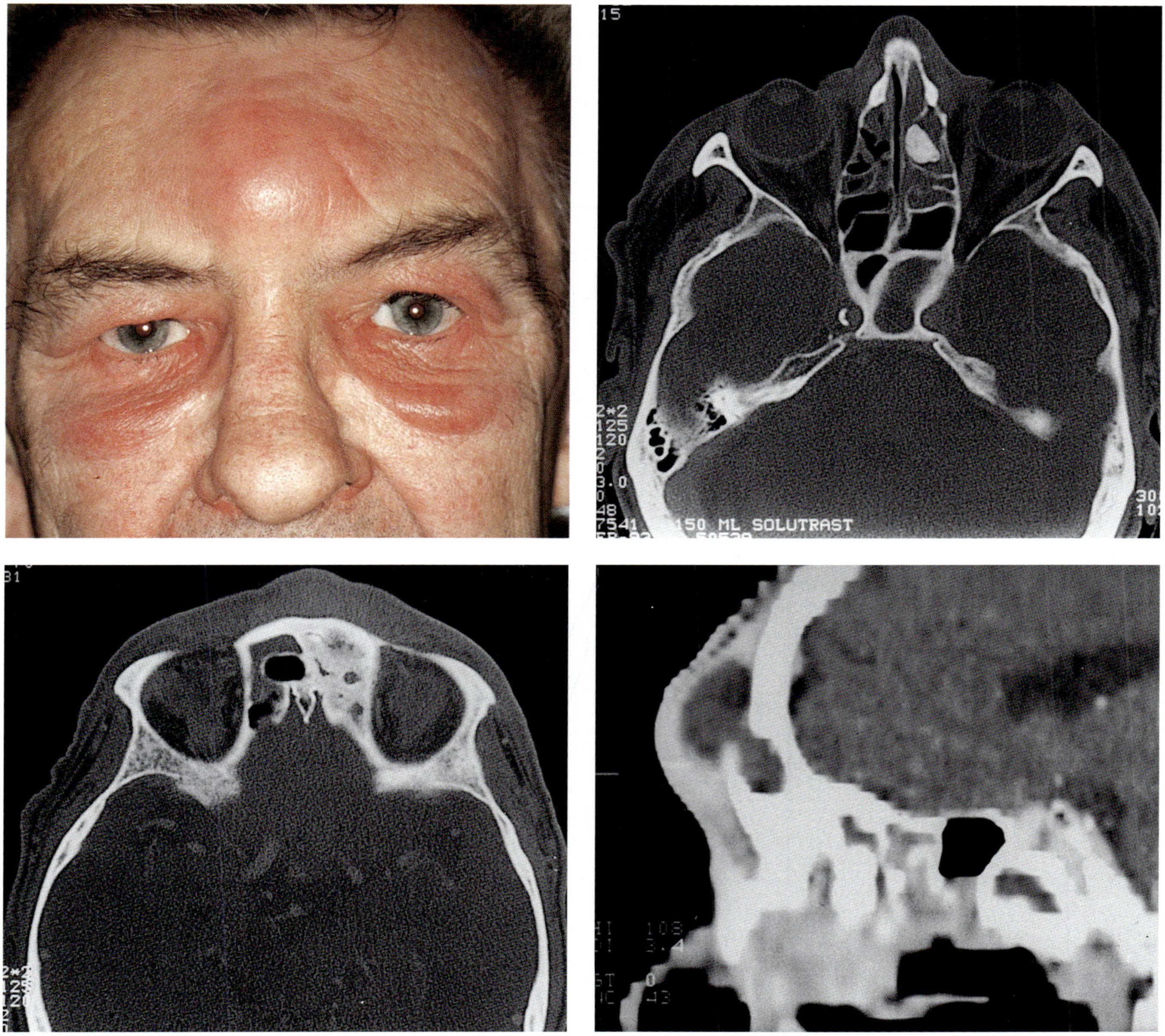


A B C D

**FIGURE 23.5.** Forehead abscess with major destruction of the left anterior frontal sinus wall from mucopyocele, chronic polypoid pansinusitis, and osteoma of the left ethmoid with concomitant bony obstruction of the frontal sinus outflow tract. **A:** Macroscopic view of the forehead abscess and periorbital swelling on both sides. **B:** Preoperative axial computed tomography (CT) scan shows opacification of the ethmoid cell system bilaterally and an osteoma on the left side. **C:** Preoperative axial CT scan shows total bony obstruction of the left frontal sinus drainage. **D:** Preoperative sagittal CT scan shows the forehead abscess with destruction of the anterior frontal sinus wall.

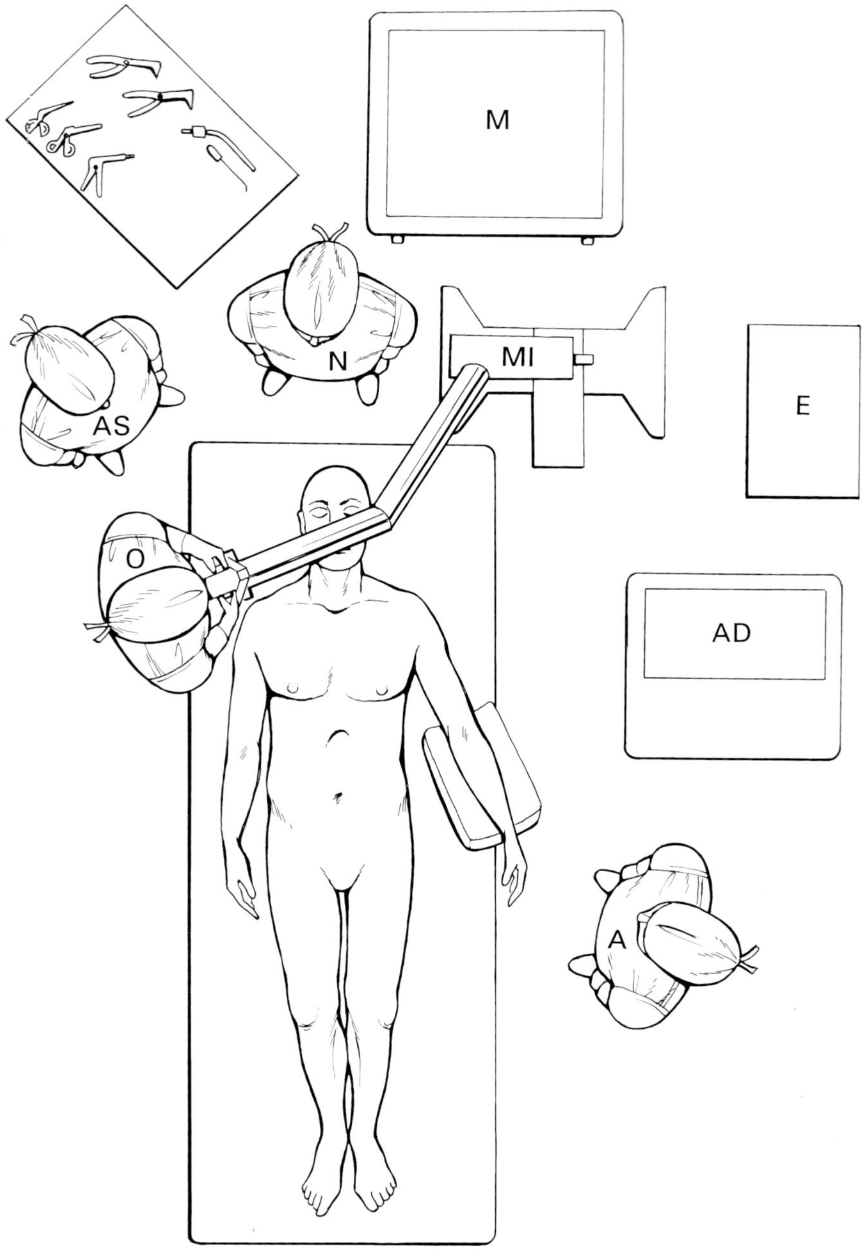


**FIGURE 23.6.** Operating room layout for endonasal micro–endoscopic frontal sinus surgery. *A,* anesthesiologist; *AD,* anesthesia device; *AS,* assistance; *E,* electrocoagulation; *M,* monitor; *MI,* microscope *N,* nurse; *O,* operator.

The operating room layout for endonasal micro–endoscopic frontal sinus surgery is shown in Figure 23.6.

## ANESTHESIA

The combined micro–endoscopic technique is carried out under general anesthesia (i.e., intubation) combined with local anesthesia. We infiltrate the nasal mucosa with lidocaine and 1:120,000 epinephrine. We first insert oxymetazoline-saturated strips, and 5 minutes later, we insert other Cottonoid strips that have been soaked in a 10% cocaine solution (maximum single dose of 2 mL, equivalent to 200 mg). The patient's blood pressure should be 80 to 100 mm Hg. Placement of a hypopharyngeal pack is recommended for preventing aspiration of blood immediately after removal of the orotracheal tube and for preventing gastric ingestion.

## OPERATIVE TECHNIQUE

For the first part of the operation, we use the Zeiss microscope with a 250-mm objective. Surgeons with very long arms should use the 300-mm lens. A Cholewa self-retaining speculum is held by an assistant.

***Step 1:*** Using the microscope, the middle turbinate is first carefully mobilized medially with the septal scissors. In cases of a concha bullosa or a polypoid-distorted turbinate, it is resected partially.

***Step 2:*** The uncinate process is removed.

***Step 3:*** If only the frontal sinus is diseased, it is possible to preserve the bulla ethmoidalis. The ethmoid cells in front of it are removed toward the frontal sinus outflow tract. This provides sufficient space for type I drainage.

***Step 4:*** Removal of the frontal sinus floor between lamina papyracea and middle turbinate or nasal septum (depending on the individual anatomic situation) results in type II drainage (Fig. 23.7). Important landmarks are the agger nasi cells and the frontal process of the maxilla, which must be reduced in most cases. In revision cases, it may be necessary to expose the lacrimal sac for anatomic orientation. Depending on the thickness of the bone, a punch, curette, or diamond burr is used, and as much mucosa as possible should be preserved.

***Step 5:*** Performing a type II drainage procedure on both sides requires identification of the anterior border of the cribriform plate by seeing the first olfactory fiber with the microscope at the anterior part of the middle turbinate bone (Fig. 23.7C). Removing the upper part of the nasal septum and the lower part of the frontal sinus septum results in a type III drainage procedure, allowing drainage and ventilation of both sinuses from both nasal sides. For

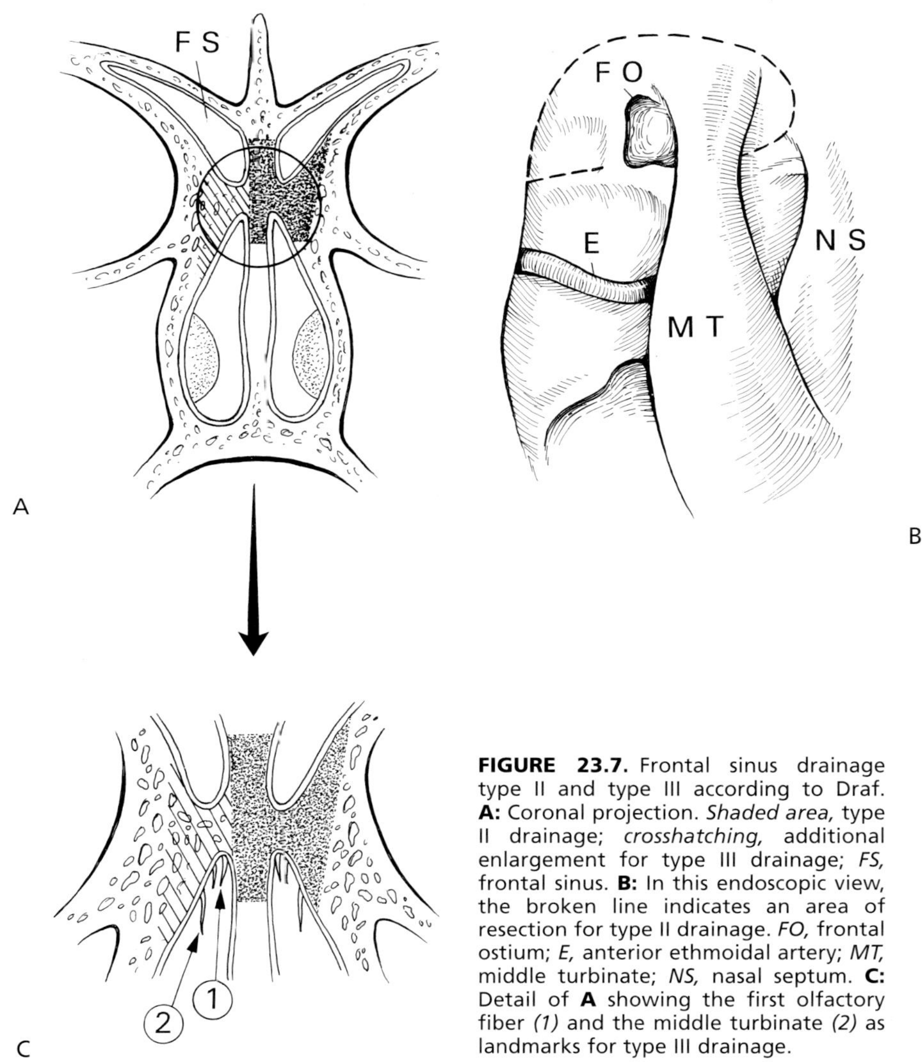


**FIGURE 23.7.** Frontal sinus drainage type II and type III according to Draf. **A:** Coronal projection. *Shaded area,* type II drainage; *crosshatching,* additional enlargement for type III drainage; *FS,* frontal sinus. **B:** In this endoscopic view, the broken line indicates an area of resection for type II drainage. *FO,* frontal ostium; *E,* anterior ethmoidal artery; *MT,* middle turbinate; *NS,* nasal septum. **C:** Detail of **A** showing the first olfactory fiber *(1)* and the middle turbinate *(2)* as landmarks for type III drainage.

this, the burr has to be used, and in some cases, special punches are useful. Complementary use of the microscope and endoscope improves the likelihood of successful opening of the sinus and complete removal of the pathologic process.

***Step 6:*** If an ethmoidectomy is needed, step 3 can be changed, and the bulla can be opened. The anterior ethmoid cells are removed, and the surgeon can identify the anterior skull base, including the anterior ethmoidal artery. Some millimeters anteriorly, the opening of the frontal sinus can be found.

***Step 7:*** At the end of the procedure, rubber finger packing (Rhinotamp, Vostra, Aachen, Germany) is inserted into the nose and ethmoidal cavity for 3 to 5 days to stop bleeding, to maintain a moistened wound, and to hasten re-epithelization. In special cases, one rubber finger is placed into the neo-ostium for 1 week.

## SPECIAL POINTS

The insertion of stents into the frontal sinus outflow tract for 6 months in special cases may significantly improve the postoperative patency of the frontal sinus neo-ostium (36). In our study, a prototype made of soft silicone was used (Vostra, Aachen, Germany), which is not yet commercially available. The frontal sinus stent designed by Rains (Smith & Nephew, Memphis, TN) is an alternative. Clear indications have to be formulated, but it should be considered when trying to avoid using a major external approach in special cases.

## POSTOPERATIVE CARE

Postoperative care includes local mechanical cleaning with instruments. This should be performed cautiously to prevent damaging the regenerating tissue. The nose should not bleed after the procedure. The crust is removed only if it obstructs nasal breathing or hinders sinus drainage.

Topical steroids are used to reduce postoperative edema and hasten the healing process (33,45–48). They should be applied until the mucosa is well healed or for at least 6 months. In some cases, application is necessary for years.

Saline solution irrigation is used for moistening tissues and for atraumatic cleaning of the nose. The use of a special nasal douche (Rhinocare, Siemens & Co., Bad Ems, Germany) is recommended for effective irrigation (49). It is performed if the patient complains of crusts and feels irrigation improves the local condition in the nose.

Systemic steroids are prescribed in cases of recurrences of nasal polyps, major eosinophilia as determined by histologic examination of the sinus mucosa, bronchial asthma, and analgetic hypersensitivity. We combine a steroid with an antihistamine, using dexamethasone (6 mg for 4 weeks, 3 mg for 1 week, 1.5 mg for 1 week) plus an agent such as Cetirizine (10 mg, given once daily for 6 weeks).

Systemic antibiotics are not used routinely at our institution. We administer antibiotics in cases of acute sinusitis or superinfection of chronic sinusitis and in cases of significantly increased yellowish secretion in the postoperative period. The exact prescription should be adapted to results of a nasal smear. In many cases, we give cefuroxime or amoxicillin–clavulanic acid.

## COMPLICATIONS

There are no major studies regarding complications after endonasal frontal sinus surgery. Most surgeons report results but not complications after frontal sinus surgery, and all major studies consider more or less complete pansinus operations (20,22,50). A summary of possible complications is provided in Table 23.3 (35,50–56). Cerebrospinal fluid (CSF) leak can be successfully managed endonasally (57). Orbital lesions may require immediate decompression because of hematoma. We perform this intervention endonasally in most cases by resection of the lamina papyracea. We seldom use an external fronto-orbital approach with closure of the anterior or posterior ethmoidal artery, as necessary (58). Another late complication after frontal sinus surgery is the development of mucoceles. Exact data about the frequency are not available. The occurrence of mucopyoceles due to scarring can be minimized by preserving mucosa at the neo-ostium or least at the posterior wall.

## ADVANTAGES AND LIMITATIONS OF THE MICRO–ENDOSCOPIC TECHNIQUE

The microscopic technique can be employed in cases of major intraoperative bleeding, with the procedure completed with the use of an endoscope. Limitations consist only of situations in which a long-term opening will not be achieved and recurrence is probable.

## LITERATURE REVIEW

Hosemann and colleagues (22) summarized the results of extended endonasal frontal sinus surgery according to Draf type II and III drainage procedures (Table 23.4).

We have carried out three studies. In the first retrospective study (16), we evaluated patients who underwent endonasal frontal sinus drainage (471 type I, 125 type II, 52 type III). From these, random samples were taken, and the patients were examined (42 type I, 43 type II, 47 type III). In each case, the indication was a chronic polypoid sinusitis, with an orbital complication of acute sinusitis in

**TABLE 23.3. COMPLICATIONS IN ENDONASAL ETHMOID SINUS SURGERY WITH THE MICROSCOPE**

| Study | No. of Patients (P) and Sides (S) | Procedure and Optical Aids | Major Complications: % P and S | Minor Complications: % P and S |
|---|---|---|---|---|
| Bagatella and Mazzoni (51) | 155 (P)<br>290 (S) | Ethmoidect.<br>Microscope | 6 CSF fistulae<br>3.9% (P); 2.1% (S) | 13 adhesions<br>8.4% (P); 4.5% (S) |
| Silverstein and McDaniel (52) | 31 (P) | Pansinus<br>Microscope | 2 hemorrhages<br>1 meningitis<br>1 possible CSF fistula<br>13% (P) | 1 reversible diplopia<br>1 hemorrhage<br>6% (P) |
| Amedee et al. (53) | 325 (P) | Pansinus<br>Microscope | 0% | 0% |
| McFadden et al. (54) | 25 (P)<br>64 (S) | Partly with microscope<br>Partly with endoscope | 2 CSF fistulae<br>1 hematoma<br>12% (P); 5% (S) | 1 bronchospasm<br>4% (P); 1.6% (S) |
| Ilberg et al. (55) | 221 (P) | Various procedures<br>Micr./End. | 3 CSF fistulae<br>1.4% (P) | 3 lid hematomas<br>2 hemorrhage<br>1.8% (P) |
| Teatini et al. (56) | a) 78 (P)<br>b) 22 (P) | a) Microscope<br>b) Micr./End. | a) 0%<br>b) 0% | a) 15 lid hematomas, 19% (S)<br>b) lid hematomas, 14% (S) |
| Weber et al. (35) (15 surgeons) | 170 (P)<br>340 (S) | Pansinus<br>Micr./End. | 12 hemorrhages<br>15 dural injuries<br>2 carotid artery injuries<br>17% (P); 9% (S) | 2 periorbital injuries<br>1 dental or lip numbness<br>2.2% (P) |
| Weber and Draf (50) | 1,178 (S) | Pansinus<br>Micr./End. | 30 injuries to dura (2.55%)<br>2 injuries to carotid artery (0.17%) | 40 periorbital injuries (3.4%) |

CSF, cerebrospinal fluid; Ethmoidect., extensive (complete) ethmoidectomy; Micr./End. = combined use of microscope and endoscope; Pansinus, pansinus operation.
From Hosemann W, Weber R, Keerl R, et al. *Minimally invasive endonasal sinus surgery.* New York: Thieme Medical Publications, 2000, with permission.

**TABLE 23.4. RESULTS OF EXTENDED ENDONASAL FRONTAL SINUS SURGERY USING DRAF TYPE II OR TYPE III TECHNIQUE**

| Study | Technique | No. of Operations | Follow-up Period | Healing of Frontal Sinus Ostium | Complications | Remarks |
|---|---|---|---|---|---|---|
| Close et al. (15) | Median drainage | 11 | 5.8 mo | 100% | 1 CSF leak | Additional small external incision in 5 of 11 patients |
| Draf et al. (16) | a) Extended drainage (type II)<br>b) Median drainage (type III) | a) 128<br>b) 57 | 5 yr | Normal/polyps/ pathological:<br>a) 61.7%/14.8%/23.5%<br>b) 67%/ 9.1%/ 23.9% | ? | |
| Har-El and Lucente (18) | a) Simple drainage<br>b) Extended drainage<br>c) Median drainage | a) 16<br>b) 5<br>c) 1 | 10–50 mo | Ostium occlusion in 1 of 22 patients<br>2 of 22 patients with CT opacification but patent ostium | — | Additional small external incision in 1 of 22 patients |
| Gross et al. (17) | Median drainage ("modified Lothrop procedure") | 10 | 7 mo | 100% | — | |
| Weber et al. (34) | a) Extended drainage<br>b) Median drainage | a) 96<br>b) 43 | 51 mo<br>34 mo | 70% reventilation<br>76% reventilation | | |
| Weber et al. (36) | a) Extended drainage | 21 | 12–16 mo | 33% endoscopically patent, 71.4% aerated frontal sinus | — | |
| | b) Extended drainage with silicone spacer for 6 mo | 15 | 12–16 mo | 80% endoscopically patent, 93.3% aerated frontal sinus | — | Prospective study, statistically significant difference |
| Rudert et al. (59) | Type II and type III drainage | 40 | 1–3 yr (?) | Restenosis in 3 cases | | |
| Simmen (32) | Type II and type III drainage | 55 | 23 mo (mean) | 62% symptom-free<br>29% improved | | No data on endoscopic result |

CSF, cerebrospinal fluid; CT, computed tomography.
From Hosemann W, Weber R, Keerl R, et al. *Minimally invasive endonasal sinus surgery.* New York: Thieme Medical Publications, 2000, with permission.

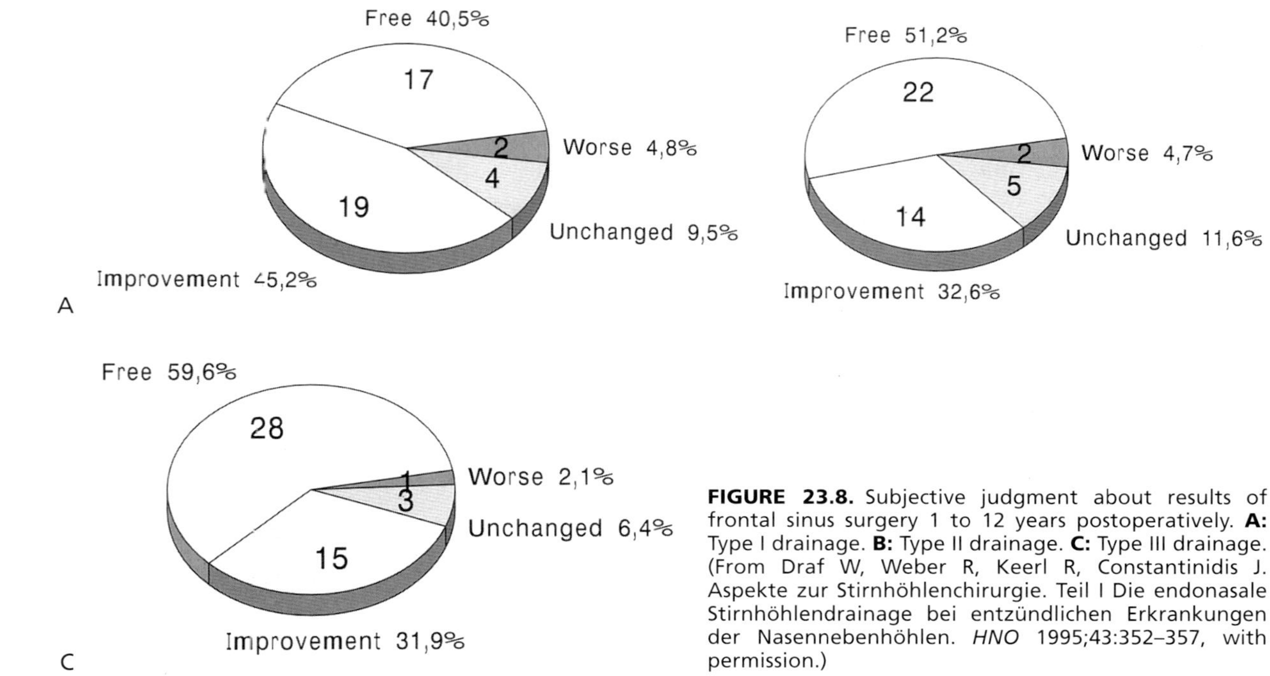


**FIGURE 23.8.** Subjective judgment about results of frontal sinus surgery 1 to 12 years postoperatively. **A:** Type I drainage. **B:** Type II drainage. **C:** Type III drainage. (From Draf W, Weber R, Keerl R, Constantinidis J. Aspekte zur Stirnhöhlenchirurgie. Teil I Die endonasale Stirnhöhlendrainage bei entzündlichen Erkrankungen der Nasennebenhöhlen. *HNO* 1995;43:352–357, with permission.)

five cases (type III). The follow-up period was 1 to 12 years, with an average period of 5 years.

The patients' subjective estimations of the operative results are shown in Figure 23.8. Individual symptoms had improved to various degrees. It is notable that the tendency of the mucosa for increased secretion could not be satisfactorily dealt with by surgery, and additional medical treatment (e.g., topical corticosteroids) was necessary. The fact that only a Yes or No answer was possible must be taken into account in evaluating the responses. Subjective and

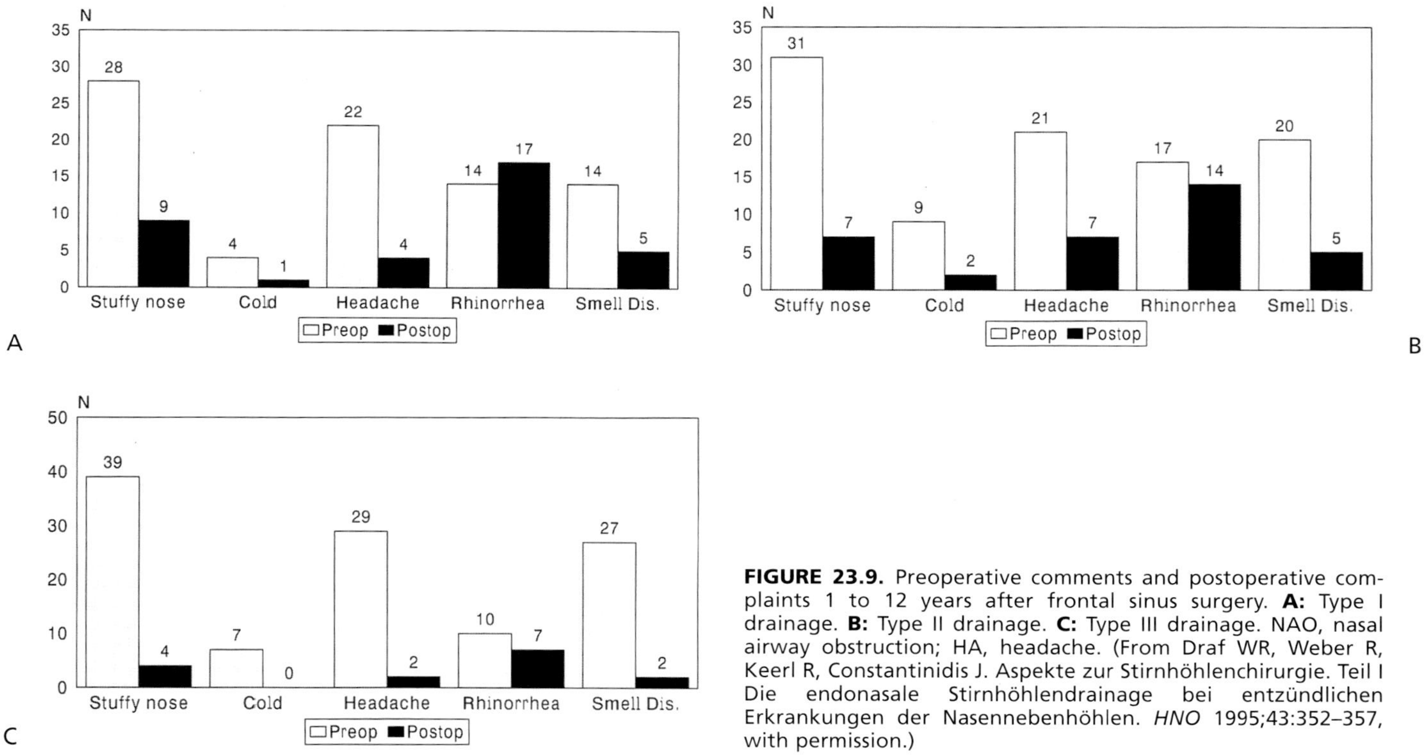


**FIGURE 23.9.** Preoperative comments and postoperative complaints 1 to 12 years after frontal sinus surgery. **A:** Type I drainage. **B:** Type II drainage. **C:** Type III drainage. NAO, nasal airway obstruction; HA, headache. (From Draf WR, Weber R, Keerl R, Constantinidis J. Aspekte zur Stirnhöhlenchirurgie. Teil I Die endonasale Stirnhöhlendrainage bei entzündlichen Erkrankungen der Nasennebenhöhlen. *HNO* 1995;43:352–357, with permission.)

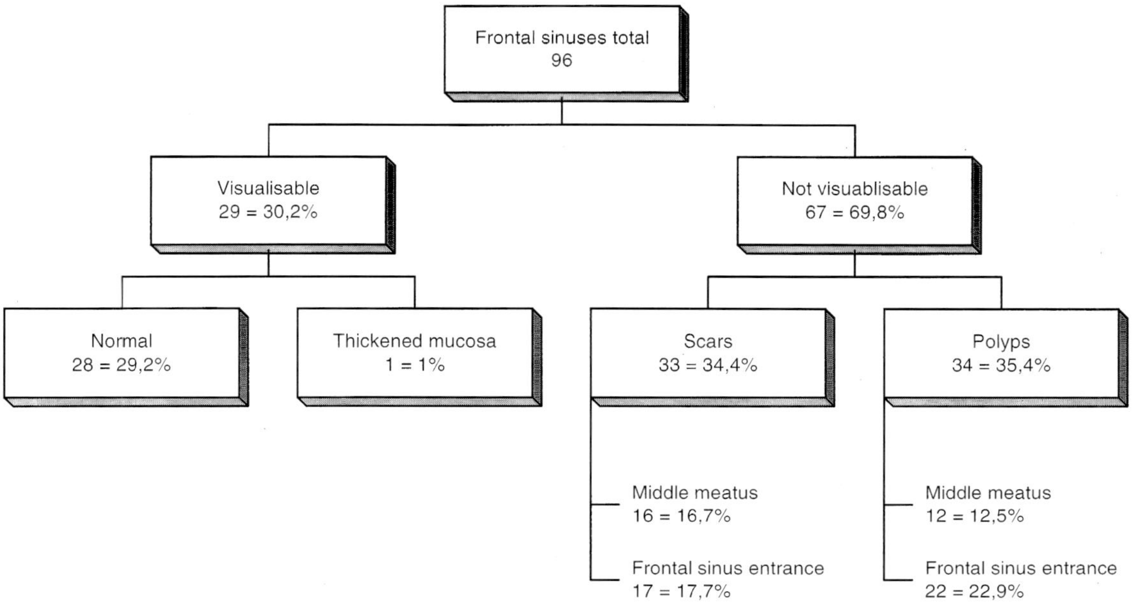


**FIGURE 23.10.** Endoscopic findings 12 to 98 months after type II drainage. (From Weber R, Draf W, Keerl R, et al. [Long-term results of endonasal frontal sinus surgery]. *HNO* 1996;44:503–509, with permission.)

objective criteria can be combined to evaluate the success of endonasal frontal sinus drainage: grade 1, endoscopically normal mucosa without subjective complaints; grade 2, subjective freedom from symptoms with endoscopically visible inflammatory mucosal changes present; grade 3, no improvement subjectively and pathologic changes in the mucosa (i.e., failure). Applying these subjective and objective criteria to determine the results of endonasal frontal sinus drainage, we were able to achieve a success rate of 83.4% for type I drainage, 83.7% for type II drainage, and 89.4% for type III drainage (Fig. 23.9). This means that, despite the choice of prognostically unfavorable cases, the type III drainage produced the best results.

In a second study, endoscopic and CT examinations were systematically carried out for patients who had undergone type II or type III drainage procedures (34) (Figs. 23.10–23.13). Twelve to 98 months after type II drainage, we found that 58% of 83 frontal sinuses were ventilated and normal. A ventilated frontal sinus with hyperplastic mucosa was seen in 12%. Scarred occlusion with total opacification on CT was obvious in 14%. In 16%, total opacification was caused by recurrent polyposis. Seventy-nine percent of patients were free of symptoms or had only minor problems. Twelve to 89 months after type III drainage, 59% of 81 frontal sinuses were ventilated and normal. A ventilated frontal sinus with hyperplastic mucosa was seen in 17%.

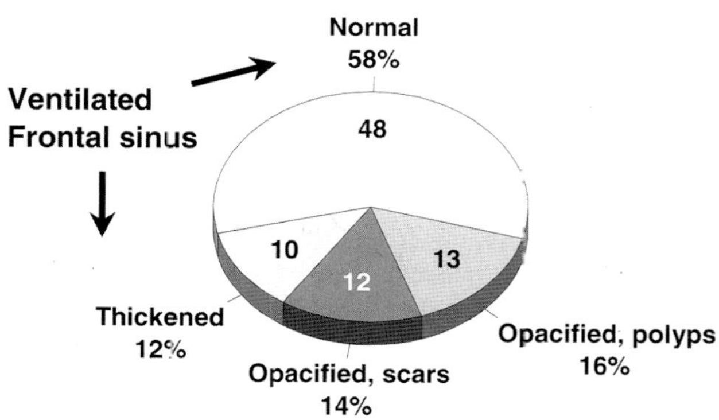


**FIGURE 23.11.** Synopsis of computed tomography and endoscopy 12 to 98 months after type II drainage. (From Weber R, Draf W, Keerl R, et al. [Long-term results of endonasal frontal sinus surgery]. *HNO* 1996;44:503–509, with permission.)

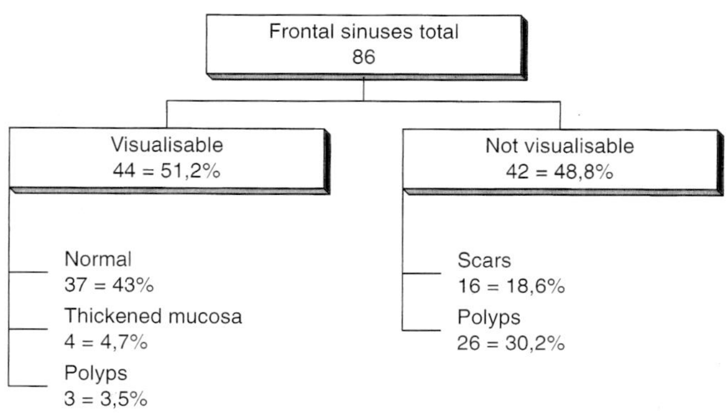


**FIGURE 23.12.** Endoscopic findings 12 to 98 months after type III drainage. (From Weber R, Draf W, Keerl R, et al. [Long-term results of endonasal frontal sinus surgery]. *HNO* 1996;44: 503–509, with permission.)

**TABLE 23.5. RESULTS AFTER ENDONASAL TYPE II DRAINAGE USING FLEXIBLE ENDOSCOPY, CT, AND MRI**

| Results | With Stenting (N=15) | Without Stenting (N=21) |
|---|---|---|
| Endoscopically open | 12 (80%) | 7 (33,3%) |
| Normal | 9 (60%) | 7 (33,3%) |
| Edematous swelling only at the frontal sinus opening | 3 (20%) | 0 |
| Thickening of frontal sinus mucosa, minor polyposis | 0 | 0 |
| Occlusion of frontal sinus due to scarring | 1 (6,7%) CT: completely opacified | 10 (47,6%) |
| Occlusion of frontal sinus due to polyps | 2 (13,3%) MRI: completely aerated, no mucosal thickening | 4 (19,0%) |

CT, computed tomography; MRI, magnetic resonance imaging.
From Weber R, Hosemann W, Draf W, et al. [Endonasal frontal sinus surgery with permanent implantation of a place holder.] *Laryngorhinootologie* 1997;76:728–734, with permission.

Scarred occlusion with total opacification seen on CT was obvious in 7%. In 16%, total opacification was caused by recurrent polyposis. Ninety-five percent of patients were free of symptoms or had only minor problems.

In a prospective survey, Weber and coworkers (36) found that long-term stenting of the frontal sinus significantly reduced the rate of restenosis of the frontal sinus neo-ostium (Table 23.5). They performed endonasal sinus surgery with Draf type II extended drainage (nasofrontal approach II according to May) because of chronic polypoid sinusitis, with or without long-term stenting of the neo-ostium for 6 months using a silicone spacer. Twelve to 16 months postoperatively, with the use of a stent, the neo-ostium was endoscopically patent in 80%, and the frontal sinus was aerated in 93.3%. In the group without stenting, the neo-ostium was endoscopically patent in 33%, and the frontal sinus aerated in 71.4%. The difference was statistically significant ($p = 0.0416$).

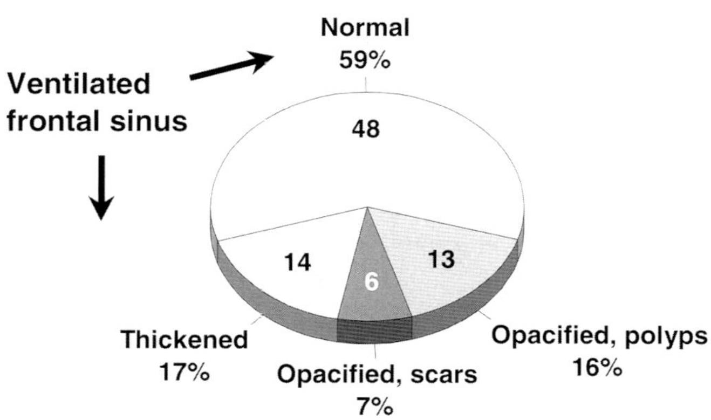


**FIGURE 23.13.** Synopsis of computed tomography and endoscopy 12 to 98 months after type III drainage. (From Weber R, Draf W, Keerl R, et al. [Long-term results of endonasal frontal sinus surgery]. *HNO* 1996;44:503–509, with permission.)

Endonasal frontal sinus surgery has been established as effective treatment for most frontal sinus diseases requiring surgery. The microscope allows successful surgery with optimal vision in difficult cases with severe bleeding. The use of microscope *and* endoscope combines the advantages of both optical aids and has been recommended by us since 1979.

## REFERENCES

1. Schaeffer M. Zur Diagnose und Therapie der Erkrankungen der Nebenhöhlen der Nase mit Ausnahme des Sinus maxillaris. *Dtsch Med Wochenschr* 1890;16:905–907.
2. Spiess G. Die endonasale Chirurgie des Sinus frontalis. *Arch Laryngol* 1899;9:285–291.
3. Ingals EF. New operation and instruments for draining the frontal sinus. *Ann Otol Rhinol Laryngol* 1905;14:515–519.
4. Halle M. Externe und interne Operation der Nebenhöhleneiterungen. *Berl Klin Wochenschr* 1906;43:1369–1372, 1404–1407.
5. Good RH. A simple and safe operation on the frontal sinus by the intranasal route. *JAMA* 1907;49:753–754.
6. Good RH. An intranasal method for opening the frontal sinus establishing the largest possible drainage. *Laryngoscope* 1908;18: 266–274.
7. Halle M. Die intranasalen Operationen bei eitrigen Erkrankungen der Nebenhöhlen der Nase. *Arch Laryngol* 1915;29:73–112.
8. Heermann H. Über endonasale Chirurgie unter Verwendung des binocularen Mikroskopes. *Arch Ohr Nase Kehlkopf Heilk* 1958; 171:295–297.
9. Draf W. [Surgical treatment of the inflammatory diseases of the paranasal sinuses. Indication, surgical technique, risks, mismanagement and complications, revision surgery]. *Arch Otorhinolaryngol* 1982;235:133–305.
10. Draf W. Endonasal micro-endoscopic frontal sinus surgery: the Fulda concept. *Otolaryngol Head Neck Surg* 1991;2:234–240.
11. Draf W, Weber R. Endonasal micro-endoscopic pansinus operation in chronic sinusitis. I. Indications and operation technique. *Am J Otolaryngol* 1993;14:394–398.

12. Kennedy DW. Functional endoscopic sinus surgery: technique. *Arch Ototaryngol* 1985;111:643–649.
13. Kennedy DW, Zinreich SJ, Rosenbaum AE, Johns ME. Functional endoscopic sinus surgery: theory and diagnostic evaluation. *Arch Otolaryngol* 1985;11:576–582.
14. Stammberger H. Endoscopic endonasal surgery—concepts in treatment of recurring rhinosinusitis. Part I. Anatomic and pathophysiologic considerations and endoscopic endonasal surgery—concepts in treatment of recurring rhinosinusitis. Part II. Surgical technique. *Otolaryngol Head Neck Surg* 1986;94:143–156.
15. Close LG, Leach JL, Lee NK, Manning SC. Endoscopic resection of the intranasal frontal sinus floor. *Ann Otol Rhinol Laryngol* 1994;103:952–958.
16. Draf W, Weber R, Keerl R, Constantinidis J. Aspekte zur Stirnhöhlenchirurgie. Teil I die endonasale Stirnhöhlendrainage bei entzündlichen Erkrankungen der Nasennebenhöhlen. *HNO* 1995;43:352–357.
17. Gross WE, Gross CW, Becker D, et al. Modified transnasal endoscopic Lothrop procedure as an alternative to frontal sinus obliteration. *Otolaryngol Head Neck Surg* 1995;113:427–434.
18. Har-El G, Lucente FE. Endoscopic intranasal frontal sinusotomy. *Laryngoscope* 1995;105:440–443.
19. Hoffmann DF, May M. Endoscopic frontal sinus surgery: frontal trephine permits a "two-sided approach." *Otolaryngol Head Neck Surg* 1991;2:257–261.
20. Hosemann W. [Endonasal surgery of the paranasal sinuses—concepts, techniques, results, complications and revision interventions]. *Eur Arch Otorhinolaryngol Suppl* 1996;1:155–269.
21. Hosemann W, Kühnel T, Held P, et al. Endonasal frontal sinusotomy in surgical management of chronic sinusitis: a critical evaluation. *Am J Rhinol* 1997;11:1–9.
22. Hosemann W, Weber R, Keerl R, Lund V. *Minimally invasive endonasal sinus surgery*. New York: Thieme Medical Publications, 2000.
23. Kennedy DW. Prognostic factors, outcomes and staging in ethmoid sinus surgery. *Laryngoscope* 1992;102[Suppl 62]:1–18.
24. Loury MC. Endoscopic frontal recess and frontal sinus ostium dissection. *Laryngoscope* 1993;103:455–458.
25. Lund VJ. Endoscopic surgery for fronto-ethmoidal mucoceles. *Otolaryngol Head Neck Surg* 1995;6:221–225.
26. May M, Schaitkin B. Frontal sinus surgery: endonasal drainage instead of an external osteoplastic approach. *Otolaryngol Head Neck Surg* 1995;6:184–192.
27. Metson R. Endoscopic treatment of frontal sinusitis. *Laryngoscope* 1992;102:712–716.
28. Perko D. Endoscopic surgery of the frontal sinus without external approach. *Rhinology* 1989;27:119–123.
29. Rudert H. Endonasal microscopic frontal sinus surgery. In: Tos M et al, eds. *Rhinology—a state of the art*. New York: Kugler, 1995:59–62.
30. Schaefer SD. Endoscopic frontal sinusotomy. *Otolaryngol Head Neck Surg* 1990;1:128–130.
31. Schaefer SD, Close LG. Endoscopic management of frontal sinus disease. *Laryngoscope* 1990;100:155–160.
32. Simmen D. [Endonasal, microscopically controlled frontal sinus surgery]. *Laryngorhinootologie* 1997;76:131–136.
33. Weber R, Draf W, Constantinidis J, Keerl R. [Current aspects of frontal sinus surgery. IV: On therapy of frontal sinus osteoma]. *HNO* 1995;43:482–486.
34. Weber R, Draf W, Keerl R, et al. [Long-term results of endonasal frontal sinus surgery]. *HNO* 1996;44:503–509.
35. Weber R, Draf W, Keerl R, et al. Endonasal micro–endoscopic pansinus operation in chronic sinusitis. II. Results and complications. *Am J Otolaryngol* 1997;18:247–253.
36. Weber R, Hosemann W, Draf W, et al. [Endonasal frontal sinus surgery with permanent implantation of a place holder]. *Laryngorhinootologie* 1997;76:728–734.
37. Wigand ME. Endoscopic surgery of the paranasal sinuses and the anterior skull base. New York: Thieme Publications, 1990.
38. Wigand ME, Hosemann WG. Endoscopic sinus surgery for frontal sinusitis and its complications. *Am J Rhinol* 1991;5: 85–89.
39. Weber R, Draf W, Constantinidis J. Osteoplastic macroscopic and microscopic frontal sinus surgery. *Am J Rhinol* 1994;8: 247–251.
40. Weber R, Draf W, Keerl R, Constantinidis J. [Current aspects of frontal sinus surgery. II: External frontal sinus operation—osteoplastic approach]. *HNO* 1995;43:358–363.
41. Weber R, Draf W, Keerl R, Constantinidis J. [Aspects of frontal sinus surgery. III: Indications and results of osteoplastic frontal sinus operation]. *HNO* 1995;43:414–420.
42. Weber R, Draf W, Kahle G, Kind M. Obliteration of the frontal sinus—state of the art and reflections on new materials. *Rhinology* 1999;37:1–15.
43. Draf W. *Die Endoskopie der Nasennebenhöhlen: Technik, Typische Befunde—Therapeutische Möglichkeiten*. Berlin: Springer, 1978.
44. Draf W. Endoscopy of the paranasal sinuses. Verbesserte amerikanische Auflage der 1978 erschienenen Endoskopie der Nasennebenhöhlen. Berlin: Springer, 1983.
45. Weber R, Keerl R, Jaspersen D, et al. Computer-assisted documentation and analysis of wound healing of the nasal and oesophageal mucosa. *J Laryngol Otol* 1996;110:1017–1021.
46. Weber R, Keerl R, Schick B, et al. [Effects of postoperative care on wound healing after endonasal paranasal sinus surgery]. *Laryngol Rhinol Otol* 1996;75:208–214.
47. Weber R, Keerl R, Huppmann A, et al. Investigation of wound healing after paranasal sinus surgery with time lapse video—a pilot study. *Am J Rhinol* 1996;10,4:235–238.
48. Weber R, Keerl R. Applications of modern image data processing in clinico-rhinologic research. *Eur Arch Otorhinolaryngol Suppl* 1996;1:271–296.
49. Keerl R, Weber R, Müller C, Schick B. [Effectiveness and tolerance of nasal irrigation following paranasal sinus surgery]. *Laryngorhinootologie* 1997;76:137–141.
50. Weber R, Draf W. [Complications of endonasal micro-endoscopic ethmoid bone operation]. *HNO* 1992;40:170–175.
51. Bagatella F, Mazzoni A. Microsurgery in nasal polyposis transnasal ethmoidectomy. *Acta Otolaryngol Suppl* 1986;431: 1–19.
52. Silverstein H, McDaniel AB. Microsurgical sphenoethmoidectomy. In: Goldman JL, ed. *The principles and practice of rhinology*. New York: J Wiley, 1987:435–442.
53. Amedee RG, Mann WJ, Gilsbach JM. Microscopic endonasal surgery: clinical update for treatment of chronic sinusitis with polyps. *Am J Rhinol* 1990;4:203–205.
54. McFadden EA, Kany RJ, Fink JN, Toohill FJ. Surgery for sinusitis and aspirin triad. *Laryngoscope* 1990;100:1043–1046.
55. Ilberg C, May A, Weber A. [Microsurgery of the nasal cavity and paranasal sinuses]. *Laryngorhinootologie* 1990;69:52–57.
56. Teatini GP, Stomeo F, Bozzo C. Transnasal sinusectomy with combined microscopic and endoscopic technique. *J Laryngol Otol* 1991;105:635–637.
57. Weber R, Keerl R, Draf W, et al. Management of dural lesions occurring during endonasal sinus surgery. *Arch Otolaryngol* 1996; 122:732–736.
58. Keerl R, Weber R, Draf W, Maran AG. *Endonasal sinus surgery*, CD-ROM. Germany: Giebel Eiterfeld, 1998.
59. Rudert H, Maune S, Mahnke CG. [Complications of endonasal surgery of the paranasal sinuses: incidence and strategies for prevention]. *Laryngorhinootologie* 1997;76:200–215.

# 24

# ENDOSCOPIC SURGICAL MANAGEMENT OF PEDIATRIC RHINOSINUSITIS

TODD A. LOEHRL
TIMOTHY L. SMITH

## INDICATIONS AND HISTORICAL PERSPECTIVE

Chronic rhinosinusitis in the pediatric population is increasing in frequency. It represents a frustrating problem for the patient, family, and their physicians. Evidence also indicates pediatric acute or chronic rhinosinusitis is associated with significant morbidity and health care costs. Some estimates indicate that acute sinusitis complicates 5% to 10% of upper respiratory tract infections in children (1). The larger number of children in day care may play a role in the increasing incidence of pediatric rhinosinusitis. Wald and colleagues prospectively examined children 1 to 3 years old and found that day care enrollment doubled the incidence of rhinosinusitis, defined as an upper respiratory infection persisting beyond 15 days, from 6.5% to 13.1% per year (2). Other contributing factors include advances in sinus imaging and endoscopic techniques that have improved physicians' ability to diagnose and treat rhinosinusitis.

The incidence of pediatric rhinosinusitis generally peaks at age 3 and gradually tapers thereafter (3) for unknown reasons. It is possible this represents the natural maturation of immune function. However, there can be a great variability in the disease course among patients, and treatment therefore must be tailored to the individual. Chronic rhinosinusitis may adversely affect the overall health of the child by aggravating underlying disease processes, such as pulmonary problems and underlying immunodeficiencies.

Abnormalities in anatomy, mucociliary clearance, immune function, or some combination thereof may predispose to the development of chronic rhinosinusitis. Ostial patency, mucociliary clearance, appropriate mucous viscosity or quantity, and an intact immune system are required to maintain sinonasal health. A deficiency in any of these can result in compromised sinonasal ventilation, retained secretions, and bacterial overgrowth.

Endoscopic sinus surgery for the pediatric population remains controversial even after being reported as an effective option for patients failing medical therapy (4). Two main issues drive the controversy. The first is that pediatric rhinosinusitis tends to be self-limited and often spontaneously resolves. For patients that require treatment, appropriate medical therapy can resolve the situation in most cases (5). Alternatively, good outcomes are reported in a high percentage of patients undergoing functional endoscopic sinus surgery (FESS) (6–8), which is advocated when medical therapy has been exhausted. Children with an underlying immune deficiency, cystic fibrosis, allergy, asthma, or mucociliary dysfunction are more likely to require surgical management of rhinosinusitis (9).

The second issue is the potential effect of FESS on facial skeletal growth in children. Preliminary findings in a piglet model and ethmoid bone specimens from 84 children who underwent FESS reveal a potential affect on sinus and facial growth in children undergoing even a very limited endoscopic sinus procedure (10). The decision to proceed with endoscopic sinus surgery in children should be made with great deliberation. Absolute and relative indications for endoscopic sinus surgery are listed in Table 24-1 (9).

## ANATOMY

The frontal and sphenoid sinuses are largely undeveloped at birth. Newborns have relatively large, bulky turbinates that tend to constrict the inferior, middle, and superior meatus; these areas are not a functioning part of the sinonasal cavity. The ethmoid sinuses are approximately 1 to 3 mm wide, 1 to 5 mm high, and 10 mm long. The ethmoid cells are almost completely present in number, but they are smaller, with a fair amount of connective tissue found between the cells. The uncinate process, hiatus semilunaris, and bulla ethmoidalis are present and can be consistently found under the middle turbinate. The maxillary sinus tends to be spherical or pyramidal, 10 mm long, 3 mm wide, and 4 mm high. The frontal sinuses are not present, but bony cells

**TABLE 24.1. SIGNS AND SYMPTOMS OF PEDIATRIC RHINOSINUSITIS**

| Signs or Symptoms | Nonsevere | Severe |
|---|---|---|
| Rhinorrhea | Yes | Yes: frank, purulent |
| Nasal congestion | Yes | Yes |
| Headaches, facial pain | May be present | Yes |
| Fever | None or low grade | High grade |
| Frequent cough | Yes | Yes |
| Postnasal discharge | Mild | Mild |

Adapted from Lusk RP, Stankiewicz JA. Pediatric sinusitis. *Otolaryngol Head Neck Surg* 1997;117:S54, with permission.

originating from the ethmoidal infundibulum (i.e., cellulae ethmoidales) are seen pneumatizing toward the frontal bone. The sphenoid sinus is not developed, although the ostium can sometimes be identified with a probe.

Between the ages of 1 and 4 years, the inferior meatus develops, and by age 4, approximately one half of it is integrated into the sinonasal cavity. The ethmoid sinus rapidly expands, measuring 12 to 21 mm long, 8 to 16 mm high, and 5 to 11 mm wide. The frontal bones start to pneumatize and ranges in size from 4 to 8 mm long, 6 to 9 mm high, and 11 to 19 mm wide. The maxillary sinuses rapidly enlarge, pneumatizing laterally to the infraorbital nerve and inferiorly to the attachment of the inferior turbinate. At this age, it measures 22 to 30 mm long, 12 to 18 mm high, and 11 to 19 mm wide. The sphenoid sinus also starts to pneumatize and measures 4 to 6 mm long, 3 to 5 mm high, and 6 to 8 mm wide.

Between the ages of 4 and 8 years, pneumatization continues to progress in all directions. The ethmoid sinus system is 18 to 24 mm long, 10 to 15 mm high, and 9 to 13 mm wide. The frontal sinus is 6 to 10 mm long, 15 to 16 mm high, and 8 to 10 mm wide. The maxillary sinus has pneumatized laterally past the infraorbital canal and assumed a tetrahedral shape. The maxillary sinus is 34 to 38 mm long, 22 to 26 mm high, and 18 to 24 mm wide. The sphenoid sinus is 11 to 14 mm long, 7 to 11 mm high, and 9 to 11 mm wide.

By age 12, the sinonasal cavity is almost completely developed and has reached adult proportions (11).

A few comments are appropriate with regard to paranasal sinus development and safe pediatric sinus surgery. The floor of the maxillary sinus is not necessarily at the level of the nasal cavity floor. Care must be taken, especially if surgery is performed through the inferior meatus or canine fossa. Damage may occur to the tooth buds, spongiotic bone under the floor of the sinus, the lateral wall of the sinus, or the inferior turbinate.

The inferior turbinate tends to be positioned higher on the lateral nasal wall, resulting in the anterior margin of the uncinate process being closer to the lamina papyracea. If this relationship is not respected, penetration of the orbital cavity during uncinectomy is possible (11).

## PREOPERATIVE EVALUATION

### Signs and Symptoms

Rhinosinusitis can manifest with a variety of signs and symptoms, depending on the age of the patient and severity of the disease. The diagnosis of acute rhinosinusitis requires signs and symptoms persisting for more than 10 days. Chronic rhinosinusitis is associated with low-grade symptoms lasting 12 weeks or more. Patients with chronic rhinosinusitis may have periods of acute exacerbation. Another variety is recurrent acute rhinosinusitis, which consists of repeated acute episodes with complete resolution in between.

Younger patients with rhinosinusitis tend to have nasal obstruction, cough, and purulent anterior rhinorrhea as primary symptoms. Daytime cough is a more reliable indicator of underlying rhinosinusitis, although nighttime cough is a more common complaint. The association of cough with chronic rhinosinusitis may indicate contamination of the lower airways by sinonasal secretions or result from a reflex arc from the sinuses to the lower respiratory tract (12). Patients with associated reactive airway disease may have worsening of their pulmonary status, which fluctuates in parallel with exacerbations of sinonasal disease. Headaches, fever, postnasal discharge, irritability, and halitosis may also be associated with rhinosinusitis (9). Patients with acute rhinosinusitis tend to have severe symptoms and are more likely to develop infectious complications compared with individuals with chronic disease. Toddlers commonly insert foreign bodies in the nose and typically present with unilateral purulent nasal discharge and halitosis. Other causes of unilateral nasal purulence or obstruction to consider include neoplasms, central nervous system herniation, nasal stenosis, and choanal atresia.

### Physical Examination

In many children, anterior rhinoscopy using an otoscope to visualize the middle meatus is all that can be accomplished. Septal deflection, size and character of the inferior turbinates, mucopurulence, presence or absence of polyps, masses, and foreign bodies should be documented. In a cooperative patient, the flexible endoscope may be used as well. The posterior choanae and adenoid pad can be assessed using the flexible endoscope. If possible, it is often helpful to topically decongest and anesthetize the nasal cavity with a 1:1 combination of 0.05% oxymetazoline and 4% lidocaine.

### Imaging

Plain film radiography has been found to underestimate and overestimate the amount of sinus disease compared with computed tomography (CT) and is not thought to be a reliable screen for chronic sinus disease (13). However, plain film radiographs may be helpful in the diagnosis of acute sinusitis in which air-fluid levels are commonly seen.

CT in the coronal plane is considered the standard radiologic modality for diagnosing chronic sinus disease. It provides much more information at approximately the same cost as a plain series of sinus radiographs. CT imaging is indicated to document the existence and extent of chronic rhinosinusitis. It is also helpful for identifying anatomic deformities, such as concha bullosa and septal deflections, that may predispose to the development of chronic rhinosinusitis. A patient's CT scans should be present during surgery and reviewed for any anatomic deformity that may place the patient at increased risk for intraoperative complications. In addition to the location and extent of disease, the relationship of the cribriform plate to the ethmoid roof, course of the optic nerve, and location of the ethmoid arteries should all be assessed on the preoperative CT scan. Other indications for CT include facial pain or headaches, evaluation of potential infectious complications, and assessment of central nervous system (CNS) herniation or neoplastic processes. Any child with a unilateral nasal mass should be considered to have CNS herniation until proven otherwise.

### Additional Evaluation

The workup should include evaluation for allergy, immune deficiency, cystic fibrosis, ciliary disorders, and gastroesophageal reflux disease (14). All pediatric patients with nasal polyps should be evaluated for cystic fibrosis.

## NONENDOSCOPIC SURGERY

Many physicians advocate adenoidectomy in children with chronic rhinosinusitis manifested by moderate to severe nasal obstruction caused by adenoid hypertrophy (9). The degree of symptomatic improvement corresponds to the size of the adenoid pad (15). Although adenoidectomy is considered the first line of surgical therapy and is thought to be beneficial in children with chronic rhinosinusitis, the procedure has not been shown to be beneficial in a statistically valid manner (16).

Antral lavage is no longer considered a viable method of treating chronic rhinosinusitis because it involves only the maxillary sinus and not the ethmoid, where most rhinosinusitis originates (17). However, in patients with isolated maxillary sinus disease or in an immunocompromised patient, this remains an important means to obtain culture material for directing antibiotic therapy.

Inferior meatal antrostomy (i.e., nasal antral window) is not a proven method of treating rhinosinusitis in most pediatric patients. It is prone to failure because the cilia continue to carry secretions to the natural ostium, resulting in a circular flow of secretions from the natural ostium to the inferior antrostomy. The procedure is also compromised because the antrostomy cannot be made large enough in most pediatric patients to maintain patency (18). One exception for the placement of an inferior antrostomy is in patients with ciliary dyskinesia in whom the cilia do not function properly and gravity may play more of a role in sinus drainage.

## CASE EXAMPLE

A 10-year-old child presented with a history of chronic rhinosinusitis with six to eight recurrent acute exacerbations per year manifested by bilateral purulent rhinorrhea and nasal obstruction. The patient also complained of bilateral frontal headaches during the acute episodes. The allergy evaluation result was negative. Medical management included nasal steroids, prolonged courses of antibiotics (3- to 6-week courses on numerous occasions), decongestants, nasal saline, and gastroesophageal reflux disease evaluation and management. A sweat chloride test result was negative.

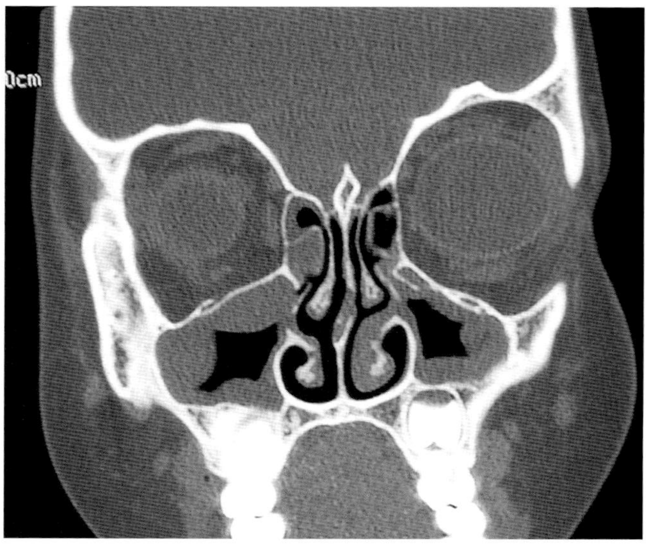

**FIGURE 24.1.** Preoperative coronal computed tomography scan of the sinuses. The patient had been maximally medically treated.

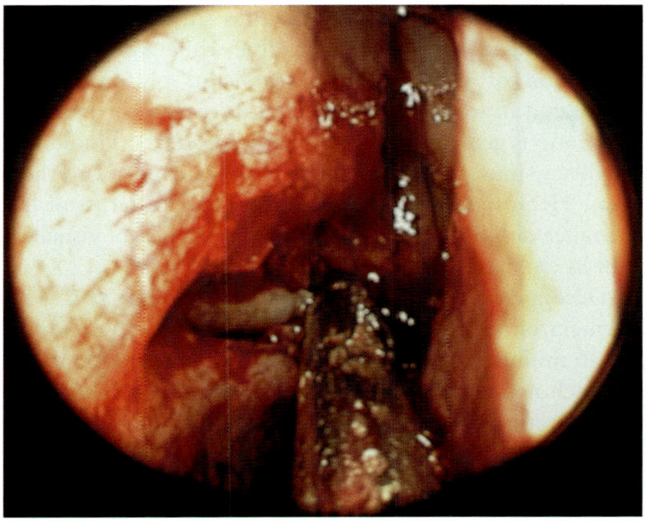

**FIGURE 24.2.** Right middle meatus. The microbackbiter had been used to create an "edge" for the microdebrider and to define the anterior extent of the uncinate process. The superior portion of the uncinate process is left intact to prevent frontal recess stenosis. The middle turbinate is not well visualized because of a septal deflection.

The patient had asthma, which was exacerbated by her chronic sinus difficulties. She had previously undergone adenoidectomy and maxillary sinus irrigation and aspiration, which failed to resolve the problem. A CT scan was obtained (Fig. 24.1) and revealed anterior ethmoid, maxillary, and frontal recess mucosal thickening. The posterior ethmoids and sphenoid had no evidence of disease.

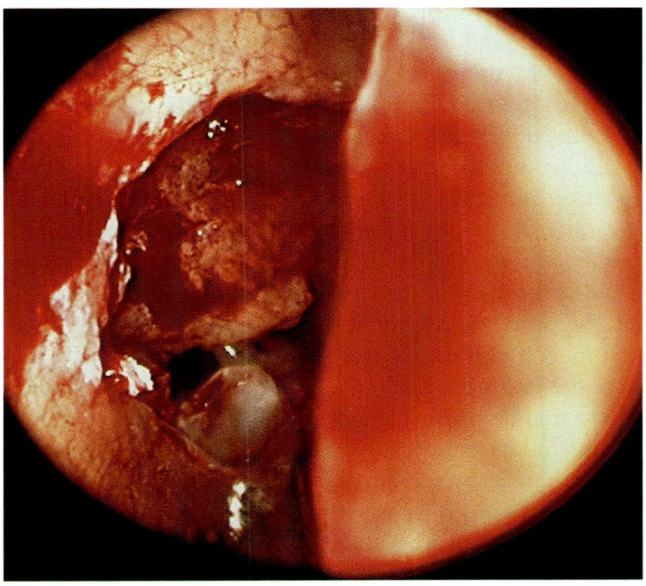

**FIGURE 24.3.** Completed uncinectomy. Notice the exposure of the natural maxillary sinus ostium.

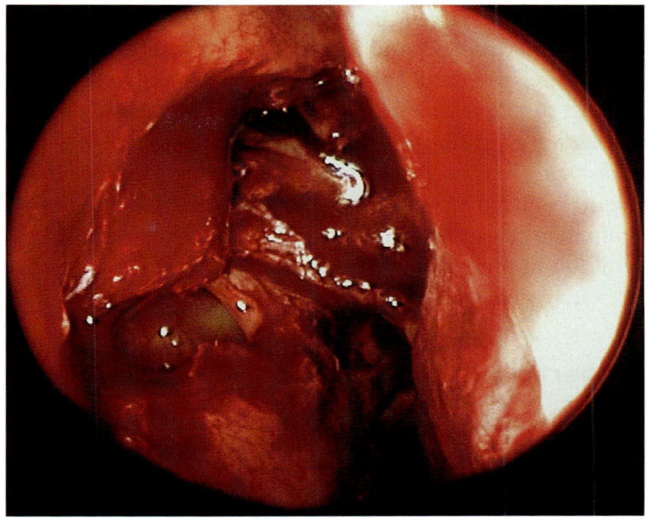

**FIGURE 24.4.** Completed anterior ethmoidectomy.

The patient subsequently underwent FESS incorporating an anterior ethmoidectomy and maxillary antrostomy (Figs. 24.2–24.4).The patient has done well since, with no episodes of acute rhinosinusitis after recovering from surgery. Her asthma has been much less symptomatic.

## INSTRUMENTATION

### Traditional

Traditional instrumentation includes the Blakesley cup forceps in straight, 45°, and 90° angulations. Curved sinus seekers are useful for identification of the maxillary sinus natural ostium and frontal recess. The J-curette is a useful instrument for controlled entrance into sinus cells within the sphenoethmoidal complex, and a microbackbiter is a useful instrument for uncinate removal.

The instrumentation for pediatric sinus surgery is similar to that for adults, but smaller pediatric instrumentation is often required for safe endoscopic sinus surgery. Both pediatric and adolescent instrumentation is available. The adolescent instrumentation should generally be considered in children older than 8 years of age, although the smaller pediatric instrumentation may still be required.

Endoscopes consist of 2.7- and 4.0-mm-diameter Hopkins rod-lens telescopes. The 4.0-mm device provides superior illumination and visualization and should be chosen whenever possible. Alternatively, the 2.7-mm endoscope provides the surgeon with less light and a smaller image, making visualization more challenging. However, technologic advances continue to narrow the gap between the two sizes. The endoscopes come in 0°, 30°, 45°, and 70° angles. We prefer to use the 0° endoscope as much as possible throughout the case. The 30° and 45° endoscopes are useful for precise identification of the maxillary sinus ostium and when working in the frontal recess. The 70° endoscope is rarely required and can be disorienting. Only very experienced surgeons should use forceps with this endoscope.

Suction-irrigation devices are available for the 4.0-mm endoscopes, but they add considerable diameter to the instrument. In the narrow pediatric sinonasal cavity, this makes trauma to the septum and lateral nasal wall more likely, resulting in more bleeding and compromise in visualization. We rarely find them useful in treating this group of patients.

### Powered Instrumentation

Soft tissue shavers (i.e., microdebriders) are a relatively new advance in endoscopic sinus surgery instrumentation. They were originally developed for arthroscopic joint surgery and have been adapted for sinonasal surgery. Their use was first reported by Setliff and Parsons (19) in 345 patients, 90 of whom were children. Powered instrumentation offers the advantage of precise soft tissue resection, and the continuous suction helps to maintain a clear surgical field.

Several manufacturers produce soft tissue shavers. We have chosen to use the Xomed microdebrider system (Jacksonville, FL). All systems consist of a power source, a handpiece, and disposable, sheathed shaving blades. The mechanics of soft tissue shavers have been well described and are beyond the scope of this chapter (20).

Soft tissue shavers are advantageous in patients with and without nasal polyps. In both cases, they allow precise removal of obstructing tissue or structures while potentially preserving adjacent normal mucosa. This results in less bleeding, which is critical for safe and effective sinus surgery in the constricted anatomy of the pediatric sinonasal cavity. Preservation of the normal mucosa results in more rapid healing and less chance for obstructive scar formation. Continuous suction allows for longer uninterrupted periods of dissection in a clear field. This can reduce operative time and allow for more thorough ventilation of the involved sinuses. This is especially important in children with profuse sinonasal polyposis. The intraoperative use of powered instrumentation is described in the surgical technique section of this chapter.

## ANESTHESIA

General anesthesia is the only appropriate choice in most children.

## OPERATIVE TECHNIQUE

Endoscopic sinus surgery is a last resort and should only be considered when all medical options have been exhausted and after a thorough preoperative evaluation has been carried out. Another caveat is that sinus surgery in children should be as conservative as possible while accomplishing ventilation of the diseased sinuses and preservation of undiseased mucosa. Most sinonasal disease in the pediatric age group is generally confined to the anterior ethmoid and maxillary sinuses. Most surgery should be confined to these areas. Hemostasis is of critical importance in terms of less tolerance of blood loss and greater compromise of visualization in children.

Decongestion is initiated in the holding area with oxymetazoline spray (0.05%), with two sprays in each nostril 30 minutes before surgery. Once in the operating room, 0.5-inch neurosurgical pledgets soaked with oxymetazoline (0.05%) are placed atraumatically in the sinonasal cavity. No attempt is made to place the pledgets in the middle meatus to minimize destabilization of the middle turbinate. Great care is taken throughout the entire case to minimize any trauma to the septum, lateral nasal wall, or any uninvolved structures.

The injection of the local anesthetic is carried out using a 25-gauge spinal needle that is bent at the tip approximately 10° toward the bevel. Under endoscopic guidance, using the 0° endoscope, 1% lidocaine with 1:100,000 epinephrine is injected initially at the posterior attachment of the middle turbinate. This injection is crucial in blocking the sphenopalatine artery, and the entire middle turbinate often blanches with this one injection if performed correctly. The inferior border of the middle turbinate is subsequently injected in a posterior-to-anterior direction. The final injection is carried out just superior to the anterior attachment of the middle turbinate. All the injections are placed just below the mucosal surface. The 0.5-inch neurosurgical pledgets soaked in 0.05% oxymetazoline are replaced atraumatically while the powered instrumentation is being set up. We prefer to start the case with the 4-mm-diameter, 0° endoscope, although the 2.7-mm endoscope is required to minimize trauma in many cases. The entire sinonasal cavity is examined initially in a posterior-to-anterior direction. The size of the adenoid pad is observed, and decisions regarding the adenoidectomy can be made. The sphenoethmoidal recess and middle meatus are evaluated for inflammatory or infectious processes that require surgical ventilation. Destabilization of the middle turbinate is avoided throughout the entire case.

The posterior edge of the uncinate process is identified, and the 3.5-mm microdebrider or microbackbiter is used to start the resection. Demucosalization of the lateral portion of the middle turbinate is avoided. This is facilitated with the microdebrider because the oscillating blade is guarded, preventing unwanted mucosal injury. Superiorly, 2 to 3 mm of uncinate are left to prevent frontal recess stenosis. Complete removal of the uncinate is facilitated using the microbackbiter (Fig. 24.5) to define the anterior edge of the uncinate and to create an edge for the microdebrider to work on (Fig. 24.6). Removal of the uncinate usually cre-

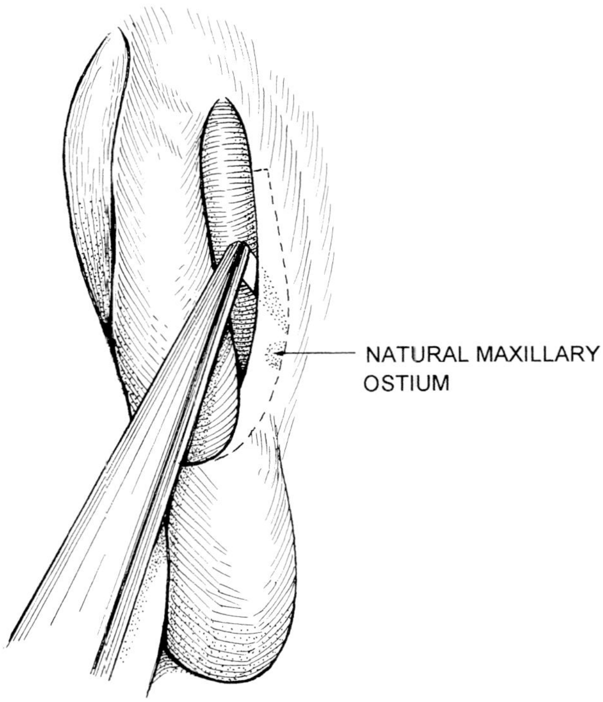


**FIGURE 24.5.** Use of the microbackbiter to initiate uncinate process removal. This creates an "edge" for the microdebrider and defines the anterior extent of the uncinate process.

ates adequate space to work in the ethmoid and maxillary sinuses without resection of the middle turbinate. Thorough removal of the uncinate allows visualization of the natural ostium of the maxillary sinus. A 30° endoscope and maxillary sinus seeker are helpful in identification of the natural maxillary sinus ostia. If necessary, a maxillary antrostomy is performed by opening into the posterior fontanel, taking great care to include the natural ostium. The maxillary antrostomy may be done before or after the anterior ethmoidectomy. Anteriorly and superiorly, the mucosa is left intact to prevent circumferential mucosal denudement and injury to the nasolacrimal apparatus.

Subsequently, the ethmoid bulla is entered inferiorly. A J-curette may be used to fracture the anterior face, but we prefer the microdebrider (Fig. 24.7). The use of the microdebrider minimizes instrument removal and reinsertion, avoiding injury to adjacent mucosa and structures. The superior portion of the ethmoid bulla is left intact to prevent compromise of the frontal recess (Figs. 24.8 and 24.9). After removal of the bulla ethmoidalis, the basal lamella is exposed. If indicated, the basal lamella is penetrated at the level of maxillary sinus ostium to enter the posterior ethmoid cells. Before entering the posterior ethmoids, it is helpful to visualize the posterior attachment of the middle turbinate, the location of the natural maxillary sinus ostium, and your overall position within the sinonasal

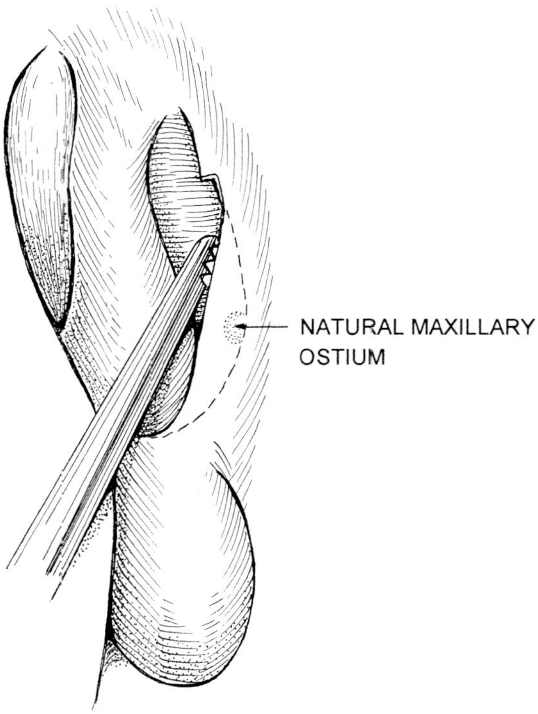


**FIGURE 24.6.** Removal of the uncinate process using the microdebrider.

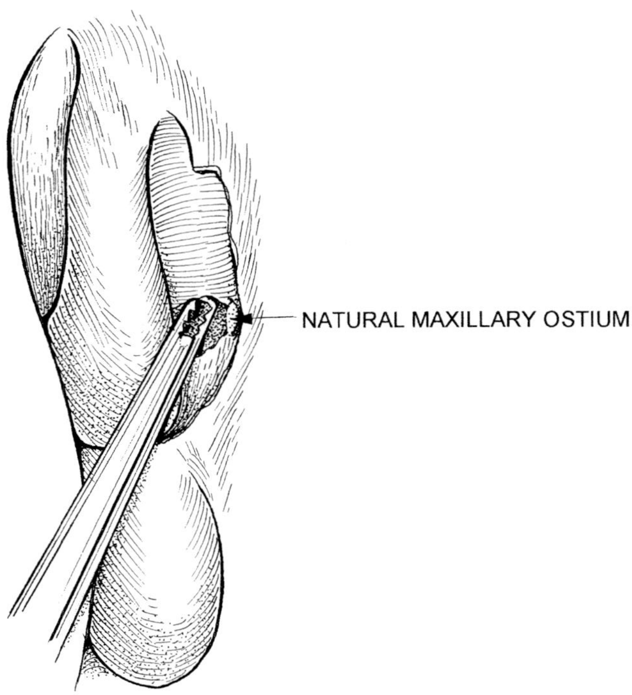


**FIGURE 24.7.** Opening into the bulla ethmoidalis with the microdebrider. Care is taken to maintain stability of the middle turbinate.

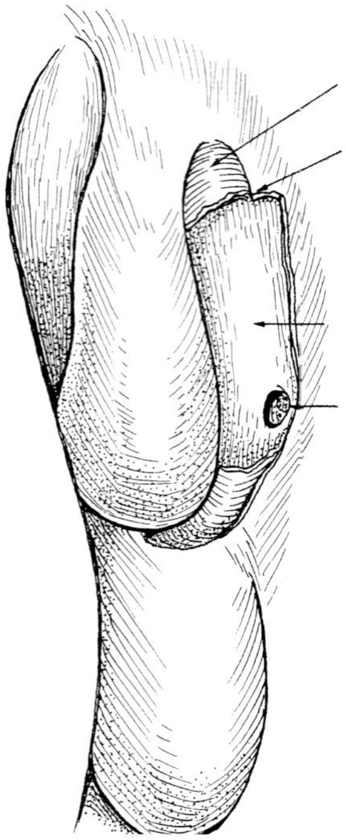


**FIGURE 24.8.** Completed anterior ethmoidectomy.

cavity. This helps to maintain the surgical orientation and avoids penetration of the skull base or the orbital cavity. If the sphenoid sinus is diseased and requires surgical ventilation, the dissection is carried medially to identify the superior turbinate. The superior turbinate is an excellent landmark and usually is present even in revision cases. This requires that the posterior portion of the middle turbinate be fenestrated for access. If care is taken with the middle turbinate and an adequate amount of the inferior basal lamella is left intact, the middle turbinate will remain stable. The sphenoethmoidal recess is then readily accessible, and the sphenoid ostium can be identified (21). This may require minimal resection of the inferior portion of the superior turbinate. In patients with profuse sinonasal inflammatory disease, visualization may not be possible, and gentle probing with a blunt instrument, such as a J-curette, is helpful. The probing should start low, and after the sinus is identified, the J-curette can be used to gently dilate the sphenoid ostium. Keeping in mind the parasphenoidal structures and using direct endoscopic visualization, the face of the sphenoid may be gently outfractured and removed. After the sphenoidotomy, the skull base is readily apparent and dissection can be carried anteriorly, gently curetting and removing the bony lamella of the ethmoidal cells. The microdebrider is helpful in precise removal of obstructive soft tissue. The dissection should not extend into the frontal recess. The sinonasal cavity can then be

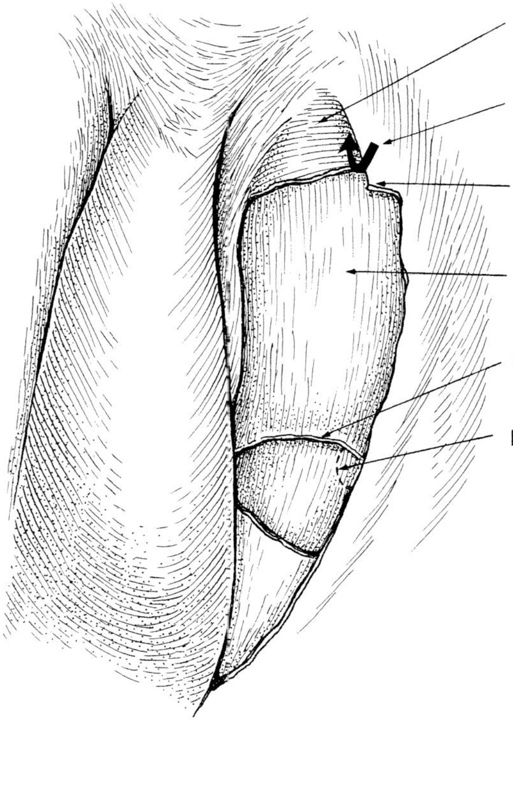


**FIGURE 24.9.** Completed anterior ethmoidectomy and maxillary antrostomy. Notice the inclusion of the natural maxillary sinus ostium.

gently irrigated with saline, and the entire dissection site should be inspected for evidence of intracranial or orbital injury. The position and stability of the middle turbinate is assessed as well. If necessary, rolled Gelfilm may be placed in the middle meatus to maintain middle turbinate position. Packing is rarely required.

## POSTOPERATIVE CARE

Most children are resistant to postoperative manipulation of the nose. If possible, nasal saline misting is instituted to facilitate crust resolution, which is thought to help with postoperative healing and prevention of scar formation. Postoperative antibiotics are prescribed for 10 days, and nasal steroid sprays are restarted on postoperative day 2 or 3.

There is some controversy regarding a second-look procedure. We make a decision regarding the necessity of a second-look procedure on a case-by-case basis. When there is some concern about the position of the middle turbinate and Gelfilm is placed, a second look at 2 weeks postoperatively is helpful to remove the Gelfilm and remove any associated crusts or debris. In patients who undergo a very limited procedure, a second look is unnecessary. We think meticulous attention to surgical technique, minimizing unnecessary trauma and mucosal injury to adjacent structures, is probably the most important determinant in postoperative healing. A retrospective review of 100 pediatric patients without systemic disease who underwent endoscopic sinus surgery was carried out. The review revealed no difference in the postoperative result between the 50 patients who underwent second look and 50 patients who did not (22). However, patients with associated systemic disease, including cystic fibrosis, immotile cilia syndrome, and immunoglobulin deficiency and those undergoing revision surgery should strongly be considered for a second-look operation.

## COMPLICATIONS

The prevention and management of orbital, intracranial, and olfactory complications associated with endoscopic sinus surgery are outlined fully elsewhere in this textbook, but a few caveats are appropriate here. Given that most pediatric sinus surgery is limited in scope, complications are unusual. However, all complications reported in the adult population may occur in the pediatric population. As with all surgery, thoughtful preoperative evaluation, an intimate knowledge of the anatomy and its potential variations, meticulous attention to detail, and maximizing hemostasis all facilitate a thorough, safe procedure. Intraoperatively, the surgeon should be constantly vigilant of his or her position within the sinonasal cavity and the dissection's relationship to the patient's skull base and orbit. If hemostasis becomes a problem during a procedure, especially if there is compromised visualization, the procedure should be aborted.

## REFERENCES


1. Wald ER. Chronic sinusitis in children. *J Pediatr* 1995;127:339–347.
2. Wald ER, Guerra N, Byers C. Upper respiratory tract infections in young children: duration of and frequency of complications. *Pediatrics* 1991;87:129–133.
3. Otten FW, Van Aarem A, Grote JJ. Long-term follow-up of chronic maxillary sinusitis in children. *Int J Pediatr Otorhinolaryngol* 1991;22:81–84.
4. Gross CW, Gurucharri MJ, Lazar RH, et al. Functional endonasal sinus surgery (FESS) in the pediatric age group. *Laryngoscope* 1989;99:272–275.
5. Poole MD. Pediatric sinusitis is not a surgical disease. *Ear Nose Throat J* 1992;71:622–623.
6. Muntz HR, Lusk RP. Surgical management of chronic sinusitis. In: Lusk HR, ed. *Pediatric sinusitis.* New York: Raven Press, 1992:77–125.
7. Lazar RH, Younis RT, Gross CW. Pediatric functional endonasal sinus surgery: review of 210 cases. *Head Neck* 1992;14:92–98.
8. Manning SC, Wasserman RL, Silver R, et al. Results of endoscopic sinus surgery in pediatric patients with chronic sinusitis and asthma. *Arch Otolaryngol Head Neck Surg* 1994;120:1142–1145.
9. Lusk RL, Stankiewicz JA. Pediatric rhinosinusitis. *Otolaryngol Head Neck Surg* 1997;117:S53–S57.
10. Mair EA, Bolger WE, Breisch EA. Sinus and facial growth after pediatric endoscopic sinus surgery. *Arch Otolaryngol Head Neck Surg* 1995;121:547–552.
11. Wolf G, Anderhuber W, Kuhn F. Development of the paranasal sinuses in children: implications for paranasal sinus surgery. *Ann Otol Rhinol Laryngol* 1993;102:705–711.
12. Wald ER. Epidemiology, pathophysiology and etiology of sinusitis. *Pediatr Infect Dis J* 1985;4:S61.
13. McAlister WH, Lusk RP, Muntz HR. Comparison of plain film radiographs and coronal CT scans in infants and children with recurrent sinusitis. *AJR Am J Roentgenol* 1989;153:1259.
14. Zacharisen MC, Kelly KJ. Allergic and infectious pediatric sinusitis. *Pediatr Ann* 1998;27:759–766.
15. Kay NJ, Setia RN, Stone J. Relevance of conventional radiography in indicating maxillary antral lavage. *Ann Otol Rhinol Laryngol* 1984;93:37–38.
16. Lusk RP. Surgical modalities other than ethmoidectomy. *Allergy Clin Immunol* 1992;90:538–542.
17. Maes JJ. The usefulness of irrigation of the maxillary sinus in children with maxillary sinusitis on the basis of the Water's x-ray. *Rhinology* 1987;25:259–264.
18. Lund VJ. Inferior meatal antrostomy: fundamental considerations of design and function. *J Laryngol Otol Suppl* 1988;15:1.
19. Setliff RC, Parsons DS. The "Hummer": new instrumentation for functional endoscopic sinus surgery. *Am J Rhinol* 1994;8:275–278.
20. Becker DG. Technical considerations in powered instrumentation. *Otolaryngol Clin North Am* 1997;30:421–434.
21. Bolger WE, Keyes AS, Lanza DC. Use of the superior meatus and superior turbinate in the endoscopic approach to the sphenoid sinus. *Otolaryngol Head Neck Surg* 1999;120:308–313.
22. Mitchell RB, Pereira KD, Younis RT, et al. Pediatric functional endoscopic sinus surgery: is a second look necessary? *Laryngoscope* 1997;107:1267–1269.

# 25

# REVISION PARANASAL SINUS SURGERY

**HOWARD L. LEVINE**

## INDICATIONS

Revision endoscopic sinus surgery (RESS) is considered for all patients who have undergone sinus surgery and continue to have symptoms despite adequate medical management. The type of medical management depends on the cause, pathologic findings, and symptoms. If allergic or vasomotor rhinitis is present, it is managed with nasal steroid sprays, nasal anticholinergic sprays, antihistamines (with or without decongestants), or desensitization. If infection is present, an endoscopically guided culture sample is obtained and drug sensitivities determined, and based on the results, an appropriate antibiotic chosen. The antibiotic is frequently continued for 3 to 6 weeks. If sinus or nasal polyposis is present, nasal topical, systemic steroids, or both agents are used to reduce the polyposis.

There are several reasons for failure of the primary endoscopic sinus surgery (ESS). Understanding the clinical reasons for and categories of failure and need for revision allows the rhinologist to tailor the treatment to specific causes. The patient with sinus or nasal polyps may have a systemic cause, and despite the best nasal surgical treatment, cure is not possible. It is not always obvious why nasal and sinus polyposis recurs. Some systemic causes include asthma, aspirin sensitivity, and nasal polyposis (i.e., triad asthma, also known as Samter's triad) or cystic fibrosis. Failure in the removal of nasal polyps may result from inability to surgically access the sinus or identify all of the sinuses. This may occur if there are retained ethmoid sinus air cells or polyps in the frontal or sphenoid sinus.

A missed accessory maxillary ostium can lead to recurrent or subacute maxillary sinusitis. Mucus flows out from the natural ostium and enters the infundibulum of the osteomeatal complex and then flows back into the maxillary sinus through the accessory ostium. This leads to retained secretions in the sinus, stasis, and secondary infection.

After endoscopic maxillary antrostomy, the maxillary sinus ostium may scar and contract. This response leads to retained secretions and secondary infection.

Retained infection may occur in any of the sinuses that are not opened surgically because of inaccessibility, improper identification, or postoperative obstruction of the sinuses. This occurs most often in retained ethmoid sinus air cells at the fovea ethmoidalis and the frontal or sphenoid sinuses. When well pneumatized, a lateral extension of the frontal or sphenoid sinus also predisposes to infection.

Adhesions can occur between the middle turbinate and the lateral nasal wall even with the most careful of surgical procedures. These are often asymptomatic but occasionally may obstruct the outflow from the sinus into the nose. Stasis of secretions behind adhesions can lead to infection in the nasal and sinus cavities.

Even the best of operations sometimes fail, and revision is needed. There are numerous reports of successes, ranging from 76% to 98% for primary ESS (1–4). May found that 11% of his 609 patients required revision surgery (5). I found that 15% of his patients (160 of 1,100) required revision surgery (5).

It is not clear whether previous sinus surgery alters the outcome for revision surgery. Matthews and colleagues found that prior sinus surgery had no predictive value for the success of a revision sinus procedure (6). Kennedy determined that prior ethmoid sinus surgery adversely affected the outcome but demonstrated no significant prognostic value when adjusted for extent of disease (1). It seems reasonable to think that, by preserving the ciliated mucous membrane, turbinate function of warming and humidifying, and normal nasal airflow, nasal and sinus function will be improved. Previous surgery that has been destructive alters this function, and revision surgery will never restore the nose and sinus to its previous role.

Although a few articles discuss the results of RESS, there is little in the literature discussing technique.

## CONTRAINDICATIONS

There are no specific sinus or nasal contraindications to RESS other than the general medical contraindications to surgery. Associated medical problems such as severe cardiovascular disease, severe pulmonary disease (e.g., asthma out of control, bronchiectasis, respiratory failure), and uncontrolled diabetes are relative contraindications to RESS in an ambulatory surgery center. However, each patient's general medical condition must be assessed and a determination made about the type of facility and type of anesthetic for the particular operation to be performed.

## PREOPERATIVE EVALUATION

As with any patient undergoing ESS, RESS requires preoperative testing to ensure that the patient is fit for safe surgery. The type of preoperative evaluation varies with the institution, ambulatory surgery center, and anesthesiologist. A coronal computed tomographic (CT) scan of the sinuses is obtained. Occasionally, there is value in reviewing the CT scans from the previous operations and compare them with the new scan. This helps in understanding the fluctuating nature of disease, especially for the patient with recurrent acute and subacute rhinosinusitis. An axial scan provides additional valuable data if there is frontal or sphenoid sinus disease. It helps define the anterior-posterior dimension of the frontal sinus to localize the posterior wall. It provides a view of the depth and configuration of the sphenoid sinus; its lateral, posterior, and superior walls; and the location of the optic nerves and internal carotid arteries. For patients undergoing image-guided surgery, a helical CT scan is obtained that is used with the InstaTrak VTI (Visualization Technology, Inc., Woburn, MA) navigational sinus surgical system. Based on the patient's history, allergy testing, pulmonary function testing, and immunologic testing looking for immune deficiency states are obtained.

## CASE EXAMPLES

A 16-year-old boy presented with right facial and eye pressure. He had had three previous ESS procedures, but his symptoms persisted. A coronal CT scan of the sinuses revealed a high nasal septal deviation to the right and opacified agger nasal air cells and frontal sinus on the right. His senses of taste and smell were good. His symptoms had been managed with mucolytics, antibiotics, and decongestants on numerous occasions but failed. His health was good other than severe asthma and allergies. His nasal endoscopic examination revealed an extremely narrow nasal cavity with a markedly narrow frontal recess. The nasal septum was deviated high on the right, and scar tissue was present between the nasal septum and lateral nasal wall in this area obstructing the outflow from the anterior ethmoid and frontal sinuses.

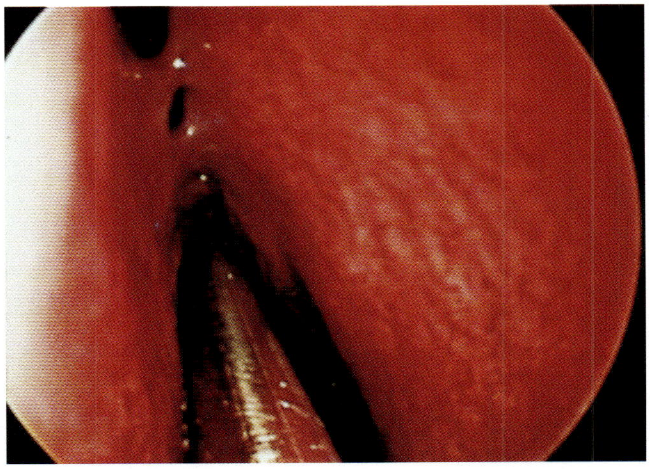

**FIGURE 25.1.** Endoscopic view of the right nasal cavity with synechia between the nasal septum and lateral nasal wall.

Because of the narrow frontal recess and multiple previous operations, an image-guided triplanar localization approach was used. The synechia between the nasal septum and lateral nasal wall was removed (Fig. 25.1). A section of the superior nasal septum was removed to gain access into the frontal recess during surgery and for postoperative management. Using triplanar localization, the agger nasi air cells were removed and the frontal sinus opened (Fig. 25.2). The thick mucoid secretion found in the frontal sinus was suctioned from it. Postoperatively, the patient did well and was discharged from the ambulatory surgery unit on the day of surgery. Two months after surgery, he was free of symptoms, and the frontal recess remained open based on results of the endoscopic examination.

## INSTRUMENTATION

Although traditional ESS instruments are used for RESS, additional technology is used to minimize the complications, make the surgery technically easier, and improve the results. Powered surgical instrumentation helps remove diseased soft tissue, bone, and scar while preserving much of the normal mucosa. Various straight and angled blades and burrs (e.g., 0°, RAD 40°, RAD 60° blades, 55° burr) (Xomed Surgical Products, Inc., Jacksonville, FL) are used to gain access to the various spaces and recesses of all of the sinuses. Several different blades of varying aggressiveness are available. Powered instrumentation can be used in a con-

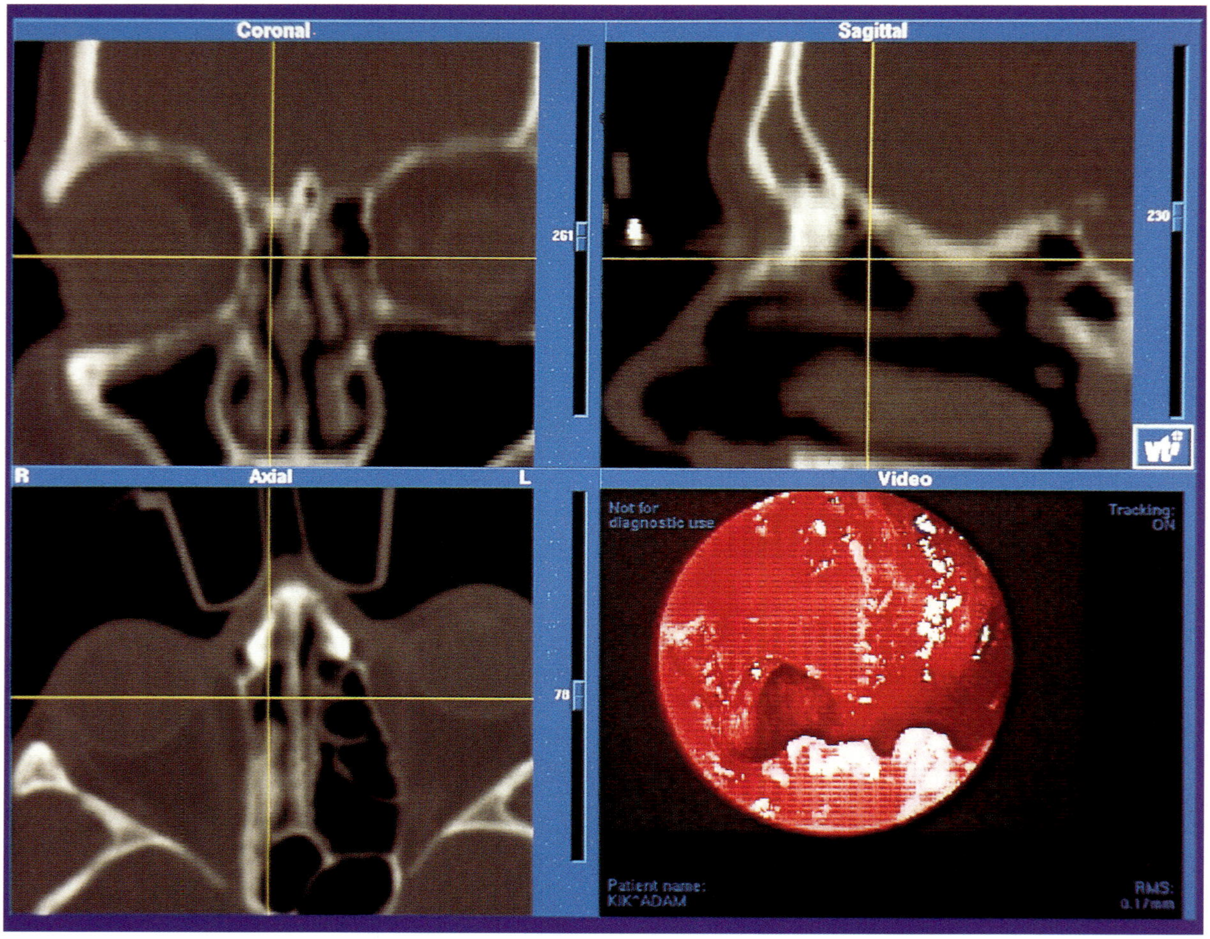


**FIGURE 25.2.** Triplanar view of the opacified frontal sinus and surgically created opening into the right frontal sinus.

tinuous mode at 6,000 rpm for bony work or oscillating mode 1,500 rpm for soft tissue. The slower speed allows the suction portion of the powered instrument to draw soft tissue into the blade. Microendoscopic sinus instruments and through-cutting forceps allow for precision bony and soft tissue removal without undo trauma to the adjacent tissue.

Revision surgery is often associated with nasal and sinus cavities that are devoid of landmarks, such as the middle and superior turbinates, uncinate, and basal lamella. Image-guided surgery with InstaTrak VTI using straight, 45°, 60°, and microshaver couplers allow for triplanar localization of nasal and paranasal sinus anatomy and persistent pathology.

## OPERATING ROOM LAYOUT

The operating room is organized in a way VTI to that for traditional ESS procedures. The surgeon stands to the side of the patient. The scrub nurse (i.e., operating room technician) is positioned opposite the surgeon. The Mayo stand with the most frequently used instruments is at the head of the operating table, and the video cart is just behind this. The image-guided (VTI) equipment is positioned next to the video cart. The CT scan is readily visible to the surgeon throughout the procedure.

## ANESTHESIA

General anesthesia is used for nearly every RESS. Most patients, having had previous sinus surgery, have moderate to significant scar tissue. This makes it difficult or impossible to obtain good local and topical anesthesia. Scar tissue frequently prevents the flow or absorption of injectable topical anesthesia. The use of image-guided triplanar technology necessitates lack of movement by the patient that can disrupt the positioning and calibration of the patient's headset. General anesthesia with intubation protects the airway from aspiration of blood. This is often a greater problem in RESS because of increased bleeding from scar tissue and the potential of bronchospasm in the patient with reactive airway disease. Patients with asthma frequently require revision surgery because the systemic disease has caused recurrent sinus disease.

Intubation is generally accomplished with an ultrashort-acting barbiturate (usually thiopental) or propofol. A muscle relaxant facilitates intubation. Succinylcholine often is used, but an intermediate-acting, nondepolarizing muscle relaxant (i.e., atracurium, cisatracurium, mivacurium, rocuronium, or vecuronium) can be used. A small dose of glycopyrrolate (0.005 mg/kg up to 0.2 mg) is given before induction to prevent excessive salivary secretion. The anesthetic maintenance is accomplished with small, intermittent doses of a narcotic (i.e., fentanyl or alfentanil) or a continuous drip infusion of propofol. Any of the major inhalation anesthetics agents (i.e., halothane, enflurane, isoflurane, sevoflurane, and desflurane) are used. Emergence and extubation is monitored carefully, because excessive coughing before extubation can cause increased bleeding.

There are no data to correlate increased intraoperative bleeding with increased blood pressure, but this has been observed on numerous occasions. Attempts are made to keep the intraoperative blood pressure at 80% of the normal pressure.

## OPERATIVE TECHNIQUE

The 0°, 4-mm endoscope is used to visualize the nasal and sinus cavity. A complete nasal endoscopic examination is performed to orient the surgeon to the specific idiosyncrasies of the particular nasal or sinus cavity and to visualize the pathology. Landmarks that remain from previous operations are identified. If the middle turbinate is present, it is medialized. Any remaining ethmoid sinus air cells are removed, identifying and preserving the lamina papyracea and fovea ethmoidalis.

The front face of the sphenoid sinus is identified by one of several techniques. The choana of the nasal cavity is on the same vertical plane as the front face of the sphenoid sinus. The choana can be followed to its superior margin, and the bony wall superior to it that represents the front face of the sphenoid sinus is identified. The sphenoid sinus is entered medially and inferiorly, and the front face is opened. Another technique to identify the sphenoid sinus is used when the posterior attachment of the middle turbinate is present. The attachment is at the front face of the sphenoid sinus. The middle turbinate or its remnant is medialized and the bony wall opened medially and inferiorly to enter the sphenoid sinus. A third method of identifying the sphenoid sinus is to find the natural ostium of the sinus and enlarge it inferiorly. Each method of entering the sphenoid sinus mandates that the sinus be opened inferiorly and medially away from the optic nerve, internal carotid artery, and superior wall.

Any remnant of uncinate process is removed to be certain that the infundibulum is wide open and that there is no obstruction to anterior ethmoid, maxillary, or frontal sinus drainage.

When frontal sinus disease is present in a previously operated patient, image-guided triplanar VTI localization is used. Any retained agger nasi air cells are opened using the 30° or 70° endoscope, the RAD 40 or RAD 60 microshaver blade, and if extensive scar or bone is present, the 55° microshaver burr. The frontal sinus is opened, inspected, and irrigated.

## SPECIAL POINTS

Many patients having RESS experience greater intraoperative and postoperative bleeding, probably because of scar tissue that prevents blood vessel constriction. For this reason, Oxycel (i.e., oxidized cellulose) (Becton Dickinson and Company, Franklin Lakes, NJ) is inserted into the nasal and sinus cavity. Small strips of the Oxycel are lightly rolled in mupirocin ointment (Bactroban, Smith, Kline, Beecham Pharmaceuticals, Philadelphia, PA) and layered into the nasal and sinus cavities. This provides a light dressing, aids hemostasis, and minimizes postoperative bleeding. Especially for the asthmatic patient, this reduces the postoperative nasal drainage and seems to reduce bronchospasm.

A small piece of Telfa covered in mupirocin ointment is inserted into the nose and left in place for about 1 hour. It is removed before discharging the patient from the ambulatory surgery center.

## POSTOPERATIVE CARE

Postoperative care is similar to the care provided for any patient undergoing ESS. Patients are discharged on the same day and sent home with 2 × 2 gauze nasal dressings, 0.5-inch nonallergic tape, and saline nasal spray. The nasal dressing is worn only if there is nasal drainage. The saline nasal spray is used four to five times each day beginning on the first postoperative day. This helps to moisturize the nose, thin any blood and mucus, and liquefy the Oxycel. Patients are instructed not to blow the nose until after their first postoperative visit. They are seen at about 5 or 6 days after their RESS.

At the first postoperative visit, the nose is topically anesthetized and examined endoscopically. Any mucus, old blood, loose eschar, or partially dissolved Oxycel is removed with suction and microforceps. Patients are allowed to gently blow the nose and return to all activity, and they are continued on the saline nasal spray. If excessive mucus, blood, eschar, or dressings are still present; the patient is seen 1 week later for a second endoscopic débridement. If minimal material is found, the patient is seen in 2 to 4 weeks. For patients who had extensive polyposis, a nasal steroid spray is started after the sinus and nasal mucous membranes are reasonably well healed.

## COMPLICATIONS

The types of potential complications after RESS are the same as those for ESS. Distortion or absence of landmarks could lead to an increase rate of complications for RESS patients. Image-guided surgery with triplanar localization and surgical experience should minimize the chances of complication.

Minor complications include periorbital emphysema, periorbital ecchymosis, dental or lip pain or numbness, adhesions, epistaxis, bronchospasm, infection, and anosmia. Major complications include orbital hematoma, loss of vision, diplopia, cerebrospinal fluid leak, meningitis, brain abscess, focal brain hemorrhage, hemorrhage requiring transfusion, carotid artery injury, epiphora requiring dacryocystorhinostomy, and death. All of the complications occurring from RESS are managed the same as those from ESS.

## ADVANTAGES AND LIMITATIONS OF ENDOSCOPIC TECHNIQUE

Revision sinus surgery done endoscopically has several advantages over conventional sinus surgery. CT scanning and nasal endoscopy can localize the sinus disease and often identify the cause. This allows the surgeon to correct the residual disease and its cause. Endoscopic approaches allow for direct visualization of the disease and permit correction of the disease alone without disruption of other nasal and sinus function. Because previous surgery has often removed some of the normal structures (e.g., turbinates, nasal or sinus mucosa), RESS should attempt to preserve as much of the remaining function as possible.

Use of various angled endoscopes, microendoscopic sinus instruments, and image-guided technology permits accurate, safe, and thorough management of sinus disease involving all of the sinuses. Healing is faster. Morbidity is lower. Return to work, school, family, and social activities occurs sooner.

## LITERATURE REVIEW

RESS fails in 9% to 59% of cases (2,3,7–10). In a review of RESS, King and colleagues (2) attempted to evaluate the reasons that ESS might fail. They examined typical features of sinusitis that are usually refractory to medical or surgical management, such as the presence of nasal polyps, asthma, systemic steroid use, and various types of prior surgery. Of their 295 patients undergoing ESS, 43 (14.6%) underwent RESS. Of these 43, 33 (76.7%) had prior traditional sinus surgery, and 10 (23.3%) had previous FESS. Most patients requiring RESS were women presenting with facial pain, purulent rhinorrhea, and nasal obstruction. Most patients who failed ESS had a history of oral steroid use, asthma, and prior nonendoscopic sinus surgery. Patients with aspergillosis sinusitis were more likely to fail RESS.

In another review of RESS, Moses and coworkers (11) evaluated 90 patients (36 men, 54 women) undergoing RESS from a group of 753 consecutive primary FESS patients. Twenty (22%) RESS patients had undergone previous conventional sinus surgery, 17 (19%) had undergone conventional sinus surgery and ESS, and 53 (59%) were managed by ESS alone. Among the RESS patients, 51 (57%) had deviated nasal septum, 50 (55%) had polyposis, 37 (41%) had frontal sinus disease, 35 (39%) were asthmatics, 33 (37%) had allergy, 16 (18%) were systemic steroid users, 7 (8%) had Samter's triad, and 3 (3%) had *Aspergillus* sinusitis. They found that some factors were statistically significant. A history of previous traditional sinus surgery and the presence of nasal polyps were associated with less favorable RESS results. Male gender and allergy were associated with less favorable RESS outcomes, but these factors were not statistically significant. Asthma was prevalent among RESS patients but did not affect outcome.

## REFERENCES

1. Kennedy DW. Prognostic factors, outcomes, and staging in ethmoid sinus surgery. *Laryngoscope* 1992;102[Suppl 57]:1–18.
2. King JM, Calderelli DD, Pigato JB. A review of revision functional endoscopic sinus surgery. *Laryngoscope* 1994;104:404–408.
3. Schaitken B, May M, Shapiro A, et al. Endoscopic sinus surgery: 4-year follow-up on the first 100 patients. *Laryngoscope* 1993; 103:1117–1120.
4. Levine HL. Functional endoscopic sinus surgery: evaluation, surgery, and follow-up of 250 patients. *Laryngoscope* 1990;100: 79–84.
5. May M, Levine HL, Schaitken B, Mester SJ. Results of surgery. In: Levine HL, May M, eds. *Endoscopic sinus surgery.* New York: Thieme Medical Publishers, 1993:176–192.
6. Matthews BL, Smith LE, Jones R, et al. Endoscopic sinus surgery: outcome in 155 cases. *Otolaryngol Head Neck Surg* 1991; 104:244–246.
7. Eichel BS. Revision sphenoethmoidectomy. *Laryngoscope* 1985; 95:300–304.
8. Wigand ME, Hosemann WG. Endoscopic surgery for frontal sinusitis and its complications. *Am J Rhinol* 1991;5:85–89.
9. Lazar RH, Younis RT, Long TE, et al. Revision functional endonasal sinus surgery, *Ear Nose Throat J* 1992;71:131–133.
10. Ng M, Rice DH. Revision sinus surgery. *Ear Nose Throat J* 1994; 73:44–46.
11. Moses RL, Cornetta A, Atkins JP, et al. Revision endoscopic sinus surgery: the Thomas Jefferson experience. *Ear Nose Throat J* 1998;77:190–202.

# 26

# ENDOSCOPIC APPROACH TO BENIGN TUMORS OF THE PARANASAL SINUSES

**BRENT A. SENIOR**

The past 15 years have brought a revolution in the surgical management of inflammatory paranasal sinus disease. With greatly increased understanding of sinus anatomy and physiology, combined with excellent visualization and minimal morbidity, sinus surgery using Hopkins rod endoscopes has been a significant advance for otolaryngologists in terms of excellence of surgical outcome as well as safety. Although Mosher's (1) admonition in 1929 that surgery of the ethmoid "should be easy, but has proved the easiest way to kill a patient," remains pertinent today, use of the endoscope has minimized this risk such that intranasal procedures using the endoscope are commonplace and safe.

Exponentially increasing since these techniques were introduced in the United States in 1985 (2), it is only natural to see endoscopic approaches extended to applications other than treatment of inflammatory sinus disease. This chapter focuses on our experience with management of benign tumors of the paranasal sinuses, including tumors with intracranial and orbital extension, using endoscopic techniques evolving from our experience with management of inflammatory disease. Numerous other tumor types have been reported in the literature to be successfully managed endoscopically, including juvenile nasopharyngeal angiofibroma, cholesterol granulomas, plasmacytomas, and triton cell tumors (2). In this chapter, we focus on the more common tumors, including mucoceles, inverted papillomas, fibro-osseus lesions, and pituitary adenomas. In certain exceptional situations, endoscopic approaches may be considered for malignant lesions, but craniofacial resection remains the standard approach in nearly all situations and is not discussed in this chapter.

## INVERTED PAPILLOMA

One of the most common tumors involving the paranasal sinuses is the inverting papilloma, also called villiform cancer, Schneiderian papilloma, Ewing's papilloma, transitional cell papilloma, and papillary sinusitis. Noted for its propensity for recurrence and aggressive growth, these tumors were first described by Ward in 1854 (3). The approximate 10% risk of concomitant malignancy is also well known. Traditional approaches to removal originally involved simple polypectomy, but very high rates of recurrence showed this to be ineffective. As a result of this, lateral rhinotomy or midface degloving with en bloc resection of the medial maxilla became the procedure of choice. In 1900, Phillips and coworkers emphasized this point by comparing 112 cases of inverted papilloma treated between 1944 and 1987 (4). Recurrences were reported for lateral rhinotomy with medial maxillectomy (14%), transnasal with sinus exenteration (35%), and transnasal alone (58%). Others have reported similar low rates of recurrence when managed with medial maxillectomy (approximately 7%).

In 1992, Waitz and Wigand performed the first large assessment of the usefulness of endoscopic techniques for the removal of inverting papillomas (5). Comparing endoscopic with extranasal, open approaches, they found a 17% (6 of 35) recurrence rate for the endoscopically treated group versus a 19% (3 of 16) recurrence rate for the extranasally treated group. There was, however, a difference in severity of disease between the two groups. Specifically, the endoscopically treated group was made up of 77% with T2 or T3 lesions, 4% had T4 lesions, and the remainder had T1 lesions. Conversely, the extranasally treated group tumors were larger; 44% were T3 and T4 lesions, with no T1 and the remainder T2. Despite this difference, the investigators successfully emphasized the usefulness of the endoscopic approach with its concordant reduced morbidity in the properly selected patient.

Others, including Dolgin and colleagues in 1992 (6), have also supported a graded approach to management of these tumors. In two papers, Lawson and coworkers (7,8) compared conservative techniques for tumors limited to the inferior turbinate or middle turbinate with limited extension into the ethmoid sinuses or maxillary antrum to more radical en bloc resection for more extensive tumors, including involvement of the supraorbital air cells, perilacrimal cells, frontal sinus, or cribriform plate. With an average follow-up of 6 years, recurrence in the limited procedures group was 20% compared with 13.8% in the en bloc resection group.

In 1993, Stankiewicz and Girgis (9) retrospectively analyzed 15 patients treated with endoscopic approaches, including five recurrent tumors after previous medial maxillectomy. Three of 10 tumors recurred after primary endoscopic management. Three of five of the patients who had undergone previous medial maxillectomy were successfully managed with endoscopic approaches, emphasizing the utility of the endoscopic approach even in the setting of recurrent disease.

## MUCOCELES

First described by Langenbeck in 1818 (10), mucoceles are epithelial cell–lined, mucus-filled cysts occurring most commonly in the frontoethmoid region, followed by the sphenoid and maxillary sinuses. Frequently occurring after trauma (including after previous sinus surgery) or in the setting of chronic sinus disease, the origin of these cysts involves sinus obstruction with gradual buildup of mucus until the bony limits of the cavity are reached. With continuous slow growth, expansion and erosion of the surrounding bony walls frequently occur, yielding dehiscences in critical areas such as the lamina papyracea with orbital extension and the fovea ethmoidalis or posterior table of the frontal sinus with intracranial extension (Fig. 26.1). Intraorbital extension may lead to the dramatic findings of proptosis and diplopia, whereas intracranial extension may yield temporary or permanent cranial nerve deficits, including blindness. Infection of a mucocele may require emergent need for surgery because of the propensity of such infections to spread to adjacent structures. Intraorbital spread may occur, as well as intracranial spread through the foramina of Breschet; spread through the face of the frontal sinus results in a Pott's puffy tumor. Traditional approaches to treatment have depended on the location of the involved sinus: frontal involvement resulted in a Lynch procedure or an osteoplastic flap with sinus obliteration; ethmoid involvement mandated an external, transnasal, or transantral ethmoidectomy; maxillary involvement called for a Caldwell-Luc procedure; and sphenoid involvement was addressed with a transnasal or transseptal sphenoidotomy.

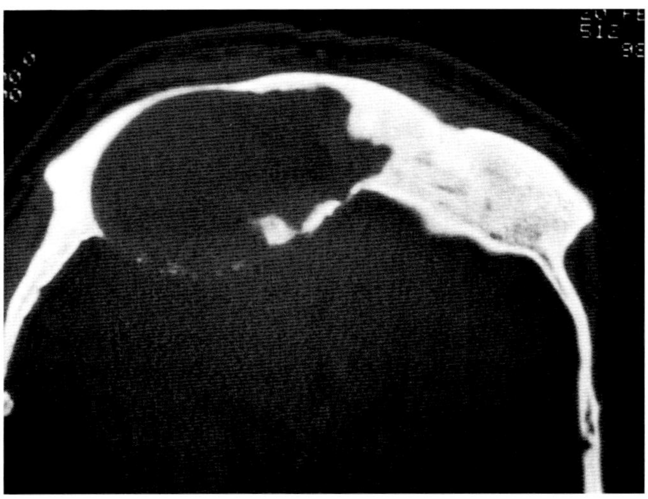

**FIGURE 26.1.** Bone-windowed, axial computed tomography image through the frontal sinuses shows a homogeneous lesion occupying the left side and erosion of the posterior table.

However, since the description in 1989 by Kennedy and colleagues of the successful use of the endoscopic approach for the management of mucoceles (11), including those with intracranial and intraorbital extension, endoscopic approaches have been widely used for management of these lesions. In that initial paper, the investigators reported that 16 of 18 patients were successfully approached endoscopically, and two required open approaches. Of the 16 treated endoscopically, at an average follow-up of nearly 18 months, no recurrences or complications were identified. Since then, many others have reported similar, excellent outcomes. Benninger and Marks (12), reviewing 15 ethmoid and sphenoid mucoceles treated endoscopically (11 with intracranial or intraorbital involvement) reported only two recurrences. Both were ultimately successfully treated with an endoscopic approach. Similarly, Moriyama and colleagues (13) reviewed 25 patients with sphenoid and ethmoid mucoceles and visual disturbances, including 20 who had been previously managed with nonendoscopic approaches, who were successfully managed endoscopically. Hartley and Lund (14) published their results using endoscopic techniques in the management of mucoceles in children. Seven children with mucoceles involving the anterior ethmoid (5), posterior ethmoid (1), and sphenoid (1) were reviewed, including those with orbital involvement. With a minimum of 1-year follow-up, no recurrences have been identified.

## BONY AND FIBRO-OSSEUS TUMORS

Bony and fibro-osseus tumors comprise primarily osteomas and include fibrous dysplasia, nonossifying and ossifying fibromas, and osteoblastoma. The tumors are typically characterized by asymptomatic, slow, progressive growth over many years. Two large series reported that facial pain was the most common presenting symptom for these types of tumors (15,16). Morbidity is most commonly related to obstruction of affected sinuses with infection, mucocele, or mucopyocele, particularly in the frontoethmoid region, where a preponderance of these tumors occur. With time, these tumors may grow to cause facial deformity and, with direct compression and involvement of the adjacent orbit, proptosis, diplopia, or visual loss. Pneumocephalus, first reported by Dandy in 1925, may be a presenting feature when these bony tumors involve the skull base and extend intracranially (17). Here, tiny microfissures at the edge of the skull base defect allow for passage of air at high pressure (e.g., a sneeze) to pass intracranially with resultant morbidity such as a seizure and change in mental status.

The traditional approach to tumors of this type has varied significantly, depending on the exact location, ranging from the Lynch procedure or transantral procedures to frontal sinusotomy through osteoplastic flap to frontal craniotomy. Despite successful application of endoscopic techniques to other tumors of the paranasal sinuses, application to bony tumors has been slow. Reasons for this include distortion of sinus anatomy in the presence of these tumors, the frequency with which these tumors involve the skull base or the posterior table of the frontal sinus (thereby resulting in large skull base defects after resection), and limitations in instrumentation limiting removal of a large, bony mass transnasally.

In the past several years, many of these problems have begun to be overcome. Techniques have improved, and surgeons have become quite proficient with endoscopic methods to repair large cerebral spinal fluid leaks (CSF) with cranial base defects, yielding excellent efficacy with limited morbidity (18). Similarly, newer powered instrumentation and drills have made it possible to resect and deliver large bony tumors transnasally. Use of intraoperative three-dimensional computed tomography (3D CT) image guidance has been a significant aid for endoscopic resection of tumors of this type, allowing careful endoscopic intraoperative localization in a setting of distorted anatomy (19) (Fig. 26.2).

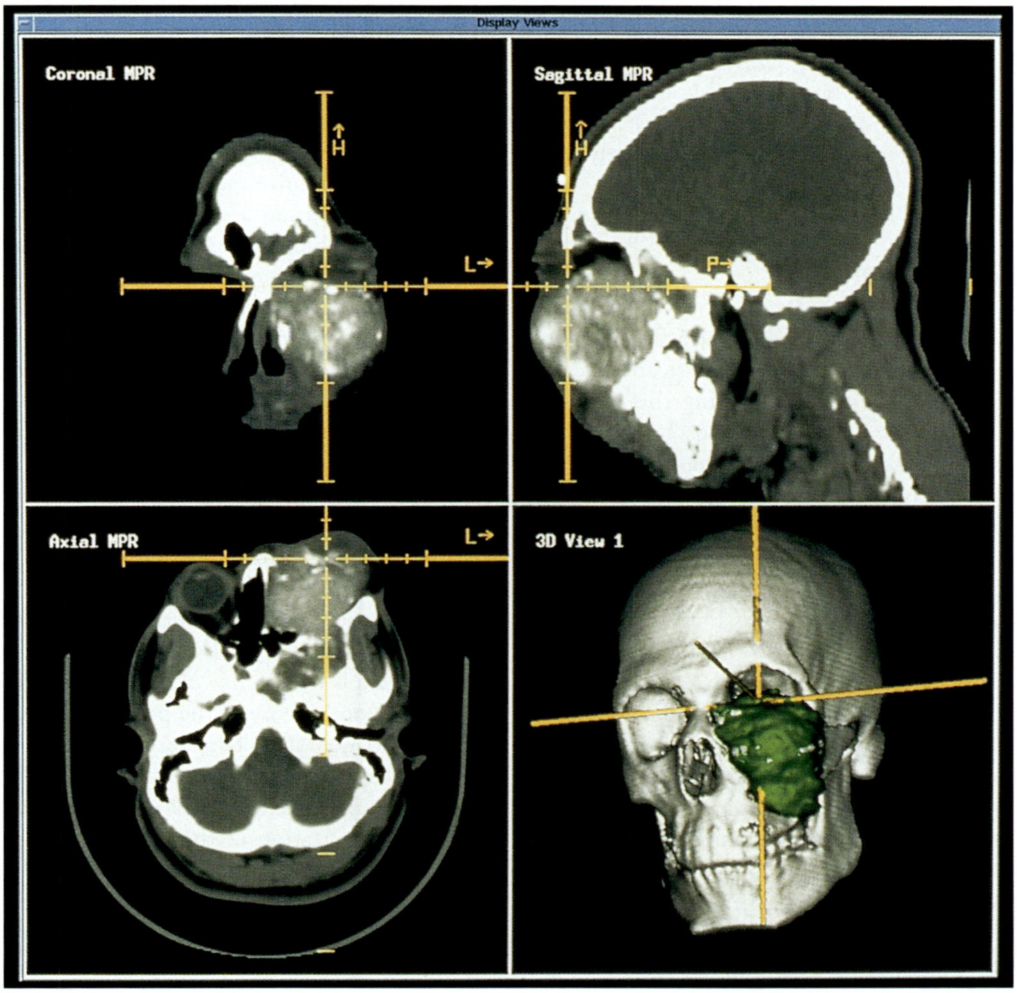


**FIGURE 26.2.** Intraoperative, three-dimensional (3D) computed tomography (CT) image of a large fibrous dysplasia of the left maxilla. The 3D CT was useful in determining normal landmarks in a setting of distorted anatomy and for estimating the depth of resection to create a symmetric postoperative appearance in this combined endoscopic-open procedure.

After solving these problems, investigators began to report during the past 6 years on the utility of endoscopic approaches for management of tumors of this type. In 1994, Menezes and Davidson provided the first report in the English literature with their description of the endoscopic removal of a sphenoethmoid osteoma in a 33-year-old woman (20). At the 1-year follow-up examination, no recurrence was identified. Seiden and Hefny used a combined approach with an endoscope to remove an osteoma involving the frontal sinus through a 3-cm infrabrow trephine incision (21). Kennedy and associates expanded on this work by reporting in 1996 on the application of endoscopic techniques for management of bony tumors with intracranial and intraorbital involvement without need for craniotomy or external incisions (10). Similarly, we have reported on the utility of endoscopic techniques in isolation and combined with open approaches for approaching bony tumors with frontal sinus involvement (22).

Limitations of the endoscopic approach to resection of bony and fibro-osseus tumors, as with inverted papillomas, primarily involve the location of the tumor. Tumors high in the frontal sinus, particularly those involving the posterior table of the frontal sinus, may be inaccessible through the frontal infundibulum alone and are probably best treated with a traditional open approach or a combined open and endoscopic approach.

## INTRACRANIAL TUMORS

Often working in conjunction with the neurosurgeon, the endoscopic surgeon has begun to take a significant role in the resection of intracranial tumors involving the anterior and middle cranial fossae. Although most commonly applied to the resection of pituitary adenomas, endoscopic transnasal approaches have begun to show their usefulness as a diagnostic technique for other intracranial tumors, yielding minimal morbidity.

The transsphenoidal approach to resection of pituitary microadenomas and macroadenomas was first described in 1907 (23), but it fell into disfavor with the high incidence of associated complications. Subsequently, introduction of the operating microscope with its magnification and improved lighting, combined with fluoroscopy in the 1950s renewed interest in the transnasal transsphenoidal approach (24), making it the favored approach today. Until recently, options for performing this kind of procedure involved only open approaches such as the sublabial approach, the external rhinoplasty decorticating approach, or the alotomy approach. Although significant improvement in the overall morbidity compared with frontal or temporal craniotomy has been seen, morbidity related to these transsphenoidal approaches is not insignificant, including numbness over the upper lip and nasal tip, septal perforation, nasal tip collapse, and rarely, septal collapse.

Although initially reported in the 1970s (25), during the past 5 years, many investigators have begun to report on the endoscopic transsphenoidal approach to these tumors. Sethi and coworkers reported the first comprehensive use of the endoscope for management of lesions of the sella turcica in 1995 (26), and they subsequently reported successful application in 100 patients with pituitary neoplasms (27). Although they specifically used an endoscopic transseptal approach, Carrau and Jho (28) and others (29,30) have reported successful application of a transnasal approach, directly accessing the sphenoid sinus through its natural ostium and bypassing the need for septal flaps, thereby eliminating the risk of septal perforation. With increasing acceptance among neurosurgeons of endoscopic approaches to management of intracranial tumors, expansion of these techniques will continue.

## TECHNIQUES: GENERAL PRINCIPLES

Preoperatively, a thorough endoscopic evaluation is necessary to define the anatomy and evaluate the lesion about which there is concern. If infection is present or in the setting of coexistent sinusitis, aggressive treatment is initiated with broad-spectrum antibiotics and possibly also with steroids to minimize the risk of intracranial infection complicating the tumor resection, particularly in cases where intraoperative skull base dehiscence is expected.

Proper imaging is essential when planning endoscopic approaches to tumors of the paranasal sinuses and skull base. CT with a minimum of 3-mm sections in axial and coronal planes helps to delineate tumor and adjacent anatomy; usually, contrast is not required. Magnetic resonance imaging (MRI) is helpful at differentiating tumor mass from adjacent retained secretions, thereby more accurately estimating tumor size and exact location. MRI is necessary in the setting of any dehiscence of the skull base to delineate tumor from possible encephalocele or meningoencephalocele.

Delineation of the vascular anatomy with magnetic resonance angiography (MRA) or arteriography is necessary when there is dehiscence of the lateral sphenoid sinus with opacification because of the possibility of carotid aneurysm or pseudoaneurysm. It is recommended in the setting of large encephaloceles or meningoencephaloceles to exclude the presence of a large vessel in the herniated brain. Preoperative embolization of the tumor may be required in the setting of vascular lesions such as a juvenile nasopharyngeal angiofibroma. Typically, this is performed about 24 hours before the surgery. This allows for maximal hemostatic effect, precluding the possibility of neoangiogenesis, while avoiding the masking of neurologic sequelae resulting from the embolization by the surgical anesthetic.

If 3D CT is expected to be used, preoperative imaging with fiducials or a headpiece in place is needed. Using infrared energy or magnetic energy to localize an instrument in the surgical field to the preoperative CT scan, this technology has proven beneficial at clarifying paranasal sinus and skull base anatomy when distorted by the presence of a tumor (Fig. 26.2). It helps to provide an intraoperative guide to the degree of tumor resection while eliminating the need for other intraoperative radiologic imaging techniques such as fluoroscopy. Limitations of this technology include the placement of a registration device (i.e., headpiece or fiducials) over the face or anterior skull that may get in the way if open approach or combined approach is being considered.

For tumors with intraorbital involvement, preoperative vision evaluation is needed, and preoperative ophthalmologic consultation should be considered. For those with intracranial involvement, neurosurgical consultation should be considered. If a large skull base repair is expected, consideration for the placement of a lumbar drain is also helpful.

Intraoperatively, the greatest consideration is to minimize bleeding. Although serious bleeding is extremely rare, the excellent visualization and lighting that is paramount to performing endoscopic resection of nasal tumors is greatly hindered by the presence of even a small amount of blood in the field. Key to minimizing bleeding is the use of excellent technique with avoidance of undue trauma to adjacent nasal structures. Because bleeding from a small abrasion in the anterior nose or a frayed edge of ethmoid mucosa spills down the lateral nasal wall or the shaft of the scope into the operative field, obscuring visualization of the area, it must be avoided. Similarly, thought should be given to the order of débridement and the location of endoscopic incisions, working primarily posterior to anterior to minimize the dripping into the field.

Bleeding may also be minimized by injection of a vasoconstricting solution, typically 1% Xylocaine with 1:100,000 epinephrine, into the region of the uncinate anteriorly and the region of the sphenopalatine posteriorly. These are usually supplemented with an injection in the greater palatine foramen on the appropriate side using a 25-gauge needle bent at 2.5 cm and inserted into the foramen located adjacent to the second molar, with 1.5 mL of solution injected here. If opening of the sphenoid is anticipated, the face of the sphenoid is injected as well. Similarly, if middle turbinate resection is planned, the head of the turbinate is injected with the same solution.

For tumors located anteriorly along the skull base, ligation of the anterior ethmoid artery and vein should be considered. Injury to these vessels may result in intraorbital or intracranial bleeding. Coagulation may be easily accomplished endoscopically using an endoscopic bipolar forceps (Aesculap Werke, Tuttlingen, Germany) under guidance with an angled endoscope (Figs. 26.3 and 26.4). Similar consideration should be given to ligation of the sphenopalatine or the posterior ethmoid posteriorly.

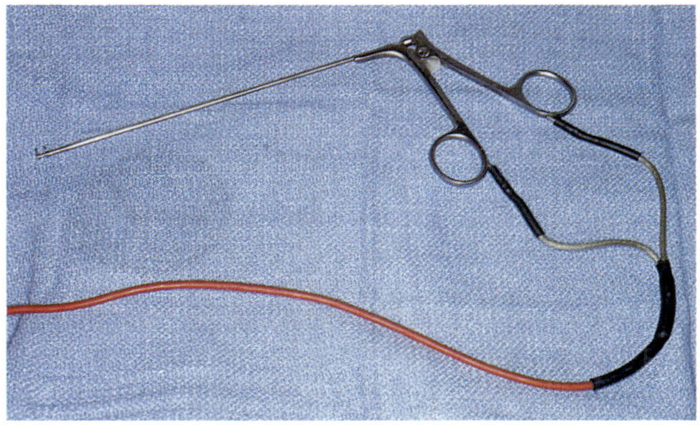

**FIGURE 26.3.** Endoscopic bipolar forceps (Aesculap Werke, Tuttlingen, Germany).

As with any endoscopic procedure, ascertaining the anatomy early in the dissection is essential. The surgeon should attempt to identify the lamina papyracea and the skull base as anatomic constants. Thorough dissection of normal tissue around the tumor is performed to widen the surgical field. When tumor at the skull base is encountered, defects of bone and dura may occur and require careful closure to prevent postoperative CSF fistula. Endoscopic closures of such defects have been found to be effective in more than 90% of cases. Briefly, our technique involves ensuring that all the edges around the defect are freshened, similar to a tympanoplasty. For smaller defects, an overlay graft of

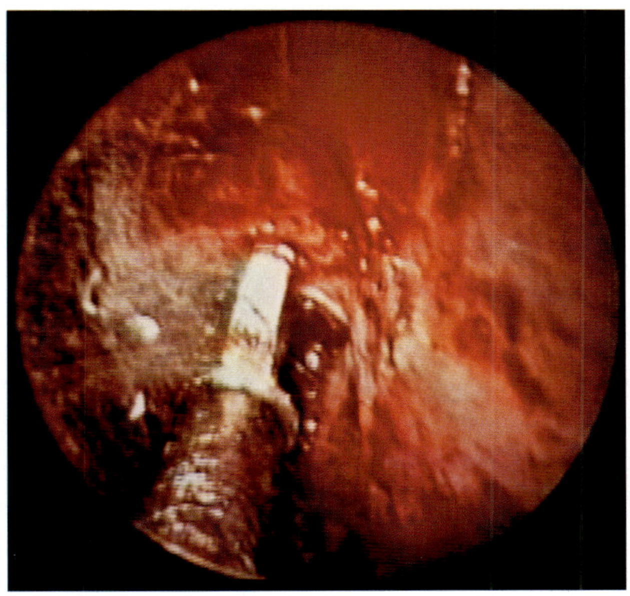

**FIGURE 26.4.** The endoscopic bipolar forceps is used to cauterize the anterior ethmoid vessels under visualization with a 45° endoscope.

mucoperichondrium (Fig. 26.5) or temporalis fascia is placed, followed by multiple alternating layers of absorbable material, including microfibrillar collagen (Avitene, Alcon, San Juan, PR) and Gelfoam (Upjohn, Kalamazoo, MI). Larger defects may benefit from an additional layer of cartilage or bone placed intracranially. Ultimately a nonabsorbable pack (Merocel, Medtronic, Jacksonville, FL) coated in mupirocin ointment is placed below to support the repair.

Resection of a tumor extending into the orbit through the lamina papyracea generally does not require reconstruction. Occasionally, slight enophthalmos or diplopia may occur if significant orbital periosteum is removed; this is avoided if possible.

Postoperatively, patients are maintained on antibiotics providing good antistaphylococcal activity while packs remain in place. They may be removed in 2 to 5 days, usually being left longer if significant skull base repair was performed. Nasal saline spray is used to moisten the nose and encourage dissolution of the absorbable packing material. Sinus débridement is usually delayed until about 4 to 6 weeks after surgery. Lumbar drains, when placed, are usually allowed to remain for about 3 to 5 days, draining 10 mL per hour. Before removal, the lumbar drain is usually clamped for 24 hours to ensure no residual leaking.

In the setting of leak repair, patients are encouraged to avoid stooping, straining, bending, coughing, and nose blowing. Appropriate stool softeners, antitussives, and other drugs are prescribed. Patients are confined to bed rest with the head of bed elevated in the immediate postoperative period, and activity level gradually is increased with the removal of drains and packs.

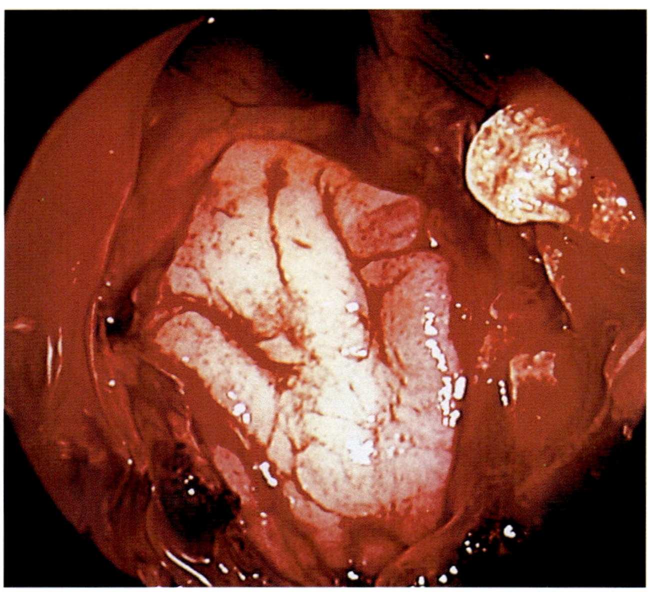

**FIGURE 26.5.** Intraoperative intranasal endoscopic view of an overlay graft of mucoperichondrium used to cover the skull base defect to provide water-tight closure and prevent cerebrospinal fluid leak. Notice that the free graft is oversized by about one third and that all edges are placed tightly against the edges of the defect without tenting.

Essential for all patients with tumor removal is regular and long-term surveillance. The ability to identify residual disease or early recurrence of disease through endoscopic examination is helpful for the patient who has undergone surgery through traditional techniques or endoscopic approaches. Arguably, this is the greatest advantage of the endoscope in the management of patients with paranasal sinus tumors.

## Mucoceles

The surgical approach for mucoceles is determined by the position of the lesion and the presumed cause, but the overriding goal of the procedure is marsupialization of the lesion. For example, in the frontoethmoid region for a mucocele of presumed traumatic origin, an anterior ethmoidectomy with marsupialization may be all that is required. More commonly for lesions occurring in a setting of chronic sinus disease, a complete ethmoidectomy with wide marsupialization may be required. In this case, the walls of the mucocele are made flush with the surrounding preserved tissue so that a wide opening from the mucocele into the sinus cavity is accomplished.

The course of the operation is similar to that of a typical ethmoidectomy with sphenoidotomy, frontal sinusotomy, and maxillary antrostomy, as needed. The details of this procedure have been elaborated previously, but briefly, local anesthetic with vasoconstrictor is administered as described earlier. This is followed by complete uncinectomy with the microbackbiter forceps or microdebrider. The bulla ethmoidalis is opened and the lamina papyracea identified. Dissection is carried posteriorly into the posterior ethmoid cells in a medial and inferior direction to the face of the sphenoid sinus, where the skull base can then be confidently identified. If the sphenoid is to be opened, it is approached in the manner described by Lanza (31) through the superior meatus. A thin strip of the inferior aspect of the superior turbinate is removed, allowing visualization of the sphenoethmoid recess and the ostium of the sphenoid sinus through the posterior ethmoid. The ostium is then enlarged with a sphenoid punch forceps (Medtronic-Xomed, Jacksonville, FL) (Figs. 26.6 and 26.7), taking down the face of the sinus to make it confluent with the posterior ethmoid. Removal of persistent septations and cells along the skull base and the lamina papyracea is performed with cutting forceps (Fig. 26.8), minimizing damage to the preserved mucosa over these areas. Dissection continues into the frontal recess, focusing on mucosal preservation, while at the same time removing all ethmoid septations in this area.

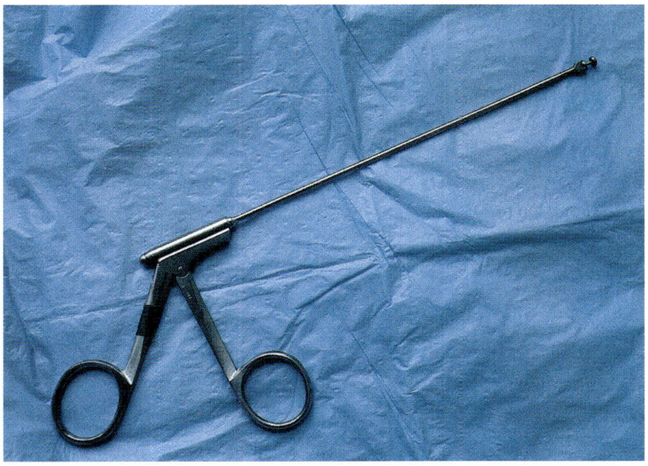

**FIGURE 26.6.** Sphenoid punch (Medtronic-Xomed, Jacksonville, FL) is used to create a wide sphenoidotomy.

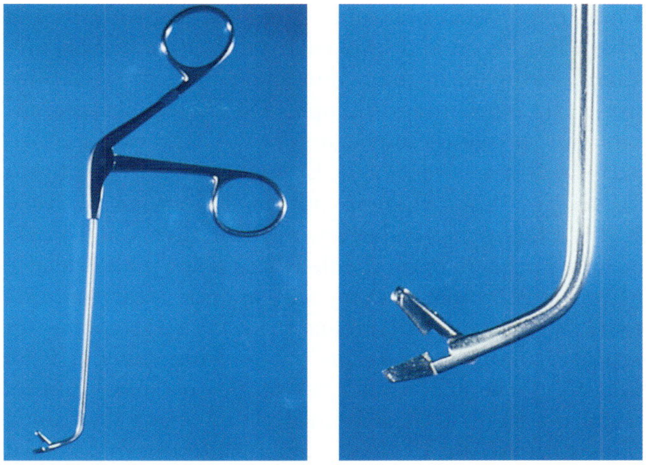

**FIGURE 26.8.** Frontal cutting instrumentation (SSI, Nashville, TN) is helpful for mucosal preservation in the frontal recess.

After the mucocele is encountered, the thickened lining or rind is opened using a cutting instrument such as a sickle knife or a through-cut forceps. Typically, the surgeon encounters a thick, clear fluid filling the cavity. The opening is enlarged to make it confluent with the adjacent mucosa. Just as within the sinuses themselves, great care is taken to not strip the lining of the mucocele but to preserve it and make it confluent with the adjacent sinus cavities.

Postoperatively, patients are followed very closely with frequent sinus débridement, usually on a weekly basis. Old mucus and blood in the cavity is suctioned away, taking great care to remove as much of the fibrinous debris as possible. It is this debris that functions as a latticework for migrating fibroblasts, ultimately resulting in cavity scarring and possible recurrence of the mucocele. Patients should be followed long term because sinus stenosis may progress over years, and the physician must ensure that the mucocele cavity remains patent.

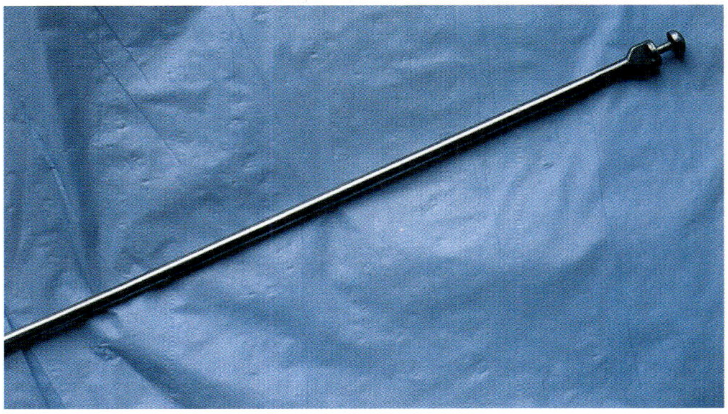

**FIGURE 26.7.** Close-up view of the head of the sphenoid punch (Medtronic-Xomed, Jacksonville, FL) shows the cutting action.

This technique has proved valuable for mucoceles involving all regions of the paranasal sinuses, including the frontal sinuses, even frontal sinuses that have previously undergone fat obliteration (10). Such history does not preclude an endoscopic approach, although it may require novel adaptations such as a modified Lothrop-type approach in which the entire floor of the frontal sinus is removed. More difficult is the mucocele located high in the frontal sinus or laterally in the frontal sinus (Fig. 26.9). In some situations, these can be managed endoscopically, although many require an open approach or possibly a combined endoscopic-open approach.

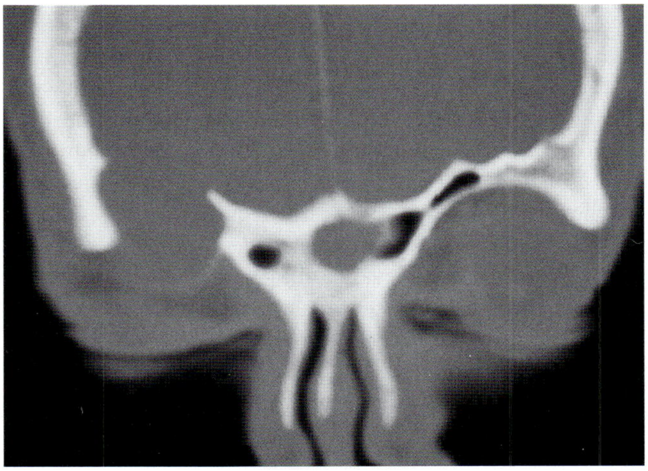

**FIGURE 26.9.** Coronal, bone-windowed computed tomography scan shows mucoceles occupying midline of the frontal sinus and left lateral frontal sinus. The lateral position of the left mucocele combined with the hard bone forming its border precluded an isolated endoscopic approach in this case.

***Case 1:*** A 58-year-old woman presented with a history of ciliary dyskinesia and associated pulmonary disease presented with pain in the region above her left eye accompanied by intermittent diplopia. Her history was significant for previous sinus surgery for chronic sinusitis performed many years ago. Examination was significant for no significant diplopia and no diminution of visual acuity. Endoscopic evaluation revealed edema and thick, opaque mucus in both middle meati, along with evidence of previous ethmoidectomy and inferior meatal antrostomy. Ophthalmologic evaluation was significant for an extrinsic compressing lesion compressing superiorly on the left globe. CT evaluation of the paranasal sinuses revealed a large, left-sided mucocele involving the frontal sinus with erosion of the posterior table and intracranial extension (Fig. 26.1).

She was taken to the operating room, where a revision endoscopic sphenoethmoidectomy with middle meatal antrostomy and frontal sinusotomy was performed. Marsupialization of the mucocele was accomplished with an 8-mm frontal sinusotomy. Two years after surgery, following a period of postoperative care, she remains free of recurrence with a wide frontal sinusotomy confirmed on office endoscopy.

## Inverted Papilloma

Endoscopic resection of inverted papilloma may be successfully performed for primary and recurrent tumors. Most surgeons agree that small tumors involving the ethmoid or middle turbinate are well managed endoscopically. Similarly, tumors that are larger with skull base involvement or involvement of the sphenoid for which traditional approaches may require craniofacial resection can be well managed endoscopically. Under endoscopic guidance, the bone of the skull base or the sphenoid may be drilled with a diamond burr, taking it down to the dura without violation and creation of a CSF leak. More controversial is the tumor that may be removed en bloc through a midface degloving or lateral rhinotomy approach. With accumulating experience in the hands of the skilled endoscopist, even these can be successfully managed in a minimally invasive technique.

In all cases, an en bloc procedure is performed to the greatest extent possible, including removal of underlying bone and soft tissue. Accompanying this is a cuff of normal tissue surrounding the tumor to reduce the chance of recurrence. Adjacent preserved bone is ground down with the drill. For tumors involving the lamina papyracea, the bone may be taken, but care is taken to preserve the underlying orbital periosteum. Similarly, along the skull base, bone may be removed, but the underlying dura is preserved.

Limitations of the endoscopic approach to removal of inverted papilloma primarily involve the location of the tumor. Specifically, tumors located high in the frontal sinus, although rare, are difficult to reach through the frontal infundibulum with an endoscopic approach. Such tumors are probably best managed with a traditional approach such as osteoplastic flap or with a combined endoscopic-open approach, avoiding obliteration of the frontal sinus (Fig. 26.10). Similarly, tumors located laterally in the maxillary sinus may be difficult to reach with an endoscopic approach alone, requiring the addition of a Caldwell-Luc approach to remove en bloc adjacent normal tissue and to drill the bone of the effected area (Fig. 26.11).

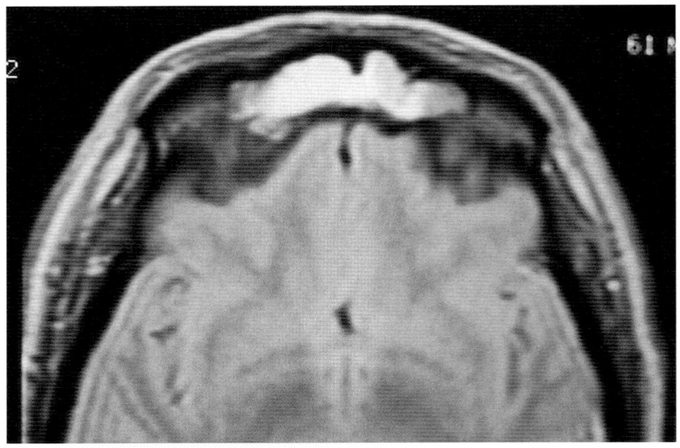

**FIGURE 26.10.** Axial, T1-weighted magnetic resonance image of the frontal sinus shows a heterogeneous lesion occupying the midline area. Because of the location, this inverted papilloma required an open approach to ensure complete removal.

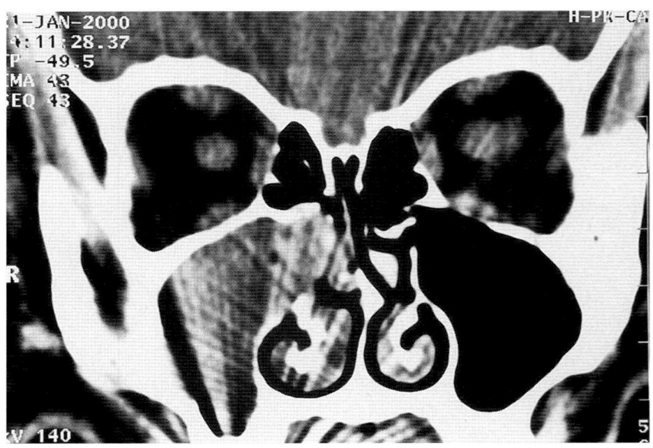

**FIGURE 26.11.** Coronal, soft tissue–windowed computed tomography scan of the paranasal sinuses through the region of the mid-ethmoid and the maxillary sinuses. A heterogeneous lesion fills the right maxillary sinus. Because of tumor extension into the lateral aspects of the maxillary sinus, this inverted papilloma was resected using a combined endoscopic and Caldwell-Luc–type approach.

***Case 2:*** A 44-year-old woman was referred for evaluation of a known inverting papilloma of the right maxillary sinus. She had presented to her referring surgeon with a history of facial discomfort and congestion on the right side of 1 year's duration. Without improvement on medical therapy and with CT and endoscopic evidence of disease, endoscopic sinus surgery was performed. Pathology findings were significant for inverted papilloma without evidence of malignancy. She was subsequently referred for further management.

On presentation, she complained of pain but was experiencing no bleeding and no tearing. On examination, she was found to have intact sensation over the upper lip and intact extraocular motion. Endoscopic evaluation identified a polypoid mass occupying the right maxillary sinus medially and along the floor and anteriorly to the limits of the scope examination. The roof of the sinus and the adjacent ethmoid were not involved.

CT examination revealed a mass filling the right maxillary sinus without evidence of bone erosion, extending into the middle meatus (Fig. 26.11). She was taken to the operating room, where a combined endoscopic and open approach to removal of the tumor was performed. The procedure was begun endoscopically. The middle meatal antrostomy was enlarged superiorly to the junction of the maxillary sinus roof and the ethmoid and posteriorly to the back of the maxillary sinus. Next, the inferior turbinate was cut posteriorly at approximately the back of the maxillary sinus and anteriorly at the face of the sinus. Using a 4-mm osteotome, a cut was made along the floor of the nose into the maxillary sinus, and this cut was completed anteriorly and posteriorly with the through-cut forceps. A small scalpel was used to incise the mucosa superiorly and posteriorly in the maxillary sinus. A sublabial incision was made, and the face of the sinus opened, allowing exposure of the tumor anteriorly, laterally, and superiorly in the sinus. Cuts were made in all these areas, connecting them to the previous endoscopic incisions (including transection of the nasolacrimal duct), and the en bloc mass was removed through the sublabial incision. The drill with cutting burr was used to burr down residual bone, and the cavity was inspected endoscopically transnasally and sublabially for evidence of persistent disease. Without any sign of disease, the sinus was packed with Gelfoam coated in mupirocin cream, and the sublabial incision was closed.

Packing was débrided in the office 2 weeks after surgery, and endoscopic surveillance carried out at regular intervals. Three years postoperatively, there was no evidence of recurrence.

## Bony and Fibro-Osseus Tumors

In some cases, bony tumors are small and easily removed from the sinus cavity (Fig. 26.12). However, they often have enlarged to the point that the drill is required to debulk the tumor and remove it transnasally (Fig. 26.13). Even when large and escaping the confines of the nose and sinuses, they are frequently loosely attached to the surrounding tissue and can be gently dissected away.

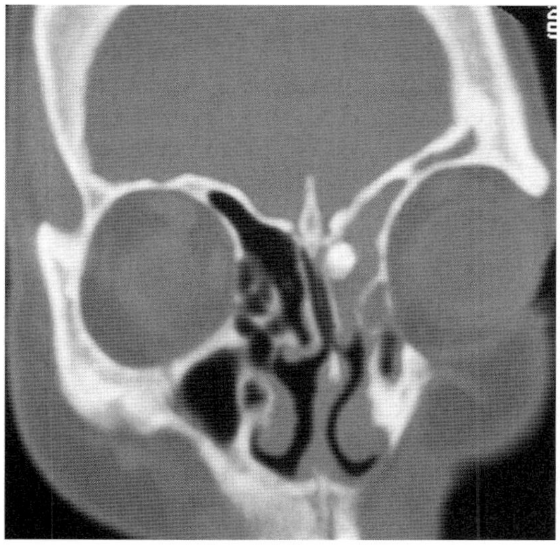

**FIGURE 26.12.** Coronal computed tomography scan of the paranasal sinuses with bone windowing illustrates a small, right-sided boney mass in the anterior ethmoid with an associated frontoethmoid mucocele. This osteoma was easily removed using an endoscopic approach.

The initial endoscopic approach is to completely remove adjacent sinuses to allow for careful inspection of the skull base and the lamina papyracea around the tumor given the propensity of these to exhibit intracranial and intraorbital extension. If located in the frontoethmoid region, the anterior ethmoid artery and vein is cauterized using the endoscopic bipolar forceps (Aesculap Werke, Tuttlingen, Ger-

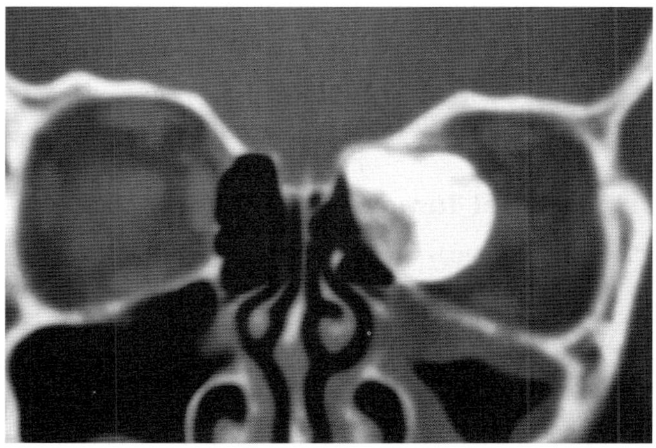

**FIGURE 26.13.** Coronal computed tomography scan of the paranasal sinuses with bone windowing illustrates a large, heterogeneous bony mass of the left ethmoid with intraorbital extension and extension to the skull base. It was removed using only endoscopic techniques.

many) (Figs. 26.3 and 26.4). The endoscopic drill with cutting burr (TPS Hummer, Stryker, Kalamazoo, MI) is used to debulk the tumors by shelling them out and cutting them as appropriate until they are small enough to be safely delivered through the nose. The advantage of this type of drill is that suction and irrigation are contained within one unit, and the sleek profile lends itself to rhinologic application. Mastoid drills, although effective, require an assistant to help with suction and irrigation. Regardless of the drill used, drilling of these tumors tends to be a tedious process, with smoke forming in the nose or bone dust and foam from blood in the field being thrown onto the scope, requiring frequent cleaning. Patience is key. After the tumor has been shelled and debulked, it may be gently rocked and teased away from adjacent structures with the Lusk ball-tipped seeker or the Kuhn-Bolger frontal recess curette and delivered into the nose.

***Case 3:*** A 19-year-old man was referred for evaluation of progressive left-sided proptosis occurring over 1.5 years with two discreet episodes of brief left eye blindness and subsequent complete resolution. Examination revealed 4 mm of left proptosis with diplopia on extreme right and left gaze. Visual acuity was normal. Endoscopic evaluation revealed no abnormalities of the infundibulum or the bulla ethmoidalis. The CT scan showed a large, bony mass extending from the ethmoid through the lamina papyracea and into the left orbit, abutting the optic nerve (Fig. 26.13).

He was taken to the operating room, where left-sided total ethmoidectomy, middle meatal antrostomy, and debulking of the intraorbital tumor was performed. Intraoperative CT localization was used, allowing on-going assessment of the depth of resection in the orbit. The bony tumor was shelled out as described earlier, although the portion of tumor adjacent to the optic nerve was not removed. A large lamina papyracea defect resulted and was not reconstructed; care was taken not to remove orbital fat nor to enlarge defects in the orbital periosteum.

Pathologic analysis revealed fibrous dysplasia. Postoperatively, vision returned to normal and proptosis resolved.

## Intracranial Tumors

Pituitary adenomas may be approached endoscopically in several ways, depending on the preference of the otolaryngologist–head and neck surgeon and the neurosurgeon. Options include a midline approach in which a typical hemitransfixion incision is made and mucoperichondrial flaps are elevated. Septal bone and cartilage are displaced laterally, providing ready access to the rostrum of the sphenoid. Mucosa on the rostrum of the sphenoid is lifted laterally beyond the sphenoid ostium, and bone is removed at the ostium with the endoscopic curette. The intersinus septum is also removed, allowing excellent midline visualization of the region of the sella and the adjacent carotid arteries and optic nerves. A self-retaining nasal speculum is then placed, maintaining the lateral position of the septal flaps and allowing the neurosurgeon greater access to the pituitary.

We use a unilateral approach with excellent success and even less morbidity. In this approach, the side with easier access to the sphenoethmoid recess and the ostium of the sphenoid sinus is chosen. The nose is decongested with 1% oxymetazoline on 0.5 × 3 inch neurosurgical cotton patties placed deep into the sphenoethmoid recess under endoscopic guidance. Although this provides excellent decongestion of the membranes, it also gently dilates the space, allowing for easier access into the sphenoethmoid recess. One percent Xylocaine with 1:100,000 epinephrine is injected in the posterior septum at the rostrum of the sphenoid. Greater palatine injections and sphenopalatine injections are similarly performed. The sphenoid ostium is cannulated with the Frazier suction and the ostium enlarged with the J-curette. Subsequently, the sphenoid punch (Medtronic-Xomed, Jacksonville, FL) (Figs. 26.6 and 26.7) is used to enlarge the ostium, ultimately followed by the Hajek rotating sphenoid sinus punch. Great care is taken to open the ostium medially beyond the septum so that a more midline perspective is maintained for the neurosurgeon. The intersinus septum is removed with through-cutting forceps. After an adequate opening is achieved, a long, self-retaining nasal speculum is placed into the nose, allowing the neurosurgeons greater ease of scope placement while resecting the tumor. This also minimizes bleeding into the field by gentle tamponade and helps prevent abrasion of adjacent nasal tissues by the repeated in-and-out action of the instruments.

Mucosa is then removed from the posterior wall of the sphenoid over the sella turcica using the suction cautery. The scope is secured in the scope holder, allowing a two-handed approach for the rest of the procedure. A curette is used to remove bone from the posterior wall of the sphenoid, followed by use of the small Kerrison forceps. With an adequate opening (usually at least 8 mm), the tumor is removed using ring curettes in the usual fashion. After removal, we have had great success using a small piece of abdominal fat placed in a dumbbell fashion through the opening with or without CSF leak. The sphenoid is not packed, and no intranasal packing is performed. Postoperatively, urine specific gravity is monitored, and patients are discharged on day 2 or 3.

***Case 4:*** An 8-year-old boy was referred for evaluation of precocious puberty without other neurologic deficit. The MRI scan revealed a large, midline mass compressing the horns of the lateral ventricles and extending down into the anterior superior sella turcica (Fig. 26.14). A biopsy was attempted externally by the neurosurgeons using endoscopic technique but was unsuccessful.

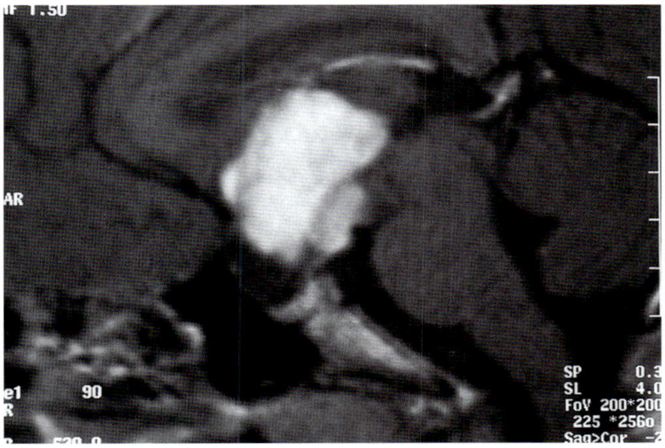

**FIGURE 26.14.** Sagittal, T1-weighted magnetic resonance image shows a large, midline tumor occupying the sellar and suprasellar regions. A transnasal transsphenoidal endoscopic approach was successfully used for biopsy of this pilocytic astrocytoma.

The child was subsequently brought to the operating room, and a transnasal transsphenoidal endoscopic biopsy of the mass through the left nares using the technique described previously was performed. With opening of the posterior superior wall of the sphenoid, as suspected from the MRI, a large, cystic cavity filled with CSF was encountered. The 0°, 30°, and 45° scopes were then used to explore the cavity, and multiple biopsies were obtained using endoscopic small through-cut forceps. Bleeding was controlled with neurosurgical patties soaked with 1% Xylocaine with 1:100,000 epinephrine. The large CSF leak was repaired with "dumbbell fat," and no other packing was performed (Fig. 26.15). Pathologic analysis revealed pilocytic astrocytoma.

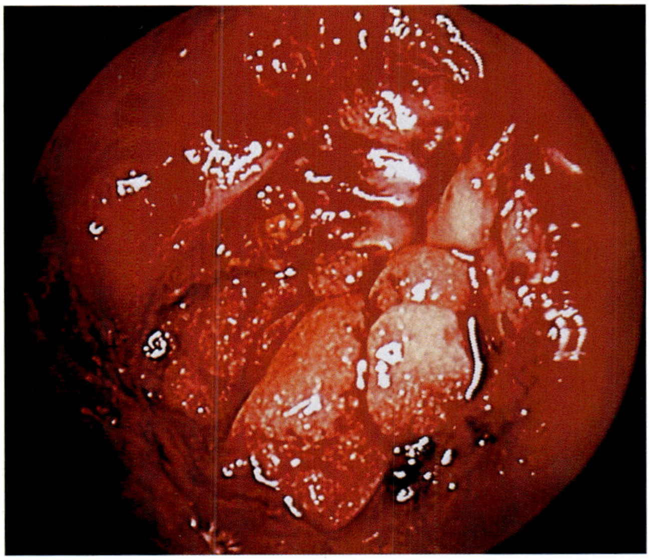

**FIGURE 26.15.** Endoscopic view of the posterior wall of the sphenoid shows fat placed through the wall and into the sella, successfully sealing the cerebrospinal fluid leak.

## BASIC INSTRUMENTATION FOR ENDOSCOPIC RESECTION OF PARANASAL SINUS AND NASAL TUMORS

1. Hopkins rod telescopes: 0°, 30°, 45°, and 70°
2. Endo Scrub (Medtronic-Xomed Surgical Products, Jacksonville, FL)
3. Standard endoscopic sinus instrumentation, including upbiting and straight Blakesley forceps
4. Frontal Recess instruments, including Kuhn-Bolger curette (Karl Storz, Culver City, CA) and giraffe punches (SSI, Nashville, TN) (Fig. 26.8)
5. Sphenoid punches (Medtronic-Xomed, Jacksonville, FL) (Figs. 26.6 and 26.7)
6. Microbipolar endoscopic forceps: 45° and 90° (Aesculap Werke, Tuttlingen, Germany) (Figs. 26.3 and 26.4)
7. Endoscopic microdebrider or drill with cutting burrs (TPS Hummer, Stryker-Leibinger, Kalamazoo, MI)
8. Standard otologic set with various picks and knives

## STEP-BY-STEP TECHNIQUES

### Cerebrospinal Fluid Leak Repair

1. *(Optional)* Lumbar drain is placed with instillation of 0.1 mL of 10% intravenous fluorescein mixed in 10 mL of the patient's CSF and reinstilled over several minutes.
2. Sinus surgery is completed with wide exposure of the defect area, including sphenoidotomy and frontal sinusotomy as needed as described in the section on Endoscopic Sphenoethmoidectomy with Frontal Sinusotomy, Sphenoid Sinusotomy, and Middle Meatal Antrostomy.
3. Edges of the defect are freshened with a curette or otologic instruments similar to those for tympanoplasty. Endoscopic bipolar is used to fulgurate the edges of the mucosa and the bed of the defect (Fig. 26.4).
4. For smaller defects, a graft of mucoperichondrium from the contralateral septum or temporalis fascia is placed in overlay fashion, taking great care to prevent tenting of the graft at the edges of the defect (Fig. 26.5). Larger defects may benefit from an additional layer of cartilage or bone placed intracranially.
5. Multiple alternating layers of absorbable material, including microfibrillar collagen (Avitene, Alcon, San Juan, PR) and Gelfoam (Upjohn, Kalamazoo, MI), are placed under the graft for support. Ultimately, a nonabsorbable pack (Merocel, Medtronic-Xomed, Jacksonville, FL) coated in 2% mupirocin ointment is placed below to support the repair.

### Endoscopic Sphenoethmoidectomy with Frontal Sinusotomy, Sphenoid Sinusotomy, and Middle Meatal Antrostomy

1. 1% Xylocaine with 1:100,000 epinephrine injection:
   a. 1.5 mL in each greater palatine foramen
   b. 1.4 mL in the region of the sphenopalatine foramen posteriorly
   c. 1.5 mL in the region of the uncinate process
2. The uncinectomy is completed with the microbackbiter forceps or microdebrider.
3. Bulla ethmoidalis is opened and the lamina papyracea identified; mucosa is spared over the lamina papyracea by using cutting instrumentation or microdebrider.
4. Basal lamella is opened, and dissection is carried posteriorly into the posterior ethmoid cells in a medial and inferior position to the face of the sphenoid sinus, where the skull base can then be confidently identified
5. The superior meatus is identified medially. A thin strip of the inferior aspect of the superior turbinate is removed, allowing visualization of the sphenoethmoid recess and the ostium of the sphenoid sinus through the posterior ethmoid.
6. The sphenoid ostium is then enlarged with a sphenoid punch forceps (Medtronic-Xomed, Jacksonville, FL), taking down the face of the sinus to make it confluent with the posterior ethmoid.
7. Removal of persistent septations and cells along the skull base and the lamina papyracea is performed with cutting forceps, minimizing damage to the preserved mucosa over these areas.
8. Dissection continues into the frontal recess, focusing on mucosal preservation, while at the same time removing all ethmoid septations in this area, allowing for wide opening of the frontal sinus.

### Mucoceles

1. Complete sinus surgery provides wide exposure adjacent to the mucocele as described in the section on Endoscopic Sphenoethmoidectomy with Frontal Sinusotomy, Sphenoid Sinusotomy, and Middle Meatal Antrostomy.
2. After the mucocele is encountered, the thickened lining or rind is opened using a cutting instrument such as a sickle knife or a through-cut forceps.
3. The opening is enlarged to make it confluent with the adjacent mucosa. Just as within the sinuses themselves, great care is taken to not strip the lining of the mucocele but to preserve it and make it confluent with the adjacent sinus cavities using through-cut or punch-type instrumentation (Fig. 26.8).

### Inverting Papilloma

1. Complete sinus surgery provides wide exposure adjacent to the inverted papilloma as described in the Endoscopic Sphenoethmoidectomy with Frontal Sinusotomy, Sphenoid Sinusotomy, and Middle Meatal Antrostomy section.
2. Mucosal and bone incisions are fashioned in a posterior-to-anterior direction, performing an en bloc procedure to the greatest extent feasible with an accompanying cuff of normal tissue surrounding the tumor.
3. Adjacent preserved bone is ground down with the endoscopic drill using cutting and diamond burrs (Hummer, Stryker-Leibinger, Kalamazoo, MI). For tumors involving the lamina papyracea, the bone may be removed, but care is taken to preserve the underlying orbital periosteum. Similarly, along the skull base, bone may be removed, but the underlying dura is preserved.
4. Caldwell-Luc and osteoplastic flap procedures are performed as needed for appropriate exposure.

### Bony and Fibro-Osseus Tumors

1. Complete sinus surgery provides wide exposure adjacent to the bony tumor as described in the Endoscopic Sphenoethmoidectomy with Frontal Sinusotomy, Sphenoid Sinusotomy, and Middle Meatal Antrostomy section. This allows careful inspection of the skull base and the lamina papyracea around the tumor given the propensity of these to exhibit intracranial and intraorbital extension.
2. If tumor is located in the frontoethmoid region, the anterior ethmoid artery and vein are cauterized using the endoscopic bipolar forceps (Aesculap Werke, Tuttlingen, Germany) (Fig. 26.3).
3. The endoscopic drill with cutting burr (Hummer, Stryker, Kalamazoo, MI) is used to debulk the tumors, shelling them out and cutting them as appropriate until they are small enough to be safely delivered through the nose. Patience is key.
4. After the tumor has been shelled and debulked, it may be gently rocked and teased away from adjacent structures with the Lusk maxillary ostium seeker or the Kuhn-Bolger curette and delivered into the nose.

### Pituitary Adenoma

1. The side with easier access to the sphenoethmoid recess and the ostium of the sphenoid sinus is chosen.
2. The nose is decongested with 1% oxymetazoline on 0.5 × 3 inch neurosurgical cotton patties placed deep into the sphenoethmoid recess under endoscopic guidance.

3. One percent Xylocaine with 1:100,000 epinephrine is injected in the posterior septum at the rostrum of the sphenoid. Greater palatine injections and sphenopalatine injections are similarly performed.
4. The sphenoid ostium is cannulated with the Frazier suction, and the ostium is enlarged with the J-curette.
5. The sphenoid punch is used to enlarge the ostium (Medtronic-Xomed, Jacksonville, FL), ultimately followed by the Hajek rotating sphenoid sinus punch. The ostium is opened medially beyond the septum.
6. The intersinus septum is removed with through-cutting forceps.
7. A long, self-retaining nasal speculum is placed into the nose.
8. Mucosa is removed from the posterior wall of the sphenoid over the sella turcica using the suction cautery.
9. The scope is secured in the scope holder, allowing a two-handed approach for the rest of the procedure.
10. A curette is used to remove bone from the posterior wall of the sphenoid, followed by the small Kerrison forceps, creating an opening of at least 8 mm.
11. The tumor is removed using ring curettes in the usual fashion.
12. A small piece of abdominal fat placed in a dumbbell fashion through the opening with or without CSF leak. The sphenoid is not packed, and no intranasal packing is performed.

## CONCLUSIONS

Endoscopic sinus surgery has been a major development in the management of inflammatory sinus disease. However, with the excellent lighting, detail, and resolution provided, it was only natural that these techniques be applied to management of benign nasal and sinus tumors as well. In the past 5 years, with the remarkable improvement in instrumentation, including punches, microdebriders, and drills, along with the evolution of intraoperative CT localization systems, excellent outcomes are being seen, and such procedures are becoming commonplace for the management of mucoceles, bony tumors, and inverted papillomas. These techniques are being applied successfully to tumors escaping the nasal or sinus cavity and extending into the orbit or intracranially and to brain tumors such as pituitary adenomas.

Education and training are key. An intimate understanding of the anatomy and the techniques analogous to otologic and skull base surgery are required before embarking on these procedures. Similarly, skill and expertise in the setting of repair of large CSF leaks are needed. In the hands of the skilled otolaryngologist–head and neck surgeon, results can be excellent while minimizing facial incisions, the need for craniotomy, and their accompanying morbidity.

## REFERENCES


1. Mosher H. The symposium of the ethmoid—a surgical anatomy of the ethmoidal labyrinth. Presented at the 34th Annual Meeting of the American Academy of Ophthalmology and Otolaryngology. 1929;34:376–410.
2. Kennedy DW, Zinreich SJ, Rosenbaum AE, et al. Functional endoscopic sinus surgery. *Arch Otolaryngol* 1985;111:576–582.
3. Ward N. A mirror of the practice of medicine and surgery in the hospitals of London: London Hospital. *Lancet* 1854;2:480–482.
4. Phillips P, Gustafson R, Facer G. The clinical behavior of inverting papilloma of the nose and paranasal sinuses: report of 112 cases and review of the literature. *Laryngoscope* 1990;100:463–469.
5. Waitz G, Wigand M. Results of endoscopic sinus surgery for the treatment of inverted papillomas. *Laryngoscope* 1992;102:917–922.
6. Dolgin S, Zaveri V, Casiano R, et al. Different options for the treatment of inverting papilloma of the nose and paranasal sinuses: a report of 41 cases. *Laryngoscope* 1992;102:231–236.
7. Lawson W, Ho B, Shaari C, et al. Inverted papilloma: a report of 112 cases. *Laryngoscope* 1995;105:282–288.
8. Lawson W, Le Benger J, Som P, et al. Inverted papilloma: an analysis of 87 cases. *Laryngoscope* 1989;99:1117–1124.
9. Stankiewicz J, Girgis S. Endoscopic surgical treatment of nasal and paranasal sinus inverted papilloma. *Otolaryngol Head Neck Surg* 1993;109:988–995.
10. Kennedy D, Keogh B, Senior B, et al. Endoscopic approach to tumors of the anterior skull base and orbit. *Otolaryngol Head Neck Surg* 1996;7:257–263.
11. Kennedy D, Josephson J, Zinreich S, et al. Endoscopic sinus surgery for mucoceles: a viable alternative. *Laryngoscope* 1989;99:885–895.
12. Benninger M, Marks S. The endoscopic management of sphenoid and ethmoid mucoceles with orbital and intranasal extension. *Rhinology* 1995;33:157–161.
13. Moriyama H, Hesaka H, Tachibana T, et al. Mucoceles of the ethmoid and sphenoid sinus with visual disturbance. *Arch Otolaryngol Head Neck Surg* 1992;118:142–146.
14. Hartley B, Lund V. Endoscopic drainage of pediatric paranasal sinus mucoceles. *Int J Pediatr Otorhinolaryngol* 1999;50:109–111.
15. Aarabi B, Leibrock L. Neurosurgical approaches to cerebrospinal fluid rhinorrhea. *Ear Nose Throat J* 1992;71:300–305.
16. Atallah N, Jay M. Osteomas of the paranasal sinuses. *J Laryngol Otol* 1981;95:291–304.
17. Dandy W. Pneumocephalus (intracranial pneumocele or aerocele). *Arch Surg* 1926;12:949–983.
18. Senior B, Jafri K, Benninger M. Safety and efficacy of endoscopic management of encephaloceles and CSF leaks. *Am J Rhinol* 2000;15:21–25.
19. Senior B, Lanza D, Kennedy D, et al. Computer-assisted resection of sinonasal tumors with skull base and orbital extension. *Arch Otolaryngol Head Neck Surg* 1997;123:706–711.
20. Menezes C, Davidson T. Endoscopic resection of a sphenoethmoid osteoma: a case report. *Ear Nose Throat J* 1994;73:598–600.
21. Seiden A, el Hefny Y. Endoscopic trephination for the removal of frontal sinus osteoma. *Otolaryngol Head Neck Surg* 1995;112:607–611.
22. Senior B, Lanza D. Benign lesions of the frontal sinus. *Otolaryngol Clin North Am* 2000;34:253–267.
23. Schloffer H. Erfolgreiche operation eines hypophysen-tumors auf nasalem wege. *Wein Klin Wochenschr* 1907;20:621–624.

24. Hardy J. Microneurosurgery of the hypophysis: a subnasal transsphenoidal approach with television magnification and televised radiofluoroscopic control. In: Rand R, ed. *Microneurosurgery*. St. Louis: CV Mosby, 1969:87–103.
25. Halves E, Bushe K. Transsphenoidal operation on craniopharyngiomas with extrasellar extensions: the advantage of the operating endoscope. *Acta Neurochir* 1979;28:362.
26. Sethi D, Pillay P. Endoscopic management of lesions of sella turcica. *J Laryngol Otol* 1995;109:956–962.
27. Sethi D, Pillay P. Endoscopic pituitary surgery: a minimally invasive technique. *Am J Rhinol* 1996;10:141–148.
28. Carrau R, Jho H, Ko Y. Transnasal transsphenoidal endoscopic surgery of the pituitary gland. *Laryngoscope* 1996;106:914–918.
29. Sheehan M, Atkinson J, Kasperbauer J, et al. Preliminary comparison of endoscopic transnasal versus sublabial transseptal approach for clinically nonfunctioning pituitary macroadenomas. *Mayo Clin Proc* 1999;74:661–670.
30. Heilman C, Shucart W, Rebeiz E. Endoscopic sphenoidotomy approach to the sella. *Neurosurgery* 1997;41:602–607.
31. Bolger WE, Keyes AS, Lanza DC. Use of the superior meatus and superior turbinate in the endoscopic approach to the sphenoid sinus. *Otolaryngol Head Neck Surg* 1999;120:308–313.

# 27

# ENDOSCOPIC DACRYOCYSTORHINOSTOMY

RALPH METSON

## INDICATIONS

Endoscopic dacryocystorhinostomy (DCR) provides the surgeon with a safe and effective technique for opening an obstructed lacrimal sac without the need for an external incision. Patients with obstruction of the lacrimal drainage system usually present with epiphora. They complain of excessive tearing of the affected eye, which interferes with vision and can be socially unacceptable. Continued blockage of the sac leads to chronic dacryocystitis with drainage of purulent material from the canaliculi at the corner of the eye. Inflammation of the skin in the region of the medial canthus overlying the obstructed sac may occur, particularly during acute infections.

Although intranasal DCR was described by West (1) almost a century ago, it never gained widespread popularity because of problems with limited visibility and poor exposure of the lacrimal sac within the narrow confines of the superior nasal cavity (2). These problems have been overcome by the introduction of nasal endoscopes that provide excellent visualization for surgical manipulation within the depths of the nasal cavity. Surgeons who have developed expertise with endoscopic treatment of sinus disease are applying similar skills for endoscopic treatment of lacrimal obstruction (3,4).

## CONTRAINDICATIONS

Endoscopic DCR is not recommended in patients with acute dacryocystitis who present with periorbital fluctuance. These patients should be treated with conventional external DCR, as well as incision and drainage of any subcutaneous fluid collections. External DCR is also recommended for patients who are found on dacryocystogram to have diverticula of the lacrimal sac that cannot be adequately drained through an intranasal approach.

## PREOPERATIVE EVALUATION

Preoperative evaluation for endoscopic DCR includes nasal endoscopy to look for signs of sinusitis or anatomic abnormalities that could contribute to lacrimal obstruction. After installation of a topical decongestant and anesthetic (e.g., 0.5% phenylephrine HCl and 4% lidocaine HCl), an endoscope is introduced into the nasal cavity. I prefer a nasal endoscope with a 2.7 mm diameter and a 30° angle of view for patient examination in the office. This scope provides good visualization with a maximum of patient comfort. The inferior meatus is inspected for any masses that could cause obstruction the nasolacrimal duct orifice. The middle meatus is examined for the presence of polyps or mucopurulent drainage. A septal deviation or enlarged middle turbinate may need to be addressed at the time of DCR.

Before endoscopic DCR, patients should have an ophthalmologic examination to document the results of visual acuity, visual fields, and slit-lamp examination. The patency of the lacrimal drainage system can be accessed by irrigation of the canaliculi with saline or fluorescein dye to determine ease of flow into the nose or the presence of reflux. Canalicular stenosis, which may indicate the need for placement of a Jones tube to relieve epiphora, can be assessed by probing the puncta with a lacrimal probe.

Computed tomography of the paranasal sinus can be performed before endoscopic DCR to delineate sinus anatomy and identify any disease not recognized on physical examination. Axial and coronal scans are preferred. Anterior ethmoid air cells, which overlie the lacrimal sac and need to be opened at time of surgery, are found in more than 90% of patients. Magnetic resonance scans are not generally obtained because they are unable to image the thin bony sinus partitions.

Although many surgeons do not routinely obtain a dacryocystogram before DCR, others think it is helpful to identify the location and degree of lacrimal obstruction. Radiopaque contrast media is injected into the canaliculi while a radiograph is obtained. Normally, the media should been seen to flow freely into the inferior meatus. When obstruction is present, dye flows only to the site of obstruction and does not reach the nasal cavity. The most common site of obstruction is just distal to the lacrimal sac, which may be dilated. Filling defects representing lacrimal stones may also be seen.

## INSTRUMENTATION

- Routine endoscopic instruments used for sinus surgery
- Lacrimal dilator and probes
- Drill or microdebrider for removing bone overlying lacrimal sac
- Guibor or Crawford tubes: lacrimal probes with attached Silastic catheter used to stent the DCR ostium at conclusion of surgery (Guibor Canaliculus Intubation Set, Concept, Inc., Largo, FL)
- Fiberoptic light pipe, 20 gauge—optional, used to transilluminate the lacrimal sac at the start of surgery (Endoilluminator, Storz Instruments, St. Louis, MO)

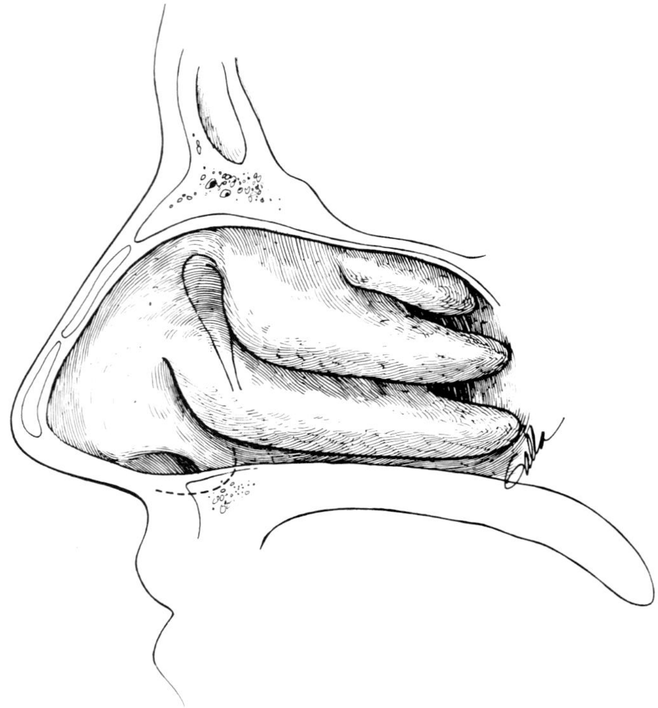

**FIGURE 27.1.** View of the right lateral nasal wall demonstrates the relationship of the lacrimal sac and the nasolacrimal duct to the turbinates. Notice how a portion of the sac may extend beneath the middle turbinate, requiring turbinate resection for adequate exposure. (From Metson R. Endoscopic diagnosis and treatment of lacrimal obstruction. In: Lucente F, ed. *Highlights of the instructional courses 1994*, vol 7. St. Louis: Mosby–Year Book. 1994:255–265, with permission.)

## OPERATING ROOM LAYOUT

The operating room layout is similar to that used for routine endoscopic sinus surgery. The surgeon is seated to the patient's right, with the instruments and video monitor at the head of the operating table. The scrub nurse and anesthesiologist are positioned to the patient's left. The operation is performed with a video camera attached to the endoscope, so that the assistant surgeon can observe the entire procedure on the video monitor.

## ANESTHESIA

Endoscopic DCR may be performed under local or general anesthesia, depending on condition of the patient and preference of the surgeon. I perform most endoscopic DCRs under general anesthesia to ensure patient comfort.

Before draping the nose and affected eye in the operative field, the nasal cavity is sprayed with a 0.05% oxymetazoline HCl solution to initiate vasoconstriction. With the head slightly elevated to decrease venous pressure at the operative site, submucosal injections of 1% lidocaine HCl with epinephrine 1:100,000 are placed along the lateral nasal wall just anterior to the attachment of the middle turbinate under endoscopic visualization with a 4-mm-diameter, 0° nasal endoscope.

## OPERATIVE TECHNIQUE

The lacrimal sac is located beneath the bone of the lateral nasal wall, just in front of the anterior attachment of the middle turbinate (Fig. 27.1). In many patients, agger nasi cells of the anterior ethmoid sinus overlie the sac, producing a bulge in the lateral nasal wall in this location. The superior border of the sac may extend above the level of the turbinate attachment. The posterior end of the sac often extends beneath the middle turbinate, behind a landmark referred to as the maxillary line.

The maxillary line is an important landmark for endoscopic DCR. It is readily identified as a curvilinear eminence along the lateral nasal wall (Fig. 27.2), which runs from the anterior attachment of the middle turbinate to the root of the inferior turbinate. Its location corresponds to the suture line between the maxillary and lacrimal bones that runs in a vertical direction through the lacrimal fossa. Exposure of the posterior half of the sac typically requires removal of the uncinate process and underlying lacrimal bone located posterior to the maxillary line. In contrast, exposure of the anterior sac necessitates removal of thicker bone located just anterior to the maxillary line.

An optional step at the start of surgery involves the use of a 20-gauge fiberoptic light probe that is passed through a canaliculus into the lacrimal sac. This probe transilluminates the lateral nasal wall and provides confirmatory information as to the location of the lacrimal sac. The area of maximal brightness corresponds to the posterior end of the

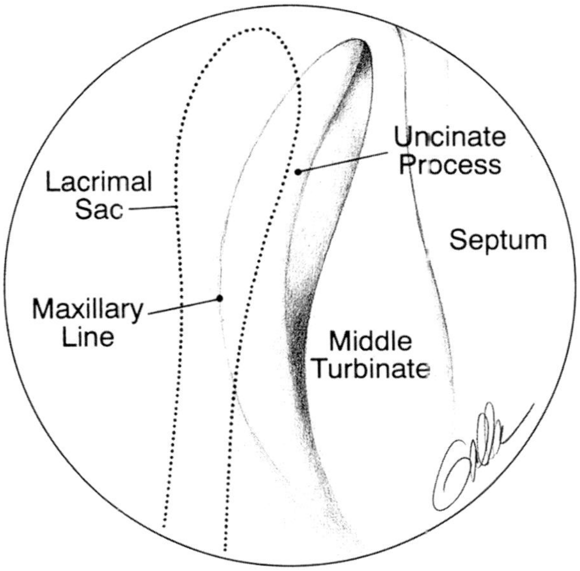


**FIGURE 27.2.** Endoscopic view of the right nasal cavity demonstrates the location of the lacrimal sac *(dotted line)* underlying the lateral nasal wall. The maxillary line, a bony eminence that originates at the middle turbinate attachment, is a reliable anatomic landmark for location of the sac. (From Metson R. Endoscopic diagnosis and treatment of lacrimal obstruction. In: Lucente F, ed. *Highlights of the instructional courses 1994*, vol 7. St. Louis: Mosby–Year Book. 1994:255–265, with permission.)

lacrimal sac, where the overlying bone is thinnest, not the center of the sac.

Surgical dissection begins with removal of an approximately 1-cm-diameter circle of mucosa along the lateral nasal wall anterior to the maxillary line (Fig. 27.3). The upper portion of the uncinate process located posterior to the maxillary line is similarly incised. An air space is often entered that corresponds to the infundibulum or an anterior ethmoid air cell overlying the lacrimal sac. As dissection is carried more anteriorly, agger nasi cells overlying the lacrimal sac may be entered. Removal of the thin underlying lacrimal bone exposes the medial wall of the lacrimal sac. Exposure of the sac is confirmed by movement of a lacrimal probe that has been passed by the assistant through a canaliculus into the sac.

The frontal process of the maxillary bone that forms the anterior aspect of the lacrimal fossa must be removed. Removal of this relatively thick bone is technically the most difficult step of the surgery. Bone removal may be accomplished with a curette, bone-biting forceps, microdebrider, or drill (Figs. 27.4 to 27.6). Although the surgical laser has also been used for endoscopic DCR, it is not recommended for bone removal because of difficulty in monitoring the depth of thermal destruction, which can result in bony sequestra and scar formation (5). After

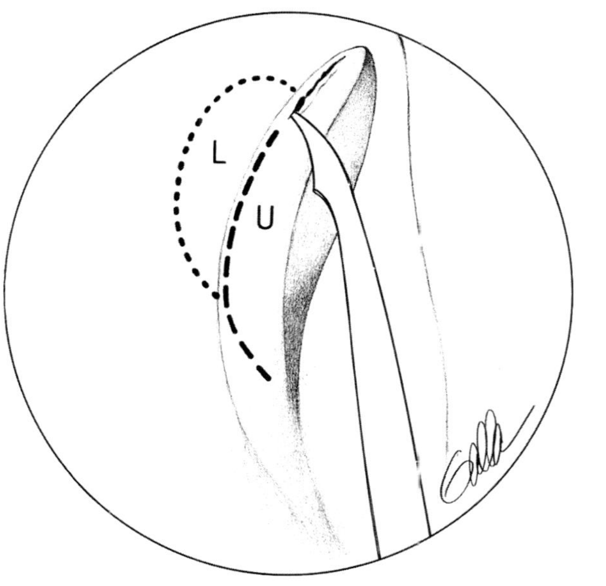


**FIGURE 27.3.** After submucosal injections to promote hemostasis, the uncinate process *(U)* is incised just posterior to the maxillary line and removed. An area of mucosa along the lateral nasal wall *(L)* is similarly incised and removed to expose bone that overlies the anterior portion of the lacrimal sac. (From Metson R. Endoscopic dacryocystorhinostomy—an update on techniques. *Operative techniques in otolaryngology–head and neck surgery.* 1995;6:217–220, with permission.)

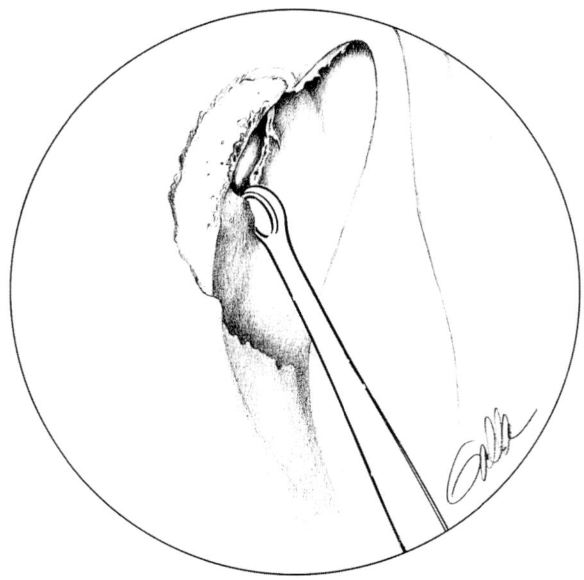

**FIGURE 27.4.** A spoon curette is used to expose the posterior lacrimal sac by removing remnants of the uncinate process and the underling lacrimal bone. Bone removal and sac identification can be facilitated by the use of a fiberoptic light pipe. This pipe is passed through a canaliculus into the lacrimal sac to transilluminate the lateral nasal wall in the region of the sac. (From Metson R. Endoscopic dacryocystorhinostomy—an update on techniques. *Operative techniques in otolaryngology–head and neck surgery.* 1995;6:217–220, with permission.)

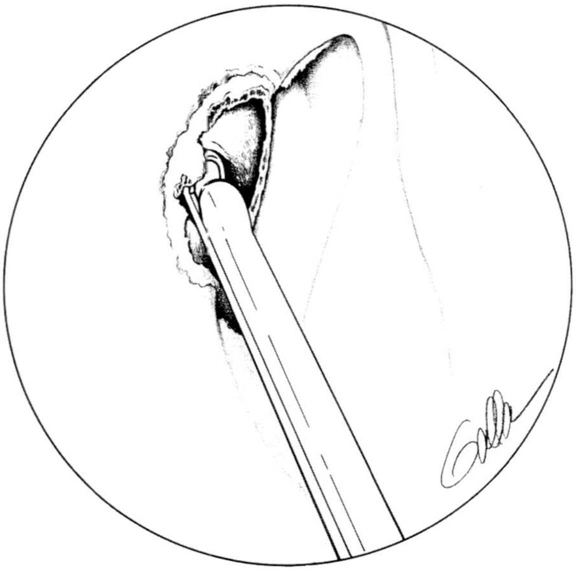

**FIGURE 27.5.** Thick bone of the frontal process of the maxilla is removed with a bone-biting rongeur to expose the anterior portion of the lacrimal sac. (From Metson R. Endoscopic dacryocystorhinostomy—an update on techniques. *Operative techniques in otolaryngology–head and neck surgery.* 1995;6:217–220, with permission.)

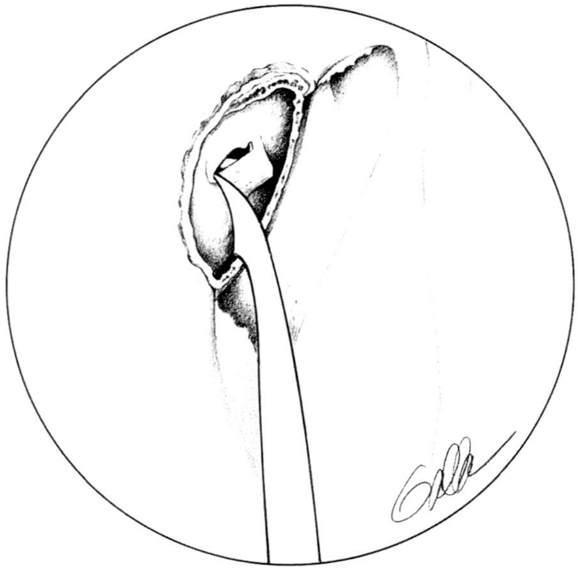

**FIGURE 27.7.** The lacrimal sac is opened with a sickle knife. This maneuver is facilitated by tenting the exposed medial sac wall with the probe, which has been passed into the sac through a canaliculus. Entrance into the sac is confirmed by identification of the bare probe within the sac interior. (From Metson R. Endoscopic dacryocystorhinostomy—an update on techniques. *Operative techniques in otolaryngology–head and neck surgery.* 1995;6:217–220, with permission.)

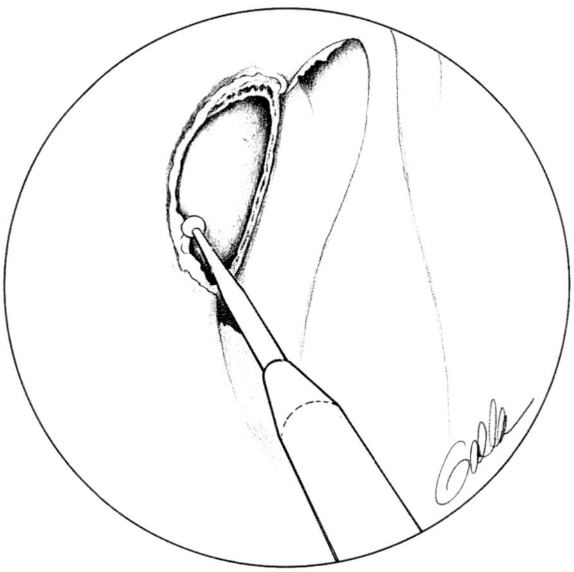

**FIGURE 27.6.** The drill is a useful tool for removal of thick bone overlying the lacrimal sac. (From Metson R. Endoscopic dacryocystorhinostomy—an update on techniques. *Operative techniques in otolaryngology–head and neck surgery.* 1995;6:217–220, with permission.)

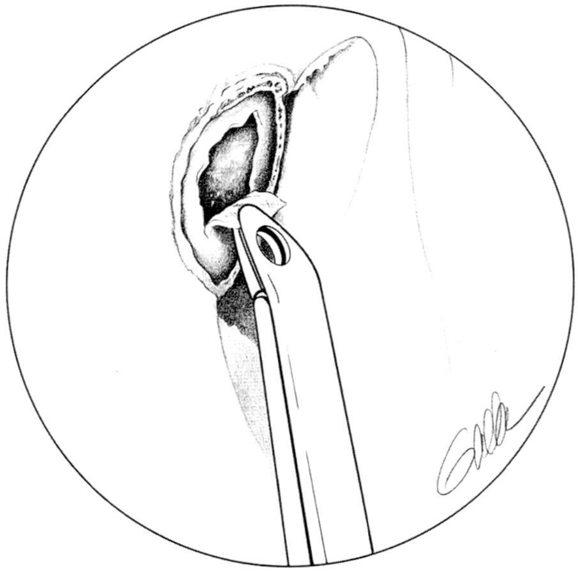

**FIGURE 27.8.** The opening into the lacrimal sac is enlarged with an angled Blakesley forceps. The medial sac wall is removed, and no attempt is made to create mucosal flaps. (From Metson R. Endoscopic dacryocystorhinostomy—an update on techniques. *Operative techniques in otolaryngology–head and neck surgery.* 1995;6:217–220, with permission.)

the entire medial sac wall has been exposed, it is entered with an angled Blakesley forceps. It is often helpful to use the lacrimal probe within the sac to tent up the medial sac wall as it is opened (Fig. 27.7). This maneuver isolates the medial wall and prevents inadvertent injury to the underlying structures. After the sac is entered, the probe is visible.

The opening into the lacrimal sac is enlarged to a diameter of approximately 10 mm (Fig. 27.8). Its inferior edge should extend to the level of the sac-duct junction. No attempt is made to create mucosal flaps. The location of the common punctum is verified by passing stents attached to a Silastic tubing (i.e., Guibor or Crawford tubes) through the superior and inferior canaliculi. The stents are grasped with a Blakesley forceps (Fig. 27.9), withdrawn from the nasal cavity, and cut from the tubing. The ends of the tubing are then tied and trimmed within the nasal cavity to form a continuous loop around the canaliculi (Fig. 27.10). This tubing stents the surgical ostium during the postoperative healing period. Unless bleeding is a problem or a concurrent septoplasty has been performed, no nasal packing is used.

Endoscopic revision DCR is performed in a similar fashion to endoscopic primary DCR; however, bone of the lateral nasal wall overlying the lacrimal sac has already been removed (6). Revision DCR is therefore usually easier to perform than primary DCR. This factor makes revision DCR patients who have already failed an external DCR approach very appropriate initial candidates for the surgeon who wishes to learn endoscopic DCR techniques.

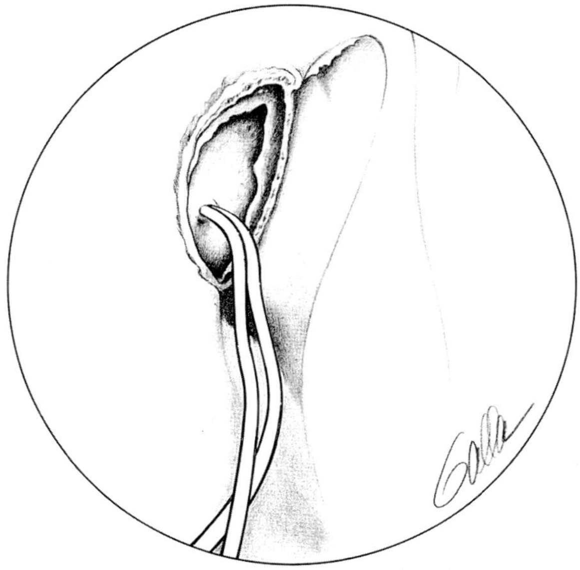

**FIGURE 27.10.** View of the tubing that stents the intranasal opening into the lacrimal sac during the healing period. (From Metson R, et al. Endoscopic dacryocystorhinostomy. *Head and neck surgery: An update on techniques.* 1995;6:217–220, with permission.)

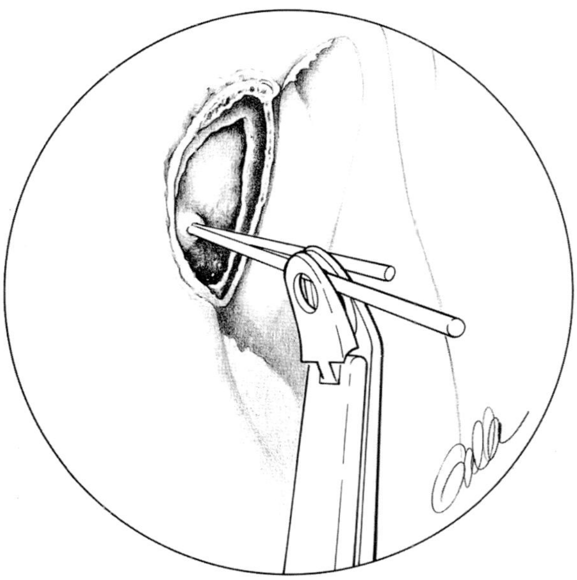

**FIGURE 27.9.** Lacrimal probes threaded with Silastic tubing are passed through the canaliculi, grasped with forceps, directed out of the nasal cavity, trimmed, and tied. Notice the opening of the internal common punctum, through which the catheters enter the sac interior. (From Metson R, et al. Endoscopic dacryocystorhinostomy. *Head and neck surgery: An update on techniques.* 1995;6:217–220, with permission.)

## HIGHLIGHTS

1. Exposure of the entire medial wall of the lacrimal sac, which requires removal of thick bone anterior to the maxillary line
2. Passage of lacrimal probes through the canaliculi into the lacrimal sac to verify location of the sac and provide countertraction when opening into the sac
3. Removal of the entire medial wall of the lacrimal sac; visualization of the internal common punctum with a 30° endoscope ensures that an adequate portion of the superior sac has been opened
4. Stenting of the surgical ostium with a Silastic catheter, which remains in place during the postoperative healing period

## POSTOPERATIVE CARE

If nasal packing is placed at the conclusion of surgery, it is removed the next morning. Patients are discharged with

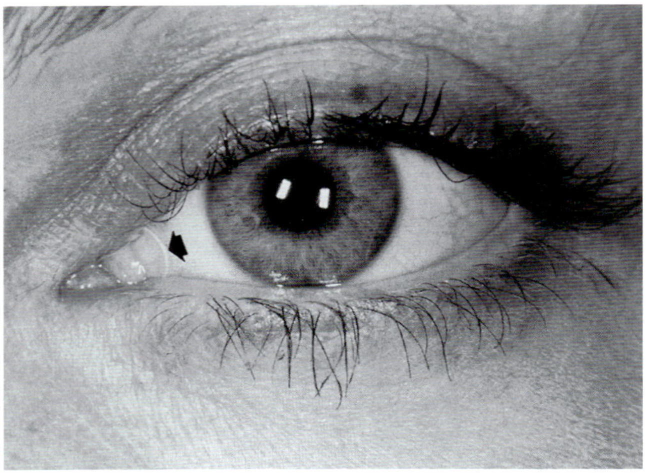

**FIGURE 27.11.** The extranasal course of the catheter used to stent the surgical ostium during the healing period is shown *(arrow)* as it passes between canaliculi. The ends of this catheter pass through the lacrimal sac and into the nasal cavity, where they are tied to form a continuous loop. (From Metson R. Endoscopic diagnosis and treatment of lacrimal obstruction. In: Lucente F, ed. *Highlights of the instructional courses 1994*, vol 7. St. Louis: Mosby–Year Book. 1994:255–265, with permission.)

instructions to begin twice-daily nasal saline irrigations with a bulb syringe. Any remaining intranasal debris is removed from the operative site at the first postoperative visit 1week after surgery.

The Silastic tubing used to stent the surgical ostium is typically removed 2 months after surgery by cutting the exposed tubing at the medial canthus and withdrawing it through the nose (Fig. 27.11). It may be removed sooner if excessive granulation tissue formation occurs around the tube at the ostium. In revision cases in which postoperative scarring has been a problem, stents may be left in place for 6 months or longer. Patency of the lacrimal drainage system is verified by irrigation of the canaliculi and by endoscopic observation of fluorescein dye flowing from the eye through the surgical ostium into the nose (Figs. 27.12 and 27.13).

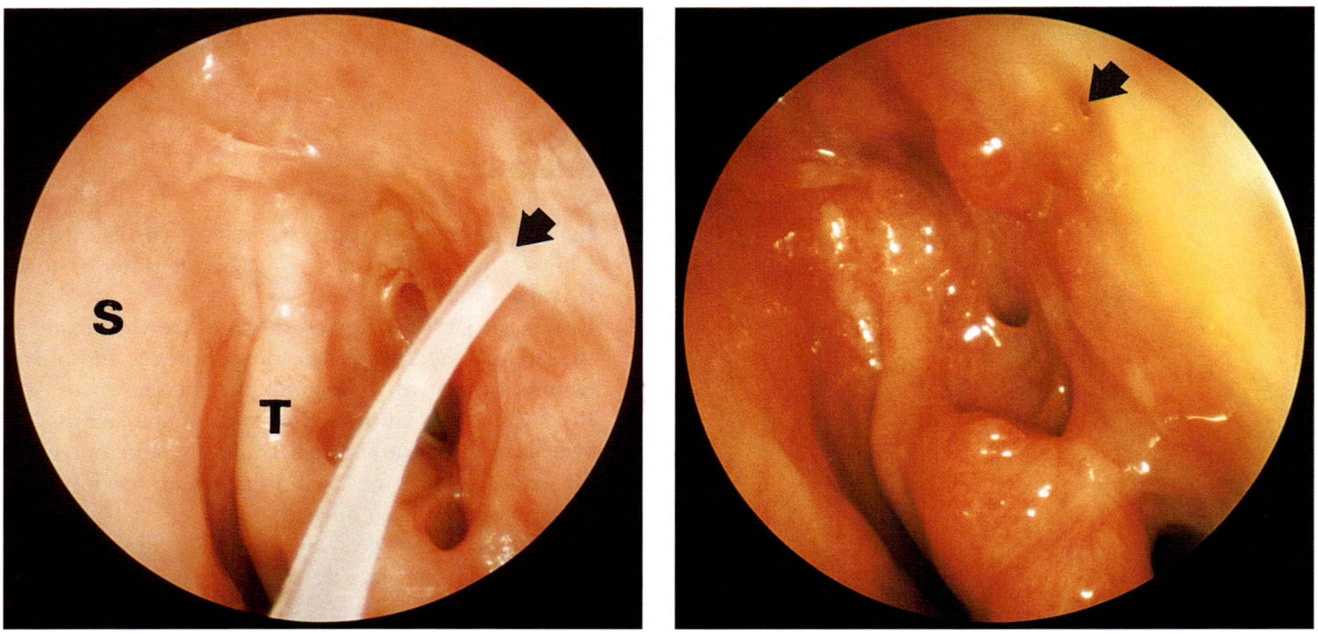


A B

**FIGURE 27.12. A:** Endoscopic view of the left nasal cavity in a patient shown in Figure 27.11 demonstrates the Silastic catheter *(arrow)* passing through the lateral nasal wall into the lacrimal sac *(S)*. The remaining posterior portion of a resected middle turbinate *(T)* is visible behind the catheter. **B:** After the Silastic catheter has been removed, fluorescein dye from the eye flows into the nose through the healed ostium and is visible along the lateral nasal wall *(arrow)*. An opening into the ethmoid sinus is seen in the center of the field just lateral to the middle turbinate remnant. (From Metson R. Endoscopic diagnosis and treatment of lacrimal obstruction. In: Lucente F, ed. *Highlights of the instructional courses 1994*, vol 7. St. Louis: Mosby–Year Book. 1994:255–265, with permission.)

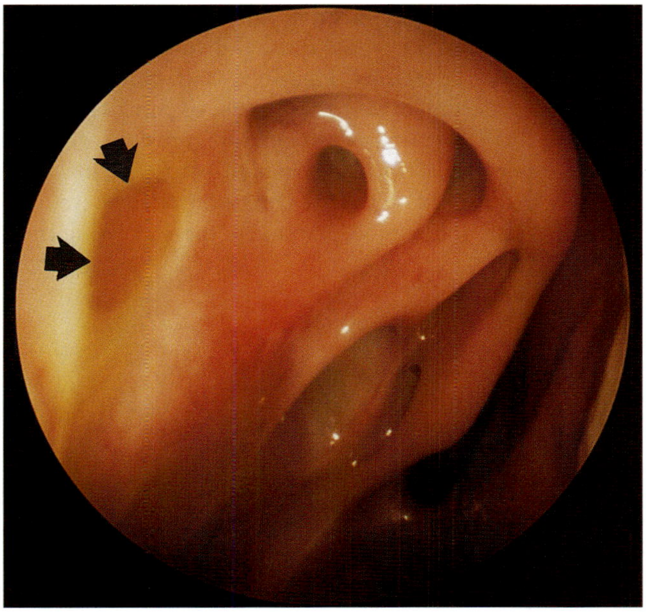

**FIGURE 27.13.** Endoscopic view of the right lateral nasal wall shows fluorescein dye flowing through the surgical ostium *(arrows)* into the nose. The variation in sizes of healed ostia is demonstrated by comparing this relatively large lacrimal opening with the small one shown in Figure 27.12. Prominent structures *(center)* are openings into the ethmoid sinuses in this patient, who has undergone an ethmoidectomy and middle turbinate resection. (From Metson R. Endoscopic diagnosis and treatment of lacrimal obstruction. In: Lucente F, ed. *Highlights of the instructional courses 1994*, vol 7. St. Louis: Mosby–Year Book. 1994:255–265, with permission.)

## COMPLICATIONS

Endoscopic DCR should be performed only by those who are experienced in endoscopic intranasal techniques. If excessive bleeding occurs during surgery, the procedure should be terminated or converted to an open DCR. Occasionally, orbital fat is exposed while removing bone to uncover the lacrimal sac. Care must be taken not to disturb this fat to prevent injury to underlying orbital structures. Damage to the adjacent medial rectus and superior oblique muscles can lead to diplopia. Blindness can result from laceration of intraorbital vessels with subsequent hemorrhage or by direct injury to the optic nerve itself.

Postoperative epistaxis severe enough to require nasal packing occurs in less than 5% of cases. Postoperative infection involving the nose or orbit after DCR is rare. Perioperative antibiotics are administered in an attempt to avoid this complication.

Postoperative adhesions are one of the most common causes of surgical failure for external (7,8) and endoscopic (4) DCR. These adhesions usually span the lateral nasal wall and middle turbinate or septum, causing obstruction of the surgically created ostium. The incidence of this complication can be reduced by avoiding surgical trauma to the turbinate mucosa or resecting the anterior half of the turbinate so that it is not in the proximity of the ostium. Correction of a deviated septum also reduces the likelihood of postoperative adhesion formation, as does meticulous cleaning of debris from the intranasal operative during the postoperative period.

## ADVANTAGES AND LIMITATIONS OF ENDOSCOPIC TECHNIQUE

Instead of replacing external DCR, endoscopic DCR is an alternative approach for the treatment of lacrimal obstruction in selected patients. For the younger patient with epiphora who wishes to avoid a surgical scar on the face, endoscopic DCR offers an excellent alternative to conventional techniques.

Endoscopic DCR also appears to have a place for revision surgery in the patient who has already failed an external DCR. Endoscopic instrumentation provides excellent visualization within the nasal cavity for the identification and removal of adhesions, which are a common cause of DCR failure. Other intranasal factors that contribute to DCR failure, such as middle turbinate hypertrophy, septal deviation, and ethmoid sinusitis, also lend themselves to endoscopic correction.

Endoscopic DCR has the potential to reduce patient morbidity through improved intraoperative hemostasis, greater use of local anesthesia, and shorter hospitalization compared with conventional techniques. Alternatively, the issues of increased operative time and cost associated with a new surgical procedure, particularly if a laser is used, must also be considered. As clinical expertise with endoscopic DCR techniques increases, these considerations become less of a factor.

## LITERATURE REVIEW

Reports have demonstrated a greater than 90% success rate for endoscopic DCR (9–11). In a series of 30 patients with lacrimal obstruction, Onerci (9) reported relief in epiphora in 93% of patients who underwent endoscopic DCR. A group of 152 patients who underwent endoscopic DCR by Sprekelsen (10) observed "good" or "very good" results 1 year after surgery. No major complications occurred in either series.

Hartikainen (11) compared a group of 32 patients who underwent endoscopic DCR for lacrimal obstruction with a group of 32 others who underwent conventional external DCR. The success rate at 1 year after surgery was higher for the external procedure (91% versus 75%). This difference was not statistically significant and can be readily explained by the fact that patients who underwent endoscopic surgery were not seen for postoperative cleaning until 1 month after surgery. The investigator recognized this deficiency and stated "the most important modification necessary to improve the success rate for [endoscopic DCR] is a weekly postoperative intranasal cleaning of debris and mucus at the rhinostomy site." The success rate after secondary surgery was 97% in both groups.

Earlier reports of endoscopic DCR describe success rates ranging from 82% to 86% for primary procedures and reflect the learning curve associated with the development of a new surgical technique. Gonnering (12) and Massaro (13) first described laser-assisted endoscopic DCR in 16 patients with no initial failures, although seven patients still had lacrimal stents in place at time of publication. Woog (5) reported a long-term ostial patency rate of 82% for 40 laser-assisted DCR procedures performed on 37 patients. Follow-up periods ranged from 6 to 91 weeks. Surgical failure, defined as the inability to perform lacrimal irrigation through the DCR ostium, was evident within 14 weeks of surgery in all cases.

Metson (14) described 46 endoscopic laser DCRs performed on 40 patient who were followed for more than 1 year and found that surgery relieved nasolacrimal duct obstruction in 85% of cases. Most surgical failures were the result of gradual closure of the surgical ostium. In one case, a subsequent external DCR revealed an inadequately drained diverticulum of the lacrimal sac as a cause of recurrent dacryocystitis. Revision laser DCR in patients who had already failed a primary laser DCR was not found to be beneficial.

Mannor and Millman (15) suggested that lacrimal sac anatomy on reoperative dacryocystogram is an important prognostic factor for successful endoscopic DCR. In a series of 18 nonlaser endoscopic DCRs, they found that those patients with a normal or dilated lacrimal sac had a success rate of 82%, whereas those with a scarred sac had only a 29% likelihood of success. In 1992, McDonogh (3) reported successful relief of lacrimal obstruction in 20 (86%) of 23 transnasal endoscopic DCR cases followed for 4 to 26 months.

Revision endoscopic DCR (6) with or without a laser has been found to be a worthwhile surgical endeavor for those patients who have failed a primary conventional DCR. Metson (4) reported a 75% success rate for patients who had persistent epiphora or dacryocystitis after external DCR. Common causes of DCR failure, such as intranasal adhesions, concurrent ethmoiditis, and an enlarged middle turbinate, can be readily identified and corrected with endoscopic instrumentation. In the case of patients who fail repeated DCR attempts, consideration must be given to missed causes of lacrimal obstruction, such as canalicular scarring that would require a conjunctivodacryocystorhinostomy with Jones tube placement for successful treatment.

## REFERENCES

1. West JM. A window resection of the nasal duct in cases of stenosis. *Trans Am Ophthalmol Soc* 1914;12:654.
2. Jokinen K, Karja J. Endonasal dacryocystorhinostomy. *Arch Otolaryngol* 1974;100:41–44.
3. McDonogh M. Endoscopic transnasal dacryocystorhinostomy—results in 21 patients. *S Afr J Surg* 1992;30:107–110.
4. Metson R. Endoscopic surgery for lacrimal obstruction. *Otolaryngol Head Neck Surg* 1991;104:473–479.
5. Woog JJ, Metson R, Puliafito CA. Holmium:YAG endonasal laser dacryocystorhinostomy. *Am J Ophthalmol* 1993;116:1–10.
6. Metson, R.. Endoscopic revision dacryocystorhinostomy. *Laryngoscope* 1990;100:1344–1347.
7. Welham RAN, Henderson PH. Results of dacryocystorhinostomy: analysis of causes for failure. *Trans Ophthalmol Soc U K* 1973;93:601–609.
8. McLachlan DL, Shannon GM, Flanagan JC. Results of dacryocystorhinostomy: analysis of reoperations. *Ophthalmic Surg* 1980;11:427–430.
9. Onerci M, Orhan M, Erdener U. Intranasal endoscopic surgery with silicone intubation for lacrimal obstruction. *Am J Rhinol* 1996;10:93–95.
10. Sprekelsen MB, Barberan MT. Endoscopic dacryocystorhinostomy: surgical technique and results. *Laryngoscope* 1996;106:187–189.
11. Hartikainen J, Antila J, Varpula M, et al. Prospective randomized comparison of endonasal endoscopic dacryocystorhinostomy and external dacryocystorhinostomy. *Laryngoscope* 1998;108:1861–1866.
12. Gonnering RS, Lyon DB, Fisher JC. Endoscopic laser-assisted lacrimal surgery. *Am J Ophthalmol* 1991;111:152–157.
13. Massaro BM, Gonnering RS, Harris GJ. Endonasal laser dacryocystorhinostomy: a new approach to nasolacrimal duct obstruction. *Arch Ophthalmol* 1990;108:1172–1176.
14. Metson R, Woog JJ, Puliafito CA. Endoscopic laser dacryocystorhinostomy. *Laryngoscope* 1994;104:269–274.
15. Mannor GE, Millman AL. The prognostic value of preoperative dacryocystography in endoscopic intranasal dacryocystorhinostomy. *Am J Ophthalmol* 1992;113:134–137.

28

# ENDOSCOPIC ORBITAL AND OPTIC NERVE DECOMPRESSION

RICHARD E. GLIKLICH

Minimally invasive techniques for decompressing the orbit and optic nerve have dramatically improved with the advent of the nasal endoscope. The surgeon's comfort with the anatomy of the orbit and the optic nerve are developed through progressive experience with endoscopic ethmoidectomy and sphenoidotomy. Non–minimally invasive techniques for these procedures are gradually falling out of favor as the advantages of the endoscopic approach are recognized. Graves' orbitopathy and trauma are the two most common reasons for orbital decompression, optic nerve decompression, or both procedures.

## ORBITAL DECOMPRESSION

*Dysthyroid orbitopathy* refers to the ocular manifestations of Graves' disease in which there is orbital congestion because of enlargement of the extraocular muscles and fat, leading to exophthalmos, corneal exposure, lid retraction, and optic neuropathy in severe cases. The progression of dysthyroid orbitopathy is independent of changes in or treatments of the thyroid gland. There is a progression from no signs or symptoms to eyelid retraction, lid lag, and edema to soft tissue signs and symptoms to proptosis to involvement of the extraocular movement to corneal involvement and to visual loss from optic neuropathy (1). Graves' orbitopathy is typically bilateral (80% to 90%).

Dysthyroid orbitopathy occurs in two distinct phases. The acute phase is associated with inflammation of orbital contents, which leads to an increase in soft tissue volume and intraorbital pressure, usually resulting in anterior displacement of the globe. As a result, lid closure is poor, and exposure keratitis may threaten the cornea. At the same time, stretching of the optic nerve and posterior pressure may result in optic neuropathy. This phase can last 6 to 18 months. Corticosteroids, which control inflammation, are the first line of therapy. Another option is low-dose radiation therapy (20 to 35 Gy), which may limit the lymphocytic infiltrates in many cases.

A chronic phase is reached 18 to 36 months after onset of the orbital findings. Enlargement of the intraorbital contents becomes permanent. It is in this stage that surgery is most often used to treat this disease. There are three elements to surgical management: orbital decompression, strabismus surgery, and eyelid surgery. Orbital decompression, which involves removal of part of one to four walls of the orbital cavity, is used to decrease exophthalmos and its consequences, including exposure keratopathy and optic neuropathy. After a period of stabilization, strabismus surgery is performed to treat the diplopia that may arise from the congestive process and is often worsened by the decompression. Strabismus surgery is always performed after decompression. Lid retraction and excess eyelid fat are subsequently addressed.

## SURGICAL INTERVENTION

Surgical procedures are ideally performed in a stable orbit. The goal is to enlarge the confining space of the orbit. This is achieved through removal of one to four walls of the bony orbit and incision of the periosteum to allow the orbital soft tissues to prolapse into the adjacent spaces. Theoretically, up to 15mm of decompression can be achieved by removing all four walls of the orbit. However, surgery usually achieves 3 to 7 mm of posterior displacement. Significant complications, including intractable strabismus and hypoglobus may result from excessive decompression.

### Indications

Indications for surgical decompression are severe exophthalmos, globe prolapse anterior to the lids, exposure keratitis, and optic neuropathy. Cosmesis is a relative indication that should be balanced against potential complications. Patients with exophthalmos in excess of 24 mm are more common candidates for decompression. Those with less proptosis may benefit from eyelid procedures alone.

## Approaches

Multiple surgical approaches to orbital decompression have been popularized. Before the endoscopic approach, each technique has been described by the number of involved walls and the major innovator associated with the technique. These are lateral (Kronlein), inferior (Hirsch-Urbanek), superior (Naffziger [transcranial]), medial (Sewall), and medial-inferior (Ogura [transantral]). The endoscopic technique described in this chapter refers to removal of the medial and inferior walls (medial aspect). The approach can be tailored to the amount of decompression desired.

Decompression in the horizontal plane (i.e., medial, inferomedial, and lateral walls) theoretically reduces the risk of vertical dystopia. Such an approach can be achieved through a medial decompression combined with a lateral or Kronlein procedure. The portion of the orbital floor medial to the infraorbital nerve can also be removed without significant change of the globe in the vertical plane. Five millimeters or more of decompression, similar to that reported for the Walsh-Ogura technique, can be achieved by combining a medial orbital decompression, including the orbital floor medial to the infraorbital nerve, and a lateral decompression when necessary. Medial decompression through a transethmoid approach provides on average more than 3 mm of decompression alone while giving excellent access to the orbital apex in cases of optic neuropathy.

The nasal or sinus endoscope provides unsurpassed visualization of the medial orbital wall to the orbital apex. The endoscopic transethmoid approach avoids an external incision, has limited morbidity, provides excellent access to the optic nerve at the orbital apex, and may even be performed under local anesthesia. For these reasons, endoscopic transethmoid orbital decompression, combined when necessary with lateral decompression, is the approach of choice in our institution.

## Preoperative Evaluation

Preoperative evaluation includes a full ophthalmologic examination with Hertel exophthalmometry to assess the degree of proptosis. Visual acuity, visual fields, and color saturation are assessed to exclude optic neuropathy. Nasal endoscopy is performed to diagnose nasal and sinus problems, such as septal deviation, nasal polyps, or infection, which may complicate surgical management. Axial and coronal computed tomography (CT) scans are obtained and reviewed.

## Endoscopic Technique

The patient is placed on the operating table in a slight reverse Trendelenburg position (Fig. 28.1). Oxymetazoline spray is used for initial decongestion. Both eyes are left uncovered in the surgical field, with scleral shells used for corneal protection if lid closure is poor. Pledgets soaked in 4 mL of 4% cocaine solution are placed in the nasal cavity. If the patient is under general anesthesia, submucosal injections of 1% lidocaine with 1:100,000 epinephrine are begun along the lateral nasal wall and along the middle turbinate.

A standard uncinectomy is performed with a sickle knife just posterior to the maxillary line, a bony prominence that extends from the anterior attachment of the middle turbinate to the root of the inferior turbinate. A large maxillary ostium is created, and a 30° telescope is used to identify the position of the infraorbital nerve bundle in the roof of the maxillary sinus. A total ethmoidectomy is completed, and the sphenoid ostium is identified and enlarged. The lamina papyracea is skeletonized. The position of the anterior and posterior ethmoid arteries is noted. The middle turbinate is resected before exposure of the periorbita. This facilitates exposure and postoperative cleaning. A spoon curette is used to crack the lamina in its thin midportion. A Cottle elevator is used to bluntly elevate bone away from the periosteum. Care is taken to preserve the periosteum so that orbital fat does not herniate into the field and obstruct the view. Bone fragments are meticulously removed. Bone is removed superiorly to the roof of ethmoid, which is confirmed by the position of the ethmoidal arteries. Posteriorly, bone is removed to the face of sphenoid. Inferiorly, bone is removed to the maxillary ostium and anteriorly to the maxillary line. The last portion of bone to be removed is the orbital floor medial to the infraorbital nerve. Downward pressure on the remaining bony rim of the maxillary ostium with a large spoon curette accomplishes this maneuver. The bone typically fractures along the cleavage plane of the infraorbital canal.

A sharp sickle knife is used to incise the periorbita. This is begun posteriorly to avoid fat prolapse obscuring visualization. The tip of the knife must be kept superficial to avoid injury to the extraocular muscles, which are enlarged in patients with Graves' disease. Multiple cuts through periosteum or removal allow herniation of orbital fat into the ethmoid and maxillary sinuses.

### *Local Anesthesia*

In some cases, local anesthesia may be preferred to general anesthesia. These situations include patients with a sole seeing eye, those with significant medical comorbidities, or those with a strong preference for local anesthesia. Ideal sedation is achieved with an intravenous bolus of propofol at 0.4 to 0.8 mg/kg before local injection, followed by a maintenance infusion of 25 to 75 μg/kg during the procedure. Supplemental midazolam may be used to achieve an appropriate level of sedation. Submucosal infiltration of 1% lidocaine with 1:100,000 epinephrine is performed exactly

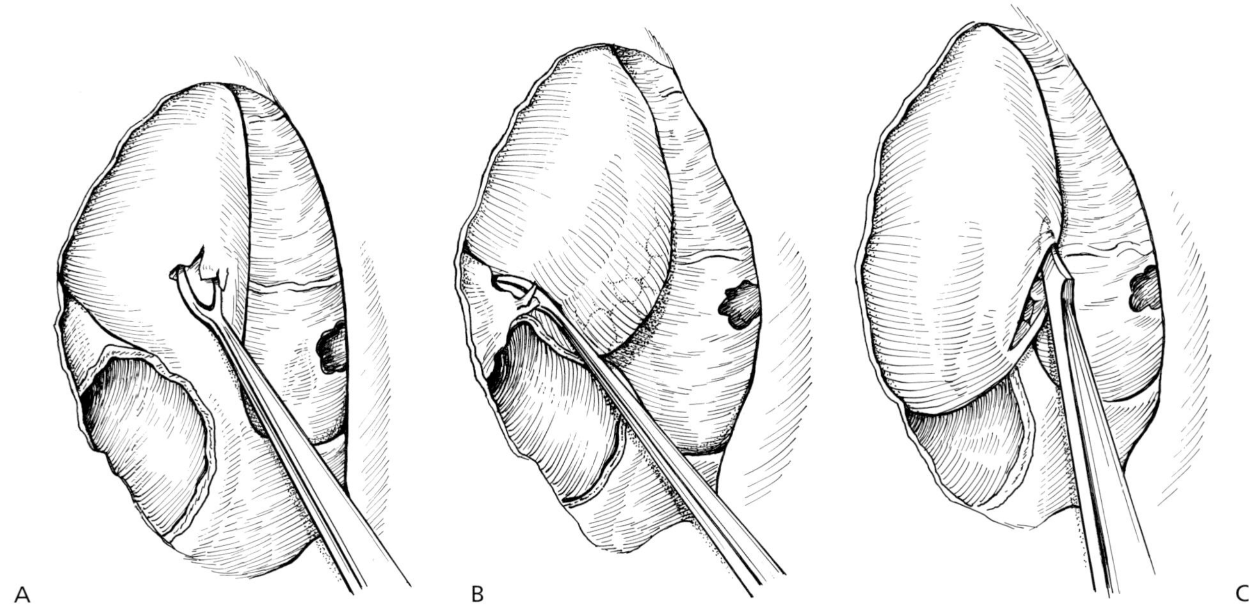


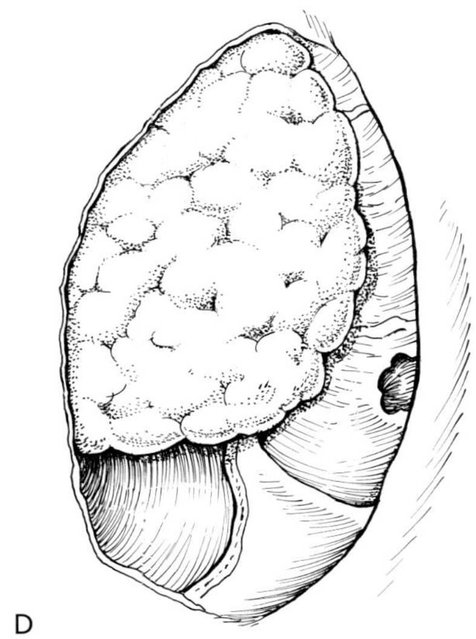


**FIGURE 28.1. A:** After completion of a total sphenoethmoidectomy, removal of the middle turbinate, and skeletonization of the lamina papyracea, the thin bone of the medial orbital wall is removed. **B:** A larger spoon curette is used to downfracture the orbital floor medial to the infraorbital nerve. **C:** After bone has been removed as far posteriorly as the face of sphenoid, the periorbital fascia is incised with a sickle knife. **D:** At the end of the procedure, herniated fat bulges freely into the ethmoid and maxillary sinuses.

as in the procedure under general anesthesia. Regional blocks are usually unnecessary. Patients may report discomfort during removal of the lamina papyracea, and this may require a small additional infiltration of anesthetic solution into the periorbita.

### *Lateral Decompression*

Lateral decompression through a standard Kronlein or an upper eyelid crease incision is performed after medial decompression. This allows retraction of the orbital contents in a medial direction, providing excellent exposure for the lateral bony wall to be excavated or removed. To approach the lateral orbit through the upper lid, the skin is marked as for upper blepharoplasty. The incision is carried laterally enough to gain exposure of the rim. Infiltration is performed with lidocaine 1% with 1:100,000 epinephrine. The lateral rim is exposed from the reflection of the zygomatic arch to the frontozygomatic suture. A deep subperiosteal dissection is created into the orbit to expose the lateral wall, roof, and floor. The canthus is left intact. A high-speed cutting burr is used to excavate the lateral orbital wall while a malleable retractor protects the orbital fat. Bone is removed to the level of the lateral periosteum, the fascia of the temporalis muscle, and to the dura superiorly while leaving the orbital rim intact. Excess orbital fat may be trimmed through this incision as well.

### Reduction in Proptosis

Endoscopic medial decompression results in an average reduction in proptosis of 3.5 mm, whereas combining endoscopic medial and external lateral decompression yields an average reduction of 5.4 mm.

### Postoperative Course

When surgery is completed, visual acuity and extraocular movements are assessed. Nasal packing is avoided. Patients may be discharged in less than 24 hours on oral antibiotics and nasal irrigations with saline. Postoperative cleaning is performed under endoscopic visualization as in routine sinus surgery. In general, bilateral orbital decompressions are performed as a staged procedure at an interval of 1 week.

## Case Example

A female patient with a history of dysthyroid orbitopathy was referred for orbital decompression after failure of radiation therapy to stop progression of optic neuropathy and exposure keratopathy. The two eyes were staged 1 week apart. A medial and medial-inferior wall decompression was performed through an endoscopic transethmoid approach. A lateral modified Kronlein procedure was also performed. Figure 28.2 is a CT scan that demonstrates the ethmoid sinuses and orbital cavities after decompression of the left orbit but before decompression of the right orbit. One week later, these procedures were repeated on the contralateral orbit. Figure 28.3 demonstrates the patient before her initial surgery. Figure 28.4 is the same patient after bilateral decompression and subsequent repair of lid retraction.

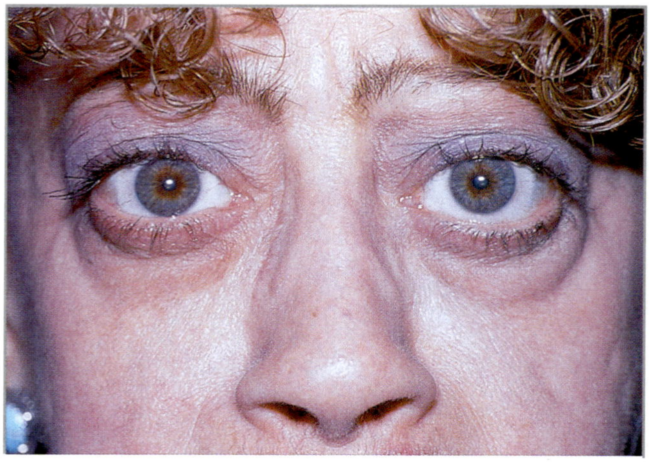

**FIGURE 28.3.** Preoperative photograph of patient with Graves' orbitopathy.

## Complications

There are many potential complications of orbital decompression; most are fortunately rare. Visual loss can occur from hemorrhage or direct optic nerve injury. Poor visualization may lead to infraorbital nerve injury or direct muscle injury. Transient infraorbital nerve paresthesias may follow aggressive downfracture of the medial orbital floor. It is common for strabismus to worsen after any orbital decompression procedure. However, it is difficult to correct secondary enophthalmos from excessive decompression, and this should be avoided. The risk of postoperative epistaxis or cerebrospinal fluid leak are the same as in standard endoscopic sinus procedures. Delayed sinusitis may occur in patients in whom extensive decompression is required. Cre-

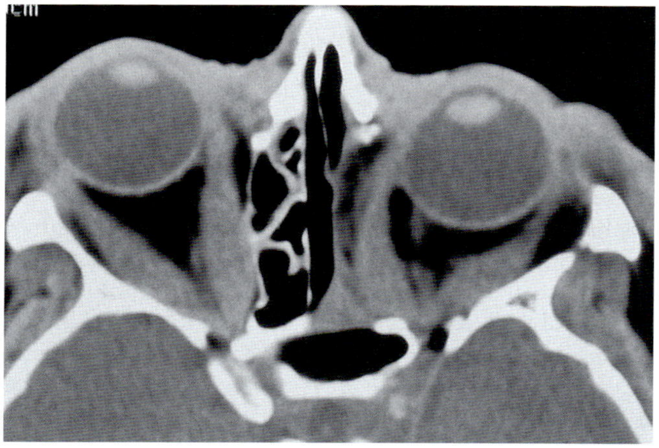

**FIGURE 28.2.** Computed tomography scan of a patient with Graves' orbitopathy after endoscopic decompression of the left orbit but before decompression of the right orbit. Notice the difference in globe proptosis and position of orbital contents.

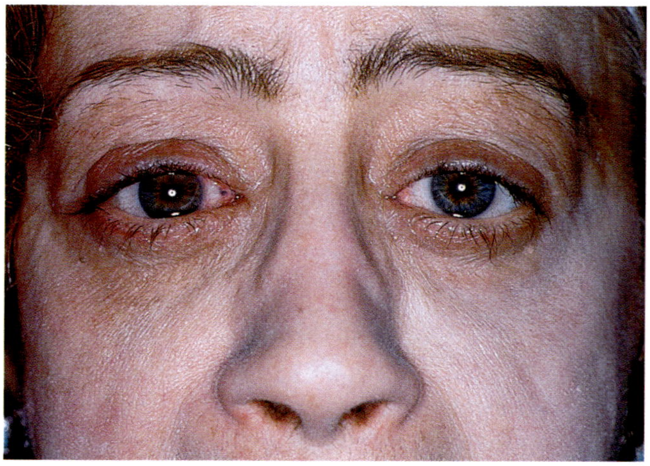

**FIGURE 28.4.** Postoperative photograph of the patient shown in Figure 28.3 after staged bilateral orbital decompression using an endoscopic transethmoid approach for the medial and inferior walls combined with a lateral approach.

ating a large maxillary antrostomy, particularly in its inferior aspect and sparing bone in the lateral frontal recess, may help avoid these difficult problems.

## OPTIC NERVE DECOMPRESSION

Indications for optic nerve decompression are traumatic blindness unresponsive to high-dose steroids and progressive optic neuropathy from fibrous dysplasia or other hyperplasia or neoplasia around the optic canal. Mucoceles, aspergillomas, and allergic fungal sinusitis of the sphenoid sinus can produce gradual bone loss and, rarely, visual loss. Optic nerve decompression is achieved by merely draining the sphenoid. Dysthyroid orbitopathy is associated with optic neuropathy in many cases, but there is disagreement in the literature about whether optic nerve decompression is necessary if adequate orbital decompression is performed. In patients who have suffered trauma with visual loss but without evidence of direct ocular injury, damage to the optic nerve should be considered. Fine-cut CT scans and neuro-ophthalmologic evaluation are necessary components of the workup. Management of the optic nerve in these cases remains controversial. At my institution, surgical optic nerve decompression for traumatic optic neuropathy is considered in patients who have a likely compressive neuropathy that is unresponsive or worsening on megadose steroid therapy or in whom an obvious bone fragment is seen impinging on the optic nerve.

### Endoscopic Approach

The endoscopic approach to optic nerve decompression is largely a continuation of the orbital decompression procedure. After the lamina papyracea has been removed to the level of the face of sphenoid, the optic nerve can be seen in its canal passing toward the opticocarotid recess, which appears as a dimple in the lateral wall of the sphenoid sinus. The fibrous annulus of Zinn begins at the orbital apex. The ophthalmic artery lies inferolateral to the nerve in the bony canal. It gives off the central retinal artery about 10 mm behind the globe. Sofferman (2) has recommended that adequate decompression of the optic nerve requires removal of one half of the circumference of the osseous canal in its entire length. Although in cases of thin bone it is possible to lift the bone from the optic nerve with a curette, a long-handled microdrill with copious irrigation is usually necessary, especially in the anterior portion of the canal. Several new drill burrs with protected shafts are commercially available for this purpose. It is critical to positively identify the position of the carotid artery before drilling begins. The technique my colleagues and I use is largely an endoscopic adaptation of the external procedure described by Joseph (3). The use of an image-guidance system may be helpful in identifying landmark and should be mandatory in cases of fibrous dysplasia in which the nerve and carotid landmarks may be significantly obscured. After the bone has been removed, there is controversy about whether the sheath should be incised. In general, we do not split the sheath.

### *Advantages of the Endoscopic Approach*

The endoscopic approach to optic nerve decompression offers several advantages over the traditional neurosurgical or craniotomy approach and the external orbital and ethmoid approaches. Morbidity is decreased. There is preservation of olfaction, more rapid recovery time, and an acceptable cosmetic result. In a dry field, I think the endoscope provides better visualization of the critical annulus region than an external transethmoid approach because the angle of visualization is less tangential.

Results for surgical optic nerve decompression are generally based on nonrandomized studies. However, the many reports of dramatic results in patients who have failed megadose steroids for 48 hours are compelling reasons to consider this approach in traumatic blindness until a more formal clinical trial is completed.

### Complications

The complications of optic nerve decompression include permanent blindness and injury to the carotid artery within the sphenoid sinus. Deaths have been reported.

## ENDOSCOPIC DECOMPRESSION FOR TRAUMATIC BLOW-OUT FRACTURES

Another reason to use the endoscope in an orbital decompression is in the repair of orbital fractures. The endoscope provides excellent visualization for repair of orbital fractures with or without other incisions such as the transconjunctival approach (4). The use of the endoscope in medial orbital wall fractures is particularly promising. Although blow-out fractures of the orbit are common, entrapment of the medial orbital wall are rare. The recommended approach for these fractures when clinically significant entrapment is present is a limited external ethmoidectomy. An endoscopic approach provides several potential advantages, including avoidance of a medial orbital skin incision, specific localization of the area of entrapment, and a very limited decompression in that zone without additional volume loss. Since January 1995, I have performed this technique for more than a dozen medial orbital blow-out fractures with entrapment.

### Case Example

A 19-year-old college student was struck in the left orbit with a lacrosse ball during athletic practice. The patient suf-

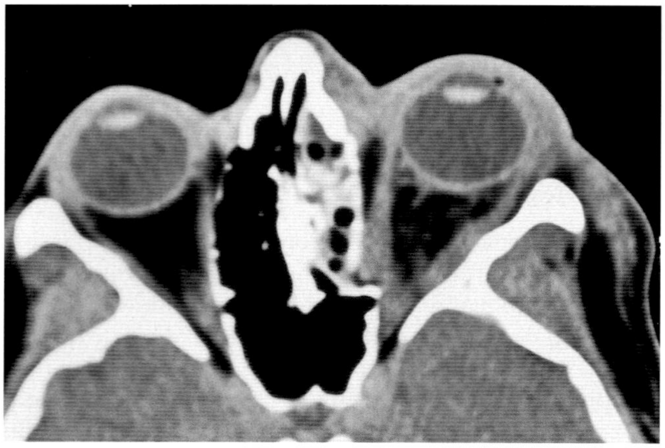

**FIGURE 28.5.** Computed tomography scan of a patient after a medial orbital blow-out fracture with impingement on the medial rectus muscle by a posterior bone fragment. This patient recovered completely after endoscopic decompression of the bone fragment.

fered orbital ecchymosis and edema, but visual acuity was 20/20. She presented 10 days after the initial injury with complaints of horizontal gaze diplopia. Examination revealed limitation predominantly in lateral gaze, with the left globe stopping abruptly while the right eye continued approximately 20 additional degrees. Vertical diplopia was not present, although the left eye was clearly enophthalmic on examination. CT scanning revealed a posterior medial blowout fracture with a bone spicule impacting the medial rectus muscle (Fig. 28.5). A concomitant but separate orbital floor fracture was present.

The patient had no improvement and was taken to the operating room. A large bony fragment of the lamina papyracea crossed the cavity in an oblique manner, pressing directly into the superior aspect of the dehiscent muscle. A blunt elevator was used to separate the bone spicule from the muscle and then the bone was removed. Immediately, the degree of freedom of the medial rectus muscle palpably and visually improved. The floor fracture was repaired through a transconjunctival approach. Forced duction testing was normal at the conclusion of the procedure. The patient was discharged to home the next morning. Postoperatively, the patient has had normal range of extraocular motion without diplopia, and orbital volume is symmetric.

### Complications

Endoscopic limited orbital decompression for entrapment is a more difficult procedure than standard orbital decompression because of the disruption of landmarks, medialization of the orbital wall, and bone fragments that may be in the region of the optic nerve. Extensive experience with standard orbital decompression is recommended before performing this procedure.

## CONCLUSIONS

The nasal endoscope provides an excellent means to approach the orbit for decompression of the orbital walls and the optic nerve. As indications expand for this approach, it is important to remember that the danger associated with these surgeries is high and that the endoscopist must have a comprehensive understanding of the anatomy of the sinus-orbital interface. The advantages of the endoscopic approach to the orbit for the purposes described earlier are clear, and it will likely replace traditional techniques in the future.

## REFERENCES

1. Werner SC. Classification of the eye changes of Graves' disease. *Am J Ophthalmol* 1969;98:646–648.
2. Sofferman RA. Sphenoethmoid approach to the optic nerve. *Laryngoscope* 1981;91:184–196.
3. Joseph MP, Lessell S, Rizzo J, et al. Extracranial optic nerve decompression for traumatic optic neuropathy. *Arch Ophthalmol* 1990;108:1091–1093.
4. Woog JJ, Hartstein ME, Gliklich R. Paranasal sinus endoscopy and orbital floor fracture repair. *Arch Ophthalmol* 1998;116: 688–691.

## SUGGESTED READING

Dallow RL, Netland PA. Management of thyroid ophthalmolopathy (Graves' disease). In: Albert DM, Jacobiec FA, eds. *The principles and practice of ophthalmology*. Philadelphia: WB Saunders, 1993.

Kennedy DW, Goodstein ML, Miller NR, et al. Endoscopic transnasal orbital decompression. *Arch Otolaryngol Head Neck Surg* 1990;116:275–282.

Kountakis SE, Maillard AA, Urso R, Stiernberg CM. Endoscopic approach to traumatic visual loss. *Otolaryngol Head Neck Surg* 1997;116:652–656.

Luxenberger W, Stammberger H, Jebeles JA, Walch C. Endoscopic optic nerve decompression: the Graz experience. *Laryngoscope* 1998;108:873–882.

Metson R, Dallow RL, Shore JW. Endoscopic orbital decompression. *Laryngoscope* 1994;104:950–957.

Metson R, Shore JW, Gliklich RE, Dallow RL. Endoscopic orbital decompression under local anesthesia. *Otolaryngol Head Neck Surg* 1995;113:661–667.

Wilson WB, Manke WF. Orbital decompression in Graves' disease: the predictability of reduction of proptosis. *Arch Ophthalmol* 1991;109:343–345.

# 29

# AVOIDANCE AND MANAGEMENT OF COMPLICATIONS OF ENDOSCOPIC SINUS SURGERY

TIMOTHY L. SMITH
MICHELLE M. SMITH
STEVEN D. SCHAEFER
PATRICIA A. HUDGINS

## AVOIDING COMPLICATIONS

Preparation is a key to avoiding complications. The history and physical examination should be thorough, thoughtful, and well documented. Tools to assist in clinical evaluation such as endoscopy and imaging procedures should be readily available. Review of previous pathology reports, operative reports, and consultation with neuroradiology should be performed in anticipation of surgical intervention. Revision surgical cases require special attention because loss of landmarks and severe disease are present in many of these cases. Computed tomography (CT)-guided (computer-aided) surgery systems may be useful in these cases but require further study before conclusions about prevention of complications can be drawn.

The radiologist plays an important role in the preoperative evaluation of patients undergoing endoscopic sinus surgery. The preoperative CT scan evaluates distribution of disease within the sinuses and obstruction of the ostia of the sinuses. In addition to identifying disease, the radiologist must alert the referring surgeon to the presence of anatomic variations that may predispose the patient to injury at the time of surgery. After endoscopic surgery, imaging may aid in the evaluation of persistent or recurrent disease and in identification of surgical complications. Many minor complications may be managed conservatively with close clinical observation. Severe complications, particularly those involving the orbits and anterior skull base, may require radiographic evaluation.

## PREOPERATIVE EVALUATION

Medical therapy is maximized in patients with chronic sinus disease. Antibiotic therapy should be given for at least 3 to 4 weeks before the patient is considered a treatment failure. Maximum medical treatment is described elsewhere in this textbook, but topical and systemic steroids, decongestants, antihistamines, and mucolytic agents should each be considered in the management of chronic rhinosinusitis. Recalcitrant rhinosinusitis raises the specter of extraesophageal manifestations of gastroesophageal reflux disease, and antireflux medications should be considered. Ulualp and colleagues demonstrated a higher occurrence of pharyngeal reflux of gastric acid by 24-hour, three-site pH monitoring in patients with chronic sinusitis compared with normal controls (1). These patients frequently have no preceding chronic nasal or sinus symptoms. This study supports a high degree of suspicion for reflux disease in selected patients with recalcitrant chronic rhinosinusitis when no other obvious cause is found.

Preoperatively, culture-directed antibiotics are continued to the day of surgery. In patients with significant mucosal inflammation, systemic steroids are initiated at least 1 week preoperatively. Patients are educated regarding the surgeon's desire to medically reduce mucosal inflammation for the day of surgery.

Nasal endoscopy using 0° and 30° endoscopes allows identification of anatomic variants and other obstructions (2,3). Endoscopically guided cultures can also be obtained to maximize medical therapy. Although preoperative sinus CT scanning is generally performed in the coronal plane, axial plane scanning can be helpful in imaging the frontal sinuses, sphenoid ostia, sphenoid septa configurations, sphenoethmoid (Onodi) cells, and carotid artery and optic nerve relationships with the lateral sphenoid wall. Bone dehiscence of the ethmoid roof, frontal sinus, and sphenoid walls requires further evaluation with magnetic resonance imaging (MRI) because encephaloceles, carotid artery aneurysms, and other structures that are unsafe for biopsy may be located adjacent to such defects. Normal anatomy and anatomic variants of the sinuses are further discussed in Chapter 19.

## ANESTHESIA AND HEMOSTASIS

General or local anesthesia can be used for endoscopic sinus surgery and depends on the preferences of the surgeon and patient. For some disease processes, more extensive manipulation of the sinuses is required, and general anesthesia is necessary. Local anesthesia is thought by some surgeons to result in less bleeding, thereby improving visualization. The skull base and orbital contents are difficult to anesthetize, and the patient under local anesthesia usually describes pain during any attempt to breach these barriers. Regardless of local or general anesthesia, excellent hemostasis is critical. Topical vasoconstrictive agents are used, and injections with 1% lidocaine with 1:100,000 epinephrine are used in all cases. Our technique is as follows:

***Step 1:*** Oxymetazoline spray (0.05%) is applied in the holding area. This begins the decongestion process.

***Step 2:*** Cottonoids saturated with oxymetazoline spray (0.05%) are placed intranasally. It is critical that atraumatic technique is used. An attempt is made to place one pledget in the middle meatus. Pledgets are left undisturbed for 10 minutes while the surgeons scrub and the endoscopic instrumentation is prepared. The pledgets are removed, and injections are performed using a 25-gauge spinal needle on a control syringe containing 8 mL of 1% lidocaine with 1:100,000 epinephrine. The tip of the needle is bent to an angle of 30° from parallel.

***Step 3:*** The first injection is near the posterior attachment of the middle turbinate at the site of the sphenopalatine artery (Fig. 29.1). Slow, gentle infusion of 3 mL produces significant blanching of the lateral nasal wall and posterior aspect of the middle turbinate. Alternatively, in cases where the posterior attachment of the middle turbinate cannot be visualized (e.g., polyps, extensive edema), injection of the greater palatine foramen may be necessary. This is performed transorally with an angled, 22-gauge spinal needle. The foramen is most often located medial to the second maxillary molar and may often be palpated with the finger as a depression in the palatal mucosa. Aspiration is required to avoid intraarterial injection. Although this technique is proven and safe, temporary blindness has been reported.

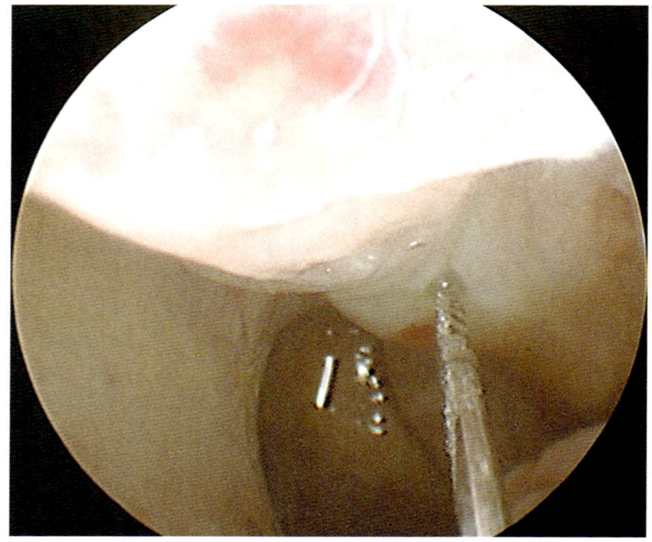

**FIGURE 29.1.** Injection at the posterior attachment of the left middle turbinate.

***Step 4:*** The second injection is to the inferior aspect of the middle turbinate approximately 1.5 cm posterior to the head of the middle turbinate (Fig. 29.2). An attempt is made to direct the needle slightly laterally so that the lateral mucosa of the turbinate receives the agent. A dose of approximately 1.5 to 2 mL is administered.

***Step 5:*** The final injection is to the anterior-superior attachment of the middle turbinate. Slow infusion results in blanching of the anterior aspect of the middle turbinate and the uncinate process (Fig. 29.3).

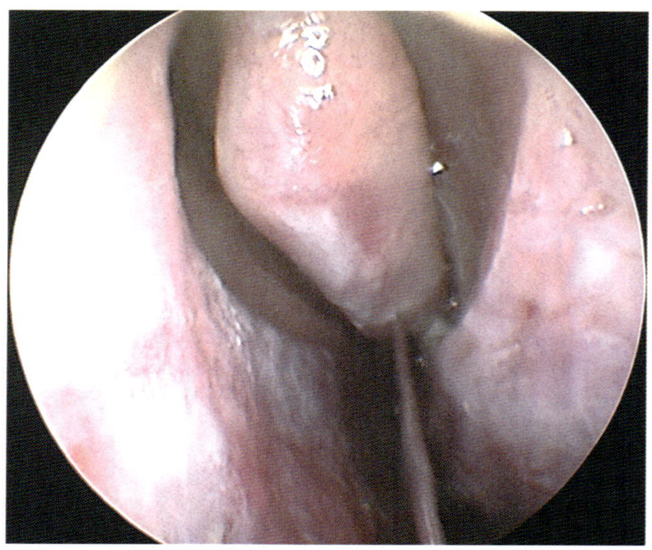

**FIGURE 29.2.** Injection in the middle aspect of the left middle turbinate.

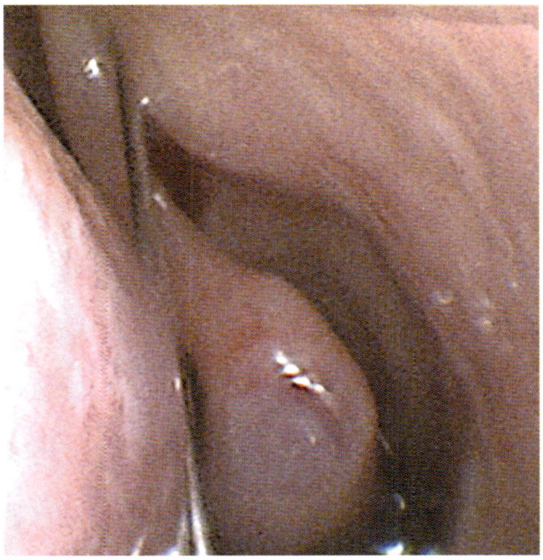

**FIGURE 29.3.** Injection of the anterior-superior attachment of left middle turbinate.

## POSTOPERATIVE CARE

At the conclusion of the operation, all bone fragments are removed, and devitalized bone and mucosa are resected. No packing, sponge, or absorbable materials are required in most cases. Nasal saline irrigations are recommended several times per day, and we routinely reinstitute nasal steroid sprays on the first postoperative day. Antibiotics are directed by culture results from the preoperative period and are adjusted accordingly when microbiology reports from the operation are available. Steroid tapers, initiated at least 1 week before surgery, are continued as dictated by mucosal disease observations at the time of surgery.

The postoperative follow-up for the endoscopic sinus surgery patient is very labor intensive to prevent synechiae and help restore mucociliary clearance. The routine patient is seen on postoperative days 6 and 13 for endoscopic débridement in the office. Crusting, devitalized mucosa, and bone are resected, and any synechiae are lysed. Patients demonstrating signs of adverse scarring, extreme crusting, or ostial stenosis are seen more frequently. Patients generally require weekly follow-up for the first 6 to 8 weeks and then every 1 to 2 months for the first year.

## COMPLICATIONS

### Hemorrhage

In the context of endoscopic sinus surgery, hemorrhage generally occurs in one of three forms: bothersome mucosal oozing, significant hemorrhage from a named vessel, and life-threatening hemorrhage from the carotid artery.

The most common bleeding seen is the bothersome mucosal oozing that may limit visualization and increase operative time occasionally requiring termination of the procedure (4). Prevention and planning are critical to avoiding hemorrhage. Patients should be maximally medically treated preoperatively, including topical and systemic steroids and antibiotics, when indicated to help reduce mucosal inflammation. We educate the patient regarding the risks of bleeding and the implications of bleeding in the context of endoscopic sinus surgery. This helps to improve compliance with preoperative medications that many patients would rather avoid. Patients are informed of the reasons to avoid aspirin and nonsteroidal antiinflammatory drugs 2 weeks before surgery. On the day of surgery, maximum mucosal decongestion is obtained before injections as outlined earlier.

During endoscopic surgery, the surgeon must remember that blood drains along the mucosa from superior to inferior and from anterior to posterior. Atraumatic technique with every endoscopic maneuver and mucosal preservation is paramount.

Significant hemorrhage may occur in sinus surgery because of bleeding from the anterior ethmoid artery, sphenopalatine artery, posterior ethmoid artery, internal carotid artery, or their branches. Careful penetration of the basal lamella at the appropriate level generally avoids injury to the sphenopalatine artery. If the surgeon's approach is too inferior and lateral, the branching sphenopalatine artery may be encountered. Pressure and topical vasoconstrictors followed by judicious use of suction electrosurgery may be sufficient to stop the hemorrhage. Bipolar electrosurgical devices are preferable because heat generation is more localized. Endoscopic ligation of the sphenopalatine artery is effective in recalcitrant cases but is rarely necessary (5,6). Other sites where bleeding may be encountered are where the posterior ethmoid artery traverses the skull base and in the mucosa inferior to the sphenoid ostium where the nasoseptal division of the sphenopalatine artery is located (7). The anterior ethmoid artery may be injured in surgery of the anterior ethmoid cells, most commonly in the frontal recess approach. Avoidance is the rule. These arteries are most commonly within the skull base but may occasionally hang in a sling inferior to the roof of the ethmoid. Transection can result in vigorous hemorrhage. Application of gentle pressure and hemostatic material can be successful. Bipolar electrosurgery may be required in some cases. Suction (unipolar) electrosurgery should not be used to control ethmoid artery bleeding because of the risk of cerebrospinal fluid cerebrospinal fluid (CSF) fistula.

Internal carotid artery injury is devastating and often not survivable. The endoscopic surgeon should approach the sphenoid sinus (or sphenoethmoid cell) with the assumption

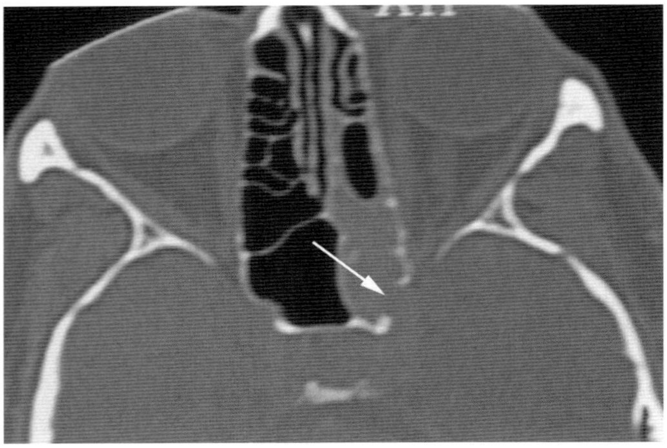

FIGURE 29.4. Axial computed tomography image in a patient after endoscopic surgery. The bone overlying the internal carotid artery *(arrow)* was inadvertently removed during sphenoid surgery.

that the bone covering the internal carotid artery is dehiscent and that any tissue or disease within the sinus is attached to the artery (Fig. 29.4). In the case of carotid artery injury, the "carotid drill" should be used as a guideline for management (8). When significant posterior ethmoid or sphenoid surgery is required, packing material should be readily available in case of severe hemorrhage. In case of carotid injury, quick action and cooperation with neurosurgery and neuroradiology colleagues may save the patient.

Severe postoperative hemorrhage that does not respond to nasal packing and usual management requires diagnostic angiography. Selective contrast injections of the external and internal carotid arteries as well as the internal maxillary artery should be performed. If active bleeding from the internal maxillary artery is identified, the vessel can be temporarily or permanently occluded endovascularly using a variety of thromboembolic agents. Injury to the internal carotid artery itself may occur at the skull base or within the intracranial cavity. Carotid cavernous fistula after endoscopic sinus surgery has been reported (9–11). These injuries should be evaluated with angiography to identify the exact site of injury. If the injury cannot be corrected surgically, sacrifice of the vessel can be performed with permanent occlusion performed endovascularly after a temporary balloon-occlusion test (Fig. 29.5).

## Cerebrospinal Fluid Fistula

CSF leak generally results from injury to the lateral lamella of the cribriform plate, roof of the ethmoid, attempted entry superior to the sphenoid sinus, aggressive superior enlargement of the sphenoidostomy, or avulsion of the superior turbinate with resultant skull base injury. The relationship of the cribriform plate and roof of ethmoid can be quite variable, and careful review of the coronal CT is indicated before surgery. The cribriform plate is lower and is separated from the roof of ethmoid by the vertical insertion of the middle turbinate. The roof of ethmoid slopes inferiorly moving from anterior to posterior. For this reason, dissection in the ethmoid sinuses requires identification of the roof of ethmoid posteriorly and proceeds from posterior to anterior, keeping the skull base under direct view. In the endoscopic approach to the frontal recess, the ethmoid roof and lamina papyracea

A

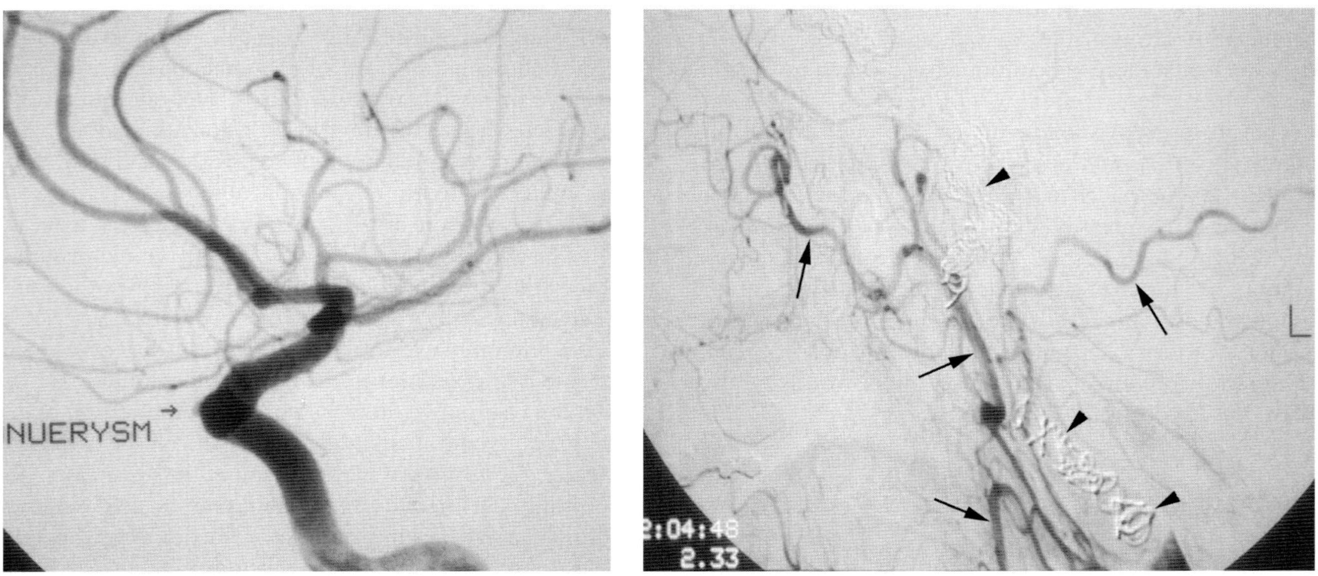


B

FIGURE 29.5. **A:** Lateral projection of a digital subtraction arteriogram during internal carotid artery injection shows a small pseudoaneurysm *(arrow)* projecting anteriorly. **B:** Lateral projection of a digital subtraction arteriogram during common carotid artery injection after coil occlusion of the internal carotid shows filling of the external carotid branches only *(arrows)*. Coils are seen filling the occluded internal carotid artery *(arrowheads)*.

are identified posteriorly, and dissection proceeds from posterior to anterior and medial to lateral. The skull base is quite thin at the lateral lamella of the cribriform plate, particularly where the anterior ethmoid artery penetrates it. Limited dissection in a medial to lateral direction may help prevent injury. Many iatrogenic injuries occur in patients with a deep olfactory fossa (Keros type 3) at the junction of the lateral lamella of the cribriform plate and frontal bone that forms the roof of the ethmoid sinus (12). Care must be taken to avoid injury to the anterior ethmoid artery or breach the posterior and superior boundary of the frontal recess.

Intraoperative recognition of the classic CSF washout of blood in the region of dural injury allows immediate repair without the need for lumbar drainage in most cases. After identifying the location of CSF leakage, the mucous membrane, fragments of bone, and arachnoid must be débrided from around and within the fistula site. Less than meticulous débridement of the fistula results in failure of closure because the graft cannot adhere to the roof of the sinus or because of arachnoid growth into the fistula with preservation of the fistulous tract. Various otologic instruments, including round knives, canal wall elevators, and dissectors, are particularly useful for débriding the fistula. We prefer a free mucosal graft from the contralateral septum bolstered with Surgicel and Gelfoam packing. A nonabsorbable sponge may be placed beneath these absorbable materials for 3 to 5 days. If the middle turbinate must be partially resected for access to the leak, its overlying mucosa makes excellent graft material and can be harvested with a Cottle elevator and fine forceps. These donor sites also provide bone that can be used in larger defects (>6 mm). After harvesting and thinning the graft, the graft is placed in the bone-dura pocket with the mucosal surface facing the nose. Tissue glue or Avitene paste (prepared by mixing Avitene with a small quantity of water) are helpful in adhering the graft to the recipient site. The graft is further held in place by Gelfoam and absorbable packing, such as Surgicel or Oxycel. Intrasphenoid CSF leaks may be treated with fibrin glue with or without mucosal or adipose tissue grafts (13). CT of the head is performed postoperatively to evaluate for intracranial complications, and the patient is placed on bed rest for 48 hours with the head elevated 30°. Stool softeners are used in all cases, and antibiotics are prescribed if nonabsorbable packing is placed.

If the leak is discovered postoperatively and is not profuse, it should be treated conservatively with bed rest and head elevation for several days. If the leak is recognized early in the postoperative period and fails to close with these conservative measures, placement of a lumbar drain may allow for healing and closure. Should spontaneous closure fail to occur, the dural tear may be approached endoscopically in most cases.

Postoperative leaks may occur from a day to several years after the procedure. In patients without obvious rhinorrhea, evidence of a fistula can be elicited by placing the patient in the provocative position, which consists of having the patient place his or her head immediately above the knees while sitting in a chair. After 5 minutes, most patients with clinical CSF rhinorrhea should show evidence of drainage from the nose. Any clear fluid draining from the nose can be collected and analyzed. The simplest form of analysis is to place several drops of the fluid on filter paper or a paper tissue. Cerebrospinal fluid is relatively devoid of the protein present in blood and mucus and should leave a clear, homogeneous ring as the fluid spreads on the paper. When CSF is mixed with blood, a series of concentric rings appear as the fluid is absorbed by the paper. This "ring sign" is problematic because mucus and other body fluids mixed with blood can give a false-positive sign (14). A much more specific test for CSF rhinorrhea is $\beta_2$-transferrin analysis. $\beta_2$-transferrin is only found in CSF, and the presence of this protein in nasal fluid is a definite confirmation of a CSF leak (15). The wide spread use of this test suffers from the lack of laboratories that perform the analysis and from delays in receiving the results (16).

Persistent CSF leaks that do not respond to conservative measures may be evaluated radiographically. In most patients with postoperative CSF leak, the patient has rhinorrhea, and the side of the leak is clinically apparent. Initially, thin-section coronal CT imaging at 2- to 3-mm slice thickness is performed. Identification of a bony defect, particularly if there is fluid or opacification of the sinus or nasal cavity adjacent to the defect, is highly suggestive of the leak site (Fig. 29.6). Scanning after injection of intrathecal contrast administration through lumbar puncture is not neces-

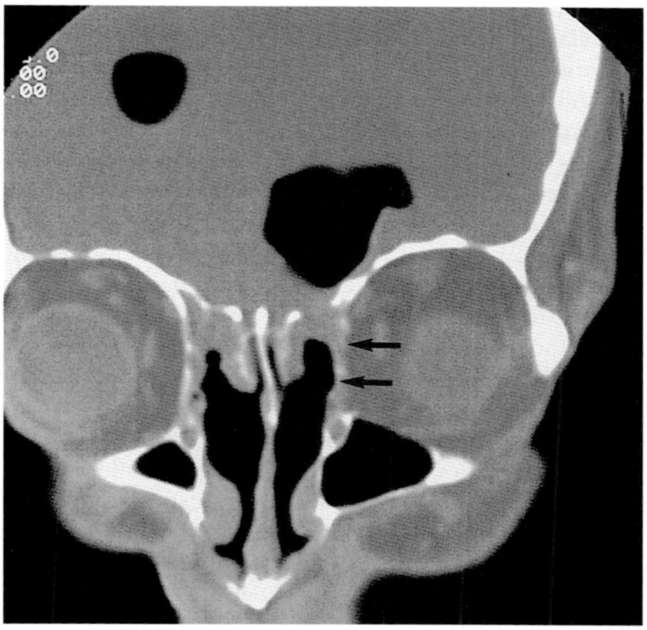

**FIGURE 29.6.** Several hours after endoscopic sinus surgery, this man complained of severe headache. Notice the large, bony dehiscence in the fovea ethmoidalis on the left and the massive pneumocephalus. The lamina papyracea on the left is interrupted (*arrows*), but the patient had no orbital symptoms.

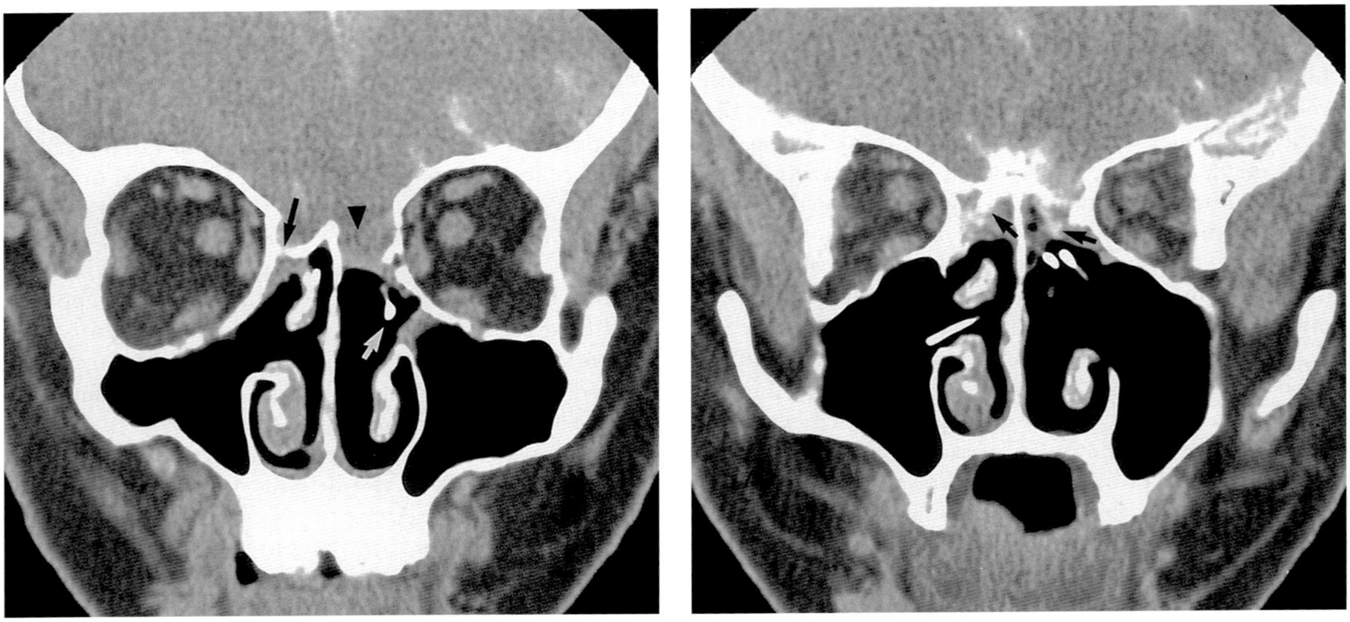


**FIGURE 29.7.** Three months after endoscopic sinus surgery, this man complained of headaches and rhinorrhea. A computed tomography cisternogram was obtained. **A:** At the level of the fovea ethmoidalis, notice the bony dehiscence on the left and the soft tissue filling the roof of the ethmoid complex *(arrowhead)*. The left middle turbinate has been resected, and a pledget *(white arrow)* fills the middle meatus. The fovea ethmoidalis on the right is low lying, with only a small region of bony dehiscence *(black arrow)*. No contrast is seen extravasating into the nasal cavity. **B:** Several millimeters posterior to the site in A, notice the high-density contrast *(arrows)* accumulating in the ethmoid complex, confirming bilateral cerebrospinal fluid leaks at the level of the fovea ethmoidalis.

sarily needed for these patients (17). If clinical symptoms are nonspecific or a clear bony dehiscence is not identified on unenhanced CT, thin-section CT cisternography may be performed. Intrathecal contrast injection (3 to 5 mL of 300 mg I/mL) by means of lumbar puncture is performed, and the patient is placed in a head-down position on the fluoroscopy table. The patient is encouraged to perform any provocative maneuvers that may encourage the leak. Repeat thin-section coronal and axial CT images are then obtained and should be filmed at an intermediate window setting. Contrast accumulation within a sinus or traversing a bony defect is consistent with site of CSF leak (Fig. 29.7). In addition to administration of intrathecal contrast, radionuclide tracer material can be administered intrathecally at the time of lumbar puncture. The radioisotopes used may include radioiodinated human serum albumin (RIHSA) labeled with $^{131}$I-, $^{99m}$Tc-, or Yb-DTPA. Intranasal pledgets are placed by the otolaryngologist before cisternography. After completion of the CT cisternogram, the pledgets are removed and counts are obtained using a gamma camera. Gamma camera images of the patient's head may also be obtained to help localize the side and location of the leak, but spatial resolution is quite limited compared with CT. The iodinated contrast and radionuclide cisternogram techniques require that the patient be actively leaking at the time of the study.

## Intracranial Injury

Intracranial injuries are rare and occur when the anterior skull base is breached. These injuries result in pneumocephalus, extraaxial hemorrhage, cerebral parenchymal hematoma, intracranial arterial injury, ventricular perforation, encephaloceles, cerebritis, and cerebral abscess formation (Fig. 29.8). In patients suspected of having pneumo-

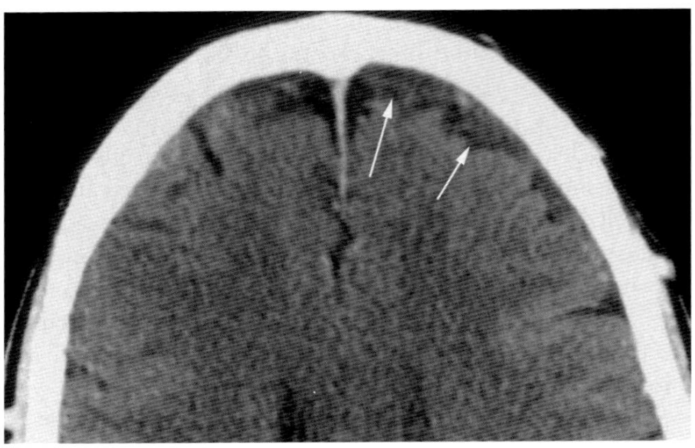

**FIGURE 29.8.** Computed tomography scan of a patient shows subdural blood *(arrows)* adjacent to the left frontal lobe after a breach of the sphenoid roof during endoscopic surgery.

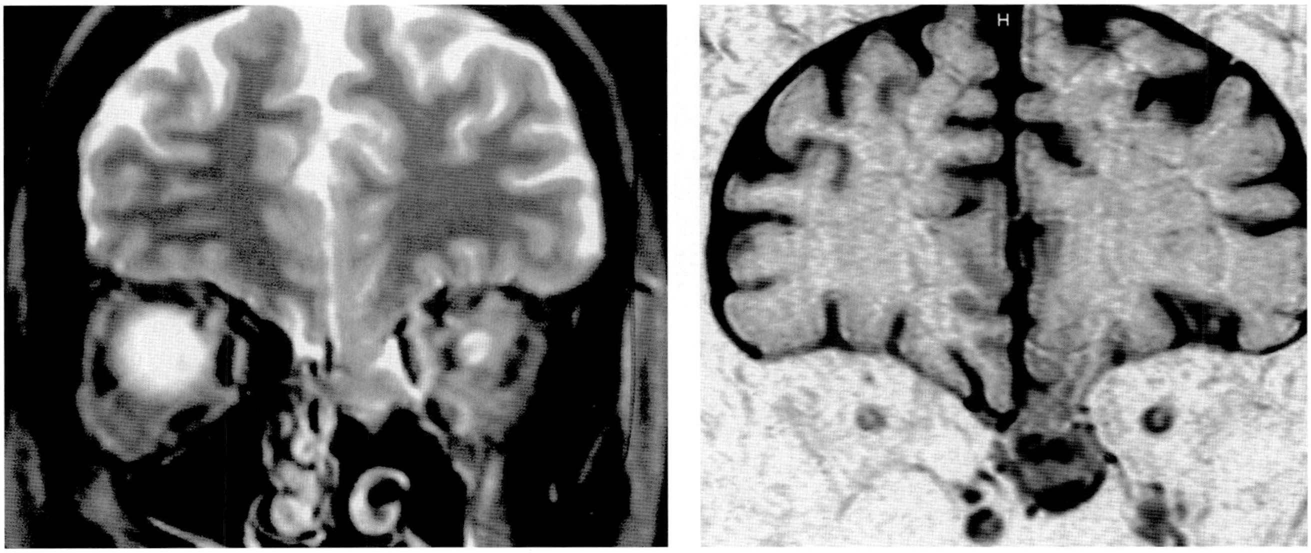


**FIGURE 29.9.** This adult complained of rhinorrhea a year after endonasal sinus surgery. Magnetic resonance imaging (MRI) was performed to characterize signal intensity of soft tissue seen on a computed tomography scan of the left fovea ethmoidalis. **A:** On fast spin-echo T2-weighted, coronal MRI, the soft tissue filling the left ethmoid complex is isointense to brain. Meningoencephalocele was confirmed at surgery. **B:** Fluid-attenuated inversion recovery image shows downward herniation of the frontal gyri.

cephalus or intracranial hemorrhage, unenhanced CT imaging of the head is recommended. If subarachnoid or parenchymal hemorrhage is identified on this study, cerebral angiography should be performed to exclude an arterial injury. MRI is recommended for the evaluation of postoperative infection and to exclude the presence of an encephalocele or meningocele (Fig. 29.9).

The anterior communicating artery lies in the anterior aspect of the suprasellar cistern, and injury results in significant hemorrhage. These injuries are likely to cause death. If cranial vault penetration occurs, immediate neurosurgical consultation is indicated.

In all injuries of the skull base, the patient should be instructed to avoid nose blowing and sneezing, because pneumocephalus may occur (Figs. 29.10 and 29.11).Fortunately, pneumocephalus most often resolves spontaneously, but tension pneumocephalus requires immediate neurosurgical consultation.

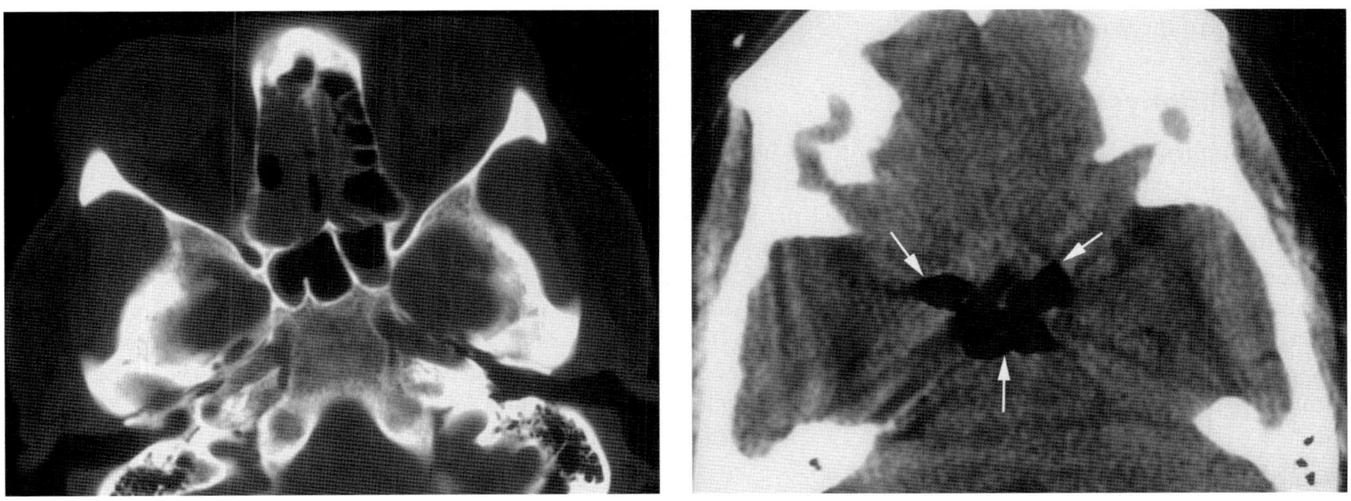


**FIGURE 29.10. A:** Axia computed tomography (CT) with bone window technique shows changes after a right ethmoidectomy. Fluid and mucosal disease nearly opacifies the ethmoidectomy cavity. **B:** Axial CT of the head with soft tissue technique shows pneumocephalus within the suprasellar cistern *(arrows)* that resulted from a breach of the skull base during surgery.

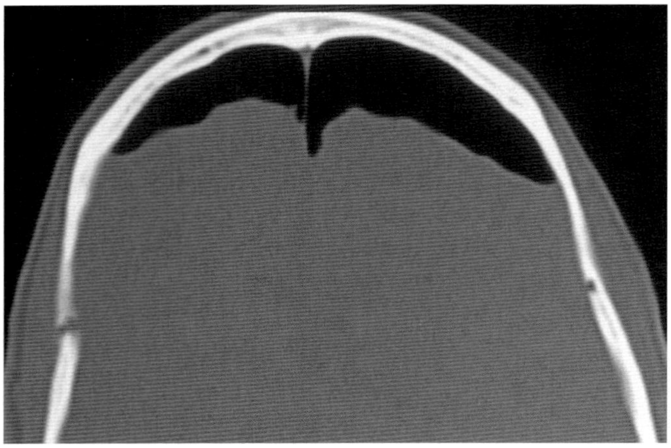

**FIGURE 29.11.** Axial computed tomography shows bifrontal pneumocephalus afte· a breach of the fovea ethmoidalis occurred during endoscopic ethmoidectomy.

## Orbital Hemorrhage

Orbital hemorrhage generally occurs in one of two forms: slow venous or rapid arterial bleeding. Slow venous hemorrhage may take several hours to fully develop and generally responds to medical management with ophthalmology consultation, removal of any packing, orbital massage, intravenous mannitol (1 to 2 gm/kg over 30 to 60 minutes) and acetazolamide (500 mg) (18).

Arterial bleeding results in rapid proptosis and orbital tension. Immediate action is required to prevent permanent sequelae. An immediate ophthalmology consultation is initiated along with the medical therapy described for slow venous hemorrhage. Surgical management may be necessary if excessive orbital pressures continue and includes lateral canthotomy. Orbital decompression along with incision of the periorbita is done with the approach most comfortable to the surgeon.

## Orbital Emphysema

Orbital emphysema results from breach of the lamina papyracea with entrance of air into the orbit because of a Valsalva maneuver, nose blowing, or anesthesia masking. The patient and anesthesiologist must be carefully instructed to avoid maneuvers that result in worsening of the emphysema. This complication generally resolves spontaneously over 7 to 10 days. Anecdotal reports of severe subcutaneous emphysema extending to the abdomen have required several weeks to completely resolve.

## Nasolacrimal Duct Injury

Identification of the natural ostium of the maxillary sinus is critical to success in endoscopic sinus surgery. The natural ostium is typically located 1 cm posterior to the nasolacrimal duct, but it can be as close as a few millimeters. If the natural ostium requires enlargement, it is most safely enlarged posteriorly into the fontanelle. If anterior enlargement is necessary, the relatively hard bone of the nasolacrimal duct may be encountered and accidentally injured or transected. Especially in the early years after the introduction of endoscopic sinus surgery in the United States, nasolacrimal duct injury occurred more often than realized (19). Most of these injuries result in fistulization and proper function of the duct. Stenosis or obstruction of the duct typically presents with epiphora or dacryocystitis. Probing and dilation of the duct may remedy the situation, but dacryocystorhinostomy may be required (20).

## Extraocular Muscle Injury

Extraocular muscle injury may occur during endoscopic sinus surgery from disruption of the lamina papyracea with breach of the periorbita during ethmoidectomy or in patients with posttraumatic or congenital dehiscence of the bone. Movement of the globe during endoscopic surgery can be seen during manipulation of these muscles. Patients typically present with diplopia that may have resulted from direct muscle injury (primarily the medial rectus) or injury to nerves or blood vessels of the extraocular muscles by instrumentation or lasers and electrosurgical devices. CT and MRI can be used to assess injury to the extraocular muscles and to evaluate the presence of orbital hematoma that may occur in these cases (Fig. 29.12). Swelling of the muscle, increased density within the muscle belly, stranding in the adjacent fat, and frank disruption of the muscle belly are all radiographic indicators of extraocular muscle injury. Intraorbital fat may protrude through the defect in the lamina papyracea and orbital emphysema may be detected at CT.

These injuries can be temporary in some cases, with only edema of the muscle. Persistent symtoms require early ophthalmology evaluation before fibrosis and calcification occur.

## Orbital Abscess or Phlegmon

Orbital abscess or phlegmon is uncommon after surgery and can manifest with proptosis, decreased motility, or cavernous sinus thrombosis, if progressive. Contrast-enhanced CT or MRI can be used to evaluate postoperative intraorbital infection and its complications (Fig. 29.13). Phlegmon and abscess can have similar imaging appearances. Strandy enhancement within the orbital fat, extraocular muscle enlargement from myositis, or a frank rim-enhancing collection are findings seen in patients with postoperative orbital infection.

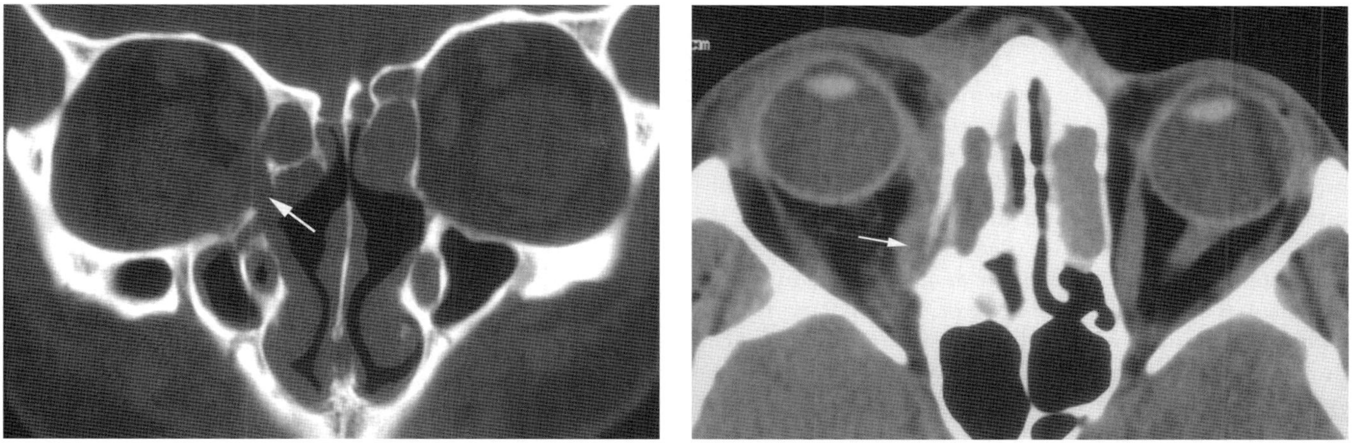

A B

**FIGURE 29.12. A:** Coronal computed tomography with bone window technique shows a focal dehiscence in the right lamina papyracea *(arrow)* (after endoscopic ethmoidectomy). **B:** Axial soft tissue image in the same patient shows a small hematoma *(arrow)* at the site of the bony defect.

## Optic Nerve Injury

Postoperative blindness may be the result of acute intraorbital hematoma or direct injury of the optic nerve. Acute orbital hematoma resulting from injury to the anterior ethmoidal artery is usually quite apparent clinically. It is a surgical emergency requiring immediate intervention without the need for imaging. Transection of the optic nerve is a rare complication of endoscopic sinus surgery. CT or MRI may show frank disruption of the nerve. If the nerve is not completely transected, imaging findings may be subtle, particularly with CT. MRI with gadolinium and fat-saturation technique is recommended in these cases to identify subtle enhancement within the nerve. On MRI, increased T2 signal within the nerve consistent with edema can indicate injury.

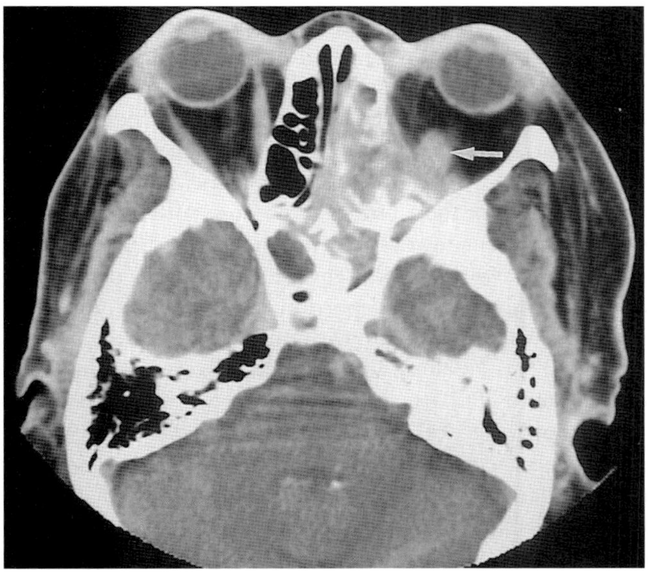

**FIGURE 29.13.** Contrast-enhanced, axial computed tomography of a patient after ethmoidectomy shows a breach in the left lamina papyracea and orbital phlegmon. There is ill-defined enhancement of soft tissue *(arrow)* in the left orbital apex and inflammatory changes in the surrounding fat. Inflammatory disease persists within the left ethmoid labyrinth.

Although the optic nerve is more likely injured in the posterior ethmoid region, surgical trauma may also occur when the lateral sphenoid wall is instrumented. Immediate ophthalmology consultation is critical, and optic nerve decompression may be necessary (21).

## Temporary Blindness from Injection

Injection of the greater palatine foramen has resulted in rare instances of temporary visual deficits. Although frightening for the patient and surgeon, all episodes have reversed within 2 hours after surgery. It is critical to distinguish this self-limiting blindness from that caused by direct optic nerve injury or orbital hematoma. As with all orbital complications, it is desirable to have a good working relationship with ophthalmology colleagues before performing difficult endoscopic cases.

## Olfactory Impairment

Olfactory impairment may result from overresection of the superior turbinate or avulsion of olfactory neuroepithelium from the olfactory cleft. If superior turbinate resection is required, the resection should be minimized and through-cutting instruments should be used to prevent stripping of olfactory neuroepithelium (22,23).

### Turbinate Destabilization and Lateralization

The anatomic attachments of the middle turbinate must be well understood to avoid destabilization and subsequent lateralization. Careful penetration of the basal lamella with preservation of the middle turbinate's lateral attachment can prevent destabilization in most cases. Despite this, at the conclusion of the case, the surgeon should verify turbinate stability. Two options are available for an unstable turbinate. The first is placement of a temporary spacer within the middle meatus (the medial mucosa of the turbinate and opposing septal mucosa are scored to allow synechiae formation in some cases). The second option is partial resection of the middle turbinate (24).

## SPECIAL POINTS

The patient's eyes should be left uncovered during endoscopic surgery to allow orbital movement or changes to be immediately recognized. Penetration of the lamina papyracea typically results in orbital fat protrusion (Fig. 29.14). When orbital fat is recognized, it should be avoided and left untouched. No attempt should be made to remove the fat or reduce the orbital contents back into the orbit. If there is a question about whether the tissue is orbital fat, endoscopic visualization of the tissue while palpating the globe with the other hand can reveal protrusion and reduction of the orbital fat in most cases. If there is any question, the tissue should not be manipulated and assumed to be orbital fat. In this situation, the patient almost always has a small amount of ecchymosis in the medial canthal area, but unless there is gross herniation or bleeding, there will be no other sequelae. If there is any concern about potential hemorrhage into the orbit, the globe should be carefully inspected. If there is significant hemorrhage or if it is uncertain, an immediate ophthalmologic consultation should be obtained. If there is definite hemorrhage with progressive proptosis, an immediate lateral canthotomy should be performed.

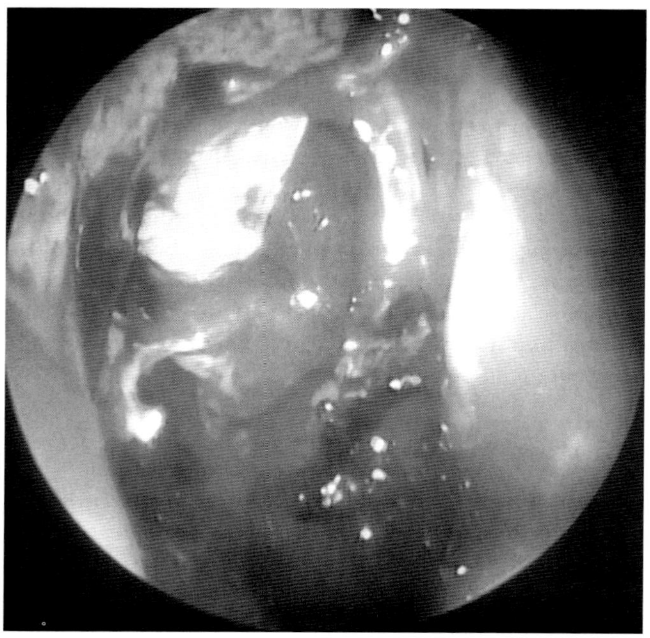

**FIGURE 29.14.** Right ethmoid sinuses with adipose tissue protruding from the lamina papyracea.

When dissecting posterior to the basal lamella in the posterior ethmoid sinus or in the sphenoid sinus, there is potential for injury to the medial rectus muscle and the optic nerve. No dissection should be performed, except where visualization is excellent.

Unless the natural ostium of the sphenoid sinus is directly visualized, opening of the anterior wall of the sphenoid sinus should always be preceded by measurement with a beaded probe or other instrument to confirm appropriate measurements. The most constant relationship is the fact that the distance from a fixed point such as the nasal spine to the posterior wall of the nasopharynx is greater than the distance from that point to the face of the sphenoid at an angle of 30°.

Disease and soft tissue within the sphenoid sinus can be instrumented and removed after a wide sphenoidostomy is created. However, many surgeons think that polypoid disease that is adherent to the superior, lateral, and posterior walls is better left unresected rather than risk injury to the carotid artery.

Vital structures such as the carotid artery and optic nerve tend to be more exposed in well-pneumatized sinuses (25). In a cadaver study of 30 specimens, the carotid produced an identifiable bulge in the lateral wall in 93% (26). The optic nerve protruded into the superolateral aspect of the sphenoid in 100%. In 3% to 5% of specimens, there was no bony covering of these critical structures. Although the rate of true dehiscence varies in a number of studies, the findings of a "very thin bony covering" and true dehiscence occur in a significant proportion of patients. Bony septa may deviate and insert into the bony covering of the carotid artery (13% to 40%) or into the bony covering of the optic nerve (3% to 7%).

Ethmoid cells can pneumatize lateral and to some extent superior to the sphenoid sinus. In these cases, these posterior ethmoid cells are known as sphenoethmoid cells or Onodi cells (27). The optic nerve and carotid artery are often exposed in these cells, and attempts to locate the sphenoid sinus posterior to these cells can place these critical structures in harms way. The optic nerve may be prominent within the lateral wall of other posterior ethmoid cells as well. Many experienced endoscopic surgeons feel that the optic nerve is at greater risk during ethmoid surgery than sphenoid surgery.

## CONCLUSIONS

Prevention of complications begins in the preoperative evaluation period using maximum medical management and resources available to the surgeon such as endoscopy and advanced imaging techniques. Thorough review of all available information allows the surgeon to devise a thoughtful plan of surgical treatment with recognition of potential complications. Despite our best efforts, all surgeons experience complications. Successful management requires early recognition and treatment, with involvement of our colleagues in related specialties when indicated.

## REFERENCES


1. Ulualp SO, Toohill RJ, Hoffmann R, et al. Possible relationship of gastroesophagopharyngeal acid reflux with pathogenesis of chronic sinusitis. *Am J Rhinol* 1999;13:197–202.
2. Sethi DS, Lau DPC, Chee LWJ, et al. Isolated sphenoethmoid recess polyps. *J Laryngol Otol* 1998;112:660–663.
3. Sethi DS. Isolated sphenoid lesions: diagnosis and management. *Otolaryngol Head Neck Surg* 1999;120:730–736.
4. Stankiewicz JA. Complications of endoscopic sinus surgery and malpractice. In: Stankiewicz JA, ed. *Advanced endoscopic sinus surgery*. St. Louis: Mosby–Year Book, 1995:151–160.
5. Snyderman CH, Goldman SA, Carrau RL, et al. Endoscopic sphenopalatine artery ligation is an effective method of treatment for posterior epistaxis. *Am J Rhinol* 1999;13:137–140.
6. Bolger WE, Borgie RC, Melder P. The role of the crista ethmoidalis in endoscopic sphenopalatine artery ligation. *Am J Rhinol* 1999;13:81–86.
7. Lang J. *Clinical anatomy of the nose, nasal cavity, and paranasal sinuses*. New York: Thieme Medical Publishers, 1989.
8. Sofferman R. Complications: prevention and management-carotid artery and optic nerve injury. Presented at the First International Symposium on Contemporary Sinus Surgery, Pittsburgh, Pennsylvania, November 4–6, 1990.
9. Hudgins PA, Browning DG, Gallup J, et al. Endoscopic paranasal sinus surgery: radiographic evaluation of severe complications. *AJNR Am J Neuroradiol* 1992;13:1161–1167.
10. Maniglia AJ. Fatal and major complications secondary to nasal and sinus surgery. *Laryngoscope* 1989;99:276–283.
11. Stankiewicz JA. Complications of endoscopic sinus surgery. *Otolaryngol Clin North Am* 1989;22:749–758.
12. Keros P. [Problem.] [Serbo-Croatian (Roman)]. *Lijec Vjesn* 1969; 91:921–923.
13. Stankiewicz JA. Cerebrospinal fluid fistula and endoscopic sinus surgery. *Laryngoscope* 1991;101:250–254.
14. Dula DJ, Fales W. The "ring sign": is it a reliable indicator for cerebral spinal fluid? *Ann Emerg Med* 1993;22:718–720.
15. Irajala K, Suoupaa J, Laurent B. Identification of CSF leakage by immunofixation. *Arch Otolaryngol* 1979;105:447–448.
16. Skedros DG, Cass SP, Hirsch BE, et al. Beta-2 transferrin assay in clinical management of cerebral spinal fluid and perilymphatic fluid leaks. *J Otolaryngol* 1993;22:341–344.
17. Hudgins PA. Complications of endoscopic sinus surgery: the role of the radiologist in prevention. *Radiol Clin North Am* 1993;31: 21–32.
18. Jones KR. Complications of endoscopic sinus surgery. In: Weissler MC, Pillsbury HC, eds. *Complications of head and neck surgery*. New York: Thieme Medical Publishers, 1995:90–93.
19. Bolger WE, Parsons DS, Mair EA, et al. Lacrimal drainage system injury in functional endoscopic sinus surgery: incidence, analysis, and prevention. *Arch Otolaryngol Head Neck Surg* 1992; 118:1179–1184.
20. Rice DH. Endoscopic intranasal dacryocystorhinostomy results in four patients. *Arch Otolaryngol Head Neck Surg* 1990;116: 1061.
21. Luxenberger W, Stammberger H, Jebeles JA, et al. Endoscopic optic nerve decompression: the Graz experience. *Laryngoscope* 1998;108:873–882.
22. Bolger WE, Keyes AS, Lanza DC. Use of the superior meatus and superior turbinate in the endoscopic approach to the sphenoid sinus. *Otolaryngol Head Neck Surg* 1999;120:308–313.
23. Orlandi RR, Lanza DC, Bolger WE, et al. The forgotten turbinate: the role of the superior turbinate in endoscopic sinus surgery. *Am J Rhinol* 1999;13:251–259.
24. Fortune DS, Duncavage JA. Incidence of frontal sinusitis following partial middle turbinectomy. *Ann Otol Rhinol Laryngol* 1998; 107:447–453.
25. Cheung DK, Attia EL, Kirkpatrick DA, et al. An anatomic and CT scan study of the lateral wall of the sphenoid sinus as related to the transnasal transethmoid endoscopic approach. *J Otolaryngol* 1993;22:63–68.
26. Sethi DS, Stanley RE, Pillay PK. Endoscopic anatomy of the sphenoid sinus and sella turcica. *J Laryngol Otol* 1995;109: 951–955.
27. Elwany S, Elsaeid I, Thabet H. Endoscopic anatomy of the sphenoid sinus. *J Laryngol Otol* 1999;113:122–126.

# 30

# MINIMALLY INVASIVE NONENDOSCOPIC SINUS SURGERY

**WILLIAM LAWSON**
**ANTHONY J. REINO**

The spectrum of sinus surgical procedures includes external, transantral, endonasal, and transcranial procedures. Although the trend is toward endoscopic procedures because of their less invasive nature, they have not totally supplanted traditional surgery for sinus disease, similar to what has occurred in other surgical disciplines. The advantages of the endoscope, which include intense illumination, magnification, and an angular field of vision, have led to its use to render the traditional procedures less invasive. Examples of the adjunctive use of the endoscope modifying traditional procedures are the external frontoethmoidectomy and the Caldwell-Luc operation. Selection of a surgical procedure is often based on the training and experience of the surgeon, the disease process encountered, and medical conditions and other factors idiosyncratic to the individual patient. Consequently, the indications for a particular procedure or operative route are highly variable. The procedures to be discussed can be performed through incisions approximately 1 inch long with no or minimal cosmetic or functional deficits. These procedures provide a margin of safety, afford direct exposure, and permit a two-portal approach using endoscopic enhancement. The latter may employ eyepiece or television screen visualization.

## EXTERNAL FRONTOETHMOIDECTOMY

### Historical Background

Throughout the past century, the surgical management of frontal sinus disease has shifted between external and intranasal approaches. In the late nineteenth century, Ogston (1) advocated external trephination of the frontal sinus with placement of a drainage tube into the nose. Shortly thereafter, Hinkel (2) reported the successful application of this procedure in a patient with frontal sinusitis.

The transorbital approach to the frontal sinus through its inferior wall was first employed in Europe by Jansen (3) in 1902 and by Ritter (4) in 1911. In 1908, Knapp (5) described the procedure in the American literature virtually in its present form; however, other workers have received eponymic credit for it.

More aggressive external approaches to the frontal sinus involved obliteration of part or the entire sinus by collapsing its anterior wall. This invariably resulted in severe cosmetic deformity (6–9). Using an external approach, Lothrop (10) attempted to circumvent a nonfunctioning nasofrontal duct on one side by removing the intersinus septum and sinus floor, providing ventilation and drainage through the healthy contralateral sinus.

The lack of success with these external approaches led for a brief period to intranasal surgery to open the frontal recess. However, this was criticized by Mosher (11) and Lynch (12), and the trend returned to external operations.

In 1921, Lynch (12) in the United States and Howath (13) in England simultaneously reported their experience with the transorbital frontal sinusotomy and ethmoidectomy. In his 15 cases, Lynch (12) partially removed the sinus floor, curetted all the mucosa, and stressed drainage of the sphenoid sinus. Howarth (13), in his review of more than 200 cases, resected the entire floor of the sinus, did not remove the mucosa, and stressed the importance of a preliminary intranasal ethmoidectomy. Both workers temporarily placed a rubber tube drain in the nose. The operative procedure has remained essentially unchanged since the early part of the century and to this day continues to have many advocates.

In the modification of the procedure proposed by Sewall (14), a portion of the lacrimal bone and frontal process was retained as an osteoplastic flap. Lillie and Williams (15) observed that, after extensive removal of bone in the Lynch operation, the soft tissue surrounding the orbit had a tendency to produce closure of the nasofrontal opening and isolation of the lateral portion of large frontal sinuses. Lillie and Williams (15) suggested that preservation of the frontal process of the maxilla would prevent this from occurring. Lillie (16) became the chief proponent of this procedure and made other modifications.

Lillie (16) advocated a two-stage operation beginning with an intranasal ethmoidectomy and removal of sinonasal disease. When an adequate intranasal operation and communication with the frontal sinus were achieved, he noticed that the disease would often resolve, eliminating the need for further procedures. If unsuccessful, an external frontal sinus operation was performed secondarily. Surgeons were urged to recognize that disease commonly occurred in the frontal and ethmoid sinuses and that the surgical procedure should be designed to eliminate pathology at both sites. Lillie (16) advocated complete removal of diseased mucosa but emphasized that total removal of the lining membrane of the frontal, ethmoid, or both sinuses was not necessary to achieve a good postoperative result. He considered the removal of all the mucosa from the frontal-ethmoid-sphenoid complex time consuming and valueless.

Subsequently, Williams and Holman (17) advocated the Lynch procedure with a mucosal rotation flap from the nasal cavity (Sewall-Hall-Boyden flap) for resurfacing the nasofrontal duct. Porto and Duvall (18) reported favorable results with this approach.

In 1987, Neel and colleagues (19) described a modification of the Lynch operation. The procedure begins with an intranasal ethmoidectomy, with the maxillary and sphenoid sinuses entered and curetted when disease was present. Through an exterior incision, the lacrimal bone is removed, as is the anterior floor of the frontal sinus. Anterior ethmoid cells are also removed to enlarge the opening so that the frontal sinus and its nasal communication can be examined. A rim of frontal sinus floor usually is spared laterally and medially.

An important difference of the Neel-Lake procedure is preservation of the frontal process of the maxilla to prevent medial collapse of the soft parts of the orbit. Other features of this procedure are preservation of the normal mucoperiosteal lining of the nasofrontal duct and the intersinus septum in unilateral disease and the middle turbinate. The newly formed frontonasal communication is stented with rolled Silastic sheeting.

## Indications

This procedure has been applied to the management of acute inflammatory disease of the frontal and ethmoid sinuses when there has been orbital extension of the process. This is especially true for a posttarsal complication, such as seen in subperiosteal and orbital abscesses and orbital cellulitis (Fig. 30.1), in which increased intraocular pressure requires rapid and complete decompression. The external approach permits removal of the sinus disease, drainage of the abscess, and decompression of the orbit by removal of bone and incision of the periorbita as required.

With chronic disease of the frontal sinus, it represents a less invasive alternative to the osteoplastic flap when previous endoscopic surgery has been unsuccessful. For small frontal sinuses in which template construction and performing a conventional osteoplastic flap may be technically difficult, the external frontoethmoidectomy procedure provides a method of removing all the diseased mucosa. However, a patent nasofrontal duct is necessary because total

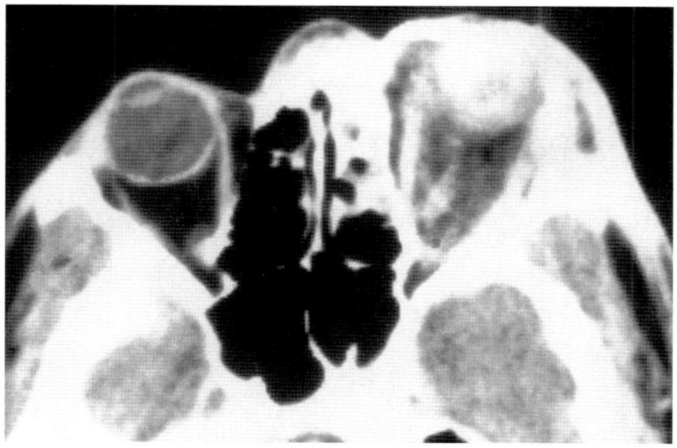

**FIGURE 30.1.** Axial computed tomography scan of orbital cellulitis. Notice the proptosis, distortion, and enhancement of the orbital contents and the opacification of adjacent ethmoid cells.

auto-obliteration of the sinus by fibrous and osseous disease does not always occur, and a secondary mucocele may result. In selected cases, the frontal sinus may be obliterated with fat from below after the cavity has been drilled out to remove any mucosal remnants. Conversely, large mucoceles with intracranial extension lend themselves to this procedure because decompression shrinks the lesion, making an osteoplastic flap less invasive and safer to perform. Some workers recommend endonasal marsupialization of mucoceles with erosion of the posterior table of the frontal sinus, but we favor isolation of the sinus by fat obliteration to shield the dura in such cases. Large frontal mucoceles with intracranial extension often are encountered in patients with allergic fungal sinusitis. This condition is characterized by the occurrence of multiple expansile mucoceles in several sinuses (Figs. 30.2 and 30.3). The external frontoethmoidectomy is a highly effective method of removing the extensive disease in the involved sinus and of providing drainage and ventilation into the nasal cavity. In patients with invasive chronic fungal sinusitis, the external approach permits the direct and safe removal of fungal elements and granulation tissue that have extended into the orbit and along the skull base. The external approach also provides a direct approach for the removal of frontoethmoidal mucoceles (Figs. 30.4 and 30.5) and osteomas (Fig. 30.6). Case selection and experience determine whether an endonasal or external approach is used. The endoscopic and external procedures require long-term patency of the opening created into the nasal cavity.

The external ethmoidectomy also provides wide-field exposure of the floor of the anterior cranial fossa for the detection and repair of cerebrospinal fluid (CSF) leaks and the resection of encephaloceles (Figs. 30.7 and 30.8). It permits bimanual instrumentation with an endoscope or a microscope through two portals in the management of these cases (Fig. 30.9). This is especially true in patients with a narrow nasal vault that may limit the introduction of the endoscope and instruments in a purely nasal approach.

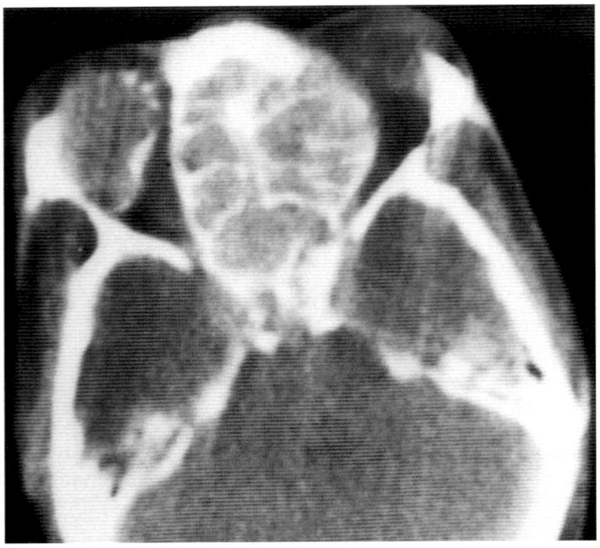

**FIGURE 30.2.** Axial computed tomography scan of a patient with fungal sinusitis who has multiple polypoid mucoceles of the ethmoid sinuses. Notice the expansion of the sinus cavities with preservation of the bony septa.

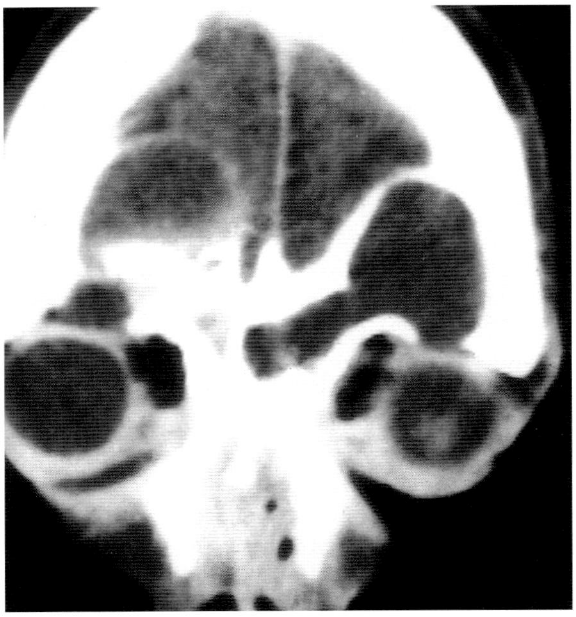

**FIGURE 30.3.** Coronal computed tomography scan of the patient in Figure 30.2 with multisinus polypoid mucoceles. Notice the intracranial extension of bilateral frontal mucoceles with remodeling of the bony walls. Bilateral mucoceles arising in supraorbital ethmoid cells have expanded into the orbits, displacing the globes.

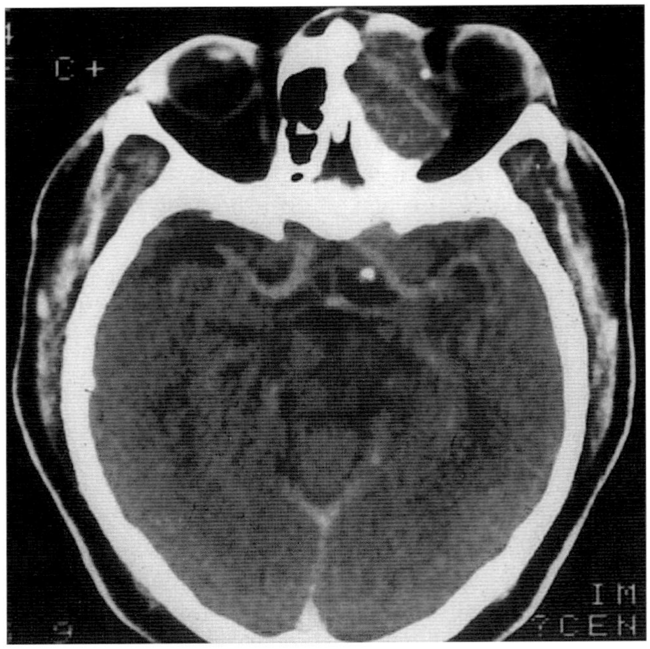

**FIGURE 30.4.** Axial computed tomography scan of a secondary ethmoid mucocele extending into the orbit after intranasal ethmoidectomy.

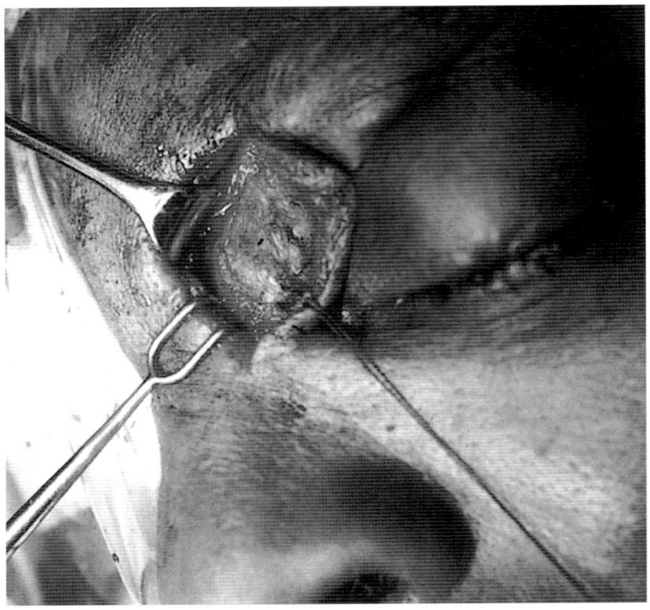

**FIGURE 30.5.** Intraoperative view of a mucocele before total extirpation.

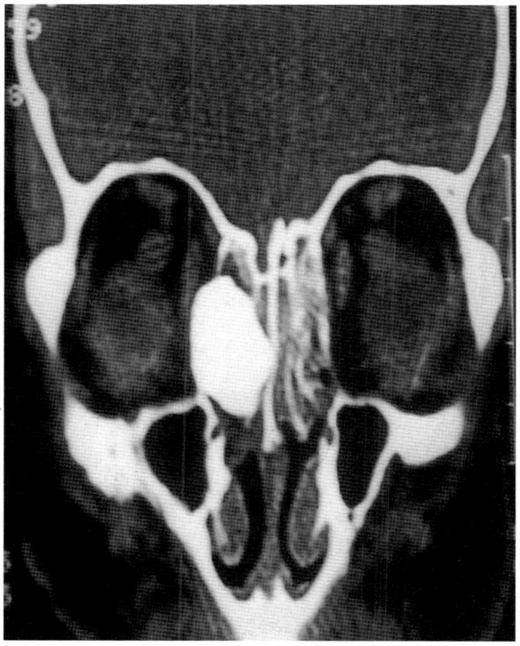

**FIGURE 30.6.** Coronal computed tomography scan of an ethmoid osteoma with intraorbital extension.

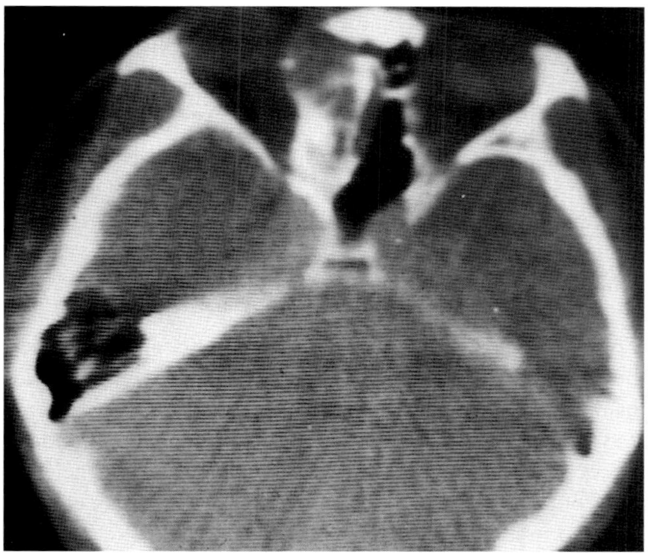

**FIGURE 30.7.** Axial computed tomography scan of a frontoethmoidal encephalocele.

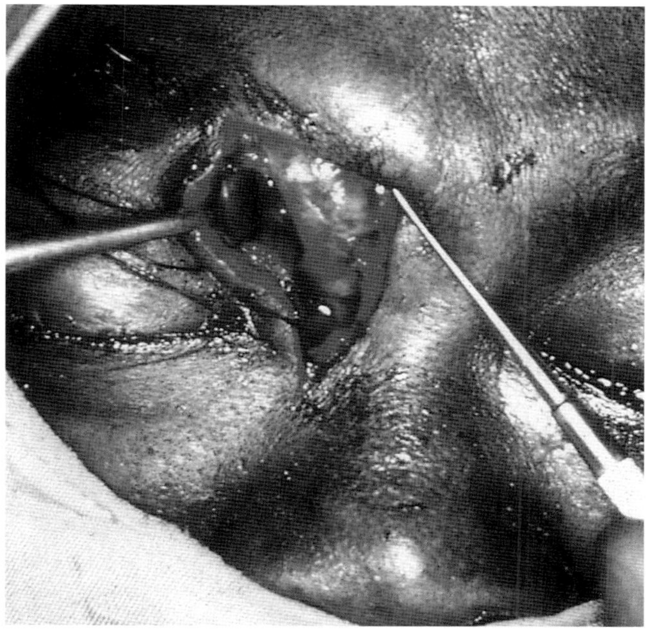

**FIGURE 30.8.** Operative exposure of a frontoethmoidal encephalocele through an external approach.

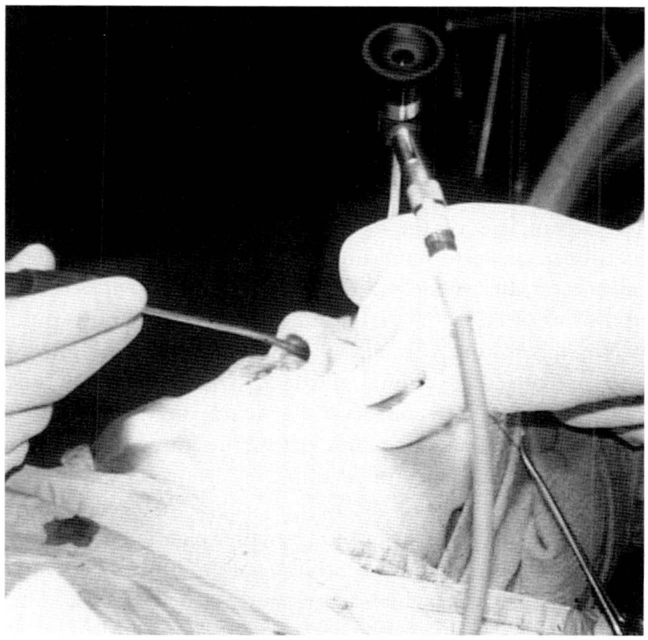

**FIGURE 30.9.** Intraoperative view of the repair of a cerebrospinal fluid leak using a combined intranasal and external approach.

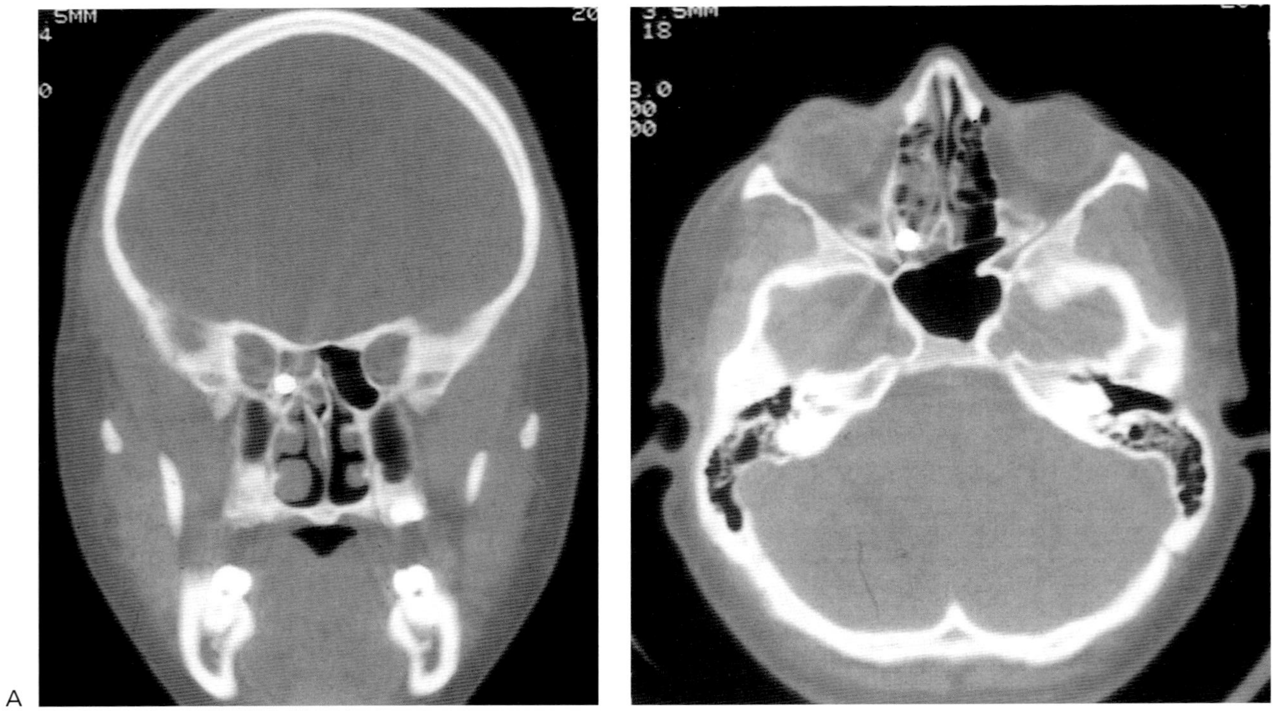


**FIGURE 30.10. A:** Coronal computed tomography (CT) scan of a pellet embedded in the ethmoid labyrinth. **B:** Axial CT scan shows the pellet in a posterior ethmoid cell adjacent to the orbital apex.

It may also be used for the removal of foreign bodies embedded in the ethmoids (Fig. 30.10).

## Advantages and Disadvantages

The advantages of the external frontoethmoidectomy are that it can be performed through a relatively small cosmetically acceptable incision (2 or 3 mm long); it provides access to the ipsilateral frontal, ethmoid, and sphenoid sinuses; and it is not deforming because the amount of bone removed does not affect the frontal and facial contours. The disadvantages of the procedure are that it can be used only for unilateral disease; it does not permit instrumentation and obliteration of a large frontal sinus; and it may result in retrograde infection from the nose or other involved sinuses into the frontal sinus or orbit. The latter effect occurs infrequently because the medial orbital wall becomes filled with dense fibrous tissue, which acts as an effective barricade. The major limiting factor to the success of this procedure is that it requires continued patency of the neoduct that is created.

The failure rate of the external frontoethmoidectomy is related to the length of time the patients are followed. Failure rates in the range of 20% to 30% have frequently been reported (17,20,21). Attempts to increase ductal patency include insertion of a variety of tubes used as stents (20,22,23). Rolled Silastic sheeting has been reported as being successful in increasing the long-term duct patency (19,24). Other attempts to maintain duct patency have involved the use of mucosal flaps rotated from the septum and lateral wall of the nasal cavity (18,24–27). It has been claimed that the external approach is less successful than the intranasal approach because it involves removal of the lamina papyracea, permitting prolapse of the orbital tissues into the newly created opening. In our experience, reexploration of such cases has not shown this to be true but rather has demonstrated that a dense wall of scar and bone forms along where the lamina papyracea had been removed, preventing herniation of the orbital soft tissues. Long-term study of unilateral cases of ductal enlargement by Draf (28) has also shown that the failure rates for endoscopic procedures reach those that have occurred with an external approach. The major complication of this procedure is closure of the recreated nasofrontal duct and the formation of a secondary mucocele. This is the success-limiting factor in all surgery on the frontal sinus in which the nasofrontal duct has been enlarged or a duct has been created unilaterally.

## Complications

Complications of the external frontoethmoidectomy may arise from injury to adjacent structures, including the ethmoidal blood vessels, lacrimal sac, trochlea, and orbital contents. An orbital hematoma may result from incomplete ligation or electrocautery of the ethmoidal blood vessels or from excessive traction on the globe with tearing of ciliary veins within the orbital fat. This may cause visual loss from retinal artery thrombosis caused by retrobulbar hemorrhage. This problem is detected intraoperatively by the development of proptosis and requires immediate orbital decompression. Visual loss may also arise from direct injury to the optic nerve from dissection or by the use of electrocautery too far posteriorly within the orbit. Injury to the lacrimal sac may result in dacryostenosis with epiphora and chronic dacryocystitis developing in the postoperative period. Failure to reattach the trochlea may result in imbalance of the superior oblique muscle, with the occurrence of diplopia. Failure of reattachment of the medial canthal ligament may produce pseudohypertelorism. It is important to reattach the ligament at its original position to avoid a disharmony with the opposite eye. Dissection should not proceed above the frontoethmoidal suture line, except anteriorly above the lacrimal fossa to avoid injury to the anterior skull base and the formation of a CSF leak.

We have not had any instance of orbital hematoma, dacryostenosis, CSF leak, or pseudohypertelorism occur with this procedure in more than 100 cases. The development of a secondary mucocele after closure of the neoduct is usually delayed for several years but may arise as long as several decades after the surgery.

## Technique

The procedure is performed under general endotracheal anesthesia. After the face is prepared and draped, a tarsorrhaphy suture of 6-0 silk is placed for corneal protection (Fig. 30.11). An incision approximately 3 cm long is out-

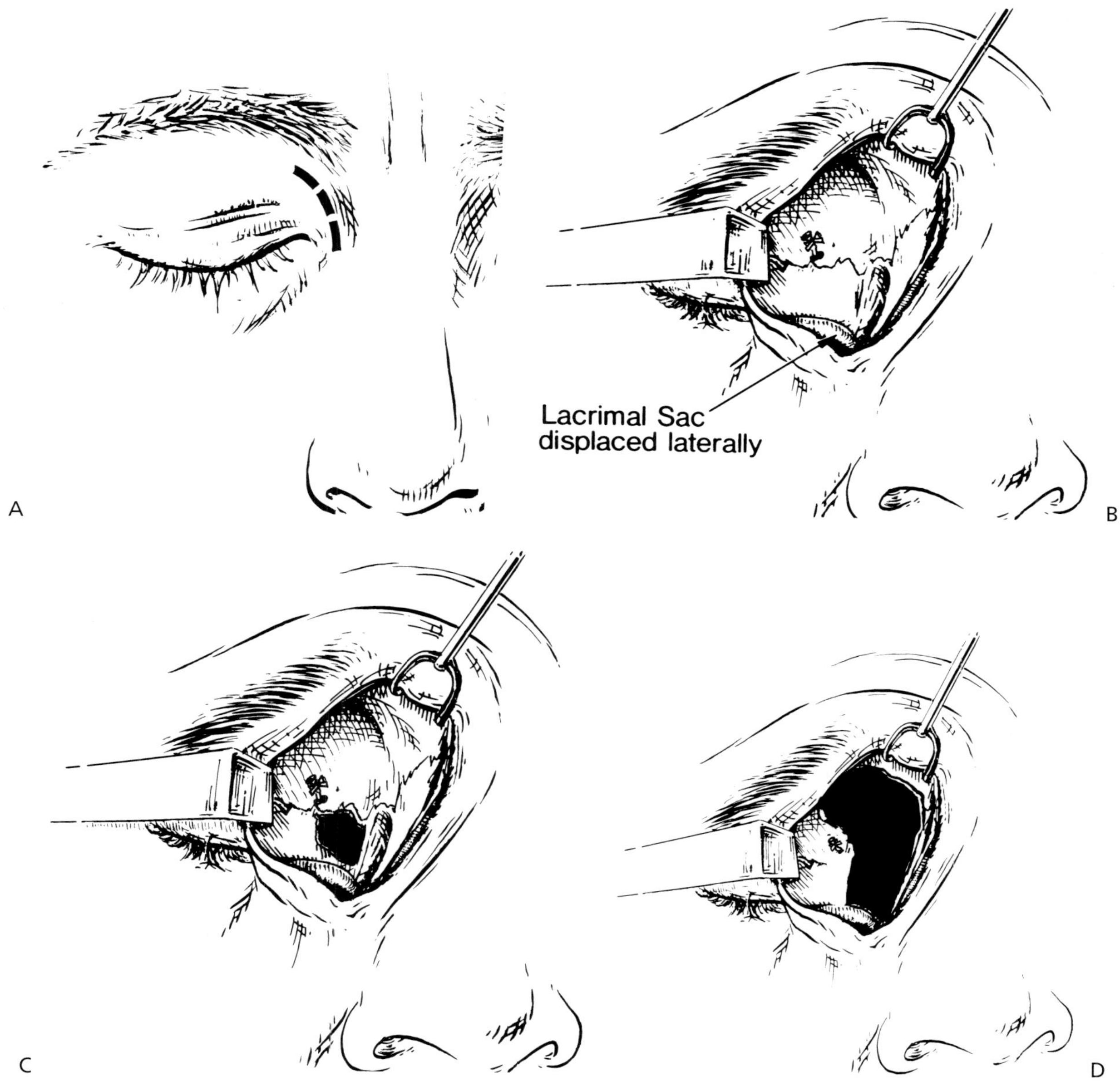


**FIGURE 30.11.** Diagram of the external frontoethmoidectomy. **A:** Incision. **B:** Exposure of the medial orbital wall. **C:** Entry into the ethmoid labyrinth through the lamina papyracea. **D:** Complete frontoethmoidectomy. (From Lawson W. The frontal sinus. In: Blitzer A, Lawson W, Friedman W, eds. *Surgery of the paranasal sinuses*, 2nd ed. Philadelphia: WB Saunders, 1991:192, with permission.)

lined with a marking pen from a point just below the medial aspect of the eyebrow to the level of the medial canthus, midway between the nasal dorsum and the inner canthus of the eye. The skin is crosshatched and stained with the marking dye to allow correct alignment and closure of the tissues at the completion of the procedure. The skin and subcutaneous tissues are divided in layers, with bleeding from transected branches of the angular blood vessels controlled with electrocautery. The periosteum is incised and raised with a Freer elevator toward the medial orbital wall. Resistance is encountered at the region of the lacrimal fossa, where additional force is required to detach the anterior and posterior limbs of the medial canthal ligament. At this point, a 4-0 silk suture is placed through the periosteum to mark the position of the medial canthal ligament and to act as a wound retractor. The lacrimal sac is displaced from the fossa and is retracted laterally. The globe is retracted atraumatically with an orbital or narrow malleable ribbon retractor exposing the lamina papyracea of the ethmoid bone. Bleeding from small diploic veins is controlled by electrocautery.

A key landmark in elevation the periorbita superiorly and posteriorly is the frontoethmoidal suture line, which marks the junction of the orbit and the anterior cranial fossa (Fig. 30.12). The suture line may be obliterated in adults, and its position can be determined by finding the anterior and posterior ethmoidal blood vessels that run through or immediately adjacent to it. Knowledge of the anatomy of these vessels is essential in performing this procedure. In the class study by Kirchner and coworkers (29) of 150 orbits, they found the anterior ethmoid foramen within the frontoethmoid suture line in 68% of the specimens and 1 to 4 mm above it in the remaining 32%. In 5 of 70 preserved orbits examined, the artery was absent. The distance from the maxillolacrimal suture line to the anterior ethmoid foramen was 14 to 18 mm in 64% of the orbits; the distance ranged from 9 to 27 mm. The distance from the anterior ethmoid foramen to the posterior ethmoid foramen averaged 10 to 11 mm. The posterior ethmoid foramen was present in the frontoethmoid suture line in 87% of the specimens and was immediately superior to it in the remainder. As with the anterior ethmoid foramen, it was never below the suture line.

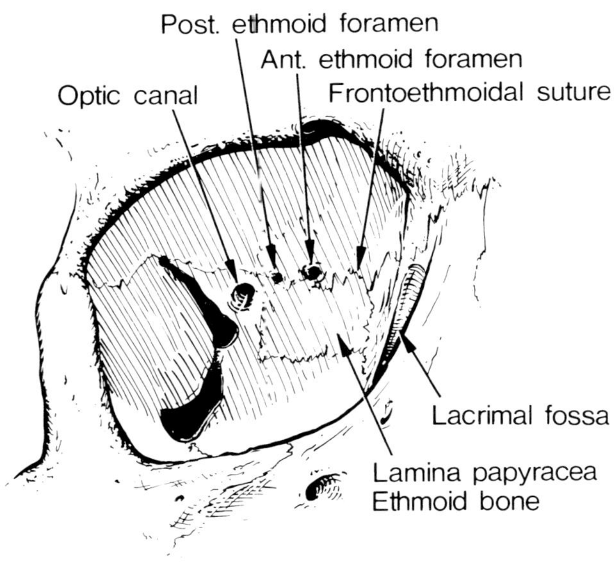


**FIGURE 30.12.** Anatomy of the medial aspect of the orbital wall. (From Lawson W. The frontal sinus. In: Blitzer A, Lawson W, Friedman W, eds. *Surgery of paranasal sinuses*, 2nd ed. Philadelphia: WB Saunders, 1991:194, with permission.)

The posterior ethmoidal artery was absent in 22 of 70 orbits studied. Although the anterior ethmoidal artery is larger than the posterior one, the opposite relationship was found in four orbits. The distance from the posterior ethmoid foramen to the optic nerve was relatively constant, being 4 to 7 mm in 84% of the skulls. However, the optic nerve enters the orbit at an acute angle to the medial orbital wall and lies 1 to 2 mm from the posterior ethmoidal artery as it passes from the orbital soft tissues to its foramen. This places the optic nerve at considerable risk for injury with dissection, ligature passage, and electrocautery of the posterior ethmoidal artery. Caution also must be exercised in attempting to ligate or clip the anterior ethmoid artery when the frontoethmoidal junction is very acute, because the risk of vessel rupture and retraction is great in these circumstances.

Keeping these distances in mind, the periorbita is elevated on a line with the superior border of the lacrimal fossa until a funnel-like evagination is seen to enter the medial orbital wall (Fig. 30.13). The periorbita is attenuated at this point, and excessive pressure can cause herniation of orbital fat. This should signal that the vessels are there and should be controlled. Continued forceful retraction will rupture the vessels, and bleeding into the orbit will ensue. We favor control of the anterior ethmoidal artery with bipolar electrocautery, which also creates a burn mark on the bone to facilitate identification of the frontoethmoidal suture line later. The periorbita is elevated superiorly to expose the floor of the frontal sinus anterior to the ethmoidal vessels and above the lacrimal fossa.

The ethmoid labyrinth is entered through the lamina papyracea with a small, straight punch forceps. The medial orbital wall is further removed with angled punch forceps. (e.g., Kerrison rongeur). The margins of the dissection are the frontoethmoidal suture superiorly, the level of the posterior ethmoidal artery posteriorly, the anterior lacrimal crest anteriorly, and the junction of the medial wall and floor of the orbit inferiorly. If extensive decompression of the orbit is necessary, bone can be removed down to the infraorbital foramen and canal. The bony septa and lining of the ethmoidal cells are removed until a large, common cavity is formed. The nasal mucosa may be preserved if it is

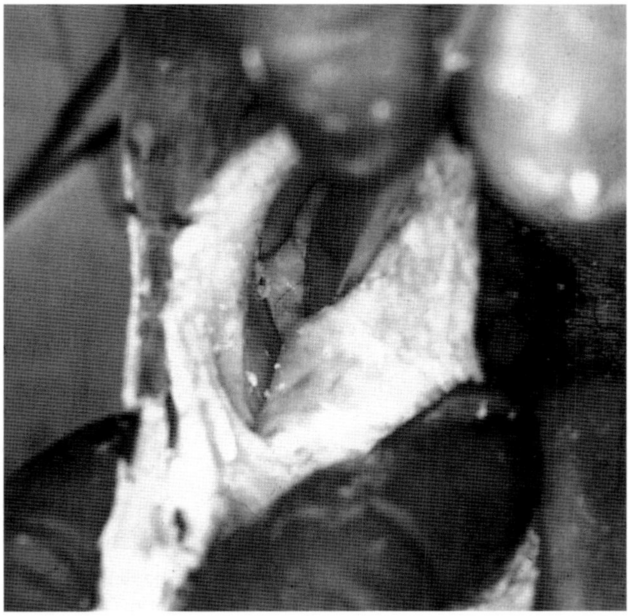

**FIGURE 30.13.** Intraoperative view of the anterior ethmoidal artery passing through the frontoethmoidal suture line.

to be used for a flap to partially resurface the reconstructed nasofrontal duct. If the frontal sinus is to be opened, bone is removed with a right-angle punch forceps superior to the lacrimal fossa. The nasofrontal duct can usually be identified and enlarged. If a supraorbital ethmoid cell is present and is creating a cul de sac, a trephine can be made in the floor of the frontal sinus medially. The intervening bone can be safely removed to create a confluent opening into the nasal cavity. The middle turbinate is partially resected intranasally with an angled scissors. The attachment of the middle turbinate is another critical landmark, because the cribriform plate is situated medial to it. At this point, it is possible to inspect the roof of the ethmoid labyrinth, the cribriform plate, and the face of the sphenoid sinus. The ostium of the sphenoid sinus may be found medially in the plane of the posterior ethmoidal artery.

We favor stenting the nasofrontal neoduct with a rolled tube of thin Silastic using the method of Neel. This tube is anchored superiorly with a 4-0 Vicryl suture placed in the deep tissues below the medial eyebrow. The tube is left in position 8 to 10 weeks and is removed in the office transnasally. After careful hemostasis, the wound is closed in layers using 4-0 Vicryl for the periosteum. This is a critical step because its approximation serves to reattach the medial canthal ligament and the trochlea. The subcutaneous tissues are closed with 4-0 chromic interrupted sutures and the skin with a continuous 5-0 nylon suture. No drain is placed, and the nasal cavity is left unpacked to provide dependent drainage. The incision is coated with an antibiotic ointment, and the eye is left uncovered to detect any evidence of intraorbital bleeding and to institute prompt decompressive measures should it occur.

## CALDWELL-LUC PROCEDURE

### Historical Background

The maxillary sinus is also known as the antrum (Latin for cave) of Highmore, acknowledging his detailed description of this structure in his anatomic text published in 1651 (30). In the preantibiotic era, the maxillary sinus was a frequent source of infection from the adjacent teeth and contiguous sinuses, often with devastating consequences. Early attempts at the management of antral disease reported in the eighteenth century consisted of drainage and lavage of the cavity by creating an opening by the extraction of a tooth (31,32) or by a puncture made in the oral cavity or the inferior or middle meatus of the nose (33). Maxillary sinus drainage and irrigation through the alveolus and the middle (34) and inferior meatus (35,36) continued to be advocated as late as the 1890s.

In 1743, Lamorier (37) reported a method of entry into the maxillary sinus by creating an opening through its lateral wall. However, this publication went unnoticed for almost 150 years. Heath (38) in 1889 and Robertson (39) in 1892 described removal of the anterior wall of the sinus and curettage of its contents; however, neither of these surgeons created an opening into the nasal cavity.

It remained for the closing years of the nineteenth century for the operation to assume its modern form by combining a canine fossa approach with the creation of a nasoantral window. In New York in 1893, Caldwell (40) reported débridement of the maxillary sinus through a canine fossa opening that was closed after the creation of an inferior meatus window. In London in 1894, Spicer (41) performed the same procedure but kept the buccal incision open with gauze packing. In Paris in 1897, Luc (42) independently described a radical antrostomy opening with a rhinostomy made through the middle meatus.

The Caldwell-Luc operation was the most common radical sinus operation performed (43–45), but its popularity has decreased since the development of endoscopic techniques. For maxillary sinus cases that were difficult to manage or that failed the Caldwell-Luc operation, the Denker procedure was proposed (46). In this operation, the bone was removed from the lateral nasal wall across the pyriform aperture and into the canine fossa. Although it allows a more complete removal of the diseased mucosa, there is risk of damage to the dental nerves and the nasolacrimal duct. This operation continued to be described in textbooks until the mid-twentieth century (47).

The procedure currently advocated is a miniantrotomy in which the oral soft tissues and the bony lateral wall of the maxillary sinus are minimally disturbed, creating a small aperture into the sinus through which endoscopic visualiza-

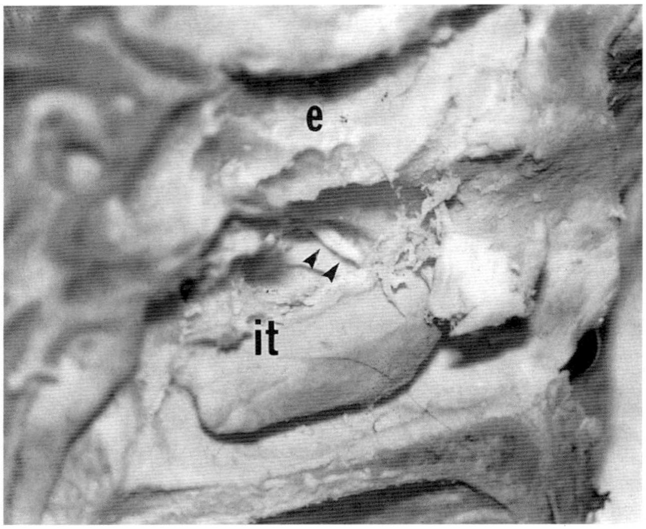


**FIGURE 30.14.** Cadaver dissection. The infraorbital nerve *(arrows)* runs outside a bony canal. *it*, inferior turbinate; *e*, ethmoid labyrinth.

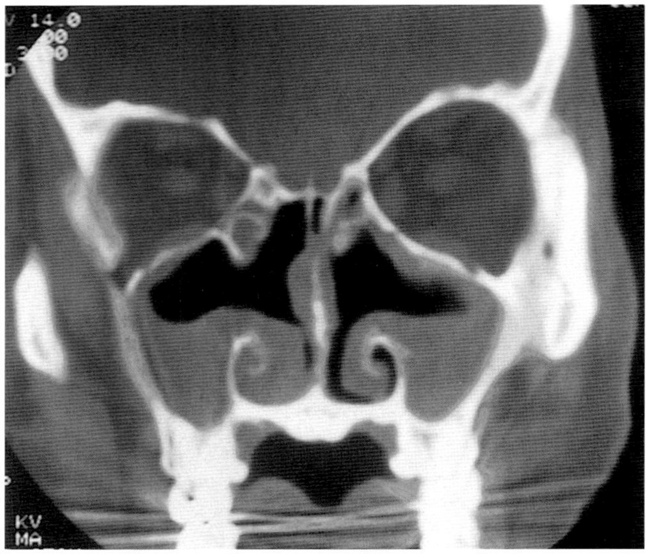

**FIGURE 30.15.** Coronal computed tomography scan demonstrates severe mucosal thickening in the maxillary sinuses bilaterally after endoscopic ethmoidectomies and middle meatus antrostomies.

tion and instrumentation can be performed. The purpose of this operative modification is to decrease the morbidity of the traditional Caldwell-Luc procedure while having the advantage of being able to remove disease in all parts of the maxillary sinus under direct vision. Cadaver dissection studies have demonstrated that the infraorbital nerve is not always encased in a bony canal and may have a slightly aberrant course when the canal is dehiscent (Fig. 30.14). This is confirmed clinically by reports of small cysts or polyps having been removed endoscopically from the antrum through a middle meatus antrostomy with permanent infraorbital nerve injury. Creating limited exposure of the lateral wall of the maxillary sinus by minimal soft tissue elevation decreases the incidence of infraorbital nerve injury by direct contact or traction. Creating a small opening in the canine fossa minimally disturbs the alveolar plexus formed by branches of the superior alveolar nerve and decreases the extent and duration of gingival and dental paresthesias. Visualizing the apices of the tooth roots and creating an opening in the canine fossa above them also decreases the possibility of developing a nonvital tooth. Having a sublabial and a transnasal portal through which the endoscope and instruments can be interchangeably placed permits direct access to every segment of the maxillary sinus. The mucosal and bone incisions are at different levels to prevent the occurrence of an oroantral fistula.

## Indications

The most common indication for the Caldwell-Luc procedure is chronic maxillary sinusitis that has proven refractory to medical management and previous endoscopic middle meatus antrostomy and ethmoidectomy when indicated. This is confirmed by computed tomography (CT) scanning, which reveals persistent and recurrent opacification of the maxillary sinus with extensive mucosal thickening and polyp formation despite a patent middle meatus antrostomy (Fig. 30.15). Patients with hypertrophic rhinosinusitis, especially those with comorbid factors such as asthma,

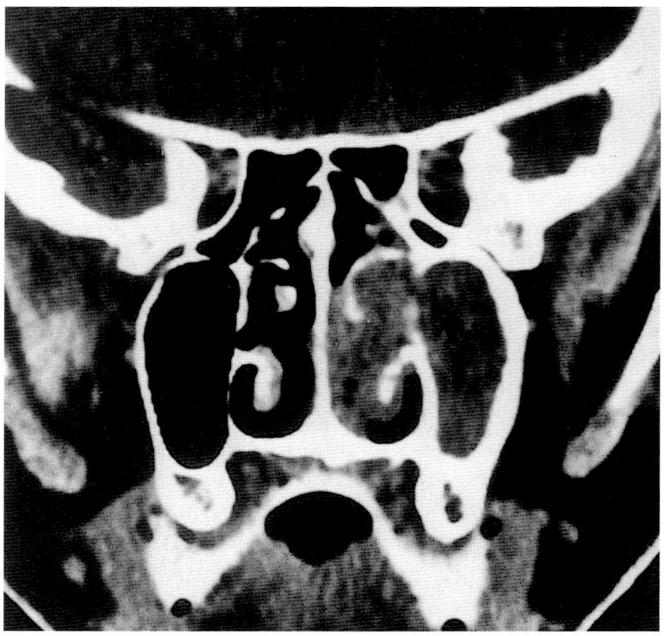

**FIGURE 30.16.** Coronal computed tomography scan of a patient with an antrochoanal polyp. Notice the antral opacification, widening of the maxillary ostium, and presence of a polypoid mass filling the middle and inferior meatus.

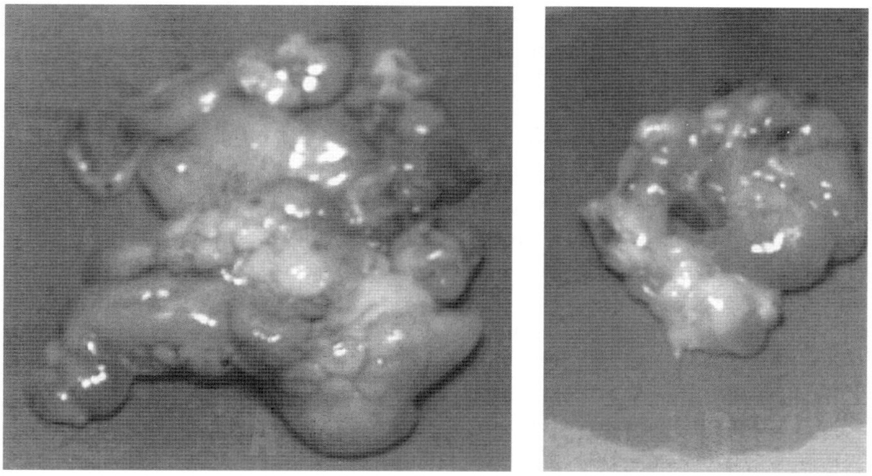

FIGURE 30.17. Specimens of the nasal and sinus components of an antrochoanal polyp. **Left:** Nasal specimen. **Right:** Maxillary sinus specimen.

aspirin sensitivity, atopy, immunodeficiency, and ciliary dysfunction, may require direct removal of the antral contents after unsuccessful, less-invasive endonasal procedures. Patients with antrochoanal polyps often have extensive polypoid degeneration within the maxillary sinus (Figs. 30.16 and 30.17). Removal of the nasal-choanal portion may result in recurrence, and the greatest success is achieved by direct and complete removal of the polypoid antral contents. Patients with fungal sinusitis may require a combined sublabial and endonasal approach to totally exenterate infected tissue and large mycetomas (Fig. 30.18). Individuals having septate maxillary sinuses may require a transoral approach to access sequestered compartments within the sinus. Mucoceles and pneumatoceles of the maxillary sinus are generally successfully treated by the creation of a large middle meatus antrostomy. Secondary mucoceles develop after trauma or previous surgery from the formation of fibrous septa that segment the antrum and trap pockets of mucosa that undergo cystic change (Fig. 30.19). They are best managed by total removal through a Caldwell-Luc procedure because their location often does not permit marsupialization into the nasal cavity.

Biopsy of maxillary sinus lesions, especially those suspected of being malignant, should be performed

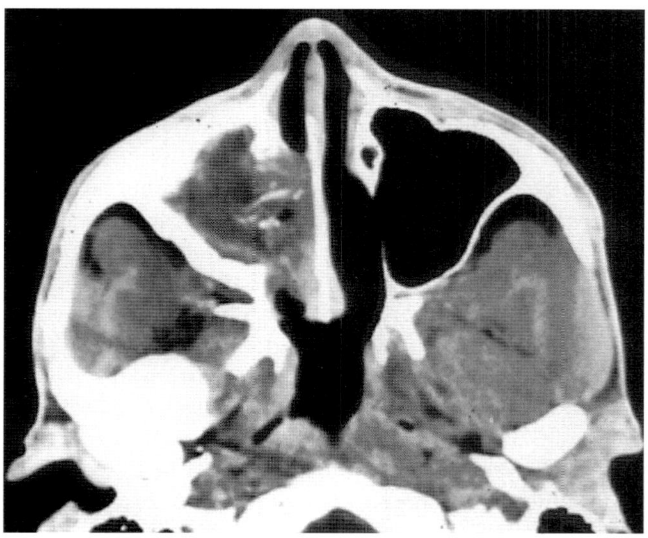

FIGURE 30.18. Axial computed tomography scan demonstrates an aspergilloma of the maxillary sinus extending into the nasal cavity. Notice the sclerosis of the bony walls of the maxillary sinus and scattered areas of high-attenuation material within the mycetoma.

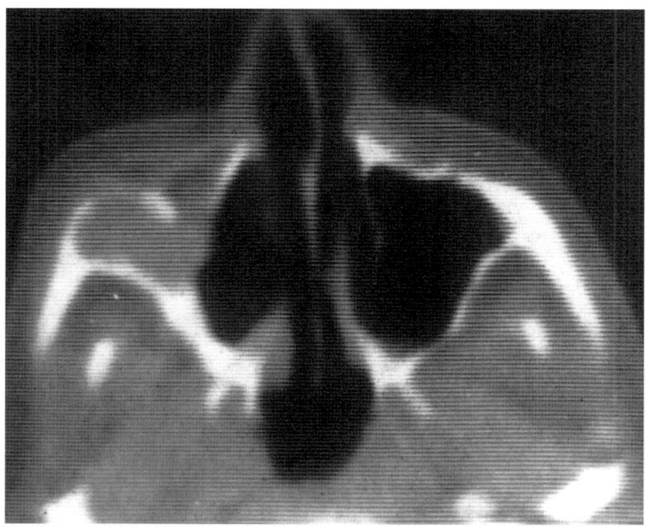

FIGURE 30.19. Axial computed tomography scan of a secondary mucocele that has developed in the lateral recess of the maxillary sinus after a Caldwell-Luc procedure.

transnasally to prevent seeding the buccal soft tissues with tumor. Rarely, a direct approach may be necessary through the canine fossa after unsuccessful endoscopic nasal biopsy. Dental cysts and tumors extending into the maxillary sinus are best managed by the sublabial approach because it permits complete removal of the lesion, including the alveolar and sinus portions (Fig. 30.20). In cases lacking secondary infection, it may not be necessary to disturb the natural ostium of the maxillary sinus and disrupt normal mucociliary clearance. The Caldwell-Luc procedure is an excellent method for the removal of foreign bodies, including teeth and tooth fragments, dental filling material, sinoliths, and traumatically implanted materials.

The repair of chronic oroantral fistulas, especially those having failed previous attempts at closure, requires removal of all infected and polypoid tissue within the maxillary sinus (Fig. 30.21). This can be accomplished by a Caldwell-Luc procedure in conjunction with an inferior meatus antrostomy and intraoral closure of the fistula by a buccal or palatal flap.

The Caldwell-Luc procedure is useful in the management of malar, orbital blow-out, and nasomaxillary fractures by exposing and aiding in the reduction of herniated orbital fat, allowing positioning and fixation of fracture segments and use of bone from the anterior maxillary wall for a graft.

Occasionally, the traditional wide-field Caldwell-Luc procedure may be necessary to perform radical orbital decompression (i.e., Ogura-Walsh procedure) (48) or for surgery of the pterygopalatine space (e.g., biopsy, internal maxillary artery ligation, vidian neurectomy, sphenopalatine or maxillary nerve section) (49). It may be employed in conjunction with other procedures (e.g., lateral rhinotomy, transpalatal

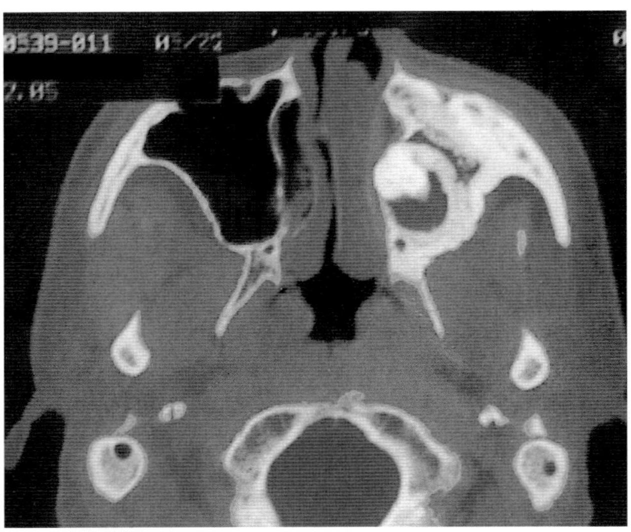

**FIGURE 30.20.** Axial computed tomography scan of a dentigerous cyst extending into the maxillary sinus. Notice the separate cyst cavity containing the crown of an unerupted molar tooth.

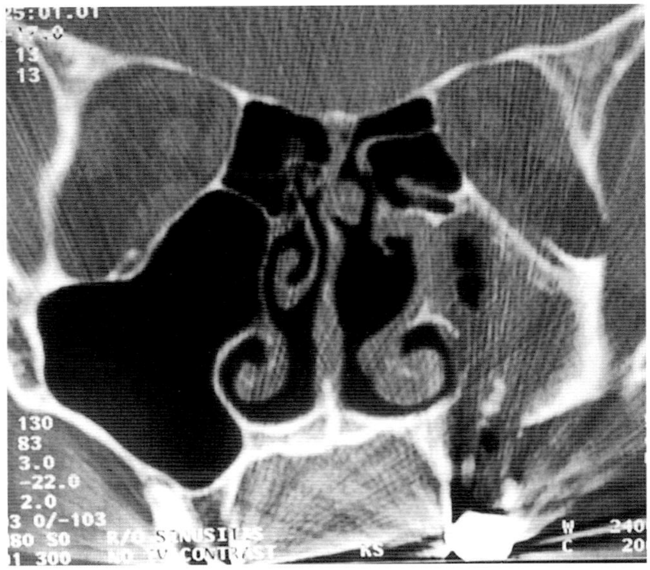

**FIGURE 30.21.** Coronal computed tomography scan demonstrates an oroantral fistula. Notice the extensive opacification of the maxillary sinus, retained radiopaque dental material along the sinus floor, and a defect in the alveolus.

approach) for the removal of large juvenile angiofibromas. The Caldwell-Luc procedure may be performed in conjunction with a transnasal endoscopic ethmoidectomy for the resection of large sinonasal inverted papillomas, eliminating the need for an external approach (50).

## Advantages and Disadvantages

The major advantage of the Caldwell-Luc procedure is that it provides direct access to all the recesses of the maxillary sinus and permits total removal of its contents. With limited antral lesions, there is no need to disturb the natural ostium of the sinus, but a small, temporary inferior meatus opening may be created for dependent drainage in the postoperative period.

Disadvantages are related to the gingivobuccal dissection, which produces facial swelling. Moreover, dental, gingival, and facial paresthesias develop from disturbance of the alveolar plexus of nerves on the lateral antral wall and pressure on the infraorbital nerve from edema or traction. This was commonly found with the traditional Caldwell-Luc procedure, with facial swelling occurring in 89% and anesthesia of the face, teeth, and gingival developing in 9.1% of 670 cases reviewed by DeFreitas and Lucente (51). The miniantrotomy procedure advocated here is designed to minimize these complications and lessen their duration.

## Complications

The facial swelling is usually self-limited and resolves in most cases within 1 week, although in a small number of patients, it may persist for several months. The occurrence of infraorbital nerve paresthesia is more troubling. In some patients, persistent pain or numbness may occur from fibrosis enveloping the infraorbital nerve as it exits its foramen or by direct injury to the nerve, causing a neuroma. Simple curettage of the floor of the maxillary sinus through a Caldwell-Luc procedure or an endoscopic intranasal procedure may result in irritation of branches of the superior alveolar nerve and may produce gingival and dental paresthesias. The infraorbital nerve may have an aberrant path, or its canal may be dehiscent, and the possibility of injury exists when removing the mucosa from the roof of the maxillary sinus. An oroantral fistula is eliminated by having the gingival incision and the bony opening at different levels so that the mucosa is always supported by underlying bone. In patients who have lost a considerable amount of bone from the lateral wall of the maxilla, the formation of a fistula is a danger, and in these patients, the use of a gingival flap should be considered. In creating or enlarging a middle or inferior meatus antrostomy, anterior dissection carries the risk of injury to the nasolacrimal duct. Dacryocystitis was present in 2.6% of the cases of DeFreitas and Lucente (51). These investigators also observed an incidence of oroantral fistula of 1.1% and of devitalized teeth in 0.4% in their series. The creation of the opening through the lateral maxillary wall into the sinus should be above the apices of the posterior teeth to eliminate devitalization of the teeth.

We have performed this limited procedure more than 100 times with no significant morbidity. The facial swelling that occurs is less severe than seen with the classic Caldwell-Luc procedure and generally resolves within 1 week. The application of ice to the face minimizes it. Gingival, dental, and facial paresthesias have been minimal, with no permanent neurologic sequelae. There has been no incidence of hematoma, infection, or oroantral fistula.

## Technique

The procedure can be done under general or local anesthesia. After the administration of intravenous sedation or endotracheal intubation, the right maxillary vestibule is infiltrated with 3 to 5 mL of 1% Xylocaine with 1:100,000 epinephrine. After adequate regional anesthesia is attained, an incision 3 cm long is made through the mucosa 1 cm above the line of the attached gingival, from the area of the canine tooth to the first molar tooth. The mucoperiosteum is elevated with a Freer elevator for a distance of only 2 to 3 cm. The infraorbital nerve is not identified. In the region of the canine fossa, an opening is made with a small, half-round gouge and mallet, and the opening is enlarged minimally with a small Kerrison punch forceps to a diameter of approximately 1 cm (Fig. 30.22). Care is taken to place this opening above the apices of the maxillary premolar teeth, whose roots can be seen bulging against the lateral wall of the maxilla. This reduced opening is adequate to insert an

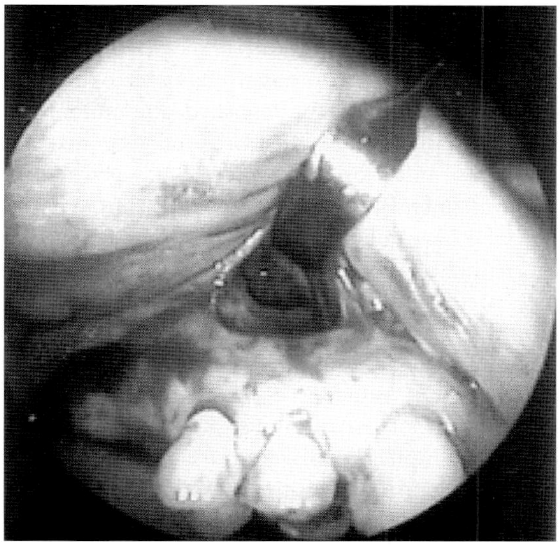

**FIGURE 30.22.** Clinical view of the miniantrotomy procedure. Notice the small mucosal incision and limited bone opening a distance above the apices of the dental roots.

endoscope and a fine grasping forceps or suction aspirator. The sinus is inspected with 0° and 30° endoscopes to visualize the status of the mucosa and to assess the nature of the lesions to be treated (Fig. 30.23). After the lesion is removed, an intranasal middle meatus antrostomy is created endoscopically. An inferior antrostomy is performed when the sinus has been totally denuded of mucosa and dependent drainage is needed as mucociliary clearance no longer exists. The incision is closed with three or four sutures. A small amount of petrolatum impregnated gauze is placed in the nose.

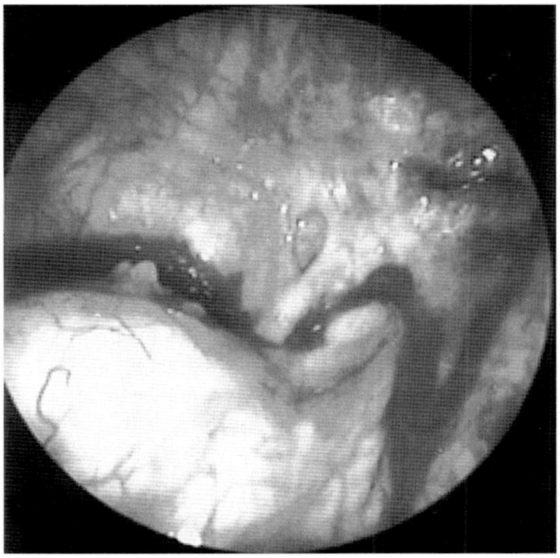

**FIGURE 30.23.** Endoscopic view through a canine fossa opening of a mass in the posterior portion of a maxillary sinus. Biopsy revealed a non-Hodgkin's lymphoma.

## CONCLUSIONS

The Caldwell-Luc procedure is still a viable operation, primarily in the modified form described, the miniantrotomy. With hypertrophic rhinosinusitis, it may be necessary to gain control of infection and provide drainage (in conjunction with an inferior meatus antrostomy) in symptomatic patients who have failed intranasal endoscopic management and lack functional mucociliary clearing. It is also a highly effective method of removing primary cyst and tumors, odontogenic lesions, foreign bodies, mycetomas, and secondary mucoceles and of accessing hidden compartments of the antrum. It provides exposure of the orbital floor, facilitates repair of oroantral fistulas, and is a route for surgery of the pterygopalatine fossa, decompression of malignant endocrine exophthalmus, and the removal of sinonasal inverted papilloma, and juvenile angiofibromas.

The transorbital approach to the sinonasal tract is applicable to the management of diverse lesions. It provides immediate drainage and decompression of postseptal infections of the orbit accompanied by increased intraocular pressure. It has a role in chronic inflammatory disease of the frontal sinus and its outflow tract in patients who have failed intranasal endoscopic surgery and is an option before obliteration by an osteoplastic flap procedure. It provides wide exposure of the anterior skull base for the detection and repair of CSF leaks and encephaloceles. Knowledge of this approach is also important for control of epistaxis from the ethmoidal blood vessels and for biopsy and removal of lesions of the lacrimal sac. The incidence of complications is low. The success-limiting factor of external frontoethmoidectomy is closure of the surgically created neoduct.

## REFERENCES


1. Ogston A. Trephining the frontal sinuses for catarrhal diseases. *Med Chron Manchester* 1884–1885;1:235–238.
2. Hinkel FW. A report of the operative treatment of several cases of frontal and maxillary sinusitis. *Trans Am Laryngol Assoc* 1899; 21:153–158.
3. Jansen A. Neue Erfahrungen uber chronische Nebenhohleneiterungen der Nase. *Arch Ohren Nasen Kehlkopfheilk* 1902;56: 110–118.
4. Ritter G. Erhaltung der vorderen Stirnhohlenwand bei der Radikaloperation. *Verh Dtsch Laryngol* 1911;628:628–635.
5. Knapp A. The surgical treatment of orbital complications in disease of the nasal sinuses. *JAMA* 1908;51:299–305.
6. Kuhnt H. Uber die entzundlichen Erkrankunge der Stirnhohlen and ihre Folgezustande. *Arch Laryngol Rhinol* 1895;24:309–325.
7. Ropke. Die Radicaloperation bei chronischen Verschleimungen und Eiterungen der Oberen Nasennebenhohlen. *Arch Laryngol Rhinol* 1898;1:199–216.
8. Riedel-Schenke H. Uber die Stirnhohlen und ihre Erkrankungen [Cited by Goodale RH]. *Ann Otol* 1955;64:470–485.
9. Killian G. Die Killian'sche Radicaloperation chronischer Stirnhohleneiterungen. II. Weiteres Kasuistisches material und Zusammenfassung. *Arch Laryngol Rhinol (Berl)* 1903;13:59–88.
10. Lothrop HA. Frontal sinus suppuration with results of new operative procedure. *JAMA* 1915;65:153–160.
11. Mosher HP, Judd DK. An analysis of seven cases of osteomyelitis of the frontal bone complicating frontal sinusitis. *Laryngoscope* 1933;43:153–160.
12. Lynch RC. The technique of a radical frontal sinus operation which has given me the best results. *Laryngoscope* 1921;31:1–15.
13. Howarth WG. Operations on the frontal sinus. *J Laryngol* 1921; 36:417–421.
14. Sewall EC. Frontal-ethmosphenoidectomy: further experience with this operation performed under local anesthesia; a new osteoplastic flap. *Arch Otolaryngol* 1928;8:144–150.
15. Lillie HI, Williams HL. The external frontoethmo-sphenoid operation: a critical review of the literature and details of the technic in use at the Mayo Clinic. *Minn Med* 1935;18:786–789.
16. Lillie HI. The surgical treatment of certain unusual conditions of the frontal sinus. *Ann Otol Rhinol Laryngol* 1932;41:59–73.
17. Williams HL, Holman CB. The causes and avoidance of failure in surgery for chronic suppuration of the frontoethmo-sphenoid complex of sinuses: with a previously unreported anomaly which produces chronicity and recurrence and the description of a surgical technique usually producing a cure of the disease. *Laryngoscope* 1962;72:1179–1227.
18. Porto DP, Duvall AJ. Long term results with nasofrontal duct reconstruction. *Laryngoscope* 1986;96:858–862.
19. Neel HB III, McDonald TJ, Facer GW. Modified Lynch procedure for chronic frontal sinus diseases: rationale, technique, and long-term results. *Laryngoscope* 1987;97:1274–1279.
20. Harris HE. The use of tantalum tubes in frontal sinus surgery. *Cleve Clin Q* 1948;15:129–134.
21. Goodale RL. Some cause for failure in frontal sinus surgery. *Ann Otol* 1942;51:648–656.
22. Wolfowitz BL, Solomon A. Mucoceles of the frontal and ethmoid sinuses. *J Laryngol* 1972;86:79–83.
23. Erich JB, New GB. An acrylic obturator employed in the repair of an obstructed frontonasal duct. *Trans Am Acad Ophthalmol Otolaryngol* 1947;51:628–663.
24. Neel HB, Whicher JH, Lake CF. Thin rubber sheeting in frontal sinus surgery: animal and clinical studies. *Laryngoscope* 1976;86: 524–536.
25. Boyden GL. Surgical treatment of chronic frontal sinusitis. *Ann Otol Rhinol Laryngol* 1952;61:558–566.
26. Sewall EC. The operative treatment of chronic frontal sinuses. *Ann Otol Rhinol Laryngol* 1935;44:307–316.
27. Dedo AH, Broberg TG, Murr AH. Frontoethmoidectomy with Sewall-Boyden reconstruction: alive and well, a 25-year experience. *Am J Rhinol* 1998;12:191–198.
28. Draf S. Endonasal micro-endoscopic frontal sinus surgery: the Fulda concept. Operative techniques. *Otolaryngol Head Neck Surg* 1991;2:234–240.
29. Kirchner JA, Yanagisawa E, Crelin ES. Surgical anatomy of the ethmoidal arteries. *Arch Otolaryngol* 1961;74:382–386.
30. Highmore N. *Corporis humani disquisitio anatomica*. Hagae Comitis: S. Brown, 1651.
31. Cowper W. Of the nose. In: Drake J, ed. *Antropologia novia*, vol 2. London, 1707:526–549.
32. Deschamps JL. Dissertations sur les maladies des fosses nasales et de leurs sinus. Paris: Veuve Richard an XII, 1804.
33. Tange RA. Some historical aspects of the surgical treatment of the infected maxillary sinus. *Rhinology* 1991;29:155–162.
34. Garel, cited in Dundas Grant J. Empyema in the nasal accessory sinuses. *Br Med J* 1894;6:1360.
35. Lothrop H (1897), cited by Weir N. *Otolaryngology: an illustrated history*. London: Butterworth, 1990.
36. Clauoe RC. Traitement des suppurations chroniques du sinus

maxillaire par la resection de la partie inferieure de la paroi nasale de sinus. *Ann Mal Oreil Larynx* 1904;30:220–230.
37. Lamorier L. Cite par Bordenave. *Mem Acad R Chir* 1768;4: 329–384, 5:225–262.
38. Heath C. Transactions of the Odontological Society of England; November 1889.
39. Robertson, cited in Spicer S. The surgical treatment of chronic empyema of the antrum maxillaire. *Br Med J* 1894;2: 1359–1361.
40. Caldwell GW. Diseases of the accessory sinuses of the nose and an improved method of treatment of the suppuration of the maxillary sinus. *N Y Med J* 1893;58:526–528.
41. Spicer SRH. Annual congress meeting of the British Medical Association; Bristol, August 1894.
42. Luc H. Nouvelle methode operatoire pour la cure radicale et rapide de l'empyeme chronique du sinus maxillaire. Communication a la Societe Francaise d'Otologie, 1897.
43. Goodman WS. The Caldwell-Luc procedure. *Otolaryngol Clin North Am* 1976;9:187–192.
44. Blitzer A. Surgery for infection and benign disease of the maxillary sinus. In: Blitzer A, Lawson W, Friedman W, eds. *Surgery of the paranasal sinus*, 2nd ed. Philadelphia: WB Saunders, 1991: 277–287.
45. Macbeth R. Caldwell, Luc and their operation. *Laryngoscope* 1971;81:1652–1657.
46. Denker A. Zur radikaloperation des chronischen Kieferhohlenempyems. *Arch Laryngol Rhinol* 1905;17:221–232.
47. Myers EN. Caldwell-Luc operation and extensions. In: Goldman JL, ed. *The principles and practice of rhinology*. New York: John Wiley & Sons, 1987:455–474.
48. Ogura JH, Walsh TE. The transantral orbital decompression operation for progressive exophthalmos. *Laryngoscope* 1962;72: 1078–1083.
49. Friedman W. Surgery of the pterygopalatine fossa. In: Blitzer A, Lawson W, Friedman W, eds. *Surgery of the paranasal sinuses*, 2nd ed. Philadelphia: WB Saunders, 1991:331–338.
50. Lawson W, Biller HF, Jacobson A, Som P. The role of conservative surgery in the management of inverted papilloma. *Laryngoscope* 1983;93:148–155.
51. DeFreitas J, Lucente FE. The Caldwell-Luc procedure: institutional review of 670 cases: 1975–1985. *Laryngoscope* 1988;98: 1297–1300.

31

# ENDOSCOPY IN POSTOPERATIVE CARE

DALE H. RICE

## INTRAOPERATIVE CARE

Postoperative care begins during the procedure itself. Several key steps should be taken during and at the termination of the procedure to minimize problems and maximize rapid, satisfactory healing. The steps vary, depending on whether the surgeon has done a limited anterior dissection or a complete sphenoethmoidectomy.

For the limited anterior dissection, the middle meatus should be as wide as possible at the termination of the procedure (1). This means thorough removal of the uncinate and bulla ethmoidalis coupled with some management of the middle turbinate. In some situations, this merely requires medialization of the middle turbinate to open the middle meatus. In patients with an especially bulbous or edematous middle turbinate, particularly if it tends to touch the top of the inferior turbinate, partial resection of the anterior-inferior portion may be prudent (2). However, resecting part of the turbinate may result in unwanted bleeding and is best prevented by taking the following steps. The middle turbinate should be grasped with a curved tonsil hemostat and crushed with this instrument slightly posterior and superior to the line of resection. Care should be taken to clamp all the way through the inferior-posterior aspect of the part to be resected, because bleeding is more troublesome here than in the anterior-superior aspect. The clamp should be left in place for 2 to 3 minutes and then removed. A distinct crushed zone is produced. The turbinate scissors should be used to resect the turbinate at the edge of the crushed zone, leaving the crushed area behind. If this is done, bleeding will not be a problem.

Hemostasis should be excellent at the termination of the procedure, regardless of the exact procedure performed. If a complete sphenoethmoidectomy is performed, bleeding can be minimized by the gentle handling of tissue and by using sharp, through-cut instruments. Occasionally, troublesome bleeding occurs from branches of the sphenopalatine artery. Usually, temporary packing with a vasoconstrictor agent suffices, but occasionally, bipolar cautery is necessary.

At this point, the question is whether to pack or not to pack. Both methods seem to get equally good results. A variety of packing materials are available. These include traditional antibiotic-impregnated gauze and other materials. Over the years, I have tried all of them and generally favor no packing. My experience with most of the commercially available packs is that they tend to cause considerable pain and bleeding on removal. Packing materials that do not appear to have this problem include Gelfoam pledgets and Acticoat dressings. For the past several years, I have been using fibrin glue in the middle meatus. This material is bacteriostatic and hemostatic and serves well as a barrier to prevent synechiae. If the middle meatus is sufficiently wide and there is no tendency of the middle turbinate to lateralize, the procedure may be completed by merely filling the middle meatus with an antibiotic ointment. My preference is povidone-iodine ointment. The base of this ointment is polyvinyl pyrrolidone, not petroleum. It tends to flow more readily and obviates the risk of lipoidosis in the tissues. This ointment can also be injected directly into any involved sinus with a syringe attached to a large, curved, olive-tipped aspirator. In patients with eosinophilic (e.g., allergic fungal) sinusitis, healing is often accelerated by mixing the povidone-iodine with a 2% hydrocortisone cream and injecting this mixture into the involved sinuses.

If the procedure has been done under general anesthesia, it is important to have the anesthesiologist extubate the patient while still deep, as is done for patients with asthma. The patient should not be allowed to buck when awakening before being extubated. This bucking may cause an instant and occasionally impressive epistaxis. This bleeding stops after the patient stops bucking and does not necessitate the placement of intranasal packs. It is, however, annoying and tends to wash out the antibiotic ointment. It is completely preventable with early extubation.

## POSTOPERATIVE CARE

There is considerable diversity of opinion about true postoperative management. The patient should be placed on an appropriate antibiotic for 1 to 2 weeks. Surgeons who use traditional packing tend to remove the packing in 48 hours or 5 to 7 days postoperatively and begin their care at that point. Those who use no packing tend to begin their postoperative care earlier. This may be done in a variety of ways. A common way is to have the patient begin intranasal saline irrigations on the second or third postoperative day (3). This may be accomplished with a nasal irrigator attachment to a Water Pick or by using a rubber bulb ear syringe or any other product designed for nasal irrigation. The patient must be very through with each irrigation, which should be performed initially two or three times daily. The patient may use purchased saline, a solution such as Alkolol, or salt water made at home by mixing 1 to 2 teaspoons of salt in 1 quart of water. The mixture should not sting when being used if it is properly made. The patient should be instructed to irrigate thoroughly but gently on each occasion. After irrigation, the patient should gently blow the nose and repeat this process until it is clear of mucus, crusts, and other debris. After the last nose blowing, the patient should spray each side with a steroid nasal spray. There is no scientific evidence that this speeds healing, but most seem comfortable using it.

An alternative to saline irrigations preferred by some is to have the patient do steam inhalations for 5 to 10 minutes, four or five times each day, beginning on the first or second postoperative day. This is continued for 1 to 2 weeks and seems equally as effective in promoting healing.

In the early postoperative period, the patient should be seen in the office and the middle meatus meticulously cleaned to prevent synechiae (Fig. 31.1) and to promote drainage of the involved sinuses. If the middle meatus is made as wide as possible, cleaning can generally be accomplished on the first postoperative visit easily with a standard

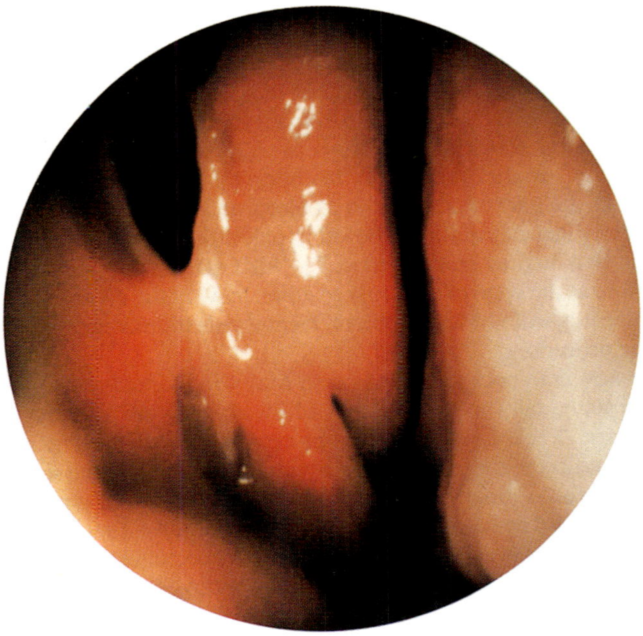

**FIGURE 31.1.** Endoscopic view of synechiae. (From Rice DH, Schaefer SD, eds. Endoscopic paranasal sinus surgery. New York: Raven Press, 1993, with permission.)

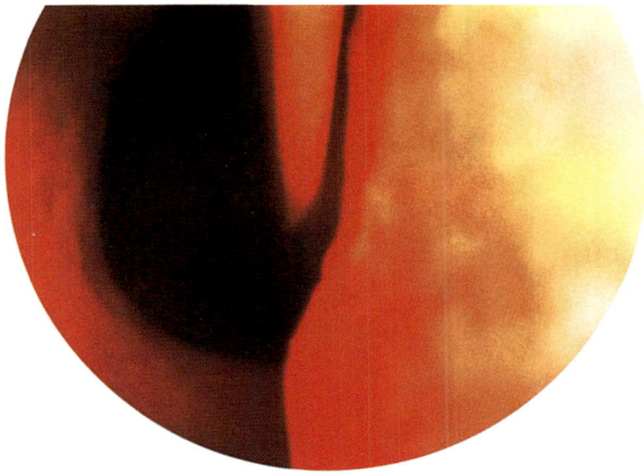

**FIGURE 31.2.** Endoscopic view of a well-healed middle meatus. (From Rice DH, Schaefer SD, eds. Endoscopic paranasal sinus surgery. New York: Raven Press, 1993, with permission.)

head mirror or headlight and a no. 5 or 7 suction tip. Occasionally, a crust requires removal with forceps, but this is the exception rather than the rule.

Further follow-up visits should be scheduled as appropriate, depending on the intranasal condition. On these visits, it is prudent to decongest the patient's nose with a mixture of any decongestant mixed with 1% Xylocaine to anesthetize the intranasal mucosa. Each operative site should be carefully inspected with a 2.7-mm endoscope, and the area should be cleaned and manipulated as necessary. Any remaining crusts should be removed, and each involved sinus should be carefully suctioned. Any synechiae that have developed should be excised. If the surgery has involved the frontal sinus ostium or the sphenoid sinus ostium, these areas should be carefully inspected and the sinuses suctioned. A sinus that shows signs of delayed healing can be filled with an antibiotic ointment or steroid cream to facilitate normalization of the mucous membranes. This careful inspection should continue until the operative site is completely healed (Fig. 31.2). This takes between 2 to 3 weeks and 2 to 3 months, depending on the extent of the dissection, the severity of the disease, and the presence or absence of underlying, aggravating conditions such as allergies or smoking.

## REFERENCES


1. Kennedy DW, Zernick SJ, Johns ME. Functional endoscopic sinus surgery. In: Goldman JL, ed. *The principles and practice of rhinology.* New York: John Wiley & Sons, 1987.
2. Toffel PH, Aroesty DJ, Weisman RH. Secure endoscopic sinus surgery as an adjunct to functional nasal surgery. *Arch Otolaryngol Head Neck Surg* 1989;115:822–825.
3. Rice DH. Basic surgical techniques and variations of endoscopic sinus surgery. *Otolaryngol Clin North Am* 1989;22:713–726.

SECTION

# IV

# HEAD AND NECK SURGERY/ PLASTIC AND RECONSTRUCTIVE SURGERY

# 32

# ENDOSCOPIC FACIAL REJUVENATION

JOHN S. RHEE
JULIO F. GALLO
PETER D. COSTANTINO

The use of endoscopes has significantly added to the armamentarium available to the facial plastic surgeon. Previously regarded major surgical procedures have been replaced with techniques that allow outpatient surgery with minimal incisions, faster recovery, and safer dissection. The use of endoscopes for facial plastic and reconstructive surgery is still evolving. The endoscopic approach has gained most popularity for rejuvenation of the forehead and brow, although endoscopic techniques have been described for midface lifts, temporal lifts, cervicoplasty, rhytidectomy, and insertion of implants.

A comprehensive compilation of facial rejuvenation procedures using endoscopic techniques is beyond the scope of this chapter. The primary focus of the chapter is on the endoscopic brow and forehead lift, a technique that has largely replaced the traditional coronal approach and is arguably the procedure of choice in most instances in addressing the aged upper third of the face.

## APPLIED SURGICAL ANATOMY

The anatomy of the forehead is ideally suited for application of endoscopic principles. The forehead is an expandable, confined cavity with avascular planes for dissection and direct visualization. Small incisions can be hidden behind the hairline, allowing bimanual endoscopic assisted dissection, broad elevation, and fixation of elevated tissue.

As in any surgical technique, the mastery of pertinent anatomy is integral to performing successful surgery. Endoscopic techniques promote and rely on excellent visualization of the surgical field; therefore, surgical dissection in relatively avascular planes is paramount. Knowledge of the fascial planes and the relevant neurovascular anatomy allow the surgeon to safely and effectively use the endoscopic assisted dissection.

### Forehead

The central forehead and scalp is composed of five distinct layers, described by the pneumonic SCALP: skin (S), subcutaneous tissue (C), galea aponeurosis (A), loose areolar tissue (L), and pericranium (P) (Fig. 32.1). The skin is thick and densely adherent to the underlying subcutaneous tissue. The galea aponeurosis is a thin, mobile, fibromuscular sheet that envelops the entire skull and splits anteriorly to encase the frontalis and procerus muscles. The galea is an extension of the superficial musculoaponeurotic system (SMAS) in the face and the temporoparietal fascia of the temple. The loose areolar tissue plane is a relatively avascular plane and the traditional layer of dissection for coronal approaches. This layer is continuous with the loose connective tissue that separates the temporoparietal fascia and the deep temporal fascia. The pericranium is a thickened layer of connective tissue adherent to the skull and is continuous with the periorbita at the level of the supraorbital ridges (1).

The sensory innervation of the forehead and scalp is supplied by the supraorbital and supratrochlear nerves, which are extensions of the ophthalmic branch of the trigeminal nerve. Both nerves exit the frontal bone through a notch or foramen, pierce the orbital septum, and turn upward to pierce the corrugator muscle and travel on the superficial aspect of the frontalis muscle (Fig. 32.2).

The actions of the muscles of the brow and forehead are listed in Table 32.1. The temporal branch of the facial nerve innervates all of these muscles. The mimetic actions of these muscles produce the wrinkles and furrows in the skin of the forehead and glabellar areas. The corrugator and procerus muscles are usually surgically weakened in the correction of the aging brow and forehead.

### Temporal Fossa

The transition from the forehead to the temporal fossa occurs at the superior temporal line, demarcated by the conjoint fascia, a condensation of the pericranium and the deep temporal fascia. The temporal fossa is bounded inferiorly by the zygomatic arch and anteriorly by the frontal process of the zygomatic bone. The fascial layers of the temporal fossa have been prone to confusing and conflicting nomenclature (Fig. 32.1).

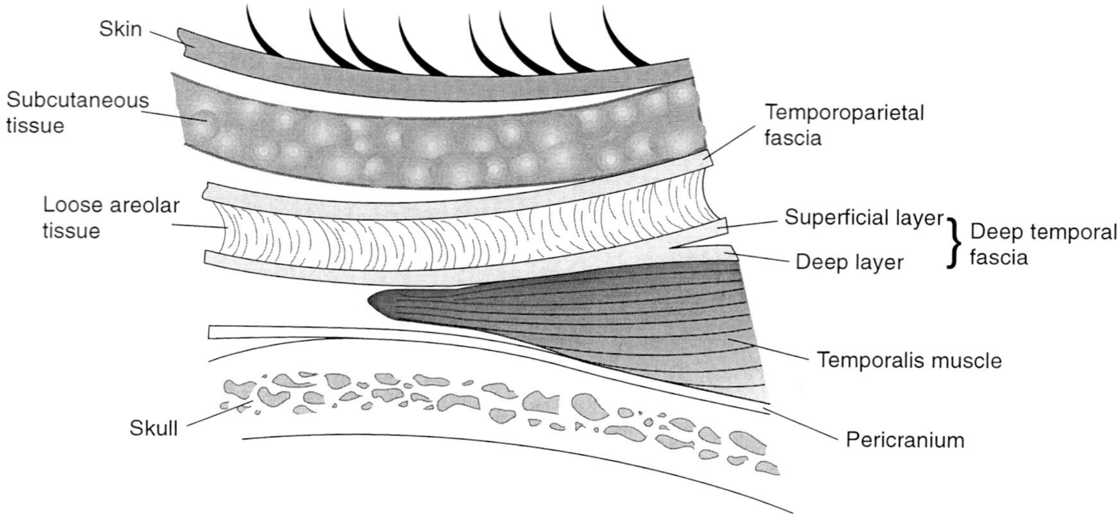


**FIGURE 32.1.** The layers of the scalp and temple.

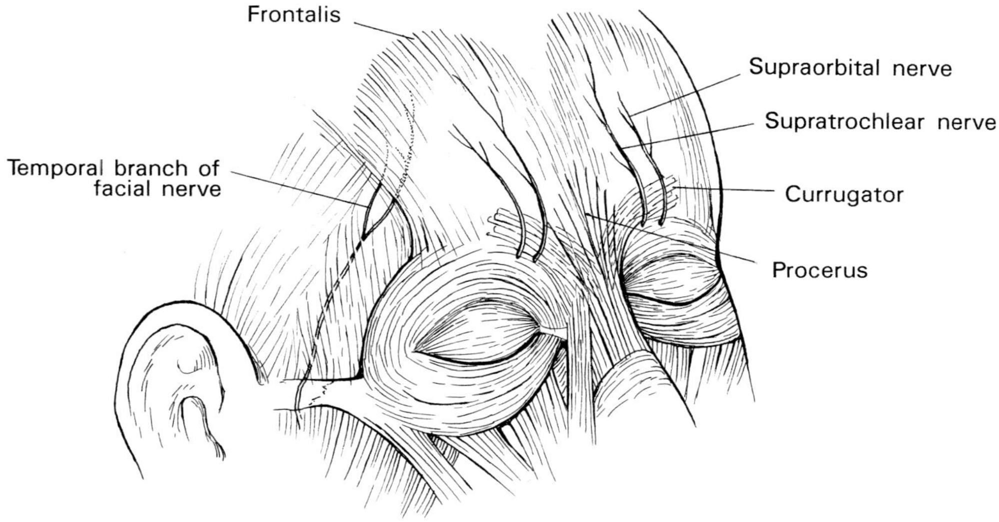


**FIGURE 32.2.** The nerves and expressive muscles of the forehead and temple.

**TABLE 32.1. MUSCLES OF THE UPPER THIRD OF THE FACE**

| Muscle | Action | Result |
|---|---|---|
| Frontalis | Elevates brow | Forehead rhytids |
| Orbicularis oculi | Depresses brow; closes eyelids | Crow's-feet |
| Procerus | Depresses medial brow | Transverse glabellar rhytids |
| Currugator | Depresses brow; medializes brow | Vertical glabellar rhytids |

The temporoparietal fascia is a thin, vascular layer that is densely adherent to the overlying skin and subcutaneous tissue. This layer is continuous with the galea aponeurosis of the scalp and SMAS of the face. The deep temporal fascia envelops the temporalis muscle and divides into a superficial and deep layer at approximately 2 cm above the zygomatic arch. The arch and the temporal fat pad are ensheathed by the superficial and deep layers of the deep temporal fascia.

Understanding the course of the temporal branch of the facial nerve is critical to safe dissection in this area. The nerve enters the temporal fossa by crossing superficially over the midportion of the zygomatic arch. It travels in the temporoparietal fascia layer and then exits the temporal fossa to course along the deep aspect of the frontalis muscle, supplying the muscles of the brow and forehead (Fig. 32.2).

## AESTHETIC CONSIDERATIONS OF THE BROW AND FOREHEAD

The shape of the eyebrow is one of a graceful and gentle arch. The ideal position and shape of the eyebrow is quite subjective and varies according to gender, ethnicity, and current fashion trends. As a general rule, the medial brow has a clubhead configuration and begins at a point tangent to a vertical line drawn through the medial canthus and lateral nasal ala margin (Fig. 32.3). The brow gradually tapers to a handle shape, with the lateral third of the brow coursing above the superior orbital rim in women and at the rim in men. It terminates laterally at a point tangent to an oblique line drawn from the lateral nasal ala to the lateral canthus (2). Depending on a person's aesthetic sense, the apex of the brow arch should coincide with the lateral limbus of the eye or the lateral canthus (3).

The upper third of the face is a focal point for expression and emotions. With the aging process, there is loss of tissue elasticity, decrease in the bulk of the subcutaneous tissue, and an increase in skull bone resorption. Excessive displacement of the medial portion of the eyebrows along with deep glabellar furrows may project expressions of anger or malice. A similar lateral hooding or drooping of the eyebrows suggests a fatigued or sad appearance (4).

Some surgeons have turned to more objective parameters when assessing harmony of the upper third of the face. McKinney and colleagues (5) described the existence of brow ptosis when the distance from the midpupil to the top of the brow was less than 2.5 cm (Fig. 32.3). He also observed that the female forehead should measure 4 to 6.2 cm (mean, 4.8 cm). Farkas and Kolar (6) found that the most attractive women had a relatively smaller upper third of the face compared with the middle and lower third of the face. It is important to remember that the endoscopic technique does raise the hairline, although not to the degree as with the traditional coronal lift.

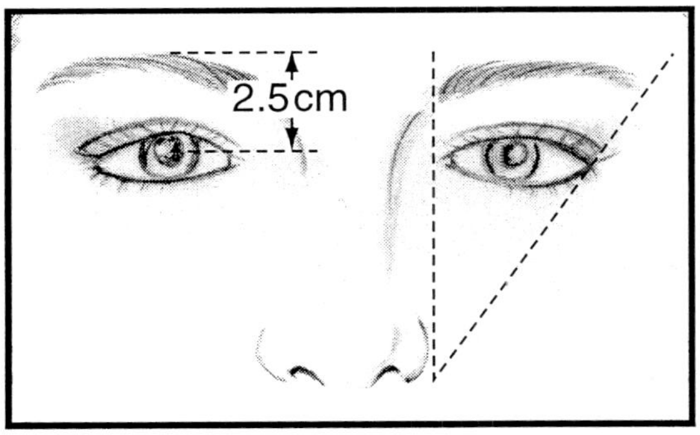


**FIGURE 32.3.** Ideal eyebrow position and proportion. The medial brow begins at a point tangent to a vertical line drawn through the medial canthus and lateral nasal ala margin and terminates laterally at a point tangent to an oblique line drawn from the lateral nasal ala to the lateral canthus. The apex of the brow arch should lie between the lateral limbus and the lateral canthus. Brow ptosis exists when the distance from the midpupil to the top of the brow is less than 2.5 cm.

## PREOPERATIVE EVALUATION

Careful patient selection and appropriate surgical goals help to ensure optimal results. In evaluating candidates for rejuvenation of the upper third of the face, it is important to consider the aesthetics of the brow and the upper third of the face. The need for an upper lid blepharoplasty may be obviated by a brow lift or markedly reduce the requirements for skin excision. The entire orbital complex, brow position, frontal hairline, hair density, forehead contour, forehead rhytids, and furrows caused by the actions of the underlying musculature should be considered in the preoperative assessment.

### Indications

Indications for the endoscopic brow and forehead lift are ptosis of eyebrows and the existence of glabellar frown lines. The ideal candidate has the following characteristics: female, low hairline, abundant hair, flat contour of the forehead, normal or thin forehead skin, and moderate brow ptosis.

### Contraindications

There are no absolute contraindications for the endoscopic approach; however, there are patient factors that make this approach less favorable. Patients requiring extensive bone recontouring may be better treated with an open procedure. Patients with thick, heavy sebaceous skin and severe brow ptosis are less favorable candidates and may be better served with conventional skin excision techniques. Similarly, the use of the endoscopic approach for patients with facial paralysis has been abandoned by most surgeons because of severity of the brow ptosis associated with the complete loss of frontalis muscle function (7). Patients with high hairlines, sparse hair, male pattern baldness, and rounded foreheads are less ideal candidates for the endoscopic approach.

## CASE EXAMPLES

### Case 1

This 52-year-old woman complained of "looking angry and tired all the time." She exhibited many of the classic manifestations of the aging upper third of the face (Fig. 32.4). In Figure 32.4, the brows are ptotic resulting in hooding of the

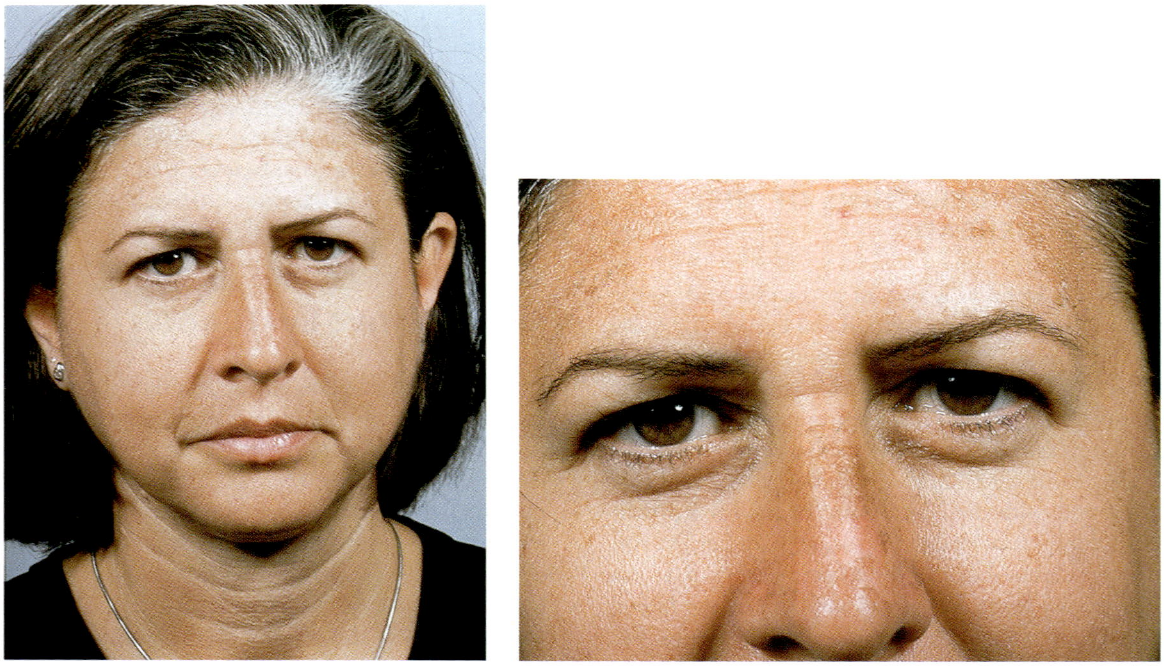

A B

**FIGURE 32.4. A,B:** Preoperative views of patient with brow ptosis and an overactive procerus muscle.

upper eyelids. An overactive procerus muscle further accentuates the medial brow ptosis. She is a good candidate for the endoscopic approach, given her hairline position, abundant hair, normal forehead skin thickness, and flat contour of forehead.

The patient underwent an endoscopic assisted forehead and brow lift as the sole procedure. At 9 months postoperatively, she exhibits improvement in the aesthetics of her orbital complex and upper third of face (Fig. 32.5). In Figure 32.5, notice the reemergence of her own supratarsal lid creases, without the need for upper lid blepharoplasties. Although the hairline has been raised slightly, the proportions of her face remain in a harmonious relationship.

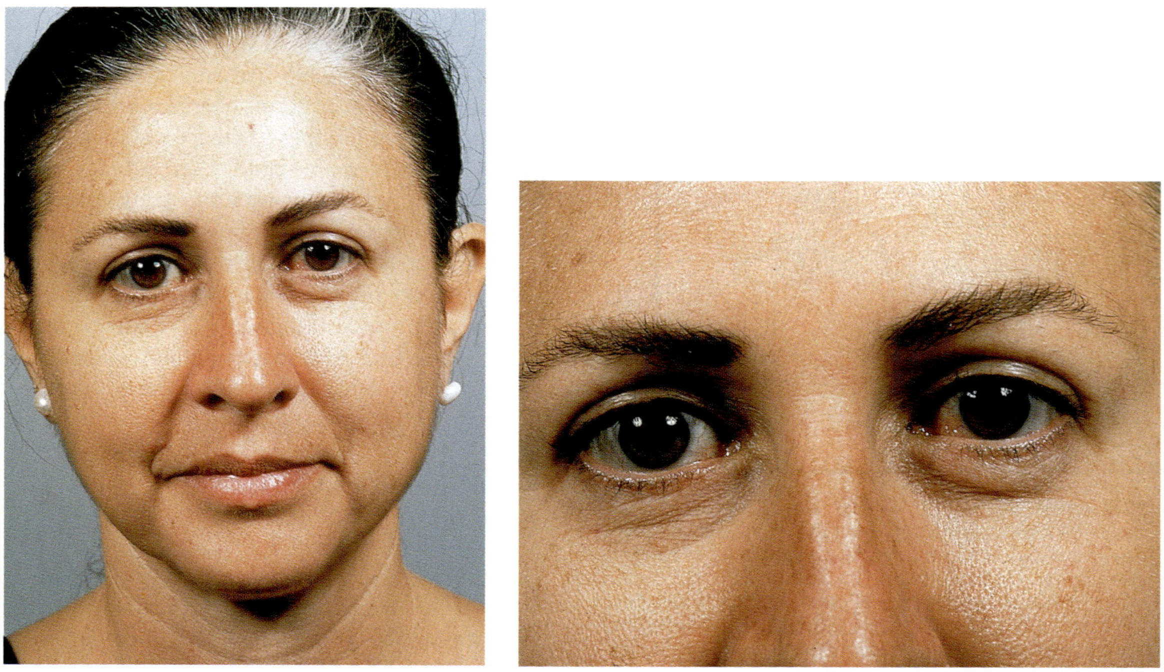

A B

**FIGURE 32.5. A,B:** Views 9 months after endoscopic brow and forehead lift. Notice the improvement of the orbital complex without the need for upper lid blepharoplasties.

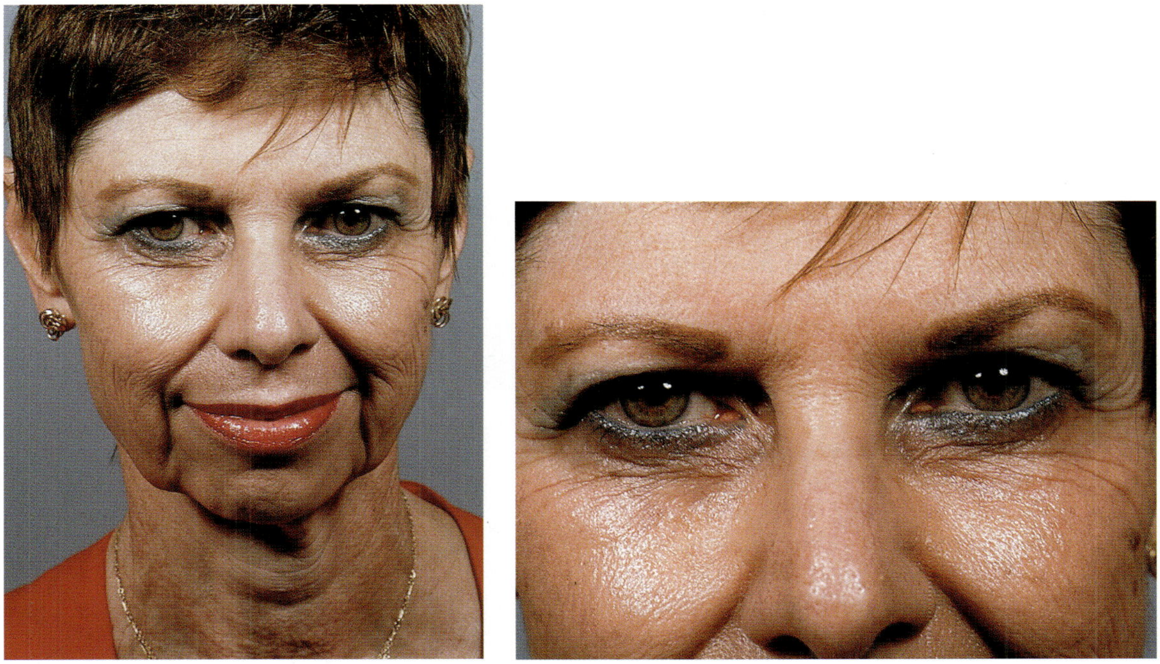

A B

**FIGURE 32.6. A,B:** Preoperative views of a patient with brow ptosis, overactive procerus and corrugator muscles, and associated aging of the lower face.

## Case 2

This 55-year-old woman complained of "looking too serious and tired." She exhibited moderate brow ptosis along with an aging lower face (Fig. 32.6). The procerus and corrugator muscles were overactive. She was a good surgical candidate for the endoscopic approach.

Patient underwent an endoscopic assisted brow and forehead lift, upper and lower lid blepharoplasties, and a cervicofacial rhytidectomy (Fig. 32.7). At 6 months postoperatively, she states that her "eyes are much brighter." Concomitant upper lid blepharoplasties were needed in this instance because of the persistent hooding after the completion of the brow and forehead lift.

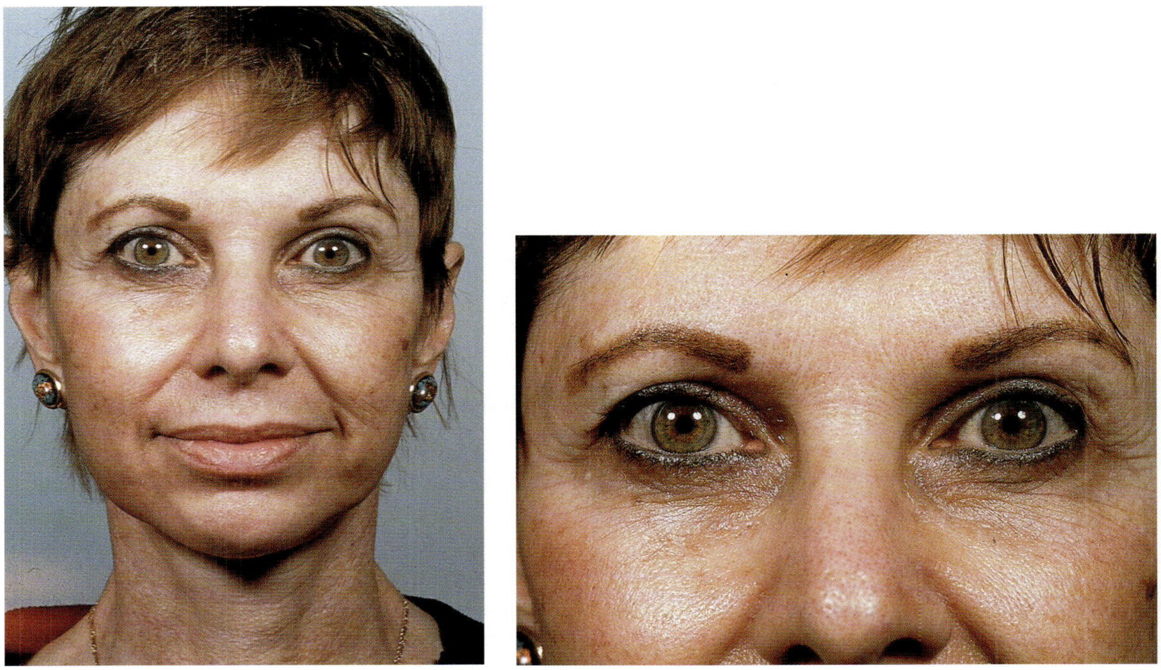

A B

**FIGURE 32.7. A,B:** Views 6 months after an endoscopic brow and forehead lift, upper and lower lid blepharoplasties, and cervicofacial rhytidectomy.

## INSTRUMENTATION AND OPERATING ROOM LAYOUT

The necessary specific instruments are relatively few, and the essential equipment should be familiar to most otolaryngologists who perform endoscopic sinus surgery. A video recorder, xenon light source, video camera, and high-resolution video monitor (>400 lines) are standard equipment. These pieces should be housed in a mobile cart that can be easily moved about the operating room.

The most common type of endoscopes used in facial plastic surgery is the 4- or 5-mm, 0° and 30° Hopkins-type rigid endoscopes. A protective sheath locks onto the endoscope, preventing accidental bending and damage. The sheath provides additional ports for suction, irrigation, and cautery. The end of the sheath extends 0.5 to 1.0 cm beyond the tip of the scope and gently slopes away from the tip. This feature provides retraction of the overhanging tissue, allowing better visualization (Fig. 32.8).

The available surgical instrumentation for endoscopic procedures has greatly expanded in recent years. A basic set of essential instrumentation is shown in Figure 32.9. The dissecting elevators are available in different arcs of curve to allow easier dissection over rounded or prominent convexities of the frontal bone. The elevator ends come in various shapes and degrees of sharpness. Graspers, scissors, and hooks are helpful when operating around the glabellar muscles and the supratrochlear and supraorbital nerves. These instruments are also available insulated for electrocautery.

The operating surgeon should be seated at the head of the table, with the first assistant to the patient's right and the scrub nurse to the left. The anesthesiologist and the anesthesia cart are situated to the patient's left. The Mayo stand is placed over the patient and the video cart is placed at the right foot of the bed. In this way, anesthesia monitoring lines do not entangle with the endoscopic cables, and the surgeon has an unobstructed view of the monitor.

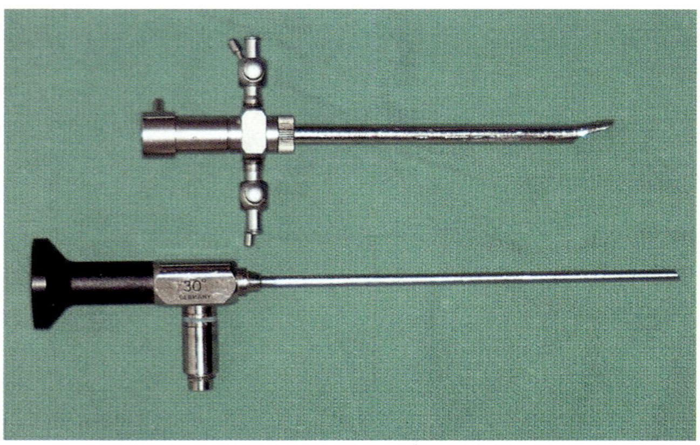

**FIGURE 32.8.** A 4-mm, 30° rigid endoscope and protective cannula with two ports (Smith & Nephew Richards, Memphis, TN).

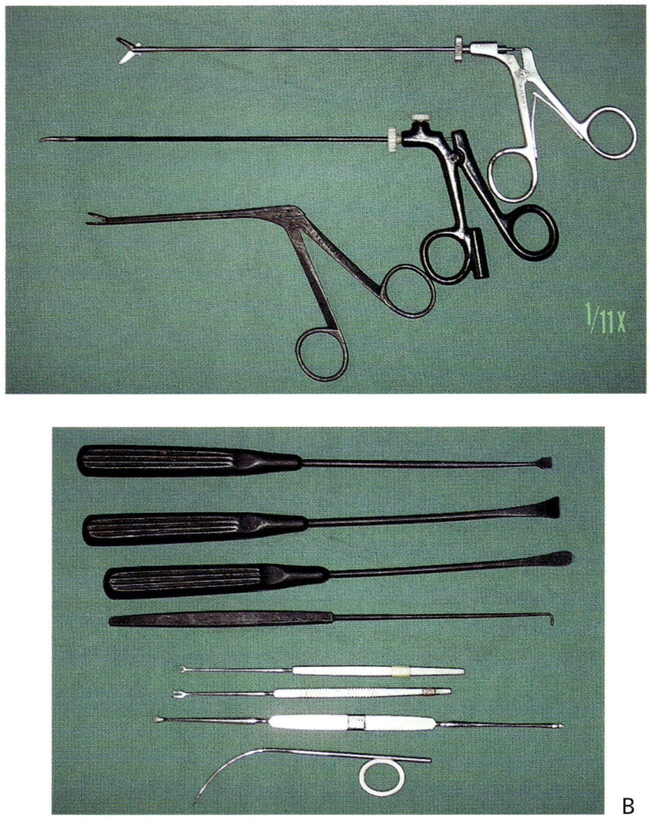


A

B

**FIGURE 32.9. A,B:** Endoscopic instrumentation with various angled elevators, scissors, graspers, nerve hooks, electrocoagulators, and a Wright needle (Smith & Nephew Richards, Memphis, TN).

## OPERATIVE TECHNIQUE

### Overview

There are four steps in executing the endoscopic brow lift: placement of small but precisely placed incisions, dissection and adequate release of the scalp and forehead, myotomy of the desired facial expressive muscles, and elevation and fixation of the forehead to the desired level.

### Preoperative Markings

The patient is evaluated in an upright sitting position, observing the glabellar frown lines at rest and during forceful muscle contraction. The midline vertical incision is marked, as well as the course of the supraorbital and supratrochlear nerves (Figs. 32.10 and 32.11). The two paramedian incisions are marked at the desired high point of the brow arch. The temporal incisions are determined by manually elevating the lateral brow in a vector drawn from the

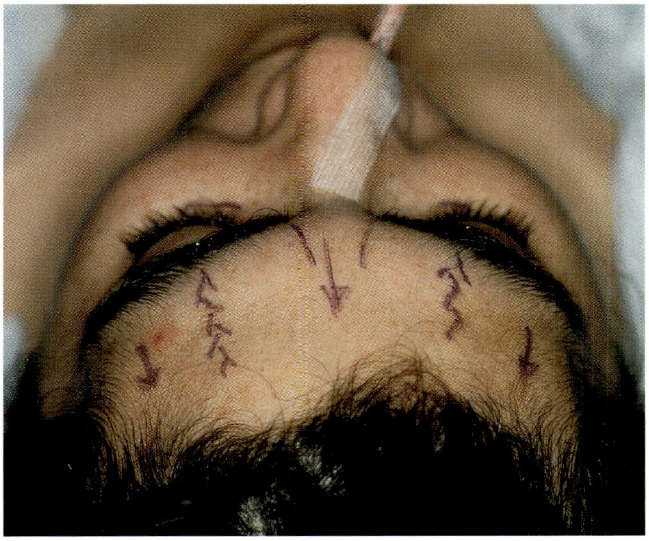

**FIGURE 32.10.** The course of the supraorbital-supratrochlear neurovascular bundle is marked according to the desired vectors of lift.

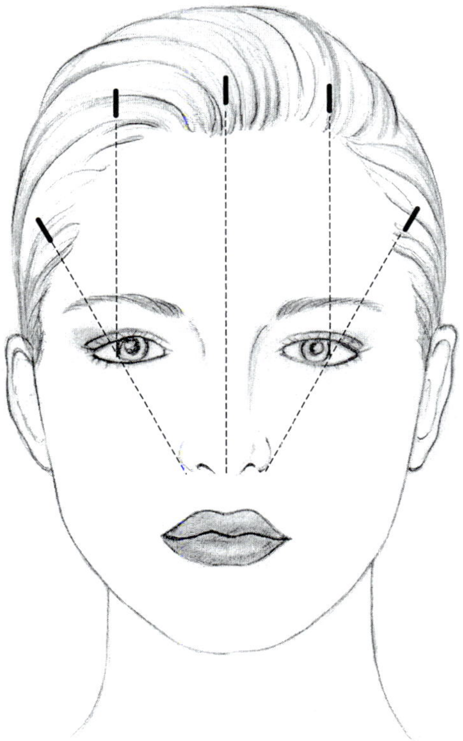

**FIGURE 32.11.** Placement of the incisions for the endoscopic brow lift. The paramedian incisions should be tangent to the lateral limbus of the eye. The temporal incisions should be tangent to the lateral limbus of the eye and the lateral alar base. The temporal incisions may be placed more laterally, depending on individual aesthetic desires and goals.

alar base to the lateral canthus. This determines the optimal vector of elevation of the lateral brow.

## Anesthesia

The endoscopic procedure can be done under general anesthesia or intravenous conscious sedation. Local infiltration with 0.5% lidocaine with 1:200,000 epinephrine allows anesthesia, hydrodissection, and vasoconstriction. The tip of the needle is inserted down to bone, and the anesthetic is injected in the subperiosteal plane. The injection over the temporal region is less precise. The injection is done deep to the temporoparietal layer.

## Incisions

The endoscopic forehead lift has been described using four, five, or six incisions placed 2 to 3 cm behind the hairline. We prefer using five vertical incisions, each about 2 cm long and placed approximately 2 cm behind the hairline (Fig. 32.11). The central incision marks the midline and is the main endoscopic port. The two paramedian incisions are placed at the level of the lateral limbus or canthus. The two temporal incisions are needed for dissection over the temporalis fossa and to allow better positioning the lateral portion of the brow.

## Dissection

The plane of dissection over the skull for the endoscopic forehead lift can be subperiosteal or subgaleal. We prefer the subperiosteal dissection because it is a safe and easily dissected area with minimal bleeding. The dissection is done "blindly" with a large, square elevator over the skull down to approximately 3 cm above the orbital rim (Fig. 32.12).

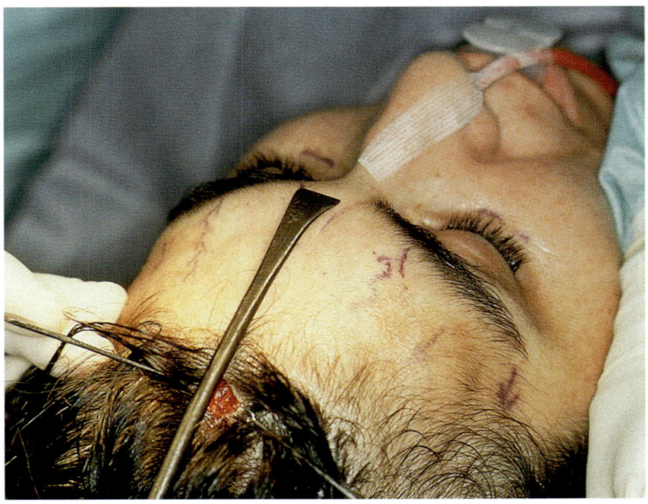

**FIGURE 32.12.** A wide elevator is used to elevate an initial subperiosteal pocket in the central forehead.

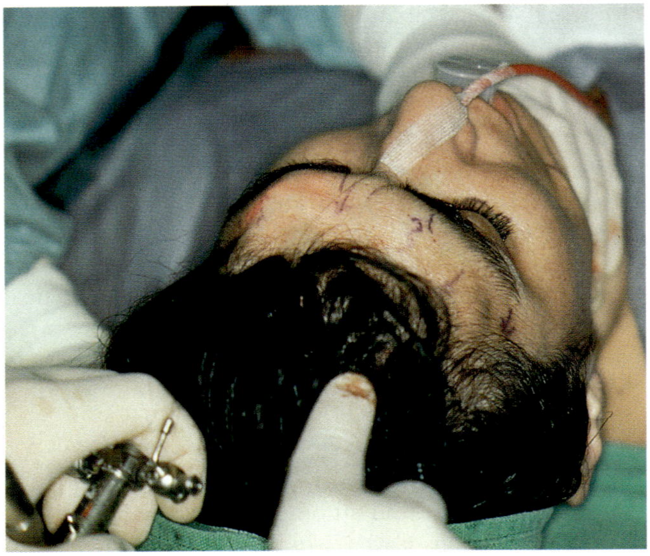

**FIGURE 32.13.** Endoscope is introduced into the central incision. A small, square elevator is placed through the paramedian incision.

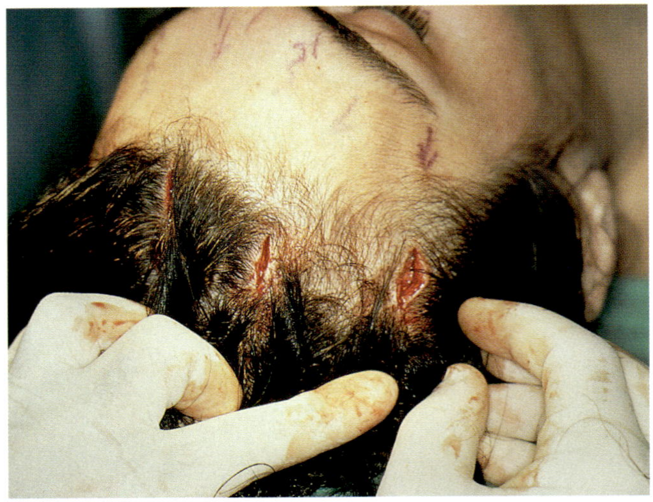

**FIGURE 32.15.** The temporal incision is placed at the desired vector pull of the lateral brow.

This blind dissection allows rapid elevation of the forehead tissue and provides the necessary optical cavity for the endoscope. The 30° endoscope is then inserted in the central incision, and dissection is continued under direct endoscopic visualization down to the orbital rim (Figs. 32.13 and 32.14).

The temporal incision is made down to the deep layer of the deep temporalis fascia (Fig. 32.15). Using a Freer elevator, the dissection is continued along this plane and connected to the paramedian incision. Under endoscopic visualization, the temporal dissection is connected to the subperiosteal plane of the forehead by sharply dissecting the transition zone at the temporal crest line with a curved, round-tipped elevator (Fig. 32.16).

The temporal dissection is continued to the level of the zygomatic arch and the zygomaticofrontal suture line. If the dissection is in the correct plane, the temporal fat pad in the levated flap should become visible as the surgeon nears the zygomatic arch (Fig. 32.17). A branch of the zygomaticotemporal communicating vein is often encountered when

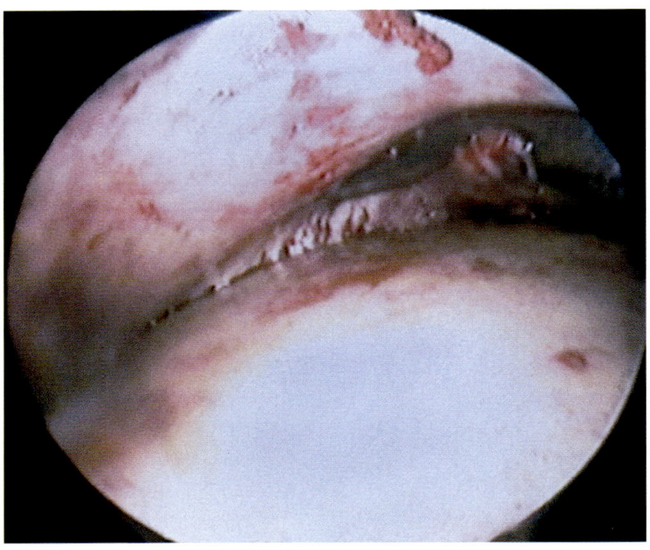

**FIGURE 32.14.** A small, square elevator is used to release the periosteum at the supraorbital rim. Adequate release of the entire superior arcus marginalis is essential for brow elevation.

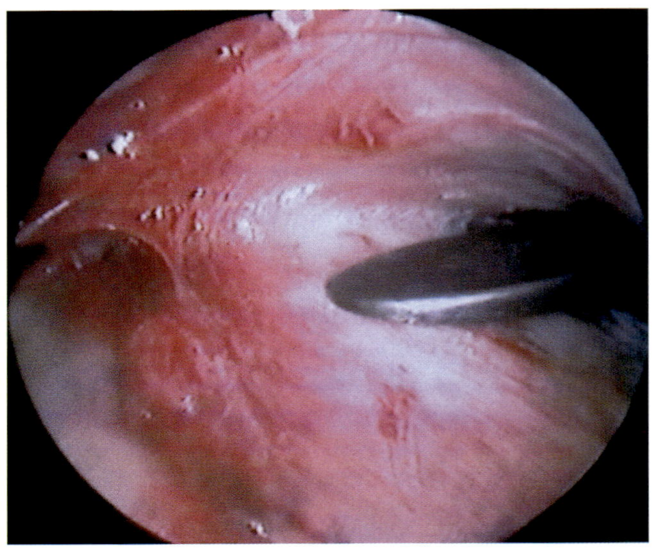

**FIGURE 32.16.** Connection of the temporal dissection with the subperiosteal plane of the forehead.

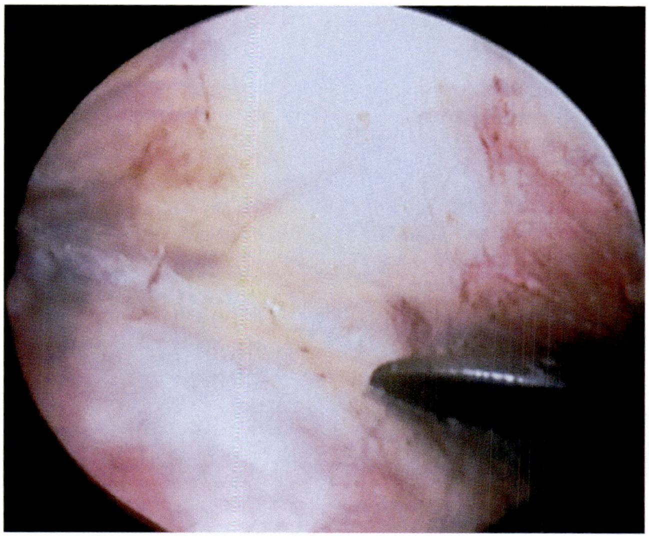

**FIGURE 32.17.** Temporal dissection taken down to the zygomatic arch. Notice the yellow color of the temporal fat pad in the elevated flap.

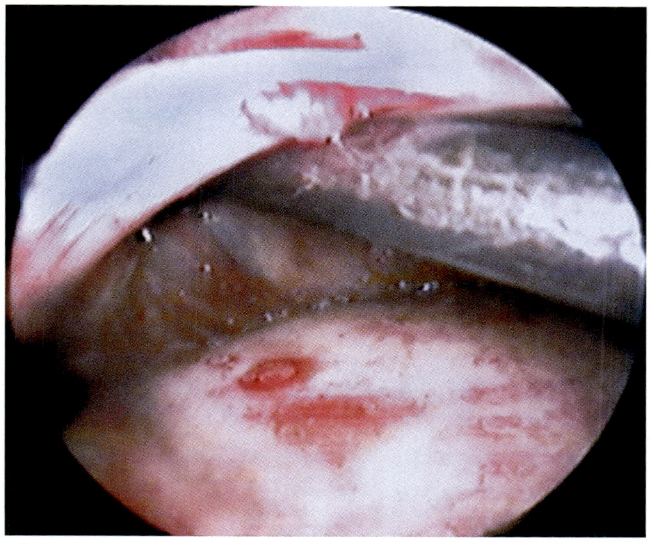

**FIGURE 32.19.** View of the corrugator muscle after incising the periosteum and galea. Notice the oblique orientation of the muscle fibers.

dissecting near the zygomaticofrontal suture line. The vein can be cauterized with a bipolar cautery or gently dissected from the surrounding tissue. One of the temporal branches of the facial nerve runs close to the vein. Bleeding caused by injury to this vein can lead to poor visualization, with possible inadvertent injury to the nerve by cauterization or further dissection. It is important to avoid overzealous upward lifting over the temporal area, which may cause traction neuropraxia of the frontal branch of the facial nerve.

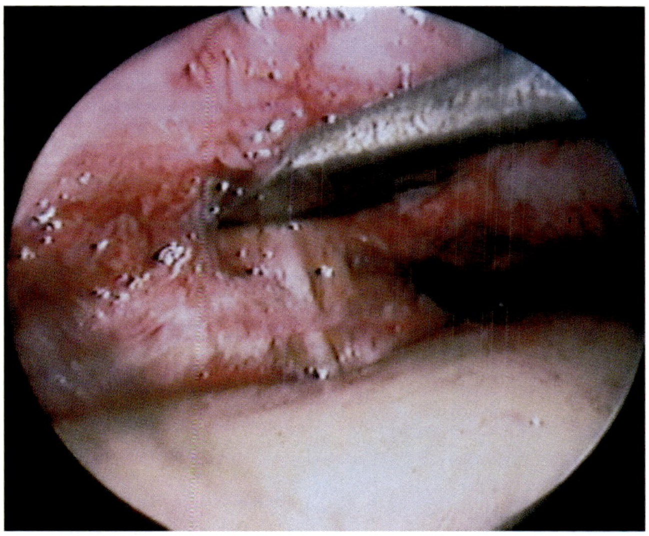

**FIGURE 32.18.** The supraorbital bundle emanating from the supraorbital foramen.

After the temporal cavity and the forehead cavity are freely communicated, a large optical cavity exists for the finer points of dissection. Using the small, square elevator, flap elevation is continued down to the orbital rim. It is important to fully release the entire length of the superior arcus marginalis to achieve adequate brow elevation. The periosteum and galea is horizontally scored at this point, exposing the corrugator muscle, procerus muscle, supraorbital nerve, and supratrochlear nerve (Figs. 32.18 and 32.19). For patients in whom glabellar muscle modification is desired, the supratrochlear and supraorbital nerves are dissected from the corrugator muscle by using a gentle vertical spreading motion with Takahashi forceps.

After the nerves are safely separated from the corrugator muscle, the muscle is resected by gentle avulsion. If desired, the procerus muscle, too, can be resected by using the same avulsion technique. These muscles may also be ablated using a carbon dioxide ($CO_2$) laser. The advantage of the $CO_2$ laser is the hemostasis coupled with the precision of the ablation. The subcutaneous fat becomes visible on removal of the muscle. Care should be used not to remove any subcutaneous tissue, because dimpling or contour irregularities can occur. It is not necessary to remove all of the muscle fibers to achieve the desired result; the extent of the resection should be tailored to the preoperative assessment of the severity of the glabellar frown lines.

## Fixation

Perhaps the greatest discrepancy in the endoscopic approach is in the method of fixation of the elevated forehead. Several techniques have been described including the

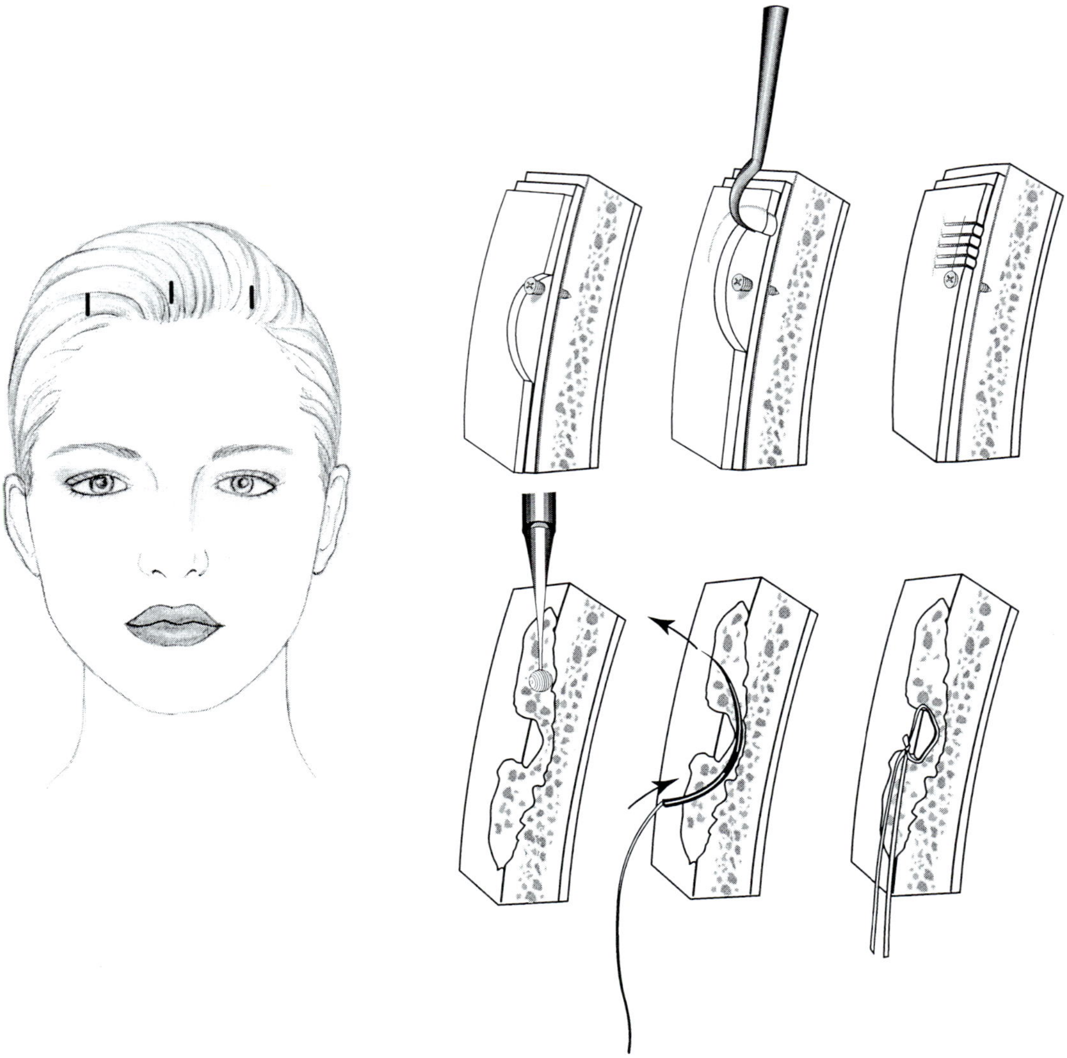

**FIGURE 32.20.** Fixation techniques. **Top row:** Variation on the external screw technique. A screw is placed at the posterior extent of the vertical incision, and the scalp complex is advanced posteriorly. Surgical staples are placed behind the protruding screw. **Bottom row:** Creation of an outer cortex bone bar with a cutting burr. The suture is secured from the galeal-periosteal layer to the bone bar.

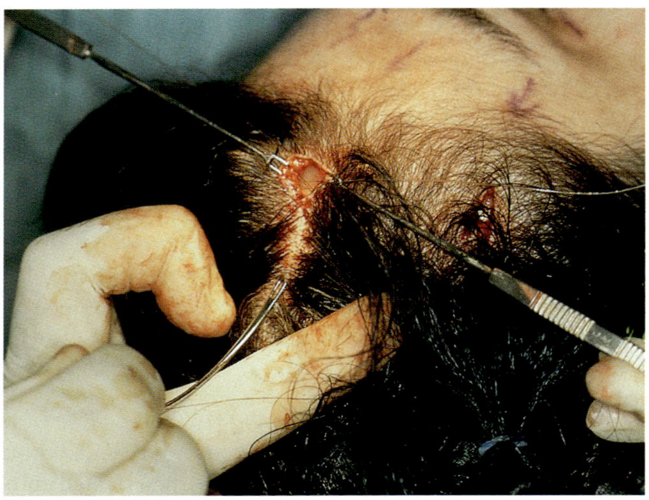

**FIGURE 32.21.** Demonstration of the use of the Wright needle for the periosteal-galeal suture.

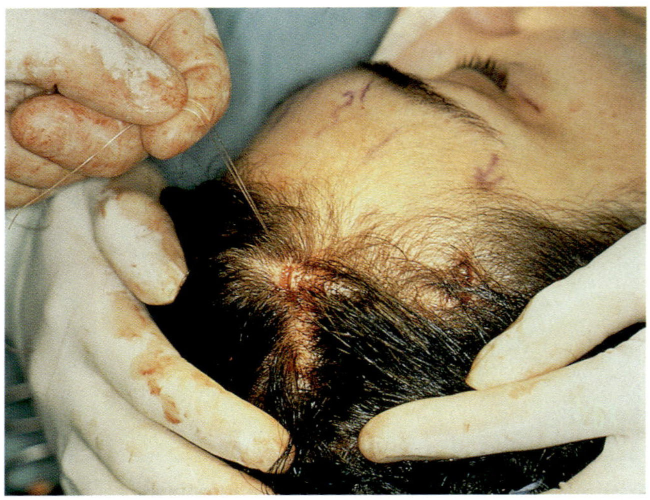

**FIGURE 32.22.** Bunching of the scalp after fixation of the elevated tissue with the periosteal-galeal suture. The bunching resolves in 2 to 3 months.

use of miniplates, screws, bone bars, and suture techniques (8,9) (Fig. 32.20). Regardless of the method of fixation, adequate dissection and mobilization of the forehead tissue is paramount for successful brow elevation.

We prefer the use of a modified periosteal-galeal suture technique (10) for the central and two paramedian incisions. We have found this suture technique reliable and lasting, with the advantage of not having to use miniplates, drills, or screws. An incision is made approximately 7 to 8 cm directly posterior to the original incisions. The anterior corner of the original incision is secured with a 2-0 Maxon suture, engaging the galea and the periosteum. A Wright needle is directed through the posterior stab incision in a subcutaneous plane to exit at the posterior corner of the original incision (Fig. 32.21). The needle end of the suture is threaded through the Wright needle. The Wright needle is then brought back to the posterior stab incision, directed deep to the galea, and again exited at the posterior corner of the original incision. The suture is tied, and the scalp bunches as the elevated forehead is raised to the desired level (Fig. 32.22). The bunching of the scalp generally resolves in 2 to 3 months.

The temporal fixation determines the final position of the lateral brow. Using a 3-0 PDS suture, the anterior corner of the incision is engaged and secured to the desired point on the deep layer of the temporalis fascia, determined by the desired vector pull. The scalp is then closed with stainless steel staples.

## HIGHLIGHTS

1. In evaluating candidates for rejuvenation of the upper third of the face, it is important to keep in mind the aesthetics of the brow, the entire orbital complex, and the dynamic actions of the facial musculature.
2. The need for an upper lid blepharoplasty may be obviated by a brow lift or markedly reduce the requirements for skin excision.
3. The ideal candidate has the following characteristics: female, low hairline, abundant hair, flat contour of the forehead, normal or thin forehead skin, and moderate brow ptosis.
4. The correct plane of dissection in the temporal fossa is integral in safeguarding the frontal branch of the facial nerve.
5. The subperiosteal dissection of the central forehead must be connected with the temporal dissection for adequate elevation of the lateral brow.
6. Adequate release of the arcus marginalis is integral for successful brow elevation.
7. The periosteum and galea must be incised to expose the corrugator and procerus muscles. These muscles do not need to be totally excised; weakening and attenuating the muscle can achieve the desired effect.
8. The methodology of fixation of the elevated forehead is less important than the adequate release and mobilization of the forehead.

## POSTOPERATIVE CARE

A mild compression dressing that is wrapped around the head and chin is applied. Elastic tape of Coban is used to prevent the formation of a hematoma and to facilitate adhesion of the newly elevated tissues to the bone. Drains are generally unnecessary. The dressing is removed the next day, and the staples are removed on the fifth postoperative day.

Periorbital ecchymosis and swelling is not uncommon for the first week. However, the rapidity of recovery of the endoscopic technique is unmatched by the traditional coronal approach.

## COMPLICATIONS

The incidence of complications for this procedure is quite low. Hypesthesia over the forehead and scalp due to traction neuropraxia of the sensory nerves is usually temporary and returns to normal in 6 to 10 weeks. There have been some anecdotal reports of temporary weakness of the frontal branch of the facial nerve after the procedure. Permanent facial nerve paralysis has not been reported.

Imprecise surgical technique may result in asymmetrical brows, excessive brow elevation, or more commonly, recurrence of brow ptosis. Sufficient release of the brow at the level of the orbital rim and adequate fixation can prevent the recurrence of brow ptosis. There may be some temporary local alopecia at the incision sites, and bunching of the skin resolves in 2 months.

## CONCLUSIONS

The traditional coronal incision for rejuvenation of the upper third of the face has been largely replaced with endoscopic techniques, which require minimal incisions, broad elevation, and fixation of tissue. Situations necessitating direct skin excisions or open surgical exposure are relatively infrequent. An appreciation of brow aesthetics and the pertinent surgical anatomy helps to ensure optimal surgical outcomes.

## REFERENCES

1. Larrabee W, Makielski K, Sykes J. Surgical anatomy for endoscopic facial surgery. In: Keller GS, ed. *Endoscopic facial plastic surgery.* St. Louis: Mosby, 1997:3–33.
2. Sullivan MJ. Brow and forehead aesthetics. *Facial Plast Surg Clin North Am* 1997;5:95–98.

3. Cook TA, Brownrigg AJ, Wang TD, et al. The versatile midforehead browlift. *Arch Otolaryngol Head Neck Surg* 1989;115: 163–168.
4. Sullivan MJ. Endoscopic facial surgery. In: Cheney ML, ed. *Facial surgery: plastic and reconstructive.* Baltimore: Williams & Wilkins, 1997:913–926.
5. McKinney P, Mossie RD, Zubowsi ML. Criteria for the forehead lift. *Aesthetic Plast Surg* 1991;15:141–147.
6. Farkas LG, Kolar JC. Anthropometrics and art in the aesthetics of women's faces. *Clin Past Surg* 1987;14:559–616.
7. Freeman MS, Graham HD. Endoscopic surgery of the forehead and midface. *Facial Plast Surg Clin North Am* 1997;5: 113–132.
8. Graham HD. Methods of soft-tissue fixation in endoscopic surgery. *Facial Plast Surg Clin North Am* 1997;5:145–154.
9. Bostwick J, Eaves F, Naha F. Forehead lift and glabellar frown lines. In: Bostwick J, ed. *Endoscopic plastic surgery of the head and neck.* St. Louis: Quality Medical Publishing, 1995:166–230.
10. Maloney BP. Endoscopic forehead lifting. In: *Facial plastic surgery.* Stamford: Appleton & Lange, 1997:167–176.

# 33

# ENDOSCOPIC-ASSISTED REPAIR OF FACIAL FRACTURES

JOHN S. RHEE

Management of facial fractures is based on the concepts of open reduction and rigid internal miniplate or screw fixation. Advances have been made in smaller fixation systems, bioresorbable plates and screws, and new bone substitutes. However, all of these rely on traditional techniques of wide exposure.

As in other surgical subspecialties, the application of endoscopic surgical techniques have revolutionized the approach to various clinical problems. The use of minimally invasive incisions have greatly reduced the morbidity associated with open repair. The use of endoscopes for facial fractures may be the next exciting frontier. Scientific papers have described endoscopic techniques to assist in repair of mandible, midface, and frontal sinus fractures. This chapter discusses the current state of the art for endoscopic management of facial fractures, the limitations of this approach, and future directions.

## INDICATIONS AND CONTRAINDICATIONS

### Frontal Sinus Fracture

The endoscopic approach has largely replaced the conventional coronal incision for rejuvenation of the brow and forehead (see Chapter 32). A logical extension of this technique is its application for repairing frontal sinus fractures. The use of this minimally invasive technique has been limited to noncomminuted anterior table fractures that do not involve the nasofrontal duct (1). These injuries tend to occur in relatively low-energy impact settings. Endoscopic-assisted obliteration of the frontal sinus is not a feasible option with the currently available instrumentation. It is not possible to adequately remove all of the frontal sinus mucosa, especially for largely pneumatized sinuses. Fractures of the posterior table, nasofrontal duct, or severely comminuted anterior table fractures are best treated with traditional open approaches.

The technique basically consists of exposing the fracture segments using a subperiosteal dissection under endoscopic guidance. Additional small stab incisions are made in the brow and along forehead mimetic lines. These incisions allow for bimanual fracture reduction and miniplate fixation with screws (2) (Fig. 33.1).

### Orbital Floor Fractures

Fractures of the orbital floor may occur as part of a zygomaticomaxillary complex (ZMC) fracture or as an isolated blow-out fracture. The endoscope can be used as a diagnostic tool and a surgical adjunct to open repair.

Coronal computed tomography (CT) scans are extremely useful for evaluation of the orbital floor. Unfortunately, coexisting injuries such as cervical spine injury may preclude obtaining this imaging technique. CT scans also are susceptible to artifacts from dental fillings or other metallic objects, which may obscure important views of the orbit. Preoperative CT sizing of the orbital floor fracture is not always accepted as the definitive assessment of injury. For all of these reasons, exploration of the floor is frequently performed for diagnosis, with reports of a 40% to 65% incidence of nontherapeutic orbital floor explorations (3).

Patients with suspected orbital floor fractures whose conditions prohibit radiographic assessment are candidates for bedside sinus endoscopy, as illustrated later in the case example. The pulse test can be used to determine orbital floor integrity by transantrally inserting a 30° rigid endoscope into the maxillary sinus. When a significant orbital fracture exists, retropulsion of the globe results in fat herniation into the maxillary sinus antrum (Fig. 33.2).

Intraoperative use of endoscopes for repair of orbital floor fractures has been shown to have some useful applications (4,5). The posterior portion of the orbital floor is sometimes difficult to assess by standard examination through a periorbital approach. This area lies behind the equator of the globe and assumes a superior angulation of 15° as is proceeds from the orbital rim to the orbital apex (6) (Fig. 33.3). Endoscopic visualization using a transantral approach allows accurate determination of the size and

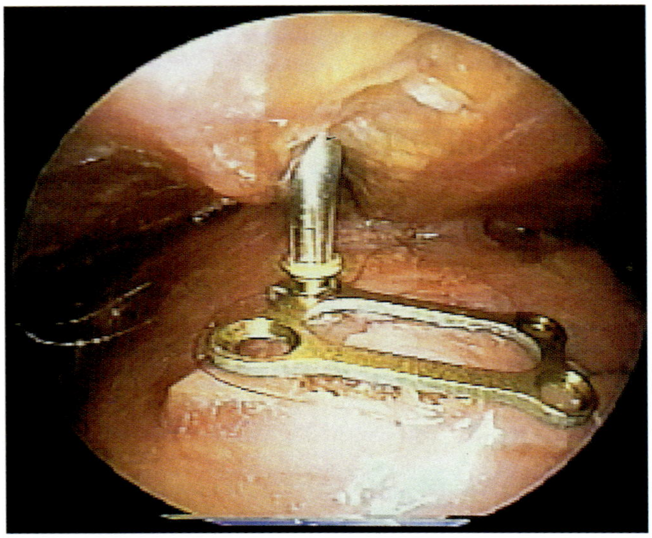

**FIGURE 33.1.** Endoscopic view of a frontal sinus anterior table fracture. A self-drilling screw is being applied to the titanium plate through the stab brow incision.

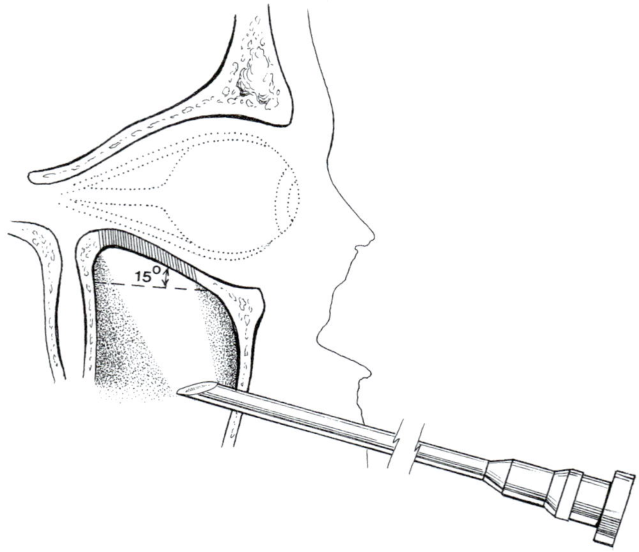


**FIGURE 33.3.** Endoscopic transantral visualization of the posterior portion of the orbital floor. Angulation of the orbital floor makes for difficult direct inspection through a conventional periorbital incision.

location of the floor fracture and ensures appropriate positioning after orbital floor reconstruction with bone grafting or alloplastic material. Often, a fracture-induced antral window already exists with ZMC fractures, and the scope can be easily introduced through this portal. In a pure orbital blow-out floor fracture, a trocar can be used to enter the maxillary sinus. The endoscope can then be introduced through the trocar cannula for evaluation of the orbital floor (Fig. 33.4).

There are no absolute contraindications to the use of the endoscope for orbital floor fractures. However, it may not be needed when obvious exploration and repair is indicated or when surgical repair is deemed satisfactory with direct inspection.

## Medial Orbital Wall Blow-out Fractures

In the past, medial orbital wall blow-out fractures had been given relatively less attention; however, later studies showed that the incidence of orbital fractures of the medial wall may be higher than that for fractures of the floor (7). These studies suggested that enophthalmos may be worse from nonrepaired medial orbital wall blow-out fractures than

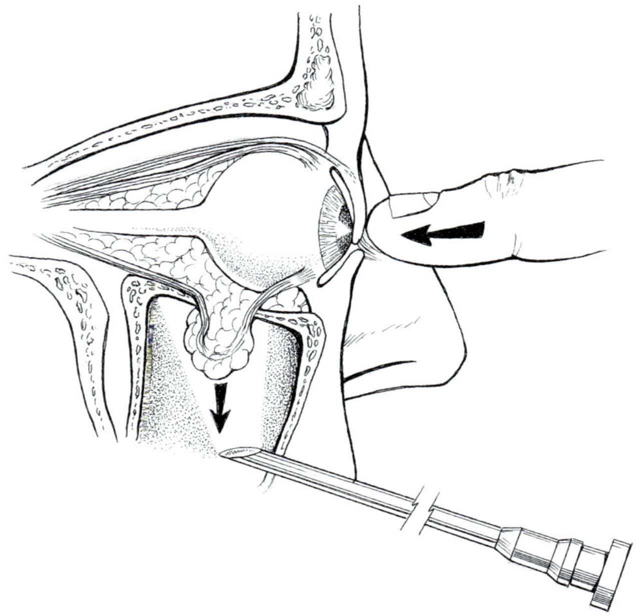

**FIGURE 33.2.** The pulse test is used to determine orbital floor integrity. Retropulsion of the globe result in fat herniation into the maxillary sinus, as visualized transantrally with a 30° endoscope.

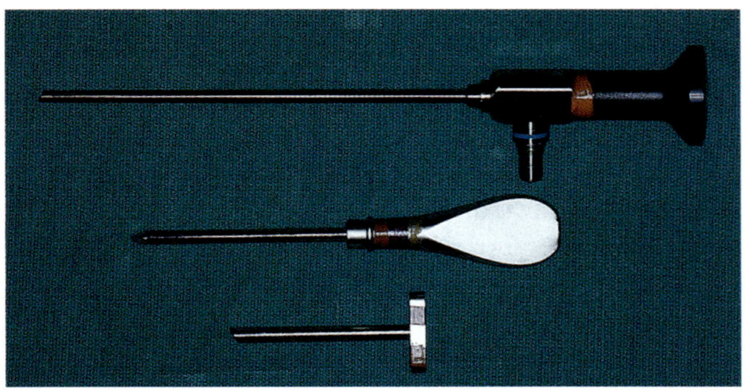

**FIGURE 33.4.** Sinus trocar, cannula, and 30° rigid endoscope.

from blow-out fractures of other walls (8). We have developed a technique that allows for endoscopic assistance in reduction of the orbital contents and in placement of the alloplast or graft for reconstitution of the medial orbital wall (see section on Operative Technique for Medial Orbital Wall Fracture) (9).

## Zygomaticomaxillary Complex Fractures

Lee and colleagues (10) described an endoscopic method of zygomatic arch repair obviating the need for the bicoronal incision. However, the application for this approach is somewhat limited, because only a minority of cases require zygomatic arch exposure. Three-point fixation at the frontozygomatic suture, zygomaticomaxillary buttress, and inferior orbital rim is sufficient in most ZMC fractures. The endoscopic technique may be most beneficial in those cases with isolated severely comminuted zygomatic arch fractures that cannot be elevated to anatomic position with a Gillestype approach.

The most useful application of the endoscope in ZMC fractures is the ability to transantrally inspect the orbital floor to confirm the absence or presence of a significant floor fracture. If the pulse test result is negative, and there is no evidence of entrapment or enophthalmos, no orbital floor exploration needs to be performed and the orbital rim may be fixated through the gingivobuccal incision, obviating the need for a periorbital incision.

## Subcondylar Fracture

Endoscopic techniques have been described for the repair of subcondylar mandible fractures (11,12). Conventional open approaches for subcondylar fractures have not gained universal acceptance because of risk of facial nerve injury, impaired fracture visualization, and difficult dissection and fixation.

Lee and coworkers (11) treated the largest series of patients using this technique. The endoscopic approach has been used for displaced subcondylar fractures of the mandible. Intracapsular, comminuted, and pediatric fractures are considered to be contraindications to the endoscopic technique. The fracture is approached through an intraoral buccal sulcus incision sited over the oblique line of the mandible. The endoscope allows visualization of the fracture, aids in the reduction, and confirms correct anatomic fixation of the screws that are introduced through a trocar located in the preauricular region.

# CASE EXAMPLES

## Orbital Floor Fracture

A 25-year-old man was involved in a severe motor vehicle accident. He had sustained significant intracranial and visceral injuries and a questionable cervical spine fracture. Consultation was requested by the trauma service for evaluation of his facial fractures seen on the axial CT scans. The patient was nonresponsive, intubated, and in a hard cervical collar. The ophthalmologist had diagnosed a left-sided traumatic optic neuropathy. Physical examination revealed marked swelling of the left cheek and periorbital region. A slight step-off along the left orbital rim was palpated. The left pupil was fixed and dilated, with moderate subconjunctival hemorrhage. The forced duction test result was negative for entrapment. Axial CT scans revealed a nondisplaced ZMC fracture. Coronal CT scans for evaluation of the orbital floor could not be obtained because of the patient's coexisting injuries.

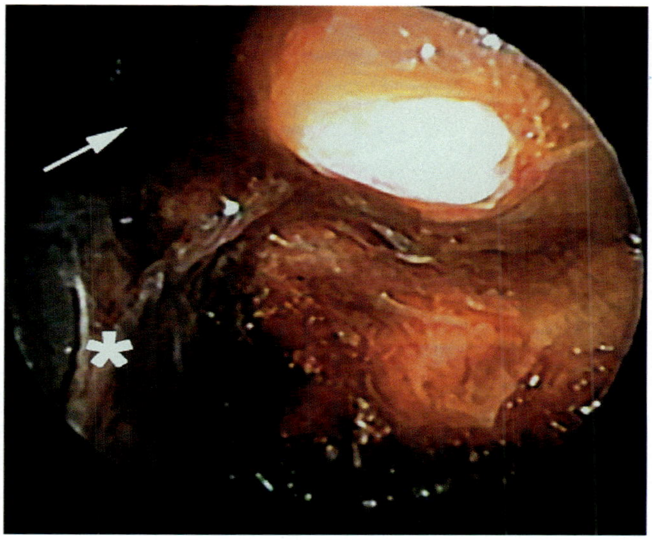

**FIGURE 33.5.** Endoscopic transantral view of a left-sided orbital floor fracture with herniation of the orbital contents into maxillary sinus. The *asterisk* marks the maxillary sinus wall for orientation, and an *arrow* designates the true maxillary sinus ostia.

The gingivobuccal sulcus was injected with 1% lidocaine with epinephrine. A trocar was placed in the left maxillary sinus. Old blood was suctioned from the maxillary sinus cavity. A 4-mm, 30° rigid endoscope was introduced into the trocar cannula (Fig. 33.4). Inspection of the orbital floor revealed a significant orbital floor defect with a positive Pulse test (Fig. 33.5). A single chromic suture was used to close the trocar site. Orbital floor fracture repair was recommended because of risk of delayed enophthalmos.

## Medial Orbital Wall Fracture

A 29-year-old man was referred for consultation 1 week after an assault. He had sustained blows to the right periorbital region with fists. He complained of orbital pain and diplopia on upward gaze. Visual acuity was measured at 20/25 OS. Intraocular pressure was within normal limits.

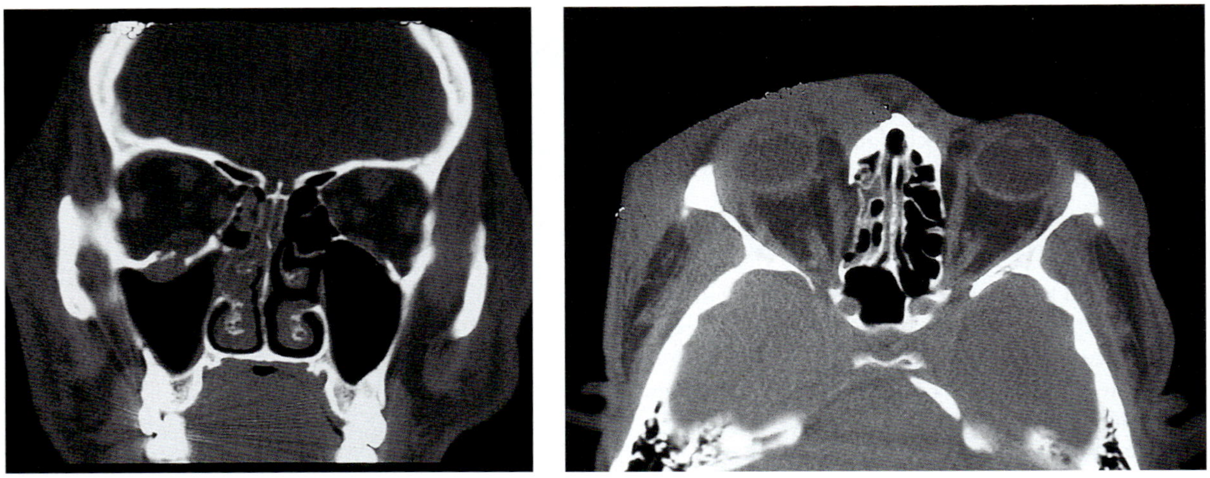

A B

**FIGURE 33.6. A,B:** Coronal and axial computed tomography scans of a displaced combined orbital floor and medial wall fracture.

Extraocular movements were normal. There was decreased sensation along the $V_2$ nerve on the right cheek. CT scans of the orbits revealed a combined fracture of the floor and medial wall, without evidence of entrapment (Fig. 33.6). Because of the risk of delayed enophthalmos from increased orbital volume, the patient underwent an endoscopic-assisted repair of the medial orbital wall and floor (Figs. 33.7 and 33.8). By the fourth postoperative week, the patient's diplopia had resolved, and there was no evidence of enophthalmos. The operative technique is detailed later in this chapter.

## INSTRUMENTATION

The necessary specific instruments are relatively few, and the essential equipment should be familiar to most otolaryngologists who perform endoscopic sinus surgery. A video recorder, xenon light source, video camera, and high-resolution video monitor (>400 lines) are standard equipment. These pieces should be housed in a mobile cart that can be easily moved about the operating room.

The repair of frontal sinus fractures requires the use of equipment designed for endoscopic forehead and brow lifts

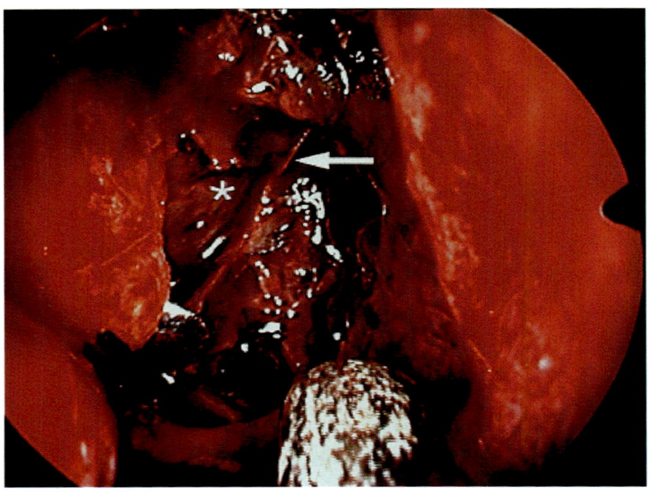

**FIGURE 33.7.** Endoscopic intranasal view of a medial orbital wall fracture. The *arrow* delineates the posterior ledge of the displaced lamina papyracea, and the *asterisk* marks the exposed periorbita.

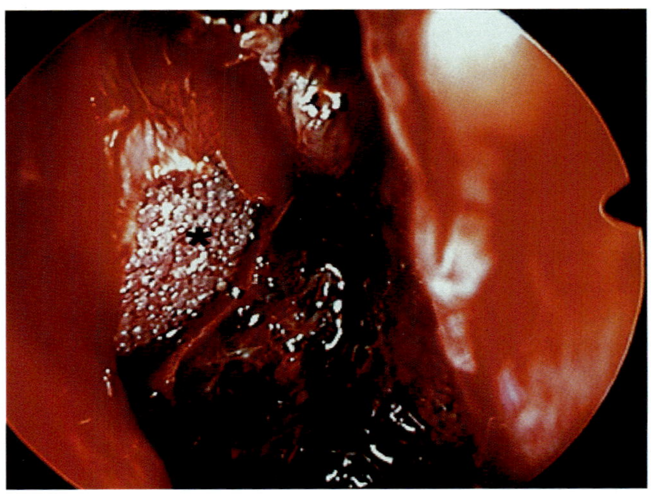

**FIGURE 33.8.** Endoscopic intranasal view of the medial orbital wall fracture after repair with a Medpor barrier sheet (Porex Surgical, Inc., College Park, GA). The *asterisk* marks the alloplast.

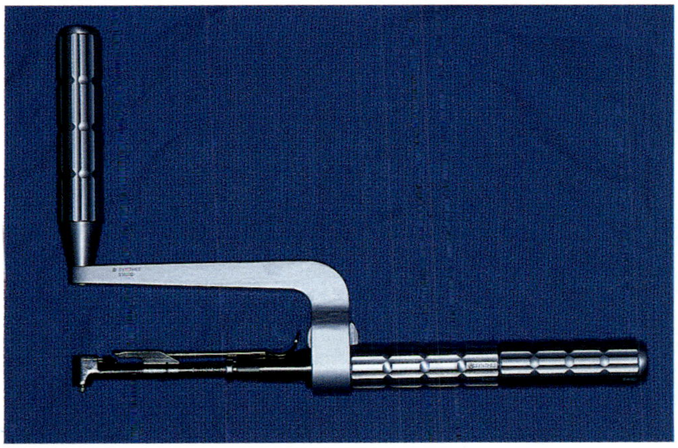

**FIGURE 33.9.** Commercially available right-angle screwdriver (Synthes Maxillofacial, Paoli, PA).

(see Chapter 32). These instruments allow creation of an optical cavity and dissection along the curved forehead contour. Additional equipment includes power drills and titanium plates and screws (e.g., Stryker-Leibinger craniomaxillofacial modular system). With the development of more sophisticated equipment, the additional incisions in the forehead and brow may not be necessary in the future. Several companies have developed a right-angle screwdriver that can be used with self-drilling screws (Fig. 33.9). However, these screwdrivers are still quite bulky and need to be modified to mimic the curvature of the endoscopic browlift equipment to be used effectively for frontal sinus fractures. Prototype equipment for rigid fixation using the endoscopic approach is under development (13).

Evaluation of the orbital floor requires the use of a standard 4-mm, 30° rigid endoscope. A sinus trocar and cannula system is useful for entry into the maxillary sinus with relatively minimal morbidity (Fig. 33.4).

Standard sinus instrumentation is needed to complement an oculoplastic soft tissue tray for repair of medial orbital wall fractures. I use an alloplastic implant for repair of orbital floor and medial wall fractures: Medpor orbital implant barrier sheet (38 × 50 × 1 mm, Porex Surgical, Inc.).

## OPERATIVE TECHNIQUE FOR MEDIAL ORBITAL WALL FRACTURE

The techniques for endoscopic-assisted repair of frontal sinus, ZMC, subcondylar, and orbital floor fractures have been previously described by other investigators and are too numerous to include in this chapter. The technique for endoscopic-assisted medial orbital wall fracture is elucidated below. Preoperative and postoperative CT scans from a cadaver specimen with a medial orbital wall fracture illustrate the result that can be achieved with this approach (Figs. 33.10 and 33.11).

The operation is performed under general anesthesia and with the patient in a supine position. A corneal protector is placed in the affected eye. The periorbital region is injected in the preseptal plane with 1% lidocaine with 1:100,000 epinephrine. Decongestion of the sinonasal cavity is initiated in the preoperative holding area with topical 0.05% oxymetazoline spray. The 4% topical cocaine pledgets are placed in the operating suite. Injections are carried out with a 25-gauge spinal needle, using 1% Xylocaine with 1:100,000 epinephrine. Under endoscopic guidance, the following sites are injected in this order: the posterior attachment of the middle turbinate, the inferior border of the middle turbinate, and the anterior attachment of the middle turbinate to the lateral nasal wall.

The orbital floor is approached by a transconjunctival incision with a canthotomy and cantholysis or a subciliary incision. A preseptal dissection is carried down to the

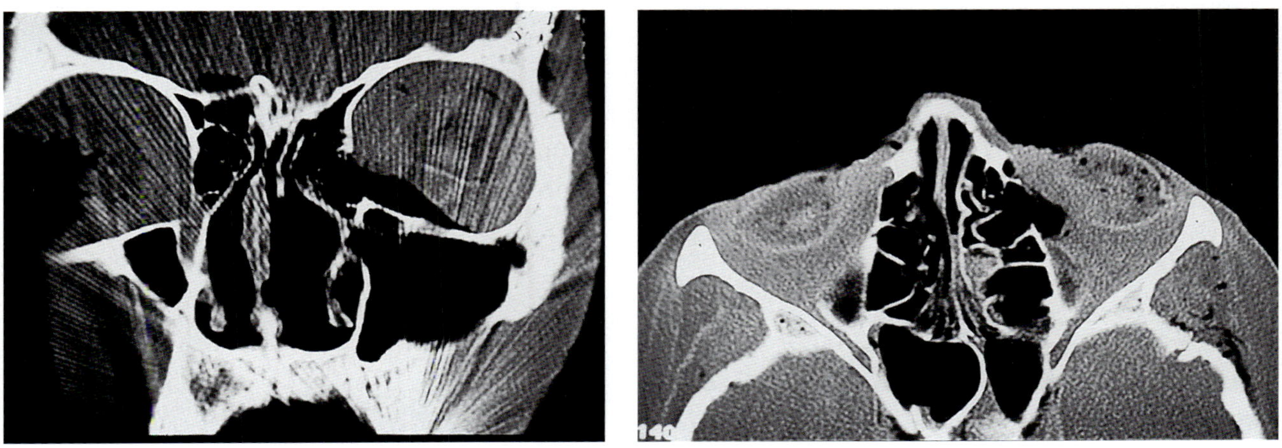

A B

**FIGURE 33.10. A,B:** Coronal and axial computed tomography scans of an experimentally created medial orbital wall fracture in a cadaver.

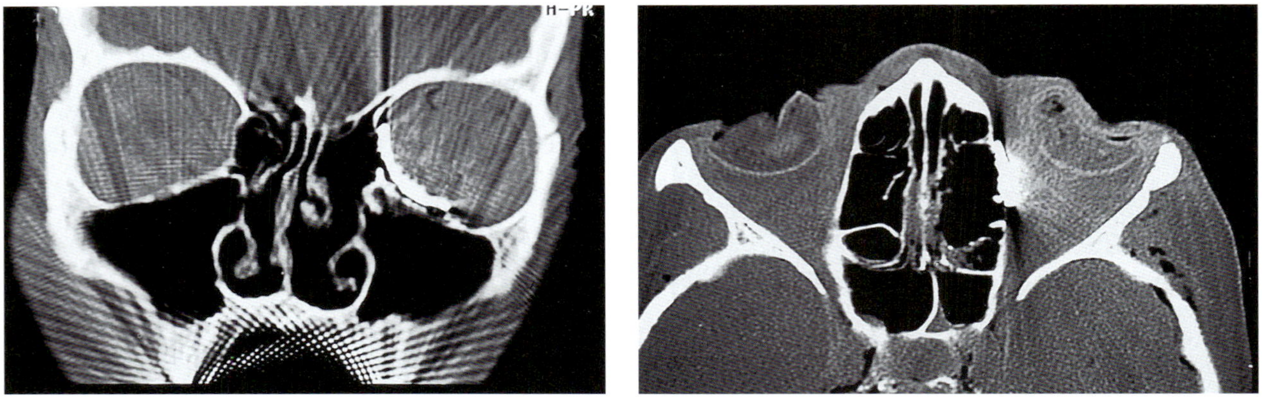

A B

**FIGURE 33.11. A,B:** Coronal and axial computed tomography scans after repair of the medial orbital wall fracture with alloplast. Alloplast impregnated with radiopaque material for illustrative purposes.

orbital rim. The arcus marginalis is sharply incised at the orbital rim. Dissection is continued along the orbital floor, deep to the periorbita. If a concomitant orbital floor defect exists, the orbital contents are gently reduced from the maxillary sinus. Before the manipulation of the medial orbital contents, the medial orbital wall is approached intranasally.

After decongestion is accomplished using a 4.0-mm endoscope, the uncinate process is identified and resected. Approximately 3 to 4 mm of uncinate is left superiorly to prevent frontal recess stenosis. This exposes the natural ostium of the maxillary sinus, and an antrostomy is performed in a posterior and inferior direction. The maxillary antrostomy prevents the development of chronic maxillary sinusitis due to traumatic obstruction of the sinus ostia. Injury to the orbital contents is unlikely during the endoscopic maxillary antrostomy because the orbital floor contents have already been reduced through the external incision. However, because of the possibility of orbital herniation into the sinonasal cavity, the use of powered instrumentation is avoided in these cases. The bulla ethmoidalis is then entered medially and resected to expose the lamina papyracea defect. The herniated orbital contents are apparent at this stage and great care should be taken to prevent further injury (Fig. 33.12). If necessary, the dissection is carried posteriorly through the grand lamella to fully expose the defect in the lamina papyracea.

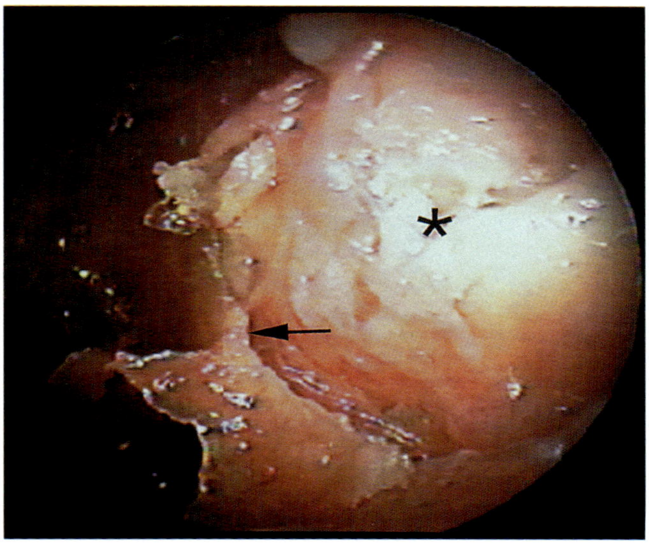

**FIGURE 33.12.** Endoscopic intranasal view of the lamina papyracea defect. The *asterisk* marks the herniated periorbita and orbital fat, and the *arrow* delineates the intact posterior ledge of the lamina papyracea.

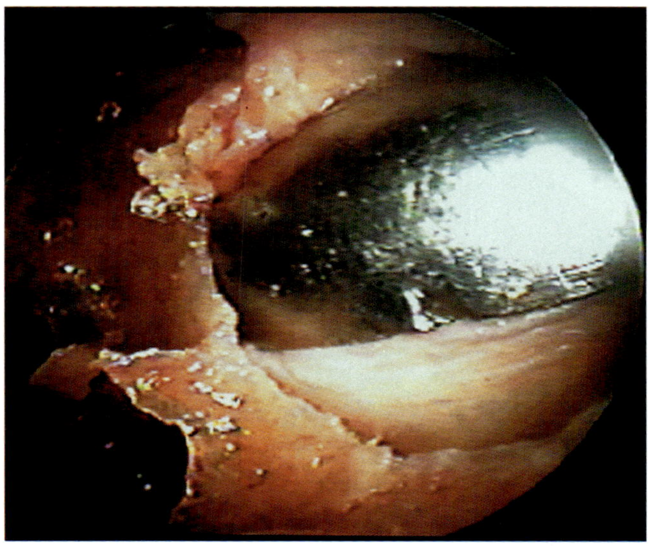

**FIGURE 33.13.** Endoscopic intranasal view of the orbital contents being reduced with a retractor.

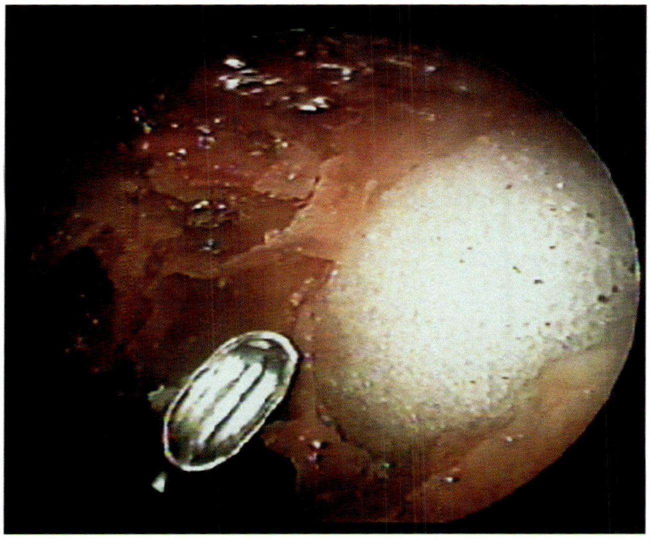

**FIGURE 33.14.** Endoscopic intranasal view of the orbital implant in position. Notice the ability to confirm the correct posterior placement of the implant and to ensure that no orbital contents are impinged by the implant.

From the external incision, the orbital contents are reduced and held in place with a malleable retractor (Fig. 33.13). Adequate reduction is confirmed from the intranasal endoscopic and external approaches. The endoscope is most helpful in visualizing the most posterior extent of the fracture. An appropriately shaped implant that covers the defect and rests on relatively stable bony fragments of the orbit is then placed through the external incision and guided into position using the endoscope for visualization. While an assistant holds the endoscope in proper position, the implant is bimanually manipulated from the sinonasal and external approaches into proper position (Fig. 33.14).

Nasal packing is unnecessary. The periorbital incision is closed in standard fashion. Postoperatively, the patient is placed on nasal saline irrigations and is seen every 7 to 14 days for endoscopic débridement until the ethmoid cavity is mucosalized. Débridement should be performed with care, because crusts may firmly adhere to the implant, and inadvertent dislodgement of the implant may result.

## ADVANTAGES AND LIMITATIONS

The techniques of endoscopic-assisted repair of facial fractures represent a refinement of standard open reduction and internal fixation approaches. Its widespread application is limited by the currently available technology that allows for accurate reduction and rigid fixation. However, the usefulness of the endoscopic technique lies in its ability to maximize and expand the view through currently used minimal access incisions and approaches. It is hoped that the use of these techniques can facilitate the management of facial fractures and stimulate surgeons and engineers to create new designs and applications for endoscopic equipment and techniques.

## REFERENCES


1. Lappert PW, Lee JW. Treatment of an isolated outer table frontal sinus fracture using endoscopic reduction and fixation. *Plast Reconstr Surg* 1998;102:1642–1645.
2. Onishi K, Osaki M, Maruyama Y. Endoscopic osteosynthesis for frontal bone fracture. *Ann Plast Surg* 1998;40:650–654.
3. Ellis E III, el-Attar A, Moos KF. An analysis of 2,067 cases of zygo-matico-orbital fracture. *J Oral Maxillofac Surg* 1985;43: 417–428.
4. Sandler NA, Carrau RL, Ochs MW, et al. The use of maxillary sinus endoscopy in the diagnosis of orbital floor fractures. *J Oral Maxillofac Surg* 1999;57:399–403.
5. Saunders CJ, Whetzel TP, Stokes RB, et al. Transantral endoscopic orbital floor exploration: a cadaver and clinical study. *Plast Reconstr Surg* 1997;100:575–581.
6. Woog JJ, Hartstein ME, Gliklich R. Paranasal sinus endoscopy and orbital fracture repair. *Arch Ophthalmol* 1998;116:688–691.
7. Burm JS, Chung CH, Oh SJ. Pure orbital blowout fracture: new concepts and importance of medial orbital blowout fracture. *Plast Reconstr Surg* 1999;103:1839–1849.
8. Whitehouse RW, Batterbury M, Jackson A, et al. Prediction of enophthalmos by computed tomography after "blow-out" orbital fracture. *Br J Ophthalmol* 1994;78:618–620.
9. Rhee JS, Lynch J, Loehrl T. Intranasal endoscopy–assisted repair of medial orbital wall fractures. *Arch Fac Plast Surg* 2000;2: 269–273.
10. Lee CH, Lee C, Trabulsy PP, et al. A cadaveric and clinical evaluation of endoscopically assisted zygomatic fracture repair. *Plast Reconstr Surg* 1998;101:333–345.
11. Lee C, Mueller RV, Lee K, et al. Endoscopic subcondylar fracture repair: functional, aesthetic, and radiographic outcomes. *Plast Reconstr Surg* 1998;102:1434–1443.
12. Chen CT, Lai JP, Tung TC, et al. Endoscopically assisted mandibular subcondylar fracture repair. *Plast Reconstr Surg* 1999; 103:60–65.
13. Shumrick KA. Endoscopic management of facial fractures. *Facial Plast Surg Clin North Am* 1997;5:185.

34

# ENDOSCOPIC SURGERY OF THE PARATHYROID GLANDS

GREGG H. JOSSART
MICHEL GAGNER

## INDICATIONS AND CONTRAINDICATIONS

The first parathyroidectomy was performed by Mandl in Vienna in 1925, and the first subtotal parathyroidectomy for renal hyperparathyroidism was performed in 1960 (1). Since the late 1980s, minimally invasive surgical techniques have been applied to all surgical specialties. Practical experience in endoscopic surgery has been limited to procedures performed in the abdomen or thorax, because these areas have a preexisting cavity or space in which to work. The advent of preperitoneal and retroperitoneal laparoscopy through balloon or blunt dissection has expanded our ability to create and then work in a potential space. We developed the new technique of endoscopic parathyroidectomy, and the first patient underwent a subtotal parathyroidectomy in November 1995 (2,3).

Indications for endoscopic parathyroidectomy are potentially the same as for open surgery, but current technology mandates careful patient selection. Endoscopic removal should mostly be limited to first-time explorations, single-gland disease, benign disease, and glands weighing less than 3 g in patients without significant thyroid enlargement. We have performed bilateral endoscopic exploration for multiple gland disease, but it is technically more demanding and time consuming and should be limited to select cases.

### Preoperative Evaluation

The diagnosis of primary hyperparathyroidism is made by documenting an elevated serum intact or two-site parathyroid hormone (PTH) level in a patient with hypercalcemia (i.e., serum calcium >10.5 mg/dL) and normal or increased urinary calcium concentration (4). Patients with benign familial hypocalciuric hypercalcemia are hypercalcemic with an inappropriately high PTH, however, these patients have a low urinary calcium level (<100 mg/24 hours). Most other patients with hypercalcemia (e.g., malignancy, multiple myeloma) have a suppressed serum PTH level. Other laboratory findings consistent with primary hyperparathyroidism include a low serum phosphorus level (<2.5 mg/dL), elevated serum chloride concentration (>107 mmol/L), and elevated serum chloride-phosphate ratio (>33) (4). Most patients with normocalcemic hyperparathyroidism have recurrent kidney stones or osteoporosis, and the diagnosis is confirmed by documenting ionized calcium and increased serum PTH levels (5).

Secondary and tertiary forms of hyperparathyroidism are diagnosed by elevated calcium and PTH levels in the setting of renal failure or after kidney transplantation, respectively. These patients have multiple gland disease and require subtotal thyroidectomy (4).

After the biochemical diagnosis of hyperparathyroidism is made, the surgeon must determine whether the patient is likely to have single-gland or multiple-gland disease. Patients with secondary hyperparathyroidism, tertiary hyperparathyroidism, multiple endocrine neoplasia type 1 (MEN1), MEN2A, and familial hyperparathyroidism all require bilateral exploration because of the likelihood of multiple-gland disease and the need for subtotal parathyroidectomy. The role of preoperative localization studies in these patients is limited to persistent or recurrent disease. Most patients with sporadic primary hyperparathyroidism have single-gland disease and are candidates for unilateral exploration. We prefer preoperative localization with a sestamibi scan followed by endoscopic unilateral exploration and intraoperative PTH assay for these patients. For patients with multiple-gland disease, endoscopic subtotal parathyroidectomy is possible but technically demanding and time consuming.

## PREPARATION

Patients referred for hypercalcemia and hyperparathyroidism should be evaluated with a complete history and physical. Symptoms related to hypercalcemia, including kidney stones, pancreatitis, and peptic ulcer disease, are sought. A history of malignancy and familial endocrinopathies is carefully ascertained. The neck is examined carefully for masses. Laboratory evaluation includes serum calcium, phosphorus, and intact parathormone levels. A chest radiograph is routinely obtained, and a technetium 99m sestamibi scan is used to identify the hyperfunctioning gland. Occasionally, additional radiologic studies may be preferred including cervical ultrasonography, computed tomography (CT), or magnetic resonance imaging (MRI).

If the patient has had any hoarseness or a previous neck operation, indirect or direct laryngoscopy is essential to be sure the vocal cords are functioning normally. Patients should otherwise be prepared as for any procedure requiring general anesthesia. Patients with profound hypercalcemia (12.5 mg of calcium/dL) or with mild to moderate renal failure should be well hydrated before surgery. Rarely, other treatment is also necessary in patients with profound hypercalcemia, such as treatment with diphosphonates, mithramycin, or calcitonin. Electrolyte abnormalities such as hypokalemia or hypomagnesemia should be corrected.

## INSTRUMENTATION

Endoscopic neck procedures are performed using 5-mm, 0° and 30° scopes and a 2-mm, 0° scope. The 2.3-mm trocars are inserted using a retractable needle device (Autosuture, US Surgical, Norwalk, CT) and are equipped for gas insufflation. The instruments used in endoscopic parathyroidectomy are specially designed for minimally invasive cervical exploration (Fig. 34.1). They are designed to fit through 2.3-mm ports and are shorter than those used for abdominal operations. Additional instruments include needlescopic scissors, hooks, probes, and irrigation devices. Bipolar cautery can be connected to the scissors and hook (US Surgical).

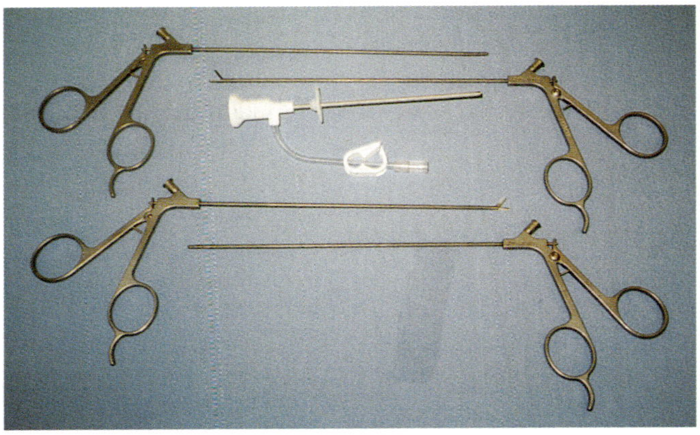

**FIGURE 34.1.** Instruments for minimally invasive cervical exploration. The short, 2-mm graspers and scissors fit through the 2.3-mm miniports (i.e., autosuture).

## OPERATING ROOM LAYOUT AND ANESTHESIA

The patient is placed under general anesthesia in a supine position with minimal extension of the neck. Full extension should be avoided, because tautness of the cervical skin precludes creation of the operative space. The patient's arms are tucked at the sides, and the monitors are placed above each shoulder. The surgeon stands on the side contralateral to the lesion, and the first assistant stands on the opposite side.

## OPERATIVE TECHNIQUE

Step 1 is port placement and exposure. The neck area is prepared and draped in the fashion typical for conventional surgery. A 5-mm skin incision is made just above the sternal notch in the lower midline of the neck. A small hemostat is used to dissect through the subcutaneous tissue and the platysma to reach the plane beneath the strap muscles at the midline. A 5-mm trocar is inserted, and a pursestring suture is placed around the trocar to prevent gas leakage and the trocar from slipping out of the wound. Carbon dioxide ($CO_2$) is then insufflated to 15 mm Hg. The 0°, 5-mm scope is inserted, and the tip is used to bluntly dissect the tissues beneath the strap muscles, moving cephalad and lateral to clear the space underneath the anterior border of the sternocleidomastoid muscles. A 2.3-mm trocar is then inserted midway along the sternocleidomastoid muscle, approximately 1 cm medial to the muscle border. The scope is exchanged for a 30° or a 45° angled scope. The pressure is decreased to 8 to 10 mm Hg. Needlescopic scissors are used to further enlarge the ipsilateral space, creating a 5 × 7 × 3 cm area of dissection. One or two additional needle ports are inserted to facilitate the location of the abnormal glands; usually one port is placed contralateral to the first needle port. Another port may also be placed along the upper third of the sternocleidomastoid muscle.

Step 2 is dissection. The creation of cervical space is continued until the ipsilateral omohyoid muscle is exposed. The anterior carotid sheath is seen medial to the omohyoid. The lateral side of the ipsilateral thyroid is exposed. If deemed necessary, the middle thyroid vein is isolated and clipped, allowing the mobilization of the lateral edge of the thyroid lobe. This maneuver exposes the most likely location of the superior parathyroid gland medial to the carotid sheath. To visualize the inferior gland, a 3-mm scope may need to be placed through one of the ports in the upper neck.

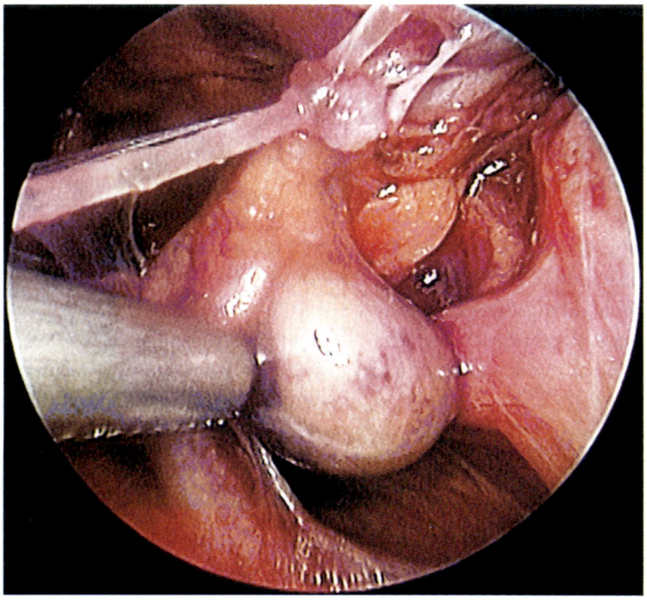

**FIGURE 34.2.** An inferior parathyroid gland with a chromic tie around the branch of the inferior thyroid artery that supplies it.

Step 3 is extraction. The branch of the inferior thyroid artery supplying the gland is isolated and clipped (Fig. 34.2). The areolar tissues holding the gland are divided. The abnormal parathyroid is removed by placing it into a makeshift bag fashioned from the thumb of a sterile surgical glove with a Prolene pursestring suture placed along its opening (Fig. 34.3).

Step 4 is closure. Most of the $CO_2$ is evacuated through the ports before their removal. The platysma and skin are closed with absorbable sutures at the 5-mm trocar site, and needle ports are reapproximated using Steri-Strips (Fig. 34.4).

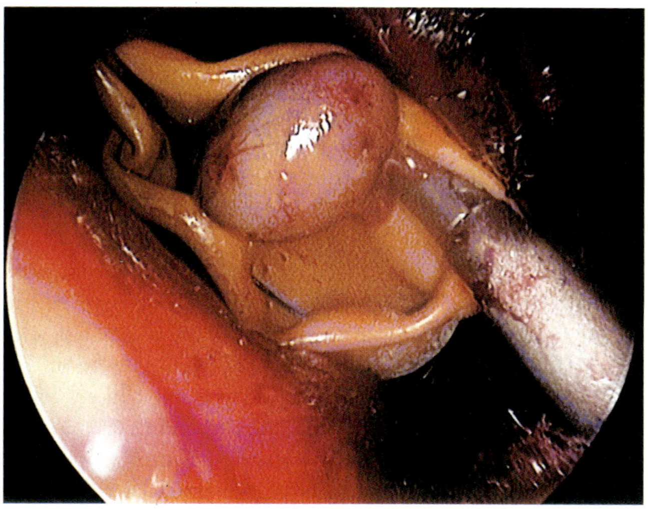

**FIGURE 34.3.** The parathyroid gland is being placed into the pouch created from the thumb of a brown glove.

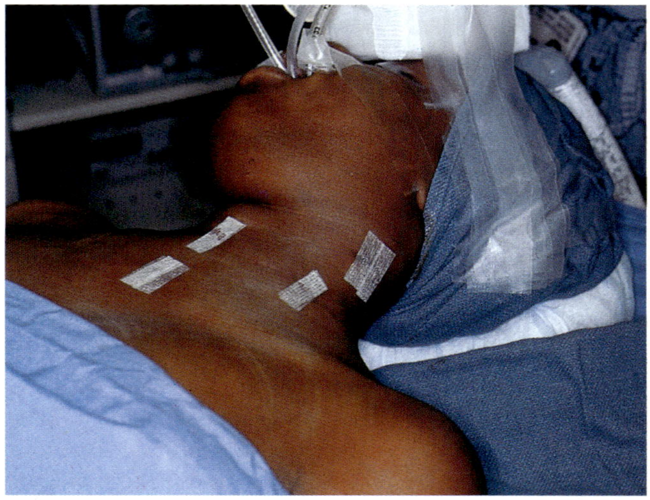

**FIGURE 34.4.** Steri-Strips on the port site incisions.

## SPECIAL POINTS

When the neck is extended as for conventional surgery, the extra tension on the skin limits the creation of an adequate operative space. Moving the neck into a more neutral position relaxes the cervical skin and facilitates the creation of an adequate operative space.

The endoscopic approach provides satisfactory access to ectopic sites, including the carotid sheath, the superior pole of the thyroid, the esophagus, and the thymus. The magnification provided by the scope results in superior clarity and aids identification of the adenoma, atrophic parathyroids, and the recurrent laryngeal nerve.

Strict maintenance of insufflation pressure below 8 to 12 mm Hg prevents subcutaneous emphysema and hypercarbia. Close monitoring of the end-tidal $Pco_2$ is necessary to prevent hypercarbia. This is more likely during a longer operation.

## POSTOPERATIVE CARE

Postoperatively, the patient's head is slightly elevated to maintain negative pressure in the veins. The patient typically resumes eating within 3 to 4 hours. Most patients do not require any analgesics. Serum calcium, phosphorus, and PTH levels are obtained the morning after surgery. If the calcium concentration is below 7.5 mg/dL or if the patient experiences perioral numbness or tingling, calcium supplements are given.

## COMPLICATIONS

Patients with very high serum alkaline phosphatase levels and osteitis fibrosa captiva are prone to profound hypocalcemia after parathyroidectomy. A low postoperative serum phosphate level (<2.5 mg/dL) is usually a sign of so-called bone hunger and suggests that there is little reason to be concerned about permanent hypoparathyroidism. On the other hand, a high postoperative serum phosphate level (>4.5 mg/dL) indicates that the physician should be concerned about permanent hypoparathyroidism (4,5). In the event that calcium supplements are ineffective, alfacalcidol (vitamin D derivative) should be added to the oral medication. Symptoms of muscular cramps and tetany must be promptly countered with administration of intravenous calcium. In some patients, symptoms of tetany may develop while the serum calcium level is normal. This condition probably occurs because of a rapid decrease in serum calcium after removal of the parathyroid tumor, causing an increased neural excitability, but it may also persist after calcium replacement resulting from an accompanying hypomagnesemia.

Recurrent laryngeal nerve injury occurs in about 1% of open parathyroidectomies and thyroidectomies. Unilateral injury may result in hoarseness. Bilateral injury may result in vocal cord paresis and stridor and may have to be treated with a tracheostomy (4). Recurrent laryngeal nerve injury has not been reported in endoscopic parathyroidectomy.

A small hematoma can develop at the trocar sites, but we have not seen any major hemorrhage or respiratory compromise caused by a neck hematoma. Subcutaneous emphysema is usually limited to the anterior neck and resolves within 48 hours.

## LITERATURE REVIEW

The conventional bilateral approach to parathyroid exploration entails a cervical collar incision at least 5 cm long, creation of subplatysmal flaps, exploration of both sides to localize all parathyroid glands, and excision of the hyperactive glands. Proponents of bilateral exploration cite a success rate as high as 96% to 98% for primary hyperparathyroidism without localization tests and when all parathyroid tissue is identified (6,7). Preoperative localization tests are considered insensitive, nonspecific, and not cost effective. The morbidity of this approach is minimal, with a recurrent laryngeal nerve injury rate of less than 1% to 3% (6). Although the success rate of 96% to 98% is admirable, it takes longer than a unilateral approach, necessitates multiple frozen sections, and often requires an overnight stay in the hospital, all of which contribute to the cost. A meta-analysis demonstrated that the average cost of bilateral exploration was $650 more than a unilateral exploration (7). Because 80% to 90% of patients have a single parathyroid adenoma (6,7), most patients are subjected to a more extensive operation than is necessary. The longer anesthetic time and larger incision result in longer recovery, more nausea and vomiting, and a higher risk for hematoma and keloid formation.

Unilateral exploration has gained popularity because of advancements in preoperative localization and intraoperative parathyroid hormone (iPTH) monitoring (8–10). In 1991, based on a review of ultrasound, thallium-technetium subtraction scanning, CT, and MRI, a National Institute of Health consensus panel concluded that preoperative localization was not cost effective (11). However, the advent of technetium 99m sestamibi scintigraphy with planar and single photon emission computed tomography (SPECT) has improved the results of localization, with a sensitivity of 90.7% and a specificity of 98.8%.

The specificity of sestamibi scanning allows a unilateral exploration to identify a solitary adenoma with a less than 1% failure rate. The sestamibi scan is especially accurate for identifying parathyroid adenomas in ectopic locations. SPECT imaging with lateral and anterior views can determine whether the tumor is in the anterior or posterior mediastinum. This is important, because most parathyroid tumors situated in the anterior mediastinum can be removed through a Kocher transverse collar incision or endoscopically through a cervical incision. Parathyroid tumors in the aortopulmonary window require left thoracoscopic removal and those in the posterior mediastinum right thoracoscopic removal (12). Sestamibi scanning does not give a precise anatomic localization, nor does it define contiguous structures; a CT scan of the chest or an MRI with T1 or T2 weighting and gadolinium can confirm the presence of an abnormal mass and provide valuable information about surrounding or contiguous structures.

The main disadvantage of sestamibi scanning is that it is poorly sensitive in patients with multiple abnormal parathyroid glands (i.e., multiple adenomas or hyperplasia). Multiple-gland involvement ranges from 4% to 30% in several series, and it is multiple-gland disease that can yield a false-negative result on sestamibi scanning (6,13–16). Other reasons for incorrect localization include adenomatous goiter, hyperplastic lymph nodes, or concentration of isotope in tissue without recognizable pathologic characteristics. The isotope fails to concentrate in all hyperfunctioning parathyroid glands in patients with multiple-gland disease (6,14–16). This has proven to be its major weakness as a reoperative localization study. However, because most sporadic primary hyperparathyroidism results from a single adenoma and the sestamibi scanning has a specificity of almost 100%, the surgeon can almost always proceed with the operation assured of locating the adenoma based on the sestamibi scan. The surgeon should realize that a false-negative sestamibi scan is not so much a failure of the technique as it is an indication for bilateral exploration and careful consideration of thyroid pathology, because the patient is more likely to have multiple-gland disease or thyroid disease.

The addition of iPTH measurements provides the surgeon with quantitative assurance that all hyperfunctioning glands are removed at the time of parathyroidectomy. Irvin and colleagues demonstrated that iPTH monitoring was successful in 41 patients (9). Patel and coworkers has demonstrated that iPTH monitoring was successful in 84 of 85 patients (17). We prefer a combination of sestamibi scanning for preoperative localization combined with unilateral neck exploration and iPTH measurements. By limiting the extent of dissection, this approach has the potential to decrease the risks of recurrent laryngeal nerve damage and hypocalcemia, and it avoids scarring and obliteration of tissue planes that may hinder future neck operations. As experience is gained, the operative times should diminish, and the procedure can be done on an outpatient basis.

The technique of iPTH measurements involves a two-site antibody immunochemiluminometric assay (Nichols Institute Diagnostics, San Juan Capistrano, CA), using a luminometer (MGM Electronics, Hamden, CT) (8,9,17). The assay can be done in the operating room and takes about 10 minutes. A decline in the iPTH level to 50% or less of the preexcision level indicates that no other hyperfunctioning parathyroid tissue is present and the operation was a success. Because the half-life of circulating PTH is 3 to 4 minutes, a blood sample for iPTH should be drawn within 7 to 10 minutes of excision of the abnormal parathyroid. However, a delayed decline at 5 minutes occurs in up to 10% of patients, and a second sample may need to be drawn to predict excision of all hyperfunctioning tissue in some patients (8,17).

In addition to preoperative localization and iPTH levels, a thorough understanding of parathyroid embryology and anatomy is crucial to the conduct and success of the operation. The superior parathyroids originate from the fourth branchial pouch, and the inferior parathyroids originate from the third branchial pouch. During embryogenesis, the third and fourth pouches become separated and form pairs on either side of the midline. The superior and inferior parathyroids receive their blood supply from the inferior thyroid artery (18).

The superior parathyroid glands originate from the dorsal tips of the fourth pharyngeal pouch. The ultimobranchial body, which is incorporated into the lateral thyroid and supplies the parafollicular (C cells) cells, arises from the ventral portion of the fourth pharyngeal pouch (19). This common embryologic origin of the lateral part of the thyroid and the upper parathyroids accounts for the occasional intrathyroidal location of the upper parathyroids. The most common location of the superior gland is just superior and posterior to the junction of the inferior thyroid artery and the recurrent laryngeal nerve at the level of the cricoid cartilage. It can also be found in the tracheoesophageal groove and retroesophageal space. This retroesophageal space is the site where upper parathyroids can descend to the posterior mediastinum (20).

The inferior parathyroid glands and the thymus arise from the third pharyngeal pouch. Because they descend as a complex in a plane ventral to the fourth pharyngeal pouch, they are usually found in a more anterior position than the superior parathyroids. However, the descent of this complex can vary widely. Normally, the inferior parathyroid usually dissociates from the thymus and is located near the lower pole of the thyroid. In the case of no migration, the inferior parathyroid gland is found cranially to the upper pole of the thyroid, mimicking a superior parathyroid. Thymic tissue surrounding the undescended parathyroid can clarify the true origin of the ectopic parathyroid gland. The absence of thymic tissue caudal to the thyroid is another indicator of an undescended inferior parathyroid. When the inferior parathyroid remains attached to the thymus during its descent, it becomes positioned in the anterior mediastinum. The most common location of the inferior parathyroid gland is anterior and inferior to the junction of the inferior thyroid artery and the recurrent laryngeal nerve. Other locations include intrathyroidal, adjacent to the thyrothymic ligament or within the thymus, anterior mediastinum, aortopulmonary window, or carotid sheath sites (19,21).

The percentage of humans with supernumerary parathyroid glands varies from 2.5% to 22%. These supernumerary parathyroids are usually located in the thymus or in relation to the thyrothymic ligament (21).

The surgical approach for unilateral or bilateral exploration should consider the previously described anatomy and the following caveats. First, explore the sites where parathyroids are usually located, near the posterolateral surface of the thyroid gland. When an inferior gland is missing, it is usually situated in the thymus, which can be identified by mobilizing the thymus from the anterior-superior mediastinum. When a superior parathyroid gland cannot be located, the surgeon should look far behind the thyroid gland superiorly and in a paraesophageal position down into the posterior mediastinum. A thyroid lobectomy or thyroidotomy should be done on the side where fewer than two parathyroid glands have been identified. The carotid sheath and the area posterior to the carotid, as well as the retroesophageal area, should also be explored. Rarely, there may be an undescended parathyroid tumor (i.e., undescended parathyroid) at the level anterior to the carotid bulb. Although we do not recommend routine biopsy of more than one normal-appearing parathyroid gland, we do recommend biopsy (not removal) and marking of normal parathyroid glands when no abnormal parathyroid tissue can be found. When four normal parathyroid glands are found in the neck, the fifth (abnormal) parathyroid gland is usually in the mediastinum (22).

## ADVANTAGES AND LIMITATIONS OF THE ENDOSCOPIC TECHNIQUE

This approach is feasible, cosmetically appealing, and leaves the neck musculature intact, and patients with primary hyperparathyroidism or parathyroid adenomas may benefit. Vessels, nerves, and nodes are highly magnified (15× to 20×), which may result in less recurrent nerve damage. This approach also may facilitate exploring the mediastinum for ectopic parathyroid glands. The routine biopsy of parathyroid glands increases the incidence of postoperative transient hypocalcemia (23), and a directed, unilateral approach therefore decreases the incidence of postoperative hypocalcemia because routine parathyroid biopsy is unnecessary.

The prolonged operating time is a disadvantage, but it does decrease with experience and improved instrumentation. The technique of endoscopic parathyroidectomy requires advanced laparoscopic skills, a detailed knowledge of parathyroid anatomy, preoperative sestamibi localization, and intraoperative PTH monitoring (1,2,24,25). This technique has the potential to access all normally located and ectopic (e.g., thymic, mediastinal) parathyroids through minimal cervical or thoracoscopic incisions. An algorithm combining these techniques with preoperative sestamibi localization and iPTH has a potential success rate of 100% with minimal morbidity.

## REFERENCES


1. Wellbourn R. *History of endocrine surgery*. New York: Praeger, 1990:217–231.
2. Gagner M. Endoscopic subtotal parathyroidectomy in patients with primary hyperparathyroidism. *Br J Surg* 1996;83:875.
3. Naitoh T, Gagner M, Garcia-Ruiz A, et al. Endoscopic endocrine surgery in the neck: an initial report of endoscopic subtotal parathyroidectomy. *Surg Endosc* 1998;12:202–205.
4. Duh QY. Surgical approach to primary hyperparathyroidism (bilateral approach). In: Clark OH, Duh QY, eds. *Textbook of endocrine surgery.* Philadelphia: WB Saunders, 1997:357–363.
5. Clark OH. Diagnosis of primary hyperparathyroidism. In: Clark OH, Duh QY, eds. *Textbook of endocrine surgery.* Philadelphia: WB Saunders, 1997:297–301.
6. Shen W, Sabanci U, Morita ET, et al. Sestamibi scanning is inadequate for directing unilateral neck exploration for first-time parathyroidectomy. *Arch Surg* 1997;132:969–976.
7. Denham DW, Norman J. Cost-effectiveness of preoperative sestamibi scan for primary hyperparathyroidism is dependent solely on the surgeon's choice of operative procedure. *J Am Coll Surg* 1998;186:293–305.
8. Kao PC, van Heerden JA, Taylor RL. Intraoperative monitoring of parathyroid procedures by a 15-minute parathyroid hormone immunochemiluminometric assay. *Mayo Clin Proc* 1994;69: 532–537.
9. Irvin GL, Sfakianakis G, Yeung L, et al. Ambulatory parathyroidectomy for primary hyperparathyroidism. *Arch Surg* 1996; 131:1074–1078.
10. Saharay M, Farooqui A, Farrow S, et al. Intra-operative parathyroid hormone assay for simplified localization of parathyroid adenomas. *J R Soc Med* 1996;89:261–264.
11. Consensus Development Conference statement. *Ann Intern Med* 1994;114:593–597.
12. Prinz RA, Lonchyna V, Carnaille B, et al. Thoracoscopic excision of enlarged mediastinal parathyroid glands. *Surgery* 1994;116: 999–1005.
13. Knight R, Ratzer ER, Fenoglio ME, et al. Thoracoscopic excision of mediastinal parathyroid adenomas: a report of two cases and review of the literature. *J Am Coll Surg* 1997;185:481–485.
14. Tezelman S, Shen W, Shaver JK, et al. Double parathyroid adenomas: clinical and biochemical characteristics before and after parathyroidectomy. *Ann Surg* 1993;218:300–309.
15. Thompson GB, Mullan BP, Grant CS, et al. Parathyroid imaging with technetium-99m-sestamibi: an initial institutional experience. *Surgery* 1994;116:966–972.
16. McHenry CR, Lee K, Saadey J, et al. Parathyroid localization with technetium-99m-sestamibi: a prospective evaluation. *J Am Coll Surg* 1996;183:25–30.
17. Patel PC, Pellitteri PK, Patel NM, et al. Use of a rapid intraoperative parathyroid hormone assay in the surgical management of parathyroid disease. *Arch Otolaryngol Head Neck Surg* 1998;124: 559–562.
18. Herrera MF, Gamboa-Dominguez A. Parathyroid embryology, anatomy and pathology. In: Clark OH, Duh QY, eds. *Textbook of endocrine surgery.* Philadelphia: WB Saunders, 1997:277–283.
19. Mansberger AR, Wei JP. Surgical embryology and anatomy of the thyroid and parathyroid glands. *Surg Clin North Am* 1993;73: 727–746.
20. Wang CA. Parathyroid re-exploration: a clinical and pathological study of 112 cases. *Ann Surg* 1977;186:140–145.
21. Bonjer HJ, Bruining HA. Technique of parathyroidectomy. In: Clark OH, Duh QY, eds. *Textbook of endocrine surgery.* Philadelphia: WB Saunders, 1997:347–356.
22. Jossart GH, Clark OH. Thyroid and parathyroid surgery. In: Wilmore D, Brennan M, Harken A, et al, eds. *Scientific American surgery.* New York: Scientific American, Spring 1996.
23. Kaplan EL, Bartlettt S, Sugimoto J, et al. Relation of postoperative hypocalcemia to operative techniques: deleterious effect of excessive use of parathyroid biopsy. *Surgery* 1982;92:827–834.
24. Yeung GH. Endoscopic surgery of the neck: a new frontier. *Surg Laparosc Endosc* 1998;8:227–232.
25. Yeung GH. The technique of endoscopic exploration for parathyroid adenoma of the neck. *Aust N Z J Surg* 1998;68: 147–150.

35

# ENDOSCOPIC NECK SURGERY

PAVEL DULGUEROV

Endoscopic neck surgery (ENS) is a new surgical procedure for removing cervical pathologic structures through small incisions with endoscopic instruments and techniques. Although the exact indications of endoscopic neck surgery must still be defined, it has the potential of spanning most of the spectrum of traditional neck surgery. A comparison can be drawn from laparoscopy. The first human abdominal procedure was an appendectomy performed by Karl Stemm, a gynecologist, in 1983 (1). Since then, the progress accomplished in endoscopic techniques and their ever-expanding indications can be witnessed in two textbooks with almost 1,000 pages each (2,3). Neither of them mentions any neck organ.

Endoscopic surgical techniques, originally developed for body cavities, have been applied to the axilla (4,5) and other body regions where cavities are not found (6–9). Results of this minimally invasive surgery appear to compare favorably with those for open surgery in terms of complications and aesthetics (4,5).

Gagner (10) was the first to report on an endoscopic procedure within the neck in 1996. He removed hypertrophic parathyroid glands for hyperparathyroidism. Since then, few reports have been published on human endoscopic thyroid (11–13) and parathyroid (12,14–16) surgery. These studies report a total of 14 thyroidectomies (11,13,17) and 96 parathyroidectomies (10,14–20) completed successfully in humans.

Endoscopically assisted surgery (21–23) is a different approach in which a relatively large incision (≥3 cm) is made and retraction is provided with various instruments, which can resemble modified laryngoscopes. The use of these instruments can be seen as a backward step from typical endoscopic surgery techniques, or as a prudent intermediate progression before adopting formal endoscopic techniques. Early publications about human (10,14,15, 24–26) and animal (25–27) thyroid and parathyroid surgery, which described serious side effects related to the high-pressure insufflation of carbon dioxide ($CO_2$) required to maintain a closed working cavity, could be a possible influence for these views.

Until recently (28), no study had directly addressed the possibility of endoscopic neck dissection (END) in animals or humans. Potential applications of ENS can be subdivided in three groups: END, thyroidectomy, and parathyroidectomy.

## INDICATIONS

In general, the indications for ENS are similar to the indications for the corresponding open surgical procedure. Certain restrictions apply, mainly regarding the size of the tissue to be extirpated.

The principal indication for neck dissection is cancer metastasis, usually from a head or neck primary tumor. For END, patients with low neck tumor burdens should be chosen for oncologic reasons and because the removed tissue must be extracted through the small trocar openings. END should be restricted to patients with N0 disease and patients with metastasis smaller than 2 cm (i.e., N1, N2b, or N2c).

An ideal application for ENS is endoscopic retrieval of labeled sentinel lymph nodes, an application which has been referred to as "a match made in heaven" (29) (Fig. 35.1). The primary tumor is labeled during panendoscopy, the tumor is resected endoscopically, and the sentinel lymph nodes are removed by ENS. Ideally, radiotherapy is withheld. This approach is only feasible for small primary tumors with little neck burden. Another potential indication is treatment of the primary tumor with some form of "organ preservation" chemoradiation while treating the neck by ENS. Benign thyroid lesions of small size are the main indication of endoscopic thyroidectomy.

The best indication for endoscopic parathyroidectomy is a single parathyroid adenoma that is clearly visualized by preoperative studies (19,20,22). Ideally, an intraoperative dosage of parathyroid hormone levels should be available and used to confirm the reduction of levels after the removal of the gland.

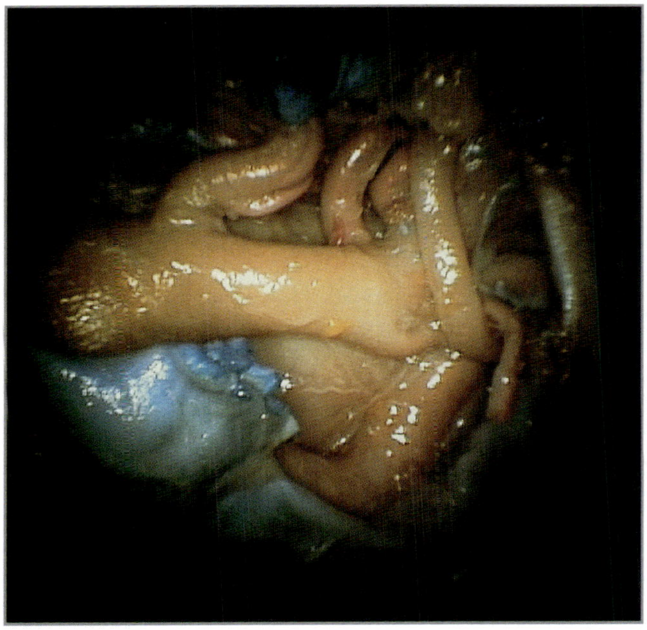

**FIGURE 35.1.** View during endoscopic neck dissection of a human cadaver. The veins and arteries were injected with blue and red colored latex, respectively, for iconographic purposes. The carotid bifurcation is well seen, as are the first branches of the external carotid artery. The internal jugular vein, vagus nerve, and hypoglossal nerve are also seen.

## CONTRAINDICATIONS

Before embarking on an endoscopic approach, the surgeon should become familiar with laparoscopic techniques through training courses and possibly through animal endoscopic neck surgery. Because conversion to an open procedure is easily done and can provide the patient the current standard of care, the main issue is the potential for serious complications.

In general, prior neck surgery or irradiation in the cervical region of interest should be considered a contraindication (16–18,20,22,23). Parathyroid or, rarely, thyroid reexplorations should be performed using traditional techniques. Other than the size of the lesion to be removed and the limitations imposed by prior treatments, no contraindications to END or thyroidectomy have been specified.

For parathyroidectomy, the presence of thyroid goiter is a relative contraindication, unless the surgeon is comfortable with the resection (16,18–20,22,23). Bilateral parathyroid exploration remains a lengthy procedure, and these cases of hyperparathyroidism are better handled through an open approach (16,18–20,22,23). Preoperative localization studies such as sestamibi scans and magnetic resonance imaging (MRI) are advised, and intraoperative rapid parathyroid hormone (PTH) assays are helpful (16,23). The best indication for endoscopic parathyroidectomy is a single parathyroid adenoma that is clearly visualized by preoperative studies (19,20,22).

In general, all these contraindications are relative and depend on the surgical expertise of the operator. As head and neck surgeons become familiar with endoscopic techniques, along with progress in instrumentation, these contraindications will probably disappear, and the limits of ENS will be extended.

## PREOPERATIVE EVALUATION

Although the possibility of missing a large neck lymph node metastasis by clinical examination is low, we recommend an imaging study such as a computed tomography (CT) scan, MRI, or ultrasound before END. Further workup of a patient with a head neck cancer is similar to that for an open neck dissection.

A detailed review of the workup for patients with thyroid and parathyroid masses and for patients presenting with hyperparathyroidism is beyond the scope of this chapter. For thyroidectomy, some form of imaging, preferably ultrasound; fine-needle aspiration of a thyroid nodule; and thyroid hormone levels are necessary. The goal is to make sure that the thyroid lesion is smaller than 3 to 4 cm. Although a small, intraglandular thyroid carcinoma could be removed endoscopically, endoscopic thyroidectomies during the surgeon's training phase should not be performed on patients with cancer.

Similarly, imaging, preferably MRI, and localization studies, most often sestamibi scintigraphy, appear necessary for treatment of hyperparathyroidism. Blood calcium, phosphate, and parathyroid hormone levels are also obtained.

Patients should be thoroughly informed about the "experimental" nature of ENS and should be aware that conversion to standard open surgery occurs for a significant proportion of patients. Ideally, initial attempts of ENS should be performed within a study protocol approved by the local ethics committee.

## INSTRUMENTATION

Usually, three openings are necessary: one for the endoscope optic that provides illumination and through which visualization of the operating field is achieved and two other for instruments. A camera (preferably three-chip charge-coupled device [3-CCD]) is attached to the end of the endoscope, and the operation is performed while looking at the monitor screen.

The endoscope should have a diameter of at least 5 mm, because the image qualities of smaller endoscopes have been reported as insufficient (18). We prefer a 10-mm endoscope to obtain better illumination and visualization. Short (20-cm) endoscopes should be used (Karl Storz AG, Tuttlingen, Germany) because traditional laparoscopic endoscopes add unnecessary weight and are cumbersome to maneuver.

Trocars with dull obturators are preferred to avoid undue bleeding during their introduction. These trocars should be light and preferably made of plastic, because they are held in position only by a thin layer tissue (i.e., skin, subcutaneous layer, and platysma). For similar considerations and until specific trocars for ENS are developed, the commercial ones should be shortened to a length of the screwing portion smaller than 3 cm. The 3-mm-diameter trocars are sufficient for ENS.

Gasless techniques of cavity maintenance seem to be preferable because they are associated with fewer risks of pneumothorax and pneumomediastinum (13,27,28,30). A gasless technique obviates the potential threat of air embolism and is not associated with extensive subcutaneous emphysema described by some investigators (14). If a gas technique is preferred, the insufflation apparatus should allow for adjusting the pressure and volume of air flow (Karl Storz AG, Tuttlingen, Germany), and the lowest satisfactory pressures and volumes should be used. Cougard and colleagues (18) reported using a pressure of 10 mm Hg and volumes of 3 L/min in 19 patients during parathyroidectomy without untoward side effects.

If gasless techniques are used, the dissection cavity is maintained with some form of external device that provides for skin lifting. Subcutaneous metal wires are passed under the skin and connected to a suspension apparatus. The best device depend on the procedure. For thyroidectomy, these wires can be passed on each side of the midline, allowing retraction of the entire central, lower neck skin (30). These wires are suspended to a lifting device (Mizuho, Bunkyo-ku, Tokyo, Japan). For END, we found that these wires are best placed more laterally and, instead of traveling in a subplatysmal plane, passed under the sternocleidomastoid muscle. This permits the laterosuperior retraction of the muscle for better access to zone V and to zones II, III, and IV. Optimal lifting is provided by three wires for END. A suspension apparatus for END and other ENS procedures is being developed by the Karl Storz Company (Tuttlingen, Germany). Another advantage of such a suspension apparatus is to alleviate the need for a holding clamp or an assistant for the endoscope.

The optimal coagulating instruments for ENS are debatable. Smoke from unipolar coagulation has proved to be a problem. The length of the exposed surface of conventional laparoscopic scissors makes them ill suited for ENS. Bipolar scissor (Metzenbaum bipolar scissors, PM 400R, Aesculap, Tuttlingen, Germany) reduce these problems by limiting the coagulation area and allowing section coagulation closer to important structures. However, available scissors are still too big and too long for ENS. The use of available bipolar coagulation forceps is cumbersome because of the repeated need to remove and insert alternatively the scissors and the coagulation forceps through the same trocar opening.

The ultrasonic device (Harmonic Scalpel, Johnson & Johnson, Cincinnati, OH) seems to offer several advantages: no electric current that can spread to nearby structures and less heat generated. However, the heat generated by the device is close to 80°C, and the potential for nerve damage remains (13,30). The smoke generated is greatly reduced relative to electric coagulation. The device has been used successfully during endoscopic thyroidectomy (13,30).

The remaining instrumentation is rather simple: several grasping forceps and a suction canula. We were not impressed with the unipolar hook instrument often used in laparoscopy because of the unipolar coagulation danger, its limited cutting possibilities, and lack of spreading space within the neck often necessary for dissection.

## OPERATING ROOM LAYOUT

The patient's position is similar to that for open neck surgery: slight contralateral head rotation and head of bed elevation to promote venous return and decrease bleeding. Maximal neck extension should be avoided because it puts tension on the strap and sternocleidomastoid muscles and skin, rendering difficult the creation of an ample working cavity difficult (14,23).

The video monitor should face the surgeon. With a suspension apparatus that incorporates and articulated holder for the optics, there is no need for an assistant. If an assistant is present, he should be at the head of the patient. The scrub nurse is positioned next to the surgeon and facing the monitor. The anesthetist and the anesthesia apparatus are located at the feet the patient.

## ANESTHESIA

ENS is performed under general anesthesia, similar to the corresponding open surgical techniques. The only potential problem that anesthetists should be aware of is the occurrence of hypercarbia during $CO_2$ insufflation. The first sign is tachycardia, and its occurrence without any other clear explanation warrants a blood gas analysis. The initial management includes hyperventilation. The case report by Gottlieb and coworkers (24) can be consulted for a detailed description.

Surgeons and anesthetists should be fully aware of the diagnosis and emergent management of air embolism. The physiopathology involves passage of air bubbles in the pulmonary circulation, pulmonary hypertension, and decreased left ventricle filling, culminating in right and left ventricle failure and decreased cardiac output (31). With air quantities above 50 mL, asystole occurs (32). The intraoperative diagnosis is made on the auscultation of a "mill wheel" cardiac murmur, sudden hypotension, and decreased end-tidal $CO_2$ levels. Treatment includes preventing further air entry by compressing the injured vein, administering 100% $FIo_2$ and a large fluid bolus (31,32). The patient's head should be lowered and the patient placed in left lateral decubitus. Right-side cardiac catheterization to aspirate air bubbles is controversial.

During the training phase of ENS, patients should be at least crossmatched because of the potential of major neck vessel injury. Lacerations of the carotid artery or internal jugular vein are difficult to handle endoscopically and may require conversion to an open procedure. Although this can be accomplished expeditiously, significant bleeding can take place in the interval.

For thyroid and parathyroid surgery, monitoring the recurrent laryngeal nerve should be considered, at least during the training phase of ENS.

## OPERATIVE TECHNIQUE

Placement of the skin incisions and therefore of the trocars requires careful planning. Usually, three openings are necessary: one for the endoscope and two other for instruments. The openings form a triangle, in the center of which should be the neck lesion to be removed. These openings should not be too close to each other to achieve a sufficient working cavity.

Aesthetic considerations suggest the lower opening should be below the collar line so the scar can be hidden by clothing. Similarly, the upper opening can be hidden under the mandible. The exact position depends of the targeted lesion. For END, we found a placement just below the chin to be adequate in most cases. The final opening is on the lateral aspect of the neck, close to the border of the sternocleidomastoid muscle. This opening is used for the endoscope (33). For thyroid and parathyroid surgery, two openings below the clavicle, one on each side, have been proposed by Shimizu and associates (30).

Blunt dissection is poorly suited for the creation of a working ENS cavity because of the resulting bleeding. Even minute amounts of blood during this step can render the procedure frustrating by the difficulty of coagulation under poor vision and by the required repeated cleaning of the endoscope tip.

We prefer to use a balloon to obtain a working cavity (PDP 1000, Origin Medical Systems, Menlo Park, CA). The dilation balloon is introduced through the endoscope opening. After the cavity is created, the remaining trocars are inserted under direct vision. Superficial neck veins and sometimes the anterior jugular vein can be lacerated by the introduction of the trocars. To circumvent the frequently encountered bleeding from the skin puncture by trocars, Henry and colleagues (23) proposed the first passage is from inside out, created by the needle of a suction drain. Before beginning dissection and tissue removal, the surgical instruments should be fully visible.

Other investigators (15,16,20) have chosen to make a larger initial incision and proceed with blunt initial dissection using traditional instruments. After creation of the cavity, the large trocar and endoscope are introduced, and a tight seal around the trocar is achieved by a pursestring suture. Miccoli and coworkers (19) used a different approach for parathyroidectomy, with initial $CO_2$ insufflation during the development of the working cavity, followed by external lifting during the remaining surgery.

The most tedious part of ENS is the initial opening, cavity creation, and exposure of the pathology to treat. Actual dissection and removal seem more gratifying and usually proceed uneventfully if proper technique is used.

Most recognizable vessels are coagulated with the bipolar scissors or sectioned with the harmonic scalpel. We have found that almost all cutting is better performed after coagulation because of difficulties in controlling bleeding once established. In case of undue bleeding, hemostasis is achieved by coagulation and, for important vessels, by endosurgical metal clips. Sometimes, the technique of packing a portion of the wound with gauze sponge (34) has been useful.

There is no shame in trying. If the endoscopic procedure is not fully successful, it is easy to convert to an open approach, as long as serious complications are avoided. Because of the lengthy initial learning curve and the cost related to operating room time, the first cases could be started endoscopically and transformed to open approach after a fixed time delay.

## POSTOPERATIVE CARE

There is little postoperative care for the endoscopic approach compared with open surgical techniques. A postoperative chest radiograph is warranted during the training phase to exclude pneumothorax. Wound drainage is seldom necessary. Sutures of these small incisions are preferably resorbing ones.

## COMPLICATIONS

Air embolism is a serious potential threat when $CO_2$ insufflation is used. With gas insufflated under pressure, the opening of a major vein can easily result in the passage of air into the systemic circulation and has resulted in a fatal outcome in an animal ENS experiment (26). Management has been previously discussed.

Other possible complications include hypercarbia resulting from $CO_2$ insufflation and subcutaneous emphysema that can be extensive (from the face to the scrotum) (10,14) and that is also related to the use of high-pressure $CO_2$ insufflation.

Injury to the recurrent laryngeal nerve in thyroidectomies and parathyroidectomies is a known problem. Recurrent laryngeal paralysis was observed in 10% of parathyroidectomies by Gauger and associates (22), Dralle and colleagues (16), and Peix and coworkers (20).

Bleeding from smaller veins such as the anterior jugular vein or thyroid vein can usually be handled endoscopically, but is often a motive for conversion to open technique.

## ADVANTAGES AND LIMITATIONS

The proposed advantages include smaller scar and better cosmesis (10,14,17–19,23), less pain (14,17–19), less tissue destruction (17), less intraoperative bleeding and therefore no need for wound drainage (18,21), and wound complications (14,19). The evaluation of these benefits has been performed quite subjectively by the investigators. In the only randomized study on ENS, Miccoli and associates (19) compared open and endoscopic parathyroidectomy. The endoscopic approach was associated with shorter operating time, less postoperative pain, shorter recovery period, better scar cosmesis, and lower costs.

Contrary to common opinion, visualization is better using an endoscopic approach (10,14,17,20,23) because of a less bloody field and magnification provided by the endoscopes. With small endoscope sizes (3 to 5 mm), certain investigators (18) have found that the color definition is less good than during an open procedure and could render parathyroid location more difficult; whether this holds true with large scopes remains to be investigated.

A disadvantage of ENS is the lack of palpation of the cervical lesion, which could be important for certain pathologies (14). The duration of the procedure, especially during the early training phase, is significantly longer than for comparable open approaches.

For thyroidectomies and parathyroidectomies, the scar benefits may not be obvious, and the complication rates of the open procedure are not high enough to justify the greater technical difficulty, equipment costs, and longer operating room time. Although the learning curve for young surgeons may not be different from that for the open surgical approach, it remains unclear whether it is worth the effort of established surgeons who are well versed in traditional neck surgery. When malignancies are involved, studies should establish the oncologic safety of ENS before a widespread popularization of these techniques.

## CONCLUSIONS

Endoscopic neck surgery is a new approach to neck surgery. Most of the published series are concerned with endoscopic parathyroidectomy. The exact indications of endoscopic neck dissections and thyroidectomy remain to be defined. Further experience with technique should extend the current indications.

Gasless techniques should be preferred because they are associated with lower complication rates. Available surgical instruments need further development before the technique becomes standardized.

## REFERENCES


1. Stemm K. Endoscopic appendectomy. *Endoscopy* 1983;15:59–64.
2. MacFadyen BV, Ponsky JL. *Operative laparoscopy and thoracoscopy*. Philadelphia: Lippincott–Raven Publishers, 1996.
3. Arregui ME, Fitzgibbons RJJ, Kathouda N, et al. *Principles of laparoscopic surgery: basic and advanced techniques*. New York: Springer-Verlag, 1995.
4. Suzanne F, Emering C, Wattiez A, et al. [Axillary lymphadenectomy by lipo-aspiration and endoscopic picking. A propos of 72 cases]. *Chirurgie* 1997;122:138–142.
5. Salvat J, Knopf JF, Ayoubi JM, et al. Endoscopic exploration and lymph node sampling of the axilla: preliminary findings of a randomized pilot study comparing clinical and anatomo-pathologic results of endoscopic axillary lymph node sampling with traditional surgical treatment. *Eur J Obstet Gynecol Reprod Biol* 1996;70:165–173.
6. Ho LCY. Endoscopic assisted transaxillary augmentation mammaplasty. *Br J Plast Surg* 1993;46:332–336.
7. Friedlander L, Sundin J. Minimally invasive harvesting of latissimus dorsi. *Plast Reconstr Surg* 1993;94:881–884.
8. Jugenheimer M, Jugenheimer T. Endoscopic subfascial sectioning of incompetent perforating veins in treatment of primary varicosis. *World J Surg* 1992;16:971–975.
9. Isse NG. Endoscopic facial rejuvenation. *Clin Plast Surg* 1997;24:213–231.
10. Gagner M. Endoscopic subtotal parathyroidectomy in patients with primary hyperparathyroidism. *Br J Surg* 1996;83:875.
11. Huscher CS, Chiodini S, Napolitano C, et al. Endoscopic right thyroid lobectomy. *Surg Endosc* 1997;11:877.
12. Yeung GH, Ng JW. The technique of endoscopic exploration for parathyroid adenoma of the neck. *Aust N Z J Surg* 1998;68:147–150.
13. Shimizu K, Akira S, Jasmi AY, et al. Video-assisted neck surgery: endoscopic resection of thyroid tumors with a very minimal neck wound. *J Am Coll Surg* 1999;188:697–703.
14. Naitoh T, Gagner M, Garcia-Ruiz A, Heniford BT. Endoscopic endocrine surgery in the neck: an initial report of endoscopic subtotal parathyroidectomy. *Surg Endosc* 1998;12:202–205, discussion 206.
15. Miccoli P, Bendinelli C, Vignali E, et al. Endoscopic parathyroidectomy: report of an initial experience. *Surgery* 1998;124:1077–1079.
16. Dralle H, Lorenz K, Nguyen-Thanh P. Minimally invasive video-assisted parathyroidectomy—selective approach to localized single gland adenoma. *Langenbecks Arch Surg* 1999;384:556–562.

17. Yeung GH. Endoscopic surgery of the neck: a new frontier. *Surg Laparosc Endosc* 1998;8:227–232.
18. Cougard P, Goudet P, Osmak L, et al. La vidéocervicoscopie dans la chirurgie de l'hyperparathyroïdie primitive. *Ann Chir* 1998;52: 885–889.
19. Miccoli P, Bendinelli C, Berti P, et al. Video-assisted versus conventional parathyroidectomy in primary hyperparathyroidism: a prospective randomized study. *Surgery* 1999;126:1117–1121.
20. Peix JL, el Khazen M, Mancini F, et al. Les opérations pour hyperparathyroïdectomie primaire en 1998: a propos de 66 patients et de trois voies d'abord. *Ann Chir* 2000;125:346–352.
21. Bellantone R, Lombardi CP, Raffaelli M, et al. Minimally invasive, totally gasless video-assisted thyroid lobectomy. *Am J Surg* 1999;177:342–343.
22. Gauger PG, Reeve TS, Delbridge LW. Endoscopically assisted, minimally invasive parathyroidectomy. *Br J Surg* 1999;86: 1563–1566.
23. Henry JF, Defechereux T, Gramatica L, et al. Minimally invasive videoscopic parathyroidectomy by lateral approach. *Langenbecks Arch Surg* 1999;384:298–301.
24. Gottlieb A, Sprung J, Zheng XM, et al. Massive subcutaneous emphysema and severe hypercarbia in a patient during endoscopic transcervical parathyroidectomy using carbon dioxide insufflation. *Anesth Analg* 1997;84:1154–1156.
25. Brunt LM, Jones DB, Wu JS, et al. Experimental development of an endoscopic approach to neck exploration and parathyroidectomy. *Surgery* 1997;122:893–901.
26. Carreno OJ, Wilson WR, Nootheti PK. Exploring endoscopic neck surgery in a porcine model. *Laryngoscope* 1999;109: 236–240.
27. Jones DB, Quasebarth MA, Brunt LM. Videoendoscopic thyroidectomy: experimental development of a new technique. *Surg Laparosc Endosc Percutan Tech* 1999;9:167–170.
28. Dulguerov P, Vaezi AE, Belenger J, et al. Endoscopic neck dissection in an animal model: comparison of nodal yield with open-neck dissection. *Arch Otolaryngol Head Neck Surg* 2000; 126:417–420.
29. Dulguerov P, Leuchter I, Costa J, et al. Endoscopic retrieval of sentinel lymph nodes in a porcine model. *Head Neck (in press).*
30. Shimizu K, Akira S, Tanaka S. Video-assisted neck surgery: endoscopic resection of benign thyroid tumor aiming at scarless surgery on the neck. *J Surg Oncol* 1998;69:178–180.
31. Muth CM, Shank ES. Gas embolism. *N Engl J Med* 2000;342: 476–482.
32. Palmon SC, Moore LE, Lundberg J, et al. Venous air embolism: a review. *J Clin Anesth* 1997;9:251–257.
33. Leuchter I, Fazel JH, Allal AS, et al. Endoscopic neck dissection in human cadavers. *Laryngoscope (in press).*
34. Yeung HC, Ng WT, Kong CK. Endoscopic thyroid and parathyroid surgery. *Surg Endosc* 1997;11:1135.

# 36

# IMAGE-GUIDED LASER PHOTOTHERAPY FOR HEAD AND NECK CANCER PALLIATION

DAN J. CASTRO
MARCOS B. PAIVA
ROMAINE E. SAXTON

Advanced head and neck cancer is a common clinical problem. Despite current treatment with surgery, radiation therapy, and chemotherapy, between one third and one half of all patients with these tumors have persistent or recurrent disease after primary therapy. Surgical access to deep tumors of the head and neck usually requires extensive dissection, with residual dysfunction and cosmetic deformities. Repeated treatment is not possible after maximum-dose radiotherapy, and chemotherapy is still limited by systemic toxicity. Interstitial laser therapy (ILT) guided by dynamic magnetic resonance imaging (MRI) or ultrasonography has been tested as a promising alternative for photothermal ablation of recurrent carcinomas in preclinical studies and in a large number of patients, with an overall 60% tumor response rate. Despite many attractive features, including minimal invasiveness and the ability to repeat ILT as an outpatient procedure, the 40% treatment failure of ILT has led to a search for more effective combined treatment modalities.

One attractive possibility for treatment of recurrent tumors is to combine ILT at low energy with a nontoxic photoenhancer dye for minimally invasive tumor destruction. However, because research on photodynamic therapy (PDT) with lasers is still focused on developing optimal laser dyes for tumor therapy, clinical applications may not occur for years.

Laser photochemotherapy is a second approach for tumor treatment that uses conventional chemotherapeutic agents injected at concentrations lower than normally used for systemic treatment but with tumoricidal effects enhanced when exposed to light by ILT. Because most standard chemotherapeutic drugs are U.S. Food and Drug Administration (FDA) approved and tested, whereas all the current laser dyes for PDT are still undergoing preclinical investigations, photochemotherapy may soon become a practical adjunct clinical technique for palliation of head and neck carcinomas.

Management of far advanced and recurrent head and neck cancer involves active treatment and supportive care. Modalities for active treatment include surgery, radiation therapy, and chemotherapy. Surgery is usually excluded in patients with disease involving the middle and posterior base of skull, the cervical spine, or major vessels within the superior mediastinum. Radiation therapy can provide effective palliation for several months using external beam therapy and implantation therapy, but treatment is time consuming and often requires daily dose fractionation for a period of several weeks. Because the total dose of radiation delivered to one site is limited, tumor treatment cannot be repeated without a high risk of soft tissue necrosis (1).

Chemotherapy for far advanced head and neck cancer remains controversial. Several protocols are being investigated, but survival benefit has yet to be definitively demonstrated. The potential benefits of chemotherapy also must be balanced against the systemic toxicity (2).

PDT with lasers and hematoporphyrins has gained popularity as a minimally invasive technique for treatment of superficial tumors (3–5). Several groups have reported that laser dyes are effective tumor sensitizers in preclinical models (6–8), but clinical applications depend on FDA approval and may be years away. Photochemotherapy is an intriguing alternative using intratumoral injections of conventional chemotherapeutic drugs followed by interstitial laser ablation for improved treatment of head and neck cancer.

The effectiveness of combined chemotherapy and radiation therapy in the treatment of human cancer provides a useful model for further development of multimodality approaches including laser photochemotherapy (9,10). Adriamycin derivatives are the most common anticancer agents that interact with light to elicit fluorescence, membrane photolabeling, laser activation, and killing of tumor cells (11–14). Several of these anthracyclines have been used to kill human leukemia cells *in vitro* by photoillumination at 20-fold decreased drug levels (15). Similar phototherapy of B16 melanoma tumors in mice with anthracenedione and red light led to prolonged median survival times (13,14).

Daunomycin has been reported to be an effective photosensitizer for argon laser treatment of human and rodent tumor cells *in vitro* (16,17). Among the most promising Adriamycin-related drugs are three anthrapyrazoles that exhibit reduced cardiotoxicity and greatly increased photosensitizing properties detected by catechol oxidation (18).

An ideal tumor targeting agent for laser fiberoptic activation would localize strongly in neoplasms after systemic administration, allowing fluorescent detection and tumor phototherapy. Rhodamines, cyanines, and hematoporphyrins all exhibit strong fluorescence and tumoricidal effects, but they localize at high levels in skin and some other normal organs in addition to neoplastic tissues (6–8). These laser dyes may diffuse poorly in tissues after intratumoral injection. Direct intratumoral injections of anticancer drugs, including Adriamycin derivatives and cisplatin, have been used to increase the therapeutic response in cerebral tumors and other neoplasms without systemic toxicity (19). This approach should increase the possibility of intratumoral drug photoactivation and photothermal enhancement through interstitial fiberoptic laser energy delivery. The concepts of interstitial laser photothermal therapy, PDT, and laser photochemotherapy are reviewed in this chapter.

## INTERSTITIAL LASER PHOTOTHERMAL THERAPY OF CANCER

### Lasers and Cancer Therapy

As early as 1965, experimental investigations on the potential of lasers to destroy malignant tumors began with studies by Minton and Ketcham (20–24) using high-energy, pulsed laser radiation for treatment of multiple intraabdominal tumor implants in experimental animals. In 1964, Goldman and Wilson (25,26) reported clinical results of the treatment of basal cell epithelioma using laser radiation. There is much interest in endoscopic laser therapy for the treatment of tumors. In 1981, Swain and colleagues (27) reported successful relief of neoplastic gastric outflow tract obstruction with the argon laser. Richey and Dixon (28) investigated a similar treatment of gastric polyps by endoscopic application of lasers. Imaoka and colleagues (29) and Iwasaki and coworkers (30) described the treatment of gastric cancers with the neodymium:yttrium-aluminum-garnet (Nd:YAG) laser. Hofstetter and Frank (31) previously reported the successful use of laser endoscopy for clinical treatment of bladder tumors. The groups led by Shapshay (32–34), Toty (35), Dumon (36), Brunctaud (37), and Carpenter and Neel (38) described in separate publications that successful management of tracheal lesions could be obtained using the Nd:YAG laser. Fleisher and colleagues (39) reported tumor palliation in a series of 14 patients with end-stage carcinoma of the esophagus treated with the Nd:YAG laser. Rontal and Rontal (40) also found that treatment of a recurrent carcinoma at the base of the skull was successful using a carbon dioxide ($CO_2$) laser. The results of these studies were encouraging as a demonstration of the clinical potential of lasers in cancer therapy, but they were also highly controversial because of the deficiency of carefully designed scientific protocols and controls.

### Image-Guided Interstitial Tumor Therapy

ILT is a promising approach being tested for minimally invasive tumor treatment using precise and controlled delivery of photothermal energy into tissues. However, this laser treatment can become clinically useful only if less invasive, accurate, and reproducible methods of dosimetry of energy delivery to tissues are developed. The invasive methods currently use thermal probes, infrared thermography, and histologic studies (41,42), which are reliable but have limited clinical usefulness. Since the mid-1970s, interstitial placement of laser fiberoptics has been applied successfully to large subcutaneous metastasis (5,43). In 1984, Svaasand (44) developed some preliminary optical dosimetry for interstitial phototherapy of malignant tumors. Bown (45) investigated the interstitial use of the Nd:YAG laser for hepatic hyperthermia in a number of ways. Matthewson (46–48) used a single Nd:YAG laser fiber at low power (1 to 2 W) to produce areas of thermal necrosis of up to 16 mm in the normal rat liver and to eradicate some induced rat colon tumors and implanted fibrosarcomas. Hashimoto (49) applied 5 to 15 W of Nd:YAG laser power with a modified diffuser fiber tip to treat liver tumors with evidence of reduction of tumor size. Godlewski (50,51) used high Nd:YAG powers of up to 100 W with a 1-second duration to produce areas of vaporization and necrosis of 16 to 22 mm in the porcine liver at great speed. However, the high power density at the distal end of the fiberoptics resulted in frequent tip damages, burning, nonuniform distribution of laser energy, and poorly reproducible tissue effects. The introduction of synthetic sapphire probes (52) that have high melting points (2,020°C to 2,050°C), greater tensile strength, and a uniform pattern of laser beam delivery from the lateral surface of the probe has allowed testing of Nd:YAG laser-induced hyperthermia in a dog model (52,53). Daikuzono (52) further developed a computer-controlled Nd:YAG system for interstitial local hyperthermia.

To increase the area of necrosis that could be produced and still use one laser as the energy source, Steger (54) used fiberoptic coupling systems to increase the number of fibers that could be inserted. This concept, while attractive, has proved difficult to achieve in practice.

In 1987, Gatenby (55,56) used computed tomography (CT)–guided laser therapy for treatment of resistant human tumors in 10 patients with favorable results. Godlewski (57) and, later, Dachman (58) stereotactically induced lesions in the liver of piglets using a Nd:YAG laser and followed these lesions for 4 months with serial ultrasound examinations and histologic correlation. These areas eventually heal with fibrosis in the center and, after their creation, could be followed with ultrasound. Steger (59) used ultrasound imaging to monitor the percutaneous interstitial Nd:YAG laser treatment of 10 patients with liver tumors and 3 with pancreatic cancers. In all, the growth of the tumors treated has been held or slowed after treatment, but the treatment did not affect overall survival. Steger (59) found ultrasound imaging to be a sensitive monitoring technique of thermal necrosis in liver. However, Dachman (58) reported changes consistent mainly with cavitation. Some studies have demonstrated that an energy density of at least 12,000 J/cm$^2$ of the Nd:YAG laser is needed (400-µm fiber, 4 W, 6 minutes) to visualize cavitation with ultrasound, as opposed to energy density as low as 1,250 J/cm$^2$ for MRI to demonstrate a similar phenomena (60). The use of ultrasound in the skull base and other areas may have limited applications. CT scanning demonstrates poor sensitivity to early tissue changes after laser exposure because is has a low contrast resolution for soft tissue.

MRI is one of the most significant advances in medical imaging in this century (61). MRI is a noninvasive and extremely sensitive diagnostic imaging system that is used to locate and guide biopsies of deep and difficult tumors and to access target tissues using needles with extremely low magnetic susceptibilities (62). MRI has the potential to become a three-dimensional, real-time, video-imaging technique that can provide accurate and detailed anatomic information during laser surgery (63). MRI has numerous advantages in evaluating the irreversible effects of laser treatment in tissues, because laser energy induces changes in the thermal motions of the hydrogen protons within the tissue and in the distribution and mobility of water and lipids (64).

The MRI signal depends on the structural dynamics of water-macromolecular interactions (64). The thermal effects of laser energy cause macromolecules to denature, which may change the number of water molecules in bound and unbound states and the amount of time spent by water in each state (64). There may also be differential absorption of light among cellular components, causing distinct alteration in their structures. These changes may be indirectly detectable by MRI because they alter the mobility of tissue water, which results in changes of relaxation times (64). T1 and T2 are relaxation parameters of the tissue that reflect normal anatomy and pathology such as edema and neoplastic transformation. T1-weighted images have image contrast that reflect hydrogen proton relaxation times of the tissue. Similarly, images with contrast that reflect the proton spin-spin values of the tissue are said to be T2-weighted.

Barroilhet (65), Fung (66), and Parker (67) demonstrated the strong temperature dependence of MR relaxation in quantitative investigations. The principal effect of a temperature rise was increased spin lattice relaxation time, T1.

However, Lewa (68) reported an irreversible decrease in T1 at temperatures greater than 40°C. This has been attributed to alteration of macromolecule-water interactions that occur before the obvious denaturation of proteins at 60°C. Parker (69), Tanaka (70), Dickinson (71), and Knuttel (72) demonstrated that MR imaging could provide three-dimensional thermal mapping with direct display of heat distribution and tissue characteristic in hyperthermia. Improved control of laser-tissue interactions may be possible by exploiting the complex and versatile capabilities of MR imaging and selected volume measurement. *In vitro* (63) and *in vivo* (60,73,74) models have been used to evaluate reversible and irreversible changes on MRI caused by interstitial Nd:YAG laser therapy. In a large series of experiments performed in *ex vivo, in vivo,* and in animals heterotransplanted with human tumors, MRI was found to be an extremely sensitive modality to visualize laser and radiofrequency (RF) energy deposition in tissues. Linear relationships were obtained for doses of laser or RF energy, thermal distribution, signal intensity changes on MRI, and histologic changes in tissue (60,73,74).

## Mechanisms of Laser-Tissue Interactions

The photobiologic effects of laser illumination can be separated into three mechanistic categories: photochemical, photomechanical, and photothermal. Photochemical effects depend on the absorption of light to initiate chemical species in PDT. This is associated with low fluency rates that do not produce a significant temperature increase in the treated tissue but do interact with a natural or exogenous photosensitizer to produce the desired reaction. Photomechanical responses occur during application of extremely high fluency rates (>10$^8$ W/cm$^2$) and short laser pulses (≤10$^{-6}$ second), which produce shockwaves and plasmas. Such effects occur, for example, when a laser operated in a Q-switch mode.

Photothermal effects result from the transformation of absorbed light energy to heat. The photothermal effects of lasers can be subdivided further into the three categories of laser hyperthermia, photoablation, and photocarbonization or photoevaporation. With hyperthermia, various cells or tissues that are heated to about 43°C to 45°C can sustain reversible injury that become irreversible (i.e., death) after exposure of 25 minutes to several hours, depending on the type of tissue and experimental or therapeutic circumstances. Systemic hyperthermia and local hyperthermia have been tested clinically with limited success, mainly because of the difficulties in delivering uniform levels of energy throughout the tumor mass. This technique is slow, cumbersome, and difficult to apply.

In photoablation, the tissue temperature is rapidly raised to a range of 60°C to 100°C, at which point visible whitening of the treated tissue is seen, indicating thermal coagulation. Thermal coagulation of tissues is defined as thermally induced, irreversible denaturation of proteins and other macromolecules, organelles, membranes, cells, and extracellular components that are observable by the naked eye or microscopic techniques. Most of these alterations are caused by thermal denaturation of structural proteins, although membrane rupture may result from alteration in lipids. By this definition, thermal tissue coagulation differs for low temperature injury in that the always lethal coagulative lesions are marked by structural changes seen immediately after heating. This process is easier, simpler, and more rapid to deliver and control in tissues.

When tissue temperature is raised above 100°C, the process of photocarbonization and photoevaporation occurs with an explosive fragmentation or tissue loss. Subsurface heating generates bubbles that eventually explode in a series of events called the *popcorn effect*. Water loss results in tissue desiccation, which rapidly changes the optical characteristics of tissues and their absorption efficiency of infrared lasers. Water loss reduces the thermal conductivity and specific heat of tissues. Black char, yellow flames, and gray smoke are the prominent phenomena characterizing the clinical use of photocarbonization.

## Clinical Experience with Interstitial Laser Photothermal Therapy

In the past 5 years, more than 50 patients with advanced cancer were treated using image-guided therapy in the UCLA the head and neck surgery program. All patients presented with recurrent or metastatic (or both), unresectable tumors that failed previous surgery, radiation therapy, chemotherapy, hyperthermia, and other treatment modalities. These patients presented with one to four recurrent tumors, and 1 to 12 palliative sessions of imaging-guided surgery were performed, with a mean of four treatments. The survival ranged between 3 months to 5 years after treatment, with a mean of 18 months. The anatomic locations of these tumors are summarized in Table 36.1, with most occurring in the head and neck area.

**TABLE 36.1. ANATOMIC LOCATIONS OF UNRESECTABLE HEAD AND NECK TUMORS**

| Location | Number |
|---|---|
| Base of skull | 2 |
| Base of tongue | 3 |
| Buccal mucosa | 5 |
| Floor of mouth | 7 |
| Lateral tongue | 3 |
| Lateral pharyngeal wall | 2 |
| Maxillary sinus | 2 |
| Nasopharynx | 2 |
| Neck | 10 |
| Nose | 2 |
| Palate (hard and soft) | 3 |
| Posterior pharynx | 1 |
| Subcutaneous sites | 4 |
| Tracheobronchial tree | 9 |

Most patients (70%) presented with pain as their major complaint. However, others presented with associated dysphagia, dyspnea, bleeding, difficulties chewing and swallowing, or cosmetic deformities. Most patients were subjected to routine clinical evaluations that included preoperative MRI, ultrasound, or positron-emission tomography (PET) studies to assess the anatomy, tumor location, volume, underlying vascular supply, and metabolic activity. Tumor volumes ranged from 2 to 80 cm$^3$, with a mean of 35 cm$^3$. Diagnosis was confirmed in all patients with a biopsy. The histology was predominantly squamous cell carcinoma (90%), but other types included melanoma, adenocarcinoma, adenoid cystic carcinoma, medullary thyroid carcinoma, adenoma, angiosarcoma, and chondrosarcoma.

Procedures were carried out in the operating room or on an outpatient basis. After obtaining appropriate informed consent, the patients were placed on continuous cardiac and pulse oximetry monitoring and then heavily sedated or placed under general anesthesia by an anesthesiologist. The surgical field was prepped and draped in a sterile fashion, and the skin overlying the tumor mass was anesthetized with 1% lidocaine with 1:100,000 epinephrine. A variable number of 16-gauge Angiocath or E-Z-EM needles with a suction port were then passed percutaneously into the tumor mass when interstitial treatment was performed (Fig. 36.1). Ultrasound was used in 50 patients to confirm the

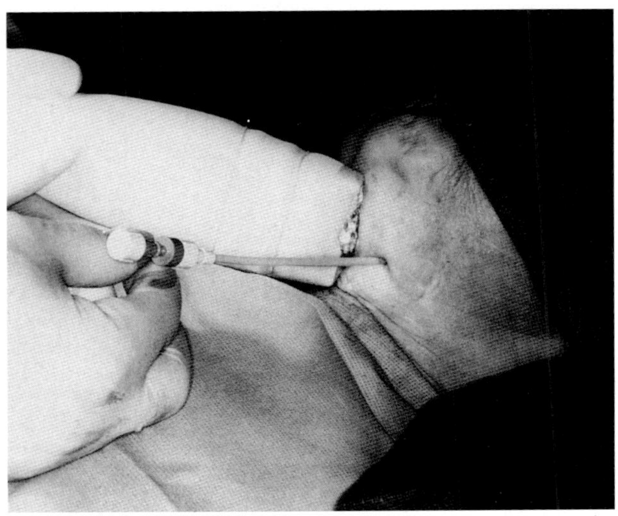

**FIGURE 36.1.** Ultrasound-guided interstitial Nd:YAG laser therapy of metastatic neck carcinoma.

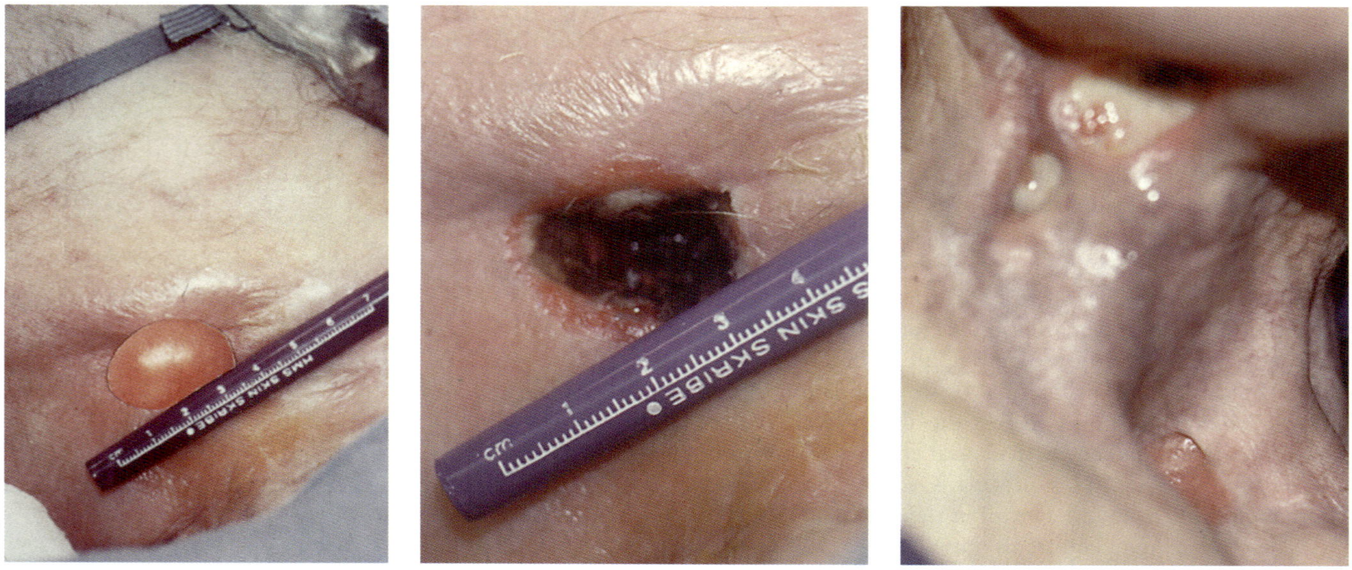

A,B C

**FIGURE 36.2. A:** Presurgical view of a patient with a submandibular squamous cell carcinoma that failed previous surgery and radiation therapy. **B:** Immediate postoperative view after ultrasound-guided interstitial Nd:YAG laser therapy. **C:** View of the submandibular area 3 months postoperatively.

position of the tip of the catheters within the tumor mass, with special attention given to the proximity to larger vessels and tumor neovascularity. The first nine patients were treated in the upgraded 1.5 T interventional MRI unit equipped with a treatment monitoring system.

The 600-μm, flexible Nd:YAG laser fiberoptic cable was then passed through the needle lumen and into the tumor mass. Nd:YAG laser energy (90% of patients) was applied interstitially (Fig. 36.2) or externally, guided by ultrasound as a monitoring technique (Fig. 36.3). Some patients (15%) with large tumor burden first underwent ultrasonic energy delivery externally or interstitially to rapidly debulk the tumor; then the bed was treated with the Nd:YAG laser.

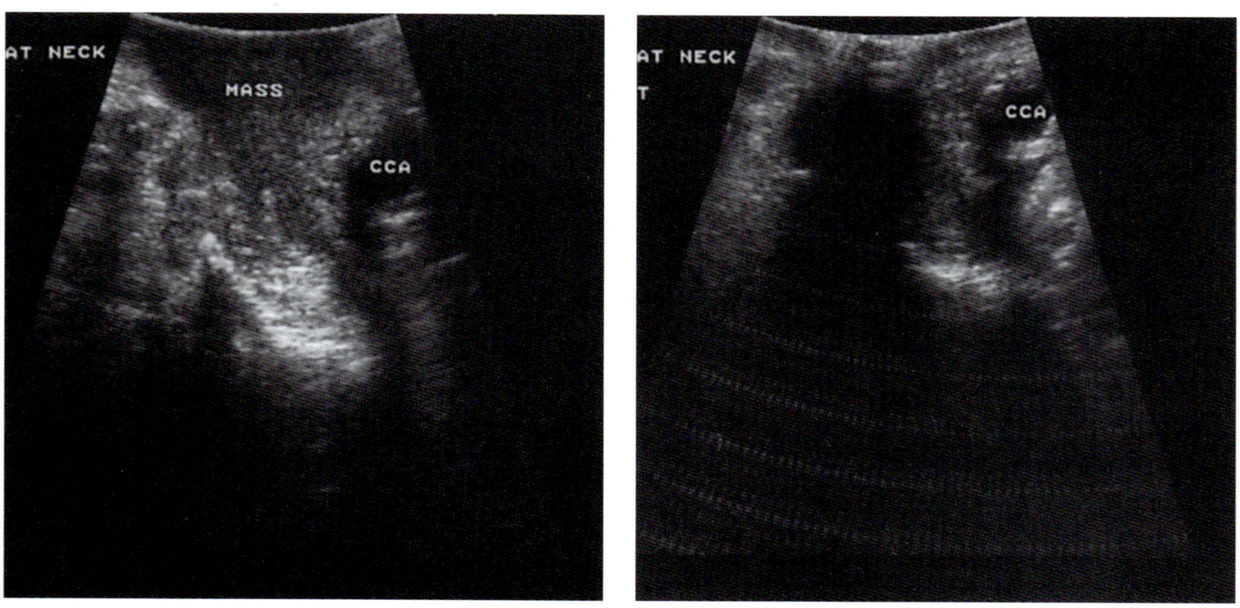


A B

**FIGURE 36.3. A:** Preoperative ultrasound image of the submandibular squamous cell carcinoma shown in Figure 36.2. **B:** Ultrasound imaging immediately after treatment shows a hyperechoic image at a previous tumor site and proximity to the common carotid artery *(CCA)*.

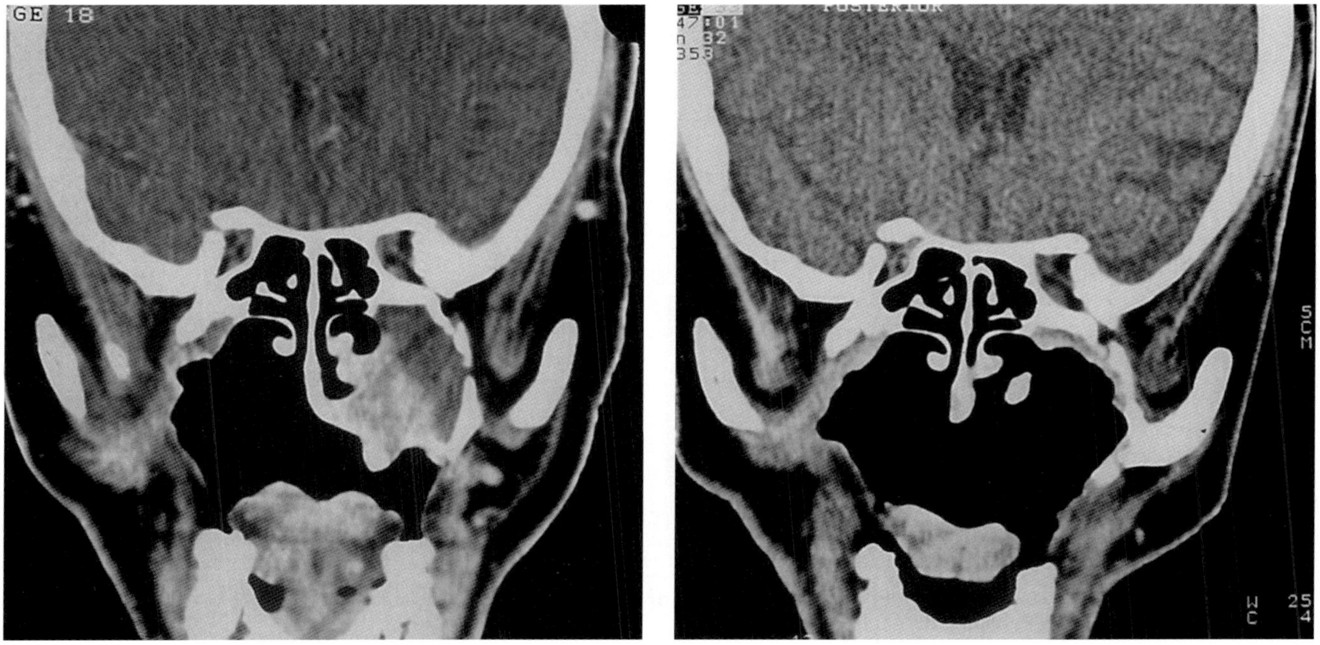


A B

**FIGURE 36.4. A:** Fourth recurrence of adenoid cystic carcinoma of the maxillary sinus. **B:** Three months after interstitial Nd:YAG laser treatment.

Most patients (91%) were treated in the operating room using ultrasound as the guiding imaging modality, and 9% were treated in the interventional MRI suite. In 90% of the cases, Nd:YAG laser was used externally or interstitially to photoablate the tumors (Figs. 36.4–36.6), and the ultrasonic energy was used in the later cases in conjunction with the Nd:YAG laser. Ninety percent of patients were treated on an outpatient basis, with 80% showing improvement or resolution of symptoms after one to five sessions, with a mean of two treatments. When stratified by the tumor site, successful laser therapy was highest in the oral cavity (85.7%) compared with other sites.

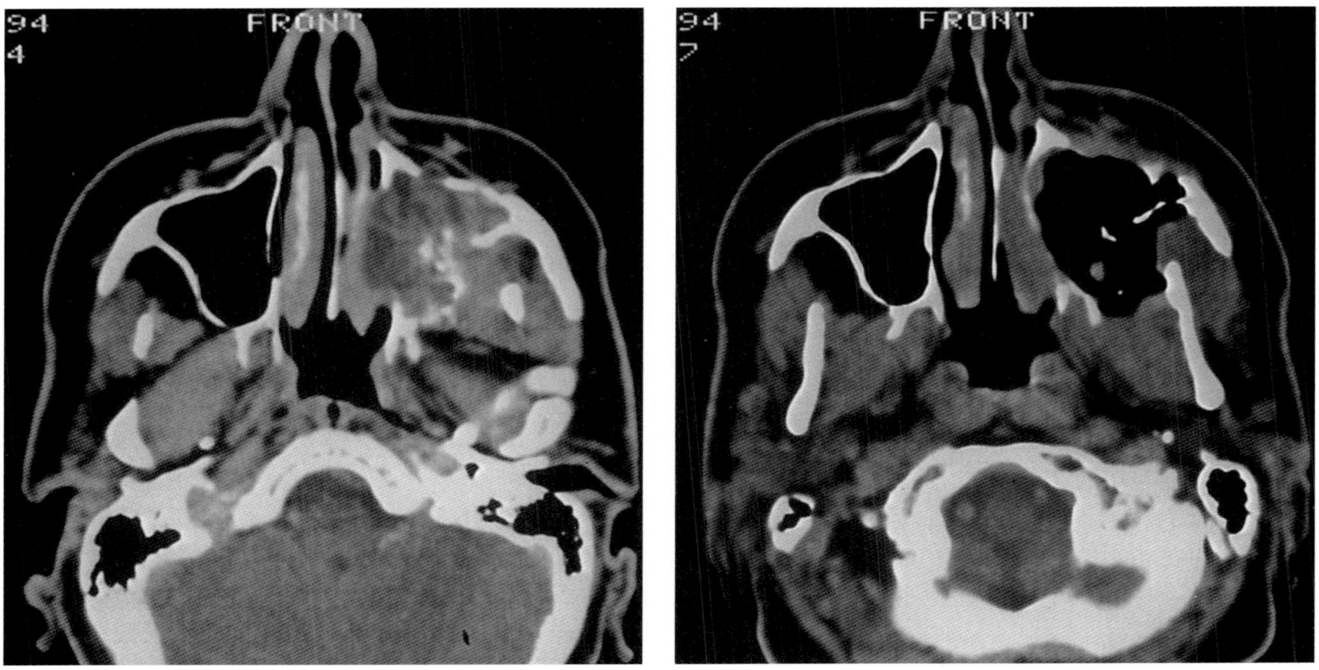


A B

**FIGURE 36.5. A:** A 54-year-old man with recurrence of an adenoid cystic carcinoma of the left maxillary sinus. **B:** Three months after interstitial Nd:YAG laser treatment.

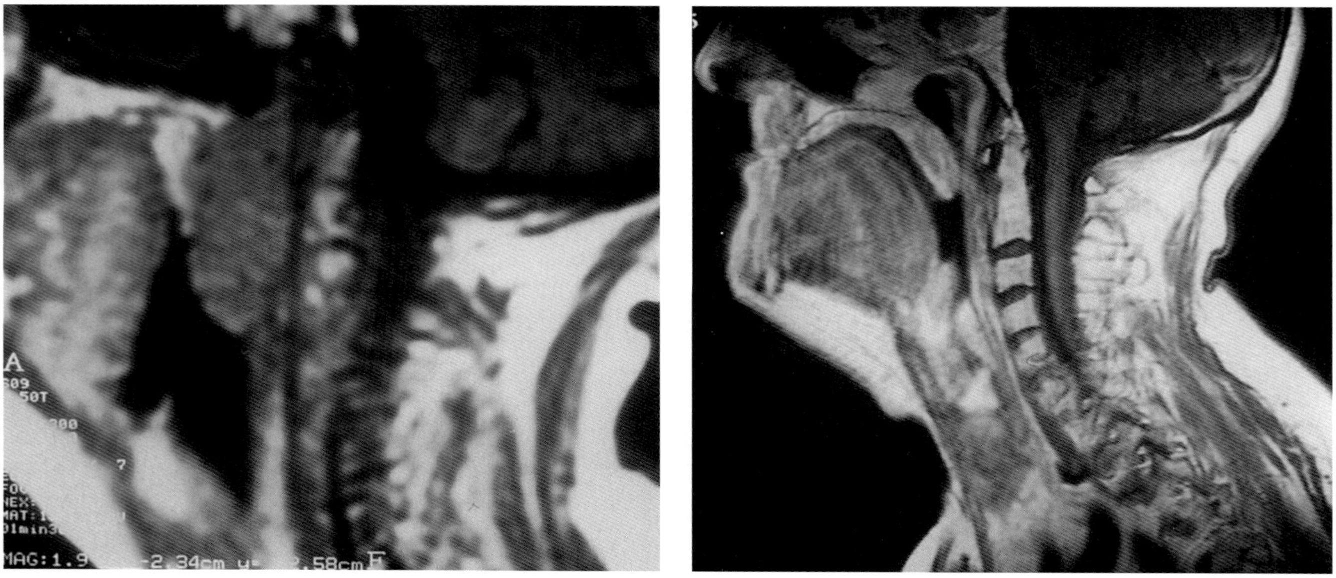

A B

**FIGURE 36.6. A:** Magnetic resonance imaging of a squamous cell carcinoma of the nasopharynx. **B:** Six weeks after Nd:YAG laser treatment.

This response was inversely related to the initial tumor volume, and it depended on tumor histology and growth rate. Smaller, slow-growing, more-differentiated tumors were palliated successfully and had a better local cure rate than rapidly dividing malignancies. More than 80% of the patients have shown significant functional and cosmetic improvement and were able to resume daily activities for periods of up to 5 years after treatment with a mean of 18 months. One major complication was observed in the second patient treated under MRI guidance. Perioperative bleeding that occurred during interstitial laser energy deposition required embolization and intubation for airway protection. This patient did well afterward and ultimately died 4 years after treatment of pulmonary metastasis. The first case was the only patient to die within 3 months postoperatively of unrelated cardiopulmonary disease; the others had a mean survival of 18 months.

Over the years, our clinical approach for image-guided palliative laser therapy of head and neck tumors has evolved, and multiple steps led to the current technique. A conservative approach was used initially with the 1.06-μm Nd:YAG laser implanted interstitially in tumors. In the first 15 patients treated, care was taken to photoablate only a small and limited volume of tumor during each treatment, leaving ample margins of untreated tumor behind, because no experience was available, and the side effects were unknown. Only one needle was implanted in the center of the tumor, and after confirmation of its position by ultrasound, a 600-μm, flexible Nd:YAG laser fiberoptic was inserted. The Nd:YAG laser was set at 25 W in a continuous mode (Fig. 36.7). A total of four Nd:YAG laser exposures, each lasting 15 seconds, were delivered to the center of the tumor while the transient hyperechoic signal generated during energy deposition was monitored by ultrasound (Figs. 36.8 and 36.9). Between each laser exposure, the Nd:YAG laser fiber was removed and its tip cleaned and reshaped. These patients tolerated the treatments well, and the only side effect observed was a transient postoperative tumor swelling due to edema. Although no infections occurred, many patients required multiple treatment sessions (up to 12) to completely ablate these tumors. The number of treatment sessions was linearly related to the

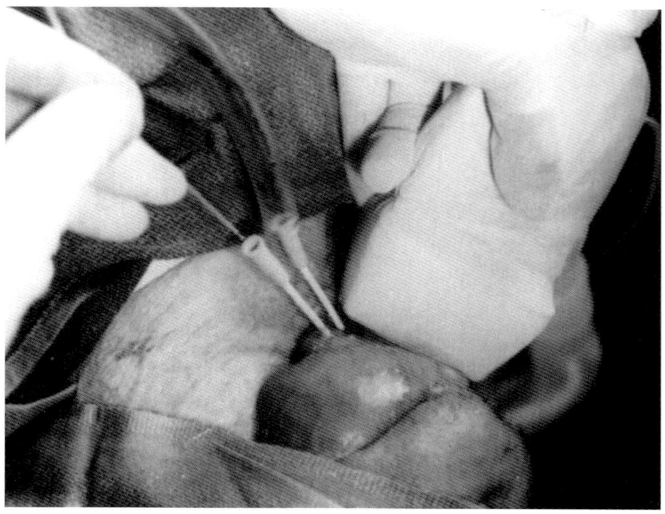

**FIGURE 36.7.** Ultrasound-guided interstitial Nd:YAG laser therapy of a recurrent submental squamous carcinoma. Notice the channels for the laser and for aspiration.

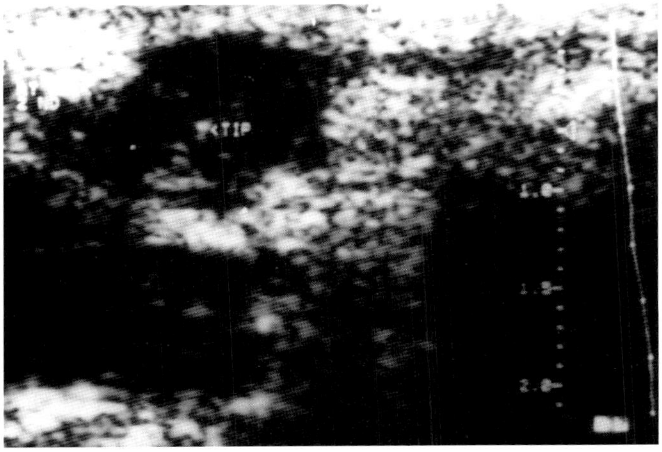

**FIGURE 36.8.** Ultrasound needle-tip localization in the tumor of the patient shown in Figure 36.6. The tumor generates a hypoechoic signal on ultrasound.

original tumor volume and its rate of regrowth. Smaller and slow-growing tumors required the least number of sessions.

A number of problems were identified in the first 15 patients treated. First, there was a transient (2 weeks) postoperative increase in tumor volume that was accompanied by worsening of the symptoms (e.g., pain, swelling). These symptoms improved gradually during follow-up. Second, no cooling of the Nd:YAG laser fiber tip was used initially, resulting in frequent damage to the laser tip, which was cleaved and reshaped multiple times during each procedure. Third, only a single major complication was seen, and this occurred in the second patient treated under MRI guidance in 1990. Perioperative bleeding occurring during interstitial Nd:YAG laser energy deposition required embolization and 24-hour intubation for airway protection. This complication was caused by poor resolution of the needle tip location under MRI guidance into the tumor site. This problem has been resolved completely by subsequent use of ultrasound for real-time needle introduction and localization and by the availability of faster MR pulse sequences. Fourth, too many treatment sessions were required to achieve local tumor control. An average of eight treatments was required per patient to obtain significant improvement of symptoms. Patients were treated every 2 to 4 weeks, and during each treatment, only a fraction of the residual tumor mass was destroyed.

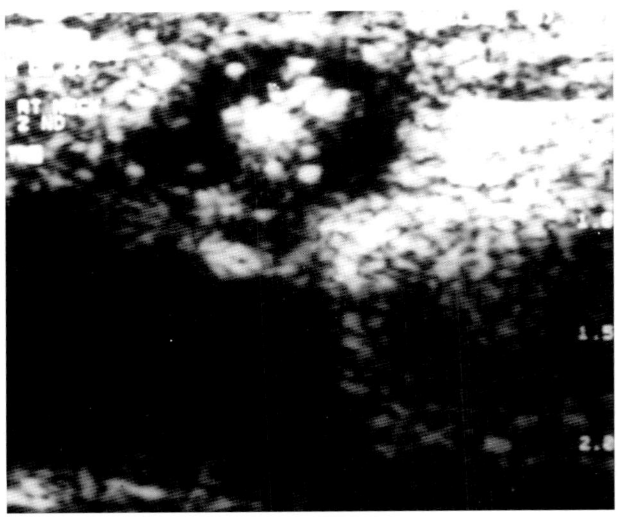

**FIGURE 36.9.** A transient hyperechoic signal is shown on ultrasound while the Nd:YAG laser remains powered.

To reduce the number of treatments per patient, avoid potential bleeding complications, and prevent damage to the Nd:YAG laser fiber tip during energy deposition, a number of changes were tested in the next five patients. First, all patients were scanned with a color Doppler ultrasound preoperatively to map the underlying tumor vasculature and its relation to surrounding major blood vessels. All patients with tumors surrounding the carotid artery in the neck or base of skull area were excluded early on from our study. However, two patients treated in the past 6 months with base of skull and carotid artery involvement were successfully palliated after carotid artery occlusion followed by ultrasound-guided Nd:YAG laser excision. Second, an irrigation-suction system was added using normal saline during interstitial Nd:YAG laser energy deposition. This measure has significantly reduced the frequency of damage to the fiber's tip and prevented charred tissue from accumulating around the fiber. Third, an attempt to photoablate an increased volume of tumor during each treatment was made by inserting multiple needles at various sites in the tumor under ultrasound guidance. Each site was then treated separately with interstitial Nd:YAG laser energy while monitoring thermal effects with ultrasound. The largest tumor treated in one session had a volume of 40 $cm^3$, measured by preoperative MRI. This patient did well postoperatively, with no significant side effects, except for a large amount of necrotic debris that drained from all the needle sites at 2 weeks. No other side effects were observed, despite the fact that follow-up included only oral antibiotics. This patient remained alive for 4 years with no evidence of a local recurrence. However, she later developed a malignant pleural effusion and died 6 months later of metastatic disease. The other patients treated using this technique did well except for a transient (2 to 4 weeks) increase in their symptoms (e.g., pain, swallowing difficulties).

The clinical symptoms were proportionally related to the changes in tumor volume. For this reason, in addition to the measures described previously, an attempt was made to suction all of the debris to rapidly debulk tumors during each treatment. This proved to be more effective because symptoms such as pain and swallowing difficulty improved dramatically within 1 to 3 days postoperatively.

This aspiration technique appeared to be safe and effective because no major complications occurred when tested on 15 patients with head and neck tumors ranging from 4 to 50 cm$^3$. However, the procedure time remained lengthy, with an average operating time of 2 hours, because the Nd:YAG laser was the only source of energy used for tumor eradication. To reduce the operating time in the later patients presenting with tumors larger than 20 cm$^3$, the CUSA ultrasonic/RF surgical aspirator (Valley Lab, Boulder, CO) was used in conjunction with the Nd:YAG laser and irrigation-suction systems. In accessible and large tumors, under ultrasound guidance, the ultrasonic aspirator is now used first to rapidly debulk the treated tumor, and the interstitial Nd:YAG laser with suction-irrigation is used to treat the underlying bed and margins. The operating time has been reduced to 45 minutes, with patients responding well to the procedure. Tumors located in the oral cavity, pharynx, hypopharynx, larynx, and esophagus were treated endoscopically with the Nd:YAG laser fiber mounted on a Frazier suction catheter, and the 10-MHz ultrasound transducer was placed externally on the neck's skin, monitoring the underlying anatomy, vascular supply, and treatment effects. To avoid the possibility of tumor cell seeding along the path of the needles during insertion or extrusion, new needles were used for each passage. The Nd:YAG laser was kept "on" while the needle was pulled out of the target, although the treated patients had no evidence of recurrences or tumor regrowth along the needle path.

The first five patients with recurrent, unresectable head and neck tumors were treated in a standard MR suite and later in an upgraded 1.5-T MR suite. Because the initial experimental results demonstrated a high sensitivity and a linear relationship between the measured MR signal intensity change with the amount of interstitial energy deposition in tumors and subsequent histologic damage, MRI was selected as the guiding modality for this laser therapy technique. However, the average procedure time in the MR interventional suite lasted 3 to 5 hours because of the slow technique of needle localization and difficulties in monitoring blood flow. The cost of upgrades of the MR interventional suite exceeded $500,000, and access to patients was still limited. Color Doppler ultrasonography was used for the last 50 patients because it was portable, easily adaptable to the operating room, and cost effective. Ultrasound was found to be the most practical imaging modality for real-time guidance and localization of interstitial needles or probes in a target. Because color Doppler ultrasonography is a very sensitive modality for noninvasive monitoring of blood flow, its use during the procedure has helped avoid neurovascular structure and any further bleeding complications. Before treatment, a tumor appears as a zone of hypoechoic signal on ultrasound that completely regresses after successful debulking with interstitial ultrasonic energy followed by Nd:YAG laser photocoagulation.

In summary, lasers have several advantages and drawbacks:

1. Lasers are versatile sources of nonionizing light that can be delivered to a target through flexible fiberoptics using a minimally invasive approach.
2. Lasers are ideal for delivery of localized photothermal energy, leading to palliative destruction of early head and neck tumor recurrences.
3. Intraoperative color Doppler ultrasonography was the most useful monitoring technique for guidance of ILT in tumors.
4. Preclinical and clinical experience demonstrated a 40% incidence of tumor regrowth, occurring mostly at the margins when the laser alone was used as a photoablative source of energy.
5. The relatively high failure of tumor thermal therapy with the laser alone led to additional investigations in the treatment by laser PDT and laser photochemotherapy.

## PHOTODYNAMIC THERAPY

PDT consists of the administration of a photosensitizer, such as a photochemical, at an extremely low and nontoxic level to the host. If this photochemical is taken up by malignant cells, the "sensitized" tumor can be exposed in the presence of oxygen to a laser beam at a matching wavelength, resulting in the ablation of the target site. Because most lasers can be transmitted through flexible fiberoptics, physicians can perform these procedures endoscopically on an outpatient basis, reducing hospitalization and reducing costs. Because lasers produce nonionizing radiation beams, these procedures can be repeated multiple times without the tissue toxicity limits seen using conventional radiation therapy. However, effective PDT can occur only when three major components are combined: efficient photosensitizers, monochromatic light sources, and minimally invasive light delivery systems.

### Photosensitizers

The field of PDT has regained popularity in recent years, particularly since the introduction of lasers by Maiman (75) and the successful use of newer hematoporphyrin derivatives for the treatment of superficial malignant tumors (76). The properties of a porphyrin photosensitizers as tumor-localizing agents include prolonged retention near malignant lesions compared with normal tissues and its detectability by virtue intense of fluorescence. Porphyrins are useful therapeutically because of photochemical oxidation activity that can be elicited using a tissue-penetrating wavelength of visible light (i.e., red) (Fig. 36.10).

The initial enthusiasm originated by the early successful results observed in patients treated with hematoporphyrin

A 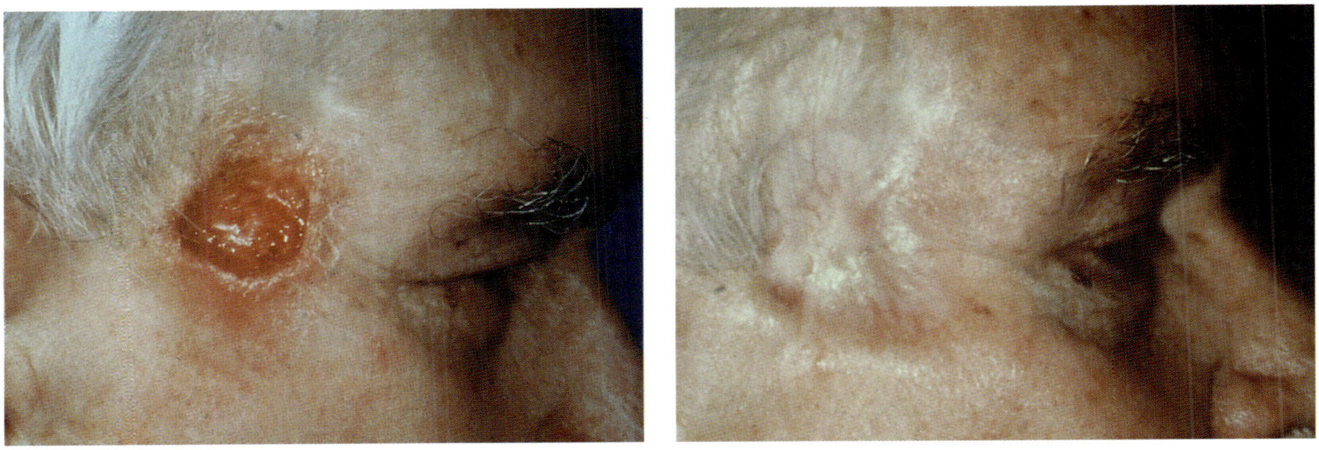 B

**FIGURE 36.10. A:** Eighth recurrence of basal cell carcinoma in a 90-year-old man. **B:** One year after photodynamic therapy using hematoporphyrin.

derivative and laser light was decreased by cutaneous side effects and limitations (77). The major side effect of hematoporphyrin derivatives is severe photosensitivity for 30 days or longer after administration of this dye (77). Patients must be protected with adequate clothing or sunscreens against any sunlight and cannot even venture outside or sit near a window during this period. Pain is another common side effect, particularly involving the calvarium, with patients frequently experiencing severe headaches after the light activation (77). Hematoporphyrin derivatives have shown a nonspecific absorption by inflammatory and traumatized tissues, which decreases its potential use as a tumor specific fluorescent dye and the advantages of the low-power milliwatt dye lasers used for PDT. These side effects and limitations of hematoporphyrin derivatives will probably remain significant in its future clinical applications, especially in attempts to treat deeply invasive tumors.

A variety of compounds, such as acridine orange, mercurochrome, nitro red, methylene blue, psoralens, rose Bengal, and sodium fluorescein, have been investigated as potential photosensitizing agents with some advantages but also frequently with side effects similar to the cutaneous photosensitivity caused by hematoporphyrin derivatives and lack of specificity for tumor cells. These potential complications also may limit their future clinical applications.

The search for improved fluorochromes that are more specific and less phototoxic or chemotoxic has stimulated investigations of new photosensitizers, including rhodamine-123 (Rh-123) (7,78–81), as a potential chemosensitizing agents for the treatment of superficial malignant tumors with the argon laser and Kodak Q-switch II dye for the Nd:YAG laser (SLT Company, Philadelphia, PA) (82). Rh-123 (Eastman Kodak Laboratories) is a lipophilic, cationic compound absorbed specifically by living mitochondria, with an absorption maximum at 511 nm and a fluorescence maximum at 575 nm. In 1980, Johnson and coworkers (83) were the first to visualize mitochondria with Rh-123. Since then, multiple investigators have used this compound in a wide variety of imaginative applications to study mitochondrial and general cellular functions. In 1981, James and Bowman (84) showed that uptake of Rh-123 and the subsequent changes in mitochondrial morphology of human fibroblasts are related to the growth of these cells. In 1982, Bernal and associates (85) used Rh-123 as an indicator of cell viability. Evenson and colleagues (86) used Rh-123 to study to motility of sperm by flow cytometry. In 1982, Clark and Shay (87) used Rh-123 as a mitochondrial marker for studying mitochondrial transformation of mammalian cells.

Two new groups of photosensitizers were synthesized by Morgan and coworkers (88). These are the purpurins and their metallo derivatives. These are all synthetic compounds that can be prepared in pure form and are of known structure. Purpurins have major absorption peaks between 630 and 715 nm, an area of the visible spectrum with excellent tissue-penetrating properties using dye lasers. From histologic studies of transplanted urothelial tumors, it is clear that purpurins and metallopurpurins are capable of causing extensive tumor necrosis when combined with visible light.

Detty (89) at the Eastman Kodak Company demonstrated the potential of a new group of photosensitizers, the chalcogenapyrylium dyes, which are water-soluble, cationic compounds with various absorption maxima between 750 and 875 nm. These dyes are compatible with commercially available gallium arsenide lasers. Pyrilium dyes appear to may be promising because their light absorption is in the so-called biologic window between 700 and 900 nm, a range that permits excellent transmissibility of light wavelengths through tissues.

Mercocyanine-540, specific for the argon laser at 514 nm, has been tested by Gulliya and Dowben (90). The cationic kryptocyanine dye, EDKC, was tested by Ara and coworkers (91), and has been shown to be preferentially taken up and retained by cancer cells of various histologies, with a dye absorption maximum at 700 nm in saline. Pheophorbide, a chlorophyll derivative with a peak absorption at 670 nm, has been tested by Segelman (92). This new field of PDT with lasers appears to hold great promise as an adjunctive modality for the diagnosis and treatment of malignant disease or connective tissue disease when fluorochromes with high tumor specificity and low systemic toxicities are developed (93,94).

## Lasers

Interest in the technology of light production, stimulated by industrial, military, and space applications, gave rise to new and medically useful light sources. In 1960, Maiman (75) first observed stimulated emission in the visible portion of the spectrum by exciting a ruby rod with intense pulses of light from a flash lamp, generating the first laser beam. In 1961, Javan and associates (95) developed the first gas laser and demonstrated the first continuously operating laser using a mixture of helium and neon. Also that year, using a neodymium-doped yttrium-aluminum-garnet (Nd:YAG) rod, Johnson (96) developed a laser that emitted energy in the near-infrared portion of the spectrum. The argon laser, emitting energy in the blue-green portion of the spectrum, was developed by Bennett and colleagues (97) in 1962. The carbon dioxide laser, emitting spectral energy in the mid-infrared portion was developed in 1964 by Patel and coworkers (98).

## Features of a Laser Dye Candidate

Effective PDT occurs only when three major components are combined: efficient photosensitizers, monochromatic light sources, and light delivery systems. When choosing a laser dye for phototherapy, many chemical properties need to be considered. First, the dye must be soluble and remain stable in aqueous solution at physiologic pH to allow circulation and selective accumulation in tumor cells. Defining these ideal characteristics and selecting appropriate photochemicals is a major area requiring cooperation between basic scientists and clinicians. For example, phthalocyanines were thought to be promising candidates for PDT (99), but the unsubstituted phthalocyanines are completely insoluble in water but have slight solubility in ethanol and dimethyl sulfoxide (DMSO). With the help of biochemists, direct sulfonation of phthalocyanines was made feasible, making it water soluble and therefore easily tested *in vitro* as a potential new photosensitizer. Another example is that of Kodak Q-Switch II dye, which has shown some promise as a fluorochrome *in vitro* (100). The natural solvent for Kodak Q-Switch dye is chlorobenzene, which by itself is extremely toxic to humans. Another nontoxic solvent was used with further dilutions of sterile water (100), making it feasible to carry out *in vitro* testing.

Some dyes such as hematoporphyrin derivatives, rhodamines, mercocyanine-540, chalcogenapyriliums, and related compounds are soluble in aqueous solution and therefore easily tested *in vitro* and *in vivo*. Many other dyes may be tested in the future, because we know that aqueous solubility and stability can be improved by the appropriate biochemical modifications.

A second important feature of a laser dye is its ability to demonstrate selectivity of uptake and retention by malignant cells, which is necessary to distinguish cancer from normal tissue. It is unrealistic to anticipate finding a chemical that is taken up only by cancer cells and not by normal surrounding tissues. It has been difficult to identify major differences between the metabolism of cancer and normal cells. The pharmacokinetics of laser dye candidates should be elucidated to define *time windows* in which the differences between normal and cancer tissues are observed in the uptake or retention phases.

In some studies (101,102), the pharmacokinetics of Photofrin II (PII) and [$^{14}$C]-Photofrin II were studied *in vivo*. No preferential tumor uptake by PII was observed (101). Normal tissue uptake of the drug occurred at about 7.5 hours after administration, with peak concentrations seen in liver, adrenal glands, urinary bladder, kidneys, and spleen. Only skeletal muscle and brain had peak concentrations of [$^{14}$C]-PII lower than the tumor tissues, and 61% of the initial level of [$^{14}$C]-PII was still present in the spleen and other tissues up to 75 days after injections. These findings may partly explain the long-term phototoxic effects seen in patients injects with PII (101).

The biodistribution of Rh-123 has been tested in normal rabbits and nude mice heterotransplanted with human tumors (103,104). No preferential uptake of Rh-123 by tumors occurred, with rapid uptake of the dye by normal tissues and peak concentrations observed in kidneys, liver, and muscle in mice. However, Rh-123 is rapidly metabolized from normal tissues, falling to 2.7% of peak concentrations at 72 hours and to undetectable levels at 7 days after injection (103,104). Tumor uptake of Rh-123 peaks between 3 and 24 hours (104), with progressive and slow washout afterward and a longer retention of up to 10 days after injection. A time window for Rh-123 can be observed between day 7 and 10 after injection in the animal model, when Rh-123 is still present in tumors but almost completely eliminated from normal surrounding tissues. This time window may provide differentiation between normal and malignant tissues with Rh-123. These two examples with Photofrin II and Rh-123 illustrate the importance of studying the pharmacokinetics of each laser dye candidate to define the optimal time window for PDT or for photodiagnostic imaging of tumors with lasers and dyes.

A third desirable feature of a laser dye is its ability to undergo passive or active transport into the cells and to have a well-known intracellular target site. For example, Rh-123 is a lipophilic, cationic dye (7,78–80,104–107) that localizes specifically in living mitochondria. Merocyanine-540 is a negatively charged dye (108,109) that localizes in plasma membranes. Rhodamine 800 and 8-methoxy-psoralen localize in nuclear DNA (110). The intracellular target sites of hematoporphyrin photosensitization is still controversial, and the plasma membrane (111), nucleus (112), microsomes (113), lysosomes (114), and mitochondria (115) have all been considered. Subcellular localization is important because dyes with different intracellular target sites may be used synergistically to optimize the tumor destructive capabilities of PDT, much like with antibiotics when penicillin and streptomycin are used together. Knowledge of the intracellular target site of each laser dye helps to clarify the mechanism of photodestruction with lasers and allows selection of other dyes with similar characteristics.

The photoprocess ability of a laser dye candidate (i.e., the singlet or triplet state quantum yield and lifetime versus its fluorescence quantum yield) is a fourth characteristic that must be elucidated (Fig. 36.11). A dye with a high yield of the singlet or triplet state is an excellent candidate for PDT in the presence of oxygen with selected laser wavelengths leading to a type I or type II photo-oxidation (116), producing free radicals (I) or singlet oxygen (II), which are instantly toxic to tumor cells.

A dye with a high fluorescence quantum may be an excellent candidate for photodiagnostic imaging of tumors, because this dye fluoresces easily when exposed to a matching, low-power laser wavelength, enabling visualization of and differentiation between malignant and normal surrounding tissues. However, tests (117) demonstrated a direct relationship between the singlet or triplet state yield of dye, its fluorescence quantum, and the systemic toxicity to the host (Fig. 36.11). A laser dye with a high yield of the singlet or triplet state, which is perfect for PDT, also demonstrates a linear increase in systemic toxicity to the host. However, a laser dye with a high fluorescence quantum that is perfect for photodetection demonstrates minimal or no PDT effects (Fig. 36.11).

Studies comparing the efficiency of Rh-123, Rh-6G, and Rh-3B *in vitro* on cancer cells illustrate these facts. Rh-6G has a higher triplet state quantum yield compared with Rh-123 (117), but Rh-123 has a higher fluorescence quantum compared with Rh-6G (117). Theoretically, Rh-6G is a better photosensitizer for PDT, and Rh-123 is a better fluorochrome for photodiagnostic imaging with lasers. The kinetics of uptake of these three dyes demonstrate higher levels and faster uptake of Rh-6G by cancer cells compared with Rh-123 (117). When these cancer cells were first sensitized with each of these three dyes and exposed to nonthermal levels of energies of the argon laser (514.5 nm), only 1 mg/mL of Rh-6G was needed to obtain significant suppression of cell proliferation (117), whereas concentrations of 1 mg/mL were required with Rh-123 to observe similar levels of suppression. When the toxicity of each of these dyes was tested on cancer cells, a reverse effect was noticed. Rh-6G demonstrated significantly greater toxicity on these cancer cells compared with Rh-123 at almost the same ratio as their photosensitizing abilities (117). This study (117) demonstrated that Rh-6G has greater potential than Rh-123 as a photosensitizer for PDT with the argon laser. However, Rh-6G alone had significantly higher toxic effects on the host compared with Rh-123. When choosing a laser dye candidate, a compromise between its efficiency as a photosensitizer for PDT and its systemic toxicity to the host may have to be determined.

An ideal sensitizer should not be oxidized or inactivated when exposed to light, and its redox properties should be compatible with the biologic environment. The control of redox potentials can be an important consideration in dye design to the extent that biologic electron transfer can destroy the dye chromophore. An illustration of this is found in the reduction of chalcogenapyrylium (89) dyes by microorganisms; for example, *Escherichia coli* reduces the dye and permanently inactivates the chromophore of these dyes.

For maximum efficiency, the absorption wavelength of a laser dye also must match the laser's emission wavelength.

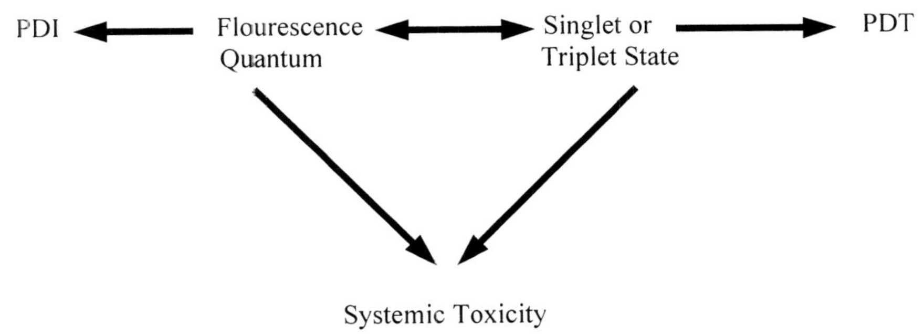


**FIGURE 36.11.** Laser dye: fluorescence quantum versus singlet staple versus system toxicity. *PDT,* photodynamic therapy; *PDI,* photodiagnostic imaging.

One example of this was seen with Rh-123, which has a peak absorption in cells at 516 nm (7,78–80,105–107), closely matching the argon laser emission wavelength at 514.5 nm. Hematoporphyrin derivatives show five major peaks of absorptions, all in the visible spectrum of light. The five peaks occur at 402, 507, 540, 573, and 624 nm (118). The least tissue penetration and the highest hematoporphyrin derivative absorption are at 402 nm, and the greatest tissue penetration and least absorption occur at 624 nm. An argon-pumped dye laser that emits at 630 nm is used to activate hematoporphyrin derivatives for the treatment of malignant lesions. The Nd:YAG laser (1,060 nm) is used to excite Kodak Q-switch II dye (1,051 nm) *in vitro* (7). Mercocyanine-540 demonstrates two absorption peaks at 502 and 532 nm, which could match the laser wavelengths of the potassium-titanyl-phosphate (KTP) laser (KTP-532) or the doubled frequency of the Nd:YAG laser (532 nm). Chalcogenapyrylium dyes are a group of new compounds (89) with various absorption maxima between 750 and 875 nm. These dyes should be compatible with commercially available gallium arsenide lasers.

The fifth requirement of a candidate laser dye is that the dye should have no toxicity or minimal morbidity to the host at therapeutic levels and be rapidly metabolized to minimize potential side effects. The major side effect of hematoporphyrin derivatives is long-term cutaneous phototoxicity observed for more than 6 weeks after injection with the dye (101). The long retention of [$^{14}C$]-Photofrin II of up to 75 days after injection in multiple organs of animals tested provides a likely explanation of this side effect (101).

Preclinical studies with Rh-123 (103,118) have demonstrated no toxicity in several animal species at therapeutic dose levels. The pharmacokinetics of Rh-123 tested in rabbits (103) and nude mice have shown rapid biodistribution of the dye in normal organs, with very efficient elimination through the kidneys and no residual dye 7 days after injection. Because Rh-123 is rapidly metabolized from normal tissues, the potential side effects and morbidity with this dye can be minimized.

## Future Directions with Photosensitizers

The field of PDT with dyes and lasers for the treatment of cancer may become clinically useful only after performing extensive drug screening, similar to antibiotic therapy for infectious diseases. There is no single effective antibiotic for all infectious processes, and by analogy, there may not be one effective dye for all malignancies. Most likely, many dyes, each with a specific affinity for various histologic types of cancer, will be required. For example, Rh-123 appears to have promising effects as a photosensitizer for argon laser treatment of squamous cell carcinomas, melanomas, adenocarcinomas, leukemia, and lymphomas cell lines but has a poor response in mesotheliomas and sarcomas cell lines (119). Mercocyanine-540 is extremely efficient in leukemias, lymphomas, and neuroblastomas, but it has poor uptake in lung and ovarian carcinomas (120).

With the collaboration of clinicians, chemists, biologists, and photochemists, laser dyes may be designed in the laboratory and then tested clinically. Laser dyes with the higher affinity to various neoplasms, rapid metabolism, and lower systemic toxicity can then be developed. Laser dyes with synergistic or antagonistic effects (or both) on various neoplasms may be found, and optimal fluorochromes for PDT and photodiagnostic imaging with lasers can then be classified. The chalcogenapyrylium dyes are a good example of a dye design system because their absorption wavelength maxima, fluorescence versus singlet yields, redox properties, and aqueous stability can be modified by changing different chalcogen atoms and substituents in the dye chromophore.

## Current Concepts of Photodynamic Therapy

Few concepts used currently in the field of PDT with lasers and dyes need to be modified in the future for successful clinical application. For example, the idea of the biologic window, which was introduced years ago, is based on the observation that a wavelength in the electromagnetic spectrum between 600 and 900 nm provides a window where light has the "deepest" tissue penetration abilities (121). In this range of wavelengths, an external laser beam can affect maximum tissue destruction to only 10 to 20 mm deep. Unfortunately, when clinically treating most recurrent tumors with external laser therapy, a 10- to 20-mm tissue destruction limit is not sufficient. Because laser wavelengths lack the ability to penetrate body tissues as effectively as x-rays, gamma rays, or neutron rays, the depth of tissue penetration of laser energy is the critical limiting factor.

It should, however, be possible to direct laser energy into tissues based on the concept of ILT, which through fiberoptics allows laser energy to be delivered directly into deeper tissues. The major advantage of ILT is that this energy can be delivered to any volume of tissue at any depth. The major drawbacks of ILT result from an absence of efficient laser delivery systems and the need for improved monitoring techniques to direct the interstitial laser beam.

## Preliminary Conclusions

A new approach for cancer diagnosis and therapy (PDT) may be developed using lasers and dyes. As with antibiotic therapy, tumor cultures may be initiated in laboratories and then tested for sensitivity to multiple photosensitizers and laser wavelengths. The optimal tumoricidal effects of laser-dye combinations for a specific tumor may be defined and then applied clinically.

With collaboration between photochemists, physicists, tumor biologists, engineers, and clinicians, many different photosensitizers and new laser wavelengths will be developed. This may result in more specific dye uptake by tumors, longer retention, lower systemic toxicity, and deeper tissue penetration, and it could lead to identification of new dyes with synergistic effects, enhancing the tumoricidal effect of lasers.

The rapid technologic revolution of MRI, laser fiberoptics, and MR-compatible needle probes will allow tumor destruction and real-time monitoring of interstitial laser phototherapy for the treatment of large and deep tumors using dyes and lasers in a wide range of the electromagnetic spectrum. PDT is still in the early clinical phases of investigation, and its usefulness and practicality must still be defined. FDA approval of any new laser dyes for PDT may be years away.

## LASER PHOTOCHEMOTHERAPY

The search for a clinically practical adjunctive technique allowing effective treatment of head and neck cancers as well as other tumors has led to the development of laser photochemotherapy. Photochemotherapy uses FDA-approved chemotherapeutic drugs that are first injected into tumors at concentrations lower than the normal treatment dose, reducing systemic effects. The "sensitized" tumor is then activated by laser photo-oxidation or photothermal levels of energies using monochromatic light that is delivered through external or interstitial fiberoptics to enhance the *killing threshold.*

### Historical Perspectives

Adriamycin and other anthracycline antibiotics, derived from organisms of the genus *Streptomyces*, continue to be the most active anticancer agents in the treatment of carcinomas, sarcomas, lymphomas, and acute leukemia (118). Chemically, the anthracyclines are composed of a tetracycline ring structure with an attached aminosugar moiety (122). The most common drugs available are doxorubicin (Adriamycin), daunorubicin (daunomycin, Cerubidine), and idarubicin (Idamycin). Anthracyclines have the ability to bind directly to DNA and RNA, but they also block topoisomerase enzymes during DNA replication and interfere with numerous other biologic activities through mechanisms that occur at the cell membrane or other intracellular sites (123). Carmichael and colleagues (124) and Li and Chignell (125) first raised the possibility of using chemotherapeutic drugs to photosensitize tumors, because many are chromophoric and absorb light at specific wavelengths of the visible spectrum, leading to energy transfer to oxygen species. Andreoni's group (9,126), Saxton and colleagues (17), Edell and Cortese (13), and Nahabedian and coworkers (14) demonstrated the enhanced phototoxic efficiency of anthracyclines using *in vitro* cell cultures after light illumination. The absorption maxima of Adriamycin and daunomycin is 493 nm (17), a blue light wavelength that corresponds closely to the 488 nm argon laser emission peak, making this laser ideal for photoactivation of these anticancer drugs. Despite the usefulness of these anthracycline antibiotics in treating a spectrum of different types of human cancer, common high-dose systemic side effects such as nausea, vomiting, myelosuppression, mucositis, alopecia, and cardiotoxicity (122) are seen at therapeutic levels. The risk of cardiac injury in cancer patients increases in frequency at cumulative doses of anthracyclines in excess of 450 to 550 mg/m (2,76,122).

Attempts to reduce cardiotoxicity of anthracyclines has led to the development of a variety of derivatives, including anthrapyrazoles such as DUP-941, possessing lower toxicity and greater clinical efficacy against breast cancer and other carcinomas (126,127). One unexpected additional property of these anthrapyrazoles is a more than 100-fold increased photo-oxidation efficiency compared with Adriamycin or daunomycin, as reported by Reszka and associates (18). Other anthracyclines have also been identified that exhibit greater photosensitizing potential and less cardiotoxicity than Adriamycin or daunomycin. Although some photochemical studies and limited *in vitro* testing of several of these Adriamycin-related agents have been reported (1,2,14,128–131), few have been evaluated so far for chemophototherapy of any human solid tumor in preclinical or clinical investigations.

Another important advantage of anthracyclines is their simultaneous role as antitumor drugs and as potential photosensitizers. Because they are effective chemotherapy agents without photoactivation, different approaches are possible to increase tumor responses. First, they can be used at maximum tolerated systemic dose, followed by intratumoral photoillumination through laser fiberoptics to obtain improved tumor palliation with minimal invasiveness. Second, improved tumor response to anthracyclines at lower dosages may be seen in tumors after laser activation compared with single-modality, high-dose systemic chemotherapy, reducing cardiotoxicity.

Lasers also can be used for thermal activation of cisplatin (*cis*-diamminedichloroplatinum) (11). Cisplatin cytotoxicity is caused by a reaction of the platinum molecule with nucleophilic sites on the DNA (132,133). Hyperthermia has been reported to enhance the cytotoxicity of various anticancer drugs, including bleomycin (134), mitomycin (135), Adriamycin (136), and cisplatin (137–140). Moreover, hyperthermia has been reported to overcome cisplatin drug resistance, which is a common cause of chemotherapy failure (140,141). Hyperthermic enhancement of tumoricidal treatment effects of cisplatin *in vitro* (135,142) and *in vivo* (137,142) has generated interest in laser chemotherapy for the treatment of malignancy. Cisplatin has been effective for patients with solid tumors, but nephrotoxicity is a major complication (143). Local hyperthermia in combination with chemotherapy (i.e., cisplatin or bleomycin) and irradiation for the treatment of patients with esophageal cancer was reported (144–147). The 2-year survival rate of patients with incompletely resected esophageal cancer was increased from 15.6% to 34.3% when local hyperthermia was added (144).

## Experimental Approach with Photochemotherapy

An alternative approach that couples standard light or heat-sensitive chemotherapeutic drugs with laser surgery was explored as a new method for improved tumor palliation. Nd:YAG laser endoscopy often is an effective treatment for obstructive tumors in airways (148) but MR-guided interstitial laser fiberoptics promises to become a more precise minimally invasive approach for treatment of unresectable head and neck malignancies (60,149–151). A number of studies have shown that anthracyclines can be activated by heat or light for increased tumoricidal effects (16,17,152).

Substantial data (16,153) indicate that cell membranes, not DNA, are the major targets for photoactivation of daunomycin in intact cells. Daunomycin and Adriamycin have similar patterns of intranuclear concentration after prolonged uptake (154,155) but completely different cytoplasmic distribution after initial exposure to tumor cells. After 2 hours' uptake, daunomycin had high cytoplasmic and low nuclear concentrations (156). This pattern suggests rapid intracellular distribution of daunomycin in membrane sites, leading to laser-activated lipid peroxidation and consequently a high effectiveness of daunomycin as a photosensitizer.

After short-term incubation of daunomycin with human carcinoma cells, the results show nonthermal laser photoactivation is highly effective when the drug is in the cytoplasm (157). Although daunomycin dark cytotoxicity was increased 10-fold after 24 hours of drug uptake, the level of tumor cell killing at low drug concentrations was improved significantly by light exposure. It might be expected that, with long-term incubation and nuclear uptake, daunomycin would potentiate laser effects by inducing DNA photo-oxidation, but significant photoenhancement seen only for low drug concentrations of 1 and 2 μg/mL. At higher daunomycin concentrations, laser light did not potentiate further cell killing (157,158).

Andreoni (9) reported that singlet oxygen was not the sole agent responsible for cell death after daunomycin exposure. Photochemical generation of many oxygen radical species (124,125,159) occurs with photobinding to DNA (160,161) and to cell surface proteins (29). Anthracyclines may be poor type II photosensitizers and do not generate significant amounts of singlet oxygen (40).

Data show the time at which the cells are illuminated during incubation with daunomycin determines the level of photocytotoxicity and suggests a correlation with drug distribution in the tumor cell (16,17,157). The contribution of membrane versus nuclear localization in daunomycin chemotherapy still needs to be clearly distinguished. In agreement with other studies (156), we observed a greater phototherapy response to daunomycin after incubation with human carcinoma cells, suggesting that laser activation is highly efficient when the drug remains in the cytoplasm. However, daunomycin cytotoxicity in the absence of light was much higher after 24 hours of drug uptake than at 2 hours (Fig. 36.12). It appears that photoactivation after long-term daunomycin incubation does potentiate the toxic effects of nuclear update, but this is significant only at lower daunomycin concentrations (1 and 2 μg/mL).

Photoactivation of some daunomycin analogues indicate red-shifted absorption spectra. Uptake of these antitumor drugs before laser photoactivation *in vivo* also may improve tumor killing, because tissue light penetration increases at with the higher wavelengths from blue to red (156). Three different light sources were compared for daunomycin photoactivation of tumor cells: a xenon lamp (300 to 900 nm), an argon laser (488 to 514 nm), and a KTP-532 (532 nm) laser. The results show longer wavelengths of light are more effective for drug activation and exhibit improved tissue transmission, indicating a need for further clinical studies with daunomycin and lasers (157,158,162). Laser light delivery through fiberoptics for *in situ* treatment of drug-sensitized tumors should lead to more effective and less invasive surgical procedures and to lower toxicity compared with systemic chemotherapy. However, the *in vivo* studies with daunomycin injections and laser treatment did not demonstrate any tumor regression, even at concentrations up to 10 μg/g of tumor weight. Future studies will increase the drug concentrations of daunomycin and time of laser treatment.

Other promising drugs for laser chemotherapy are the anthrapyrazoles, which exhibit significant clinical responses

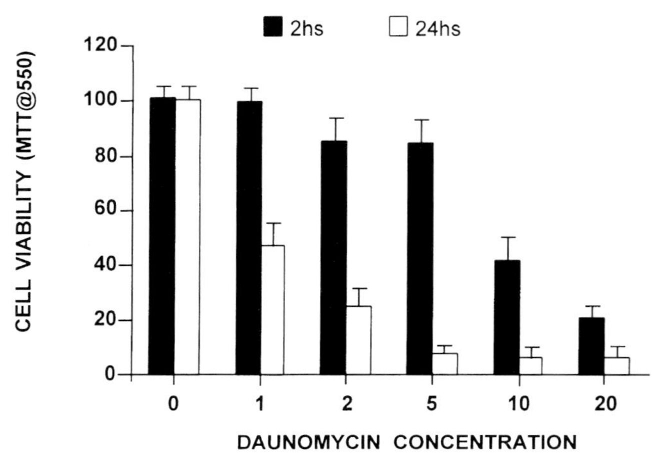


**FIGURE 36.12.** Viability of P3 squamous cell carcinoma cells incubated for 2 and 24 hours with different daunomycin concentrations as measured by the MTT assay.

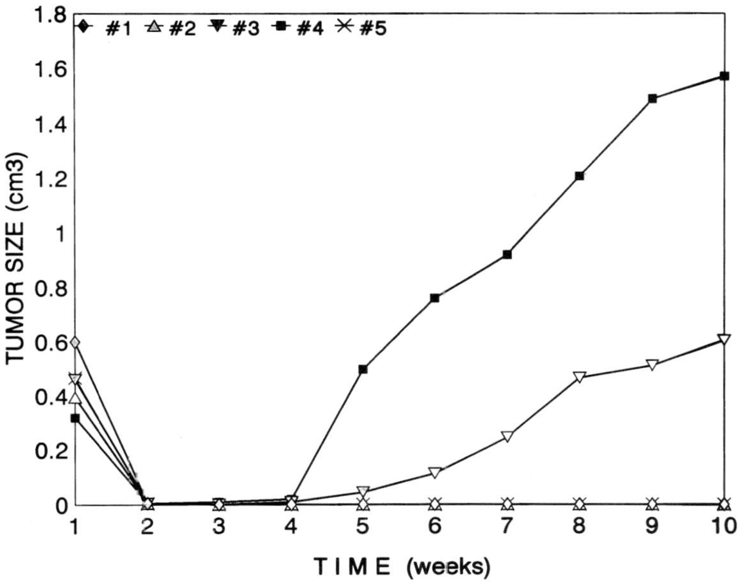


**FIGURE 36.13.** Treatment response after interstitial fiberoptic KTP laser therapy of P3 tumor transplants with 27 J/cm² per site (10 seconds at 0.8 W; average, 60 sites).

in patients with lymphoma and advanced breast cancer (121,163). Because the anthrapyrazole DUP-941 has reduced cardiotoxicity compared with Adriamycin and daunomycin as a chemotherapy agent, tumor dosage can be increased during systemic treatment. Studies by Reszka and colleagues (164) showed that anthrapyrazoles are very strong photosensitizers. Studies by Wallner (140), Alberts (137), and Overgaard (142) demonstrated the enhancement effects of cisplatin *in vitro* and *in vivo* with hyperthermia. This served as a rationale for current studies to evaluate DUP-941 and cisplatin after intratumoral injections as light- or heat-sensitive drugs for interstitial laser activation (162,165,166).

*In vivo* tumor transplantations first were performed to observe the tumor growth rate in the absence of treatment. Using human carcinoma transplants in mice, a technique for tumor palliation was developed using interstitial implantation with a 0.6 μm fiberoptic coupled to a KTP-532 laser (162,165,166) (Fig. 36.13). After establishing the laser energy threshold for optimal treatment (13.5 J/cm² per site), the energy level was lowered by one half to ensure that laser alone did not induce complete tumor regression (Fig. 36.14). Tumors were then pretreated with DUP-941 or cisplatin (Fig. 36.15) before applying reduced laser energy laser levels (13.4 J/cm² per site) to define the opti-

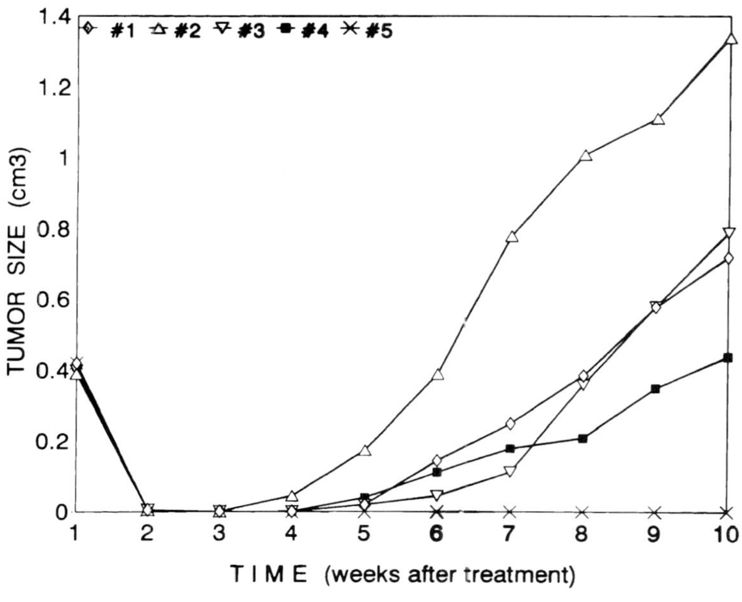


**FIGURE 36.14.** Treatment response after interstitial fiberoptic KTP laser therapy of P3 tumor transplants with 13.5 J/cm² per site (5 seconds at 0.8 W; average, 60 sites).

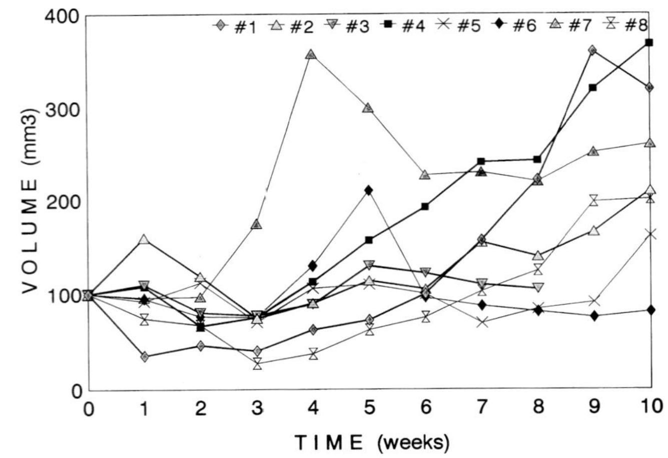


**FIGURE 36.15.** Growth curve of P3 squamous carcinoma tumors after cisplatin injections (3 mg/mL).

mal level of drug injections before laser treatment. The results suggest that a combination of intratumoral drug delivery and laser treatment can improve tumor response (158,166,167) (Fig. 36.16).

One advantage of intralesional drug injections compared with systemic chemotherapy is higher intratumoral levels of drug (168). The limitations on systemic chemotherapy for solid tumors include central necrosis (i.e., avascular area) and high pressure in the interstitial matrix. These factors impede vascular delivery and intratumoral distribution of standard chemotherapy drugs and photosensitizers. Using interstitial drug injections with a total volume of only 5% of the tumor mass allowed us to avoid reflux (169) and increase the pressure at the core of the tumor relative to the

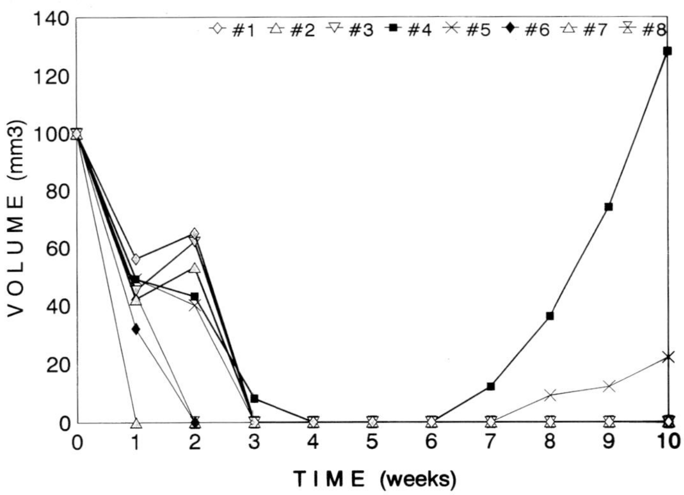


**FIGURE 36.16.** Response of P3 squamous carcinoma tumors after cisplatin injections (3 μg/g of tumor) and interstitial KTP laser therapy (13.5 J/cm$^2$ per site, 0.8 W, 5 seconds).

surrounding tumor tissue, ensuring drug diffusion from the avascular core to the periphery for more effective chemotherapy.

Because external laser light illumination is possible only for superficial malignancies, a tumor larger than a few millimeters thick is a candidate for interstitial treatment. Because light penetration in tissues decrease rapidly with increasing distance from an implanted fiberoptic, effective photochemical activation is limited to approximately 5 to 10 mm (14). Greater penetration depths can be accomplished using higher light energy levels, but the increased photothermal ablation results from thermal effects rather than a photoactivation (13). ILT also is more effective for photoablation of deep solid tumors and for treatment of metastatic masses with fibrosis and hypertrophic postoperative scars.

With the KTP laser or Nd:YAG bare fibers, it was possible to deliver reproducible energy dosages to the tumor xenografts (158,162,165–167,170). Multiple, low-energy interstitial fiber implantation also may overcome the commonly observed problem of tissue carbonization and charring of the fiberoptics, which reduces light delivery to tumors. Although a laser bare fiber may not be the ideal model for interstitial treatment compared with a diffuser tip that produces a uniformly dispersed emission of light at lower power density without carbonization, the low-energy bare fiber used in the current study was effective as a preliminary design to future studies with sapphire tips (171,172). We selected a bare 0.6 μm fiberoptic as the KTP delivery system to emulate our clinical interstitial treatment with a 600-μm flexible Nd:YAG laser fiberoptic cable. The fiber is passed through a 16-gauge Angiocath needle implanted percutaneously into the tumor mass (149,173).

Because the heat delivery is unavoidable during laser treatment of the tumors, it was not possible to separate photoactivation from hyperthermia in the study using tumor model systems (171,172). It is possible that DUP-941 and cisplatin act as thermal sensitizers similar to Adriamycin or a photosensitizer as indicated from *in vitro* experiments. Drug photoactivation, lipid peroxidation (164), or generation of oxyradicals (18), in addition to thermal effects, may contribute to the tumor response seen after DUP-941 or cisplatin injection and laser treatment. Previous studies have reported that some anticancer drugs are more effective when administered in combination with hyperthermia. The biologic aspects of thermochemotherapy have been studied rigorously by Hahn (174). Thermochemotherapy using a combination of hyperthermia and anticancer drugs has been tested in preclinical and clinical applications but is not as widely accepted as thermoradiotherapy (175). However, interest increased in thermochemotherapy (38) with the clinical response to Adriamycin and thermal enhancement reported by Matsuda (176).

For recurrent or persistent head and neck tumors after surgery, irradiation and chemotherapy are the treatment choices for one third to one half of these patients, but both methods carry a poor prognosis. The options for active palliative care are usually limited, based largely on supportive measures to control pain and improve functions such as respiration, swallowing, and speech. Ultrasound-guided ILT is a promising, cost-effective, and safe clinical approach for palliation of recurrent head and neck carcinomas. It is a minimally invasive technique that uses flexible laser delivery system to thermally ablate tumors with minimal damage to adjacent normal tissues. However, 40% tumor regrowth is observed when the laser alone is used as a source of energy.

PDT with lasers using photosensitizers such as hematoporphyrin derivatives (1,2), merocyanine-540 (MC-540), and Rh-123 (4–10) is an adjunctive treatment modality that is being evaluated in multiple preclinical and clinical trials, with encouraging results. This technique is simple, produces low morbidity, can be performed on an outpatient basis, and may be repeated as needed based on the anatomic site. However, because none of these laser dyes is FDA approved, clinical applications of PDT may be years away. Photochemotherapy with lasers is an alternative that consists of using a local source of monochromatic light to enhance the killing threshold of tumors previously sensitized with conventional chemotherapeutic drugs. Preclinical studies suggest intratumoral drug injections of DUP-941 and cisplatin allow better drug diffusion and act with photothermal interstitial laser treatment for enhanced tumor response with minimal systemic toxicity. Interstitial treatment provides more light delivery and improves drug potential in the tumor. Further studies are needed to confirm the effectiveness of this new approach to achieve local tumor control. Because these intratumoral chemotherapeutic drugs and laser treatment procedures can be used in patients with a lower likelihood of systemic or local toxicity and the possibility of improved therapeutic response, this approach of photochemotherapy with lasers should be tested in the clinic in the near future.

## REFERENCES


1. Robbins KT. Far advanced head and neck cancer. In: Gates GA, ed. *Current therapy in otolaryngology–head and neck surgery*. New York: BC Decker, 1990:251–253.
2. McQuarrie DG. Management of recurrent uncontrolled head and neck cancer. In: McQuarrie DG, Adams GL, Shons AR, eds. *Head and neck cancer: clinical decision and management principles*. Chicago: Year Book Medical Publishers, 1986: 477–484.
3. Schweitzer VG. Photodynamic therapy for treatment of head and neck cancer. *Otolaryngol Head Neck Surg* 1990;102: 225–232.
4. Feyh J, Goetz A, Muller W, et al. Photodynamic therapy in head and neck surgery. *J Photochem Photobiol* 1990;7:353–358.
5. Dougherty TJ, Kaufman JE, Goldfarb A, et al. Photoradiation therapy for the treatment of malignant tumors. *Cancer Res* 1985;38:2628–2635.
6. Delaney TF, Glatstein E. Photodynamic therapy of cancer. *Comp Ther* 1988;14:43–55.
7. Castro DJ, Saxton RE, Fetterman H, Ward PH. Rhodamine-123 as a new photochemosensitizing agent with the argon laser: "nonthermal" and thermal effects on human squamous carcinoma cells in vitro. *Laryngoscope* 1987;97:554–561.
8. Lipshutz GS, Saxton RE, Haughland RP, et al. Evaluation of four new carbocyanine dyes for photodynamic therapy with lasers. *Laryngoscope* 1994;104:996–1002.
9. Andreoni A, Colasanti A, Malatesta V, et al. Enhancement of antitumor drug cytotoxicity via laser photoactivation. *Photochem Photobiol* 1991;53:797–805.
10. Castro DJ, Soudant J, Saxton RE. The use of photodynamic therapy and photochemotherapy with lasers for palliative treatment of head and neck carcinomas: an initial human case report. *J Clin Laser Med Surg* 1992;10:367–371.
11. Myers CE. Anthracyclines. In: Chabner B, ed. *Pharmacologic principles of cancer treatment*. Philadelphia: WB Saunders, 1982: 416–434.
12. Yee G, Carey M, Tritton TR. Photoaffinity labeling of the sarcoma 180 cell surface by daunomycin. *Cancer Res* 1984;44: 1898–1903.
13. Edell ES, Cortese DA. Combined effects of hematoporphyrin derivative phototherapy and Adriamycin in a murine tumor mode. *Lasers Surg Med* 1988;8:413–417.
14. Nahabedian MY, Cohen RA, Contino MF, et al. Combination cytotoxic chemotherapy with cisplatin or doxorubicin and photodynamic therapy of murine tumors. *J Natl Cancer Inst* 1988; 80:739–743.
15. Hartley JA, Forrow SM, Souhami RL, et al. Photosensitization of human leukemia cells by anthracenedione antitumor agents. *Cancer Res* 1990;50:1936–1940.
16. Andreoni A, Colasanti A, Kisslinger A, et al. Enhanced response to daunomycin of normal tumor and metastatic rat cell lines via drug photoactivation. *Photochem Photobiol* 1993;57:851–855.
17. Saxton RE, Huang M, Plante D, et al. Laser and daunomycin chemotherapy of human carcinoma cells. *J Clin Laser Med Surg* 1992;10:331–336.
18. Reszka K, Lown JW, Chignell CF. Photosensitization by anticancer agents—10. Ortho-semiquinone and superoxide radicals produced during anthrapyrazole-sensitized oxidation of catechols. *Photochem Photobiol* 1992;55:359–366.
19. Burris HA 3rd, Vogel CL, Castro DJ, et al. Intratumoral cisplatin/epinephrine injectable gel as a palliative treatment for accessible solid tumors: a multicenter pilot study. *Otolaryngol Head Neck Surg* 1998;118:496–503.
20. Minton J, Ketcham A. The laser, a unique oncolytic entity. *Am J Surg* 1964;198:845–848.
21. Minton J, Ketcham A, Dearman J, et al. The application of pulsed, high energy laser radiation to multiple infra-abdominal tumor implants in experimental animals. *Surgery* 1965;58: 12–21.
22. Minton J, Ketcham A, Dearman J, et al. The effect of Nd:YAG laser radiation on two experimental malignant tumor systems. *Surg Gynecol Obstet* 1965;122:481–487.
23. Minton JP. A correlation of the laser wavelength absorption capabilities of experimental and human tumors. *Cancer* 1966; 19:266–272.
24. Ketcham A, Hoye R, Riggle G. A surgeon's appraisal of the laser. *Surg Clin North Am* 1967;47:1249–1253.
25. Goldman L, Wilson RC. Treatment of basal cell epithelioma by laser radiation. *JAMA* 1964;18:773–775.
26. Goldman L. The laser in skin cancer. *Int Adv Surg Oncol* 1978; 1:217–226.

27. Swain C, Brown SG, Edwards J, et al. Laser recanalization of obstructing foregut cancer. *Br J Surg* 1984;71:112–115.
28. Richey D, Dixon J. Ablation of atypical mucosa and recurrent polyps by endoscopic application of laser. *Gastrointest Endosc* 1981;27:224–228.
29. Imaoka W, Okuda J, Idak K. Treatment of digestive tract tumors with laser endoscopy. In: Atsumi K, Nimaskul N, eds. *Laser.* Tokyo: Intergroup, 1981.
30. Iwasaki M, Sasako M, Konishi T. Clinical applications of the Nd:YAG laser. In: Atsumi K, Nimaskul N, eds. *Laser.* Tokyo: Intergroup, 1981.
31. Hofstetter A, Frank F. A new laser endoscopy for treatment of bladder tumors. *Fortschr Med* 1979;97:6–10.
32. Shapshay SM, Davis RK, Vaughan CW, et al. Palliation of airway obstruction from tracheobronchial malignancy: use of the $CO_2$ laser bronchoscope. *Otolaryngol Head Neck Surg* 1983;91: 615–619.
33. Shapshay SM, Strong MS. Tracheobronchial obstruction from metastatic distant malignancies. *Ann Otol Rhinol Laryngol* 1982;91:648–651.
34. Shapshay SM, Dumon JF, Beamis JR Jr. Endoscopic treatment of tracheobronchial malignancy: experience with the Nd:YAG and $CO_2$ lasers in 506 operations. *Otolaryngol Head Neck Surg* 1985;93:205–210.
35. Toty L, Personne C, Colchen A, et al. Bronchoscopic management of tracheal lesions using the Nd:YAG laser. *Thorax* 1981; 36:175–178.
36. Dumon JR, Reboud E, Garbe L, et al. Treatment of tracheobronchial lesions by laser photoresection. *Chest* 1982;81: 278–284.
37. Brunctaud JM, Houche P, Delmotle JS. Laser in digestive endoscopy. In: Atsumi K, Nimaskul N, eds. *Laser.* Tokyo: Intergroup, 1981.
38. Carpenter RJ, Neel BH III, Sanderson DR. Comparison of endoscopic cryosurgery and electrocoagulation of bronchi. *Trans Am Ophthalmol Soc* 1977;84:313–323.
39. Fleisher DE, Haye C, Kessler F. Endoscopic palliative therapy for esophageal carcinoma with Nd:YAG laser. *Gastrointest Endosc* 1982;28:151(abst).
40. Rontal M, Rontal E. Treatment of recurrent carcinoma at the base of the skull with carbon dioxide laser. *Laryngoscope* 1983; 93:1261–1265.
41. Cummins L, Nauenberg M. Thermal effects of laser radiation in biological tissue. *Biophys J* 1983;42:99–102.
42. Welch AJ. The thermal response of laser irradiated tissue. *IEEE J Quant Electron* 1984;20:1471–1484.
43. Dougherty TJ, et al. Photoradiation in the treatment of recurrent breast carcinoma. *J Natl Cancer Inst* 1979;62:231–237.
44. Svaasand LO, Boerslid T, Oeveraasen M. Thermal and optical properties of living tissue: application to laser-induced hyperthermia. *Lasers Surg Med* 1985;5:589–602.
45. Bown SG. Phototherapy to tumors. *World J Surg* 1983;7: 700–709.
46. Matthewson K, Barr H, Tralau C, et al. Low power interstitial Nd:YAG laser photocoagulation, studies in a transplantable fibrosarcoma. *Br J Surg* 1989;76:378–381.
47. Matthewson K, Barton T, Lewin MR, et al. Low power interstitial Nd:YAG laser photocoagulation in normal and neoplastic rat colon. *Gut* 1988;29:27–34.
48. Matthewson K, Coleridge-Smith P, O'Sullivan JP, et al. Biological effects of intrahepatic Nd:YAG laser photocoagulation in rats. *Gastroenterology* 1987;93:550–557.
49. Hashimoto D, et al. In depth radiation therapy by YAG laser for malignant tumors in the liver under ultrasonic imaging. *Gastroenterology* 1985;88:1663(abst).
50. Godlewski G, Rouy S, Pignodel C, et al. Deep localized Nd: YAG laser photocoagulation in liver using a new water cooled and echo-guided handpiece. *Laser Surg Med* 1988;8:501–509.
51. Godlewski G, et al. A new device for inducing deep localized vaporization in liver with the Nd:YAG laser. *Lasers Med Sci* 1988;3:111–117.
52. Daikuzono N, Joffe SN. Artificial sapphire probe for contact photocoagulation and tissue vaporization with the Nd:YAG laser. *Med Instrum* 1985;19:173–178.
53. Panjehpour M, Overholt MF, Milligan AJ, et al. Nd:YAG laser induced hyperthermia using a long frosted contact probe. *Lasers Surg Med* 1990;10:16–24.
54. Steger AC, Bown SG. Use of multiple fibre optic systems in the medical application of lasers. In: Katzir A, ed. Optical fibres in medicine, vol IV. Bellingham, WA: Proc SPIE, 1989:256–259.
55. Gatenby RA, Hammond ND, Brown DQ. Tumor therapy with hematoporphyrin derivative and lasers via a percutaneous fiberoptic technique: preclinical experiments. *Radiology* 1987; 163:167–171.
56. Gatenby RA, Hartz WH, Engstrom PF, et al. CT-guided laser therapy in resistant human tumors: phase I clinical trails. *Radiology* 1987;63:172–175.
57. Godlewski G, Bourgeois JM, Sambuc P, et al. Ultrasonic and histopathological correlations of deep focal hepatic lesions induced by stereotactic Nd:YAG laser applications. *Ultrasound Med Biol* 1988;14:287–291.
58. Dachman AH, et al. US-guided percutaneous laser ablation of liver in a chronic pig model. *Radiology* 1989;173:425(abst).
59. Steger AC, Lees WR, Walmsley K, et al. Interstitial laser hyperthermia: a new approach to local destruction of tumors. *Br Med J* 1989;299:362–365.
60. Anzai Y, Lufkin RB, Saxton RE, et al. Nd:YAG interstitial laser phototherapy guided by magnetic resonance imagine in an ex vivo model: dosimetry of laser-MR-tissue interaction. *Laryngoscope* 1991;101:755–760.
61. Lufkin RB. *MR handbook.* Chicago: Yearbook Publishers, 1990.
62. Duckwiler G, Lufkin RB, Teresi L, et al. Head and neck lesions: MR-guided aspiration biopsy. *Radiology* 1989;170: 519–522.
63. Jolesz FA, Bleier AR, Jakab P, et al. MR imaging of laser tissue interactions. *Radiology* 1988;168:249–253.
64. Bottomley PA, Foster TH, Argersinger RE, et al. A review of normal tissue hydrogen NMR relaxation times and relaxation mechanisms from 1–100 MHz: dependency on tissue type NMR frequency, temperature, species, excision and age. *Med Phys* 1984;11:425–448.
65. Barroilhet LE, Moran PR. Nuclear magnetic resonance (NMR) relaxation spectroscopy in tissues. *Med Phys* 1975;2:191–194.
66. Fung MB, et al. The state of water in biological systems as studied by proton and deuterium relaxation. *Biochem Biophys Acta* 1975;399:191–202.
67. Parker DL, Smith V, Sheldon P, et al. Temperature distribution measurements in two dimensional NMR imaging. *Med Phys* 1983;10:321–325.
68. Lewa CJ, Majewska Z. Temperature relationships of proton spin lattice relaxation time T1 in biological tissues. *Bull Cancer (Paris)* 1980;67:525–530.
69. Parker DL. Applications of NMR imaging in hyperthermia: an evaluation of the potential for localized tissue heating and noninvasive temperature monitoring. *IEEE Trans Biomed Eng* 1984; 31:161–167.
70. Tanaka H, Eno K, Kato H, et al. Possible application of noninvasive thermotherapy for hyperthermia using NMR. *Nippon Igaku Hoshasen Gakkai Zasshi* 1981;41:897–899.
71. Dickinson RJ, Hall AS, Hind AJ, et al. Measurement of changes in tissue temperature using MR imaging. *J Comput Assist Tomogr* 1986;10:468–472.

72. Knuttel B, Juretschke HP. Temperature measurements by nuclear magnetic resonance and its possible use as a means of *in vivo* noninvasive temperature measurement and for hyperthermia treatment assessment. *Recent Results Cancer Res* 1986;101: 109–118.
73. Castro DJ, Saxton RE, Layfield LJ, et al. Interstitial laser phototherapy assisted by magnetic resonance imaging: a new technique for monitoring laser tissue interaction. *Laryngoscope* 1990;100:541–547.
74. Robinson JD, et al. MRI guided laser phototherapy: initial experience. *Radiology (in press).*
75. Maiman TH. Stimulated optical radiation in ruby. *Nature* 1960;187:493–494.
76. Policard A. Etudes sur les aspects offerts par des tumeur experimentales examinee a la lumiere de Woods. *CR Soc Biol (Paris)* 1924;91:1423–1426.
77. Gregory RO, Goldman L. Application of photodynamic therapy in plastic surgery. *Lasers Surg Med* 1986;6:62–66.
78. Castro DJ, Saxton RE, Fetterman HR, Ward PH. The effects of argon lasers on human melanoma cells sensitized with rhodamine-123 in vitro. *Am J Otolaryngol* 1988;9:18–29.
79. Castro DJ, Saxton RE, Fetterman HR, Ward PH. Phototherapy with the argon laser on human melanoma cells "sensitized" with rhodamine-123: a new method for tumor growth inhibition. *Laryngoscope* 1988;98:369–376.
80. Castro DJ, Saxton RE, Fetterman HR, et al. Rhodamine-123 as a chemosensitizing agent for argon laser therapy: a new technique for treatment of superficial malignancies. *Arch Otolaryngol* 1987;113:1176–1182.
81. Castro DJ, Saxton RE, Fetterman HR, et al. Biostimulation of human carcinoma cells with the argon laser: a previously unreported potential iatrogenic effect on lasers. *Laryngoscope* 1987; 98:109–116.
82. Castro DJ, Saxton RE, Fetterman HR, et al. Biostimulative effects of Nd:YAG Q-switch dye on normal fibroblast cultures: study of a new chemosensitizing agent for the Nd:YAG laser. *Laryngoscope* 1987;97:1454–1459.
83. Johnson LV, Walsh L, Chen LB. Localization of mitochondria in living cells with rhodamine-123. *Proc Natl Acad Sci U S A* 1980;77:990–994.
84. James TW, Bowman R. Proliferation of mitochondria during the cell cycle of human cell line (HL-60). *J Cell Biol* 1981;89: 256–262.
85. Bernal SD, Shapiro HM, Chen LB. Monitoring the effect of anticancer drugs on L1210 cells by a mitochondrial probe, rhodamine-123. *Int J Cancer* 1982;30:219–224.
86. Evenson DP, Darzinkiewicz Z, Melamed MR. Simultaneous measurement by flow cytometry of sperm cell viability and mitochondrial membrane potential related to cell motility. *J Histochem Cytochem* 1982;30:279–285.
87. Clark MA, Shay J. Long-lived cytoplasmic factors that suppress adrenal steroidogenesis. *Proc Natl Acad Sci U S A* 1982;79: 1144–1151.
88. Morgan AR, Kreimer-Birnbaum M, Selman SH. Purpurins: improved photosensitizers for photodynamic therapy. New directions in photodynamic therapy. *Proc SPIE* 1987;847: 29–35.
89. Detty MR. Rational design of properties in chalcogenapyrylium dyes. New directions in photodynamic therapy. *Proc SPIE* 1987; 847:68–73.
90. Gulliya KA, Dowben RM. Effect of free radical quenchers on dye-mediated laser light induced photosensitization of leukemic cells: new directions in photodynamic therapy. *Proc SPIE* 1987; 847:163–165.
91. Ara G, Ohuoha D, Oseroff AR. Partial inhibition of glycolysis with 2-deoxy-D-glucose enhances EDKC mediated cellular photosensitization. New directions in photodynamic therapy. *Proc SPIE* 1987;847:201–204.
92. Segelman AB. Highly purified pheophorbide as a photosensitizer in human bladder carcinoma. New directions in photodynamic therapy. *Proc SPIE* 1987;847:205–208.
93. VanderWerf QM, Saxton RE, Chang A, et al. Hypericin: a new phototargeting agent for human cancer cells. *Laryngoscope* 1996;106:1–5.
94. VanderWerf Q, Castro DJ, Nguyen RD, et al. KTP laser and neutral red phototherapy of human squamous cell carcinoma. *Laryngoscope* 1997;107:316–320.
95. Javan A, Bennett WR Jr, Herriott DR. Population inversion and continuous optical maser oscillation in a gas discharge containing a HeNe mixture [Letter]. *Physiol Rev* 1961;6:106–110.
96. Johnson LF. Optical maser characteristics of rare-earth ions in crystals. *J Appl Physiol* 1961;34:897–909.
97. Bennett WR Jr, Faust WL, McFarlane RA, et al. Dissociative excitation transfer and optical maser oscillation in $NeO_2$ and $ArO_2$ rf discharges [Letter]. *Physiol Rev* 1962;8:470–473.
98. Patel CKL, McFarlane RA, Faust WL. Selective excitation through vibrational energy transfer and optical maser action in $N_2$-$CO_2$. *Physiol Rev* 1964;13:617–619.
99. Riesz P, Kaishna CM. Phthalocyanines and their sulfonated derivatives as photosensitizers in photodynamic therapy. New directions in photodynamic therapy. *Proc SPIE* 1987;847: 15–28.
100. Castro DJ, Saxton RE, Fetterman HR, et al. Bioinhibition of human fibroblast cultures sensitized to Q-switch II dye and treated with the Nd:YAG laser: a new technique of photodynamic therapy with lasers. *Laryngoscope* 1989;99:421–428.
101. Bellnier DA, Ho YK, Pandey RK, et al. Distribution and elimination of Photofrin II in mice. *Photochem Photobiol* 1989;50: 221–228.
102. Pantelides ML, Moore VJ, Blacklock NJ. A comparison of serum kinetics and tissue distribution of Photofrin II after intravenous and intraperitoneal injection in the mouse. *Photochem Photobiol* 1989;49:67–70.
103. Castro DJ, Gaskin A, Saxton RE, et al. Photodynamic therapy using rhodamine-123 as a new laser dye: biodistribution, metabolism, and histology in New Zealand rabbits. *Laryngoscope* 1991;101:158–164.
104. Castro DJ, Haghighat S, Saxton RE, et al. Biodistribution of rhodamine-123 in nude mice heterotransplanted with human carcinomas. *Laryngoscope* 1992;102:868–874.
105. Castro DJ, Saxton RE, Fetterman HR, et al. Rhodamine-123 as a new photochemosensitizing versus toxic agent on human squamous carcinoma cells and fibroblast cultures. *J Clin Laser Med Surg* 1992;10:83–90.
106. Castro DJ, Saxton RE, Fetterman HR, et al. Photodynamic therapy using the argon laser on human carcinoma cells sensitized with rhodamine-123: a study of tumor growth rate after heterotransplantation to nude mice. *Laryngoscope* 1987;97: 512(abst).
107. Castro DJ, Saxton RE, Fetterman HR, et al. Phototherapy with argon lasers and rhodamine-123 for tumor eradication. *Otolaryngol Head Neck Surg* 1988;98:581–588.
108. Sieber F. Merocyanine 540 yearly review. *Photochem Photobiol* 1987;46:1035–1042.
109. Atzpodien J, Gulati SC, Clarkson BD. Comparison of the cytotoxic effects of merocyanine-540 on leukemic cells and normal human bone marrow. *Cancer Res* 1986;46:4892–4895.
110. Musajo L, Bordin F, Caporale G, et al. Photoreactions at 3655 Angstrom between pyrimidine bases and skin-photosensitizing furocoumarins. *Photochem Photobiol* 1967;6: 711–714.
111. Kohn K, Kessel D. On the mode of cytotoxic action of pho-

toactivated porphyrins. *Biochem Pharmacol* 1979;28:2465–2470.
112. Gomer CJ. DNA damage and repair in CHO cells following hematoporphyrin photoradiation. *Cancer Lett* 1980;11:161–167.
113. Das M, Dixit R, Mukhtar H, et al. Role of active oxygen species in the photodestruction of microsomal P-450 and associated monooxygenases by hematoporphyrin derivatives in rats. *Cancer Res* 1985;45:608–615.
114. Santus R, Kohen C, Kohen E, et al. Permeation of lysosomal membranes in the course of photosensitization with methylene blue and hematoporphyrin: study by cellular microspectrofluorometry. *Photochem Photobiol* 1983;38:71–77.
115. Gibson SL, Hilf R. Photosensitization of mitochondrial cytochrome *c* oxidase by hematoporphyrin derivatives *in vitro* and in *vivo. Cancer Res* 1983;43:4191–4197.
116. Foote CS. Singlet oxygen. In: Wasserman HH, Murray RW, eds. New York: Academic Press, 1976:244–286.
117. Haghighat S, Saxton RE, Fetterman HR, et al. Laser dyes for experimental phototherapy of cancer cells: comparison of three rhodamines. *Laryngoscope* 1992;102:81–87.
118. Castro DJ, Saxton RE, Fetterman HR, et al. New concepts in photodynamic therapy with lasers. In: Fee W, Goepfert H, Johns ME, eds. *Head and neck cancers.* New York: BC Decker, 1989:400–408.
119. Sugita K, Giuliano AE, Sugita N, et al. Tumors of diverse therapy in *vitro. Am J Otolaryngol* 1990;11:1–7.
120. Osseroff A, Wan W, Wadwa KS, et al. Sensitive selection detection of carcinomas and melanomas using fluorescent cationic dyes. *Photochem Photobiol* 1990;51[Suppl]:745.
121. Hayata Y, Dougherty TJ. Lasers and hematoporphyrin derivative in cancer [Barron P, trans]. In: Hayata Y, Dougherty TJ, eds. *Cancer.* New York: Igaku-Shoin, 1982.
122. Carlson RW. Reducing the cardiotoxicity of the anthracyclines. *Oncology* 1992;6:95–104.
123. Sartorelli C. Adriamycin-induced changes in the surface membrane of sarcoma: 180 ascites cells. *Biochem Biophys Acta* 1981;649:317–324.
124. Carmichael RJ, Mossoba MM, Riesz P. Photogeneration of superoxide by Adriamycin and daunomycin: an electron spin resonance and spin trapping study. *FEBS Lett* 1983;164:401–405.
125. Li AS, Chignell CF. Spectroscopic studies of cutaneous photosensitizing agents. X. A spin-trapping and direct electron spin resonance study of the photochemical pathways of daunomycin and Adriamycin. *Photochem Photobiol* 1987;45:565–570.
126. Andreoni A, Colasanti A, Malatesta V, et al. Fluorescence of anthracyclines from cultured cells. *Phys Med* 1989;5[Suppl 1]:46–51.
127. Talbot DC, Smith IE, Manci JL, et al. Anthrapyrazole CI-941: a highly active new agent in the treatment of advanced breast cancer. *J Clin Oncol* 1991;9:2141–2147.
128. Foster BJ, Newell DR, Graham MA, et al. Phase I trial of the anthrapyrazole CI-941: prospective evaluation of a pharmacokinetically guided dose-escalation. *Eur J Cancer* 1992;28:463–469.
129. Breasted JH. *The Edwin Smith surgical papyrus*, vol. 1. Chicago: University of Chicago, 1930.
130. Gulliya KS, Bataglino M, Mathews JL. Breast cancer and laser photoradiation therapy: an in vitro model for autologous bone marrow purging. *Prog Clin Biol Res* 1990;333:103–107.
131. Andreoni A, Colasanti A, Malatesta V, Roberti G. Phototoxicity of anthracyclines on laser excitation in their long-wave absorption bands. *Radiat Res* 1991;127:8–13.
132. Meyn RE, Corry PM, Fletcher SE, Demetriades M. Thermal enhancement of DNA damage in mammalian cells treated with *cis*-diamminedichloroplatinum (II). *Cancer Res* 1980;40:1136–1139.
133. Terheggen PMAB, Dijkman R, Begg AC, et al. Monitoring of interaction products of *cis*-diamminedichloroplatinum (II) and *cis*-diammine (1,1-cyclobutane-dicarboxylato) platinum (II) with DNA in cells from platinum-treated patients. *Cancer Res* 1988;48:5597–5603.
134. Hahn GM. Potential for therapy of drugs and hyperthermia. *Cancer Res* 1979;39:2264–2268.
135. Wallner KE, Li GC. Effect of drug exposure duration and sequencing on hyperthermic potentiation of mitomycin-C and cisplatin. *Cancer Res* 1987;47:493–495.
136. Rice GC, Hahn GM. Modulation of Adriamycin transport by hyperthermia as measured by fluorescence-activated cell sorting. *Cancer Chemother Pharmacol* 1987;20:183–187.
137. Alberts DS, Peng YM, Chen HSG, et al. Therapeutic synergism of hyperthermia-cisplatin in a mouse tumor model. *J Natl Cancer Inst* 1980;65:455–461.
138. Baba H, Siddik ZH, Strebel FR, et al. Increased therapeutic gain of combined *cis*-diamminedichloroplatinum (II) and whole body hyperthermia by optimal heat/drug scheduling. *Cancer Res* 1989;49:7041–7044.
139. Los G, Sminia P, Wondergem J, et al. Optimisation of intraperitoneal cisplatin therapy with regional hyperthermia in rats. *Eur J Cancer* 1991;27:472–477.
140. Wallner KE, DeGeorge MW, Li GC. Hyperthermic potentiation of *cis*-diamminedichloroplatinum (II) cytotoxicity in Chinese hamster ovary cells resistant to the drug. *Cancer Res* 1986;46:6242–6245.
141. Herman TS, Teicher BA, Cathcart KNS, et al. Effect of hyperthermia on *cis*-diamminedichloroplatinum (II), (rhodamine-123)2[tetrachloroplatinum (II)] in a human squamous cell carcinoma line and a *cis*-diamminedichloroplatinum (II)-resistant subline. *Cancer Res* 1988;48:5101–5105.
142. Overgaard J, Radacic MM, Gran C. Interaction of hyperthermia and cis-diamminedichloroplatinum (II) alone or combined with radiation in a C3H mammary carcinoma *in vivo. Cancer Res* 1991;51:707–711.
143. Durant JR. Cisplatin: a clinical overview. In: Prestyko AV, Crooke ST, Carrier SK, eds. *Cisplatin: current status and new developments.* New York: Academic Press, 1980:317.
144. Matsufuji H, Kuwano H, Kai H, et al. Preoperative hyperthermia combined with radiotherapy and chemotherapy for patients with incompletely resected carcinoma of the esophagus. *Cancer* 1988;62:889–894.
145. Sugimachi K, Matsuda H, Ohno S, et al. Long term effects of hyperthermia combined with chemotherapy and irradiation for the treatment of patients with carcinoma of the esophagus. *Surg Gynecol Obstet* 1988;167:319–323.
146. Vokes EE, Weichselbaum RR, Lippman SM, Hong WK. Head and neck cancer: a review article. *N Engl J Med* 1993;328:184–194.
147. Peng Q, Moan J, Kongshaug M, et al. Sensitizer for photodynamic therapy of cancer: a comparison of the tissue distribution of Photofrin II and aluminum phthalocyanine tetrasulfonate in nude mice bearing a human malignant tumor. *Int J Cancer* 1991;48:258–264.
148. Castro DJ, Saxton RE, Ward PH, et al. Flexible Nd:YAG laser palliation of obstructive tracheal metastatic malignancies. *Laryngoscope* 1990;100:1028–1214.
149. Castro DJ, Saxton RE, Soudant J, et al. Minimally invasive palliative tumor therapy guided by imaging techniques: the UCLA experience. *J Clin Laser Med Surg* 1994;12:65–73.
150. Blackwell KE, Castro DJ, Saxton RE, et al. Real-time intraop-

erative ultrasonography as a monitoring technique for laser palliation of unresectable head and neck tumors: initial experience. *Laryngoscope* 1992;103:559–564.

151. Blackwell KE, Saxton RE, Nyerges A, et al. MRI and ultrasound guided interstitial Nd:YAG laser therapy for palliative treatment of advanced head and neck tumors: clinical experience. *J Clin Laser Med Surg* 1993;11:7–14.
152. Hahn G, Braun J, Har-Kedar I. Thermochemotherapy: synergism between hyperthermia (42–43°C) and Adriamycin (bleomycin) in mammalian cell inactivation. *Proc Natl Acad Sci U S A* 1975;72:937–940.
153. Gray PJ, Phillips DR. Ultraviolet photoirradiation of daunomycin and DNA-daunomycin complexes. *Photochem Photobiol* 1981;33:297–303.
154. Peterson C, Trouet A. Transport and storage of daunorubicin and doxorubicin in cultured fibroblasts. *Cancer Res* 1978;38: 4645–4649.
155. Noel G, Peterson C, Trouet A, Tulkens P. Uptake and subcellular localization of daunomycin and Adriamycin in cultured fibroblasts. *Eur J Cancer* 1978;14:363–368.
156. Andreoni A, Colasanti A, Malatesta V, et al. Cell photosensitization by 5-iminodaunomycin activated with red light. *Biochem Biophys Acta* 1989;1014:8–13.
157. Paiva MB, Saxton RE, St Letts GA, et al. Laser photochemotherapy with anthracyclines on cultured human squamous carcinoma cells. *Laryngoscope* 1996;106:257–262.
158. Paiva MB, Saxton RE, Graeber IP, et al. Improved photochemotherapy of malignant cells with daunomycin and the KTP laser. *Lasers Surg Med* 1998;23:33–39.
159. Gray P, Phillips DR, Wedd AG. Photosensitized degradation of DNA by daunomycin. *Photochem Photobiol* 1982;36:49–57.
160. Daugherty JP, Hixon SC, Yielding KL. Direct in vitro photoaffinity labelling of DNA with daunorubicin, adriamycin and rubidazone. *Biochim Biophys Acta* 1979;565:13–21.
161. Gray PJ, Phillips DR. Ultraviolet induced binding of daunomycin to DNA. *Photochem Photobiol* 1980;32:621–627.
162. Paiva MB, Saxton RE, St Letts GA, et al. Interstitial laser photochemotherapy with new anthrapyrazole drugs for the treatment of xenograft tumors. *J Clin Laser Med Surg* 1995;13:307–313.
163. Allan SG, Cummings J, Evans S, et al. Phase I study of the anthrapyrazole Biantrazole: clinical results and pharmacology. *Cancer Chemother Pharmacol* 1991;28:55–58.
164. Reszka K, Kolodziejczyk P, Lown JW. Photosensitization by antitumor agents, 3: spectroscopic evidence for superoxide and hydroxyl radical production by anthrapyrazole-sensitized oxidation of NADH. *J Free Radic Biol Med* 1986;2:267–274.
165. Saxton RE, Graeber IP, Suh MJ, et al. Interstitial laser and chemotherapy combined for treatment of human squamous cell carcinoma. *Proc SPIE* 1997;297:158–165.
166. Paiva MB, Saxton RE, VanderWerf QM, et al. Cisplatinum and interstitial laser therapy for advanced head and neck cancer: a preclinical study. *Lasers Surg Med* 1997;21:423–431.
167. Graeber IP, Paiva MB, Eshraghi AA, et al. Anthrapyrazoles and interstitial laser phototherapy for experimental treatment of squamous cell carcinoma. *Laryngoscope* 1998;108:351–357.
168. Wenzel M, Schneider M, Bier J, et al. Cytostatica-Konzentrationen in Organen and Tumoren: Vergleich nach intravenöser and intratumoraler Injektion. *J Cancer Res Oncol* 1979;95: 147–157.
169. Gutmann R, Leunig M, Feyh J, et al. Interstitial hypertension in head and neck tumors in patients: correlations with tumor size. *Cancer Res* 1992;52:1993–1995.
170. Paiva MB, Graeber IP, Castro DJ, et al. Laser and cisplatinum for treatment of human squamous cell carcinoma. *Laryngoscope* 1998;108:1269–1276.
171. Muschter R, Hofstetter A, Hessel S, et al. Hi-tech of the prostate: interstitial laser coagulation of benign prostatic hypertrophy. *SPIE Laser Surg* 1992;1643.
172. Mäkinen K, Nuutinen P, Eskelinen M, et al. Sapphire probe versus bare fiber in interstitial laser hyperthermia (ILH): an experimental study with Wistar rats. *Anticancer Res* 1994;14: 1023–1026.
173. Paiva MB, Blackwell KE, Saxton RE, et al. Palliative laser therapy for recurrent head and neck cancer: a phase II clinical study. *Laryngoscope* 1998;108:1277–1283.
174. Hahn GM. *Hyperthermia and cancer.* New York: Plenum Press, 1982:55–86.
175. Kakehi M, Ueda K, Mukojima T, et al. Multi-institutional clinical studies on hyperthermia combined with radiotherapy or chemotherapy in advanced cancer of deep-seated organ. *Int J Hyperthermia* 1990;6:719–740.
176. Matsuda T, Shinomaya T, Ohno T, et al. Local hyperthermia combined with chemotherapy for solid tumors: analysis of joint research conducted at a number of institutions in Japan. In: Matsuda T, ed. *Cancer treatment by hyperthermia, radiation and drugs.* Washington:Taylor & Francis, 1993:175–184.

# 37

# DIAGNOSTIC ENDOSCOPY OF THE UPPER AIRWAY FOR OBSTRUCTIVE SLEEP APNEA

B. TUCKER WOODSON

## INDICATIONS

Outcomes of pharyngeal surgery for obstructive sleep apnea (OSA) are frequently disappointing. Surgical decision making requires an accurate assessment and diagnosis of the sites of upper airway obstruction. Endoscopic assessment of the airway provides important information about airway size, shape, and collapsibility. Endoscopic evaluation is indicated in all patients who are candidates for pharyngeal surgeries. It identifies patients at risk for sleep apnea. Abnormal or dysmorphic anatomy may predict OSA. In surgical patients, evaluation identifies overt pathology, selects patients who are predicted to be good surgical candidates, and identifies all segments of obstruction that need to be treated. Pathology identified may include congenital abnormalities, enlarged lymphoid tissue, or other airway masses. Overt pathology is rare in adults. Other goals of airway examination are to select patients with a high likelihood for success from limited pharyngeal procedures. Historically, results for using the examination for this purpose have been disappointing. New data using endoscopy offer the promise of better outcomes. The greatest challenge lies in identifying and more aggressively treating multiple airway segments. Multiple segments may then be surgically corrected in single or multiple procedures.

## CONTRAINDICATIONS

Endoscopic evaluation is an office procedure that is performed using only topical anesthesia without sedation. Patients who refuse to cooperate with the examination are not candidates. Relative contraindications to the endoscopic technique are the inability to place the patient supine, severe nasal or septal obstruction (which prevents nasopharyngoscopy), or an absolute contraindication to surgery that would obviate the need for evaluation. A relative contraindication is an anxious patient who is unable to relax the upper airway muscles, which would confound results.

Endoscopy must not be interpreted in isolation. Structure alone does not determine the outcome. Severity of disease (i.e., apnea and hypopnea indexes), body mass index, and other variables can also predict outcome (1).

## BACKGROUND

OSA is a common disorder. In a middle-aged, employed Wisconsin cohort, the prevalence is estimated at 2% for females and 4% for males (2). The prevalence of sleep-disordered breathing (i.e., respiratory disturbance index value greater than 15 events/hour) has an even higher prevalence, ranging from 4% to 9%.

Tracheotomy was historically the initial treatment for OSA. Such morbid therapy is inappropriate in all but the most severely apneic patients. Tracheotomy has been replaced by less morbid therapies. The most widely accepted treatment is nasal continuous positive airway pressure (nasal CPAP). However, CPAP therapy requires nightly use, and compliance with therapy is problematic, particularly for patients with mild disease. Studies of objective compliance found only 48% of American patients use CPAP for 4 hours per night (3). A large population of patients remains insufficiently treated. The most common surgical alternative has been uvulopalatopharyngoplasty (UPPP). UPPP results are discouraging, with success rates of approximately 50% or less. Theoretically, higher success rates may be achieved by improving patient selection or with better surgical techniques. Unfortunately, attempts at selecting and operating only on those patients with a good chance of success have been disappointing (1).

The goal of surgery is to enlarge, stiffen, or alter the shape of the upper airway. Surgery is effective when airway size and stiffness are increased above the threshold of obstruction when muscle tone is lost episodically during sleep (4,5). Most pharyngeal surgical procedures are postulated to increase airway size and stiffness (6–8). Matching procedures and appropriate patients is the goal of evaluation. Airway assessment is the guide. A variety of examination techniques have been used. A common tool has been nasopharyngoscopy. Nasopharyngoscopic techniques vary. Some physicians use subjective measures during wakefulness, such as Mueller's maneuver (9,10). Others subjectively assess the airway during sleep (11). An objective endoscopic technique (12,13) improves prediction of surgical results and measures airway size (14–16). Understanding the rationale for the technique provides insight into its interpretation.

Historically, endoscopy has been a tool to predict UPPP outcomes. Reported success rates for UPPP range from 10% to 80%, and an average success rate of 40% is generally accepted (1). Using selection criteria to exclude tongue or lingual obstruction improves success rates to only 50% (1). Traditionally, endoscopy has been performed using subjective techniques. Mueller's maneuver is the most common technique described. With this technique, patients are evaluated in a sitting position, with the tip of the endoscope positioned at the level of the palate and then at the level of the tongue base. At each site, patients are asked to sniff against an occluded upper airway, and the percentage of collapse is estimated. When collapse at the retrolingual segment was estimated to be less than 25% (suggesting isolated retropalatal obstruction), UPPP success was reported to be as high as 70% (9). However, subsequent studies have not replicated these results, instead finding UPPP success rates of only 50% or less (10,17,18). An explanation for higher failure rates may be less stringent criteria used for excluding patients for UPPP (i.e., excluding patients only if they demonstrate 50% retrolingual collapse). Mueller's maneuver does predict UPPP failures if greater than 75% retrolingual collapse is observed (19). Only 11% of patients with this degree of collapse are UPPP responders. The interpretation of Mueller's maneuver is further complicated because studies demonstrate that obstruction using Mueller's maneuver does not correlate to manometric or endoscopically identified obstruction during sleep (20,21). As the application of multilevel surgeries increases, the utility of Mueller's maneuver is unknown. Studies demonstrated changes in Mueller's maneuver in the retropalatal segment correlated to changes in respiratory disturbance index. In this study, Mueller's maneuver did not correlate with other polysomnographic or airway measures (22).

A second endoscopic technique is sedated endoscopy. Sedated endoscopy attempts to identify obstruction and collapse during simulated conditions of sleep, when muscle tone is relaxed (11). With this technique, sedated sleep is induced, and the airway is observed. Sites of obstruction and collapse are then subjectively assessed. Because there is no consensus about what defines obstruction or collapse during sleep, interpretations vary among observers. Sedated endoscopy is further complicated because airway patency fluctuates during sleep because of changes in muscle tone, respiration, sleep state, and body position. Breath by breath variation may also change the interpretation of sedated endoscopy, even by individuals using the same criteria (23). Outcome data showing improved results are not yet available. Further studies with clinical outcomes with this method are needed.

The reasons for surgical failures are unknown. Dogma suggests that failure occurs because of lingual obstruction. However, data suggest that obstruction often persists at palatal and nonpalatal sites (24,25). Improved outcomes are demonstrated when multiple airway segments are treated (26–32). This is insufficient proof that multiple sites cause obstruction, because objective evaluation after mandibular advancement demonstrates that retroglossal and retropalatal segments are enlarged (31). Failures postulated as caused by poor methods of airway evaluation may instead be surgical technical failures. Ultimately, the only way to sort out these confounding results is to have better tools for upper airway evaluation.

Some of the objective research methods to evaluate the upper airway for OSA have included computed tomography (CT), magnetic resonance imaging, cephalometry, manometry, acoustic reflection, and endoscopy (12,32–36). Many methods have not been exported to the clinical environment because of high costs or complexity of use and interpretation. Physical examination, endoscopy, manometry, and cephalometric radiographs are accessible at a relatively low cost. Cephalometry is considered objective and provides skeletal and craniofacial data. It is confounded by the sitting position and its two-dimensional image. This compares with endoscopy, which may be performed while supine and gives area measurement. Multiple cross-sectional views of the pharynx may be combined to assess volume. Cephalometry and endoscopy complement each other to describe the upper airway.

## ENDOSCOPIC METHOD

### Physiology

The concept of the hypotonic endoscopic method is to estimate or measure airway size while controlling muscle tone and intraluminal airway pressures (37). Endoscopy using these methods is objective and shows promise in predicting surgical outcomes of UPPP (14,15). A similar office technique that minimizes muscle tone and physiologic variability, endoscopy has predicted apnea severity and cephalometric posterior airway space (16). The goal of this chapter is to describe the scientific rationale and method for a hypotonic endoscopic evaluation of the upper airway in OSA patients.

## Rationale

OSA results from abnormalities of upper airway structures, a sleep-related loss of muscle tone, and alterations in respiratory control. Contributions of each vary by individual. The single most important factor is that the upper airway is smaller in OSA patients than nonapneics (13,38). Upper airway size imaged with CT scanning and cephalometric radiography demonstrates a smaller than average airway space in the nasopharynx, oropharynx, and hypopharynx (39). It is the goal of surgery to improve airway size. Because size at any moment in waking individuals is the combination or sum of airway size and dilating muscle tone and because dilating muscle tone is increased during wakefulness in OSA patients and not in normal subjects, many methods of measurement underestimate differences between OSA and normal persons. Incorrect assessment hampers surgical decision making.

## Upper Airway Mechanics

The anatomic location of airway pathology in OSA is poorly understood and controversial. The airway may collapse in a narrow or wide segment (24,36). Initial manometric studies suggested that a discrete segment (often as narrow as 1 cm) collapsed occurred during an event. In a collapsible tube, manometric results may be misleading, because small segments of airway obstruction may shift distally or proximally as nearby segments are corrected (40). Simple manometry may mislead, because segments that are abnormal but not 100% obstructed may be missed (23).

A major obstacle to evaluation is that the upper airway is dynamic. At any moment, airway size, shape, and compliance are the end product of multiple variable forces. Forces are anatomic and physiologic. Anatomic and structural features probably are most important for surgical decision making. The *balance of forces model* first applied to OSA by Remmers allows separation and measurement of the anatomic and physiologic forces (41).

## Balance of Forces Model

Physiologic variability must be controlled to allow measurements of pharyngeal structure. The major variables that need to be controlled are state, fluctuating upper airway muscle tone (i.e., phasic inspiratory contraction and expiratory relaxation), negative inspiratory pressure, and airflow. Negative inspiratory pressures and the Bernoulli effect of nasal airflow change luminal pharyngeal pressures and contribute to airway collapse (37). A stable state can be produced by creating pharyngeal muscle hypotonia and measuring the airway at zero airflow. Muscle hypotonia is created using pressure support (i.e., nasal continuous positive airway pressure such as nasal CPAP) and benzodiazepam-induced sleep. Benzodiazepam-induced sleep reduces muscle tone and is physiologically similar to non–rapid eye movement (non-REM) sleep. This hypotonia persists even after an abrupt decrease in CPAP pressure, causing partial or complete obstruction. In addition to suppressing muscle tone, nasal CPAP can be modified to control airway size and collapse. Nasal CPAP dilates and "splints" the airway. This airway splint may be independently adjusted to dilate or to collapse the airway. If the examiner simultaneously measures airway size, objective measurements of airway size, compliance, and closing pressures are obtained. The most accessible method to measure the airway is endoscopic. The hypotonic method was initially applied to evaluate retropalatal mechanics of the airway (12). However, all pharyngeal airway segments of the pharynx have now been studied (42).

The hypotonic method is based on a physiologic description of airway patency referred to as the balance of forces model (Fig. 37.1). In this model, airway size is determined by the balance between dilating forces ($P_{out}$) and collapsing forces ($P_{in}$). When dilating forces of a structure are less than collapsing forces, airway size decreases. The resulting distending force determines the size of the structure. This distending force is the transmural pressure ($P_{tm} = P_{out} - P_{in}$). When $P_{tm}$ increases, the airway enlarges, and when $P_{tm}$ decreases, the airway becomes smaller.

Another method describing the airway defines the transmural pressure as the difference between luminal pressure and tissue pressure ($P_{tm} = P_L - P_{ti}$). Luminal pressure ($P_L$) can be directly measured in patients. Tissue pressure cannot

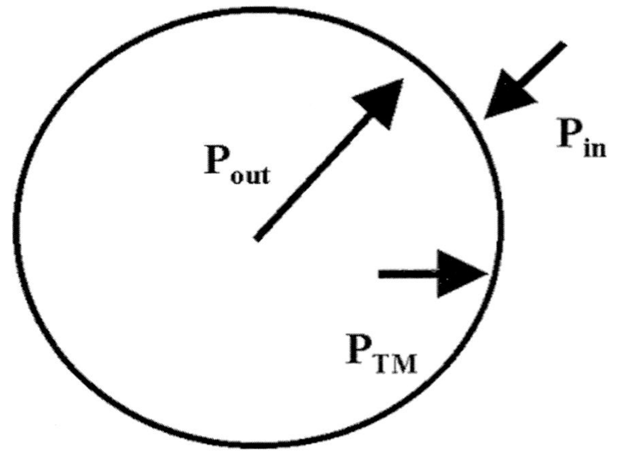


$$P_{Tm} = P_{out} - P_{in}$$

**FIGURE 37.1.** Balance of forces model. Transmural pressure ($P_{tm}$) is the resultant force that determines airway size. When $P_{tm}$ increases or decreases, airway size increases or decreases respectively. $P_{(tm)}$ may be represented as the difference between airway dilating ($P_{out}$) and collapsing ($P_{in}$) forces ($P_{tm} = P_{out} - P_{in}$). Alternatively, $P_{(tm)}$ is represented as the sum of tissue ($P_{ti}$) and luminal ($P_L$) pressures ($P_{tm} = P_{ti} + P_L$).

be directly measured. However, tissue pressure is the balance of the forces from tissue mass, tissue elastance, and neuromuscular dilating and collapsing forces. If neuromuscular tone is held constant (i.e., the hypotonic airway) and physiologic variables are controlled, $P_{ti}$ is a constant, and $P_{tm}$ may be represented by luminal pressure ($P_{tm} = P_L - k$). Application of various levels of nasal CPAP allows luminal pressure ($P_L$) to be modified as an independent variable. Upper airway size, compliance, and shape can be measured as a function of applied pressure. The $P_{tm}$ and airway plot has been described as a representation of the "tube law," and the slope of the plot measures the "compliance" (dA/dP) of the upper airway (Fig. 37.2). Other measures that may be useful include the transmural pressure at which airway area is zero. This defines the closing pressure ($P_c$) of the upper airway (area = 0, $P_{tm} = P_{close}$). Studies have indicated $P_c$ is often negative ($P_c < 0$ cm $H_2O$) in normal nonapneic patients and often positive ($P_c > 0$ cm $H_2O$) in apneic patients (43).

Studies of surgical patients demonstrate that closing pressure ($P_c$) of zero at the retroglossal segment separates and predicts successes and failures of UPPP using stringent and clinically relevant criterion of an apnea index of less than 10 events per hour (14). A larger retropalatal size and more positive closing pressure ($P_c$) also predict UPPP outcomes.

The earliest endoscopic techniques measured the hypotonic airway using the single breath test (SBT). The SBT suddenly decreases applied airway pressure during spontaneous ventilation. The lower pressure is maintained for a single breath. Measurements are taken at the end of expiration, when airflow is zero and muscles are the least active. Multiple pressure drops are necessary to evaluate the airway at different airway pressures. The SBT is a time-consuming and difficult technique. A simpler apneic method may endoscopically measure the airway during general anesthesia, sedation, and non-REM sleep (12–14,44). Apnea may be created by hyperventilation ($P_{CO_2}$ is lowered below the apnea threshold) or general anesthesia. Ventilation is paused for 20 to 40 seconds. The applied pressure is set to fully distend the pharynx ($P_{hold}$) and then lowered until airway closure occurs. During the test, airflow is minimal and the airway is measured. Ventilation is then resumed.

For both methods, the fundamental principle is that upper airway size at any point is the product of two simulta-

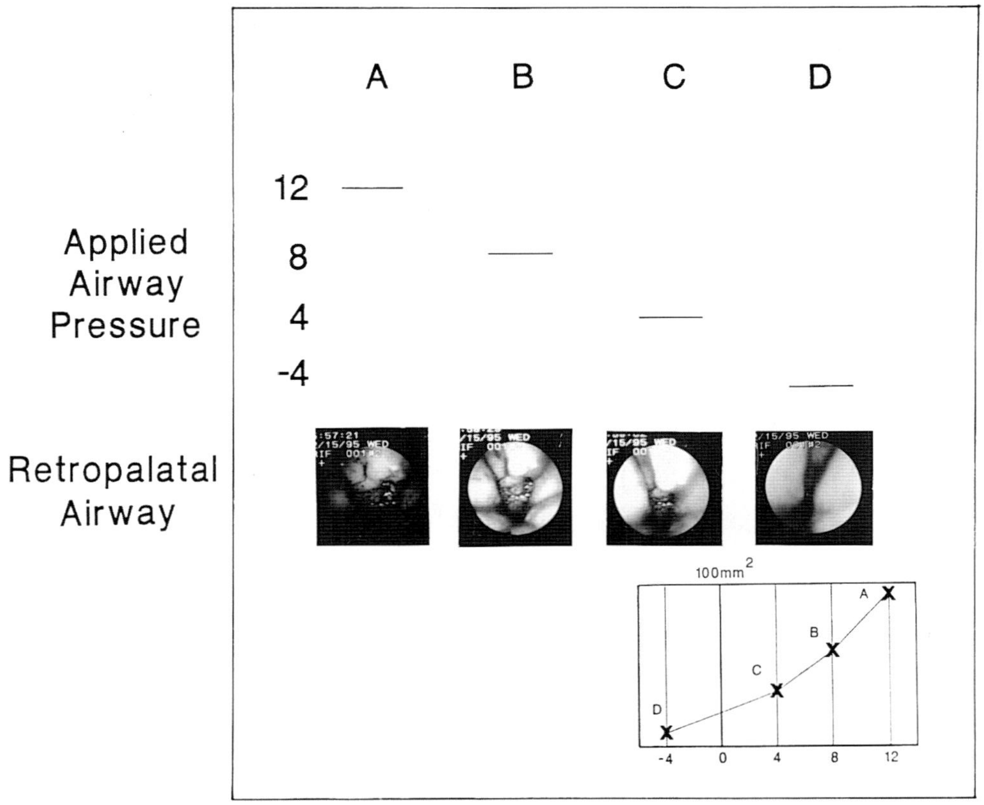


**FIGURE 37.2.** A compliance curve is shown for using sedated endoscopy with the hypnotic upper airway method. Airway size is measured endoscopically. The maximum airway size and closing pressure ($P_c$) are important variables. When $P_c > 0$ for the tongue base, uvulopalatopharyngoplasty is unlikely to be successful. Airway size at zero (ambient) pressures may be estimated using office endoscopy.

neous forces. These are structural forces, which are constant over the short term, and physiologic forces (i.e., muscle tone, vascular tone, airflow, negative inspiratory effort, and sleep or wake state), which are variable. Controlling the physiologic forces allows accurate measurement of airway structure.

## Expiratory Endoscopy Technique

How can these methods be applied to the office or clinical evaluation? To reduce physiologic variability, endoscopy is performed with the patient supine at end expiration. Muscle compensation in OSA during wakefulness augments size. During upright wakefulness, normal muscle posturing and the decreased effect of gravity result in constant upper airway size in most nonapneic persons and OSA patients. Inspiratory dilation and expiratory collapse are absent. However, when supine, the airway size decreases in OSA patients but not in nonapneics (45). In the supine position during wakefulness, phasic inspiratory dilation and expiratory collapse may be observed. The effects of posture and respiration are shown in Figure 37.3. At end expiration, multiple events occur to optimize airway measurements. First, there is a loss of phasic inspiratory muscle activation. Second, there is zero flow. Third, airway pressures may be assumed to consistently approximate zero (i.e., ambient pressure). End expiration also lessens the effects of tracheal displacement. Tracheal tug stabilizes and prevents upper airway collapse (46). By controlling body position, waking muscle tone, airway pressures, airflow, and tracheal tug, supine end-expiratory evaluation yields a consistent benchmark for measuring the pharynx.

The key points of performing passive expiratory endoscopy are the supine position, a relaxed patient, and gentle technique. The minimal required equipment includes a nasopharyngoscope and light source, an examination table or chair that allows the supine position, and topical nasal anesthesia and lubricating gel. Videoendoscopy provides a record for further evaluation and an excellent opportunity to educate the patient about the nature and sites of airway obstruction and collapse.

To begin the endoscopic evaluation, the patient is in the supine position. Anterior rhinoscopy is performed to identify any nasal septal deflection, turbinate hypertrophy, or other nasal pathologies that would affect the examination. If the nose is severely congested, a nasal topical decongestant can be applied. A topical nasal anesthetic, such as 0.5% Dyclone or a 4% lidocaine spray, is then applied. This spray usually achieves some slight degree of pharyngeal anesthesia, which assists the evaluation. If a patient has excessive gag or has discomfort, a topical oropharyngeal anesthesia may also be applied. During the examination, breathing should be by the nasal route. This reduces contraction of the levator palatini, which is activated with oral respiration.

The nasopharyngoscope is lubricated and introduced if possible into the inferior meatus. The inferior meatus is used because it is less sensitive, which allows a more relaxed patient and examination. The nasopharynx is visualized, and any overt pathology is identified. During quiet respiration, the nasopharynx is visualized. Airway shape may be critical in surgical outcomes. Airway shape is classified as coronal, circular, or sagittal (Fig. 37.4). A coronal or flat nasopharynx (with a narrow anterior posterior diameter)

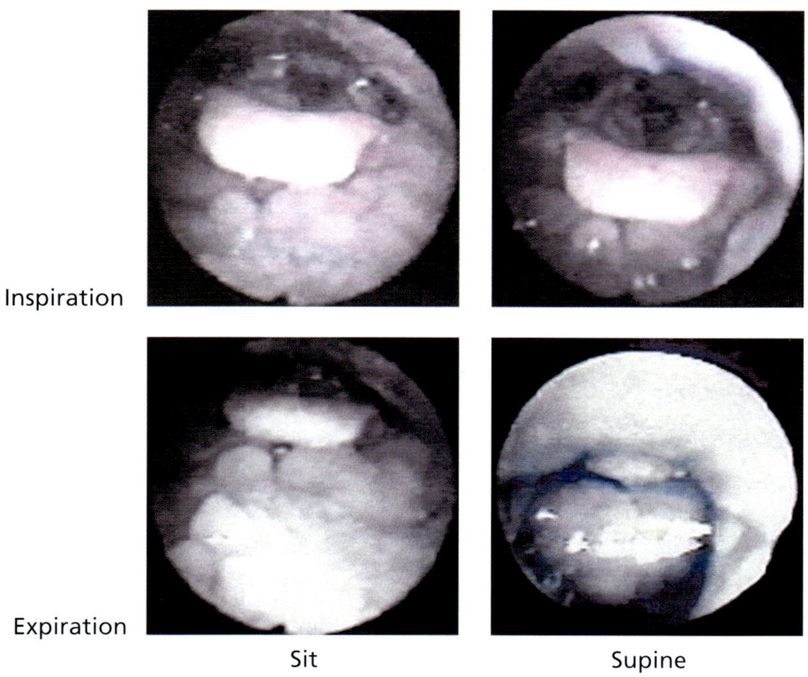


**FIGURE 37.3.** The effects of respiration and position are shown in the retroglossal segment. The airway site appears normal on inspiration while sitting, but during expiration while supine, there is complete collapse.

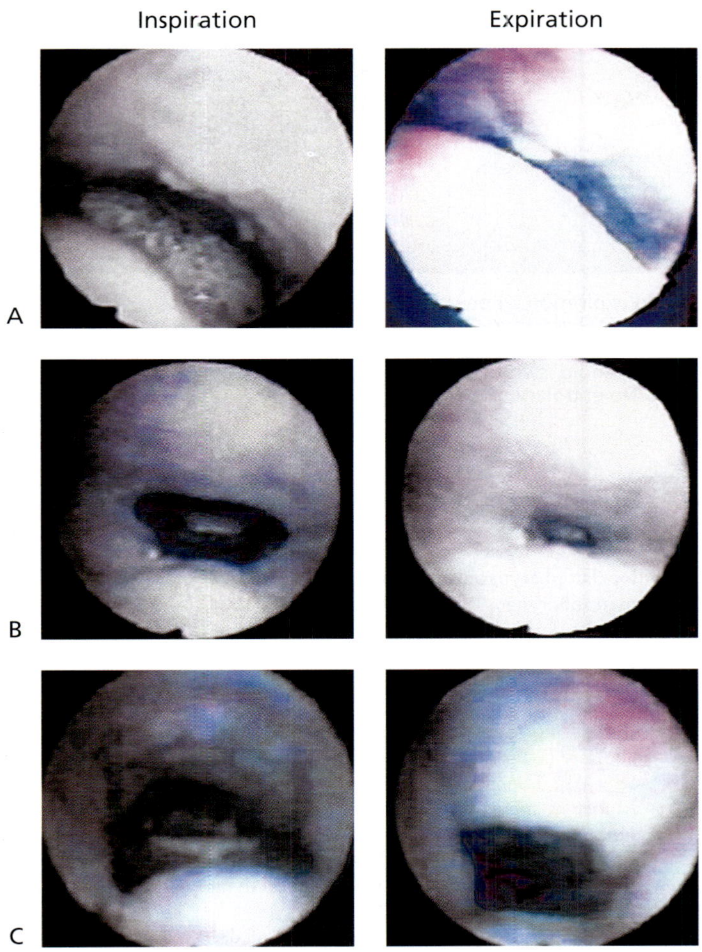


**FIGURE 37.4.** Retropalatal airway shapes are depicted as coronal (flat) **(A)**, circular **(B)**, and sagittal **(C)** for inspiration at end expiration.

suggests significant maxillary constriction. Conversely, a sagittal airway usually is caused by soft tissue from the lateral pharyngeal walls. This pattern is commonly observed in morbidly obese patients. The next maneuver is to recreate a palatal snore. This is particularly useful in patients with snoring as the primary complaint. The patient is then asked to swallow, and the pattern and adequacy of velopharyngeal closure are assessed.

Expiratory and inspiratory maneuvers are then performed. For the expiratory maneuver, the patient is asked to slowly breathe out through the nose and hold his breath. When movement of the airway has stabilized during the expiratory pause, airway size is assessed. A widely patent or normal retropalatal segment allows easy visualization of the velopharynx and oropharynx. Severe compromise is identified by complete obstruction of the airway. An intermediate pattern of collapse for the retropalatal segment is common in OSA. An inspiratory or Mueller's maneuver is then performed. At end expiration, the patient is asked to sniff against an occluded nostril, and the percentage of collapse is estimated. The two methods may often provide significantly different perspectives on the pattern of upper airway collapse (Fig. 37.5).

A lower pharyngeal examination is performed. Pathology of the lower pharynx and larynx is identified. An expiratory maneuver is performed, and the airway size is estimated (Fig. 37.6). An inspiratory Mueller's maneuver is then performed, and the percentage of collapse is estimated.

A supine examination of both segments is performed. Because in many OSA patients the airway is significantly smaller in the supine position, phasic inspiratory dilatation and expiratory collapse may occur. Expiratory and inspira-

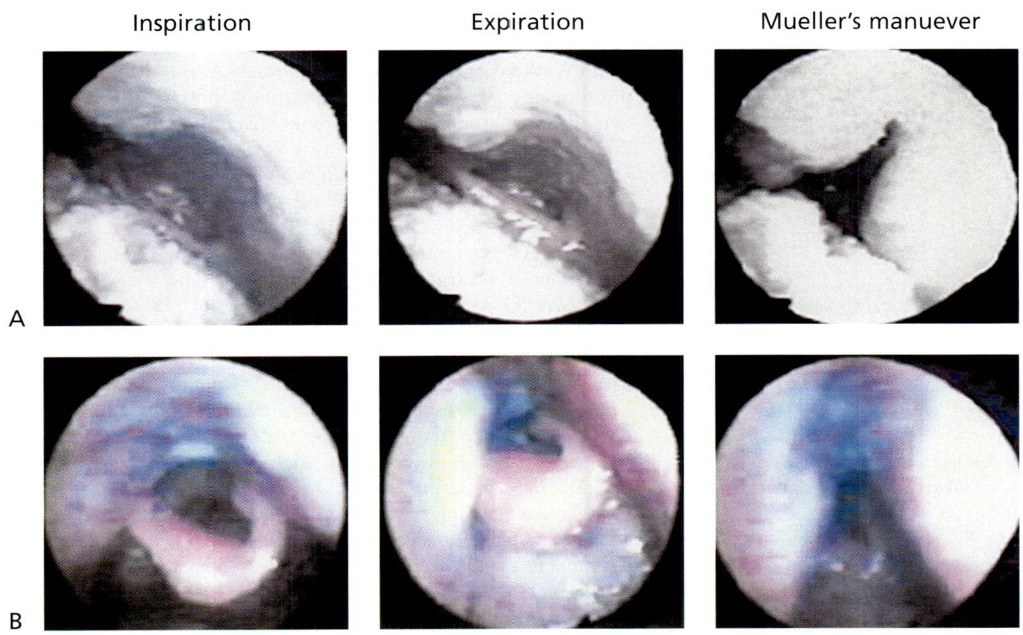


**FIGURE 37.5.** The pattern of end-expiratory collapse while supine is compared with the effect of Mueller's maneuver in two patients. Lateral wall obstruction occurs with Mueller's maneuver, whereas anterior posterior obstruction occurs on end expiration **(A)**. In the patient in **B**, lateral wall obstruction occurs with both methods.

A,B

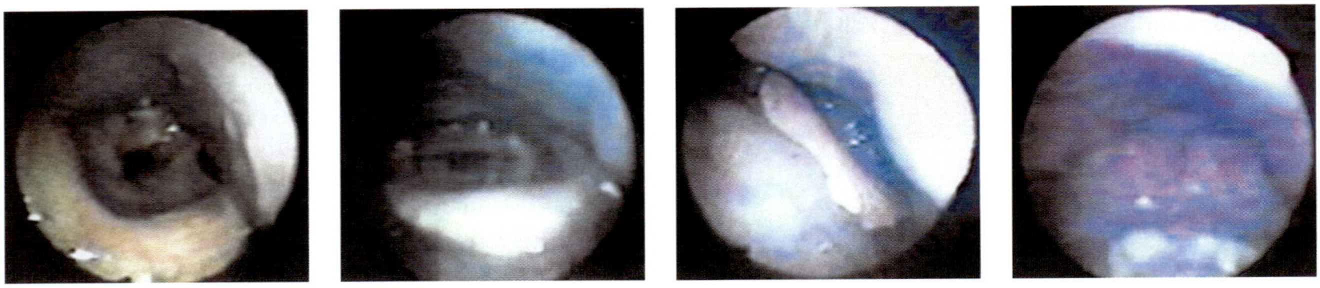

C,D

**FIGURE 37.6.** Retroglossal airway sizes are shown at end expiration when supine. **A:** Normal size (1+) is shown. The larynx is mostly visible. **B:** A small airway (2+) is shown. The arytenoid and vocal process are visible. The epiglottis does not touch the posterior or lateral wall. **C:** A very small retroglossal segment (3+) is shown. Only a portion of the arytenoid is visible. The epiglottis touches the posterior or lateral wall. **D:** Obstruction occurs (4+). No endolarynx is visible.

tory evaluations are performed. For many patients and even normal persons, it is common for the retropalatal segment to obstruct on end expiration. The significance of this is unknown. For this reason, the primary focus of supine endoscopy is directed at the lower pharynx or retroglossal segment. The retroglossal segment is visualized, and after expiration and a quiet breathhold, airway size is estimated. It is not unusual that an involuntary swallow is initiated with complete collapse of the airway. If this occurs, the maneuver is repeated.

Other airway features may also be assessed with endoscopy. Having the patient protrude his tongue and jaw during observation of tongue base movement may demonstrate the effects of limited genioglossus advancement. A submucous cleft palate, notching of the uvula, large palatal blood vessels, or poor lateral wall movement may be identified and may contraindicate UPPP.

## Limitations

Endoscopy does not measure or identify the skeletal abnormalities contributing to OSA. It also does not accurately measure airway length, which may contribute to apnea severity and predict surgical outcomes.

## REFERENCES


1. Sher AE, Schechtman KB, Piccirillo JF. The efficacy of surgical modifications of the upper airway in adults with obstructive sleep apnea syndrome. *Sleep* 1996;19:156–177.
2. Young T, Palta M, Dempsey J, et al. The occurrence of sleep-disordered breathing among middle-aged adults. *N Engl J Med* 1993;328:1230–1235.
3. Kribbs NB, Pack AI, Kline LR, et al. Objective measurement of patterns of CPAP use by patients with obstructive sleep apnea. *Am Rev Respir Dis* 1993;147:887–95.
4. Schwartz AR, Schubert N, Rothman W, et al. Effect of uvulopalatopharyngoplasty on upper airway collapsibility in obstructive sleep apnea. *Am Rev Respir Dis* 1992;145:527–532.
5. Avrahami E, Englender M. Relation between CT axial cross-sectional area of the oropharynx and obstructive sleep apnea syndrome in adults. *AJNR Am J Neuroradiol* 1995;16:135–140.
6. Woodson BT. Retropalatal airway characteristics in uvulopalatopharyngoplasty compared with transpalatal advancement pharyngoplasty. *Laryngoscope* 1997;107:735–740.
7. Wright S, Haight J, Zamel N, et al. Changes in pharangeal properties after uvulopalatopharyngoplasty. *Laryngoscope* 1989; 99:62–65.
8. Langin T, Pepin J, Pendlebury S, et al. Upper airway changes in snorers and mild sleep apnea sufferers after uvulopalatopharyngoplasty (UPPP). *Chest* 1998;113:1595–1603.
9. Sher AE, Thorpy MJ, Shprintzen RJ, et al. Predictive value of Muller maneuver in selection of patients for uvulopalatopharyngoplasty. *Laryngoscope* 1985;95:1483–1487.
10. Katsantonis GP, Maas CS, Walsh JK. The predictive efficacy of the Muller maneuver in uvulopalatopharyngoplasty. *Laryngoscope* 1989;99:677–680.
11. Pringle MG, Croft CB. A comparison of sleep nasoendoscopy and the Muller manoeuvre. *Clin Otolaryngol* 1991;16:559–562.
12. Morrison DL, Launois SH, Isono S, et al. Pharyngeal narrowing and closing pressures in patients with obstructive sleep apnea. *Am Rev Respir Dis* 1993;148:606–611.
13. Isono S, Remmers JE, Tanaka A, et al. Anatomy of pharynx in patients with obstructive sleep apnea and in normal subjects. *J Appl Physiol* 1997;82:1319–1326.
14. Isono S, Akiko S, Tanaka A, et al. Efficacy of endoscopic static pressure/area assessment of the passive pharynx in predicting uvulopalatopharyngoplasty outcomes. *Laryngoscope* 1999;109: 769–774.
15. Launois SH, Feroah TR, Cambell WN, et al. Site of pharyngeal narrowing predicts outcome of surgery for obstructive sleep apnea. *Am Rev Respir Dis* 1993;147:182–189.
16. Woodson BT, Naganuma H. Comparison of methods of airway evaluation in obstructive sleep apnea syndrome. *Otolaryngol Head Neck Surg* 1999;120:460–463.
17. Doghramji K, Jabourian ZH, Pilla M, et al. Predictors of outcome for uvulopalatopahryngoplasty. *Laryngoscope* 1995;105:311–314.
18. Petri N, Suadicani P, Wildschiodtz G, et al. Predictive value of Muller maneuver, cephalometry, and clinical features for the outcome of uvulopalatopharyngoplasty. Evaluation of predictive factors using discriminant analysis in 30 sleep apnea patients. *Acta Otolaryngol* 1994;114:565–571.
19. Aboussouan LS, Golish JA, Wood BG, et al. Dynamic pharyngoscopy in predicting outcome of uvulopalatopharyngoplasty for moderate and severe obstructive sleep apnea. *Chest* 1995; 107:946–951.
20. Skatvedt O. Localization of site of obstruction in snorers and

patients with obstructive sleep apnea syndrome: a comparison of fiberoptic nasopharyngoscopy and pressure measurements. *Acta Otolaryngol (Stockh)* 1993;113:206–209.

21. Woodson BT, Wooten MR. Comparison of upper-airway evaluations during wakefulness and sleep. *Laryngoscope* 1994;104: 821–828.
22. Yao M, Utley DS, Terris DJ. Cephalometric parameters after multilevel pharyngeal surgery for patients with obstructive sleep apnea. *Laryngoscope* 1998;108:789–795.
23. Woodson BT, Wooten MR. A multisensor solid-state pressure manometer to identify the level of collapse in obstructive sleep apnea. *Otolaryngol Head Neck Surg* 1992;107:651–656.
24. Shepard JW Jr, Thawley SE. Localisation of upper airway collapse during sleep in patients with obstructive sleep apnea. *Am Rev Respir Dis* 1990;141:1350–1355.
25. Woodson BT, Wooten MR. Manometric and endoscopic localisation of airway obstruction after uvulopalatopharyngoplasty. *Otolaryngol Head Neck Surg* 1994;111:38–43.
26. Utley DS, Shin EJ, Clerk AA, et al. A cost-effective and rational surgical approach to patients with snoring, upper airway resistance syndrome, or obstructive sleep apnea syndrome. *Laryngoscope* 1997;107:726–34.
27. Woodson BT, Fujita S. Clinical experience with lingualplasty as part of the treatment of severe obstructive sleep apnea. *Otolaryngol Head Neck Surg* 1992;107:40–48.
28. Hochban W, Conradt R, Brandenburg U, et al. Surgical maxillofacial treatment of obstructive sleep apnea. *Plast Reconstr Surg* 1997;99:619–26.
29. Hochban W, Brandenburg U, Peter JH. Surgical teatment of obstructive sleep apnea by maxillomandibular advancement. *Sleep* 1994;17:624–629.
30. Riley RW, Powell NB, Guilleminault C. Obstructive sleep apnea syndrome: a review of 306 consecutively treated surgical patients. *Otolaryngol Head Neck Surg* 1993;108:117–125.
31. Isono S, Tanaka A, Sho Y, et al. Advancement of the mandible improves velopharyngeal airway patency. *J Appl Physiol* 1995; 79:2132–2138.
32. Lyberg T, Krogstad O, Djupesland G. Cephalometric analysis in patients with obstructive sleep apnea syndrome. Skeletal morphology. *J Laryngol Otol* 1989;103:287–292.
33. Lyberg T, Krogstad O, Djupesland G. Cephalometric analysis in patients with obstructive sleep apnea syndrome: Soft tissue morphology. *J Laryngol Otol* 1989;103:293–297.
34. Kunkel M, Hochban W. Acoustic rhinometry: rationale and perspectives. *J Craniomaxillofac Surg* 1994;22:244–249.
35. Suto Y, Matsuo T, Kato T, et al. Evaluation of the pharyngeal airway in patients with sleep apnea: value of ultrafast MR imaging. *AJR Am J Roentgenol* 1993;160:311–314.
36. Katsantonis GP, Moss K, Miyazaki S, et al. Determining the site of airway collapse in obstructive sleep apnea with airway pressure monitoring. *Laryngoscope* 1993;103:1126–1131.
37. Isono S, Remmers JE. Anatomy and physiology of upper airway obstruction. In: Kryger MH, Roth T, Deent WC, eds. *Principles and practice of sleep medicine*, 2nd ed. Philadelphia: WB Saunders, 1994:642–656.
38. Galvin JR, Rooholamini SA, Standford W. Obstructive sleep apnea: diagnosis with ultrafast CT. *Radiology* 1989;171:775–778.
39. Haponik EF, Smith PL, Bohlman ME, et al. Computerized tomography in obstructive sleep apnea. Correlation of airway size with physiology during sleep and wakefulness. *Am Rev Respir Dis* 1983;127:221–226.
40. Hudgel DW, Harasick T, Katz RL, et al. Uvulopalatopharyngoplasty in obstructive apnea. Value of preoperative localization of site of upper airway narrowing during sleep. *Am Rev Respir Dis* 1991;143:942–946.
41. Remmer JE, DeGroot WJ, Sauerland EK, et al. Pathogenesis of upper airway occlusion during sleep. *J Appl Physiol Respir Environ Exercise Physiol* 1978;44:931–938.
42. Woodson BT, Feroah T, Connolly L, et al. A method to evaluate upper airway mechanics following intervention in snorers. *Am J Otolaryngol* 1997;18:306–314.
43. Gold AR, Schwartz AR. The pharyngeal critical pressure. The whys and hows of using nasal continuous positive airway pressure diagnostically. *Chest* 1996;110:1077–1088.
44. Badr MS, Toiber F, Skatrud JB, et al. Pharyngeal narrowing/occlusion during central sleep apnea. *J Appl Physiol* 1995;78:1806–15.
45. Neill AM, Angus S, Sajkov D, et al. Effects of sleep posture on upper airway stability in patients with obstructive sleep apnea. *Am J Respir Crit Care Med* 1997;155:199–204.
46. Rowley JA, Permutt S, Willey S, et al. Effect of tracheal and tongue displacement on upper airway airflow dynamics. *J Appl Physiol* 1996;80:2171–2178.

# 38

# INTERVENTIONAL SIALOENDOSCOPY

FRANCIS MARCHAL
PAVEL DULGUEROV
MINERVA BECKER
WILLY LEHMANN

Sialoendoscopy is a new procedure for visualizing the lumens of the salivary ducts and assessing their disorders. The most frequent pathology of the salivary ducts is obstruction caused by sialolithiasis, and the object of interventional sialoendoscopy is to remove the stones, thereby relieving the obstruction.

## HISTORY

The first anatomic descriptions of the salivary glands and their canals were made by Wharton, Stensen, and Bartholin in the seventeenth century. The first reported attempts to visualize the salivary ducts with an endoscope were conducted in the early 1990s (1,2).

Salivary stones (i.e., sialolithiasis) occur in the submandibular and parotid glands, and they may be located proximally or distally. For many years, the removal of proximal submandibular stones has been performed by simple anterior marsupialization. However, distal submandibular stones or parotid stones have always been problematic because they were out of reach.

The first report of a distal submandibular stone extraction was published in 1990. The procedure was performed with a wire basket during sialography (3). The first parotid stone extraction was performed in 1994 by Sharma (4). In both cases, the stone was extracted blindly. This was done before salivary stone extraction under endoscopic control was possible (5,6).

## SIALOLITHIASIS

According to most published data, salivary stones are localized in the submandibular gland in 80% to 90% of cases. In our experience, parotid glands are affected more frequently (up to 40%), a difference possibly explained by the sensitivity of the new detection methods used (7,8). Salivary stones can be unique or multiple, especially in the parotid gland. Their location can be proximal, distal, or intraglandular (Fig. 38.1). They can be round or have an irregular shape (Fig. 38.2). The annual growth rate of established salivary stones has been estimated to be 1 mm per year (9).

### Physiopathology

Although the exact physiopathologic mechanism is still unknown, sialolithiasis results from precipitation of salivary components, mainly calcium and phosphate. Several theories have been proposed. One of them suggests the presence of microcalculi in the saliva, aggregating in special conditions and leading to calculus formation (10). Another theory postulates the existence of an organic nucleus (e.g., desquamated cells, bacteria), which becomes progressively calcified when the saliva is saturated with calcium and phosphate. This second theory is supported by the fact that the submandibular glands are more often affected than the parotids because their secretion is more viscous and contains more proteins. This theory seems to be confirmed by the microscopic structure of the stone: a less dense nucleus, rich in proteins and microproteins, and a mineral cortex, rich in calcium. A third theory draws on a comparison with urinary and biliary stones, for which infectious agents have been incriminated. However, the role of microbacterial agents in sialolithiasis remains hypothetical.

The reason for calcium precipitation is also debated: lysis by proteases of salivary proline-rich proteins that naturally chelate calcium ions (11), elevated pH (in the submandibular gland) enhancing precipitation of $CaPO_4$, and a high concentration of mucins that fix calcium (11). Most probably, the cause is multifactorial.

### Consequences of Sialolithiasis

Sialolithiasis or, rarely, ductal stenosis results in mechanical obstruction of the duct, causing recurrent prandial

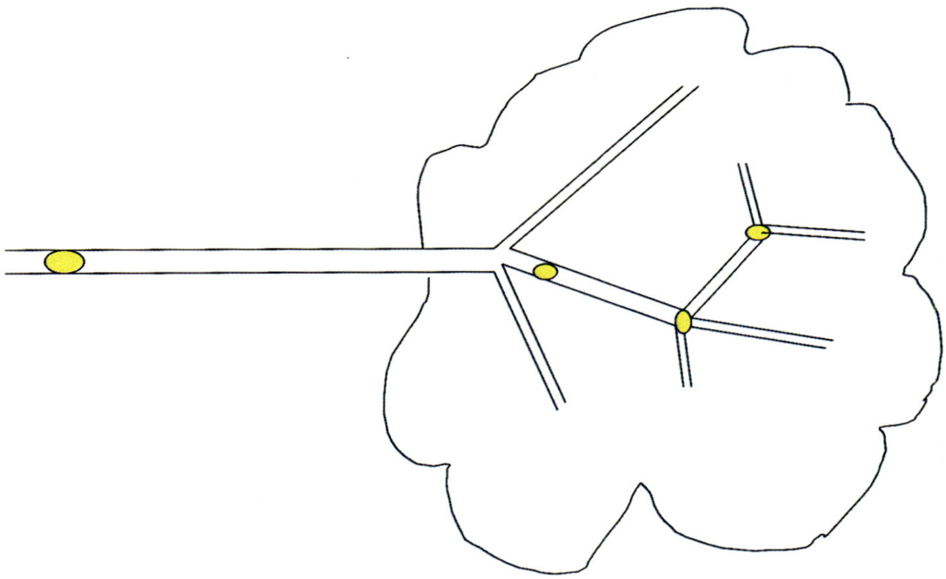

**FIGURE 38.1.** Possible location of stones in the salivary ductal system.

swellings. These swellings can be temporary but can also lead to bacterial infections. The infections are accompanied by fever, purulent discharge at the ostium, and painful swelling of the gland.

## Classic Management

The classic management approach to sialolithiasis uses an antibiotic and antiinflammatory treatment, hoping for a spontaneous stone expression through the papilla. In cases of submandibular stones located close to the Wharton duct opening, marsupialization of the papilla is performed, and the stone is removed. Although sialolithiasis is the most frequent reason for submandibular gland resection (12), the stones often are left in the remaining Wharton duct remnant (13).

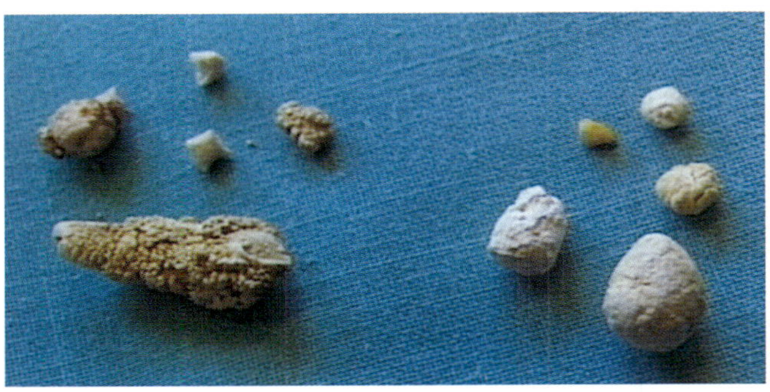

**FIGURE 38.2.** Different sizes and shapes of salivary stones.

In cases of parotid stones, a conservative approach is adopted whenever possible, because parotidectomies for infectious conditions are associated with a higher incidence of facial nerve complications (14,15). Nevertheless, in case of recurrent infections and posteriorly located stones, parotidectomy was the only option.

Because of the morbidity of both operations, the surgeon and, more often, the patients are reluctant to proceed to surgery. However, a longer delay before definitive treatment leads to stone enlargement, fibrosis of the gland, and therefore greater surgical risk.

It is commonly believed that a gland with sialolithiasis is no longer functional (16). A systematic review of 48 submandibular glands removed for sialolithiasis showed there is no correlation between the degree of gland alteration and the number of infectious episodes; there is also no correlation between the degree of gland alteration and the duration of evolution; and although our indications for submandibular gland removal were correct, almost 50% of the removed glands were histopathologically normal or close to normal (16). A conservative approach even in long-standing sialolithiasis therefore appears to be justified.

External lithotripsy has been advocated for the fragmentation of salivary stones. Initially reported by Iro and colleges in the early 1990s (17), this outpatient technique is becoming popular, with the use of the Minilith (Karl Storz, Tuttlingen, Germany), but it requires several sessions at intervals of a few weeks. Once fragmented, stones are supposed to be evacuated spontaneously because no stone extraction is described with this technique. Success rates up to 75% for the parotid and up to 40% for the submandibular gland are reported (17).

## SIALOENDOSCOPY INDICATIONS

Sialoendoscopy is a useful diagnostic procedure for any parotid or submandibular swelling of unclear origin. Because these procedures are new, the exact indications remain to be defined. It may become the investigation of choice for diseases affecting the salivary ducts, replacing the current investigations.

The main indication for interventional sialoendoscopy is the extraction of salivary stones under optical control. Its role in other ductal pathologies, such as stenosis, has been described (18) but remains to be defined.

## SIALOENDOSCOPY CONTRAINDICATIONS

There are no specific contraindications, mostly because sialoendoscopy is an outpatient procedure that is performed under local anesthesia and is minimally invasive. Even elderly or unstable patients, unable to undergo a general anesthesia, can benefit from this technique.

The main technical limitations of interventional sialoendoscopy are salivary stones too posteriorly located and a fibrosed canal wall with a reduced diameter, which renders progression of the endoscope difficult.

Manipulation of the rigid sialoendoscope is delicate, requires extensive experience, and may be hazardous because of the theoretical risks of perforation and vascular or neural damage. Progression in the canal should be performed only under adequate vision.

## PREOPERATIVE EVALUATION

Preoperative evaluation for sialoendoscopy is unnecessary because the endoscopy is minimally invasive, atraumatic, and provides direct visualization of the ductal tree. Nevertheless, sialolithiasis has been evaluated with standard radiography, sialography, magnetic resonance (MR)-sialography, ultrasound, and computed tomography (CT).

### Standard Radiography

The classic occlusal film effectively shows ductal stones, although intraglandular and small stones can be missed (19). According to the old monograph of Rauch, 20% of the sialolithiases are radiotransparent (9).

### Ultrasound

Ultrasound was first applied to the medical field in the early 1940s, head and neck applications appeared in the 1960s, and it was used for lithiasis detection in the 1970s. Ultrasound is a popular, noninvasive method of diagnosis, especially in Europe (Fig. 38.3). Unfortunately, ultrasound is operator dependent, with no directly interpretable image for the surgeon, unless the surgeon is doing the examination. Ultrasound has limitations for detection of sialolithiasis. In a study comparing ultrasound, sialography, and endoscopy, we found a sensitivity of 81%, a specificity of 94%, and an accuracy of 86% for ultrasound (8).

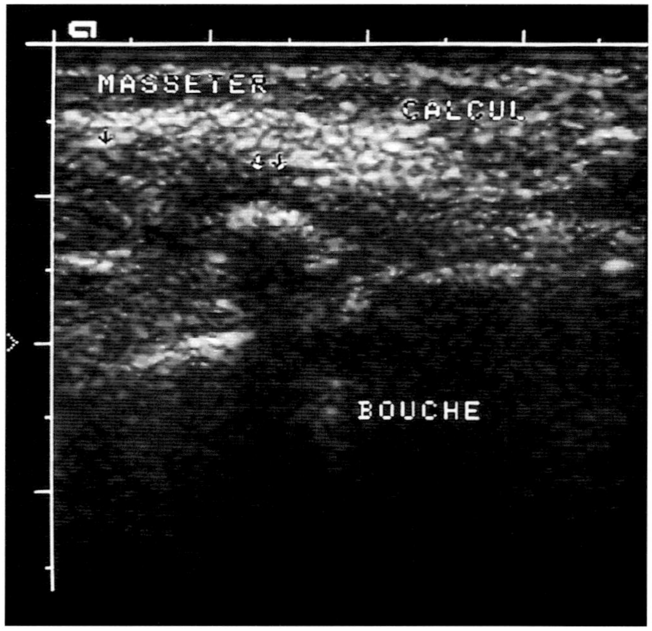


**FIGURE 38.3.** Ultrasound scan of right parotid gland sialolithiasis *(arrow)*, as discussed in case 1.

### Sialography

Sialography consists of an opacification of the Wharton and the Stensen ducts by a retrograde intracanal injection of a water-soluble radiopaque dye. Sialography is considered to be the gold standard, because it provides a clear image of the stones and of the ductal morphology (Fig. 38.4). It can also provide images diagnostic for certain disorders such as Sjögren's syndrome (20).

Sialography sometimes has the advantage of being therapeutic. The injection of dye dilates the duct and has resulted in the excretion of the stone. Nevertheless, the incidence of successful therapeutic sialography has never been documented. Disadvantages include the irradiation doses, corresponding to 20 standard chest radiographs; the pain associated with the procedure; the possibility of canal wall perforation; infection; and anaphylactic shock (21). Sialography often tends to push the stone further up the canal, a distinct disadvantage if a removal by sialoendoscopy is planned.

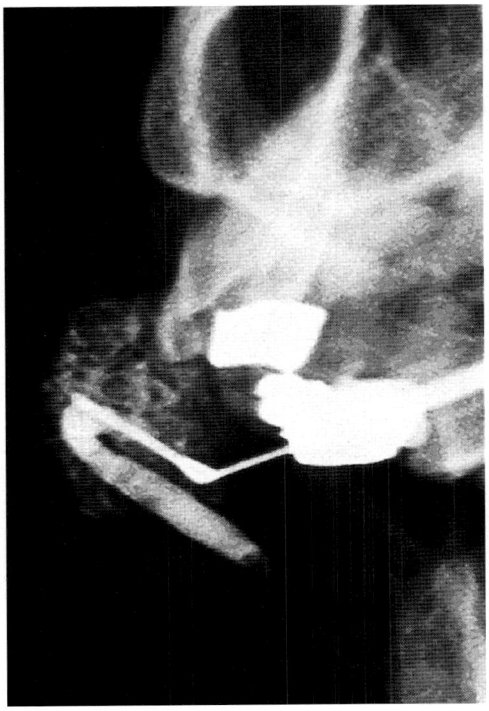

FIGURE 38.4. Sialography of case 1. The distal portion of the Stensen duct is opacified. Several stones are seen until progression of the dye is blocked by a larger stone.

## Magnetic Resonance-Sialography

MR-sialography is a newer, noninvasive diagnostic procedure, with promising results. It consists of 3-mm, T2-weighted, fast spin echo slides performed in two planes: sagittal and axial. Volumetric reconstruction is then performed, allowing a visualization of the ducts and their ramifications (Fig. 38.5). The advantages are that the technique is fast and totally noninvasive, with no dye injection, no irradiation, and no associated pain. The disadvantages are that, although the acquisition time is short (10 minutes), reconstruction requires about 45 minutes, and there are specific MRI-associated inconveniences such as equipment costs, ferromagnetic implants, and examination intolerance by claustrophobic patients. In a study of 80 patients performed in Geneva, we observed that the only limitation of this technique was that artifacts were produced by patients' dental bridges (7).

## Computed Tomography

Often performed, a CT scan is adequate for diagnosing sialolithiasis only if the stone is large or if radiologic slices of 1 mm are obtained. Among the disadvantages are the lack of precise localization of the stone and the absence of visualization of the ducts and their anomalies (22).

# CASE EXAMPLES

## Case 1: Parotid Sialoendoscopy and Extraction of Seven Stones

A 33-year-old patient presented with an acute infection of the right parotid gland, with fever, pus at the Stensen duct, and painful swelling of the gland. He received antibiotic treatment for 10 days. Ultrasound showed several aggregated stones and ductal dilatation (Fig. 38.3).

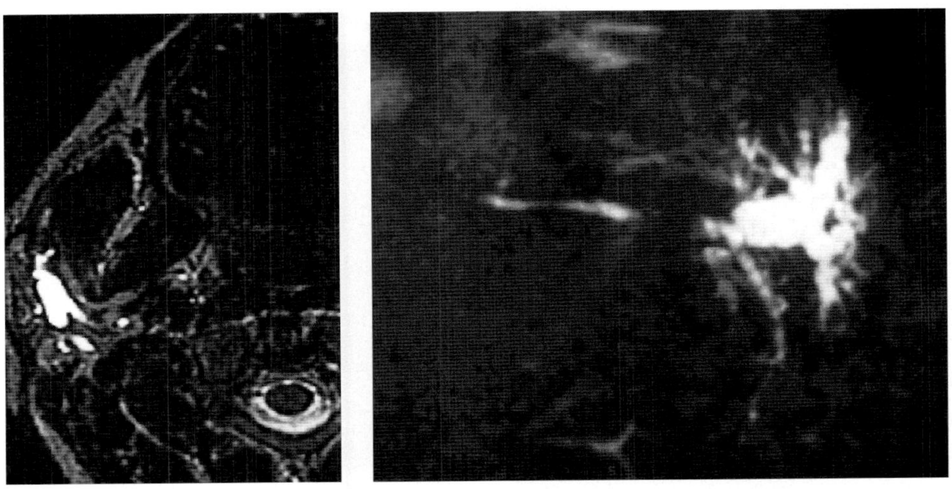

A B

FIGURE 38.5. MR-sialography of case 1. The salivary ducts are seen as bright (white) areas. Dilatation of the proximal ductal tree **(A,B)** and narrowing an irregularities of the proximal Stensen duct **(B)** can be seen.

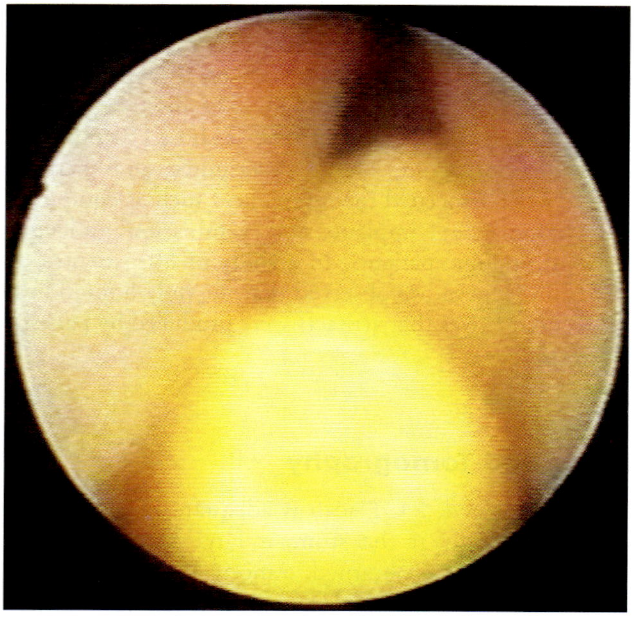

**FIGURE 38.6.** Sialoencoscopy of case 1, showing three stones partially obstructing the lumen of the Stensen duct.

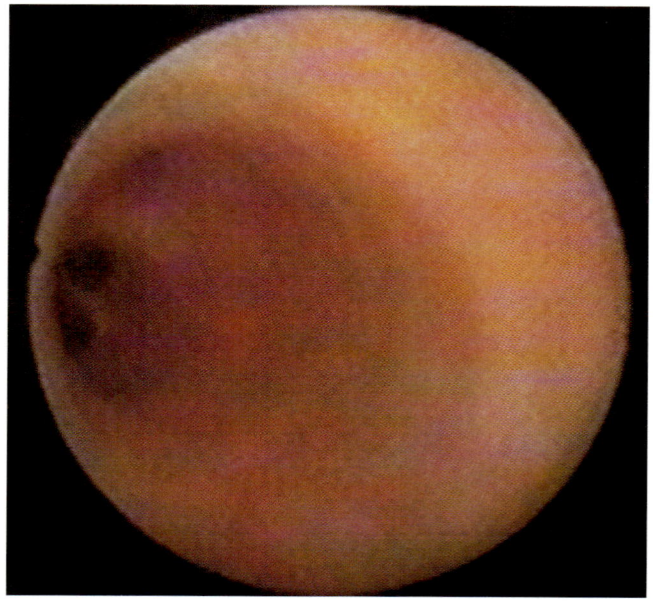

**FIGURE 38.8.** Stone-free parotid ductal system after two interventional sialoendoscopy sessions.

Sialography could only opacify the distal part of the canal, giving no information about the number of stones or their size (Fig. 38.4). MR-sialography showed only the dilated proximal ductal tree (Fig. 38.5). Sialoendoscopy of the duct was conducted 3 weeks after the acute episode. Endoscopy confirmed the presence of seven stones (Fig. 38.6). Three of them were removed during a first session (Fig. 38.7), and the other four required a second session for retrieval. Normal ductal morphology was observed at the end of the procedure (Fig. 38.8). The patient has remained free of symptoms during a follow-up period of 9 months.

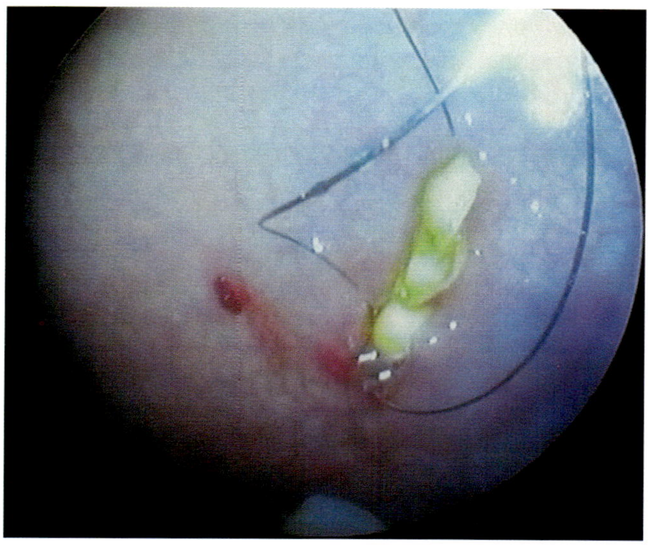

**FIGURE 38.7.** Intraora view of the three stones seen in Figure 38.6. They were extracted by interventional sialoendoscopy with a grasping basket.

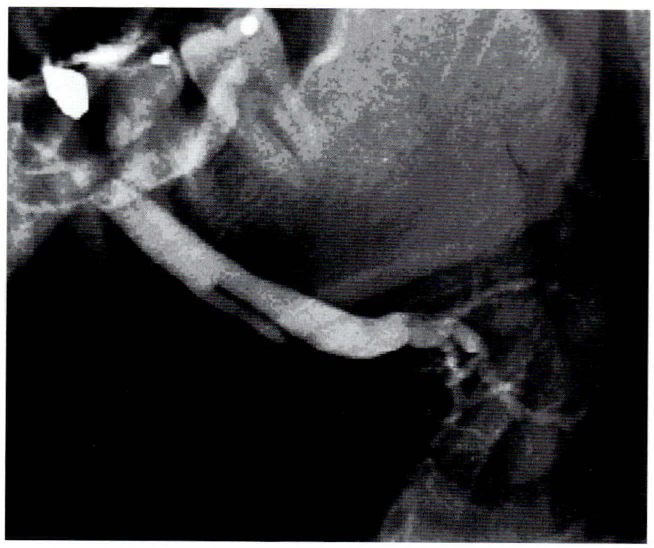

**FIGURE 38.9.** Sialography of a submandibular ductal system shows an accessory canal containing two stones (case 2).

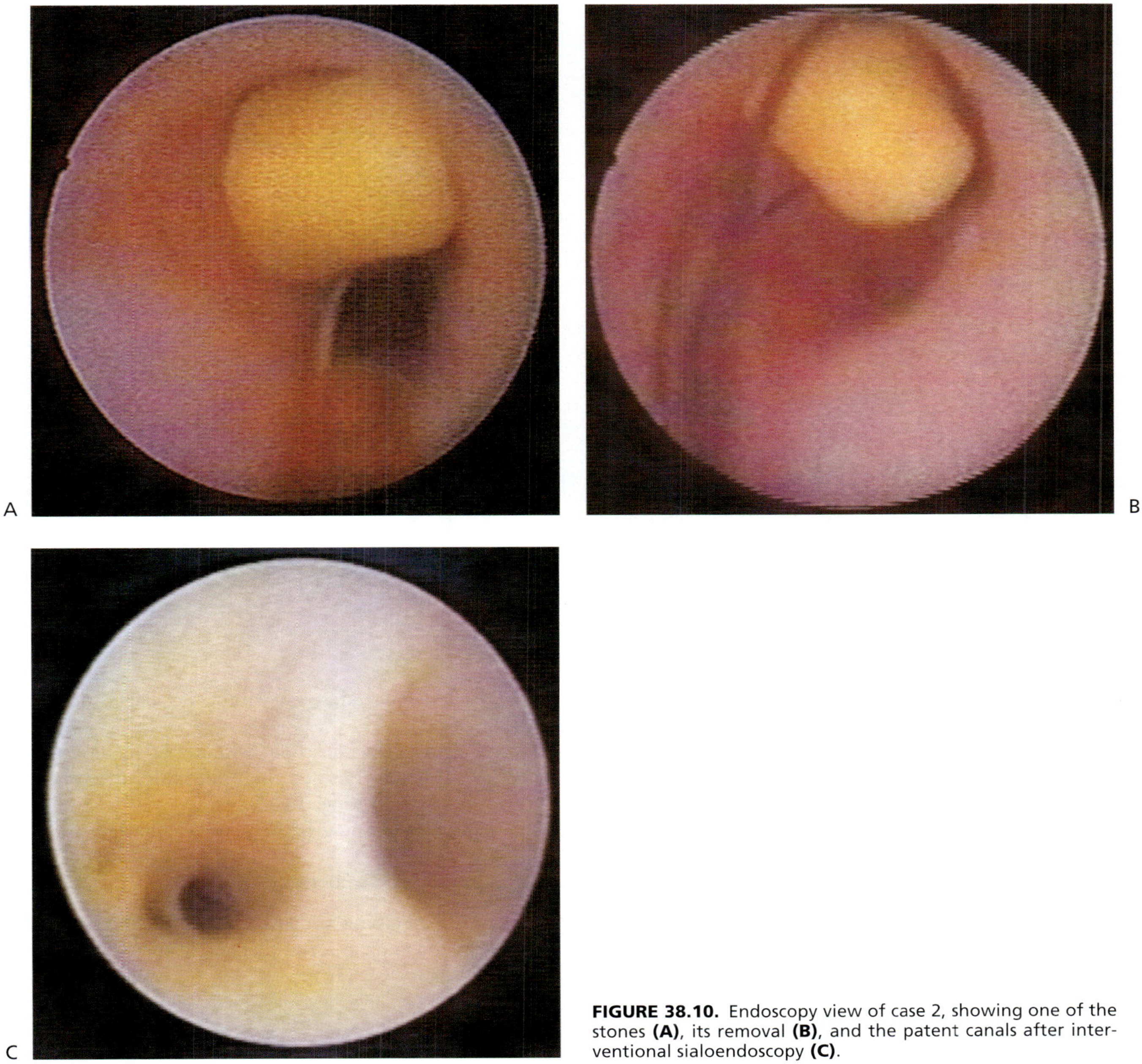

**FIGURE 38.10.** Endoscopy view of case 2, showing one of the stones **(A)**, its removal **(B)**, and the patent canals after interventional sialoendoscopy **(C)**.

## Case 2: Interventional Sialoendoscopy of a Submandibular Gland

A 22-year-old man presenting with a recurrent swelling of the submandibular gland was investigated with sialography (Fig. 38.9), showing an accessory submandibular duct containing two stones. This was confirmed by sialoendoscopy (Fig. 38.10A), and the stones were removed with a grasping basket (Fig. 38.10B). After the procedure, the accessory and main canals were patent (Fig. 38.10C). The patient has been asymptomatic for 1 year since interventional sialoendoscopy.

## Case 3: Multiple Pathologies of Wharton's Duct

An 82-year-old man presented with recurrent swellings of the right submandibular gland. A sialoendoscopy revealed a distal stone, which was removed. Careful reexamination showed a patent distal duct (Fig. 38.11A), but a stricture was found in the proximal duct (Fig. 38.11B). Dilatation of this stenosis was attempted but was unsuccessful. The patient has been free of symptoms for 4 months but may require further dilatation in the future.

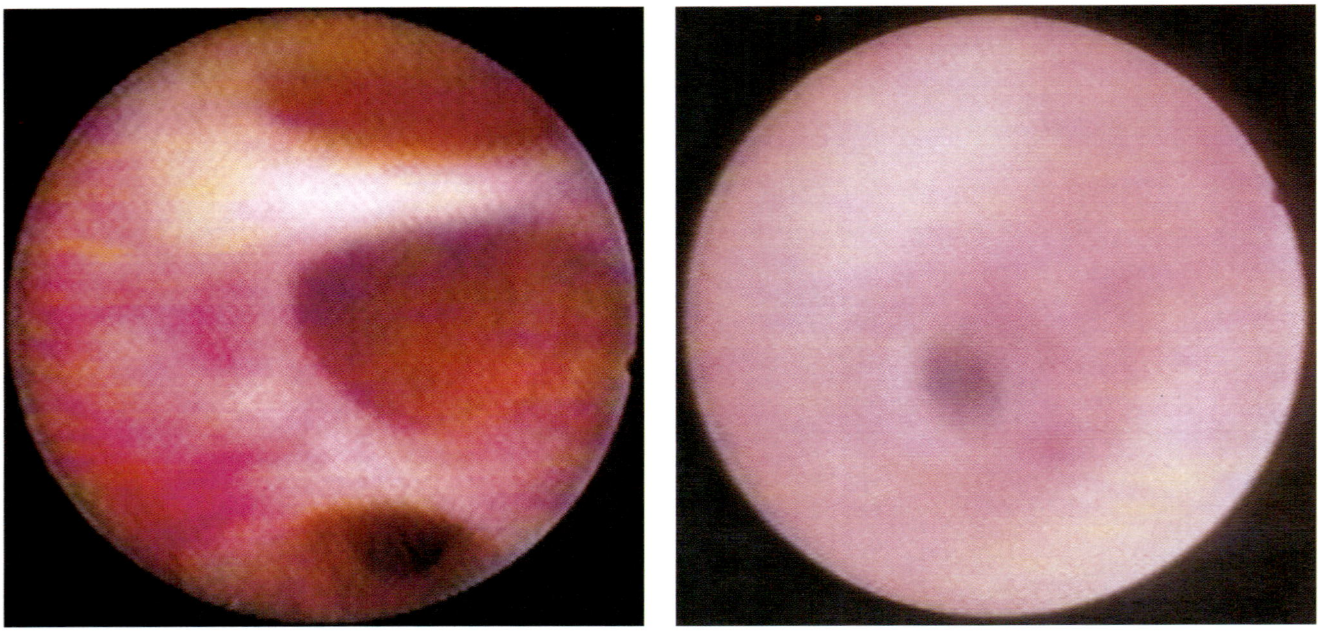

**FIGURE 38.11.** Endoscopy of a normal proximal Wharton duct **(A)** and a distal stenosis **(B)**.

## INSTRUMENTATION

The local anesthesia is performed with continuous rinsing of the ductal lumen with 20 mL of 2% Xylocaine and 20 mL 0.9% of NaCl. We use the following instrumentation for this intervention:

- Light source: any office light source
- Camera: Storz, model 20211001
- Video recorder and printer (type is unimportant but S-VHS quality is advised)
- Custom-made salivary duct dilator
- Semi-rigid sialoendoscope within the diagnostic sheath (Fig. 38.12)
- Semi-rigid sialoendoscope within the interventional sheath (one channel for the optic fiber, the other for instrumentation) (Fig. 38.13)
- Several wire grasping baskets specifically developed for this procedure
- Scalpel, forceps, smooth-tip scissors, 4-0 Vicryl suture

We are developing with G. Barki from the Karl Storz Company a complete set of diagnostic and interventional sialoendoscopy instruments.

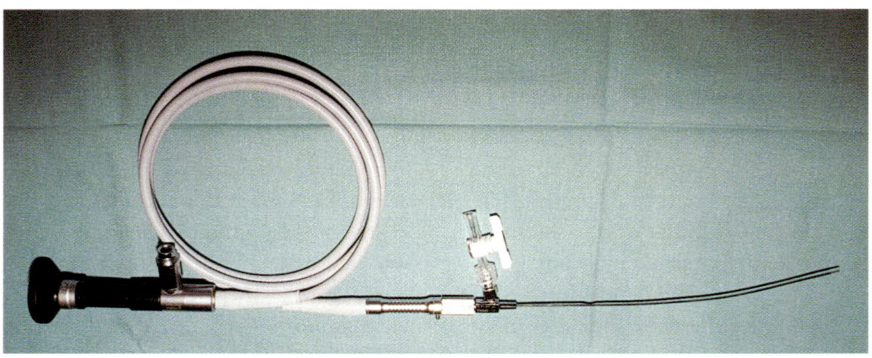

**FIGURE 38.12.** Diagnostic semi-rigid sialoendoscope.

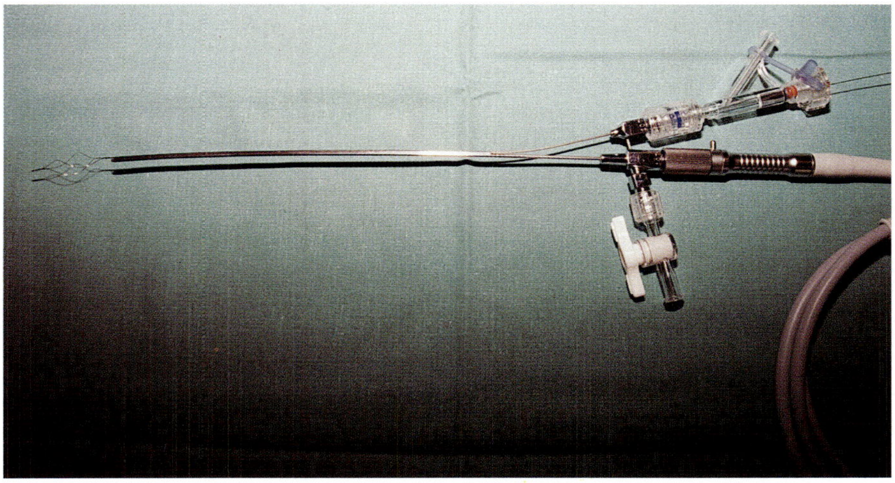

**FIGURE 38.13.** Interventional semi-rigid sialoendoscope.

## OPERATION ROOM LAYOUT

The procedure can be done on an outpatient basis in the clinic, with the patient sitting in a chair or partially recumbent. We prefer the patient sitting, which allows better mobility of the surgeon. The disadvantage is that vagal syncope may occur more frequently in the sitting position.

A cart with the connections for the camera, the TV monitor, the video recorder, and the video printer are located on the opposite side of the patient, allowing for direct observation of the manipulations by the surgeon. An assistant (i.e., physician, nurse, or technician) is located on that side and is responsible for operating the video recorder.

## ANESTHESIA

The anesthesia is purely local. If the patient is stressed, a premedication can be given, such as 0.5 mg of atropine, 6 mg of morphine given subcutaneously, or 7.5 mg of midazolam given orally. The endoscopy is performed with progressive endoluminal rinsing of the local anesthetic solution described previously.

## OPERATIVE TECHNIQUE

Contact anesthesia is performed with 10% Xylocaine. A salivary sound is introduced into the duct. Infiltration is performed with regular local anesthesia solution containing 1% Xylocaine with 1:100,000 epinephrine. Whenever possible, progressive dilatation of the duct is performed with our custom-made salivary duct dilator or salivary sounds of progressively larger diameters. Sometimes, a small papillotomy of the first 5 mm is performed, mostly for Wharton's ducts in which the papilla is narrower.

Dental absorbing tampons are placed in the posterior aspect of the vestibule and gingival-buccal sulcus for parotid sialoendoscopy and bilaterally in the lateral aspects of the floor of mouth for submandibular explorations. These tampons are replaced with new, dry ones every 5 to 10 minutes. The accumulating intraoral fluids are also aspirated intermittently. Intermittent rinsing with the local anesthetic solution is done by the assistant and produces local anesthesia, slight dilatation of the duct, cleaning of the endoscope tip, and removal of pus, debris, and (rarely) blood.

The initial procedure, especially when there are no preoperative examinations, is a diagnostic sialoendoscopy. We use the diagnostic sialoendoscope (1.33 $mm^2$ surface, 1.3 mm diameter), which allows a minimally invasive but complete exploration of the ductal system.

When a stone is located, we use the interventional sialoendoscope (1.89 $mm^2$ surface, equivalent diameter of 1.55 mm), which has two channels: one for the same optic fiber used during the diagnostic procedure and the other for the grasping basket (Fig. 38.14A) or a 400-μm laser fiber (Fig. 38.14B). When the stone has a diameter less than 5 mm, the grasping basket is passed behind the stone and subsequently deployed. When the stone is trapped, the whole device is removed. When the stone is larger, we use an endocanal laser fiber to fragment it before extraction. After the last stone is removed, the endoscope is introduced one final time to rinse the duct and verify its integrity.

Despite its apparent simplicity, interventional sialoendoscopy is a technically challenging procedure. Papillotomy should be as small as possible and should be avoided in most cases involving the parotid duct. Maneuvering within the small salivary ducts must be atraumatic because of pos-

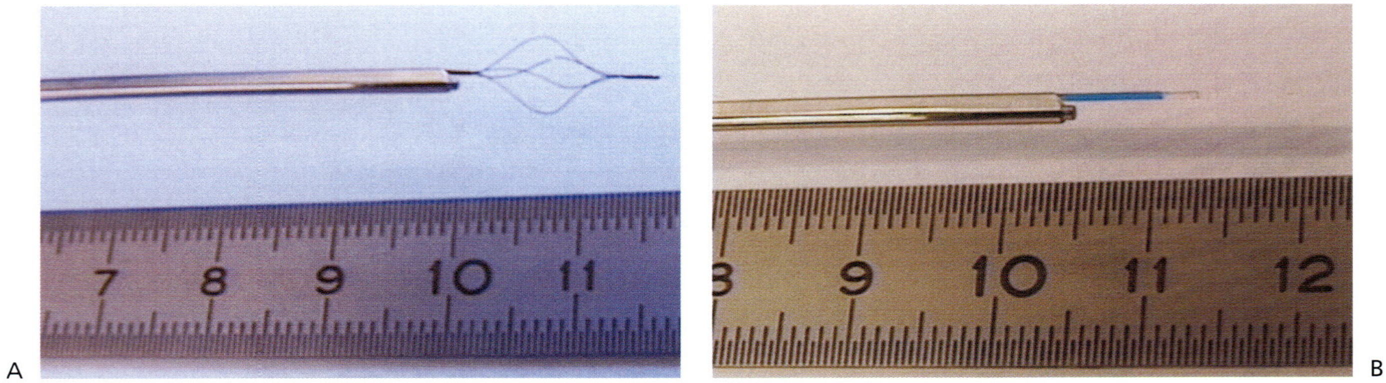


**FIGURE 38.14.** Tip of the interventional sialoendoscope with a protruding open grasping basket **(A)** and the laser fiber **(B)**.

sible ductal perforation with yet uncertain consequences. Significant trauma of the ductal wall could result in latter stenosis.

## POSTOPERATIVE CARE

The intervention is done with antibiotic prophylaxis. Antibiotics (amoxicillin–clavulanic acid or clindamycin) and corticosteroids (50 mg of prednisone per day orally) are given for 48 hours. Frequent self-massage of the gland is recommended. Follow-up assessment is performed 10 days after the procedure.

## COMPLICATIONS

In more than 100 interventional endoscopies, we have not encountered any significant complication, such as damage to the facial or lingual nerves, gross hemorrhage, or major canal wall perforations. Nevertheless, during two parotid sialoendoscopic procedures, we had blockage of the grasping basket, which could be removed by firm traction. A similar case resulted in parotidectomy (1). In three cases (two parotid and one submandibular), the stone was partially embedded in the canal wall. During the removal of the stone, a ductal perforation occurred and resulted in painful localized swellings, which resolved with a conservative treatment.

In the postoperative period, we had no serious infections requiring intravenous treatment, or postoperative strictures leading to a surgical removal of the gland.

One patient (a bassoon player) required a large sialodochoplasty of Stensen's papilla because of ductal fibrosis and the papilla's stricture. Postoperatively, repeated parotid swellings (i.e., pneumoparotitis) occurred during whistling, and recurrent intraglandular burning was experienced during meals. We had to perform a parotidectomy with ligation of the Stensen duct. Special attention should be given to minimizing papillotomy and sialodochoplasty for patients who tend to routinely increase their intraoral pressures, such as wind instrument players.

The intraoperative pain, evaluated by the patients on a 10-grade scale, has never been quantified as more than 3. Postoperative pain was usually experienced, ranging from 1 to 6 on the pain scale, depending on the duration of the procedure and on the extension of intrabuccal dissection, especially in cases requiring large sialodochoplasty of the Wharton duct.

## ADVANTAGES AND LIMITATIONS

### Diagnostic Sialoendoscopy

For diagnostic sialoendoscopy, some investigators advocate the use of simple optical fibers (1). In our experience, the difficulties of directing these fibers and of maintaining a dilated duct during the procedure result in poor visualization. We emphasize the importance of continuous rinsing, because it provides local anesthesia, cleaning of the lens, and maintenance of a dilated duct.

### Interventional Sialoendoscopy

Sialolithiases can be directly extracted or fragmented before extraction. Prior publications have focused on fragmentation.

Gundlach, in Berlin, using a 1.6-mm-diameter flexible endoscope with a working channel was the first to report intracanal lithotripsy with a laser beam (2). *In vitro* and *in vivo* studies resulted in the selection of the 504-nm dye laser, with an energy of 60 mJ, and a time setting of 0.01 second (2). Although this technique allows stone fragmentation, no stone extraction is performed, and therefore several sessions may be required to break the stones to a small enough size for spontaneous evacuation.

Electrohydraulic devices, initially described as promising (23), have been proven to have low efficiency at low voltages. At higher voltages, although we have found that destruction was possible (24), canal wall injuries have occurred (25). Our overall experience with such devices is rather negative.

Pneumoblastic devices, used routinely by urologists with satisfying results, are based on the delivery of mechanical energy to the stone. Although no clinical trials with this technique have been published for salivary stones, *in vitro* studies tend to emphasize the risks of canal wall perforations (26).

After many attempts with flexible endoscopes of various sizes and prototypes of small grasping baskets, we concluded that flexible endoscopes were very delicate, provided poor visualization, and did not allow the use of grasping baskets. We therefore developed the semi-rigid instruments.

Some investigators using rigid instruments have reported cases of submandibular and parotid endoscopy with a 2.3- or 2.7-mm endoscope (6). In our experience, even with dilatations and rinsing, we could not introduce endoscopes larger than 2.0 mm, and these endoscopes could not reach the intraglandular part of the canal. Zenk and associates (27) reported diameters of Stensen's duct between 0.5 and 1.5 mm in 25 human cadavers.

One limitation of semi-rigid sialoendoscopy is the curves of the canal, especially in the submandibular gland, where a 90° angle exists at the entrance of the gland. The main limitation remains the diameter of the interventional sialoendoscope. When the diameter of the instrument is larger than the diameter of the dilated lumen, progression within the canal becomes impossible, and the whole canal wall tends to be stripped. Marsupialization of the ductal papillae should be avoided or as small as possible to prevent retrograde passage of air and infection.

Nevertheless, the intraglandular portion of submandibular and parotid glands can be reached up to 10 cm from the papilla, and the results are already encouraging, with a rate of stone extraction as high as 75%. The size of the grasping basket was a limiting factor, because it determines the diameter of the working channel. New prototypes are being developed, and we look forward to using smaller instruments in the near future.

## CONCLUSIONS

Diagnostic sialoendoscopy is a new, minimally invasive technique, which may become the investigational procedure of choice for salivary duct pathologies. Further miniaturization of the instruments will allow deeper ductal exploration.

Interventional sialoendoscopy under local anesthesia is a new outpatient procedure, allowing stone extraction in most sialolithiasis cases and therefore preventing salivary gland excisions. Further miniaturization of the equipment will allow fragmentation of bigger stones and extraction of deeper located stones.

## REFERENCES

1. Katz P. Nouvelle therapeutique des lithiases salivaires. *Inf Dent* 1991;73:3975–3979.
2. Gundlach P, Scherer H, Hopf J, et al. Die endoskopisch kontrollierte Laserlithotripsie von Speichelsteinen. In-vitro Untersuchungen und erster klinischer Einsatz. *HNO* 1990;38:247–250.
3. Kelly I, Dick R. Technical report: interventional sialography: Dormia basket removal of Wharton's duct calculus. *Clin Radiol* 1990;43:205.
4. Sharma RK, Al Khalifa S, Paulose KO, et al. Parotid duct stone removal by a Dormia basket. *J Laryngol Otol* 1994;108:699–701.
5. Marchal F, Becker M, Vavrina J, et al. Diagnostic et traitement des sialolithiases. *Bull Med Suisses* 1997;79:1023–1027.
6. Nahlieli O, Baruchin AM. Sialoendoscopy: three years' experience as a diagnostic and treatment modality. *J Oral Maxillofac Surg* 1997;55:912–918.
7. Becker M, Marchal F, Becker CD, et al. Sialolithiasis and salivary duct stenosis: diagnostic accuracy of MR-sialography with a 3-D extended-phase conjugate-symmetry rapid spin echo sequence. *Radiology* 2000;217:347–358.
8. Marchal F, Becker M, Dulguerov P, et al. Prospective evaluation of the accuracy of ultrasound in the detection of sialolithiasis. *Eur Radiol* (submitted).
9. Rauch S. *Die Speicheldrüsen des Menschen*. Stuttgart: Thieme Verlag, 1959.
10. Weissmann GM. Imaging of the salivary glands. *Semin Ultrasound CT MR* 1995;16:546–562.
11. Fergusson DB. The physiology and biology of saliva. In: Norman J, McGurk M, eds. *Color atlas and text of the salivary glands*. London: Masby-Wolfe, 1995:40–57.
12. Goh YH, Sethi DS. Submandibular gland excision: a five-year review. *J Laryngol Otol* 1998;112:269–273.
13. Hald J, Koks Andreassen U. Submandibular gland excision: short- and long-term complications. *ORL J Otorhinolaryngol Relat Spec* 1994;56:87–91.
14. Dulguerov P, Marchal F, Lehmann W. Postparotidectomy facial nerve paralysis: possible etiologic factors and results with routine nerve monitoring. *Laryngoscope* 1999;109:754–762.
15. Bron LP, O'Brien CJ. Facial nerve function after parotidectomy. *Arch Otolaryngol Head Neck Surg* 1997;123:1091–1096.
16. Marchal F, Kurt AM, Dulguerov P, et al. Histopathology of submandibular glands removed for sialolithiasis. *Ann Otol Rhinol Laryngol* 2001;110:464–469.
17. Iro H, Waitz G, Nitsche N, et al. Extracorporeal piezoelectric shock-wave lithotripsy of salivary gland stones. *Laryngoscope* 1992;102:492–494.
18. Brown AL, Shephard D, Buckenham TM. Per oral balloon sialoplasty: results in the treatment of salivary duct stenosis. *Cardiovasc Intervent Radiol* 1997;20:337–342.
19. Schratter M, Steiner E, Imhof H. Konventionelle Rontgendiagnostik der Speicheldrusen. Immer noch klinischer Stellenwert oder "Traditionspflege"? *Radiologe* 1994;34:248–253.
20. Pfeiffer K. Present status and place of sialography. *Radiologe* 1987;27:248–254.
21. Cockrell DG, Rout P. Adverse reactions following sialography. *Dentomaxillofac Radiol* 1993;22:41–42.
22. Avrahami E, Englender M, Chen E, et al. CT of submandibular gland sialolithiasis. *Neuroradiology* 1996;38:287–290.
23. Konigsberger R, Feyh J, Goetz A, et al. Endoscopically controlled

electrohydraulic intracorporeal shock wave lithotripsy (EISL) of salivary stones. *J Otolaryngol* 1993;22:12–13.
24. Marchal F, Dulguerov P, Becker M, et al. Submandibular interventional sialoendoscopy: new procedures for ductal pathologies. *Ann Otol Rhinol Laryngol* (in press).
25. Iro H, Zenk J, Waldfahrer F, et al. Aktueller Stand minimal-invasiver Behandlungsverfahren bei der Sialolithiasis. *HNO* 1996;44:78–84.
26. Iro H, Benzel W, Gode U, et al. Pneumatische intra-korporale Lithotripsie von Speichelsteinen. In-vitro und tierexperimentelle Untersuchungen. *HNO* 1995;43:172–176.
27. Zenk J, Hosenmann WG, Iro H. Diameters of the main excretory ducts of adult human submandibular and parotid gland: a histologic study. *Oral Surg Oral Med Oral Pathol Oral Radiol Endod* 1998;85:576–580.

SECTION V

# LARYNGOLOGY AND BRONCHOESOPHAGOLOGY

# 39

# HISTORY OF MINIMALLY INVASIVE SURGERY OF THE LARYNX

STEVEN M. ZEITELS

The development of minimally invasive surgery of the larynx has been an evolutionary process that can be traced to the first attempts at mirror visualization of the larynx at the beginning of the nineteenth century. Over the 50 years after Garcia's popularization of the technique (1855), the instrumentation and the procedures for indirect laryngoscopy were improved until mirror-guided surgical manipulation of the larynx became commonplace. The origin of the field of laryngology was facilitated by laryngeal visualization and transoral laryngeal surgery. Mirror laryngoscopy provided a means to understand and treat vocal pathology. More importantly, laryngoscopy allowed visually controlled surgical interventions to alleviate airway obstruction that occurred as a result of infectious membranous laryngeal disease, a formidable problem in the nineteenth and early twentieth centuries.

Transoral surgical interventions were frequently done during the first 25 years of laryngology. The subsequent controversy surrounding the case of Crown Prince Frederick's laryngeal cancer in the late nineteenth century dissuaded many surgeons from performing these procedures. From that case, myths were perpetuated suggesting that surgical disturbance of laryngeal tissue would induce infection, malignant transformation, and metastasis. This view influenced perceptions of the laryngeal biopsy well into the twentieth century. By the time that these myths had been dispelled, direct surgical laryngoscopy had for the most part replaced indirect surgical laryngoscopy. Through the twentieth century, there were a variety of technologic developments that improved direct examination of the larynx such as improved laryngoscopes, hand instruments, and lighting, as well as the surgical microscope, the carbon dioxide laser, and general endotracheal anesthesia. During the past two decades, we have gained a greater understanding of the physiology underlying vocal fold oscillation. These principles have been joined with the technologic developments of microlaryngeal surgery and have led to current concepts of phonomicrosurgery.

## ERA OF INDIRECT MIRROR LARYNGOSCOPY

Bozzini (Fig. 39.1) was the first individual (1807) to report on mirror visualization of the larynx (1). He designed an ingenious handle (Fig. 39.2) that housed a candle with a reflector as an artificial light source. A variety of specula could be attached to the universal handle for examining different body cavities, including one speculum that had a self-contained mirror for examining the larynx (2) (Fig. 39.2). Bozzini's brilliant concept of employing an extracorporeal light source to illuminate internal body cavities is a guiding premise for all minimally invasive endoscopic surgery.

Despite multiple descriptions of the use of mirror-laryngoscopy during the subsequent 50 years, these reports had little influence on the practice of medicine at the time (3–9). However, Babington's (5) glottiscope (Fig. 39.3) and Avery's (9) laryngoscope (Fig. 39.4) attracted significant academic interest over the years. The glottiscope was composed of a mirror and a spatula that retracted the tongue anteriorly. This introduced the concept of using internal distention for enhancing laryngeal exposure (10), a concept that was further developed by Killian and colleagues (11) in the twentieth century. Avery's laryngoscope was composed of a speculum that was similar to Bozzini's and was used with artificial illumination, which was provided by a candle that was attached to a perforated concave head mirror (i.e., a headlight).

In 1855, Manuel Garcia (Fig. 39.5), the renowned classical vocal pedagogist, presented his investigations with mirror autolaryngoscopy to the Royal Society of London. In that paper, "Observations on the Human Voice" (12), Garcia made substantive contributions to the understanding of voice production. Medical historians have deduced that Garcia was unaware of the previous descriptions of mirror laryngoscopy because of his limited medical background (13,14). His independent discovery of mirror laryngoscopy stimulated new interest within the medical community in the application of this technique for the management of laryngeal disease. Unlike his medical predecessors, Garcia

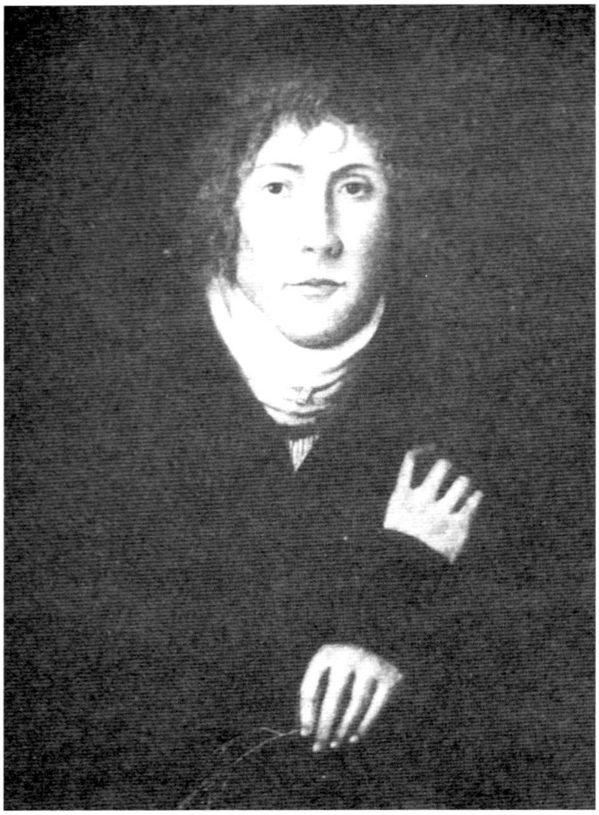

**FIGURE 39.1.** Philipp Bozzini: self-portrait (1773–1809). (From Reuter HJ, Reuter MA. *Philipp Bozzini and endoscopy in the 19th century*. Stuttgart: Max Nitze Museum, 1988.)

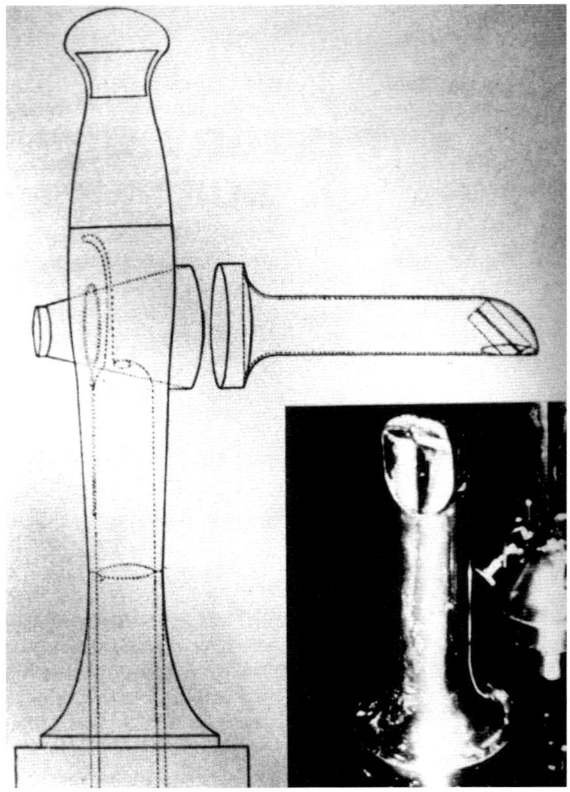

**FIGURE 39.2.** Bozzini's Lichtleiter (1807). (Courtesy of the American College of Surgeons, Chicago, IL.)

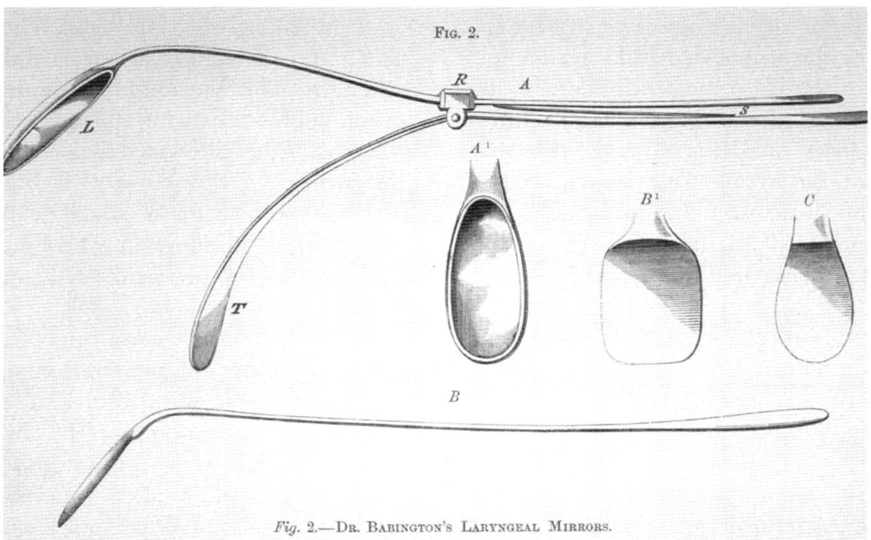


**FIGURE 39.3.** Benjamin Guy Babington's (1794–1866) glottiscope (1829). (From Mackenzie M. *The use of the laryngoscope in diseases of the throat with an appendix on rhinoscopy*. London: J&A Churchill, 1865.)

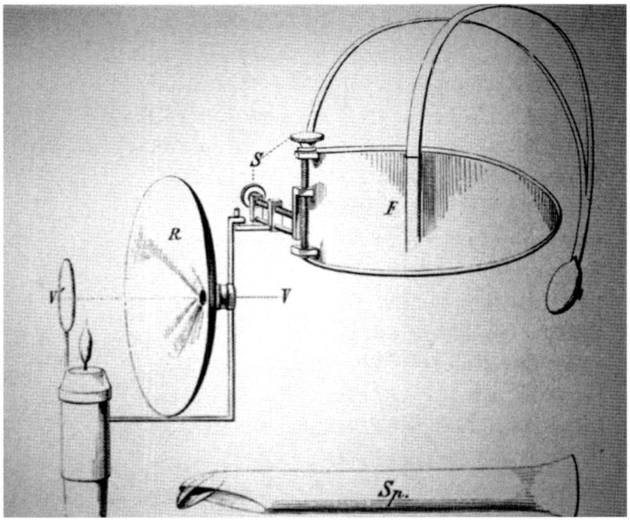


**FIGURE 39.4.** John Avery's (1807–1855) laryngoscope (1844). (From Mackenzie M. *The use of the laryngoscope in diseases of the throat with an appendix on rhinoscopy*. London: J&A Churchill, 1865.)

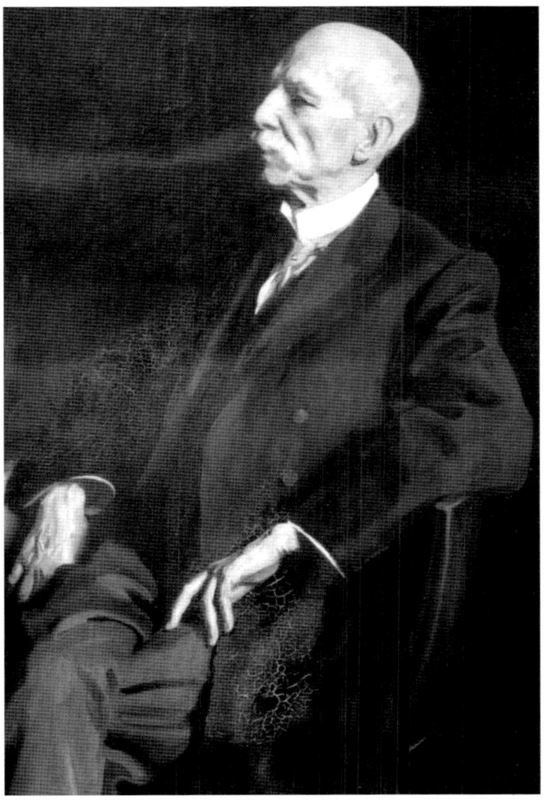

**FIGURE 39.5.** Manuel Garcia (1805–1906) at the age of 100: portrait by John Singer Sargent. (Courtesy of the Rhode Island School of Design, Providence, RI.)

primarily described what he learned about voice production from mirror laryngoscopy rather than emphasizing the instrumentation. It is believed that this was the key to the origin of laryngology (14).

## ORIGIN OF LARYNGOLOGY

Turck (15) was the first physician after Garcia's presentation to adopt mirror laryngoscopy. Depending on sunlight for illumination, he became frustrated during the cloudy autumn in Budapest and abandoned the technique. Shortly thereafter, his colleague Czermak (Fig. 39.6) borrowed the same mirrors, was more successful with their use, and reported those successes in 1858 (16,17). Czermak reintroduced the use of artificial light in conjunction with the fenestrated concave mirror (initially stabilized between his teeth), which greatly facilitated the technique. Turck also resumed his investigations. Ultimately, a rivalry developed between the two about who should receive academic recognition for introducing the broad application of mirror laryngoscopy to the mainstream of Western medicine. The rivalry stimulated much attention within and outside of the medical community, which helped stimulate interest in the fledgling field of laryngology. Czermak is recognized as influential in fostering mirror laryngoscopy and the field of laryngology in the medical community because of the innovations (i.e., artificial light and the fenestrated mirror) that he introduced (14).

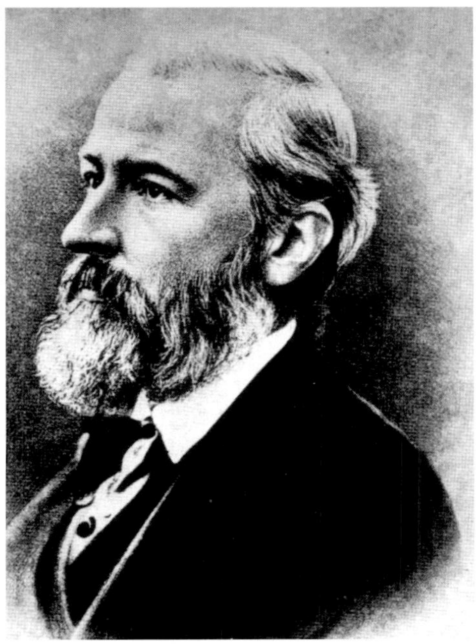

**FIGURE 39.6.** Johann Nepomuk Czermak (1828–1873).

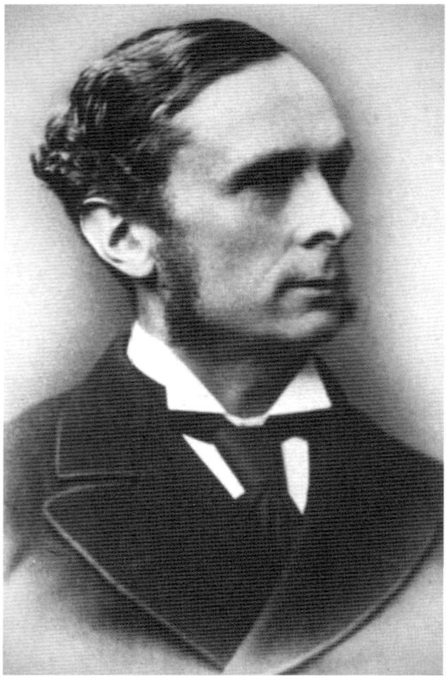

**FIGURE 39.7.** Sir Morell Mackenzie (1837–1892).

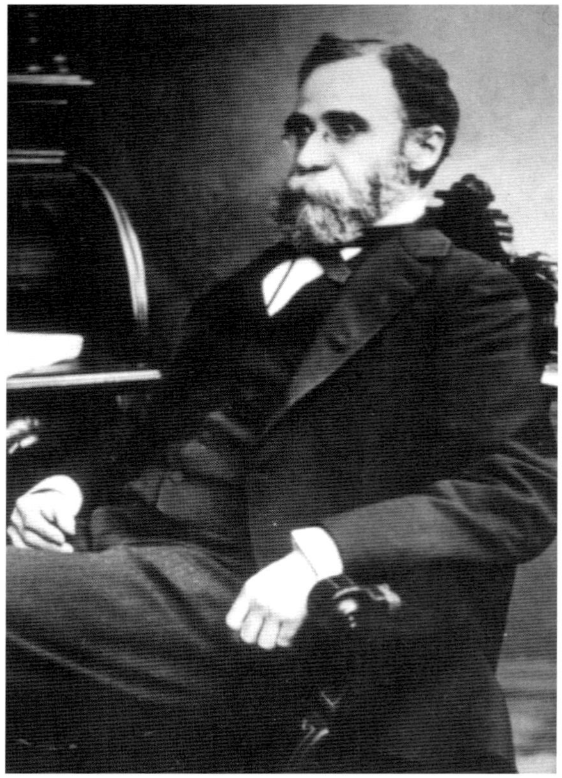

**FIGURE 39.9.** Jacob Solis-Cohen: 2nd president of the American Laryngological Association. (Courtesy of the Philadelphia College of Physicians.)

The ability to see the larynx well was catalytic for making transoral mirror-guided surgical manipulation (18) reliable and effective. Lewin (19) described the transoral management of 50 tumors in 1861. In addition to obtaining tissue for biopsy purposes, he excised three neoplasms and applied caustics to four. Mackenzie (Fig. 39.7) in Britain (20–22) and Elsberg (Fig. 39.8) in America (23,24) were key figures in improving laryngoscopic surgery and disseminating the techniques through their teachings (25). In the United States, Elsberg and, later, Solis-Cohen (Fig. 39.9) expended great effort as educators of laryngoscopy and laryngology, becoming the first and second presidents of the American Laryngological Association (14,25–27). Having served as a general surgeon during the American Civil War, Solis-Cohen was probably the first specialized head and neck surgeon. Throughout his career, he stressed that optimal management of the upper aerodigestive tract required transoral (minimally invasive) and transcervical (open) surgical skills (28).

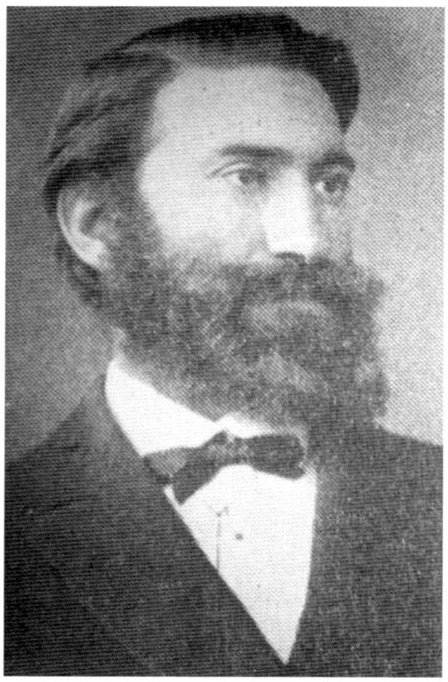

**FIGURE 39.8.** Louis Elsberg (1837–1885): first president of the American Laryngological Association.

## TRANSORAL MANAGEMENT OF LARYNX CANCER AND CROWN PRINCE FREDERICK

In Germany, Fraenkel (Fig. 39.10)was the first to report (1886) the successful transoral resection of a vocal cord cancer (29). In that article, he described performing multiple transoral excisions of recurrences in the larynx and doing a modified neck dissection, which included the removal of a

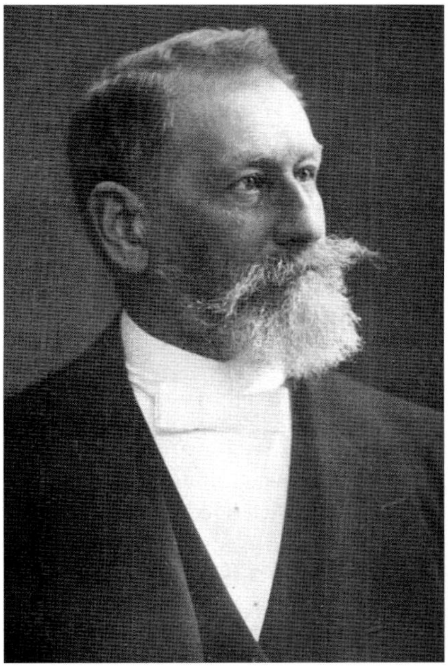

**FIGURE 39.10.** Bernhard Fraenkel (1836–1911). (From *Ann Otol Rhinol Laryngol* 15:606, with permission.)

5-cm segment of the internal jugular vein. At the time of Fraenkel's publication, more than 5 years had passed since the patient first presented with his cancer and 2 years had elapsed without a recurrence.

In that paper, Fraenkel delineated several of the current principles of laryngoscopic management of early vocal fold cancer. He observed that early vocal fold cancer was likely to arise on the superior vocal fold surface, to be small in volume, and to cause hoarseness with only minimal changes of the epithelium. The fortuitous origin of these lesions on the superior surface of the musculomembranous vocal fold makes them easily visible during laryngoscopy. Invasion at this location frequently spared the anterior commissure and the arytenoid and therefore facilitated endoscopic excision. After this publication, there were other isolated reports of the transoral removal of laryngeal cancer for cure (30–33); however, this approach did not gain significant support.

Shortly after the presentation of Fraenkel's innovative work, Crown Prince Frederick of Germany developed hoarseness, and after an initial examination, it was suspected that he had larynx cancer. Prince Frederick's primary physician insisted that there be a consulting laryngologist for the primary management. Fraenkel was practicing in Berlin, but Mackenzie was selected to be the consultant, in part because of his extensive writing on laryngology (34). The English laryngologist was summoned to Germany (35).

Based on a mirror examination, Mackenzie transorally biopsied abnormal vocal cord tissue three times during four attempts in 5 weeks (35). Virchow evaluated the specimens but could not establish the diagnosis of cancer (34,35). Mackenzie was not in favor of having the Prince undergo the perilous procedure of laryngectomy unless cancer could be documented in the specimens. Mackenzie held to this opinion despite the urging of the Prince's surgeons that he undergo the operation. The Prince had chosen Mackenzie as his primary consultant and therefore refused to have the laryngectomy. Ultimately, the Prince developed airway obstruction from the progressive growth of the clinically suspected, but pathologically undiagnosed, subglottic cancer. After a tracheotomy and further biopsies, the cancer diagnosis was established by Waldeyer (36).

Some felt that Virchow had purposely misdiagnosed the cancer because he was aware of Van Bergman's (the Prince's surgeon) abysmal survival statistics with total laryngectomy (37,38), which he had performed on seven prior occasions. The Prince did reign as the Emperor (Kaiser) for 3 months before succumbing to the disease. Had he undergone the laryngectomy, it is likely that he would not have lived to become the Kaiser.

A more likely thesis is that Virchow simply erred in the diagnosis (39). Despite creating the discipline of surgical pathology, Virchow believed that cancer arose from connective tissue and invaded toward the surface to create a mucosal irregularity. Contrary to this thesis, Waldeyer formulated the epithelial theory of carcinoma, which suggests that cancer evolves in the surface and invades into deep tissues. Waldeyer's concept is the foundation for the current theory of mucosal carcinogenesis, and because of this belief, he had little difficulty diagnosing cancer (39). Review of Virchow's detailed written accounts of the specimens that he had observed histologically from the original biopsies reveals that his descriptions are consistent with the diagnosis of cancer.

Apart from the personal and political tragedies that evolved from this unfortunate case, a damaging oncologic thesis evolved. Many believed that the Prince's cancer was precipitated by Mackenzie's biopsies. This idea, in conjunction with the international media attention attracted by the case, generated additional academic support for the thesis that a laryngeal biopsy could induce cancer (40,41) and gave rise to an exaggerated cancer phobia in many parts of the world. This concept could be extrapolated to other sites in the body.

Semon realized that the fear of transoral surgical manipulation would damage and potentially cripple the young field of laryngology. He reported an exhaustive series of more than 10,000 mirror-documented cases of laryngeal lesions (42,43). There were two groups. In one group, about 8,000 underwent biopsy, with histopathologically benign pathology found in most, and cancer ultimately diagnosed in 0.40% of the patients. In the other group, about 2,500 were observed without surgical manipulation, and 0.47% of the group developed cancer. There was no significant difference in the development of cancer between

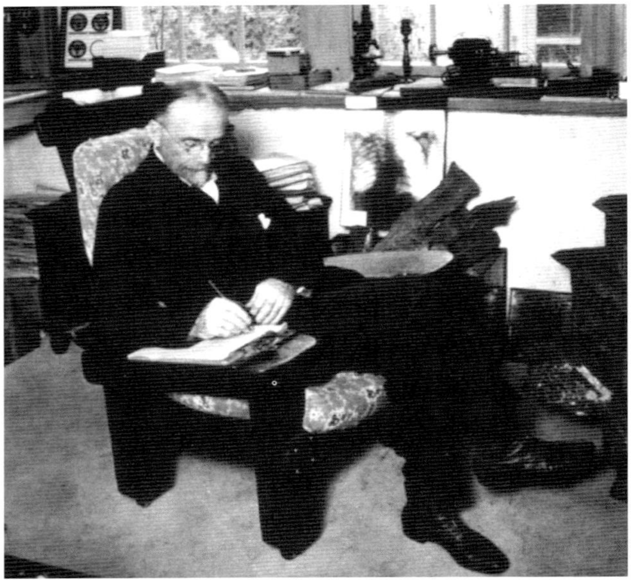

**FIGURE 39.11.** Chevalier Jackson (1865–1958). (Courtesy of the Massachusetts Eye and Ear Infirmary, Boston, MA.)

the two groups. This study was extremely helpful in clearing Mackenzie's reputation and securing the practice of laryngology for the future.

Despite the evidence in Semon's article, the controversy concerning the danger of the laryngeal biopsy persisted throughout the nineteenth century. Strong support for performing laryngeal biopsies to obtain a histopathologic diagnosis came from Butlin (44), Fraenkel (45), and Chiari (46), as well as from Solis-Cohen (47), who had previously expressed reservations about this approach. Nevertheless, misconceptions continued into the twentieth century that suggested that the laryngeal biopsy could induce infection at the biopsy site, malignant transformation of benign tissue, acceleration of cancer growth, and regional and distant metastases. Mackenzie (48,49), an American, was vehemently against the laryngeal biopsy and suggested that naked eye–mirror diagnosis should be followed by open cervical laryngectomy. Although this position was supported by Moore (50) and Mackenty (51) well into the 1920s, it did not take into account Delevan's work (52), which indicated that infectious diseases such as tuberculosis and syphilis could mimic carcinoma. Over time, based on diligent work by leaders such as Jackson (53) (Fig. 39.11), the myths surrounding the dangers of laryngeal biopsy were dispelled. This was critical to the twentieth century development of laryngology and direct surgical laryngoscopy.

## ERA OF DIRECT SURGICAL LARYNGOSCOPY

The transoral techniques used today for the management of the vocal fold evolved from the improvements that were made in direct surgical laryngoscopy. The first report of direct visualization of the laryngeal introitus was made by Horace Green (Fig. 39.12) in 1852 (54). He accomplished this by means of a bent tongue spatula (similar to an intubation spatula-blade laryngoscope) and sunlight. In his textbook, *On the Surgical Treatment of Polypi of the Larynx and Oedema of the Glottis*, Green described the visually controlled transoral excision of a polypoid mass from the ventricle region of an 11-year-old girl. The favorable elevated position that is characteristic of a child's larynx greatly facilitated the endoscopic excision of this laryngeal mass. Neither this work nor his reports of transoral application of caustics (55,56) to alleviate airway obstructive symptoms were considered credible at the time of their presentation (14,26,57). However, toward the end of Green's career, his work was broadly acknowledged (26). Seemingly unaware of Green's writings, Brunings, in his comprehensive textbook on rigid endoscopy, substantiated the concept that a bent tongue spatula could provide direct exposure of the larynx (58).

It was not until 1895, when Kirstein (Fig. 39.13) rediscovered direct examination of the larynx (59,60), that the modern era of direct surgical laryngoscopy began. Kirstein described tubular and spatula laryngoscopy, and all current laryngoscopes are derivatives of one of those designs. The design evolution of direct laryngoscopes is beyond the scope of this chapter and has been discussed elsewhere (61). Kirstein's success with the technique was facilitated by his use of the optimal head and neck position for laryngeal

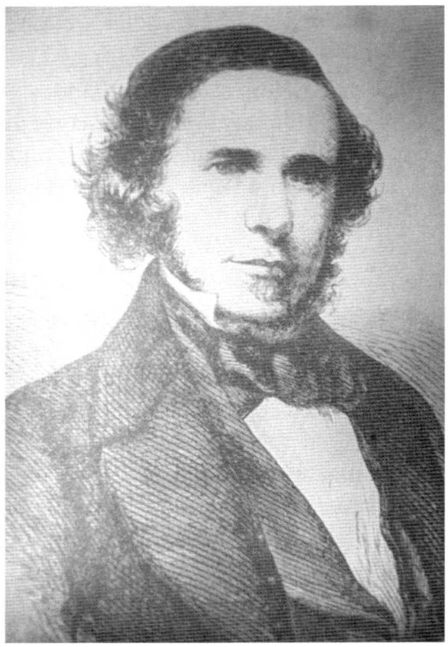

**FIGURE 39.12.** Horace Green (1802–1866): father of American Laryngology.

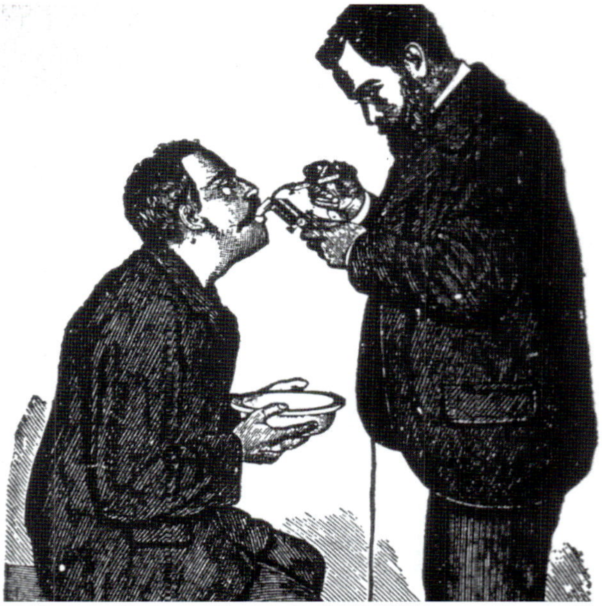

**FIGURE 39.13.** Alfred Kirstein (1863—1922). (From Jackson C. Position of the patient for peroral endoscopy. In: *Peroral endoscopy and laryngeal surgery*. St. Louis: Laryngoscope, 1915:82, with permission.)

exposure (62), his laryngoscope designs, and his use of artificial illumination in the form of a headlight. Unlike Green's earlier frustrating attempts at disseminating his technique, the widespread twentieth century adoption of direct laryngoscopy resulted from Kirstein's success in an era when interest was intense in the fledgling field of laryngology.

The primary principles for achieving and maintaining complete laryngeal exposure were developed during the 25-year period after Kirstein's presentation of direct laryngoscopy (10). These principles for exposure made effective transoral resection of laryngeal cancer possible. Several key reports promoted the development of these principles:

1. Boyce and Jackson adapted Kirstein's head and neck position for laryngeal exposure (Fig. 39.14) from sitting to supine for direct laryngoscopy (62–64).
2. Brunings (Fig. 39.15) introduced the concept of external laryngeal counterpressure (65,66).
3. Haslinger (11) described internal laryngeal distention by means of a bivalved speculum.
4. Killian (Fig. 39.14) introduced the inverted-V spatula blade to accommodate the anterior glottal commissure (66) and later joined this spatula to his suspension gallows, which freed the surgeons hands for bimanual laryngoscopic surgery (67–69).

Killian's (67–70) elaborate suspension gallows (Fig. 39.16) was an outgrowth of his 1909 cadaver studies in which the larynx was stabilized for anatomic illustration.

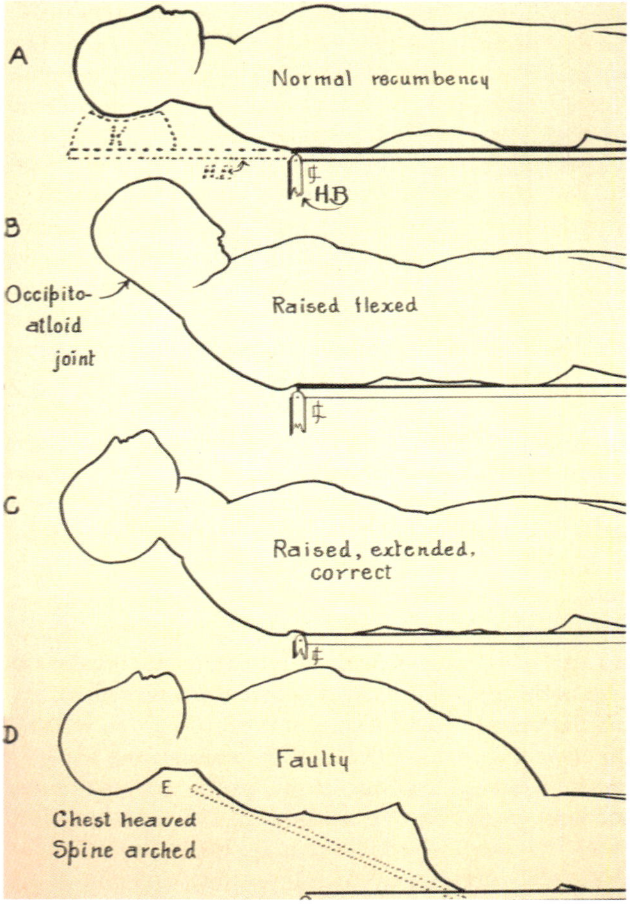


**FIGURE 39.14.** Jackson's drawings of different positions during supine direct laryngoscopy. (From Jackson C, ed. *Tracheobronchoscopy, esophagoscopy and gastroscopy. Laryngoscope,* 1907:90.)

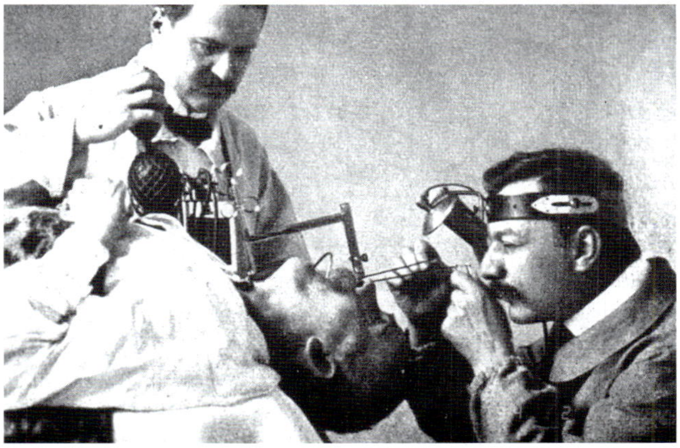

**FIGURE 39.15.** Wilhelm Brunings (1876–?). (From Brunings W. Direct laryngoscopy: criteria determining the applicability of autoscopy. In: *Direct laryngoscopy, bronchoscopy, and esophagoscopy*. London: Bailliere, Tindall, & Cox, 1912:121.)

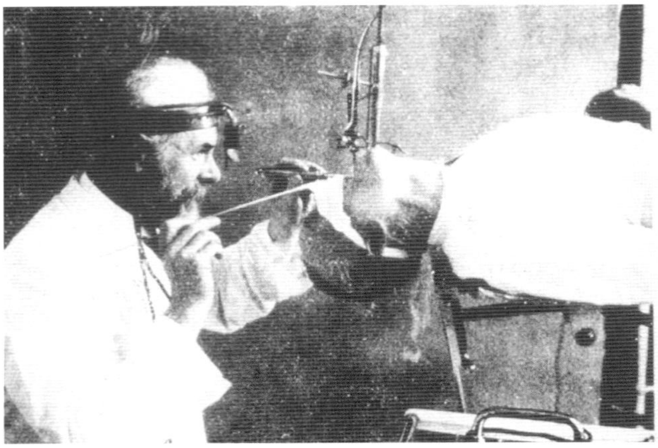

**FIGURE 39.16.** Gustav Killian (1860–1921) performing suspension laryngoscopy and applying manual external counterpressure.

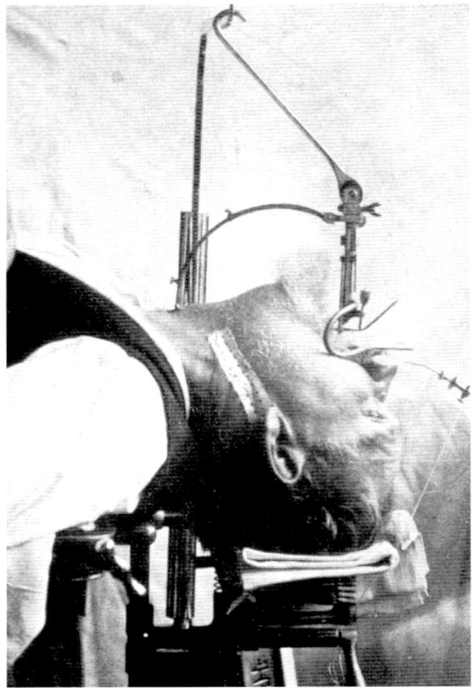

**FIGURE 39.17.** Killian's suspension laryngoscope with a retrofitted external counterpressure designed by his disciple, Brunings. (From Jackson C. Position of the patient for peroral endoscopy. In: *Peroral endoscopy and laryngeal surgery*. St. Louis: 1915:153 with permission; Courtesy of the Laryngoscope Corp.)

Jackson, inspired by Killian, authored the first textbook on rigid endoscopy and dedicated that work to Killian (71). Jackson went on to make many contributions to direct laryngoscopic method (72). In his monumental textbook, *Peroral Endoscopy and Laryngeal Surgery*, the only chapter not written by him was "Suspension Laryngoscopy" (68), which was authored by Killian. Observation of Killian working with his suspension gallows reveals that the patient is not in the Boyce-Jackson position but rather in a head-hanging extension position (Figs. 39.16 and 39.17). There was often inadequate anterior glottal exposure with the extended neck position during suspension laryngoscopy. Although exposure was improved by using Bruning's (65) extrinsic counterpressor devices to compress the lower larynx (Fig. 39.17), suspension devices that freed the surgeon's hands did not reliably expose the entire musculomembranous vocal fold.

Jackson was not in favor of using Killian's suspension technique, and there was little recognition or discussion of suspension devices or laryngoscope holders in his later textbooks (73–75). It is unclear why Jackson did not build a device that would stabilize the laryngoscope in the head and neck position that he and Boyce used. Suspension laryngoscopy done in the extended position often did not provide complete glottal exposure, but without a suspension device and two-handed tissue manipulation, successful excision of vocal fold neoplasms was not possible. Presumably, it was because of this set of conditions that Jackson did not pursue endoscopic excision of vocal fold cancer.

Lynch (76–78) furthered Killian's techniques of bimanual transoral laryngeal surgery and reported the first transoral en bloc excisions of vocal fold cancer in 1915. He designed a suspension-laryngoscope system that was a modification of Killian's. Although the modifications made it popular among some surgeons in the United States, there were disadvantages to both suspension-laryngoscope systems. General anesthesia was not used during laryngoscopic surgery and therefore mandated a high level of skill by the surgeon and the anesthesiologist. The suspension laryngoscopes did not have self-contained illumination.

About 1920, in an effort to overcome the difficulty in performing suspension laryngoscopy, Seiffert, a disciple of Killian, introduced the chest-support system (Fig. 39.18). Seiffert altered Killian's spatula suspension laryngoscope by rotating the distal arm, which initially hung on the gallows, until it was resting on the chest. This modification fundamentally transformed the suspension laryngoscope into a lever laryngoscope holder that exerted a torsion force on the upper teeth. Roberts (79,80) further modified this instrument and thoughtfully designed special pillows to support the head in the Boyce-Jackson position.

Jackson did not employ extrinsic devices to maintain his tubed laryngoscopes. In the 1950s, King (81), Sommers (82), and Lewy (83) designed holders (i.e., stabilizers) for Jackson-style laryngoscopes. They were constructed to follow the chest-support fulcrum principle. Little attention was given to laryngoscopic head position. These devices

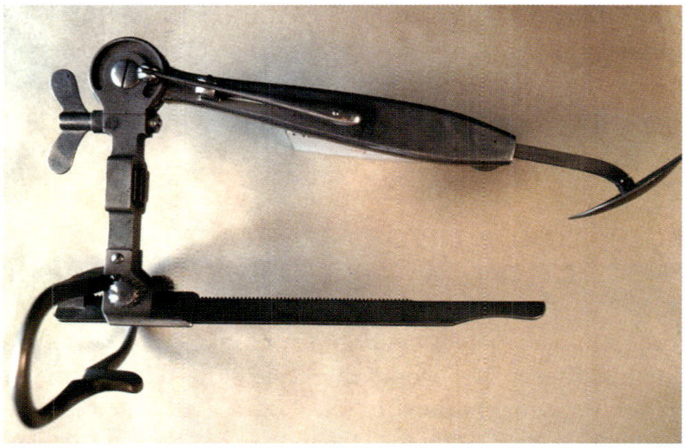

**FIGURE 39.18.** Seiffert's fulcrum chest-support spatula laryngoscope. (Courtesy of the Massachusetts Eye and Ear Infirmary, Boston, MA.)

employ a stable platform (i.e., chest wall or Mayo stand), an extension arm that creates a lever, and a fulcrum in which a torsion force is exerted on the maxilla, resulting in undesirable head and neck extension (84).

Fulcrum laryngoscope holders can precipitate iatrogenic injury because these devices produce extension forces on the neck. Cervical spine injury may occur in patients in whom degenerative kyphotic cervical fusion has occurred from osteoporosis (85). The surgeon is less aware of the force being generated and less sensitive to the resistance of a particular position because of the device's gear-power advantage. In the 1950s (86), further departure from Jackson's laryngoscopic principles was precipitated by the popularization of general endotracheal anesthesia with paralyzing agents. There was less need for orthodox laryngoscopic technique because of the use of small-lumen monocular laryngoscopes and the anesthetically induced increase in muscular compliance made possible by the neuromuscular paralyzing agents.

In 1971, Thomas (87) modified the Lewy laryngoscope holder by attaching it to a telescoping arm and an inverted U-shaped frame. His apparatus allowed for true mechanical laryngoscope stabilization in the Boyce-Jackson position. This position, in which the head and neck are lifted off the table, is referred to as elevated-vector suspension (Fig. 39.19) to distinguish it from Killian's head-hanging extension suspension. In 1975, as a modification of the Killian gallows, Grundfast and the Boston University group (88) developed an apparatus (Pilling Co., Fort Washington, PA) that also provided elevated-vector suspension (Fig. 39.19). The classic tubular laryngoscopes were fitted with extended handles to allow application of a force equal and opposite to that needed to expose the glottis; this eliminated rotation (levers) and worked in varied head and neck positions. The suspension gallows employed a simple window crank for its works.

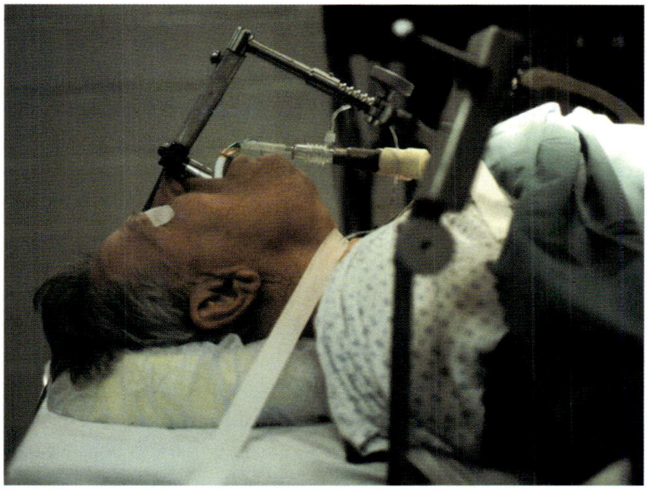

**FIGURE 39.19.** Elevated-vector suspension with the Boston University gallows and external laryngeal counterpressure facilitated by silk adhesive tape. (From Zeitels SM, Vaughan CW. "External counter-pressure" and "internal distention" for optimal laryngoscopic exposure of the anterior glottal commissure. *Ann Otol Rhinol Laryngol* 1994;103:669–675, with permission.)

## MICROLARYNGOSCOPY AND THE CARBON DIOXIDE LASER

A magnified view of the larynx was reported in 1895 by Oertel (89) in his description of the mirror-guided stroboscope. Brunings (90) also used a magnified ocular and was the first to employ magnification to enhance direct laryngoscopy. Haslinger designed a tubular laryngoscope with accompanying telescopic magnification. Kahler's panelectroscope (91) probably had magnification capabilities as well. In the early 1950s, Albrecht used a colposcope for magnified indirect vocal fold examination and for photodocumentation of keratosis. The first published report on the use of the surgical microscope during laryngoscopy was by Scalco and coworkers (92) in 1960; they employed the Lynch spatula suspension laryngoscope for the task. The surgical microscope was a monumental innovation for enhancing the precision of endolaryngeal surgery because it provided high-power magnification with a three-dimensional stereoscopic field.

Jako (93,94) in the United States and Kleinsasser (95,96) in Europe perfected surgical microlaryngoscopy. Jako (93) introduced the first set of microlaryngeal hand instruments, and Kleinsasser (96) introduced the 400-mm lens. The latter innovation increased the working distance between the microscope lens and the proximal lumen of the laryngoscope, which facilitated the placement of the long-shafted otologic instruments. Both surgeons designed wide-bore examining tubes to accommodate the optical characteristics of the surgical microscope. Strong (97,98) and DeSanto and colleagues (99) systematically discussed microlaryngeal surgery, which broadened its appeal in the United States.

Kleinsasser (96,100) designed his own hand instrumentation and established the foundations for cold-instrument microlaryngoscopic technique, which has recently enjoyed renewed enthusiasm as phonomicrosurgical procedures have increased in popularity (101–110). Today, most phonomicrosurgical procedures should be performed under 6× to 10× magnification to ensure for maximal preservation of the vocal folds' layered microstructure (i.e., laminae propria and epithelium) (110–114).

Jako (115), in cooperation with Polanyi (116), Strong (117), and Vaughan (118), went on to introduce the carbon dioxide ($CO_2$) laser (Fig. 39.20) to surgery by joining it to the surgical microscope. The $CO_2$ laser enhances cold instruments when the pathology is vascular or too large to be adequately retracted within the laryngoscope (110). The laser is a valuable component of the laryngologist's armamentarium (as an energy source to manipulate tissue), and its role will probably expand again in coming years with further breakthroughs in laser technology. The $CO_2$ laser provides excellent hemostasis as well as a stable delivery system (i.e., joystick and foot pedal) for those who have difficulty maintaining dexterity with their nondominant hand under high magnification (Strong MS, personal communication).

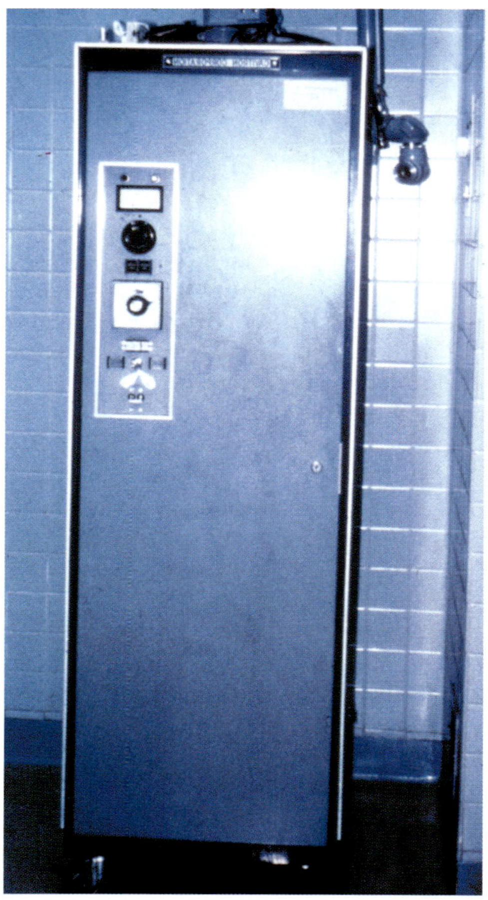

**FIGURE 39.20.** The original carbon dioxide laser. (Courtesy of S. M. Zeitels, Harvard Medical School, Boston, MA.)

## BODY-COVER THEORY OF VOICE PRODUCTION

Although a complete developmental history of voice production theory is beyond the scope of this chapter, the important contributions to the body-cover mucosal wave theory that have influenced phonomicrosurgical concepts are reviewed.

The body-cover mucosal wave theory of voice production was introduced by Bishop (119) in 1836 in his publication, *Experimental Researches into the Physiology of the Human Voice*. He stated, "The true vibrating surface of the glottis is the mucous membrane. The vocal cords confer on it the tension, resistance, position, and probably other conditions necessary for vibration." This outstanding and insightful contribution was made without the use of the mirror laryngoscope or the stroboscope; he was therefore unable to see the moving glottis.

In 1866, in his comprehensive textbook on voice, Fournie also concluded that the vocal fold mucosa was the major component of the glottal vibration.

> "The voice is a sound produced by a particular reed having walls modifiable under the influence of muscular action; the vibrating part being furnished by the mucous fold which limits the borders of the glottis. The vibrations are occasioned by the passage of air through the glottis. . . . For the membranes to vibrate, one tenses them on a frame like the skin of a drum, and they will emit their vibrations transmitting them through the air. They produce a more high pitch shrill sound according to how small and how taut they are" (120).

Hirano (102,103,121) further developed the body-cover theory of voice production by assimilating information from stroboscopy, gross anatomic evaluations, and his elegant scanning electron microscopic evaluation of the vocal fold's layered anatomy. These studies of the microanatomy of the vocal fold reveal that there is a cover (i.e., epithelium, superficial lamina propria), a transition zone (i.e., vocal ligament: medial lamina propria and deep lamina propria), and a body (i.e., muscle). The superficial lamina propria is composed of an amorphous substance with few fibroblasts and allows maximal epithelial pliability for transmission of a vibrational wave (103). It abates anteriorly as the vocal ligament and mucosa fuse with the anterior commissure tendon, and it disappears posteriorly as the vocal ligament and mucosa join the vocal process of the arytenoid. The medial lamina propria is composed primarily of elastic fibers, and the deep lamina propria is composed primarily of collagen fibers.

Precision during dissection within the superficial lamina propria has been improved by the technique of infusing saline and epinephrine into the ligament of the vocal fold (101,122,123). The infusion acts in a number of ways, including vasoconstricting the microvasculature in the superficial lamina propria, which improves visualization during cold-instrument tangential dissection. The technique was based on experiments by Hajek (124), Reinke (125,126), and Pressman (127,128). By using the subepithelial infusion technique, atypical vocal fold epithelium and selected early cancers can be resected transorally, and the patient will have a normal postoperative voice at conversational levels as analyzed by objective acoustic and aerodynamic measures (101).

Aerodynamic principles of the mucosal wave theory were discussed by Garcia in 1855. From his experiments in laryngoscopy, he described the rhythmic release of air by the vocal folds into the supraglottal vocal tract. "The voice is formed by the periodical compressions and dilations which the air experiences when, on reaching the glottis, the latter, by alternate and regular movements, stops or permits its exit" (12).

The visualization of the oscillating vocal fold was facilitated by the laryngeal stroboscope and was reported by Oertel (89,129) in 1878. In essence, a motorized, perforated pinwheel disk (Fig. 39.21) was placed between the artificial light source and the examiner's head mirror. Varying the speed of revolution of the disk allowed rhythmic interruption of the light that was transmitted from the head mirror to the laryngeal mirror. This provided the effect of slow-motion visualization of the vocal fold.

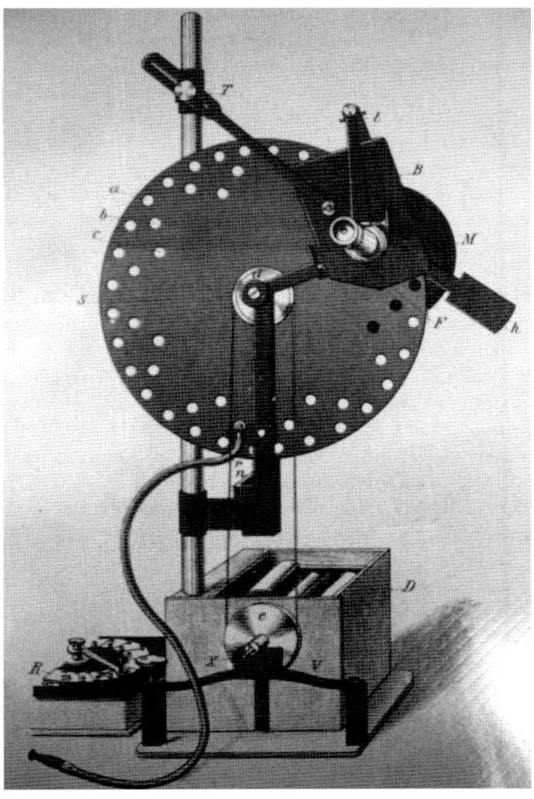

**FIGURE 39.21.** Certel's laryngostroboscope. (From *Arch Laryngol Rhinol* 2:3.)

The device initially did not gain popularity or acceptance (130) because it was necessary to train the patient to duplicate and maintain a specific pitch that was coordinated with the speed of the rotating disk and because the instrument generated considerable objectionable background noise. Whereas in Europe, speech and voice studies were frequently carried out within otolaryngology departments, in North America, these disciplines were independent and had only limited collaboration with each other (131). As a result, few laryngostroboscopic investigations (130–137) were done in North America throughout much of the twentieth century. The current increase in the number of American multidisciplinary voice and laryngologic studies emanating from centers suggests that this trend has changed.

## CONCLUSIONS

Endolaryngeal surgery, which was done through a natural passage, is one of the earliest forms of minimally invasive surgery and is fundamentally rooted in the historical development of improved visualization and surgical manipulation of the larynx. All substantive innovations in the procedures led to improved precision and continue to do so today. This rich history has served as a model for other surgical sites. There are financial rewards available to companies for the development of instrument technology for use in other minimally invasive surgical paradigms. This promise is stimulating improvements in laryngeal instrumentation, which should prove to be a major area of innovation in the first decade of the twenty-first century. The ongoing development of more successful phonomicrosurgical procedures will be driven by the interdependence among surgical technique theory, concepts of vocal fold oscillation, and principles underlying voice production.

We live in a communication-based society in which the human voice is a fundamental component of most jobs. This has led to increasing numbers of professional voice users and to more pathology. Minimally invasive surgery of the larynx has an extremely rich heritage and an exciting future.

## REFERENCES

1. Bozzini P. *Der Lichtleiter oder Beschreibung einer einfachen Vorichtung, und ihrer Anwendung zur erleucht ung inherer Hohlen, und Zwischenraume des lebenden animaschen Korpers.* Weimar, 1807.

2. Reuter HJ, Reuter MA. *Philipp Bozzini and endoscopy in the 19th century*. Stuttgart: Max Nitze Museum, 1988.
3. Cagniard de Latour C. Cited by Fournie. *Physiologie de la voix*. Journal l'Institut, 1825:350.
4. Senn. Cited by Mackenzie M. *The use of the laryngoscope in diseases of the throat*. London: J&A Churchill, 1829:11.
5. Babington BG. *London Medical Gazette* 1829;3:555.
6. Selligue. Cited by Mackenzie M. *The use of the laryngoscope in diseases of the throat*. London: J&A Churchill, 1832:17.
7. Liston R. *Practical surgery*. London: J&A Churchill, 1837.
8. Baumes. *Compte rendu des travaux de la Societe de Medecine de Lyons*. 1836–1838;19:18.
9. Avery. Cited by Mackenzie M. *The use of the laryngoscope in diseases of the throat*. London: J&A Churchill, 1844:25.
10. Zeitels SM, Vaughan CW. "External counter-pressure" and "internal distension" for optimal laryngoscopic exposure of the anterior glottal commissure. *Ann Otol Rhinol Laryngol* 1994; 103:669–675.
11. Israel S. The directoscope of Haslinger in diagnosis and surgery of the larynx. *Laryngoscope* 1923;33:945–948.
12. Garcia M. Observations on the human voice. *Proc R S Lond* 1855;7:397–410,.
13. Wright J. The laryngoscope: Manuel Garcia. In: *A history of laryngology and rhinology*, 2nd ed. Philadelphia : Lea & Febiger, 1914: 207.
14. Clerf LH. Manuel Garcia's contribution to laryngology. *Bull N Y Acad Med* 1956;32:603–611.
15. Turck L. On the laryngeal mirror and its mode of employment, with engravings on wood. *Z Gesellschaft Aerzte Wien* 1858;26: 401–409.
16. Czermak JN. Ueber den Kehlkopfspiegel. *Wien Med Wochenschr*, 1858;8:196–198.
17. Czermak JN. On the laryngoscope and its employment in physiology and medicine. *N Sydenham Soc* 1861;11:1–79.
18. Stoerk C. On the laryngoscope. *Z Gesellschaft Aerzte Wein* 1859; 46:721–727.
19. Lewin G. *Allgemeine Medizinische Zentral Zeitung* 1861;30:654.
20. Mackenzie M. *The use of the laryngoscope in diseases of the throat with an appendix on rhinoscopy*. London: J&A Churchill, 1865.
21. Mackenzie M. *Growths in the larynx*. London: J&A Churchill, 1871.
22. Mackenzie M. The laryngoscope and its accessory apparatus; laryngoscopy; autolaryngoscopy; infra-glottic laryngoscopy; the laryngoscope image; laryngeal instruments; dilators of the larynx. In: *Diseases of the pharynx, larynx, and trachea*. New York: William Wood, 1880:158–195.
23. Elsberg L. *Laryngoscopal medication or the local treatment of the diseases of the throat, larynx, and neighboring organs, under sight*. New York: William Wood, 1864.
24. Elsberg L. *Laryngoscopal surgery illustrated in the treatment of morbid growths within the larynx*. Philadelphia: Collins, 1866.
25. Elsberg L. President's address: laryngological instruction. *Trans Am Laryngol Assoc* 1880;2:4–8.
26. Elsberg L. President's address: laryngology in America. *Trans Am Laryngol Assoc* 1879;1:30–90.
27. Solis-Cohen J. President's address. *Trans Am Laryngol Assoc* 1881;3:2–4.
28. Zeitels SM. Jacob Da Silva Solis-Cohen: America's first head and neck surgeon. *Head Neck* 1997;19:342–346.
29. Fraenkel B. First healing of a laryngeal cancer taken out through the natural passages. *Arch Klin Chir* 1886;12:283–286.
30. Arslan A. Emorragia laringes. *Arch Ital* 1901;11:390–411.
31. Ingals EF. Nonrecurrent carcinoma of the larynx removed from the natural passages. *Laryngoscope* 1907;17:370–372.
32. Sendziac J. Treatment of cancer of the larynx. *N Y Med J* 1907; 86:1042.
33. Thompson SC. Intrinsic cancer of the larynx-complete excision apparently effected by the endo-laryngeal operation. *Trans Am Laryngol Assoc* 1914;36:34–44.
34. Gerhardt. Report of Dr. Gerhardt. In: *Case of Emperor Frederick III: full official reports by the German physicians and by Sir Morell Mackenzie*. New York: Edgar S. Werner, 1888:1–16.
35. Mackenzie M. The fatal illness of Frederick the noble. London: Sampson, Low, Marston, Searle & Rivington, 1888.
36. Waldeyer. Report of Dr. Waldeyer. In: *Case of Emperor Frederick III: full official reports by the German physicians and by Sir Morell Mackenzie*. New York: Edgar S. Werner, 1888:72–75.
37. Delavan DB. A consideration of the statistics of the operations for the relief of malignant disease of the larynx. *Trans Am Laryngol Assoc* 1900;22:66–74.
38. Delavan DB. *A history of thyrotomy and laryngectomy. Transactions of a commemorative meeting in the honour of Dr. John Edmund Mackenty held by the section of otolaryngology*. New York: New York Academy of Medicine, 1932.
39. Lin JI. Virchow's pathological reports on Frederick III's cancer. *N Engl J Med* 1984;311:1261–1264.
40. Browne L. The throat and its diseases. Philadelphia: Lea & Febiger, 1878.
41. Solis-Cohen J. Cited by Wright J. *A history of laryngology and rhinology*. Philadelphia, PA: 1881:330.
42. Semon F. Bezuglich des Ueberganges gutartiger Kehlkopfgeschwulste i bosartige nach intralaryngealen Operatienen [In reference to transition of benign laryngeal tumors to malignant lesions post laryngeal surgery]. *Int Zentralb Laryngol Rhinol* 1888;4:245–246.
43. Semon F. Die Frage de ueberganges gutatiger Kehlkopf-Geschwulster in bosartige, speciell nach intralaryngealen Operation. *Int Zentralb Laryngol Rhinol* 1889;4:271–279.
44. Butlin HT. *Malignant disease (sarcoma and carcinoma) of the larynx*. London: J&A Churchill, 1883.
45. Fraenkel B. The anatomopathologic diagnosis of cancer of the larynx. *Ann Otol Rhinol Laryngol* 1900;9:276.
46. Chiari O. Contributions to the diagnosis and treatment of laryngeal cancer. *Ann Otol Rhinol Laryngol* 1898;7:572–580.
47. Solis-Cohen J. The surgical treatment of laryngeal cancer. *Trans Am Laryngol Assoc* 1901;22:75–87.
48. Mackenzie J. A plea for early naked-eye diagnosis and removal of the entire organ, with the neighboring area of possible lymphatic infection in cancer of the larynx. *Trans Am Laryngol Assoc* 1900;22:56–65.
49. Mackenzie J. Remarks of the macroscopic diagnosis and general indications for treatment of cancer of the larynx. *Ann Otol Rhinol Laryngol* 1906;15:61–72.
50. Moore I. Diagnosis of intrinsic cancer of the larynx. In: *Intrinsic cancer of the larynx and the operation of laryngofissure*. London; University of London Press, 1921:13–17.
51. Mackenty J. Laryngectomy for cancer, with remarks on seventy operated cases. *Trans Am Laryngol Assoc* 1922;44:205–223.
52. Delevan DB. Recent advances in the treatment of malignant disease of the larynx. *Trans Am Laryngol Assoc* 1904;26: 150–170.
53. Jackson C, Jackson CL. A history of the laryngeal biopsy. In: *Cancer of the larynx*. Philadelphia: WB Saunders, 1939:231–240.
54. Green H. Morbid growths within the larynx. New York: GP Putnam, 1852.
55. Green H. On the subject of the priority in the medication of the larynx and trachea. *Am Med Month* 1854;1:241–257.
56. Green H. Report on the use and effect of applications of nitrate silver to the throat, either in local or general disease. *Trans Am Med Assoc* 1856;9:493–530.
57. Donaldson F. The Laryngology of Trousseau and Horace Green. *Trans Am Laryngol Assoc* 1890;12:10–18.

58. Brunings W. Direct laryngoscopy: criteria determining the applicability of autoscopy. In: *Direct laryngoscopy, bronchoscopy, and esophagoscopy*. London: Bailliere, Tindall, & Cox, 1912: 93–95.
59. Kirstein A. Autoskopie des Larynx und der Trachea (Laryngoscopia directa, Euthyskopie, Besichtigung ohne Spiegel). *Arch Laryngol Rhinol* 1895;3:156–164.
60. Kirstein A. *Autoscopy of the larynx and trachea (direct examination without mirror)*. Philadelphia: FA Davis, 1897.
61. Zeitels SM. A universal modular glottiscope system: the evolution of a century of design and technique for direct laryngoscopy. *Ann Otol Rhinol Laryngol Suppl* 1999;179:2–24.
62. Jackson C. Position of the patient for peroral endoscopy. In: *Peroral endoscopy and laryngeal surgery*. St. Louis: Laryngoscope, 1915:77–88
63. Boyce JW. Duties of the second assistant in endoscopy per os. In: Jackson C, ed. *Tracheobronchoscopy, esophagoscopy and gastroscopy*. St. Louis: Laryngoscope, 1907:145–147.
64. Jackson C, Jackson CL. The early diagnosis of cancer of the larynx: position of the patient for direct laryngoscopy. In: *Cancer of the larynx*. Philadelphia: WB Saunders, 1939:17–18.
65. Brunings W. Direct laryngoscopy: autoscopy by counter-pressure. In: *Direct laryngoscopy, bronchoscopy, and esophagoscopy*. London: Bailliere, Tindall, & Cox, 1912:110–115.
66. Killian G. Demonstration of an endoscopic spatula. *J Laryngol Rhinol* 1910;25:549–550.
67. Killian G. Die Schwebelaryngoskopie. *Arch Laryngol Rhinol* 1912;26:277–317.
68. Killian G. Suspension laryngoscopy. In: Jackson C, ed. *Peroral endoscopy and laryngeal surgery*. St. Louis: Laryngoscope, 1915: 133–154.
69. Killian G. *Die Schwebelaryngoskopie und ihre praktische Verwertung*. Wien: Urban & Schwarzenberg, 1920.
70. Killian G. Suspension laryngoscopy and its practical use. *J Laryngol Otol* 914;24:337–360.
71. Jackson C. *Tracheo-bronchoscopy, esophagoscopy and gastroscopy*. St. Louis: Laryngoscope, 1907.
72. Zeitels SM. Chevalier Jackson's contributions to direct laryngoscopy. *J Voice* 1998;12:1–6.
73. Jackson C, Jackson CL. Chronic laryngitis, benign tumors of the larynx. In: *The larynx and its diseases*. Philadelphia: WB Saunders, 1937:136–151, 315–342.
74. Jackson C, Jackson CL. *Cancer of the larynx*. Philadelphia: WB Saunders, 1939.
75. LeJeune FE. Suspension laryngoscopy. In: Jackson C, Jackson CL, eds. *Diseases of the nose, throat and ear*. Philadelphia: WB Saunders, 1945:178–180.
76. Lynch RC. Suspension laryngoscopy and its accomplishments. *Ann Otol Rhinol Laryngol* 1915;24:429–446.
77. Lynch RC. A resume of my years' work with suspension laryngoscopy. *Trans Am Laryngol Assoc* 1916;38:158–175.
78. Lynch RC. Intrinsic carcinoma of the larynx, with a second report of the cases operated on by suspension and dissection. *Trans Am Laryngol Assoc* 1920;40:119–126.
79. Roberts SE, Forman FS. Direct laryngoscopy—a simplified technique: an aid to the early detection of laryngeal cancer. *Ann Otol Rhinol Laryngol* 1948;57:245–256.
80. Roberts SE. A self retaining dual distal lighted laryngoscope with screw driven fulcrum lift. *Laryngoscope* 1952;62:215–221.
81. King NE. Direct laryngoscopy aided by a new laryngoscope "stabilizer." *Arch Otolaryngol* 1951;53:89–92.
82. Sommers KE. Direct laryngoscopy and description of a self-retaining attachment for the laryngoscope. *Arch Otolaryngol* 1952;55:484–488.
83. Lewy RE. Suspension fixation gear power laryngoscopy (with motion pictures). *Laryngoscope* 1954;64:693–695.
84. Vaughan CW. Vocal fold exposure in phonosurgery. *J Voice* 1993;7:189–194.
85. Netter FH. Osteoporosis. In: *The Ciba collection of medical illustrations: musculoskeletal system*. Summit, NJ: Ciba-Geigy, 1987: 216–227.
86. Priest RE, Wesolowski S. Direct laryngoscopy under general anesthesia. *Trans Am Acad Ophthalmol Otolaryngol* 1960;64: 639–648.
87. Thomas GK. Suspension apparatus for laryngeal microsurgery. *Arch Otolaryngol* 1971;94:258–259.
88. Grundfast KM, Vaughan CW, Strong MS, De Vos P. Suspension microlaryngoscopy in the Boyce position with a new suspension gallows. *Ann Otol Rhinol Laryngol* 1978;87:560–566.
89. Oertel M. Das laryngo-stroboskop und die Laryngo-Stroboskpische Untersuchung. *Arch Laryngol Rhinol* 1895;3:1–16.
90. Brunings W. *Direct laryngoscopy, bronchoscopy, and esophagoscopy*. London; Bailliere, Tindall, & Cox, 1912.
91. Jackson C. Instruments. In: *Peroral endoscopy and laryngeal surgery*. St. Louis: Laryngoscope, 1915:11–51.
92. Scalco AN, Shipman WF, Tabb HG. Microscopic suspension laryngoscopy. *Ann Otol Rhinol Laryngol* 1960;69:1134–1138.
93. Jako GJ. Correspondence documents between Geza Jako and the Stumar Instrument Company, 1962.
94. Jako GJ. Microscopic-laryngoscopy. Presented at the New England Otolaryngological Society, Boston, MA; 1964.
95. Kleinsasser O. Mikrochirurgie im Kehlkopf. *Arch Ohren Nasen Kehlkopfheilk* 1964;183:428–433.
96. Kleinsasser O. *Microlaryngoscopy and endolaryngeal microsurgery*. Baltimore: University Park Press, 1968:48–62.
97. Strong MS. Microscopical-laryngoscopy. *Acad Med Bull* 1968; 14:181–184.
98. Strong MS. Microscopic laryngoscopy: a review and appraisal. *Laryngoscope* 1970;80:1540–1552.
99. DeSanto LW, Carney FW. Microlaryngoscopic surgery. *Arch Otolaryngol* 1970;91:324–326.
100. Kleinsasser O. Development of microlaryngoscopy and endolaryngeal microsurgery. In: *Microlaryngoscopy and endolaryngeal microsurgery*. Baltimore; University Park Press, 1979:3.
101. Zeitels SM. Premalignant epithelium and microinvasive cancer of the vocal fold: the evolution of phonomicrosurgical management. *Laryngoscope* 1995;105:1–51.
102. Hirano M. Phonosurgery: basic and clinical investigations. *Otologia (Fukuoka)* 1975;21:239–442.
103. Hirano M. Phonosurgical anatomy of the larynx. In: Ford C, Bless D, eds. *Phonosurgery*. New York: Raven, 1991:25–41.
104. Bouchayer M, Cornut G. Instrumental microscopy of benign lesions of the vocal folds. In: Ford C, Bless D, eds. *Phonosurgery*. New York: Raven, 1991:143–165.
105. Zeitels SM. Microflap excisional biopsy for atypia and microinvasive glottic cancer. *Otolaryngol Head Neck Surg* 1993;4: 218–222.
106. Sataloff RT, Spiegel JR. Endoscopic microsurgery. In: Gould WJ, Sataloff RT, Spiegel JR, eds. *Voice surgery*. St. Louis: Mosby, 1991:227–267.
107. Sataloff R, Spiegel JR, Heuer RJ, et al. Laryngeal mini-microflap: a new technique and reassessment of the microflap saga. *J Voice* 1995;9:198–204.
108. Courey MS, Stone RE, Gardner GM, Ossof RH. Endoscopic vocal fold microflap: a three year experience. *Ann Otol Rhinol Laryngol* 1995;104:267–273.
109. Bastian RW. Vocal fold microsurgery in singers. *J Voice* 1996;10: 389–404.
110. Zeitels SM. Laser versus cold instruments for microlaryngoscopic surgery. *Laryngoscope* 1996;106:545–552.
111. Zeitels SM. Phonomicrosurgical treatment of early glottic cancer and carcinoma in situ. *Am J Surg* 1996;172:704–709.

112. Zeitels SM, Hillman RE, Bunting GW, Vaughn T. Reinke's edema: phonatory mechanisms and management strategies. *Ann Otol Rhinol Laryngol* 1996;106:533–543.
113. Zeitels SM. Phonomicrosurgical techniques. In: Sataloff R, ed. Professional voice: the science and the art of clinical care. San Diego: Singular, 1997:647–658.
114. Zeitels SM. Endoscopic management of the larynx for benign and malignant disease. In: Myers E, Bluestone CD, eds. *Advances in otolaryngology–head and neck surgery.* Chicago: Mosby, 1998:1–40.
115. Jako GJ. Laser surgery of the vocal cords. *Laryngoscope* 1972;82: 2204–2215.
116. Polanyi T, Bredermeier HC, Davis TW Jr. $CO_2$ laser for surgical research. *Meat Biol Eng Comput* 1970;8:548–558.
117. Strong MS, Jako GJ. Laser surgery of the larynx: early clinical experience with continuous $CO_2$ laser. *Ann Otol Rhinol Laryngol* 1972;81:791–798.
118. Vaughan CW. Transoral laryngeal surgery using the $CO_2$ laser: laboratory experiments and clinical experience. *Laryngoscope* 1978;88:1399–1420.
119. Bishop J. Experimental researches into the physiology of the human voice. *London & Edinburgh Philosophical Magazine & Journal of Science* 1836.
120. Fournie E. Physiologie de la voix et de la parole. Paris: Adrien Delahaye, 1866.
121. Hirano M. Structure of the vocal fold in normal and diseased states: anatomical and physical studies. *Proceedings of the Conference on the Assessment of Vocal Pathology: the American Speech-Language-Hearing Association;* 1981;11:11–27.
122. Zeitels SM, Vaughan CW. A submucosal vocal fold infusion needle. *Otolaryngol Head Neck Surg* 1991;105:478–479.
123. Kass ES, Hillman RE, Zeitels SM. The submucosal infusion technique in phonomicrosurgery. *Ann Otol Rhinol Laryngol* 1996;105:341–347.
124. Hajek M. Anatomische Untersuchungen uber das Larynxodem. *Arch Klin Chir* 1891;42:46–93.
125. Reinke F. Untersuchungen uber das menschliche Stimmband. *Fortschr Med* 1895;13:469–478.
126. Reinke F. Uber die funktionelle Struktur der menschlichen Stimmlippe mit besonderer Berucksichtigung des elastischen Gewebes [About the functional structure of the human vocal cord with special reference to the elastic tissue]. *Anat Hefte* 1897;9:103–117.
127. Pressman J, Dowdy A, Libby R, Fields M. Further studies on the submucosal lymphatics of the larynx by injection of dyes and isotopes. *Ann Otol Rhinol Laryngol* 1956;65:963–980.
128. Pressman JJ, Bertz MB, Monell C. Anatomic studies related to the dissemination of cancer of the larynx. *Trans Am Acad Ophthalmol Otolaryngol* 1960;64:628–638.
129. Oertel M. Ueber eine neues laryngostroboskopische Untersuchungsmethode des Kehlkopfes. *Zentralb Med Wiss* 1878;16:81–82.
130. von Leden H. The electronic synchron-stroboscope: its value for the practicing laryngologist. *Ann Otol Rhinol Laryngol* 1961; 70:881–893.
131. Alberti PW. The diagnostic role of laryngeal stroboscopy. *Otolaryngol Clin North Am* 1978;11:3457–354.
132. Powell LS. The laryngostroboscope. *Arch Otolaryngol* 1934;19: 708–710.
133. Kallen LA. Laryngostrobscopy in the practice of otolaryngology. *Arch Otolaryngol* 1932;16:791–807.
134. Timcke R, Von Leden H, Moore P. Laryngeal vibrations: measurement of the glottic wave: Part 1. Normal vibratory cycle. *Arch Otolaryngol* 1958;68:1–19.
135. Timcke R, Von Leden H, Moore P. Laryngeal vibrations: measurements of the glottic wave: Part II. Physiologic variations. *Arch Otolaryngol* 1959;69:438–444.
136. von Leden H, Moore P, Timcke R. Laryngeal vibrations: measurements of the glottic wave: Part III. The pathological larynx. *Arch Otolaryngol* 1960;71:16–35.
137. Morrison MD. A clinical voice laboratory, videotape and stroboscopic instrumentation. *Otolaryngol Head Neck Surg* 1984; 92:487–488.

# 40

# DIAGNOSTIC ENDOSCOPY OF THE LARYNX

PEAK WOO

Endoscopic examination of the larynx has a rich and colorful history in otolaryngology. From the genius of Jackson and Hollinger to recent contributors such as Kleinsasser, Benjamin, Yanagisawa, and Andreas, examination of the larynx by diagnostic laryngology has made major strides in this century. Today, office endoscopic examination of the larynx includes rigid and telescopic examination of the larynx, video-endoscopic examination of swallowing, videostroboscopy, and office intervention by laryngoscopy.

Operative diagnostic laryngoscopy has also seen major changes, including telescopic laryngoscopy with Hopkins rod telescopes, operating microscopes, and new microinstruments. The variety of technologic improvements in optics, video technology, and computer technology means that the larynx and its function can be examined, documented, and analyzed in detail. This chapter addresses diagnostic laryngoscopy within three main topics: office laryngoscopy and procedures, videostroboscopy, and operative diagnostic laryngoscopy. With color video prints and photographs, some of the endoscopic detail of normal tissue and pathology of the larynx is demonstrated.

## OFFICE EXAMINATION AND INDIRECT LARYNGOSCOPY PROCEDURES

Patients who present with laryngeal diseases usually have symptoms of hoarseness, dysphagia, globus (i.e., lump in the throat feeling), or breathing difficulty. Occasionally, symptoms of referred otalgia, excessive phlegm, cough, or a neck mass may prompt a consultation. Voice, airway, and swallow disorders are the primary indications for a careful office-based assessment of the larynx.

### Indications and Methods for Indirect Laryngoscopy

Indirect laryngoscopy is a fundamental procedure for examination of the larynx. Detailed diagnostic information today is often possible without the need for operative (direct) laryngoscopy. A combination of flexible fiberoptic endoscopes, rigid telescopes, and stroboscopes can be used to evaluate the larynx. Some of these procedures are complementary. For example, flexible laryngoscope examination is mandatory for evaluation of swallow, velopharyngeal insufficiency, and articulation disorders, and videostroboscopy is extremely useful when vibratory abnormalities are suspected. Examples of vibratory abnormalities are seen in vocal folds affected by scar and small vocal fold lesions.

Mirror examination is the simplest and least expensive method for examination of the larynx. Adequate illumination and position of the patient makes mirror laryngoscopy practical in most patients for a gross examination of the larynx for adequacy of laryngeal movement, lesions, and mucosal condition. The patient is asked to sit upright and protrude the chin and head toward the examiner (i.e., sniffing position). The mouth is opened, and the tongue is protruded down and out. The examiner holds the tongue with his forefinger and thumb and rolls the tongue down. The patient is asked to take a breath quietly with the tongue flaccid and immobile. The largest possible laryngeal mirror is warmed to skin temperature and placed into the oropharynx. The uvula and the soft palate are gently depressed, and the angled mirror is used to examine the reflected image of the epiglottis, arytenoid, and vocal folds. The larynx is examined during quiet respiration and phonation. The general appearance of the vocal folds and the larynx may be inspected along with the gross movements during adduction and abduction. The color of the vocal folds should be white to slightly off white, like ivory piano keys. The mucosa should be pink, with good moisture but not excessive secretions (Fig. 40.1).

The mirror examination is hampered by a lack of magnification and detail. This is where telescopic laryngoscopy with video display has a major advantage. The rigid telescope has a good depth of field and can be used in most patients who can tolerate a mirror examination. Usually, the telescope has a 70° or 90° angle. It may have a variable focus and magnification. With a video monitor, a video recorder, and a video printer coupled to a video camera, documentation and repeated review of the examination is possible. The

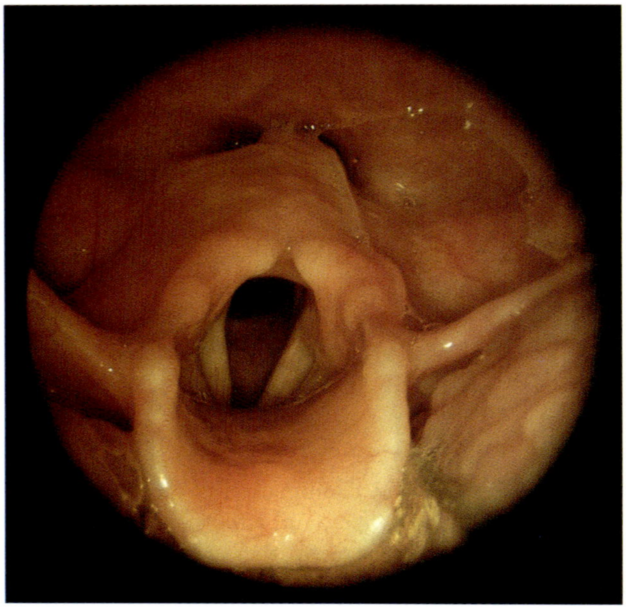

**FIGURE 40.1.** Indirect mirror examination of the normal larynx shows healthy pink mucosa and moist white to off-white vocal folds.

rigid telescopic examination offers a superior examination of the structures of the oropharynx, hypopharynx, and the larynx compared with mirror examination or flexible fiberoptic laryngoscope examination. Its main disadvantages are poor tolerance by some subjects and the requirement for extra instruments and time. Figure 40.2 shows a telescopic view of the larynx using a 70° endoscope.

Flexible fiberoptic laryngoscopy is a good instrument for examination of dynamic structural changes of the oropharynx, hypopharynx, and larynx. Some specialized flexible endoscopic examination protocols have been developed for examination of the swallow mechanism and for evaluation of obstructive apnea. In evaluation of voice disorders, flexible laryngoscopy is valuable for examination of the structural and dynamic changes of the supraglottic larynx, pharynx, and the base of the tongue. Flexible laryngoscopy is a good alternative in patients with severe gag reflex that prevents the use of rigid or mirror laryngoscopy. Children older than 4 years of age tolerate the fiberoptic examination readily provided the nose is well anesthetized. The flexible laryngoscope is able to examine the nose, nasopharynx, oropharynx, larynx, and hypopharynx in a single pass of the scope. Some physicians prefer this examination to other approaches and use it exclusively.

The flexible examination is hampered by several disadvantages. The main problem is the mosaic effect of fiberoptic bundles, which provides poor resolution of fine detail of the larynx. The image is small and does not carry light enough for stroboscopy or good video documentation. Some distortion of the fiberscope image occurs because of the wide-angled lens. To address these problems but preserve the advantages of flexible endoscopy, a videofiberscope may be used. This uses a CCD chip mounted on the end of the fiberscope. It is small enough to be passed by per nasal endoscopy. The images from this video-endoscope is superior to flexible laryngoscopy and is especially useful in patients who need close-up examination of the larynx. Detailed examination of the subglottis, going around an obstructive supraglottic lesion to assess vocal fold mobility, and office tracheal endoscopy are some of the advantages of videofiberscopes over fiberoptic endoscopes.

The equipment for diagnostic laryngology may be conveniently divided into instruments for diagnostic and interventional laryngology, rigid and flexible endoscopes, and

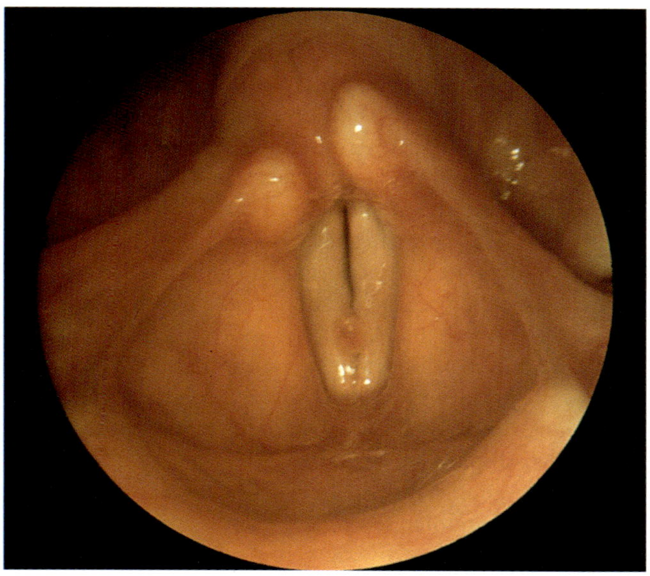

**FIGURE 40.2.** A 70° endoscopic telescope shows a magnified view of the larynx. Compared with the view provided by indirect mirror examination, it shows that a superior examination of the oropharynx, hypopharynx, and larynx is possible.

**TABLE 40.1. EQUIPMENT FOR OFFICE INTERVENTIONAL LARYNGOSCOPY**

- Laryngeal anesthesia
  - Curved tonsil suction
  - Curved cotton applicator
  - Curved instillation cannula
  - Tongue blade
  - Large particle atomizer
  - 10-mL syringe with 1.25-inch, 25-gauge needle
  - 2% Pontocaine
  - 10 mL of lidocaine (1% with 1:100,000 epinephrine)
  - Headlight or mirror
  - Cotton ball applicators with string
- Endoscopes
  - 70° rigid telescope laryngoscope
  - 150-watt light source
- Laryngeal instruments
  - Injector needle
  - Laryngeal injector (Brünning type)
  - Laryngeal biopsy forceps
- Procedure table with vacuum suction and compressed air source

**TABLE 40.2. EQUIPMENT FOR OFFICE INTERVENTIONAL FLEXIBLE LARYNGOSCOPY**

| |
|---|
| Laryngeal anesthesia |
| Same as for indirect laryngoscopy |
| Flexible laryngoscope and bronchoscope |
| Videolaryngoscope with biopsy channel |
| Fiberoptic bronchoscope with 2.0-mm channel |
| 150- or 300-watt light source |
| Laryngeal instruments |
| Endoscopic brush |
| Bronchoscopic biopsy needle |
| Endoscopic cup biopsy forceps, disposable or reusable |

**TABLE 40.3. OFFICE ENDOSCOPIC PROCEDURES**

| |
|---|
| Interventional office laryngoscopy—rigid endoscope |
| Lysis of adhesions |
| Injection of steroids |
| Office biopsy |
| Injection augmentation |
| Direct endoscopic palpation |
| Flexible laryngoscopy |
| Biopsy |
| Cytology |
| Injection of *Clostridium botulinum* toxin |
| Functional endoscopic examination of swallow |
| Videostroboscopy |
| Dynamic evaluation of voice function |
| Photodocumentation and video documentation |
| Flexible and rigid indirect laryngoscopy |

video camera and video documentation. Table 40.1 lists the equipment used for office-based laryngoscopy at our center. Table 40.2 lists the fiberoptic instruments used for interventional flexible laryngoscopy. Table 40.3 is a list of the office-based procedures done for the diagnosis and treatment of laryngeal diseases.

## Instrumentation and Office Layout

For diagnostic rigid telescopic laryngoscopy, a 70° or a 90° telescope is used. This scope also doubles as a rigid scope for videostroboscopy. A variety of scopes are available for this purpose from Japan, Germany, and the United States. The 90° telescope is placed in the oropharynx, and it is often necessary to tilt the tip of the scope to displace the soft palate to view the endolarynx. The 70° scope is the scope I prefer. This scope is placed with a downward tilt, bringing the lens of the scope close to the larynx. The endoscope follows the relaxed tongue over the epiglottis. The angulation brings the scope closer to the endolarynx and gives a better view of the vocal folds along its entire length. For general rigid endoscopic applications, a telescope with a large light-carrying capacity, clear illumination, and wide depth of focus is the most versatile. For special applications such as in singers with small lesions of the larynx, a variable-magnification laryngoscope is helpful. In children and adults who cannot tolerate the wide bore of the rigid telescope, a 70° Hopkins rod operative telescope (diameter of 4.0 mm) permits the physician to examine the larynx by rigid telescopic laryngoscopy. Office-based intervention by biopsy and injection may be done by the examiner using a headlight and mirror or with the telescope on one hand and the instrument on the other (Fig. 40.3).

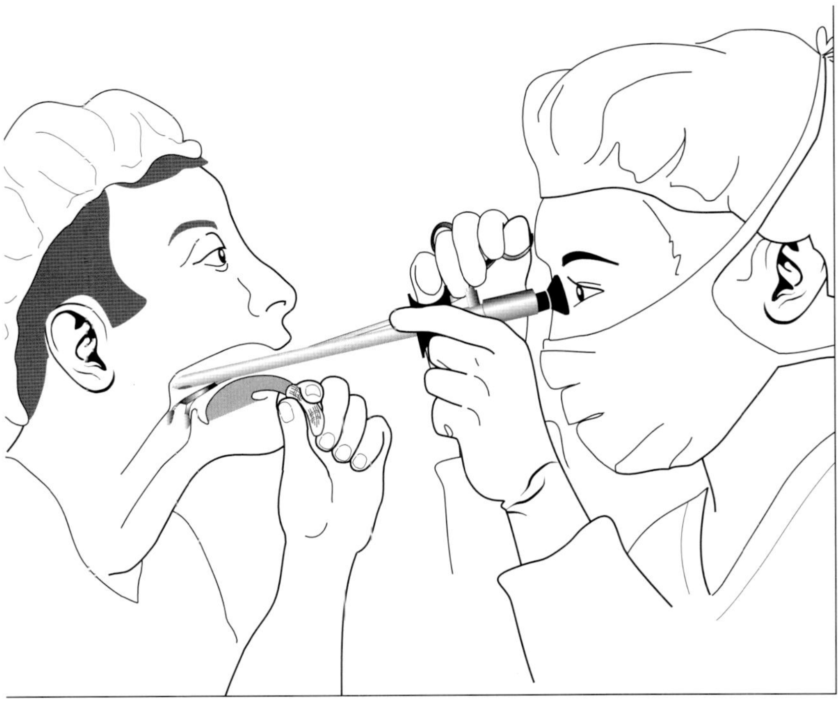

**FIGURE 40.3.** Telescope-based biopsy of a laryngeal lesion in the office. The patient holds the tongue while the physician directs the biopsy forceps with the telescope.

## Fiberoptic Diagnostic Laryngoscopy

Fiberoptic laryngoscopy is usually performed with a flexible nasopharyngoscope. The fiberoptic laryngoscope is usually well tolerated in per nasal endoscopy. Topical nasal anesthesia is helpful because the diameter is less than 4.0 mm (Olympus-ENF P3 is 3.6 mm OD). Other scopes are narrower but have a smaller field of view. A choice must often be made between illumination intensity and the size of the scope. Some of this decision is based on the patient population, whether videostroboscopy is needed, and the cost. The video-endoscope is an endoscope that has a charge-coupled device (CCD) chip incorporated into the tip of the flexible scope (Pentax video-endoscope, Hamburg, Germany). This technology is sufficiently advanced to have a nasoendoscope that is small enough to be passed through the nose without difficulty. Although it is slightly thicker than a fiberoptic nasopharyngoscope, it gives superior resolution without the moire effect.

## Fiberoptic Therapeutic Laryngoscopy

Therapeutic laryngoscopes take their design from therapeutic bronchoscopes. This type of scope operates like a fiberoptic bronchoscope having a channel for suction, biopsy forceps, laser fiber, or an injection needle. It takes practice for the endoscopist to work on the larynx because of the moving larynx, the larger-caliber scopes, and the small biopsy channels, but this skill can be mastered. Per nasal interventional laryngoscopy using fiberoptic laryngoscopes and bronchoscopes can be performed under local tracheal laryngeal anesthesia, without intravenous sedation. By passing the scope through the nasal cavity and working off the video monitor, the operator and the assistant can visualize the larynx simultaneously and work interactively.

In-office transnasal fiberoptic endoscopy techniques have been extended to pharyngoscopy, esophagoscopy, and other procedures more traditionally performed in the surgical endoscopy suite or the operating room. We have used the Pentax videobronchoscope to perform in-office biopsy of the larynx, esophagus, and trachea. Because of the larger caliber of the flexible bronchoscopes (Olympus ENF L-3 is 4.4 mm, the Pentax videobronchoscope is 5.1 mm), per nasal flexible endoscopy requires longer preparation and anesthesia. The nose must be anesthetized and vasoconstricted to permit the passage of the scope. The oral pharynx, larynx, and trachea are anesthetized by nebulized or atomized lidocaine or Pontocaine. For most office-based interventional laryngoscopy, an assistant is needed, and time must be allowed for adequate topical anesthesia.

## Rigid Telescopic Interventional Laryngoscopy

Not every otolaryngologist wishes to perform office procedures, but in-office laryngeal procedures can be mastered with practice. Examples include lysis of adhesions, injection of steroids, laryngeal biopsy, and injection augmentation.

The instruments necessary to perform such procedures include instruments for topical laryngeal anesthesia, a curved injection needle, a curved laryngeal biopsy forceps, and a Brunning syringe with a curved guarded needle. Medications necessary for indirect procedures include 2% Pontocaine, 1% lidocaine with 1:100,000 epinephrine, and topical 0.25% Neo-Synephrine. The video endoscope equipment used for rigid telescopic interventional laryngoscopy is the same as for diagnostic laryngoscopy. My approach to office procedures is shown in Figure 40.3.

## Laryngeal Photography

For most purposes, video laryngoscopy and video prints have superseded office photography because chemical-based photographs need more light for adequate exposure. This makes a flash unit for office endoscopic photography necessary. However, when exposed properly, still photographs have higher resolution than images captured by video cameras. Modern digital photography will no doubt find applications in laryngology in the near future.

Standard 35-mm photography using an endoscope coupled to a camera can be performed using a rigid telescope, endoscopic coupler, lens, and camera. Photographic exposure may be achieved using existing light or a flash unit. I use a Nikon 6006 with a 35- to 135-mm macrolens. An endoscopic coupler attaches the telescope to the lens. The through-the-lens meter has a spot meter that makes manual exposure on the center area of the larynx possible. The bright viewfinder and automatic focusing are useful adjuncts in successful office endoscopic photography. For existing-light photography, the exposure is $^{1}/_{15}$ seconds with an F stop of 4.5. When a tungsten light source is used, tungsten film must be used (tungsten ASA 160 or ASA 320 professional film). Photography using a flash unit can be accomplished with the Storz endoscope light source and a TTL cord. This requires daylight film (ASA 200) balanced for the xenon flash light source. By trial and error, the flash unit can be used to bracket the manual exposure to get the correct exposure. As with any highly technical area of photography, experience and lots of critical evaluation of the results are necessary to continuously improve the results.

Photographs during operative laryngoscopy may be accomplished through the microscope splitter. The larger the magnification, the shorter is the depth of field. Focusing is especially critical when photographing subjects through the operating microscope. To have a useful photograph, the subject must be centered through one eye and carefully focused. To avoid respiratory movements, at least $^{1}/_{15}$ seconds of exposure must be used. This means that a bright light source or a flash unit is necessary. An alternative strategy for operative laryngoscopy documentation is to use photography through a telescope passed through the laryngoscope. A distinct advantage to this method is the clear depth of field and the crisp images that can be produced. Besides the 0° telescope, other lenses such as the 30°, 70°, and 120° telescopes may be used to examine the larynx. This provides an examination of the larynx in areas that may not be visible through the operating laryngoscope.

Office documentation of laryngoscopy findings serves as a good communication tool between referring physicians and specialists. Good records are invaluable for documentation and follow-up. Objective documentation by still photographs, video recordings, or objective tests can give feedback to the surgeon about the success of his treatment.

Videolaryngoscopy, with or without stroboscopy, is the method of choice for most office laryngeal examinations. The procedure is fast, instant playback is possible, and the video preserves the motion characteristics of the examination. Patient education and review is immediate. Practically, video prints suffice for the patient charts and for referring physicians. For the traveling singer, a video tape can be easily copied and taken by the patient after the examination, providing a voice "passport" of laryngoscopic findings for the next examiner.

## Video Recording

The color video camera was revolutionized by the development of the solid-state CCD chip camera. These cameras have a remarkable low-light sensitivity and are small and durable. Image resolution has increased to near broadcast quality. Cameras that can fit in the palm are used in medical applications. The three-chip CCD camera offers further improvements in the signal-to-noise ratio and true-to-life color rendition. The illumination for a video image by the videostroboscopy light is quite excellent for rigid stroboscopic light endoscopy and is adequate for fiberoptic laryngoscopy. In application of fiberoptic stroboscopy, the fiberscope must be advanced close to the vocal folds for adequate resolution of detail. The single- or three-chip camera supplied by the equipment manufacturers may vary in resolution, signal-to-noise ratio, low-sensitivity gain, and other special features. The camera usually comes with a standard endoscope adaptor attached to a lens. The scope can have a variable- or fixed-focus lens. For general endoscopy purposes, 25- to 50-mm lenses have been used. A longer lens allows greater magnification but may make the image darker because of lack of illumination. A shorter lens has the disadvantage of a small picture on a large screen. As a compromise to reduce the number of lens changes in a busy clinic, a 35-mm lens seems to offer the best field of view for fiberoptic and rigid telescopic examinations of the larynx.

Video recorders and video capture on a personal computer may be used for storage of video data. The super-VHS tapes have superior resolution and may be copied to a VHS tape without significant loss in detail.

## Videostroboscopy

Videostroboscopy is a valuable office endoscopy tool for diagnosing patients who have voice abnormalities. Abnormal vocal fold vibration is a common cause of dysphonia, and stroboscopy can reveal subtle details that are often invaluable to the clinician.

The principle of stroboscopy is based on Talbot's law, which is the persistence of vision on the retina for 0.2 seconds after the exposure. An object moving rapidly and periodically may be slowed down or frozen by brief flashes of light synchronized to the phase of the periodic vibration. These brief but synchronized flashes of light illuminate the object and present the retina with an image of exposure during the desired phase of periodic vibration. The eye "assembles" the series of images to give the appearance of slowly vibrating vocal folds.

The modern videostroboscope unit incorporates video technology, computer integration, and signal and image processing techniques but retains the same principles of the synchronized stroboscope. The pickup microphone or electroglottograph source is used at the source to detect the frequency of vocal fold vibration. The frequency of strobe flash is synchronized to the frequency of vocal fold vibration or a fraction thereof, and the video camera is attached to the endoscope to record the image and sound. With modern refinements and the simultaneous display of waveforms, the frequency and the amplitude statistics of the sound may be displayed on screen. The fiberoptic examination gives a natural view of the vocal folds during voicing, whereas the telescopic view gives greater visual detail of the mucosal wave and other fine features of the vocal fold.

## Applications

### Documentation

Preoperative and postoperative documentation of voice and vibratory function before phonosurgery and medical therapy is essential, and videostroboscopy is an effective method of laryngeal documentation. Stroboscopy recordings may be used for clinical research, teaching, and medicolegal purposes. Videostroboscopy requires interpretation, but it nevertheless provides objective documentation of glottal function.

### Clinical Care in Laryngology and Voice Care Using Stroboscopy

Stroboscopy is most advantageously used to analyze the vibratory movement of the vocal folds during phonation. Stroboscopy can be used in clinical research to assess vocal fold vibratory function after laser surgery for recurrent respiratory papillomatosis, to evaluate glottic function before and after injection of collagen, and to detect edema or laryngitis. Stroboscopic information can influence diagnosis and treatment.

Stroboscopy has played an increasing role in the development of new phonosurgery procedures. Some researchers have investigated the variations in the glottal area and vibratory patterns during phonation using stroboscopy combined with glottographic methods. The image-analysis software incorporated into the computer-controlled stroboscopy unit allows the researcher and clinician to calculate relative changes in glottal area and amplitude. The vocal folds vibrate in a quasi-periodic fashion and are set into vibration by the air stream interacting with the unique layered structure of the vocal folds. Each vocal fold oscillation may be analyzed into the various phases of the vocal fold oscillation. Each oscillation of the vocal fold is the glottal cycle. Figure 40.4 is a single glottal cycle recorded from a stroboscopic series in a man. The various components of the glottal cycle may be divided into open and closed phases. The open phase is that portion of the glottal cycle in which the vocal folds are apart, and the closed phase is that portion of the cycle in which the vocal folds are in contact. The open phase of the glottal cycle is approximately 50% to 60% of the glottal cycle. The opening and closing phases are approximately equal for the vocal folds. The opening and closing phases of the glottal cycle should be smooth and without irregularity. The vocal folds open, reach a maximal glottal area, and then close. Each vocal fold vibrates in phase with the other. They reach approximately the same amplitude during each successive vibratory cycle. During the closed phase, the vocal folds continue to move together until the next puff of air separates them. During vibration, the vocal folds have the greatest amplitude of vibration at the mid-membranous vocal fold. The vocal folds generate the mucosal wave at the peak of glottal opening. There is a phase difference between the upper and the lower lip of the vocal fold. In normal vocal fold oscillation, the lower lip opens first and is followed by the upper vocal fold excursion. During closure, the lower vocal fold lip closes faster than the upper lip. This phase difference between the upper and lower lips is more apparent during loud voice production.

## Interpretation of Videostroboscopy

The rating of stroboscopic images is based on systematic but subjective judgment of the stroboscopic image. To achieve a level of consistent rating, it is necessary to record the stroboscopic record before and after treatment at about the same frequency and amplitude. For simplicity, the examination is most frequently done at chest or modal phonation with a comfortable loudness and pitch. For men, this is a frequency of 100 to 150 Hz with a decibel output of 70 to 75 dB. For women, this is 200 to 250 Hz with an amplitude output of 70 to 75 dB. Care should be taken to record the voice at comfortable loudness and pitch for at least 4 seconds of sustained phonation so that several cycles of vocal fold vibration may be recorded. For patients with severely disordered voices, it is especially necessary to per-

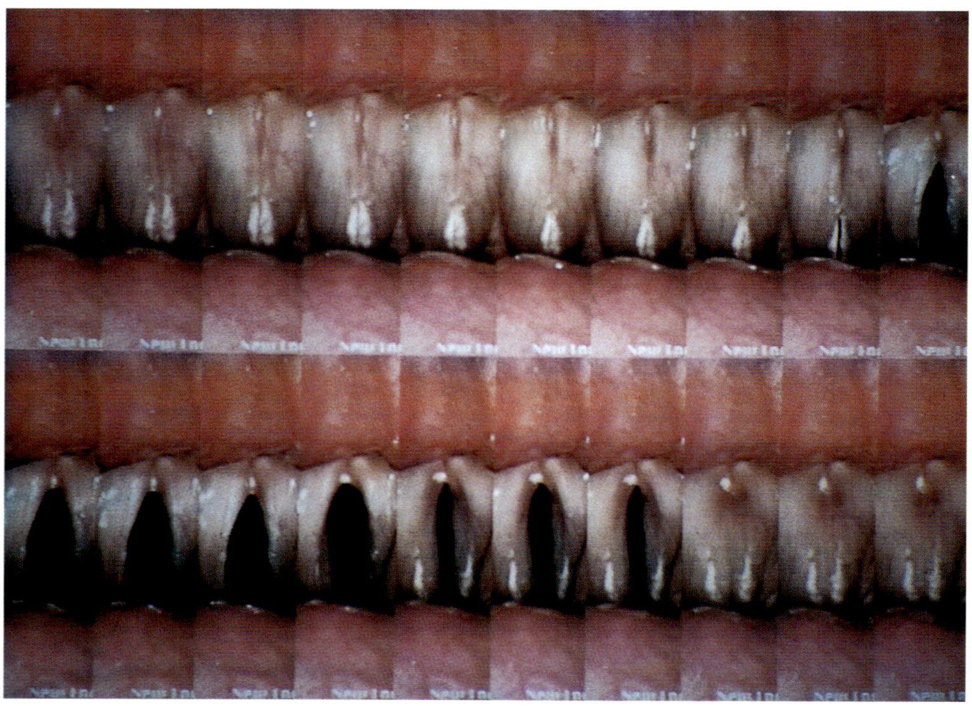

**FIGURE 40.4.** A single glottal cycle recorded from a stroboscopic examination of a man.

form the video stroboscopy while controlling for pitch and frequency.

After the recording of the videostroboscopic examination, the analysis and interpretation of the videolaryngoscopic record is based on systematic rating of parameters that have been elucidated by prior investigators. The main parameters are configuration, closure, symmetry, phase, phase shift, amplitude, mucosal wave, and nonvibratory segments. A rating form is a convenient method to report data.

### Vocal Fold Edge

The vocal folds should be smooth and straight during vocal fold vibration and during inspiration. The folds have an elliptical appearance at the maximal lateral excursion, but in normal states, they should be smooth and without irregularities The vocal fold is rated as to the degree of roughness. An irregular, rough edge that involves the entire membranous vocal fold (i.e., papilloma or cancer) is rated more severely than small thickenings in the middle cord, such as are seen in patients with early nodules.

### Glottic Closure Configuration

During maximal vocal fold closure, vocal folds are observed for their configuration and shape. Normal vocal fold configuration in men is complete closure without any air leakage. In many women, a small posterior glottal gap is normal. The normal posterior glottal gap does not extend anteriorly to cause a gap between the membranous vocal folds and is usually limited to between or posterior to the vocal processes. Some common configurations include incomplete closure (e.g., vocal cord paralysis, traumatic arytenoid dislocation), hourglass or midcord contact (e.g., vocal fold nodules, polyp with reaction of the contralateral fold), bowing of vocal folds (e.g., presbyphonia, asthenia voice), irregular closure (e.g., mass lesion, cancer, polyp, papilloma), and anterior chink or defect (e.g., scar, vocal atrophy, sulcus vocalis). When there is scarring, stiffness, and poor pliability of the vocal folds, the vocal folds often fail to obtain good closure. If complete closure can be achieved, it usually occurs with a highly strained, strident voice quality. This can be detected as high acoustic amplitude and frequency on the stroboscope monitor. The patient has difficulty producing a soft, steady, sustained vowel at a comfortable pitch.

### Phase Closure

The open or closed status of the vocal fold in the glottal cycle has important functional implications. Phase closure is an estimate of the amount of the glottal cycle spent in the open versus closed phase. The open phase of normal glottal cycle in chest phonation is approximately 50% to 70%, depending on the frequency of phonation and the loudness of the token produced. For men phonating at modal phonation, the open phase is 50% to 60% of the cycle. Women have a longer open phase.

In abnormal states, the closed phase and open phase may be abnormally short or long. In pathologic states in which masses and stiffness of the vocal folds have been altered, the vocal fold vibration pattern usually exhibits a prolonged open phase with a short or absent closed phase. Patients with spasmodic dysphonia or hyperfunctional voice disorder have a long closed phase.

### Vertical Level

The vocal folds should contact the contralateral vocal fold at the same level. Level differences are noticeable in vocal fold paralysis, vocal fold atrophy, and occasionally after vocal fold stripping.

### Amplitude of Vibration

The excursion of the vocal folds should be symmetric. The most lateral excursion should occur at the peak of the opening phase. Normal amplitude of vocal fold vibration differs according to sex, frequency, and other factors. The normal amplitude in men and women is approximately one half to two thirds of the width of the unobstructed vocal fold. Severely reduced amplitude and absent amplitude of vibration are easy to detect and imply stiffness. Severely reduced amplitude on one side is often most obvious when compared with the contralateral vocal fold. Loss of amplitude of vocal fold oscillation usually implies abnormality of the vocal fold cover due to mass, tension, or stiffness. In patients with subcordal lesions such as vocal fold cysts, the vibratory amplitude of the affected vocal fold is usually diminished. With microsurgery, speech therapy, and medical therapy, many patient shave restoration of mucosal pliability and vibration. Restoration of the vibratory amplitude is a key visual observation that accompanies restoration of vocal function in patients with organic voice disorders.

### Mucosal Wave

The mucosal wave is propagated from the subglottic larynx and travels across the glottis to the superior surface of the vocal folds. This occurs at the same time as the vocal folds are opening. The mucosal wave and the amplitude of vocal fold oscillation are often confused. The mucosal wave is a finer and more delicate epithelial disturbance that propagates across the rounded vocal folds. The mucosal wave can be seen to propagate across the superior surface of the vocal fold as the vocal folds are closing. Like ocean waves, they may be small or large and are easier to detect in male larynges. The normal mucosal wave is linear and travels uninterrupted parallel to the vocal fold edge. The wave crosses the superior surface of the vocal fold. If there is a localized area of stiffness, the mucosal wave is interrupted at the site of localized stiffness. Much as a breakwater interrupts the wave in the ocean, localized lesions of the vocal fold surface may interfere with mucosal wave propagation. The mucosal wave may propagate around a small lesion, making the site more obvious. If there is a loss of the Reinke space, the mucosal wave will be absent. In inflammatory disorders involving the vocal fold cover, the fine mucosal wave propagation is most sensitive to the disturbance. This makes observations of the mucosal wave an especially useful tool in understanding patients with subtle dysphonias.

### *Vibratory Behavior*

The vibratory behavior should be present along the membranous vocal folds. Maximal excursion is at the middle of the membranous fold. When there is a localized mass lesion or scarring, vocal fold vibratory behavior may be partially or completely absent. The partially stiffened vocal folds may show vibratory behavior at some frequency and loudness but no response with softer, less forceful attacks. This pattern gives the clinician an opportunity to estimate the degree of stiffness of a vocal fold.

### *Phase Symmetry*

Phase symmetry is the relationship of phase of vibration of a vocal fold relative to the contralateral vocal fold. Normal vocal folds open and close symmetrically. They are said to vibrate in phase. When there are level differences, mass differences, or differences in tension of the vocal folds, the vocal folds may oscillate out of phase, resulting in a less-efficient vocal fold oscillator with a prolonged open phase.

### *Periodicity*

Normal vocal fold oscillation should be quasi-periodic during sustained vowel production. This is observed on stroboscopy as a steady vibration of the stroboscopy image. An aperiodic voice is difficult to track. The statistics indicator on the strobe unit shows fluctuation of the fundamental frequency. Tremor, irregular voice breaks, and spastic voices may make it impossible to pace the stroboscopy unit to achieve steady frequency extraction. Periodicity may be mostly regular (e.g., small vocal fold nodules), mostly irregular (e.g., spasmodic dysphonia, vocal cord polyps), or always irregular (e.g., cancer). The periodicity rating describes functional severity and has no medical diagnostic significance.

## Operative Laryngoscopy

For some patients, the information from indirect laryngoscopy is inadequate to dictate accurate treatment. In these situations, diagnostic microlaryngoscopy or direct operative endoscopy becomes necessary. The surgeon must balance the risks to the patient of general anesthesia against the information to be gained by operative laryngoscopy. Although serious complication rates are low, airway obstruction, worse dysphonia, and anesthesia risks must be weighed against the potential benefits of operative endoscopy. Table 40.4 lists some of the indications for operative endoscopy and phonomicrosurgery. Operative endoscopy offers many advantages besides examination of tissue and biopsy, including the ability to examine the larynx at high magnification, use of probes and instruments for palpation, endolaryngeal examination with different

**TABLE 40.4. INDICATIONS FOR MICROLARYNGOSCOPY**

- Persistent hoarseness or airway symptoms, when the indirect examination is impossible because of gag reflex or when the anatomy is obscured by obstructing tissue that must be pushed aside
- Organic lesion of the larynx, such as polyps, cysts, and sulcus vocalis, in patients who have a voice disturbance interfering with function
- Endoscopic palpation, as in suspected arytenoid dislocation and as part of the workup of the immobile larynx
- Endoscopic exploration of the larynx by high-power magnification and palpation
- Biopsy of a suspicious lesion for histologic examination
- Gathering of endoscopic cultures for fungus, tuberculosis, or bacteria identification
- Endoscopic treatment of airway obstruction or stenosis, as in the removal of obstructing tumor before radiation therapy or endoscopic treatment of laryngeal web and stenosis
- Placement and removal of keels, stents, and prostheses
- Endoscopic arytenoidectomy or transverse cordotomy for bilateral vocal fold paralysis or arytenoid ankylosis
- Removal of benign or premalignant lesions, such as papilloma, squamous cell carcinoma, and epithelial dysplasia
- Endoscopic augmentation of vocal fold bowing or paralysis by fat, Gelfoam, or Teflon injection
- Removal of a foreign body
- Control of airway, as in adult epiglottitis

angled telescopes, and the use of intravital stains or contact microscopy.

Operative laryngoscopy has absolute and relative contraindications. Absolute contraindications for operative laryngoscopy are usually related to an anesthetic risk. If the patient is not a candidate for general anesthesia, alternative methods such as local anesthesia or indirect laryngoscopy must be considered. Occasionally, if the patient has hypotension, uncontrolled hypertension, recent myocardial infarction, or multiple systems failure, the benefits of operative laryngoscopy need to be sacrificed in favor of indirect office laryngoscopy and biopsy. Some patients have anatomy that is difficult to expose by rigid endoscopy, including scoliosis, fixation or trauma to the cervical spine, trismus, a small mandible, and a short thick neck. Some patients have a partially narrowed airway due to stenosis, trauma, tumor, or inflammation. Intubation followed by operative manipulation or treatment may worsen the airway. This can result in airway edema, which must be managed by prolonged postoperative intubation or temporary tracheotomy.

To achieve optimal voice results with phonomicrosurgery, the timing of surgery is important. A delay in surgery for benign vocal fold lesions should be considered if there is excessive edema, inflammation, or hyperemia. In the management of laryngeal stenosis and webs, poorly controlled reflux laryngitis can promote restenosis and increase the possibility of treatment failure. Reflux laryngitis is a common comorbid condition in many patients with laryngeal pathology. It should be treated by antacid therapy before endoscopic surgery. Some patients with laryngeal pathology also have poor vocal hygiene, chronic throat clearing, and voice abuse. They have thick, inspissated mucus throughout the larynx. These patients should be managed by reversal of the poor mucosal hygiene and should meet with the voice therapist to monitor voice use after the surgery. Preoperative treatment with antibiotics, mucolytics, and antitussives may be necessary before and after surgery.

There is little need to delay operative laryngoscopy when there is little hope for spontaneous resolution of the pathology. If there is suspicion of a malignancy, operative intervention is more urgent than for clearly benign lesions. Some benign lesions should be treated early. For example, cysts are much easier to treat when they are small and have little tissue reaction. Polyps or a varix of the vocal fold may become larger or stiff with repeated trauma. Untreated unilateral lesions may develop a contralateral tissue reaction such as superficial keratosis, a nodule, a varix, or ulcers. These are arguments for early intervention. In the management of the patient with laryngeal stenosis, working on immature stenosis or granulation tissue means that long-acting steroid injections or mitomycin-C applied topically may be necessary to reduce the scar and fibrosis reaction.

One of the most difficult questions to answer for the patient is about the degree of voice improvement after phonomicrosurgery. Voice results depend on the underlying vocal pathology, the preoperative severity of dysphonia, the degree and finesse of surgical treatment, the patient's healing, and the functional adaptation of the patient after surgery. Unfortunately, there is not a good staging system for the severity vocal pathology or for the degree of voice improvement. Perceptual judgment of voice by the patients may be clouded by their special needs. Objective measures of phonatory function can measure only a part of the multidimensional aspect of vocal function. Some patients have clearly favorable lesions and should have near-normal voices shortly after surgery. These lesions include soft, pedunculated polyps; obstructing granulomas; hemorrhagic varices; ventricular prolapse; and pseudocyst of the vocal folds. Voice rest for 4 to 7 days after surgery, followed by verification of healing and voice therapy, is the norm for patients with extensive or bilateral lesions, repeated surgery for removal of papillomas, and preexisting chronic laryngitis, the prognosis for return of a normal voice must be guarded. Even with the most favorable lesions, the surgeon cannot promise a normal voice in every case of surgery. This aspect should be discussed in detail with each patient. For some patients with clearly benign conditions, such as gender reassignment or voice loss due to the bowing and atrophy of aging, phonomicrosurgery should be considered a cosmetic surgery done to enhance voice. In these patients, a careful psychologic assessment of the patient's needs, expectations, and perceptions should be carried out. Objective preoperative and postoperative documentation, available from the voice centers, is an invaluable aid in this regard.

## Technique of Operative Laryngoscopy and Suspension Microlaryngoscopy

Operative laryngoscopy refers to the examination of the larynx under anesthesia. Examination is carried out with the diagnostic rigid laryngoscopes, telescopes, and laryngeal probes. Suspension microlaryngoscopy is the examination of the larynx with the patient on a suspension apparatus. A wide-bore operating laryngoscope is used to examine the larynx with the aid of binocular vision. The operating microscope and the various telescopes are used to examine the larynx under magnification. Therapeutic interventions are carried out with or without use of the laser. Each step of the procedure, from the anesthesia to the choice of laryngoscope and other instrumentation, contributes to the overall success of the examination and surgery.

### *Anesthesia*

Local anesthesia may be administered for a direct laryngoscopy. This approach is preferred in some situations, including injection of Teflon or Gelfoam, removal of a laryngeal foreign body, and patients for whom general anesthesia is contraindicated. Local administration of topical lidocaine with superior laryngeal blocks constitutes an excellent alternative to general anesthesia for brief procedures in selected cases.

Administration of anesthesia during microlaryngoscopy requires cooperation between the otolaryngologist and the anesthesiologist. The surgeon needs a quiet, relaxed patient with little movement and maximum exposure. The anesthesiologist needs a secure airway with good ventilation and total amnesia. In adults, endotracheal anesthesia with muscle relaxation and positive-pressure ventilation is preferred by most anesthesiologists. For the surgeon, the smallest endotracheal tube means the greatest working space. The choice of endotracheal tube size is often debated. Tube sizes from 4.5 to 8.0 mm have been used for artificial ventilation in adults. In most adult patients, it is possible to ventilate with a 5.0- to 5.5-mm endotracheal tube. This ensures that the tube resides posterior to the membranous vocal folds during laryngoscopy.

### Laser Surgery

Special considerations apply when a laser is to be used in the larynx. Endotracheal tube ignition with subsequent airway burn is a catastrophic complication. Laser-proof tubes do not exist, but laser-resistant tubes are available. Some of the most secure tubes, such as the Norton metal tube, are not very flexible and take up additional room in the larynx with a similar inner diameter. The Laser-flex tube on the market has a double-cuff system that can be inflated with colored saline, which serves as a warning if the cuff is penetrated. Other precautions for laser use include a high-power suction to remove steam and laser plume, use of oxygen at a concentration of less than 50%, and avoidance of nitrous oxide mixed with oxygen.

### Relaxation

Topical anesthesia using a 4% spray of lidocaine into the airway at the induction of anesthesia helps to reduce the incidence of laryngospasm after surgery. It also seems to reduce the vagal stimulatory effects of suspension laryngoscopy. Bradycardia, ectopy, and hypotension may be avoided by blocking the vagal stimulus at the beginning of the endoscopic procedure. A good muscle relaxant is one that can provide smooth relaxation throughout the endoscopic procedure but be readily metabolized or reversed. Each anesthesiologist has a preferred method for muscle relaxation. Some prefer depolarizing muscle relaxant agents such as succinylcholine or a continuous infusion drip. Others have good experience with the newer, short- or ultrashort-acting muscle relaxant such as atracurium. Anesthesia can be supplemented with the use of a short-acting barbiturate or the newer agent propofol. The surgeon should communicate the estimated duration of muscle relaxation to the anesthesiologist before the induction of anesthesia. At the end of the surgery, if there is any concern about the airway, it is mandatory that the patient has recovered his own respiratory, cough, and airway protective reflexes before extubation.

### Jet Ventilation

Venturi jet ventilation anesthesia is a technique that uses relatively high-pressure oxygen insufflation that entrains room air into the airway to ventilate the lungs. Its main advantage is that there is no endotracheal tube in the surgical field. The disadvantages are the high pressures needed in the jetting catheter, the possible risk of barotrauma, and the constant motion of the tissue during jetting. As air is blown into the airway, it dries the tissue. Two methods of delivery of jet ventilation can be used. Proximal jet ventilation places the jetting catheter above the vocal folds and is usually placed in the laryngoscope. Distal jetting uses a small catheter such as the Hunsaker or the Ben-Jet jetting catheter distal to the vocal cords. A distal jetting catheter is usually less than 3 mm in diameter and should be centered in the trachea. The operator must ensure that the catheter is not kinked or obstructed by secretions. Jet Venturi ventilation through a laryngoscope is provided by a 14- or 16-gauge needle using 40 to 50 psi driving pressure for adults. Distal jetting catheters use similar pressures. In both techniques, egress of gases must be provided during ventilation. If this is not done, the lungs may overinflate, and pneumothorax may result. When using jet ventilation, the distal airway is not protected. Any bleeding down the trachea must be monitored and managed. Blood and secretions must be evacuated before extubation.

A modification to the jet ventilation technique is the high-frequency, positive-pressure ventilation (HFPPV) method used for intraoperative ventilation. HFPPV was initially used in thoracic surgery for open ventilation during lung resections. HFPPV ventilators are readily available in the operating suites. The advantage of this approach is that the small catheter uses a much higher frequency of ventilation (100 to 150 cycles per minute) with a much lower pressure (typically 15 to 20 psi) to ventilate the patient. The advantage to the patient is a lower pressure needed for jetting and reduced risk of barotrauma. For the surgeon, the higher frequency and lower pressure are desirable because there is less movement artifact during microsurgery. During all jet ventilation procedures, the expiration of gases must be monitored. Patients with large obstructing lesions that may break off during surgery and impact the airway are not good candidates for jet ventilation.

In experienced hands, the jet ventilation technique is an invaluable tool in the management of the difficult airway. The potential complications and their management make it a tool for the experienced surgeon and anesthesiologist team trained in the potential pitfalls of this technique.

Anesthesia for pediatric endoscopy is quite different than for adults. General anesthesia without endotracheal intubation with spontaneous ventilation is the preferred method for endoscopic telescopic examination of the pediatric larynx. This technique relies on an inhalation anesthetic with spontaneous ventilation. The inhalation agents include oxygen, halothane, or another inhalation anesthetic and nitrous oxide. Topical 1% or 2% lidocaine provides added protection against laryngospasm during airway manipulation. In this way, spontaneous movements of the vocal folds and dynamic assessment of the airway may be made under general anesthesia.

### Microscopes

The operating microscope with a 400-mm objective lens is used for microlaryngoscopy. The articulating arms must be set up and balanced for suspension laryngoscopy but not for otologic surgery. A high-intensity, 300-W xenon light source for the microscope can illuminate the field without additional light from the laryngoscope. This removes one more piece of equipment from the mouth. A high-intensity xenon light also allows the beam splitter to be used for laryngeal photography.

### Telescopes

Telescopes used in conjunction with endoscopic examinations of the larynx offer additional benefits in selected situations. The Hopkins rod telescopes are 3.5 mm thick and 30 cm long. The device comes in a 0° forward view, a 30° angled view, a 70° lateral view, and a 120° retroverted view. The forward-angled scope is valuable for the inspection of the anterior commissure and the laryngeal surface of the epiglottis. The 70° lateral view is used to inspect the ventricle and the vocal fold edge. The 120° retroverted view is used to look at the subglottic larynx and the undersurface of the vocal fold. The telescopes are also extremely useful during bronchoscopy. A slim telescope can be inserted into the trachea without disturbance of spontaneous respiration. This is especially useful when the dynamic changes of the trachea and esophagus need to be visualized. When used in conjunction with the video camera and the printer, four pictures using differently angled scopes can be quickly captured and printed without undue loss in time. We do not routinely use telescopes during the performance of suspension microlaryngeal surgery, but endoscopes are routinely used during diagnostic laryngoscopy, laryngeal biopsy, vocal fold injections, and foreign body removal.

### Lasers

The carbon dioxide ($CO_2$) laser continues to be the laser of choice in laryngologic operations. Devices with other wavelengths, such as the argon, neodymium:yttrium-aluminum-garnet (Nd:YAG), and potassium-titanyl-phosphate (KTP) lasers have been used, but they have limited applications. The $CO_2$ laser can be focused down to less than 250 μm with the newest micromanipulators. A helium-neon aiming beam focuses the spot size appropriate for the lesion being treated. With the laser, a no-touch, stable platform can be used to deliver ablative laser energy to coagulate, vaporize, or cut tissue. The advantages of lasers are no-touch, continuous visualization of pathology; hemostasis; precision; and less edema. Some investigators believe there is also less operative pain. A possible disadvantage of the laser is the delay in healing and the risk of thermal damage to tissue. Some physicians object to the small area of tissue ablation by the laser, making assessment of a cancer-free margin more difficult.

Laser users may fail to appreciate the concept of power density. Tissue ablation is dictated by laser power density, not laser power. A smaller spot size means a higher power density for the same laser power output. A surgeon used to 5-W laser power with a 0.5-mm spot size must readjust the power output to a much lower level if the laser spot size is 0.25 mm. The laser power density is defined as the power delivered per square cm of tissue. To achieve the desired laser-tissue interaction, a twofold reduction in spot size means a fourfold reduction in laser power output to achieve the equivalent power density. A too-high power density results in unwanted laser penetration and energy absorption into deeper tissues. For fine ablation of tissues, milliwatt output using a superpulse mode can ensure the finest spot size with the least collateral thermal effect.

Controversies have continued about whether $CO_2$ laser is indicated in the management of benign disorders of the larynx. Concerns about excess thermal effects and the late effect of scar formation have caused some investigators to condemn the use of lasers for treating polyps, nodules, and lesions of the vocal fold edge. I feel the problem is a lack of appreciation of laser-tissue interaction and understanding of the laser instrument. Using a $CO_2$ laser as an ablative instrument for the management of an intracordal vocal cyst is misuse of the instrument. On the other hand, the use of lasers to accurately remove tissue is unparalleled. Laser cordectomy or laser ablation of small vessels on the vocal fold are good examples of the unique uses of the $CO_2$ laser. Table 40.5 lists some of the applications of the $CO_2$ laser in the larynx.

**TABLE 40.5. APPLICATION OF THE $CO_2$ LASER IN LARYNGOLOGY**

- Treatment of recurrent respiratory papilloma
- Endoscopic management of laryngeal stenosis
- Laser cordectomy for early-stage laryngeal carcinoma
- Endoscopic debulking of obstruction tumor for relief of airway obstruction
- Laser ablation of small feeding vessels causing vocal hemorrhage
- Laser arytenoidectomy or transverse cordotomy for bilateral vocal cord paralysis
- Laser debulking of granuloma and flaps
- Laser sculpting of buccal mucosal grafts

## *Laryngoscopes*

Despite the many operating laryngoscopes that are available, only a few are necessary for most procedures. Diagnostic laryngoscopes are monocular tube instruments with distal illumination that are designed to be hand held. The laryngoscopes designed by Jackson and Hollinger have stood the test of time for being a simple yet versatile, single-handed instrument for exploration of the larynx. With these instruments and the Hopkins rod telescopes, excellent visualization and biopsies of the larynx can be obtained in virtually all patients. Bimanual examination and magnification are not possible.

Operating laryngoscopes comes in different sizes and shapes. The operating laryngoscopes are designed to allow binocular visualization under the microscope. They have a wider bore to allow entrance and manipulation of microinstruments. Some have adapters for laser suction. Some of the newer modifications have side slots open to make instrument placement easier. Sometimes, the simpler tube laryngoscopes are the easiest to use. The Dedo, Jako, or Kleinsasser operating laryngoscopes have sizes for males and female larynges and are useful for most examinations and surgery of the glottis. For specialty uses, the slimline Benjamin scope, the Lindholm operating laryngoscope, and the bivalved Werda laryngoscopes should be satisfactory for most work in the larynx. The Lindholm operating laryngoscope is unique in its wide bore and distal tilt. It is placed in the vallecula to expose the epiglottis, aryepiglottic folds, the arytenoids, and the hypopharynx. With a Lindholm laryngoscope, the entire larynx may be exposed for surgery. Procedures such as laser excision of the supraglottic larynx, laser arytenoidectomy, and partial pharyngeal resections can be accomplished with this instrument. The Werda bivalve laryngoscope is useful for distention of the tissues of the larynx and is especially advantageous in laser resections of the vocal fold for larger cancers. The slimline Benjamin binocular operating laryngoscope is useful for the difficult-to-expose larynx. The anterior commissure is easier to expose with this scope than with any other operating laryngoscope. One drawback of the scope when used with the laser is the problem of parallax. Because of the smaller proximal opening, it is difficult to deliver the laser at full power to the visualized larynx. The Healy subglottiscope and the trachea scope are additions to the endoscopy cart to complete the scopes necessary for airway management.

## *Instruments*

### Instruments for Microlaryngoscopy

The instruments necessary for microlaryngoscopy are few but are delicate. Small probes, picks, and knives are the instruments that are specially designed for laryngeal surgery. These are available on an interchangeable hand grip. Suction tubes with diameters of 1 to 2 mm are very useful for microlaryngeal suction. For most tissue manipulation on the vocal fold edge, small forceps and scissors are used. The working distance is 18 to 22 cm. Developments in microinstrumentation have produced extremely delicate instruments. The cup size used is now approaching 1 mm. This makes delicate manipulation of vocal fold of tissue possible. The small cup forceps is primarily used for manipulation, not removal, of tissue. Scissors may be straight, curved to the right, or curved to the left. I use the straight scissors, the upward scissors, and the right and left curved scissors for most dissections and surgical removal of lesions. Surgical knives and probes are used to dissect the tissue deep to the vocal fold cover. Although many knives are available with different angulations, a sickle knife, straight pick, and sharp scissors of different configurations suffice for most phonosurgery procedures.

### Suction Coagulators

Electrical surgical units coupled to suction tubing are extremely helpful in the management of bleeding. During bloody procedures such as laser arytenoidectomy, having suction tubing connected to an electrical surgical unit may mean the difference between the ability to finish the procedure and aborting. The electrical coagulation units are monopolar in nature and may conduct electrocoagulation energy deep into the tissue. For patient safety, using the lowest electrocoagulation power necessary to stop the bleeding is the best.

### Topical and Injection Drugs

During microlaryngoscopy, several drugs are used topically or injected sufficiently frequently to justify their routine preparation on the operating table. For example, 1:1,000 epinephrine and Depo-Medrol (40 mg/mL) is set up with a small paddy of cotton applicators. Injection of the tissue for hemostasis before incisions and after surgery is carried out with a 25-gauge butterfly needle on a tuberculin syringe. The same arrangement is used for injections of steroids to reduce postoperative swelling and reduce granulation formation.

### Endoscopy Technique

General anesthesia is given after the anesthesiologist is certain that control of the airway is possible. The patient is intubated with a small endotracheal tube. The size of the endotracheal tube is usually 5 mm for women and 5.5 mm for men. A laser-safe tube or the jet Venturi tube is placed if jet ventilation or a laser is to be used. Even before administration of general anesthesia, the surgeon has a plan for exposure of the larynx. It includes selection of the anesthesia technique, the lasers and laser coupler, and the laryngoscope. Laryngoscope selection is based on the surgical procedure that is planned and the optimal exposure that is possible. With recognition that most of the equipment may be used in laryngoscopy and microlaryngoscopy, three distinct laryngoscopic procedures of are possible: direct laryngoscopy and biopsy, direct laryngoscopy with telescopic examination, and suspension microlaryngoscopy. These procedures are graduated in terms complexity and equipment needs.

### Position

The position of the patient is critical to exposure of the larynx. The patient should lie flat, with the head at the end of the operating table. After the patient is intubated, the table is turned 90° to the endoscopist. For the right-handed surgeon, the tube is taped to the left corner of the patient's mouth. The surgeon approaches the patient in the midline or along the left gutter of the oral cavity. To straighten out the right angle of the larynx to the oral cavity, the physician elevates the patient's head, bringing the chin forward and tilting the maxilla and upper jaw backward (Fig. 40.5). The classic Bryce-Jackson position of neck flexion and head extension is good for the initial position. Sandbags are not placed under the shoulder. The larynx is difficult to expose in some patients. They must be fully relaxed, and several trials may be needed to position the patient and bring the larynx into view. The larynx is an anterior diverticulum off the pharynx. With extreme flexion of the patient's neck while the physician's left hand moves the lower jaw in an anterior-superior direction, the larynx "drops" into view.

The tooth protector is inserted into the mouth to protect the teeth. Wet gauze or a rubber pad is used if the patient is edentulous. With the larynx exposed, topical lidocaine is sprayed into the endolarynx.

The largest possible laryngoscope is selected for laryngoscopy. A panoramic view of the larynx and pharynx is available with the wide-bore scopes operating scopes. With experience, the surgeon can select different sizes, depending on the size of the patient and the neck anatomy. The laryngoscope is introduced into the oropharynx along the dorsum of the tongue or along the lateral gutter of the floor of the mouth. Secretions are suctioned from the oropharynx and hypopharynx. The uvula, tonsil fossa, base of the tongue, vallecula, and posterior pharyngeal wall are inspected. The distal tip of the epiglottis is identified. Using the anterior lip of the laryngoscope, the opening between the tip of the epiglottis and the endotracheal tube is used to position the laryngoscope. It is important to not displace the epiglottis inward during the insertion of the laryngoscope because it reduces dramatically the view of the endolarynx and may create significant epiglottic edema. The aryepiglottic folds, the pharyngoepiglottic folds, the piriform fossa, and the postcricoid area are visualized. The laryngoscope then is passed into the endolarynx. The tip of the laryngoscope is advanced until the petiole of the epiglottis is reached. The laryngoscope should be deep enough to show both vocal folds symmetrically in the endoscope. The anterior commissure should be visible, and the false vocal folds are pushed aside to reveal the entire membranous vocal fold. The laryngoscope then may be suspended on the left hand to allow a stable platform for laryngeal biopsy, palpation, or suction. Backward tilting of the laryngoscope should be avoided because it exerts excessive pressure on the upper teeth. If the anterior commissure to the vocal fold is visible, the patient is ready for suspension laryngoscopy.

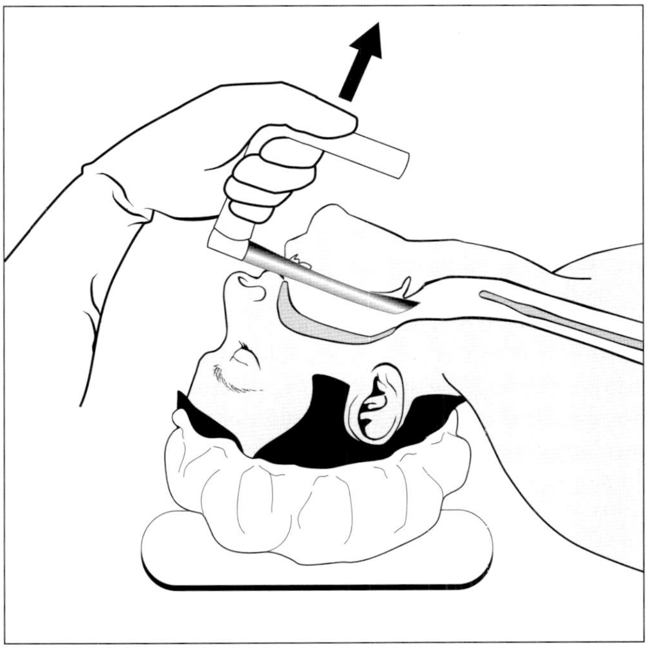

**FIGURE 40.5.** Endoscopic position and suspension. The vector of suspension is aimed superiorly to lift the jaw and head *(arrow)*.

The laryngeal surface of the epiglottis, the false vocal folds, the ventricle, and the arytenoids are inspected as part of the supraglottis examination, and the true vocal folds, the anterior and posterior commissure, the cartilagenous glottis, and the subglottis are inspected as part of the glottis and subglottis evaluation. Arytenoid palpation and inspection of the posterior larynx for intubation injuries and posterior webs are facilitated by using the laryngoscope to lift the endotracheal tube and displace it into the area occupied by the membranous vocal folds. If the area of the anterior commissure or the subglottis is difficult to visualize, external laryngeal counterpressure may be applied by the free hand to depress the larynx or to roll the larynx to better visualize the specific endolaryngeal structures. It is important to avoid injury to the true vocal folds by the tip of the laryngoscope. In no way should the laryngoscope tip splay out the vocal folds unless it is the intention of the surgeon to work on the subglottic larynx or trachea.

After the laryngoscope is in position, the suspension apparatus is applied. The vocal folds should be exposed by further turning the suspension apparatus. Tension on the vocal folds should exist but should not be excessive. Excessive tension can obscure lesions seen by preoperative stroboscopy such as vessels, Reinke's edema, and pseudocysts. This is especially important during the surgical management of small lesions of the vocal fold.

Specialty scopes are occasionally necessary. The Hollinger laryngoscope has a very narrow waist that can be very helpful in patients with small jaws and short necks. With the use of telescopes, the wide panoramic view is possible through the small channel. The Jackson laryngoscope has a broad spatula tip that can be used to lift the larynx, splay open the pyriform sinus, and inspect the upper esophageal sphincter.

**Telescopic Endoscopy**

The 0°, 30°, 70°, or 120° Hopkins rigid rod-lens telescopes offer the surgeon the chance to examine the larynx with magnification and at different angles than that possible with the laryngoscope alone. The use of the telescope may be applied during the initial laryngoscopy or after the suspension apparatus is in place. Suspension telescopic endoscopy allows the surgeon to perform suction, palpation, and tissue retraction at the same time as telescopic endoscopy. The ventricle, the subglottis, laryngeal surface of the epiglottis, and the undersurface of the vocal folds can be better visualized with the 70° and 120° telescopes. With the use of the telescopes, subtle abnormalities of the vocal fold may be visible.

## Special Operative Techniques

### Laryngeal Biopsy

The amount of tissue necessary to make a histologic diagnosis must be adequate, but the consequences of a too-large biopsy may worsen dysphonia, produce excessive scarring, and cause patient dissatisfaction after surgery. For most lesions that are clearly benign, microphonosurgery techniques that respect the layered microanatomy of the vocal folds are best. Bimanual tissue manipulation, magnification, and conservative tissue removal are the guiding principles. Even for suspected tumor, magnification allows the surgeon to take representative biopsies from the margin of the tumor. The motion of the cup biopsy after grasping the specimen should always be parallel and within the layer of the affected vocal fold. Mucosal biopsy samples should not include muscle. Injury to the vocal ligament, vocalis muscle, and conus elasticus is avoidable. Some areas are especially vulnerable to injury, such as the anterior commissure and the vocal process of the arytenoid, because the vocal ligament is much closer to the epithelium than the mid-membranous vocal fold at the anterior and posterior attachments of the vocal fold. Injury to the vocal ligament from biopsy or vocal stripping results in notching and an irregular fold, a condition that is difficult to correct.

Biopsies can be classified as diagnostic epithelial biopsies, incisional biopsies, or excisional biopsies. The excisional biopsy is recommended for small cancers, lesions of uncertain or premalignant character, and removal of lesions done to improve voice. Incisional biopsy may be necessary in patients with a normal overlying mucosa but who have bulging of tissue. Amyloidosis, chondrosarcoma, and lymphoma are examples of when an incisional biopsy is appropriate. In these cases, the laser may be used to make the initial incision down to the suspected lesion, cup forceps are used to remove tissue for frozen section, and the operative site bleeding is controlled by pressure or electrocautery. Small biopsies for frozen section from the epithelial margin may be necessary during planned endoscopic excision of squamous cell cancer. This should be sampled at the mucosal margin and the deep margin. The excised specimen should be prepared by orientation, pinned or glued onto a tissue carrier, and submitted to the pathology department with a request for multiple sections.

Vocal fold stripping as a surgery is rarely done today. Vocal fold stripping is a term that should be replaced by *vocal fold lesion excision under magnification.*

### Difficult Laryngoscopy

The difficult adult airway makes exposure for microlaryngoscopy or even laryngeal biopsy a challenge. A checklist of possible factors should be formulated to help the endoscopist to achieve maximum exposure. Some of the general factors include the relaxation of the patient, the patient's position, selection of the size of the endotracheal tube, the laryngoscope, and the skill of the endoscopy team.

Sometimes, local anatomy of the neck and jaws makes rigid endoscopic examination of the larynx impractical. Patients with an unstable cervical spine and those in a brace are not to be manipulated. Congenital dislocation of the odontoid process, craniofacial deformities, mandibular joint fixation, facial fractures, pharyngeal and floor of mouth abscesses, neck contracture, and macroglossia are but a partial list of causes that can contribute to a difficult laryngoscopy.

The most common problems of exposure encountered are the inability to expose the area because of anatomic factors of the patient. The muscular male with a short neck and prominent teeth may make exposure of anything more than the posterior larynx difficult. The anterior commissure is an especially challenging area. The larger endoscopic surgical procedures of partial supraglottic laryngectomy and laser arytenoidectomy require simultaneous exposure of the larynx and the pharynx. In the difficult exposure, greater lever action and suspension are not fruitful.

For the difficult airway, having a backup plan is prudent. Using a Hollinger laryngoscope with a 30° forward-looking rigid endoscope is one alternative. The Hollinger laryngoscope can be combined with suspension laryngoscopy. A forward telescope and an upward-biting cup forceps allow the surgeon to get a biopsy sample, even from the inaccessible undersurface of the anterior commissure. For patients who need to undergo microlaryngoscopy with excision, the Hollinger laryngoscope can be suspended, the operating microscope brought in, and using one eye, small pediatric microscissors and microcups can be introduced to permit the surgeon to perform bimanual microlaryngoscopy. This does not afford the surgeon binocular vision, but it does allow the surgeon magnification and bimanual manipulation of tissue.

Special care is necessary in the management of patients with supraglottic airway obstruction. The variable obstruction of the supraglottic by tumor, laryngocele, edema, papilloma, or cyst may make the management of the airway hazardous during the intubation and extubation. Potential compromise of the airway during induction in these patients must be anticipated. It may be safest to perform a tracheostomy under local anesthesia before operative endoscopy.

## *Mobility of the Cricoarytenoid Joint*

Operative endoscopy and palpation of the cricoarytenoid joint is indicated in some patients to differentiate between the possible causes of the immobile vocal fold. Office endoscopy may reveal an immobile vocal fold but not be able to differentiate between arytenoid dislocation, arytenoid ankylosis, or vocal fold paralysis. Mobility of the vocal folds may be compromised after prolonged intubation. Patients with rheumatologic involvement of small joints and laryngeal trauma may have joint fixation. Congenital or acquired laryngeal stenosis may mimic vocal cord paralysis. Nasogastric tube injury of the posterior cricoarytenoid muscle, myositis, muscle infiltration with tumor, fibrosis and scar after irradiation, and myasthenia gravis can cause local muscle weakness that mimics paralysis. Laryngeal electromyography, done in conjunction with a skilled electromyographer, is the best way to diagnose vocal cord paralysis without operative endoscopy. However, operative endoscopy or office endoscopy with arytenoid palpation sometimes is indicated to evaluate the mobility of the cricoarytenoid joint.

Palpation of the cricoarytenoid joint can be performed in cooperative adults after office laryngeal anesthesia. The curved laryngeal spatula or the curved laryngeal biopsy forceps is placed into the larynx under telescopic control. The joint is palpated by lateral displacement of the vocal process. Moving the spatula from the midline displaces the arytenoid cartilage and opens the glottis aperture. This is done first on the mobile vocal fold and then on the immobile vocal fold. The feel of the mobile cricoarytenoid joint is quite distinct from that of the stiff ankylosis joint.

## *Postoperative Care*

Most operative laryngoscopic surgery can be performed in an outpatient surgery center or in a hospital with day admission. Absolute voice rest after microlaryngeal surgery was the standard in the past, but for practical purposes, relative voice rest is acceptable. Relative voice rest means speaking in a confidential tone of voice. It is limited to speaking in a quiet room to an individual less than 3 feet away. If there is pain, cough, or strain, voice rest is restricted. Postoperative medication and diet restriction after microlaryngeal surgery is minimal. Antitussives, antacids, and antibiotics are usually prescribed for 7 days after surgery.

The patient is reexamined at 7 days after surgery. The physician inspects the operative site to determine whether functional rehabilitation can begin. The examiner also reviews the pathology report and medical management with the patient. In uncomplicated surgery of the vocal fold such as that for polyps, nodules, or cysts or for biopsy, the vocal fold is usually healed to permit voice use. Videostroboscopy demonstrates return of vibratory amplitude and mucosal wave. If there is persistent edema, fibrin, or erythema, medications such as steroids, antacids, and antibiotics may be needed. Early inspection and functional assessment of vibratory function enables the surgeon to better control the healing process, allows the patient to return to function earlier, and reduces complications such as scarring and compensatory vocal hyperfunction. Voice therapy is commenced after vocal fold healing, which is demonstrable as return of or improved vibratory amplitude and mucosal wave. Vigorous vocal exercises such as shouting, singing, and voice building should be avoided until the vocal fold is no longer erythematous. Many patients benefit from postoperative voice therapy. A partial list of patients who benefit from voice therapy after microlaryngeal surgery is shown in Table 40.6.

**TABLE 40.6. INDICATIONS FOR POSTOPERATIVE VOICE THERAPY**

- Vocal fold nodules
- Contact granuloma and contact ulcers
- After fat injection for vocal atrophy
- After sulcus resection
- After Reinke's edema resection
- After cordectomy or arytenoidectomy for bilateral vocal cord paralysis
- After repeated laser ablation of papilloma or vocal fold cover resection
- Excessive scar after microsurgery or biopsy

Complications are uncommon after surgery. Anesthetic complications such as urinary retention, muscle cramping, and excessive weakness may occur. These problems should be discussed with the patient before discharge from the outpatient setting.

Local complications such as dental enamel injury, lip laceration, and hematoma may occur. The use of a dental protector does not prevent such injury. Prolonged suspension laryngoscopy may result in temporary lingual nerve hypoesthesia that can last for weeks. The tip of the laryngoscope should be released periodically if the endoscopy procedure will be long. If there is discoloration of the tongue, tongue edema, or epiglottis edema, intraoperative steroids should be given, and the patient should be removed from suspension. Edema of the larynx may be observed after surgery. If the surgery is limited to the membranous vocal folds and the vocal folds are mobile, successful extubation is rarely a problem. Patients who have a limitation of vocal fold motion due to laryngeal stenosis, bilateral vocal fold paralysis, or arytenoid ankylosis are at risk for postoperative edema. These patients may need special monitoring in an intensive care setting after surgery.

Bleeding may result from trauma by a laryngoscope blade that caused tears in the base of the tongue, epiglottis, pharynx, or vocal fold. These tears are painful and may affect the recovery of oral feeding after surgery. Deeper lacerations should be treated with antibiotics, steroids, and if necessary, suture repair. Bleeding during surgery can usually be controlled by packing with epinephrine-soaked pads or with suction coagulation. Bleeding from massive tumors may be great enough to demand laryngeal or pharyngeal packing with airway control. Rarely, massive bleeding due to major vessel injury can occur with rupture of arterial venous malformation or hemangioma. These problems may demand rapid, open laryngeal surgery or surgical ligation of neck vessels to control bleeding.

Late complications of operative laryngoscopy include granulomas, scar, stenosis, and web formation. The best way to avoid late complications is by careful surgery. Avoidance of postoperative trauma by coughing or excessive throat clearing is helped by lidocaine spray during surgery and the use of cough suppressants postoperatively. This is especially true after vocal granuloma removal and after large epithelial resections. Hypertrophic scar can be managed by the early use of oral or endoscopic steroid injections. To decrease the likelihood of postoperative scar and inflammation, prophylactic use of a proton pump inhibitor is advocated to reduce reflux laryngitis.

**TABLE 40.7. PATHOLOGIC ENTITIES IDENTIFIED WITH DIAGNOSTIC LARYNGOSCOPY**

- Congenital lesions
  - Webs
  - Clefts
- Traumatic lesions
  - Intubation
  - Eustachian tube dysfunction
  - Laryngeal fracture
  - Hematoma
  - Hemorrhage
  - Granuloma
- Paralysis
  - Superior laryngeal nerve
  - Recurrent laryngeal nerve
  - Combined
  - Bilateral recurrent laryngeal nerve
- Benign mucosal lesions
  - Nodules
  - Polyps
  - Reinke's edema
  - Cysts
  - Varix
  - Sulcus
  - Granuloma
  - Keratosis
  - Varix
  - Vocal atrophy
  - Mucosal bridge
  - Scar
- Benign tumors
  - Papilloma
  - Salivary gland tumors
- Precancerous squamous lesions
  - Dysplasia and grading of dysplasia
  - Erythroplakia
- Squamous cell carcinoma
- Inflammation
  - Reflux laryngitis
    - Presentation
    - Diagnosis by endoscopy
    - Treatment
  - Acute laryngitis
  - Subacute laryngitis
  - Chronic laryngitis
  - Hyperplastic laryngitis
  - Pachydermia
- Other tumors
  - Kaposi sarcoma
  - Myeloma
  - Chondroma
  - Adenoid cystic
  - Lymphoma
- Systemic manifestations
  - Amyloid
  - Sarcoid
  - Tuberculosis
  - Human immunodeficiency viral disease
  - Systemic lupus erythematosus, rheumatoid arthritis
  - Wegener's granulomatosis

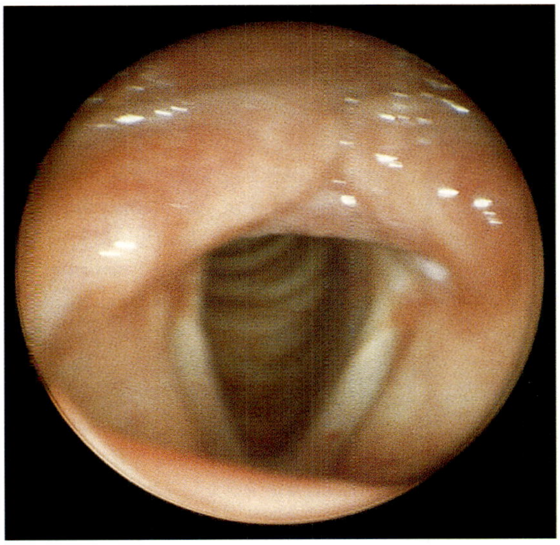

**FIGURE 40.6.** Panoramic view of the larynx and pharynx using a 70° endoscope shows the larynx, pharynx, postcricoid area, and the upper esophageal inlet.

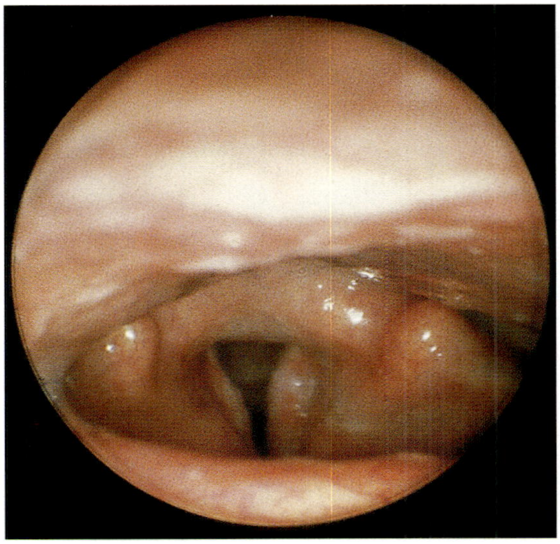

**FIGURE 40.8.** Right vocal fold abduction is greater than the left.

## SURGERY AND ENDOSCOPY

A variety of pathologic entities can be identified using diagnostic laryngoscopy (Table 40.7). In this section, examples of specific disorders are presented.

### Endoscopy

A panoramic view of the larynx and pharynx is seen with the 70° endoscope (Fig. 40.6). The larynx, pharynx, postcricoid area, and upper esophageal inlet can be seen clearly. Although the details of the vocal folds during vibration are not apparent, a panoramic view of the pharynx and larynx is important for the diagnosis of movement abnormalities, growths, and structural changes of the lower vocal tract.

Four common lesions can be appreciated by office endoscopy without other instruments, and left vocal fold paralysis can be seen in Figure 40.7. The right vocal fold is abducted more than the left (Fig. 40.8). Swelling of the right vocal fold was caused by a sizable intracordal mass or cyst (Fig. 40.9). A large, posterior glottis leukoplakia and

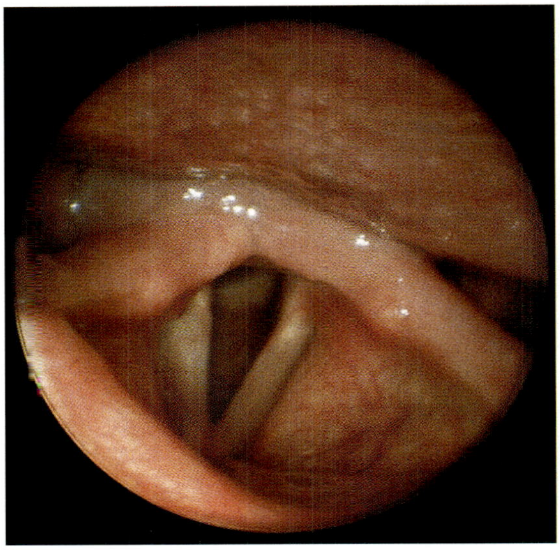

**FIGURE 40.7.** Left vocal fold paralysis.

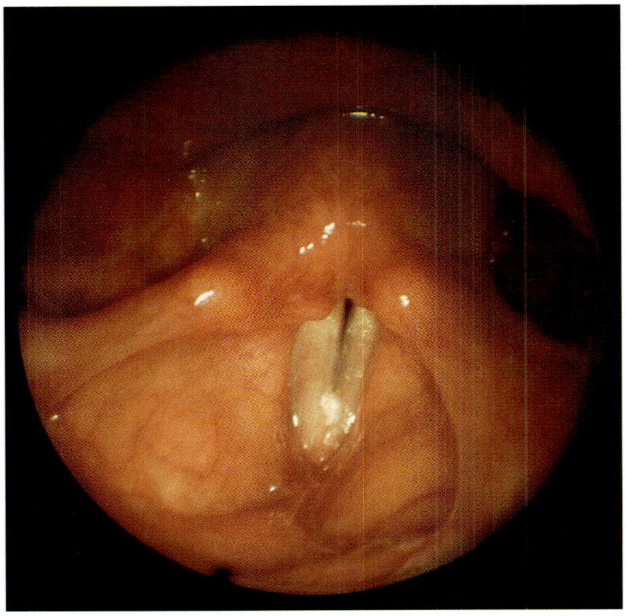

**FIGURE 40.9.** Swelling on the right vocal fold is caused by a large, intracordal mass or cyst.

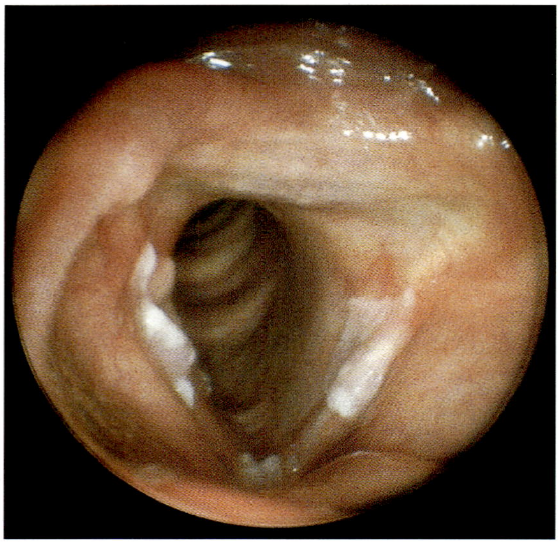

**FIGURE 40.10.** Large, posterior glottic leukoplakia and mucus retention at the anterior margin of the vocal fold in a patient with chronic laryngitis.

mucus retention are evident at the anterior margin of the vocal fold in a patient with chronic laryngitis (Fig. 40.10).

## Stroboscopy

Low, loud phonation (Fig. 40.11) at 95 Hz and 82 dB is demonstrated by a man. Vocal fold vibration patterns differ greatly depending on the frequency, loudness, and register. The vibratory pattern with the greatest amplitude and mucosal wave change is produced at low and loud phonation. High-pitched phonations of the vocal folds produce an elongated, spindle-shaped configuration.

*Unilateral vocal fold polyp* with small, contralateral keratin reaction is shown in Figure 40.12. Stroboscopic and telescopic examination of a unilateral polyp of the vocal fold is demonstrated in Figure 40.13. There is the appearance of recent hemorrhage with a hemosiderin deposit on the vocal fold. The vocal fold closure is incomplete, and there is loss of vibratory behavior in the affected vocal fold around the polyp.

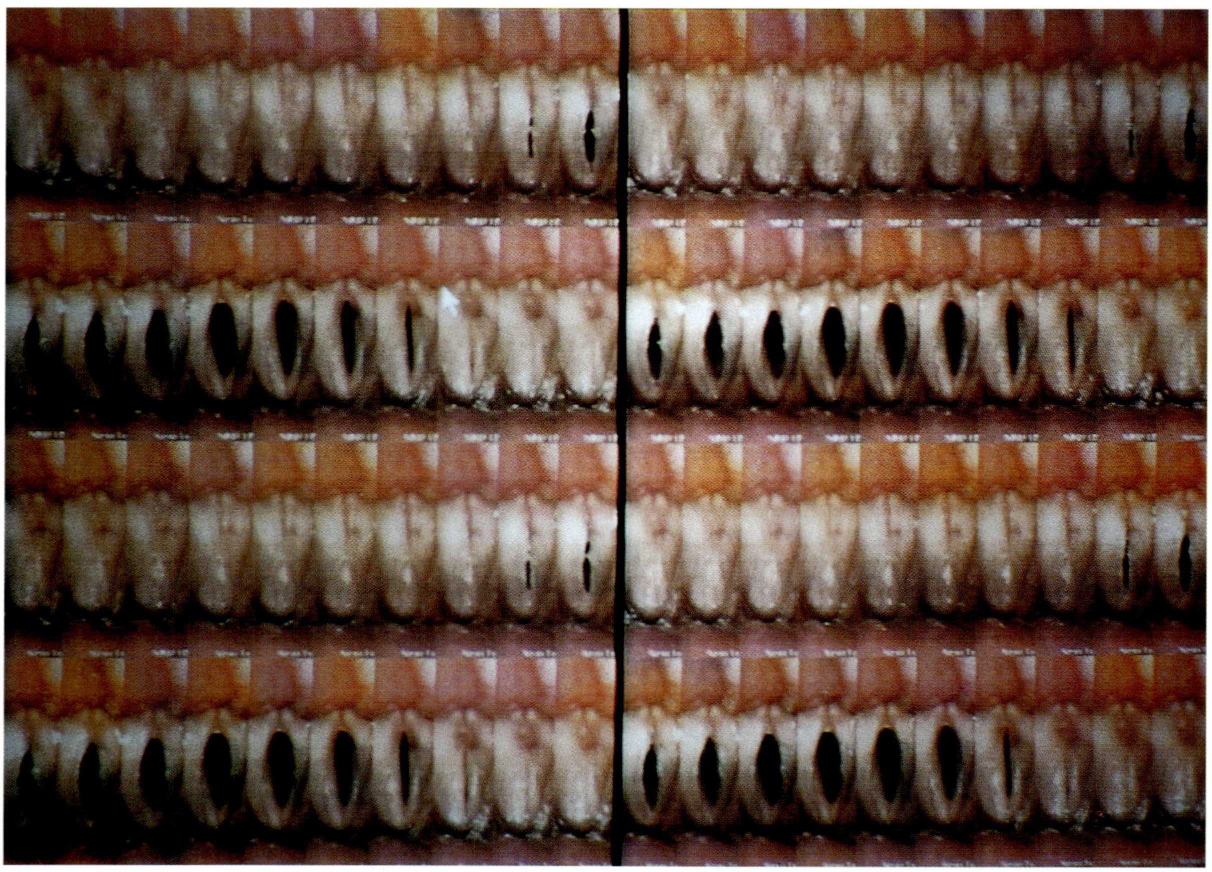

**FIGURE 40.11.** Vocal fold vibration in a man at 95 Hz and 82 dB. The vocal fold vibratory pattern with the greatest amplitude and mucosal wave change is produced at low and loud phonation.

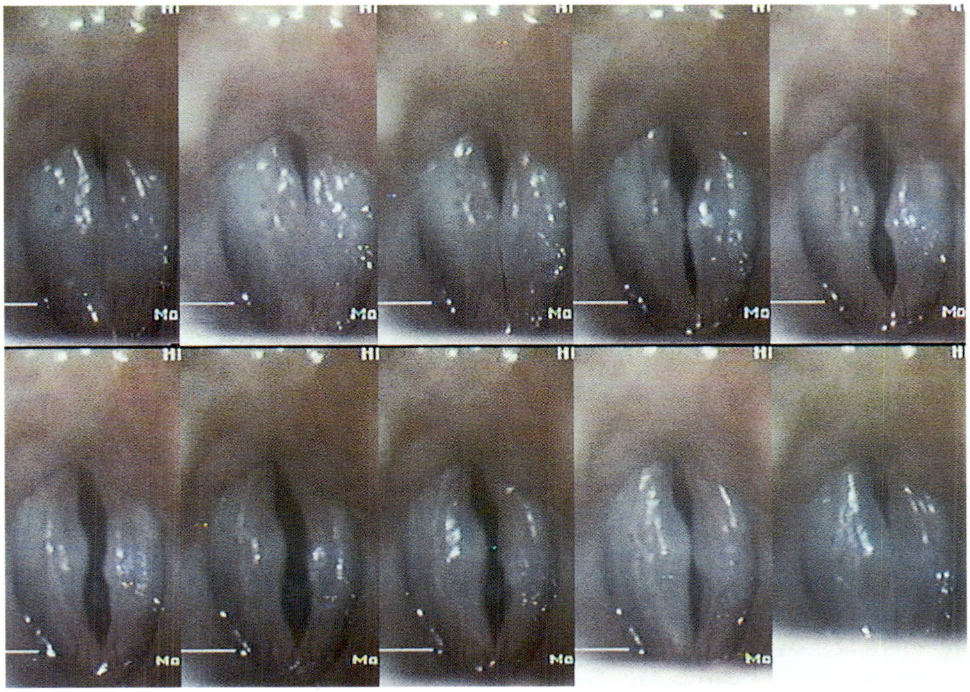

**FIGURE 40.12.** Unilateral vocal fold polyp with a small, contralateral keratin reaction.

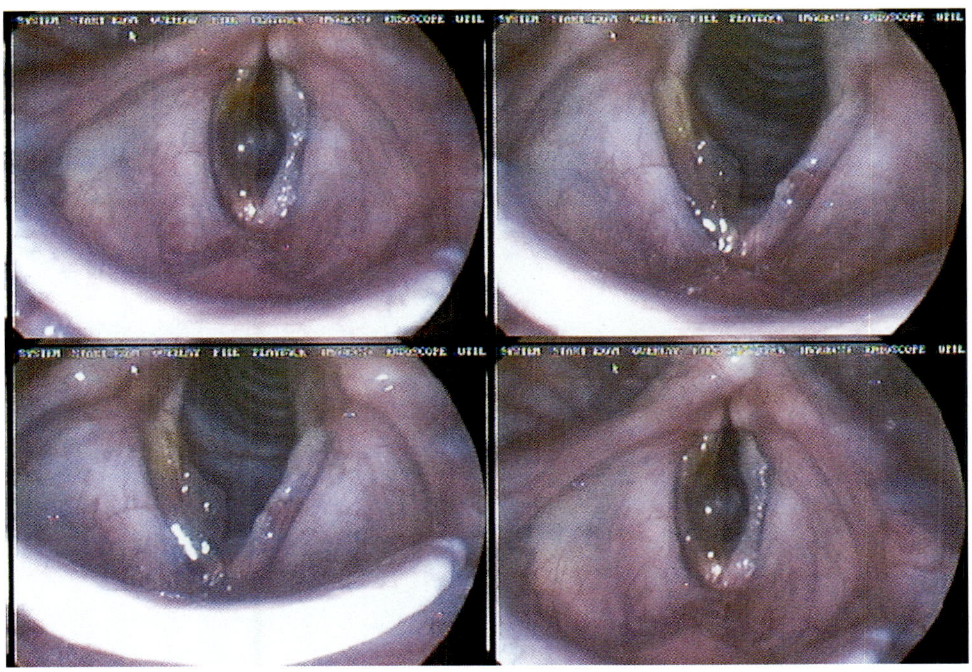

**FIGURE 40.13.** Stroboscopic and telescopic examination of a unilateral polyp of the vocal fold. Notice the recent hemorrhage, the incomplete vocal fold closure, and the loss of vibratory behavior on the affected vocal fold surrounding the polyp.

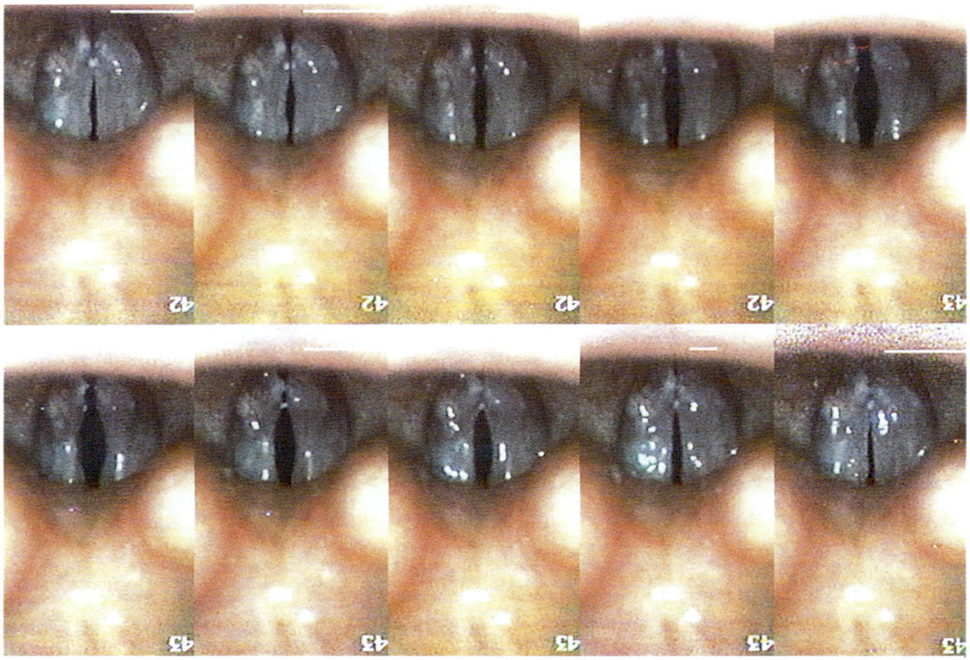

**FIGURE 40.14.** Small, intracordal cyst in a female teacher with a chronic hoarse voice.

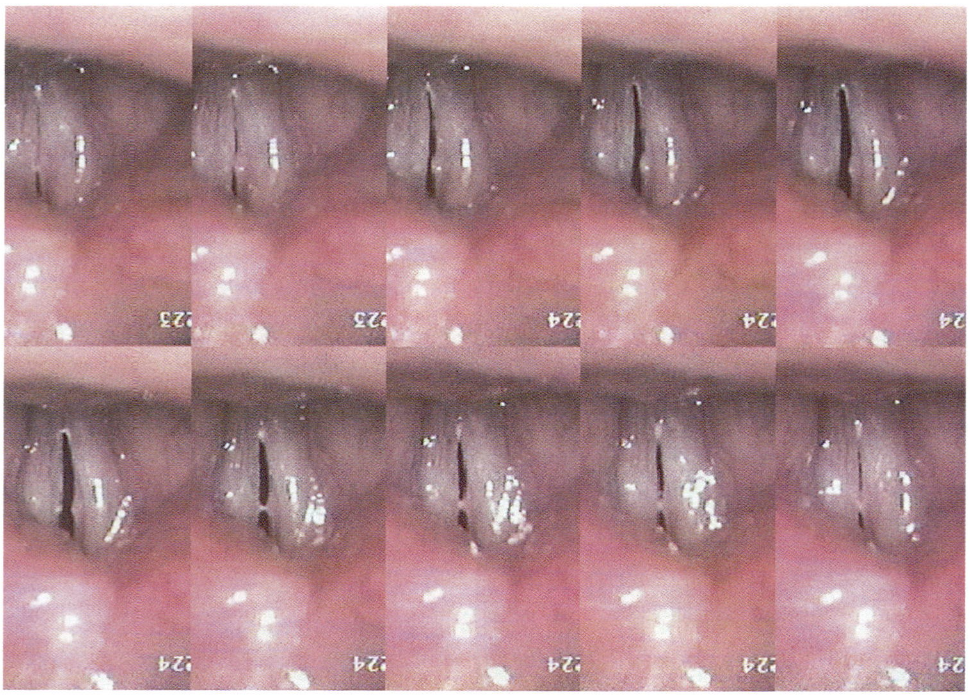

**FIGURE 40.15.** Intracordal cyst on the superior surface of the vocal fold in a patient with unexplained dysphonia.

A small, intracordal *cyst* is present in this female teacher with a chronically hoarse voice (Fig. 40.14). The vocal cords are in an open phase throughout the glottal cycle. The side with the cyst shows reduced amplitude and vibratory behavior. The mucosal wave is absent on the anterior portion of the vocal fold where the cyst lies. A more obvious cyst is seen on the superior surface of the vocal fold in a patient with unexplained dysphonia (Fig. 40.15). The glottal cycle shows a large, posterior chink, an open-phase–predominant pattern, and reduced amplitude of vibration on the side of the cyst. The cyst has caused a small, contralateral nodal reaction. Treatment is surgical.

Congenital *sulcus vocalis* is seen on videostroboscopy (Fig. 40.16). The groove on each vocal fold is apparent on inspiration and on phonation. The effect on the vibratory behavior is characterized by a spindle-shaped glottal opening, incomplete glottal closure, and loss of vibratory amplitude and wave.

A *contact ulcer or granuloma* is often confused with a cancer because of its white, keratotic appearance (Fig. 40.17). Laryngoscopic and stroboscopic findings include apparent squeezing of the false vocal folds, anterior-to-posterior squeezing of the true vocal folds, and premature vocal process contact before the onset of phonation. These are typical findings of vocal hyperfunction that lead to the development of contact granuloma (Fig. 40.18).

The stroboscopy finding in a patient with *vocal cord paralysis* is shown in Figure 40.19. The loss in the tension of the left vocal fold resulted in bowing. There is a slight phase lag of the paralyzed vocal fold relative to the innervated side. The voice was slightly breathy.

Small mid-membranous vocal fold *nodules* are seen in a male countertenor (Fig. 40.20). This condition was associated

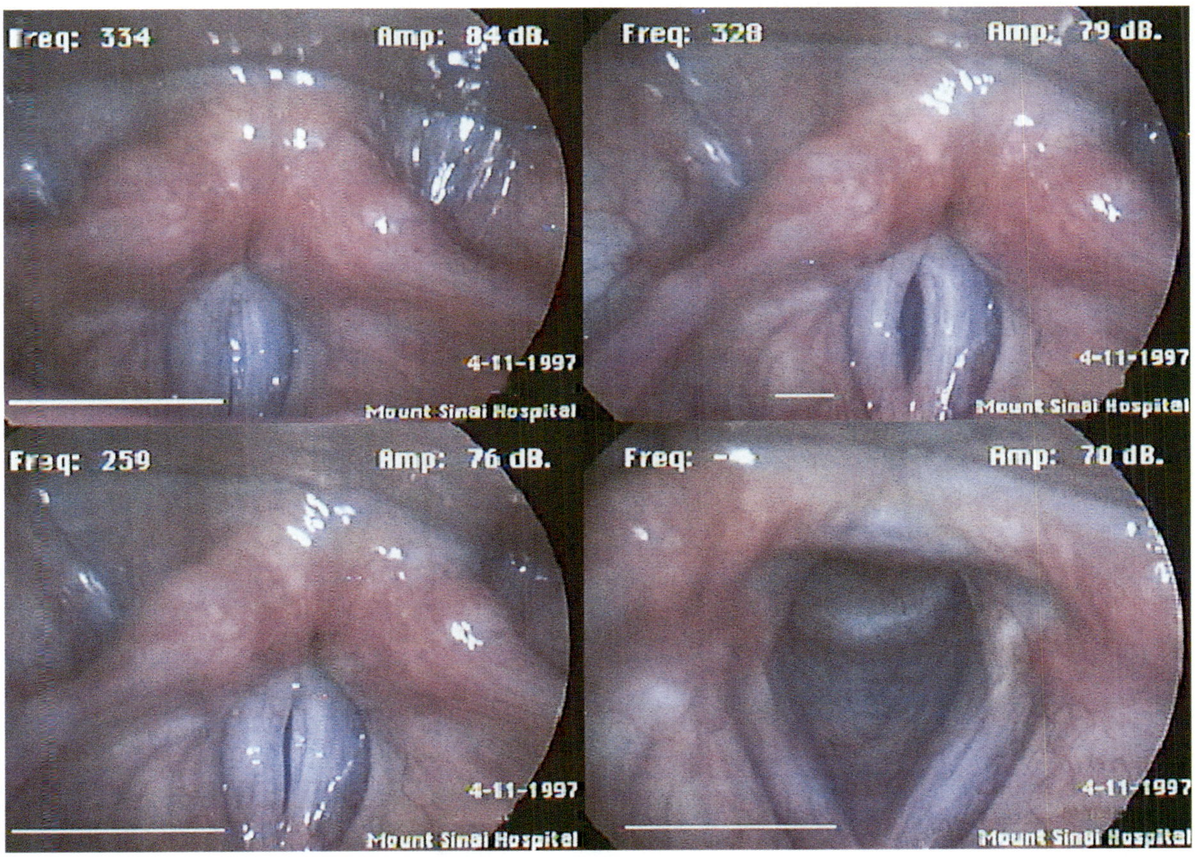


**FIGURE 40.16.** Congenital sulcus vocalis.

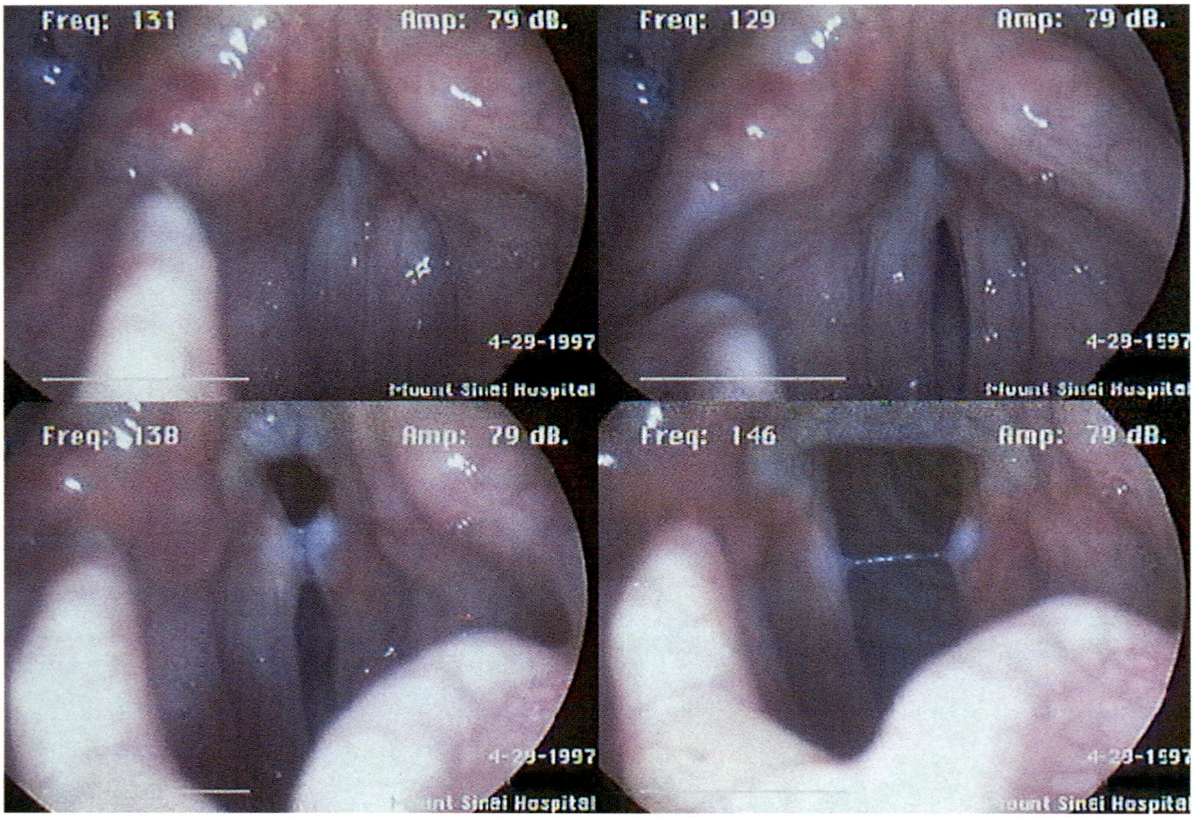


**FIGURE 40.17.** The white keratotic appearance of the contact ulcer is often confused with a cancer.

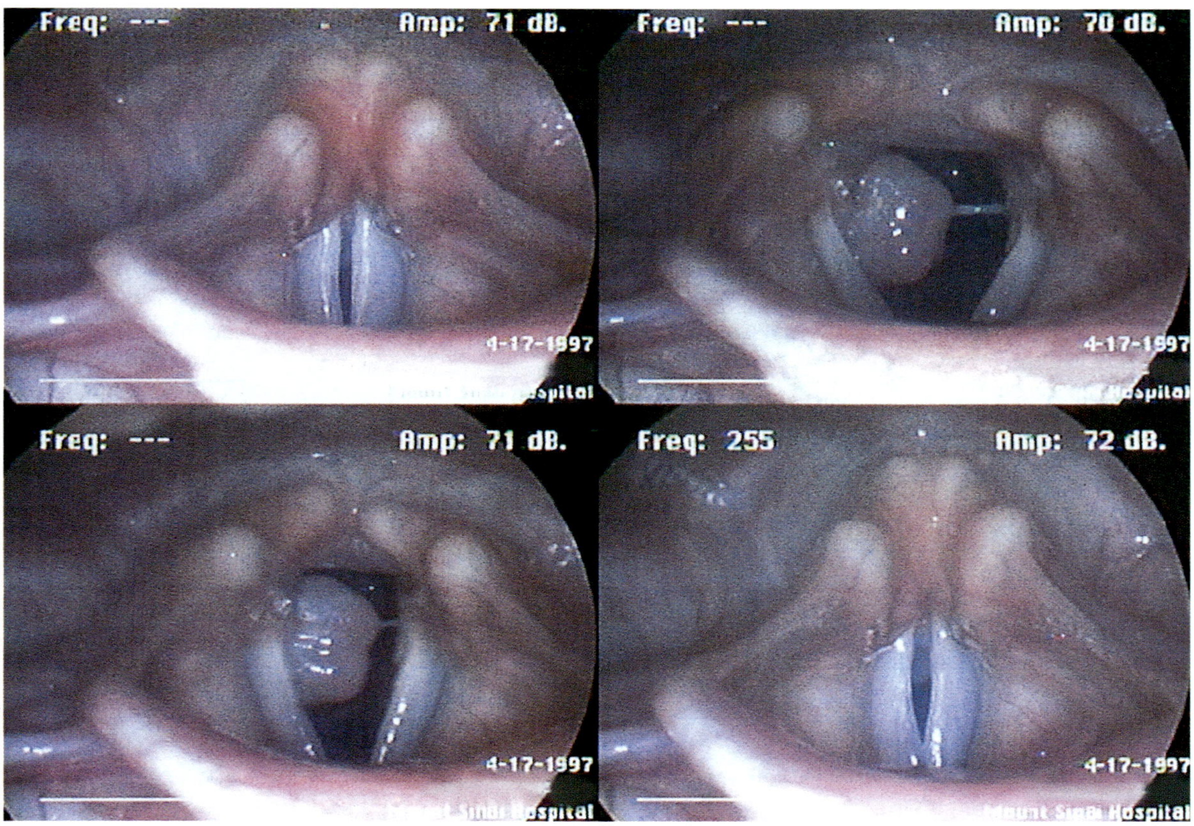


**FIGURE 40.18.** Contact granuloma.

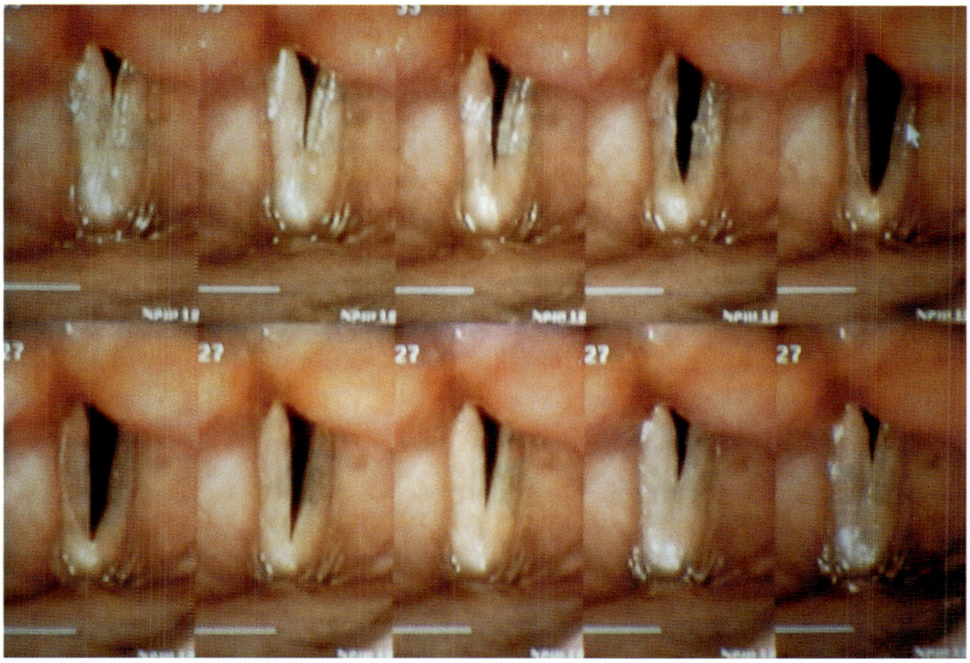


**FIGURE 40.19.** Incomplete vocal cord paralysis.

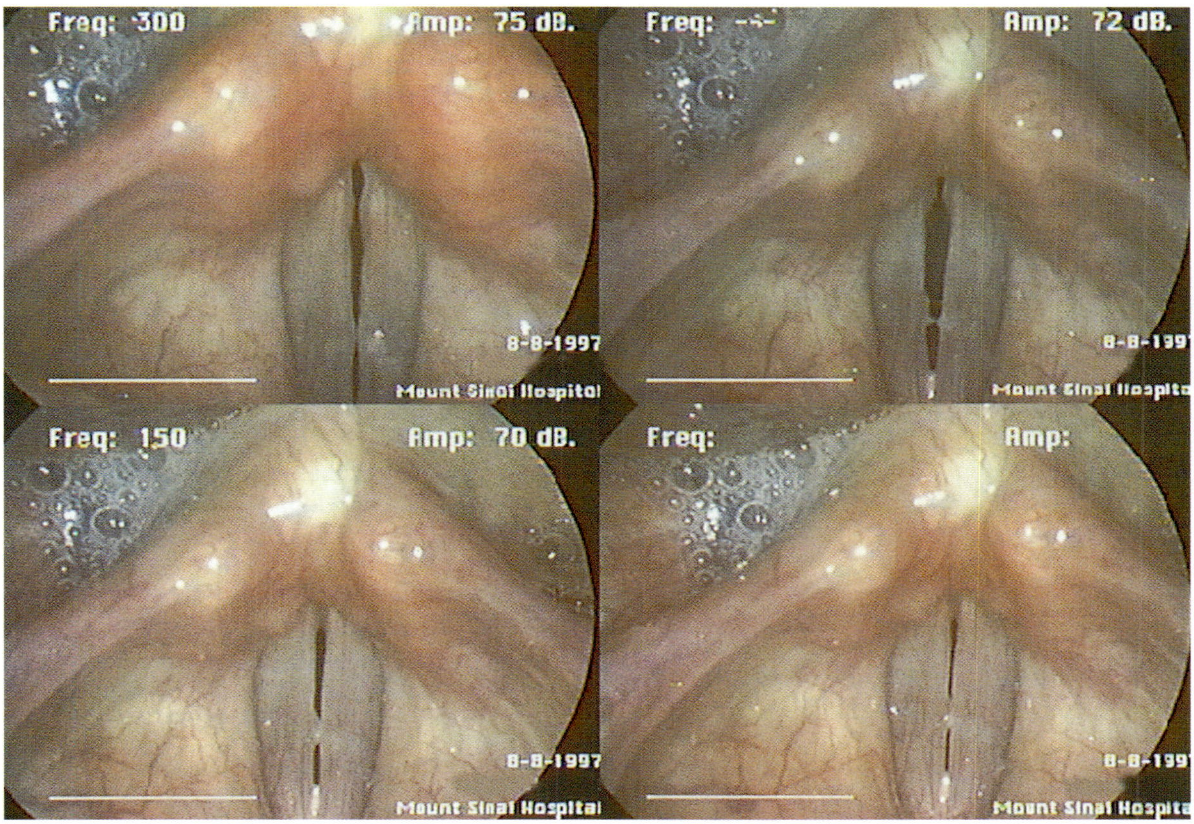


**FIGURE 40.20.** Small mid-membranous vocal fold nodules in a male counter tenor.

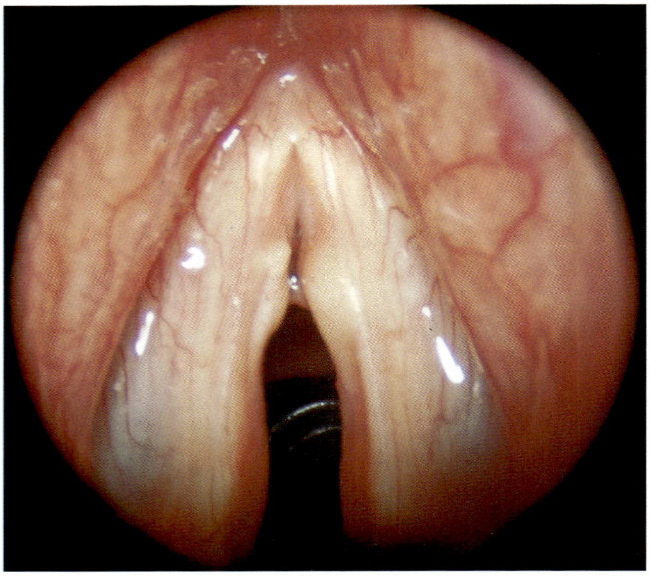

**FIGURE 40.21.** The 0° endoscopic view of the larynx. With this angle, it is not possible to see the subglottis or the extent of vocal fold involvement.

with occasional vocal fatigue but contributed to vocal style and sound. Surgery was not indicated.

## Surgical Endoscopy

### *Telescope*

In the view of a right vocal fold cyst and left keratosis through the 0° endoscope, the subglottis is not visible, nor is it possible to evaluate the extent of vocal fold involvement (Fig 40.21). The same patient is examined with a 120°, backward-looking endoscope (Fig. 40.22). The vocal fold appears inverted because of the backward view. The right and left orientations are maintained. The extent of the vocal fold cyst is clearly seen, and the contralateral epithelial reaction is minimal. The tip of the laryngoscope is visible above the vocal folds in the view into the ventricle of the larynx with the 120°, backward-looking rigid telescope (Fig. 40.23). The 70° or 120° telescope is valuable for the inspection of the ventricle for carcinoma or papilloma extension.

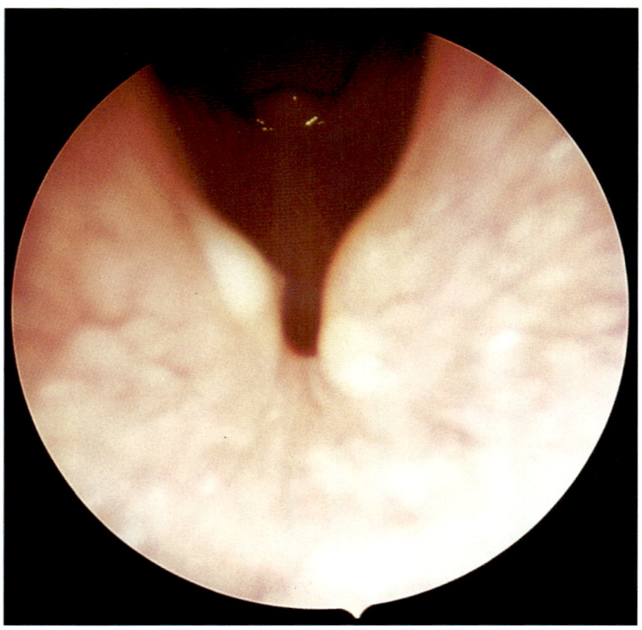

**FIGURE 40.22.** The 120° endoscopic view shows the extent of the vocal fold cyst.

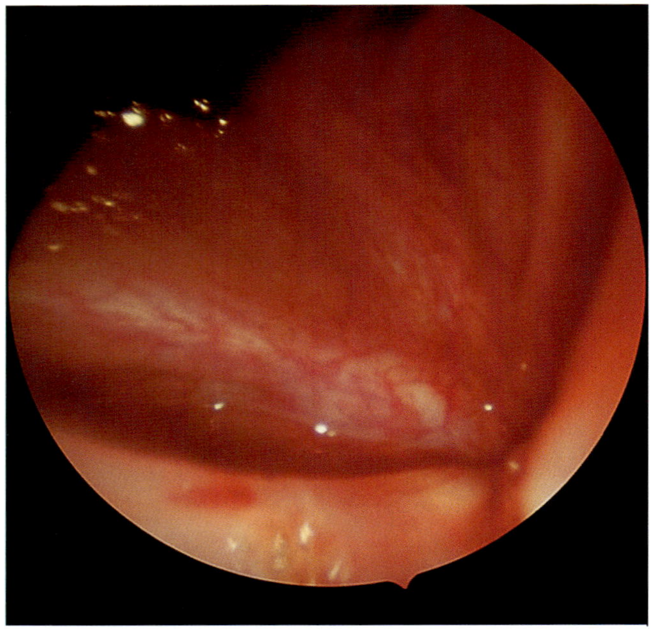

**FIGURE 40.23.** The use of a 120° backward-looking rigid telescope affords a view into the ventricle of the larynx.

### *Special Laryngoscopes*

Wide-angle view of the entire larynx and the hypopharynx is possible with the Lindholm hypopharyngoscope (Fig. 40.24). The wide view, which is available by placing the blade into the vallecula, allows the surgeon to view the larynx, piriform sinus, posterior pharyngeal wall, and the supraglottic larynx. Achieving such a view is important in the more sophisticated endoscopic resections such as endoscopic arytenoidectomy, endoscopic supraglottic laryngectomy, and laser cordectomy.

### *Anesthesia*

To maximize the exposure in tight situations, the Hunsaker jet ventilation tube (Xomed Medical, Jacksonville, FL) is used to further reduce the obstruction caused by more traditional endotracheal tubes (Fig. 40.25). The small jetting

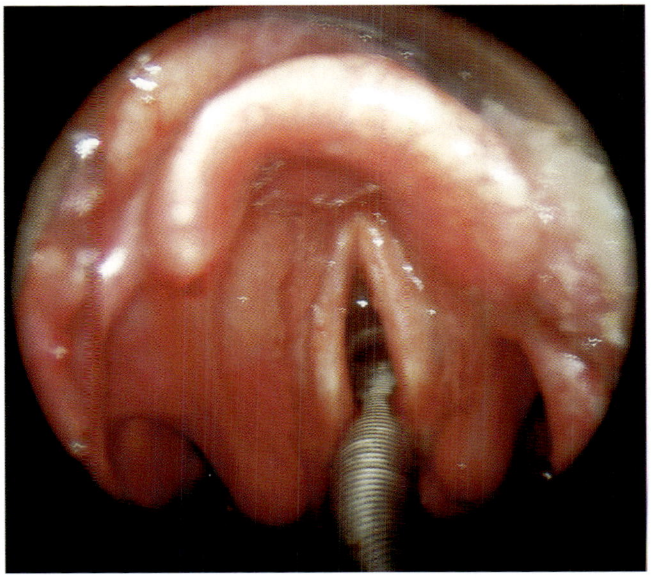

**FIGURE 40.24.** Wide-angle view of the entire larynx and hypopharynx is possible with the Lindholm hypopharyngoscope.

catheter is placed subglottically, allowing the surgeon to work around critical airways without a tracheostomy.

### *Exposure*

The Lindholm laryngoscope is used beneath the lip of the epiglottis, counterpressure is provided externally to depress the cricoid and thyroid cartilage, and hyoid suspension is used to suspend the larynx (Fig. 40.26). Using this

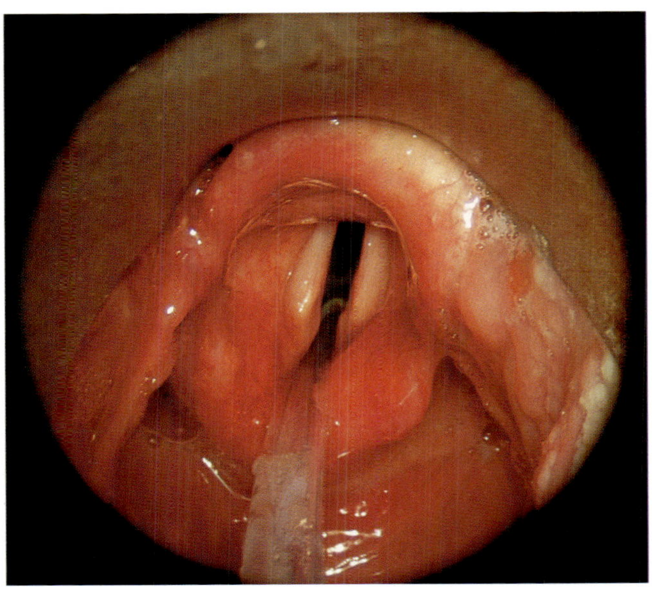

**FIGURE 40.25.** Hunsaker jet ventilation tube allows improved exposure of laryngeal structures while obviating the need for tracheostomy in many clinical situations.

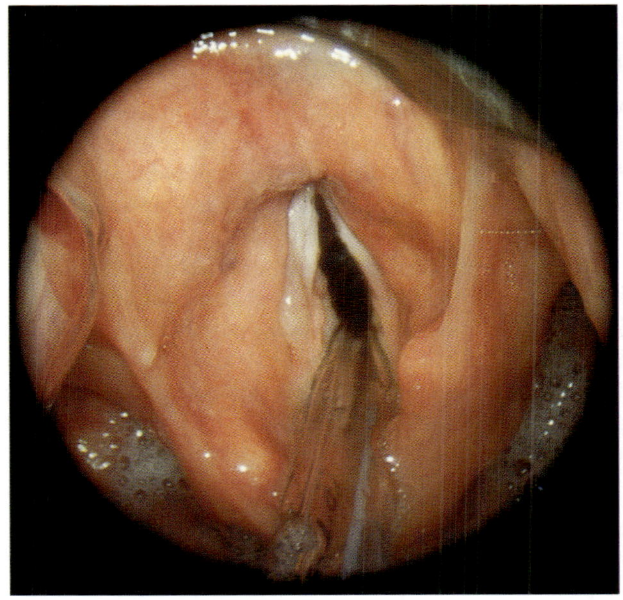

**FIGURE 40.26.** After placement of the Lindholm laryngoscope beneath the lip of the epiglottis, combined with external pressure applied to the cricoid and thyroid cartilage and thyroid suspension, the entire supraglottic larynx, membranous vocal folds, and the aryepiglottic folds can be seen.

technique, the entire supraglottic larynx, the membranous vocal folds, and the aryepiglottic folds can be visualized.

## PATHOLOGY

### Congenital Pathology

A medium-sized, anterior glottic web in a 1-year-old child with weak cry and aphonia is shown in Figure 40.27.

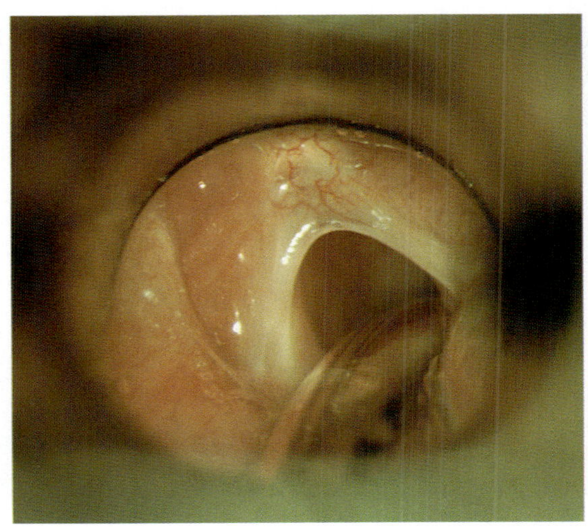

**FIGURE 40.27.** Medium-sized anterior glottic web in a 1-year-old child with aphonia and a weak cry.

## Traumatic Pathology

### Intubation and Extubation

A patient after extubation had a marked mucosal reaction, and fresh granulation tissue is seen in Figure 40.28. The site of injury was to a vocal process with exposed arytenoid cartilage underneath. This patient needed a tracheostomy because of failed extubation attempts.

A large postintubation defect resulted in aphonia (Fig. 40.29). Examination showed the large posterior glottic defect of soft tissue in the cartilage part of the larynx. This defect was difficult to visualize by traditional endoscopy because of the arytenoid rotation that covered the posterior glottic chink. Rigid endoscopy showed a defect that conformed to the endotracheal tube.

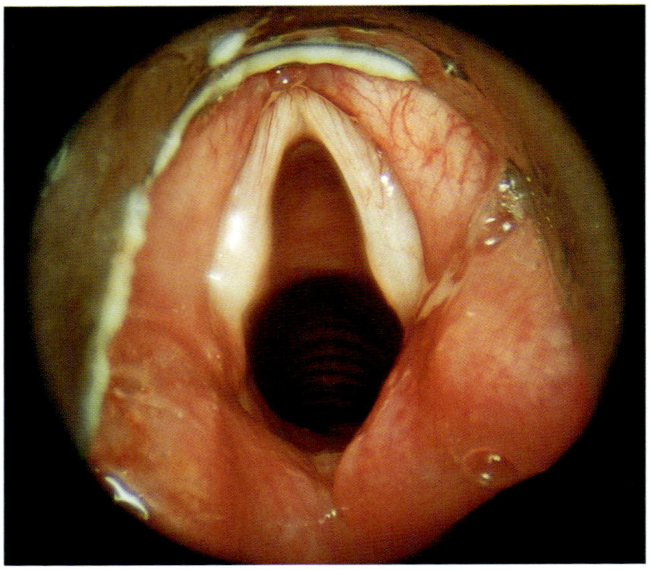

FIGURE 40.29. Postintubation aphonia. Endoscopic examination shows a large, posterior glottic soft tissue defect in the cartilagenous portion of the larynx.

### Laryngeal Fracture

An endoscopic photograph of patient with laryngeal fracture shows a mucosal tear through the membranous vocal fold (Fig. 40.30). The vocal process is dislocated anteriorly and exposed.

### Granuloma Ulcer

An early contact granuloma was identified in an executive with throat pain (Fig. 40.31). This patient had chronic clearing of the throat and cough. The voice quality was low pitched and "throaty." In these cases, laryngeal discomfort with significant pain radiating to the ear and a globus sensation are common. The possible contributing causes are voice abuse, gastroesophageal reflux, and psychosomatic manifestation of voice disorder. In the early stage, there is only hyperemia in the area of chronic irritation. Later, granuloma formation may result in a pedunculated lesion.

### Scar Web Stenosis

Anterior laryngeal stenosis after hemilaryngectomy is shown in Figure 40.32. To restore the acute angle of the anterior

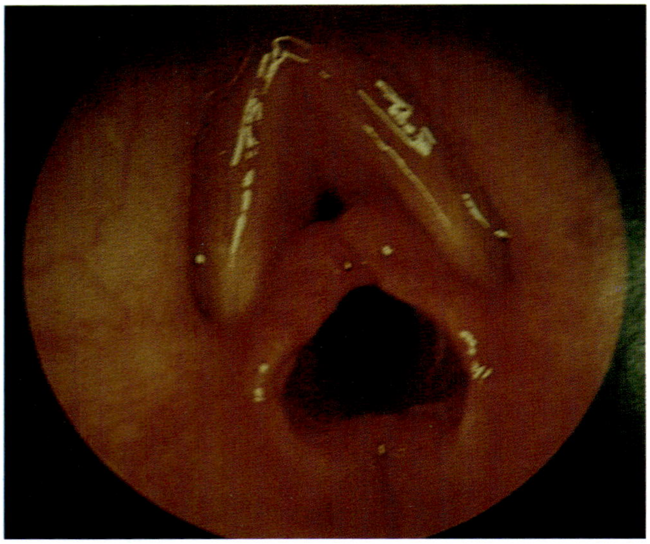

FIGURE 40.28. Intubation injury to the larynx shows a mucosal reaction and granulation tissue, as well as an injured vocal process with exposed arytenoid cartilage.

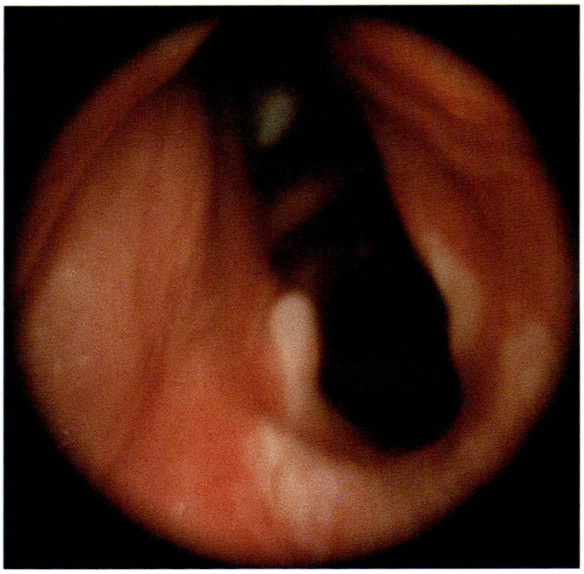

FIGURE 40.30. This patient with a laryngeal fracture was found to have a mucosal tear through the membranous vocal fold and an exposed and dislocated vocal process.

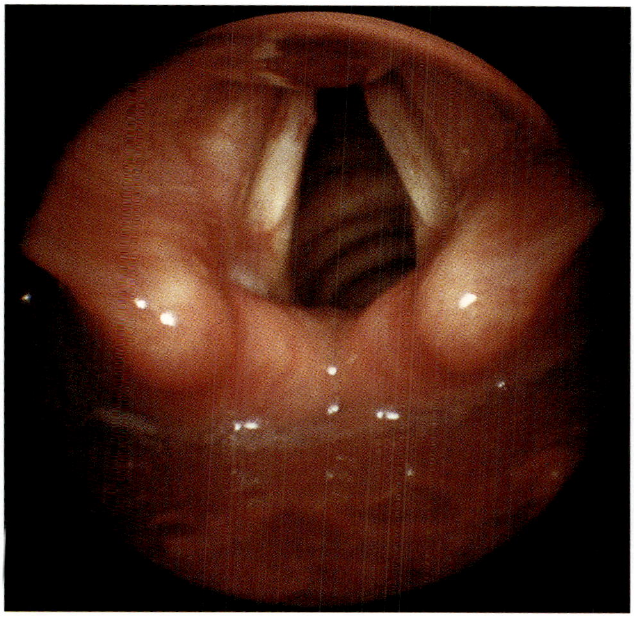

FIGURE 40.31. Early contact granuloma in an executive with throat pain.

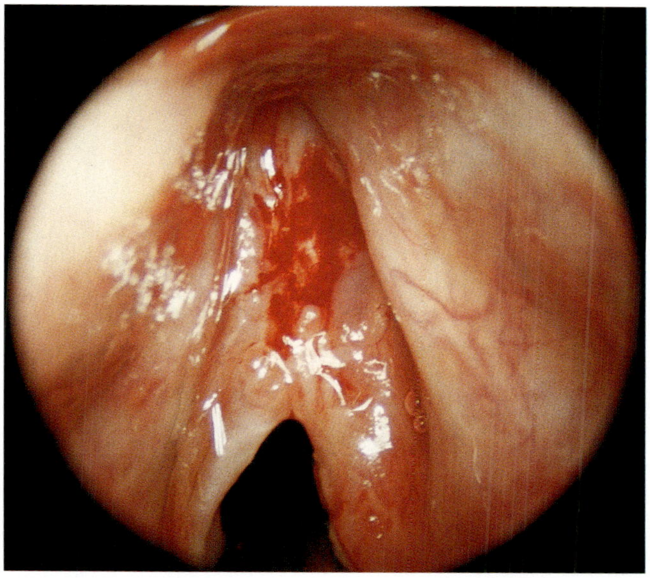

FIGURE 40.33. Large, anterior glottic web after vocal fold stripping to treat vocal cord polyps.

commissure, it is necessary to divide the stenosis. If the stenosis is thick, recurrence is likely. In examples of glottic stenosis after laryngofissure hemilaryngectomy, the laryngeal keel or mucosal graft has been used with success. Multiple-staged resections of the glottic stenosis are usually unsuccessful, although there have been promising early reports with the use of mitomycin-C application intraoperatively.

A large, anterior glottic web was detected after bilateral vocal fold stripping for vocal cord polyps (Fig. 40.33). This patient complained of dyspnea and aphonia. The condition was treated by endoscopic division followed by a buccal mucosal graft.

Obstructing glottic and subglottic stenosis was detected in a premature, 1-year-old child after prolonged intubation (Fig. 40.34). The posterior glottis was completely obliter-

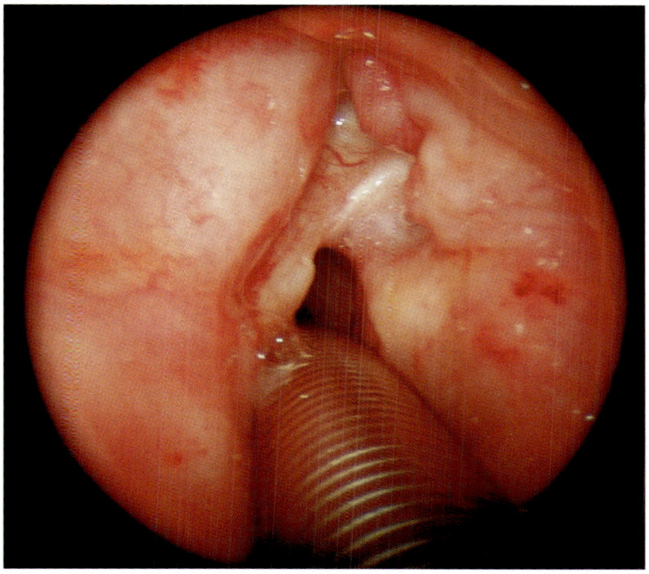

FIGURE 40.32. Anterior laryngeal stenosis (i.e., scar web) after hemilaryngectomy.

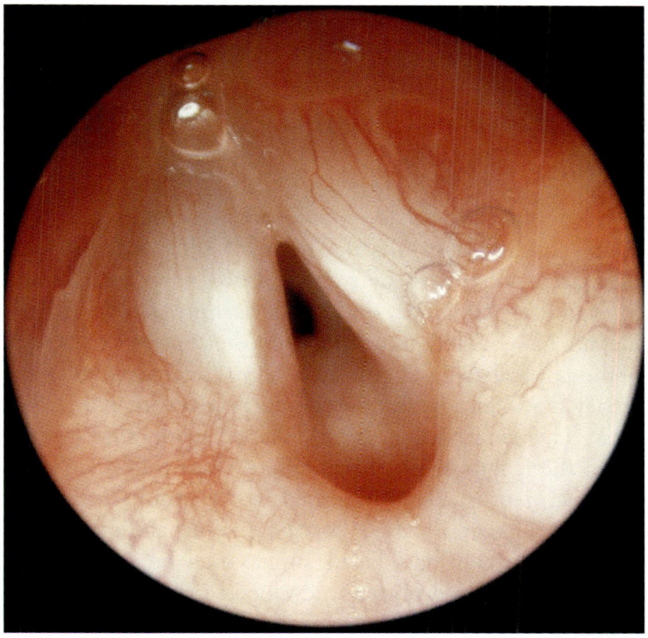

FIGURE 40.34. Prolonged intubation in a premature infant resulted in obstructing glottic and subglottic stenosis.

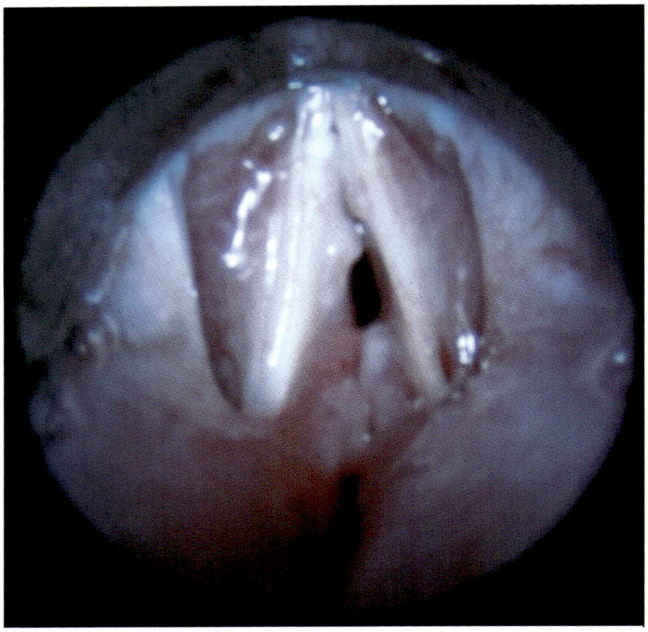

**FIGURE 40.35.** Adhesion between the vocal processes resulted in a band of scar tissue in the posterior tissue.

ated with a thick plate of fibrosis. This patient went on to have laryngeal reconstruction by laryngofissure and costal cartilage rib graft. Adhesion between the vocal processes formed a band of scar tissue in the posterior larynx (Fig. 40.35). Notice the small fistula in posterior larynx behind the vocal process. When a small fistula exists behind the interarytenoid scar, the success of laser division of the adhesion is excellent. This patient was treated with a single surgery resulting in successful decannulation.

## Benign Mucosal Lesions

### *Nodules*

Vocal nodules are predominately a disease of women and young children (Fig. 40.36). The small, soft vocal fold nodules rarely are treated by surgery. Hard vocal nodules can have an irregular surface and can be asymmetric. Vocal nodules are bilateral lesions arising from the center of the membranous vocal fold. The nodules form projections into the airway that typically give the site the appearance of an hourglass. This singer has a spindle-shaped lesion that extends along the length of the membranous vocal fold. Conservative treatment is always indicated in the treatment of vocal nodules. However, when conservative rehabilitation and medical treatment have failed, surgery may be necessary.

Small vocal fold nodules developed in a young, female singer (Fig. 40.37). Sometimes, the vocal fold nodules are not visible, but the vocal fold contact is incomplete. When this happens, this endoscopic finding is consistent with a

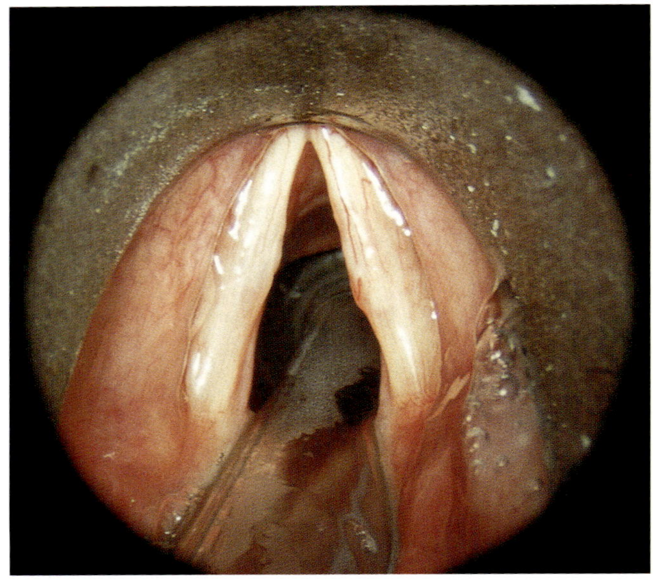

**FIGURE 40.36.** Vocal nodules.

nodular diathesis. The patients are at risk for formation of vocal nodules and should undergo voice evaluation by a speech-language pathologist.

### *Polyps and Hemorrhagic Polyps*

Vocal fold polyps are the most frequent benign lesions of the vocal folds and are thought to be caused by trauma. One explanation is hemorrhage of the blood vessel along the edges of vocal fold. They arise from the membranous portion of the vocal fold and are limited to be vocal fold itself. Unlike vocal nodules, vocal cord polyps are usually seen in men, although vocal polyps can occur in both sexes. The typical history is one of sudden onset of dysphonia

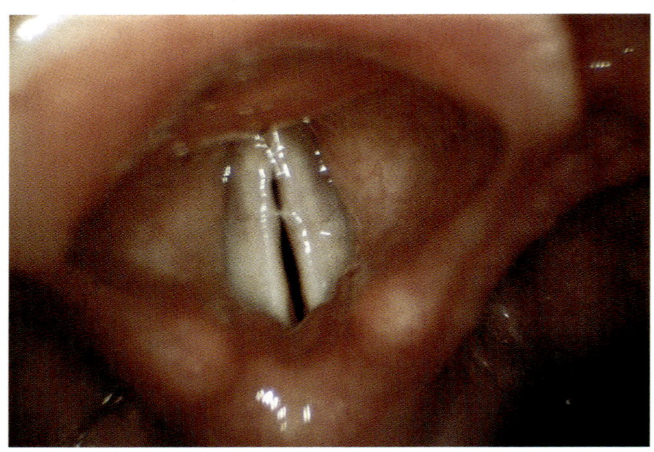

**FIGURE 40.37.** Small vocal fold nodules in a young female singer.

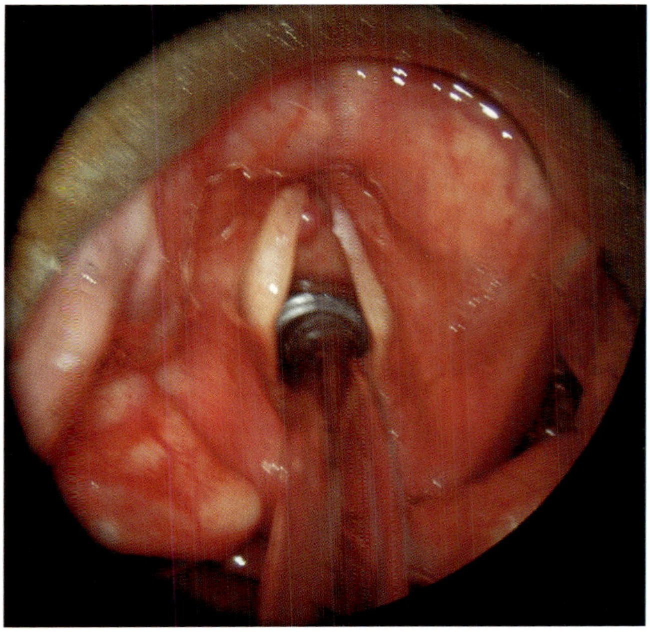

**FIGURE 40.38.** Broad, sessile hemorrhagic polyp with contralateral keratin formation.

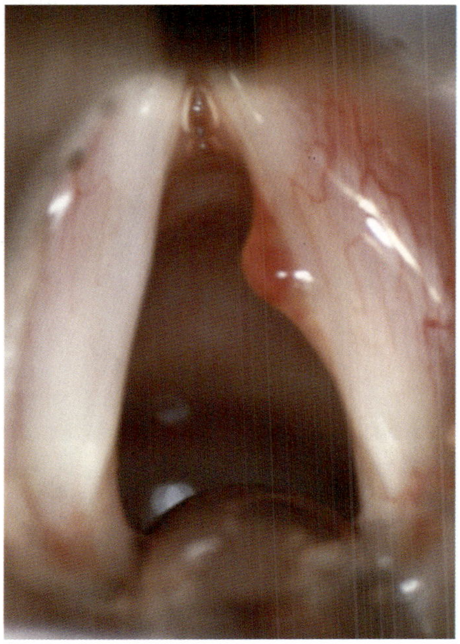

**FIGURE 40.40.** Fusiform hemorrhagic polyp on the vocal fold edge.

after violent coughing, shouting, or viral illness. After prolonged presence, they often cause contralateral vocal fold thickening. The bilateral appearance of a polyp with contralateral vocal fold reaction means that they are occasionally confused with vocal nodules. However, a careful evaluation with rigid telescopes or videostroboscopes usually can separate the polyps from nodules. Broad, sessile, hemorrhagic polyps with contralateral keratin formation are shown in Figure 40.38. A pedunculated polyp of the right vocal fold arising from near the anterior commissure is shown in Figure 40.39, and a fusiform hemorrhagic polyp on the vocal fold edge is shown in Figure 40.40.

### Reinke's Edema

Bilateral edema of the vocal folds in smoker can be seen in Figure 40.41. A more severe form of Reinke's edema is the

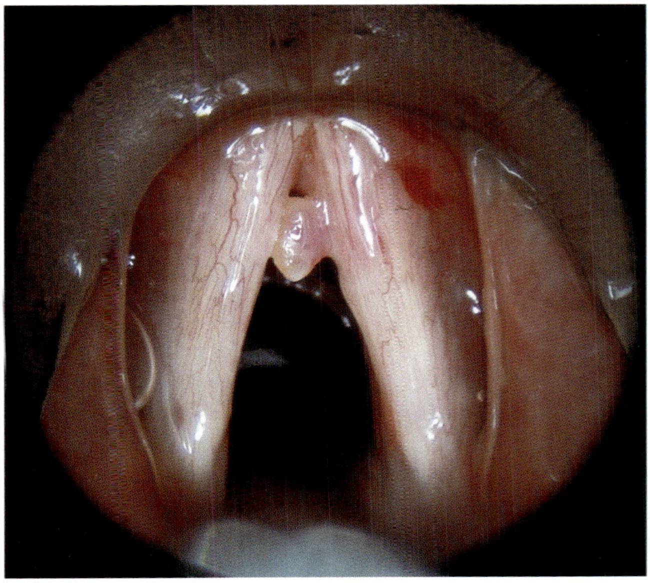

**FIGURE 40.39.** Pedunculated polyp of the right vocal fold arising near the anterior commissure.

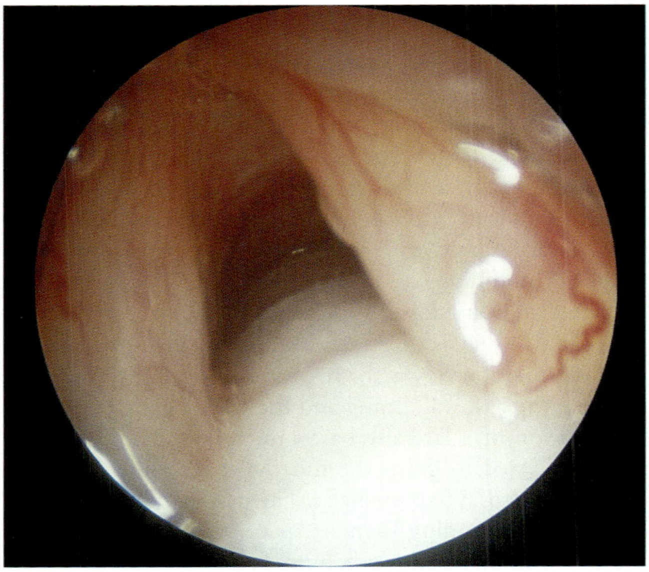

**FIGURE 40.41.** Bilateral vocal fold edema in a smoker.

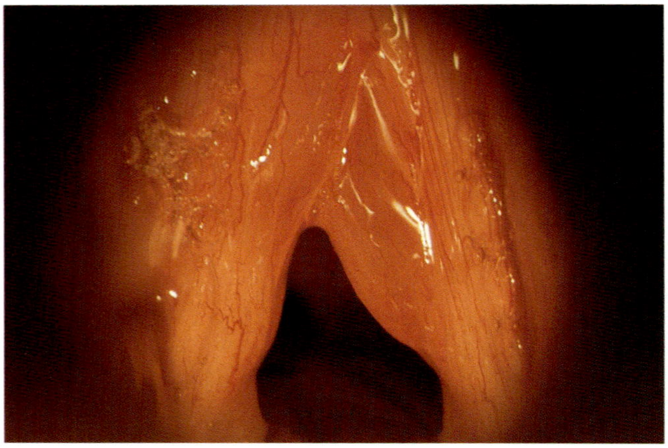

**FIGURE 40.42.** Severe Reinke's edema results in the formation of polyps (i.e., polypoid corditis).

formation of polyps (Fig. 40.42), an entity also referred to as polypoid corditis.

### *Cysts*

Vocal fold cysts are usually seen in young adults. They affect males and females equally. Most vocal fold cysts are mucus-lined cysts, but some cysts contain keratin. True vocal fold cysts always have a respiratory or squamous epithelium. The position of the cysts of the vocal fold is always within the superficial layer of the lamina propria. The size of the cyst and the surrounding tissue reaction may be highly variable, but these factors help to determine how easy it may be to dissect the cyst. Keratin cysts are usually harder to dissect than mucous cysts. Occasionally, cysts of the vocal fold are multilocular and have a complex configuration. Vocal fold cysts are completely removed by means of cordotomy. Incomplete surgical removal results in cyst recurrence and scar formation. Multiple vocal fold cysts are seen in this young female recruiter (Fig. 40.43). On the left, she has a complex vocal fold cyst with a prominent feeding vessel. The opposite vocal fold has a smaller cyst with a feeding vessel. Careful inspection and palpation of the vocal fold under anesthesia may be necessary to accurately differentiate small cysts from vocal polyps or nodules.

There are four stages in the removal of a vocal fold cyst (Fig. 40.44). A sickle knife is initially used to make a mucosal incision down to the cyst wall lining. Dissecting between the cyst wall lining and the vocal ligament enables the creation of a laterally based microflap. The microcup forceps is used to grasp the mucosal edge and reflect the cyst and mucosal flap medially. The cyst is dissected gently from the surrounding Reinke's space, and the cyst is ready for removal while leaving behind a thin vocal fold epithelium.

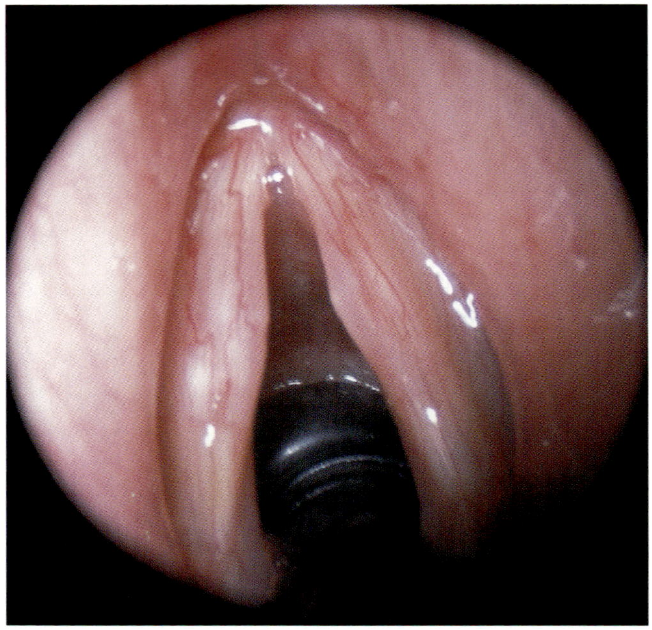

**FIGURE 40.43.** Multiple vocal fold cysts are seen in this young female recruiter.

### *Varix*

Vascular ectasia of the vocal fold is caused by trauma from vocal strain (Fig. 40.45). It affects young women more than men. The dilated capillaries may be engorged during singing and menses. Phonotrauma due to the demands of repeated and prolonged singing predispose to the development of this disorder. Microscopic varices develop from dilated vessels and go on to form tortuous vessels on the surface of the vocal folds. When prominent, they may be the cause of vocal fold hemorrhage during a performance. Occasionally, the vascular ectasia is difficult to differentiate from a small vascular polyp. Vascular ectasia and a large, solitary vascular mass are seen on the vocal fold of a male patient who had a prior vocal fold stripping followed by radiation therapy (Fig. 40.46). Notice the relative sparing by the process on the contralateral vocal fold.

### *Sulcus*

Sulcus vocalis is a furrow or groove along the longitudinal axis of the vocal fold. This white groove is the site of attachment of the vocal fold epithelium to the vocal ligament. Sulcus vergeture is a more extensive sulcus associated with vocal atrophy. At the sulcus, there is a deficiency in the superficial layer of lamina propria. The cause of sulcus vocalis is controversial. Many cases of sulcus vocalis result from the congenital presence of a glottal groove. Some believe it is the result of a ruptured cyst. Others believe the sulcus vocalis is a scarring condition caused by inflamma-

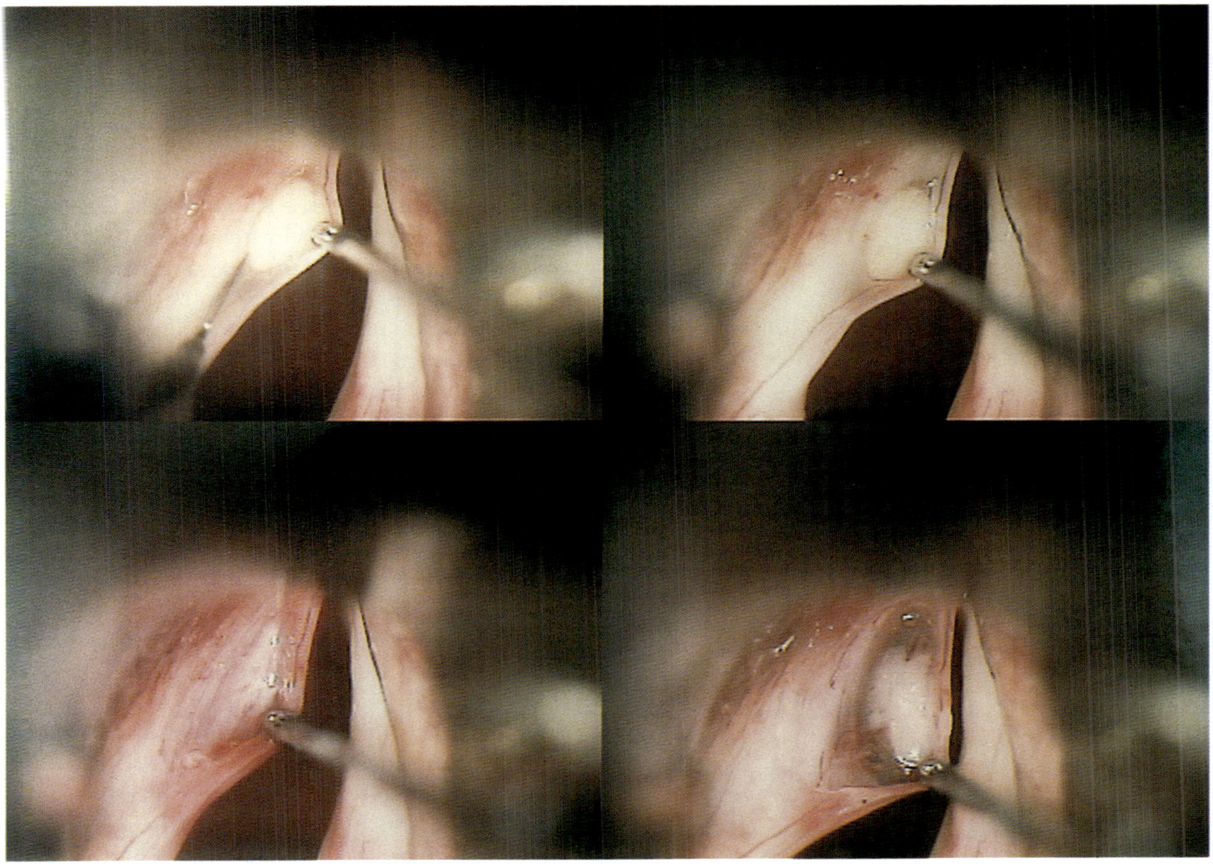

**FIGURE 40.44.** Four stages of removal of a vocal fold cyst. A sickle knife is used to make a mucosal incision down to the cyst wall lining *(top left)*. A microcup forceps is used to grasp the mucosal edge and reflect the cyst and mucosal flap medially *(top right)*. The cyst is dissected from the surrounding Reinke's space *(bottom left)*. The cyst is ready for removal from the thin vocal fold epithelium *(bottom right)*.

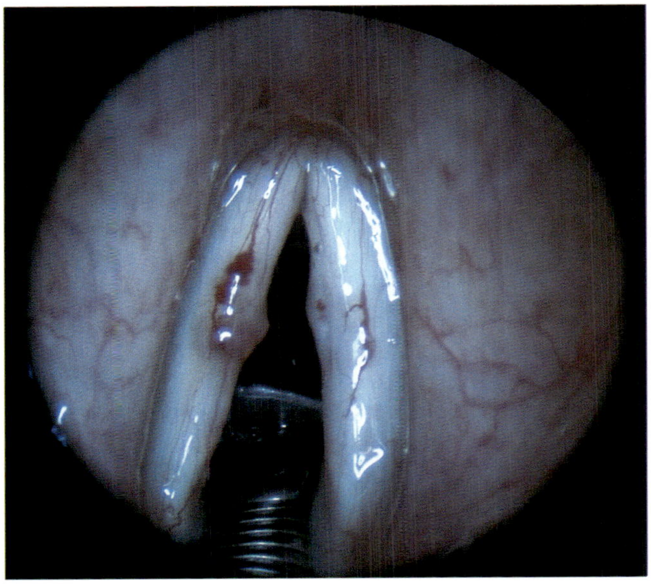

**FIGURE 40.45.** Vocal strain trauma produces vascular ectasia of the vocal fold.

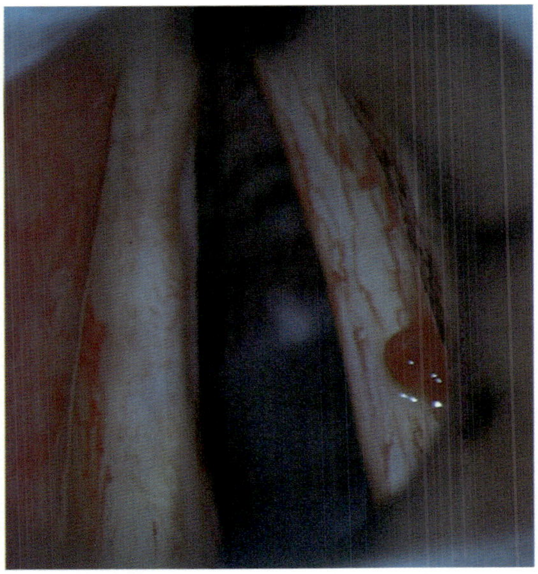

**FIGURE 40.46.** Vascular ectasia and a large solitary vascular mass on the vocal fold of a male patient who underwent vocal fold stripping followed by radiation therapy.

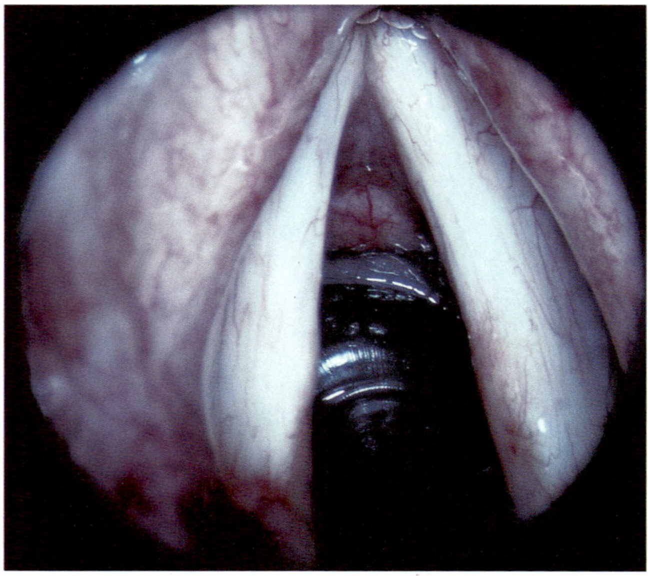

**FIGURE 40.47.** Small, right sulcus vocalis treated by microsurgical excision.

tion and attachment of the vocal ligament to the superficial epithelium. Usually, the sulcus lies on the edge of the vocal fold or just below the free edge. Because of the site of the glottal furrow, it may be exceedingly difficult to visualize by office endoscopy. The patient has a husky, rough, and breathy voice quality that is unexplained by office endoscopy findings. On videostroboscopy, there is usually a decrease in the vibratory amplitude on the affected side.

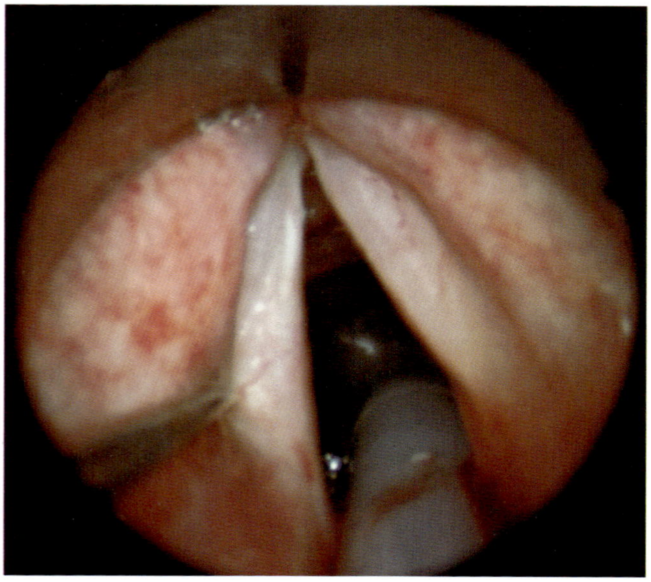

**FIGURE 40.48.** Larger sulcus vocalis on the undersurface of the left vocal fold.

The loss of Reinke's space results in vocal fold bowing with a spindle-shaped, incomplete glottis closure.

Intraoperative examination by direct laryngoscopy in a patient with suspected sulcus vocalis shows a small right vocal fold sulcus. This sulcus was treated by microsurgical excision (Fig. 40.47). A larger sulcus vocalis was identified on the undersurface of the left vocal fold (Fig. 40.48). The sulcus extended to approximately one half of the vocal fold and was not amenable to resection. It was treated by microflap formation and elevation of the vocal fold epithelium from the underlying vocal ligament, followed by steroid injection and lipoinjection. Excellent voice results are difficult to achieve for the larger sulcus vocalis and for bilateral sulcus vocalis.

### *Contact Granuloma and Teflon Granuloma*

Unlike intubation granulomas that occur at the vocal process, contact granulomas may occur above the vocal process on the arytenoid cartilage itself. The cause is aggressive and early contact of the arytenoid cartilage during speaking. The voice is characterized by an aggressive glottal attack and a low pitch (i.e., coup de glotte). The granuloma is a reddish to white, round to bilobed mass at the vocal process or just surrounding it. The throat pain on speaking is usually unilateral and radiating. A hoarse voice and early vocal fatigue also may bring the patient to examination. The diagnosis can be made by inspection followed by palpation of the cricoarytenoid area. Patients with contact granuloma have pain and tenderness on the side of the contact granuloma. The treatment focuses on re-education of the speaking habits and lifestyle. Some patients need surgery to remove large, cauliflower-like lesions. Intraoperative steroid injection, postoperative speech therapy, voice rest, and antacid treatment are also given to the patient. Despite this, patients experience a high rate of recurrence unless they are well motivated to change their underlying habits. In severe cases of recalcitrant granuloma, botulinum toxin injections can enforce a period of voice rest and allow the inflamed granuloma site to heal. A large contact granuloma above the vocal process was removed by microlaryngoscopy (Fig. 40.49). During removal of a granuloma, it is important not to injure the underlying cartilage by surgical or laser trauma. Perichondrium of the cartilage is always close to the pedicle of the granuloma, and injury can result in perichondritis and further cartilage reaction.

A Teflon granuloma is shown in Figure 40.50. Some patients have a reaction to Teflon injected for the treatment of vocal fold paralysis. Teflon causes a giant cell reaction that stiffens the tissue and makes the vocal fold bulge into the lumen. Some experience this reaction many years after successful Teflon injection. This example shows the reaction of the right vocal fold, with increased hyperemia of the right vocal fold and the glottis and the subglottis bulging characteristic of Teflon granuloma formation. Teflon gran-

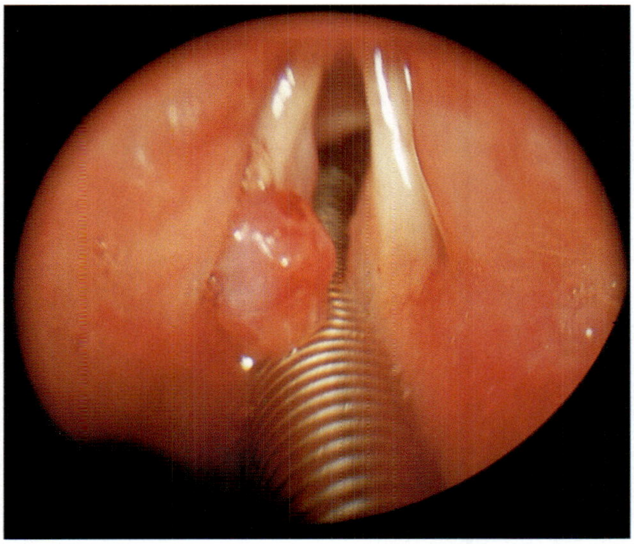

**FIGURE 40.49.** During microlaryngoscopic removal, a large contact granuloma can be seen above the vocal process.

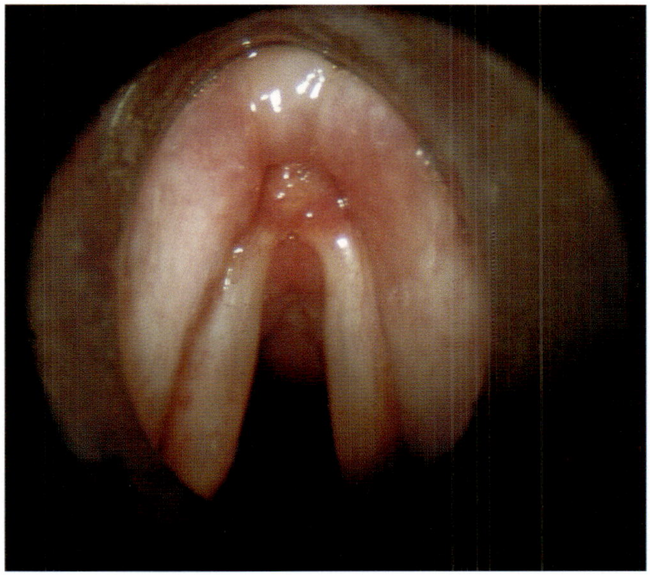

**FIGURE 40.51.** This anterior granuloma and granulation tissue mimics a malignant tumor.

ulomas are treated by laser vaporization of the offending mass or by external laryngotomy and total removal, followed by reconstruction of the larynx using laryngoplastic phonosurgery techniques.

An anterior granuloma and granulation tissue in one patient mimicked a malignant tumor (Fig. 40.51). The patient had reflux laryngitis and chronic cough. No other cause for acute and chronic granulation tissue was found.

### *Keratosis*

Chronic inflammation and irritation is thought to be the cause of epidermal metaplasia and epidermalization of the vocal fold epithelium (Fig. 40.52). The risk factors for leukoplakia of the larynx is similar to those for the development of laryngeal carcinoma. Smoking, voice abuse, and chronic irritation at work are risk factors for the development of leukoplakia of the larynx. Endoscopically,

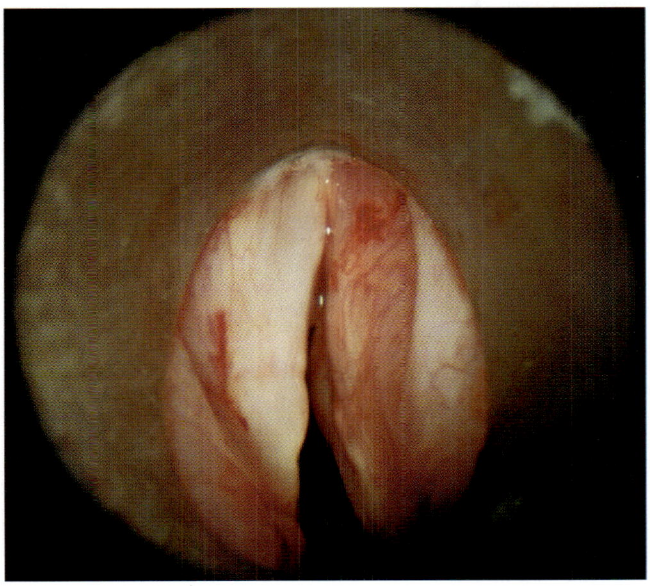

**FIGURE 40.50.** Teflon granuloma.

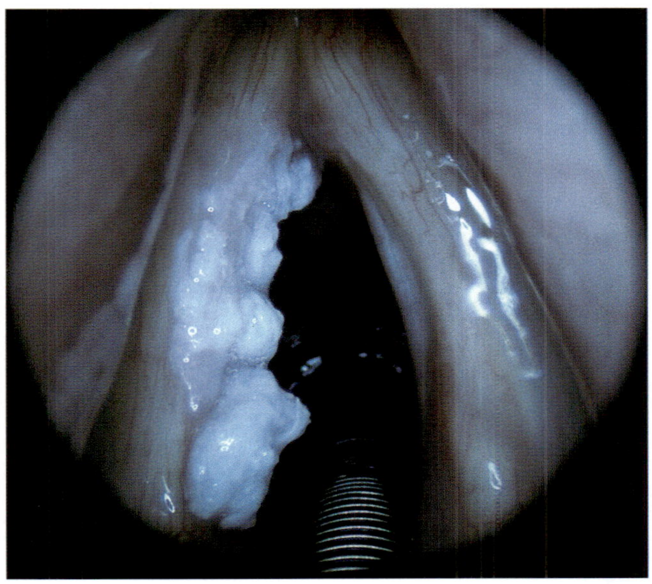

**FIGURE 40.52.** Epidermal metaplasia and epidermalization of the vocal fold epithelium result from chronic inflammation.

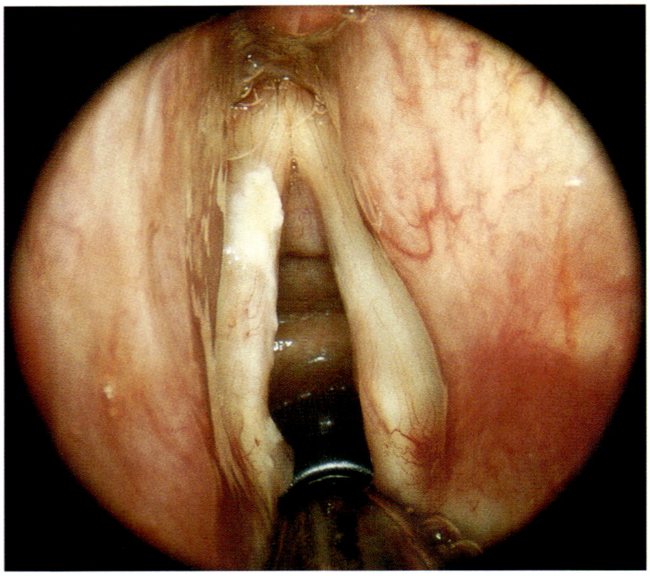

**FIGURE 40.53.** Recurrent keratosis in a patient treated 4 years earlier with vocal fold stripping.

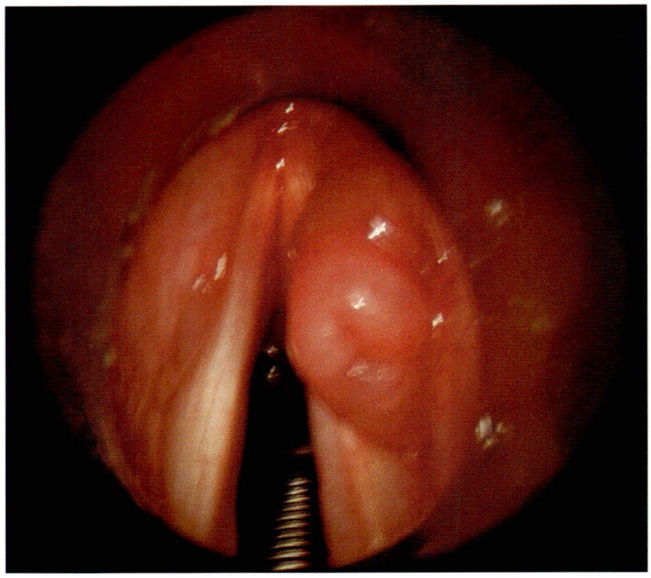

**FIGURE 40.54.** Prominent false vocal folds may represent a compensatory effort to achieve vibration when the true vocal folds are stiff and immobile.

it cannot be distinguished from well-differentiated squamous cell carcinoma. Epithelial hyperplasia followed by keratin formation is the usual route of leukoplakia formation. Early in the process, there is a ground glass appearance to the vocal fold. This is followed by frank keratin formation. The condition is frequently bilateral, and unilateral involvement may result in vocal fold stripping and poor voice quality.

Recurrent keratosis was identified in a patient treated 4 years earlier with vocal fold stripping (Fig. 40.53). Treatment by careful removal of the overlying epithelium resulted in a satisfactory voice. Occasionally, recurrent keratosis is impossible to differentiate from verrucous carcinoma or well-differentiated carcinoma based on endoscopic criteria. A careful biopsy followed by complete endoscopic removal for histologic sampling is the treatment of choice.

### *Ventricular Prolapse*

Prominent false vocal folds may be the cause of dysphonia or may be the compensatory effort to achieve vibration when the true vocal folds are stiff and immobile (Fig. 40.54). Thickening of the false vocal folds may occur in response to chronic inflammation or motor activity. Occasionally, a ventricular cyst or prolapse of the mucosa from the ventricle can result in a unilateral polypoid mass that impedes normal vocal vibratory function. In this countertenor, ventricular prolapse occurred after prolonged singing and impeded normal phonation. The treatment by laser excision of the ventricular prolapse resulted in restoration of normal vocal function.

## Benign Tumors

### *Papilloma*

Papillomas of the larynx is caused by infection of the laryngeal epithelium by the papillomavirus (Fig. 40.55). Adult papillomas occur in more men than women and have a peak in the fifth decade of life. They are not related to juvenile

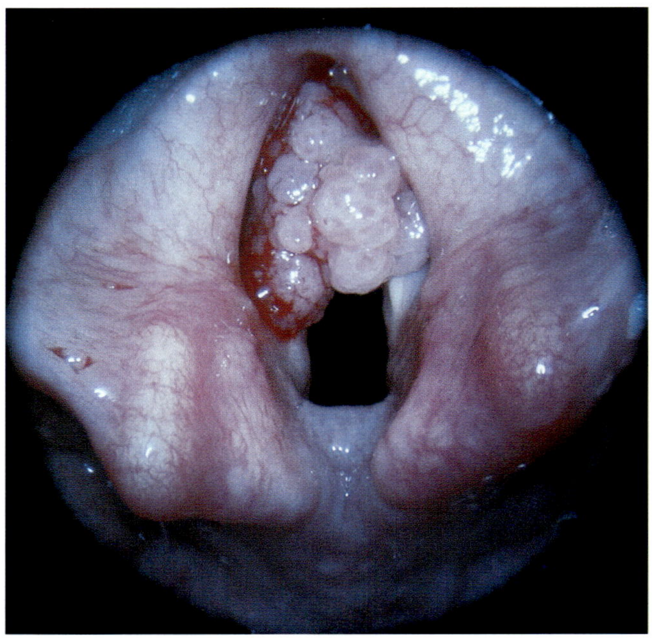

**FIGURE 40.55.** Papilloma virus infection of the laryngeal epithelium.

papillomas and are less aggressive in general than the juvenile form. The histologic appearance is characterized by squamous to cuboidal epithelium with a central vascular core. Multiple branching villi give the papilloma the typical grape-like appearance. Because active virus particles are found in surrounding normal epithelium, the recurrence rate after surgical removal is high. The management of papillomas is limited to careful surgical removal to improve symptoms, to avoid tracheostomy, and to maximize the symptom-free interval. Avoidance of surrounding tissue injury and scar is especially important when the vocal folds are involved by papillomas. Sites such as the anterior commissure, the subglottis, and the interarytenoid area makes surgical removal challenging. Because of the central vascular core, any removal by forceps or sharp instruments results in brisk bleeding from the bed, making further removal difficult.

The use of the $CO_2$ laser to debulk the tumor while sparing the surrounding normal mucosa has made the surgical management of papilloma easier. The goals of surgical therapy is to restore voice, maintain the airway, and avoid a tracheostomy. In patients with rapidly growing papillomas, the use of interferon-$\alpha$ injections as adjuvant and maintenance chemotherapy has been useful in slowing growth and reducing the number of surgeries needed to maintain a good quality of life. Adult papillomas can show dysplastic changes and may transform to squamous cell carcinoma. Periodic histologic examination of the papilloma removed during laryngoscopy is advisable.

## Precancerous Squamous Lesions

Of more concern to the otolaryngologist than the white leukoplakia of the vocal folds is the red erythroplasia mixed with keratin (Fig. 40.56). Under examination, white lesions representing keratinomas or keratosis are usually on the surface epithelium, with mobile subepithelium. The intact Reinke layer makes surgical removal of white lesions easier than surgical removal of red lesions. Early in the infiltration of cancers, there is a neovascular proliferation surrounding the abnormal tissue. There are variable degrees of inflammation. The red patch makes separation of the superficial epithelium from the deep layers difficult. Red lesions of the vocal fold are more likely to be cancer than white lesions of the vocal fold. Intravital staining with toluidine blue can be used to separate areas that take up DNA and signify nuclear atypia.

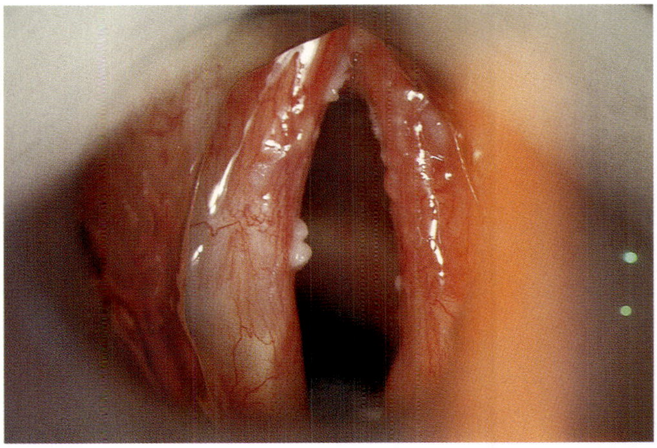

**FIGURE 40.56.** Red erythroplasia mixed with keratin represents a more ominous lesion than white leukoplakia of the vocal folds. These lesions fall along the continuum between leukoplakia and carcinoma *in situ*. The increased neovascularization in erythroplasia makes separation of the superficial epithelium from the deep layers more difficult.

## Squamous Cell Carcinoma

Carcinoma of the larynx can have superficial involvement limited to the surface epithelium. Carcinoma *in situ* (CIS) of the true vocal fold involves the surface of the vocal fold. Although many areas of biopsy show only CIS, CIS with microinvasion was documented on serial section (Fig. 40.57). The epithelium is red and thickened because of the increased vascularity to the tumor.

More ominous in terms of involvement of the vocal fold is the appearance of superficial spread of the lesion along the surface of the vocal fold. This poor delineation of the extent of tumor makes it much more difficult to obtain adequate margins during laser endoscopic removal.

Deeply invasive carcinoma with vocal fold fixation is demonstrated in Figure 40.58. The cancer is seen to invade laterally into the ventricle but is limited by the anterior commissure and is limited to the side of origin.

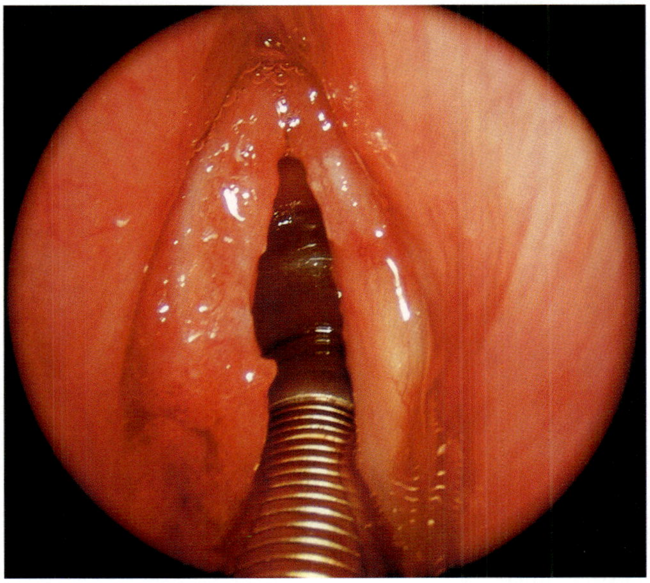

**FIGURE 40.57.** Multiple areas showed carcinoma *in situ* (CIS); however, CIS with microinvasion was seen on serial sectioning.

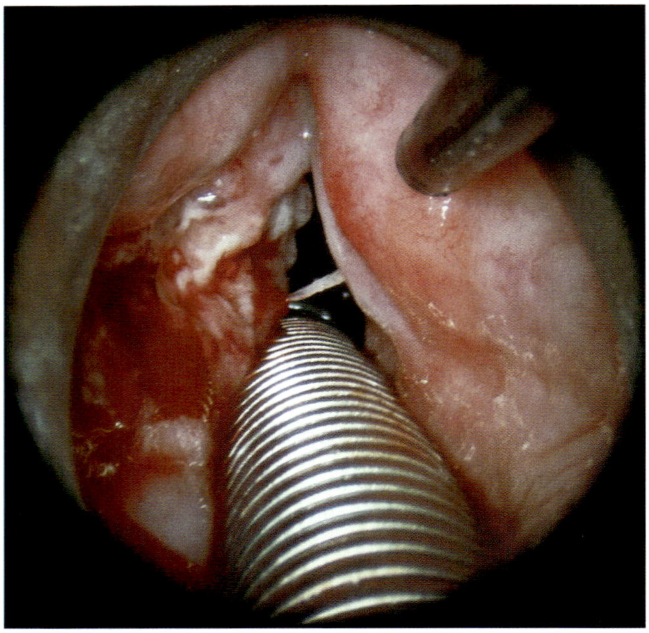

**FIGURE 40.58.** Deeply invasive carcinoma with vocal fold fixation. Notice that the cancer invades laterally into the ventricle but is limited to the side of origin and does not cross the anterior commissure.

Invasive carcinoma of the epiglottis is limited to the suprahyoid portion of the supraglottic larynx in Figure 40.59. The false vocal fold and the ventricle are free of cancer. This is an ideal patient to consider for endoscopic resection using the $CO_2$ laser.

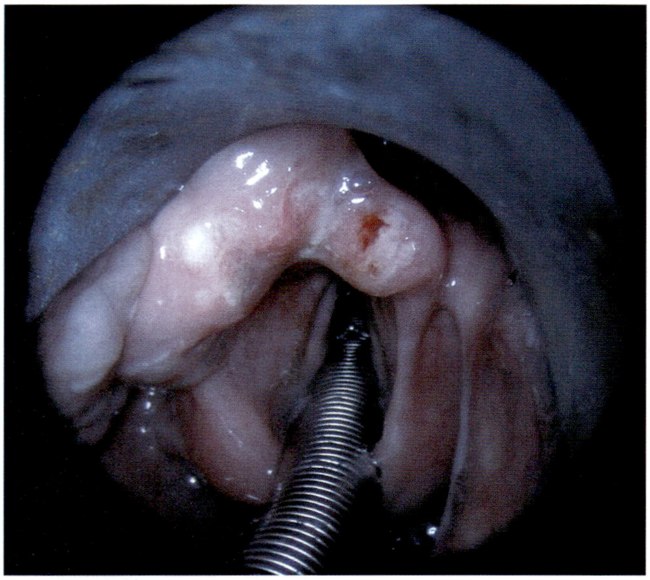

**FIGURE 40.59.** Invasive carcinoma of the epiglottis is limited to the suprathyroid portion of the supraglottic larynx. Notice that the false vocal folds and the ventricles are free of tumor.

## Presentation

In this section, examples of specific pathologic entities that can be diagnosed or treated endoscopically are provided.

### *Subacute Laryngitis*

Ulcers developed on both vocal folds in a patient with chronic, severe coughing due to pulmonary fibrosis (Fig. 40.60). These cough-related ulcers are covered with a shaggy fibrin cover and have an inflammatory infiltrate. The differential diagnosis includes chronic hyperplastic laryngitis, leukoplakia of the vocal fold, and laryngeal carcinoma. Resolution of the coughing spells and restoration of normal mucosal hygiene allowed the ulcers to heal with good functional result.

### *Chronic Laryngitis*

Interarytenoid pachydermia is seen in patients with chronic laryngitis caused by reflux or smoking (Fig. 40.61). It is a form of hyperplastic laryngitis. The differential diagnosis should include tuberculous laryngitis. Hyperplastic laryngitis with selected posterior interarytenoid involvement is seen in patients with reflux laryngitis. Unlike bacterial infection, there is little suppuration, and the mound of hyperplastic tissue can vary from white to vascular. The thickened, wrinkled tissue is sometimes alarming enough to cause a recommendation for biopsy, but it is almost always benign. Occasionally, the amount of interarytenoid pachydermia is significant enough to cause a posterior chink and interfere with clear phonation. This condition can be treated by careful $CO_2$ laser debulking.

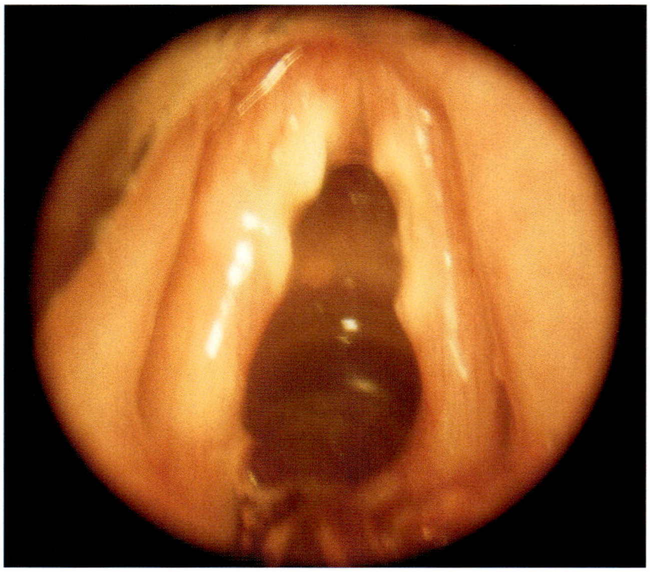

**FIGURE 40.60.** Vocal fold ulcers due to the chronic, severe coughing in a patient with pulmonary fibrosis.

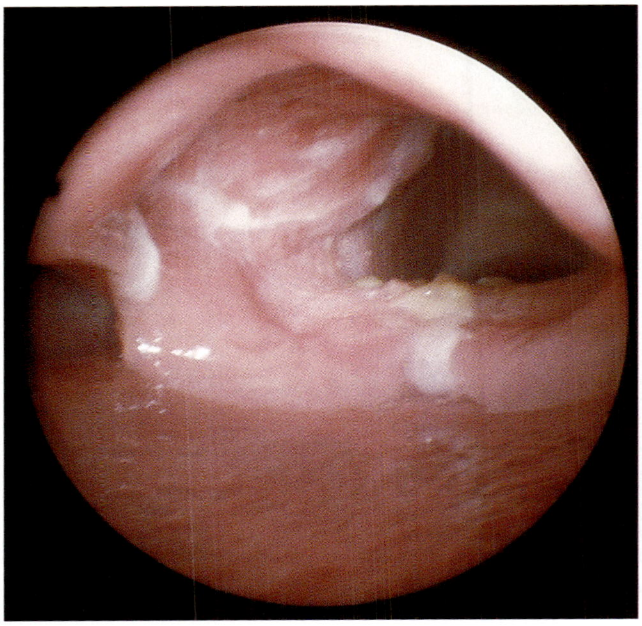

**FIGURE 40.61.** Interarytenoid pachydermia is seen in patients with chronic laryngitis due to reflux laryngitis or smoking.

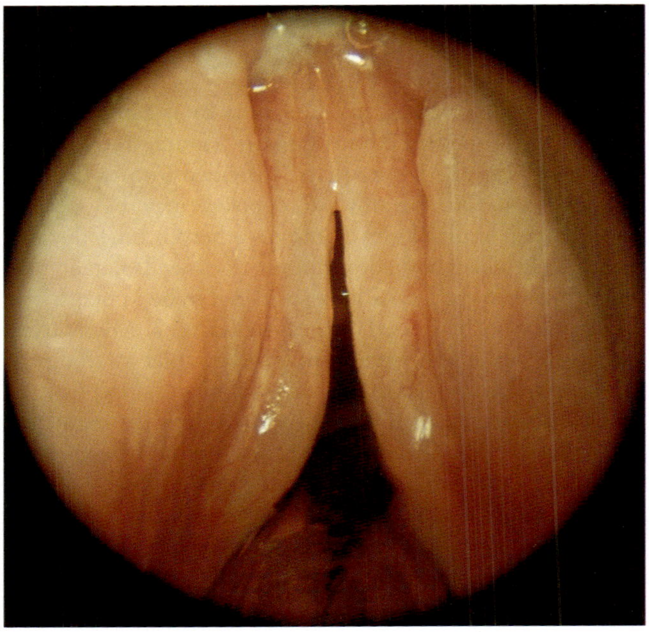

**FIGURE 40.62.** Hyperplastic laryngitis is characterized by chronically thickened vocal folds with a loss of clear, wet mucosa.

### *Hyperplastic Laryngitis*

Chronically thickened vocal folds with loss of clear, wet mucosa characterize hyperplastic laryngitis (Fig. 40.62). Patients present with a prolonged history of hoarse voice. The risk factors for chronic hyperplastic laryngitis are the same as those for squamous carcinoma of the larynx. Heavy smoking, alcohol use, reflux laryngitis, and chronic sinopulmonary infections are some of the etiologic factors. The disease is usually diffuse and involves both vocal folds. The epithelium is thickened and shows changes of hyperkeratosis, parakeratosis, acanthosis, and dyskeratosis. The thin, translucent epithelium that normally lines the vocal fold edge transforms to a thick, rough texture, much like callused skin. Multiple ridges and duplication of the vocal fold may be seen and felt. When attempts are made to move the thick epithelium from the underlying vocal ligament, there may be fibrous attachments of this layer because of inflammation and fibrosis. Sometimes, differentiation between this condition and a cancerous condition is difficult.

The hyperplastic epithelium can be managed conservatively provided cancer has been excluded. Surgery consists of conservative removal of the hyperplastic epithelium to allow a more normal mucosa to form over the surface. The surgeon should strive to remove only the hyperplastic epithelium without injury to the vocal ligament. Postoperative management of reflux laryngitis, mucosal hygiene, the environment, and voice abuse are critical to restoration of adequate vocal function.

### *Lymphangioma*

A rare case of a lymphangioma in an adult who noticed some hesitancy in her swallow function is illustrated in Figure 40.63. The lymphangioma was probably present since birth. Serial observations showed no change in the mass, and the patient was never treated.

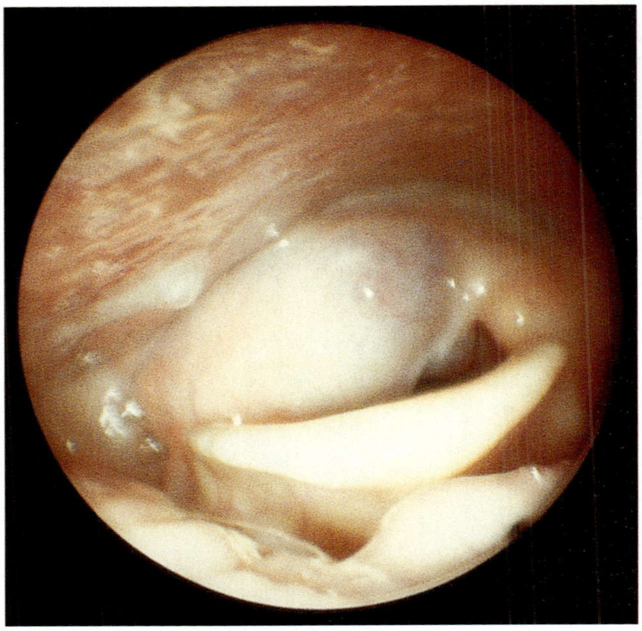

**FIGURE 40.63.** Lymphangioma.

## Systemic Manifestations

### Amyloid

Supraglottic involvement of the larynx by isolated amyloidosis of the larynx is demonstrated in Figure 40.64. Amyloid deposits of the larynx may be divided into isolated or diffuse types. Diffuse amyloid deposits may be seen in patients with multiple myeloma or other chronic diseases such as sarcoidosis and autoimmune diseases. Isolated amyloid deposits in the larynx are considered to be idiopathic in origin and may be related to localized trauma. Microlaryngoscopic examination shows multiple nodular swellings of the false vocal folds and extensive submucosal deposits of yellow, friable tissue. Amyloid deposit is easily distinguished histologically by Congo red stain and by birefringence on polarized light examination.

The process is often indolent for many years, and treatment is indicated to relieve airway obstruction and improve voice. Laser endoscopic removal of the supraglottic deposits can relieve the airway obstruction and restore the voice in many patients. Isolated amyloid deposits may manifest as a submucosal tumor with invasion of the true vocal fold (Fig. 40.65).

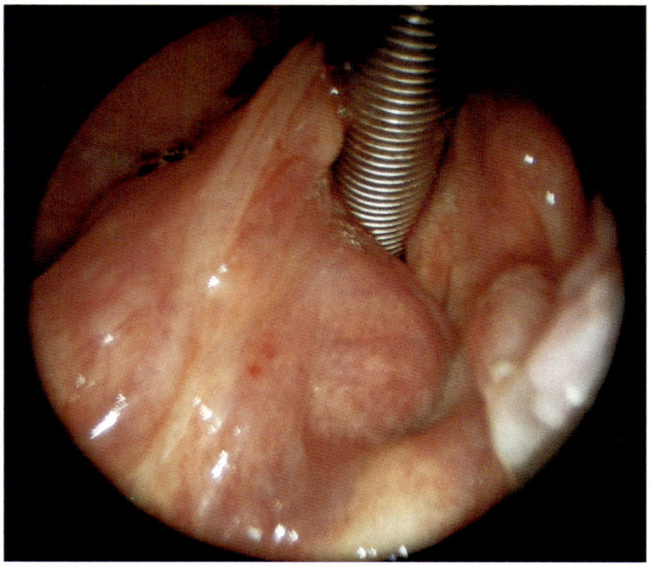

**FIGURE 40.65.** Isolated amyloid deposits manifesting as a submucosal tumor with invasion of the true vocal fold.

### Sarcoid

Laryngeal sarcoidosis can occur in men and women with or without active pulmonary disease (Fig. 40.66). Swelling of the epiglottis, supraglottis, and aryepiglottic folds while sparing the true vocal folds and the subglottis is quite characteristic of this disease. Occasionally, the surface becomes irregular and firm. Biopsy of the cobblestone areas reveals noncaseating granulomas. Treatment by systemic steroids and antimetabolite medication is usually effective. Some patients benefit by injection of steroids into the localized swollen tissue. The course of the disease is unpredictable. Some patients have periodic relapse with airway obstruction requiring tracheostomy.

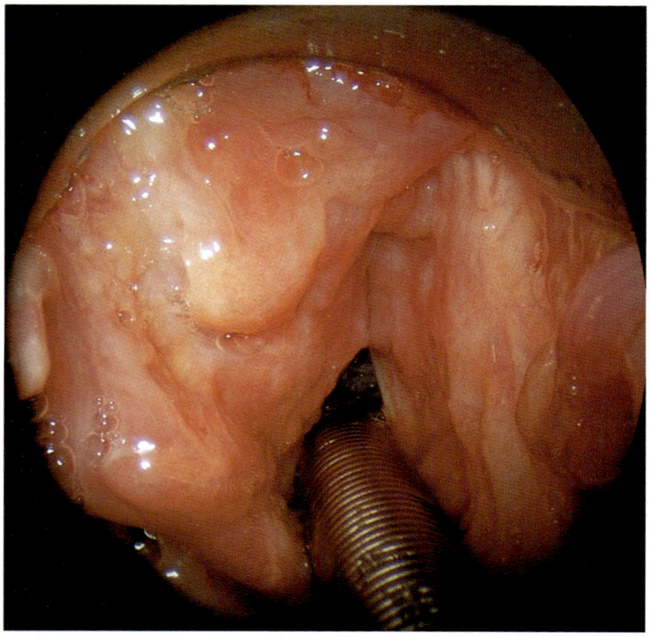

**FIGURE 40.64.** Supraglottic involvement of the larynx by isolated amyloidosis.

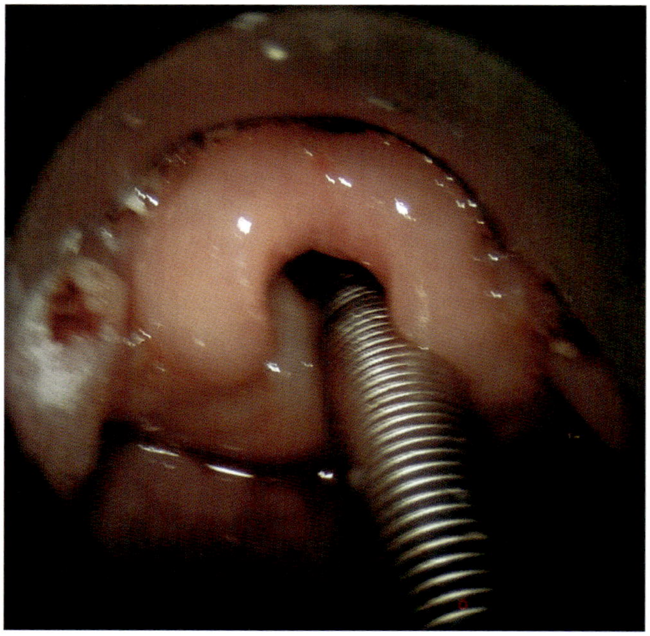

**FIGURE 40.66.** Laryngeal sarcoidosis. Notice the swelling of the epiglottis, supraglottis, and the aryepiglottic folds while the true vocal folds and the subglottis are spared.

## SELECTED READINGS


Alberti PW. Still photography of the larynx—an overview. *Can J Otolaryngol* 1975;4:759–765.

Andrea M, Dias O. *Rigid and contact endoscopy in microlaryngeal surgery–technique and atlas of clinical cases.* New York: Lippincott-Raven, 1995.

Andrea M, Dias O, Santos PT. Contact endoscopy during microlaryngeal surgery–a new technique for endoscopic examination of the larynx. *Ann Otol Rhinol Laryngol* 1995;104:333–339.

Andrews AH. Laryngeal telescope. *Trans Am Acad Ophthalmol Otolaryngol* 1962;66:268.

Andrews AH, Gould WJ. Laryngeal and nasopharyngeal indirect telescope. *Ann Otol Rhinol Laryngol* 1977;86:627.

Bastian RW. Benign mucosal and saccular disorders: benign laryngeal tumors. In: Cummings CW, Fredrickson JM, Barker LA, et al, eds. *Otolaryngology–head and neck surgery.* St. Louis: CV Mosby, 1933:1905–1906.

Becker W, Buckingham RA, Holinger P, et al. *Atlas of otorhinolaryngology and bronchoesophagology.* Philadelphia: WB Saunders, 1969.

Bell Telephone Laboratories. *High speed motion pictures of the vocal cords.* New York: Bell Telephone Bureau of Publication, 1937.

Benjamin B. Technique of laryngeal photography. *Ann Otol Rhinol Laryngol Suppl* 1984;109:1–11.

Benjamin B. *Diagnostic laryngology—adults and children.* Philadelphia: WB Saunders, 1990.

Benjamin B. Art and science of laryngeal photography. *Ann Otol Rhinol* 1993;102:271–282.

Berci G. *Endoscopy.* New York: Appleton-Century-Crofts, 1976.

Berci G, Calcaterra T, Ward PH. Advances in endoscopic techniques for examination of the larynx and nasopharynx. *Can J Otolaryngol* 1975;4:786–792.

Bless DM. Assessment of laryngeal function. In: Ford CN, Bless DM, eds. *Phonosurgery: assessment and surgical management of voice disorders.* New York: Raven Press, 1991:95–122.

Brewer DW, Gould LV, Casper J. Fiber-optic video study of the post-laryngectomized voice. *Laryngoscope* 1975;85:666–670.

Brewer DW, McCall G. Visible laryngeal changes during voice therapy—fiberoptic study. *Ann Otol Rhinol Laryngol* 1974;83:423–427.

Bouchayer M, Cornut G, Witzig E, et al. Epidermoid cysts, sulci, and mucosal bridges of the true vocal cord. *Laryngoscope* 1985;95:1087–1094.

D'Agostino MA, Jiang JJ, Hanson D. Edoscopic photography: solving the difficulties of practical application. *Laryngoscope* 1994;104:1045–1047.

Dedo HH, Jackler RK. Laryngeal papilloma: results of treatment with the $CO_2$ laser and podophyllum. *Ann Otol Rhinol Laryngol* 1982;91:425–430.

Dikkers FG, Nikkels PGJ. Benign lesions of the vocal folds: histopathology and phonotrauma. *Ann Otol Rhinol Laryngol* 1995;104:698–703.

Feder RJ. Varix of the vocal cord in the professional voice user. *Otolaryngol Head Neck Surg* 1983;91:435–440.

Feder RJ, Mitchell NF. Hyperfunctional, hyperacidic, and intubation granulomas. *Arch Otolaryngol* 1984;110:582–584.

Hirano M. Phonosurgery, basic and clinical investigations. *Otologia (Fukuoka)* 1975;21[Suppl 1]:239–440.

Hirano M. *Clinical examination of voice. Disorders of human communication,* vol 5. New York: Springer-Verlag, 1981.

Hirano M, Yoshida Y, Yoshida T, Tateishi O. Strobofiberscopic video recording of vocal fold vibration. *Ann Otol Rhinol Laryngol* 1985;94:588–590.

Hirano M. Objective evaluation of the human voice: clinical aspects. *Folia Phoniatr* 1989;41:89–144.

Hirano M, Kurita S. Histologic structure of the vocal fold and its normal and pathological variations. In: Kirchner IA, ed. *Vocal fold histopathology.* San Diego: College Hill Press, 1986:17–24.

Holinger PH. Photography of the larynx, trachea, bronchi and esophagus. *Trans Am Acad Ophthalmol Otolaryngol* 1942;46:153–156.

Holinger PH, Tardy ME. Photography in otorhinolaryngology and bronchoesophagology. In: English GM, ed. *Otolaryngology,* vol 5. Philadelphia: Lippincott, 1986.

Jako GJ. Laryngoscope for microscopic observations, surgery and photography. *Arch Otolaryngol* 1970;91:196–199.

Jako GJ. Microsurgery of the larynx with the $CO_2$ laser. *Arch Otolaryngol* 1979;3:1–20.

Kambic V, Radsel Z, Zargi M, Acko M. Vocal cord polyps: incidence, histology and pathogenesis. *J Laryngol Otol* 1981;95:609–618.

Kantor E, Berci G, Partlow E, et al. A completely new approach to microlaryngeal surgery. *Laryngoscope* 1991;101:678–679.

Kitzing P. Stroboscopy—a pertinent laryngological examination. *J Otolaryngol* 1985;14:151–157.

Kleinsasser O. *Microlaryngoscopy and endolaryngeal microsurgery.* Philadelphia: WB Saunders, 1968.

Kleinsasser O. Pathogenesis of vocal cord polyps. *Ann Otol Rhinol Laryngol* 1982;91:378–381.

Kleinsasser O. *Tumors of the larynx and hypopharynx.* New York: Thieme Medical Publishers, 1988.

Kleinsasser O, Glum H. Microcarcinoma and microinvasive carcinoma of the vocal cords. *Clin Oncol* 1982;1:479–487.

Monday LA, Cornut G, Bouchayer M, et al. Epidermoid cysts of the vocal cords. *Ann Otol Rhinol Laryngol* 1983;92:124–127.

Morrison MD. A clinical voice laboratory: videotape and stroboscopic instrumentation. *Otolaryngol Head Neck Surg* 1984;92:487–488.

Oertel MJ. Das Laryngo-strobskop und die laryngostroboskopische Untersuchung. *Arch Laryngol Rhinol (Berl)* 1985;3:1–16.

Saito S, Fukuda H, Kitahara S, Kokawa N. Stroboscopic observation of vocal fold vibration with fiberoptics. *Folia Phoniatr (Basel)* 1978;30:241–244.

Sataloff RT, Spiegel JR, Carroll LM, et al. Strobovideolaryngoscopy in professional voice users: results and clinical value. *J Voice* 1988;1:359–364.

Sawashima M, Hirose II. New laryngoscopic technique by use of fiber optics. *J Acoust Soc Am* 1968;43:168–169.

Schonharl E. *Die Stroboskopie in der praktischen Laryngologie.* Stuttgart: G Thieme, 1960.

Sercarz JA, Berke GS, Ming Y, et al. Videostroboscopy of human vocal fold paralysis. *Ann Otol Rhinol Laryngol* 1992;101:567–577.

Strong MS. Laryngeal photography. *Can J Otolaryngol* 1975;4:766–769.

Timcke R, yon Leden H, Moore P. Laryngeal vibrations: measurements of the glottic wave. Part I. The normal vibratory cycle. *Arch Otolaryngol* 1958;68:1–19.

Timcke R, von Leden H, Moore P. Laryngeal vibrations: measurements of the glottic wave. Part II. Physiologic vibrations. *Arch Otolaryngol* 1959;69:438.

Tobin HA. Office fiberoptic laryngeal photography. *Otolaryngol Head Neck Surg* 1980;88:172–173.

Von Leden H. Microlaryngoscopy: a historical vignette. *J Voice* 1988;1:341–346.

Von Leden H. The electronic synchron-stroboscope: its value for the practicing laryngologist. *Ann Otol Rhinol Laryngol* 1961;70:881–893.

Von Laden H, Moore P, Timcke R. Laryngeal vibrations: measurements of the glottic wave. Part III. The pathologic larynx. *Arch Otolaryngol* 1960;71:16–35.

Ward PH, Zwitnan D, Hanson D, Berci G. Contact ulcers and granulomas of the larynx. *Otolaryngol Head Neck Surg* 1960;88:262.

Ward PH, Berci G, Calcaterra TC. Advances in endoscopic examination of the respiratory system. *Ann Otol Rhinol Laryngol* 1974;83: 754–760.

Wendler J. Stroboscopy. *J Voice* 1992;6:149–154.

Yanagisawa E, Yanagisawa K. Stroboscopic video laryngoscopy—a comparison of fiberscopic and telescopic documentation. *Ann Otol Rhinol Laryngol* 1993;102:255–265.

Yanagisawa E, Casuccio IR, Suzuki M. Video laryngoscopy using a rigid telescope and video home system color camera. *Ann Otol Rhinol* 1981;90:346–350.

Yanagisawa E. Office telescopic photography of the larynx. *Ann Otol Rhinol Laryngol* 1982;91:354–358.

Yanagisawa E, Horowitz JB, Yanagisawa K, et al. Comparison of new telescopic video microlaryngoscopic and standard micro-laryngoscopic techniques. *Ann Otol Rhinol Laryngol* 1992;101:51–60.

# 41

# ADULT SURGICAL LARYNGOLOGY

## BENIGN LESIONS

STEVEN M. ZEITELS

## INDICATIONS

The primary indications for performing minimally invasive procedures in the larynx are for the diagnosis and treatment of a variety of lesions and diseases. Symptomatic treatment goals include restoration or improvement of the voice (i.e., phonomicrosurgery), the airway, and deglutition. Although phonomicrosurgery is the most common indication, airway restoration is the most critical one (1).

## CONTRAINDICATIONS

Contraindications for performing minimally invasive laryngeal surgery for benign lesions are primarily medical conditions or diseases that preclude reasonable risk with general anesthesia. In this scenario, the surgeon may resort to 19th century approaches (2,3) in the office setting by using local anesthesia and curved transoral instruments (4). Instead of mirror guidance, telescopic or flexible fiberoptic laryngoscopy is used. The inability to expose the larynx adequately by means of direct laryngoscopy because of a variety of anatomic characteristics (e.g., oral, pharyngeal, cervical spine, cervical soft tissue) may also require the surgeon to use this technique.

## PREOPERATIVE EVALUATION

Patients who are undergoing endolaryngeal procedures for benign lesions that result in vocal dysfunction should undergo appropriate preoperative testing for general anesthesia that is commensurate with their age and medical status. If available, strobovideolaryngoscopy should always be done at various pitch frequencies and subglottal pressures. This provides knowledge about the vibratory function of the vocal fold epithelium, which is invaluable information about what may be encountered intraoperatively and what can be expected postoperatively. Ideally, more complete objective measures of vocal function (acoustic and aerodynamic) should be obtained. If reflux laryngitis is suspected (5), it should be treated perioperatively to minimize inflammation and throat clearing. If the reflux is severe, dual-probe pH monitoring should be considered, followed by fundoplication as is appropriate.

## CASE EXAMPLES

### Vocal Polyps

Vocal polyps manifest in a variety of sizes and are typically the result of trauma to the microvasculature of the superficial lamina propria (SLP). They are most commonly found in the mid-musculomembranous region because the aerodynamically induced shearing and collision forces on the microvasculature of the SLP are greatest in this region. The lesions may be sessile (Fig. 41.1) or pedunculated (Fig. 41.2). Subepithelial infusion of saline and epinephrine enhances the precision of the resection of these lesions (6,7).

The sessile lesions can often be removed by means of an epithelial cordotomy, a microflap, and a subepithelial resection of the polyp contents (8) (Fig. 41.1C). Pedunculated lesions are optimally resected by retraction and amputation (Fig. 41.2). Care should be taken to palpate the component of the polyp that is in the SLP so that it is adequately excised. Small (0 to 3 mm) and medium-sized (3 to 6 mm) lesions can usually be removed with greater precision by cold instruments (9). When removing these lesions, a small feeding vessel may be encountered. It usually stops bleeding with application of saline with 1:10,000 epinephrine–soaked cotton. Occasionally, the carbon dioxide ($CO_2$) laser is necessary to microcauterize the vessel. Larger sessile lesions (>6 mm) are often best managed with the microspot $CO_2$ laser (9). The bleeding that occurs after incising these lesions with cold instruments can obscure the magnified operative field.

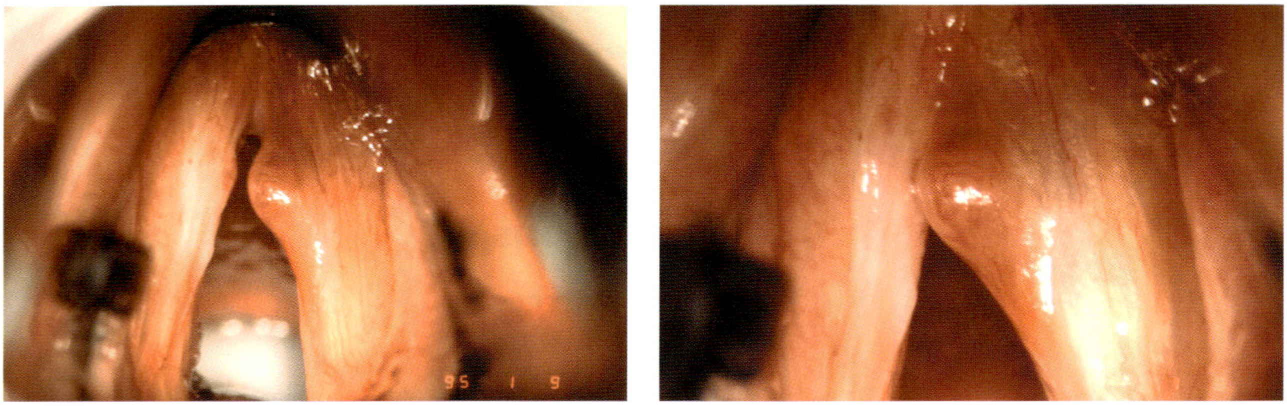

A B

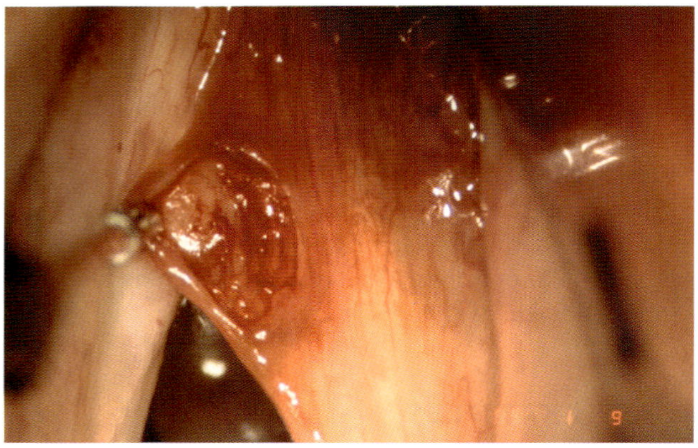

C

**FIGURE 41.1.** **A:** Sessile hemorrhagic polyp of the vocal fold. **B:** After subepithelial infusion of a 1:10,000 solution of epinephrine with saline, there is distention of the superficial lamina propria (SLP) and vasoconstriction of the microvasculature. **C:** A microflap is dissected, and the polyp contents are removed. There is maximal preservation of the normal SLP and epithelium. (Courtesy of Singular-Thomson Learning, San Diego, CA.)

## Vocal Nodules

Vocal nodules may manifest visually in a varied manner. There are divergent opinions about the value of phonomicrosurgical intervention. It is likely that the different philosophy about the efficacy of a surgical intervention is based on confusion in the literature about what constitutes vocal nodules. There is little disagreement that these lesions are the result of vocal abuse or inappropriate vocal use. Regardless of the decision to excise vocal nodules, virtually all of these patients require vocal therapy.

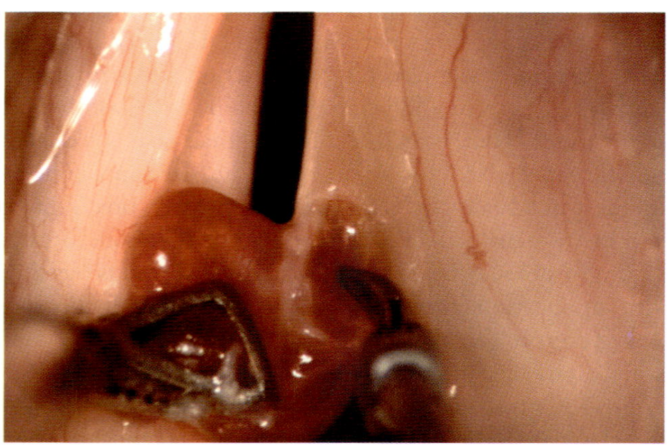

**FIGURE 41.2.** A pedunculated hemorrhagic polyp is amputated with microscissors. (Courtesy of Singular-Thomson Learning, San Diego, CA.)

In most cases, especially in performing artists, it is advantageous to employ surgery as a secondary management. An initial trial of vocal therapy should unload hyperfunctional behavior and reduce the generalized edema of the SLP that typically accompanies these lesions. Even if the nodules do not resolve and disappear visually, the patient may be satisfied with the quality and stamina of the voice such that surgical intervention is unnecessary. If further improvement is desired by the patient and clear nodules are seen, phonomicrosurgical excision may further enhance vocal quality (10) (Fig. 41.3). The prior vocal therapy can benefit the patient during the postoperative rehabilitative process in preventing injury and recurrence.

The patients who are not typically surgical candidates present with what has been called *nodular swelling*. Anatomically, these vocal folds have fusiform swelling of the SLP, which is usually bilateral and symmetric, and in the mid-musculomembranous region. A discreet mass is not seen on telescopic laryngostroboscopy. Prioritization of vocal activities and vocal therapy should adequately treat these individuals.

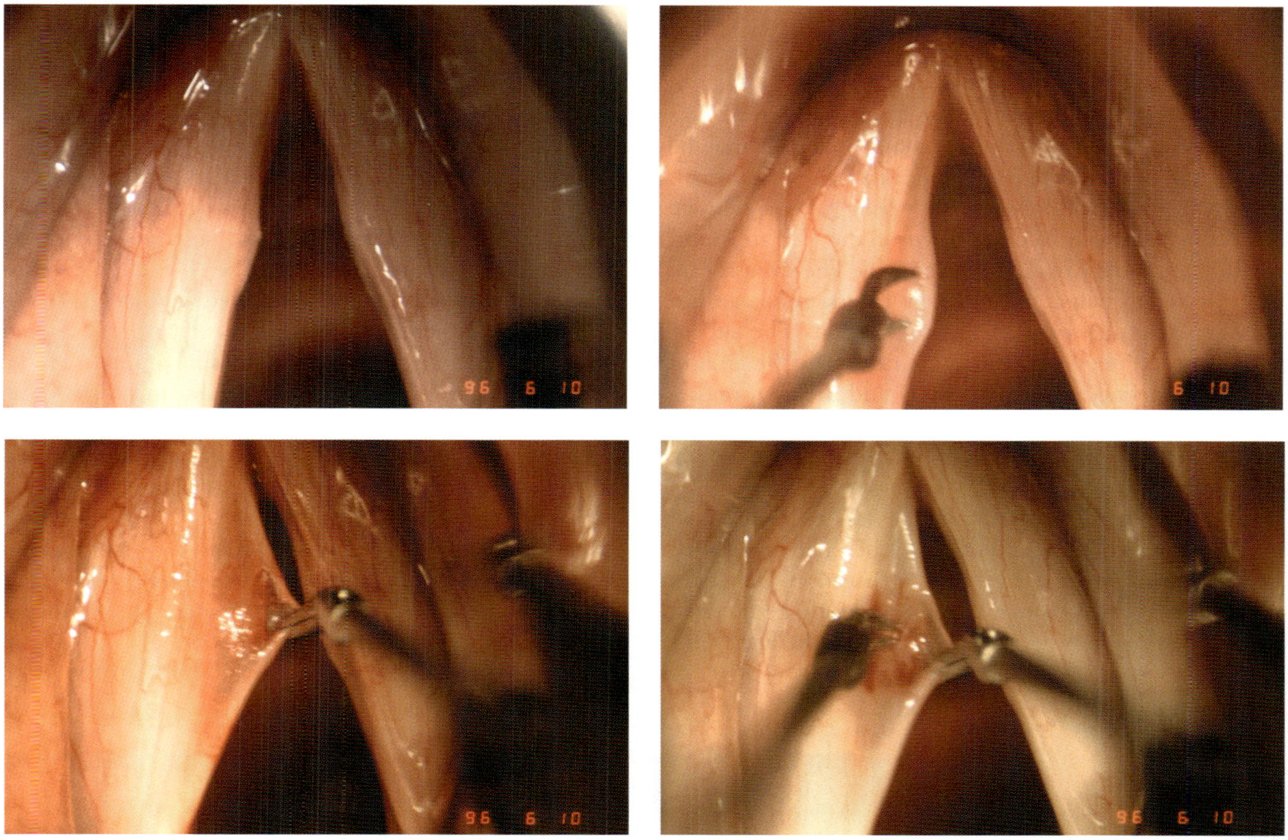

A B C D

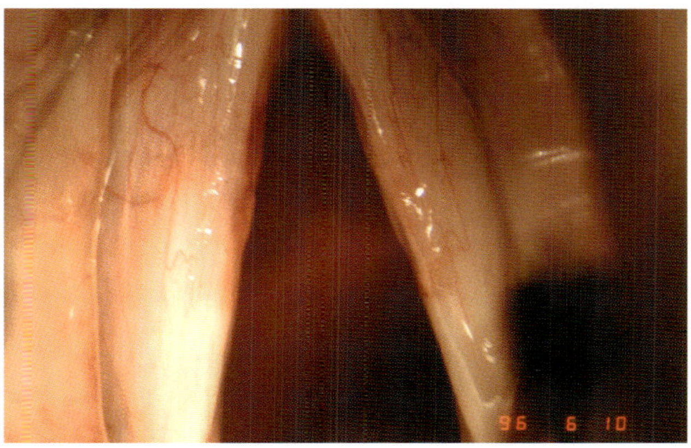

E

**FIGURE 41.3. A:** Recalcitrant vocal nodules in a classical vocalist. **B:** A curved microscissors is used to perform an epithelial cordotomy at the edge of the left lesion. **C:** A microalligator forceps is used to retract the microflap after the fibrous component has been dissected from the basement membrane. **D:** The microscissors is used to mobilize the fibrous contents of the nodule for excision. **E:** The vocal folds are now smooth and straight. (Courtesy of Singular-Thomson Learning, San Diego, CA.)

Similar to the aforementioned techniques for excising vocal polyps, phonomicrosurgical resection of vocal nodules can be performed by means of an epithelial cordotomy or by amputation. Cold instruments provide improved precision considering the small size of these lesions and the need for palpation during the procedure (9). The subepithelial infusion technique must be used selectively (6,7). Nodules that are less well defined visually and by palpation may become obscured by the infusion-induced distention of the SLP.

## Subepithelial Cysts

Subepithelial cysts arise in the SLP and manifest in a variety of sizes. They may be attached to the vocal ligament, the epithelial basement membrane, or both structures. Small cysts may also be freely suspended within the SLP. Small cysts may be confused with nodules if visual examination is performed without stroboscopy. Stroboscopic examination typically reveals a characteristic asymmetric, disordered oscillation of the mucosa because of the well-circumscribed stiffness in the area of the cyst. If the cyst protrudes from the medial surface of the glottal edge, a nodule may be observed on the contralateral vocal fold.

Subepithelial cysts probably arise from obstructed ducts within the SLP (11). They may contain mucus or may be composed of an epithelial rest (similar to a cholesteatoma). Occasionally, the small, ovoid subepithelial masses that are thought preoperatively to be cysts within the SLP are found at microlaryngoscopy to be fibrous masses. These masses are usually firmer to palpation and may be the result an old microvascular injury or a rheumatoid lesion. The subepithelial infusion technique (6,7) is extremely helpful in treating well-defined cysts (Fig. 41.4) and the firm masses within the SLP, but the infusion can obscure the boundaries of small cysts and lead to unnecessary dissection and trauma of normal SLP.

Masses within the SLP should be resected with cold instruments with few exceptions (9). The need for extremely fine, delicate tangential dissection precludes effective use of the $CO_2$ laser. Great care should be taken to minimally disturb any normal SLP and epithelium. This approach optimizes postoperative mucosal wave oscillation and vocal quality.

## Polypoid Corditis

Polypoid corditis (i.e., Reinke's edema) presents as extensive swelling of the SLP (i.e., Reinke's space) (Fig. 41.5A). The swelling is usually situated on the superior surface of the musculomembranous vocal fold (Fig. 41.5B). This entity is another manifestation of vocal fold pathology that is of multifactorial genesis. Zeitels and colleagues (12) demonstrated that these patients typically smoke extensively, have laryngopharyngeal reflux, and demonstrate vocal hyperfunction. The swelling probably occurs from the increased aerodynamic pressures that drive vocal fold mucosal oscillation in a general environment of glottal mucositis, which is caused by smoking and reflux.

Individuals with polypoid corditis have an abnormally low-pitched voice because the mass-loaded folds oscillate at an inordinately low frequency. Women present more frequently than men and undergo phonomicrosurgical man-

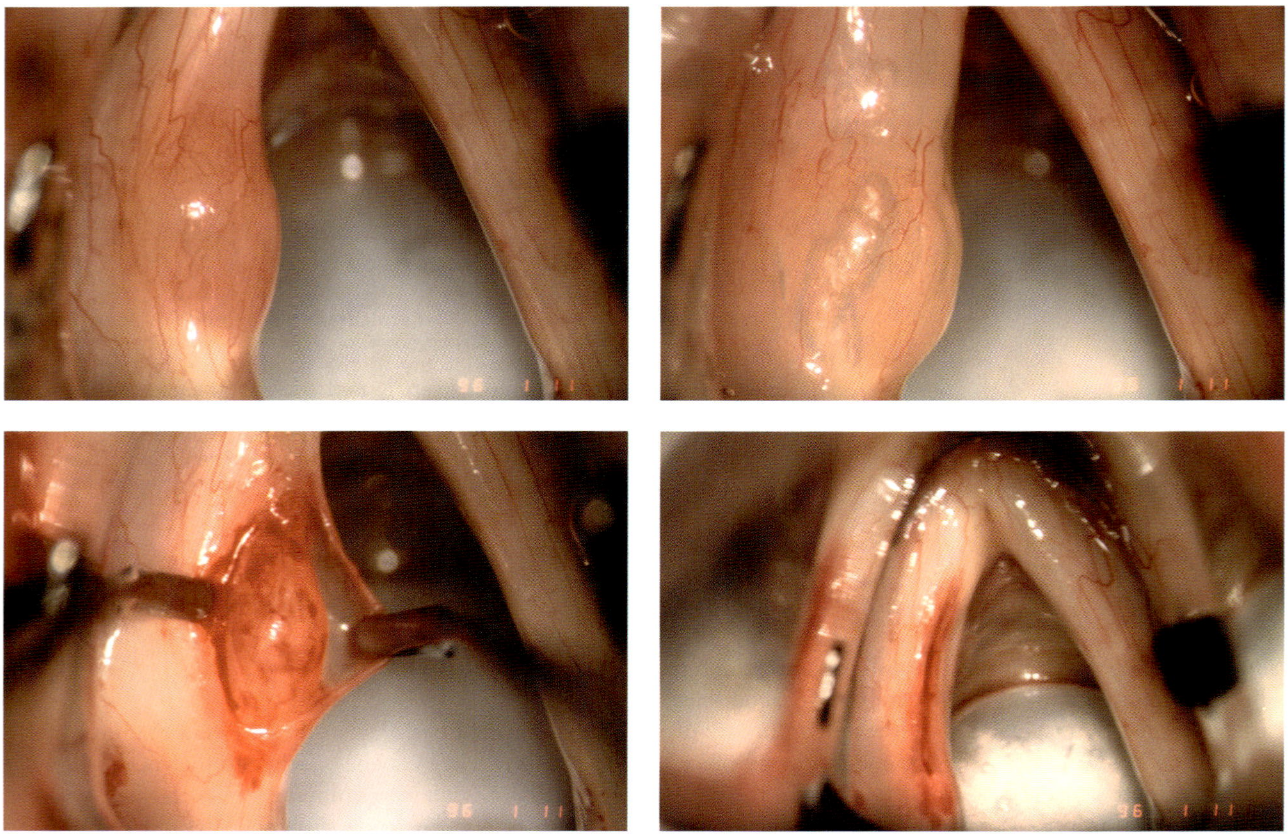

A B C D

**FIGURE 41.4.** **A:** Subepithelial cyst of the left vocal fold. **B:** After subepithelial infusion of a 1:10,000 epinephrine and saline solution, there is distention of the superficial lamina propria and vasoconstriction of the microvasculature. **C:** An epithelial cordotomy is performed, and a microflap is dissected. **D:** After excision of the cyst, there is excellent opposition of the epithelial edges. (Courtesy of Singular-Thomson Learning, San Diego, CA.)

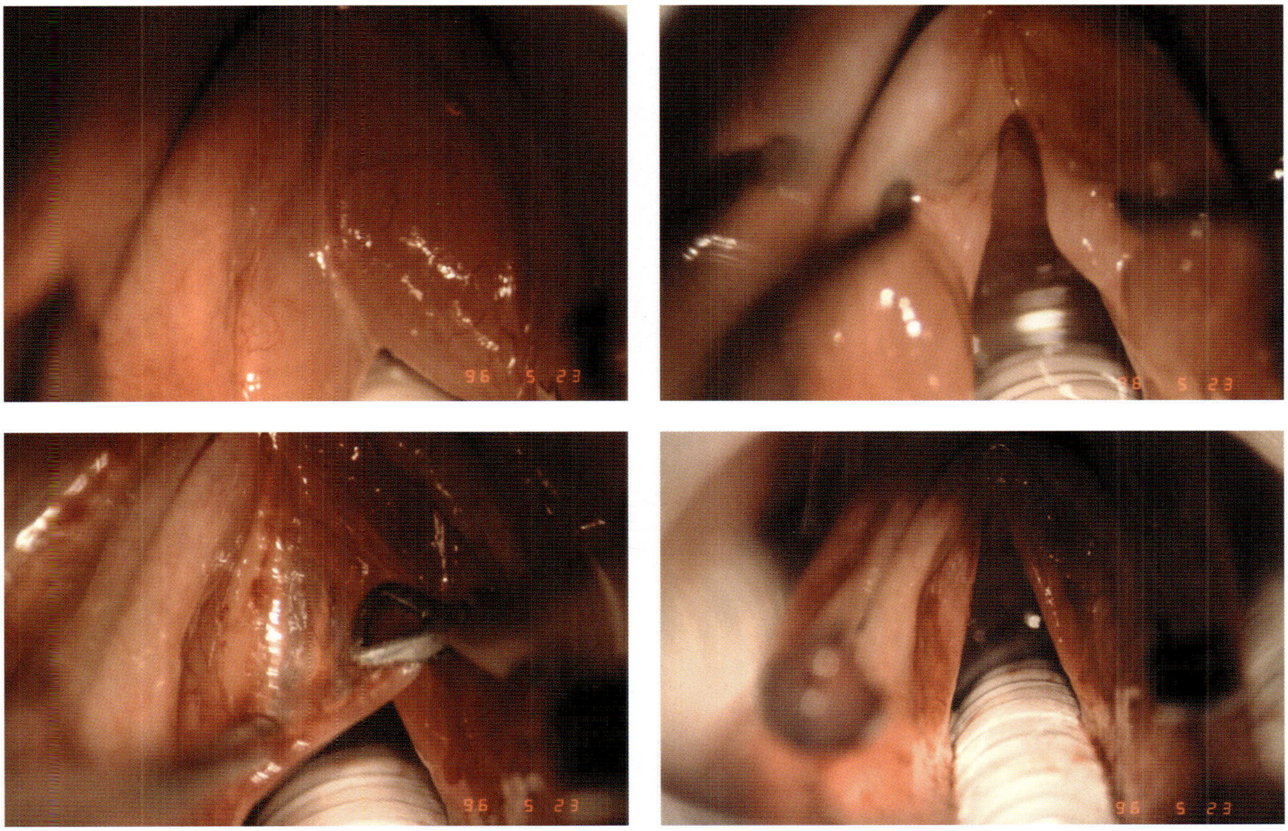


**FIGURE 41.5. A:** Massive polypoid corditis (Reinke's edema). **B:** The swelling is primarily situated on the superior surface of the vocal fold. **C:** An epithelial microflap is raised, and the superficial lamina propria (SLP) is reduced in volume. **D:** After reducing the SLP bilaterally to create a more normal glottal aperture, the redundant epithelium is trimmed so that there is good apposition of the edges. (Courtesy of Singular-Thomson Learning, San Diego, CA.)

agement more frequently because of the greater discrepancy from their normal fundamental voice frequency.

These individuals should discontinue smoking, have their reflux controlled, and should undergo preoperative vocal therapy before undergoing a procedure. The technique for the procedure is based on raising a thin epithelial microflap after incising the mucosa near the vestibular fold. A microscissors is used for the initial incision unless there is prominent subepithelial vascular injection. The gelatinous, hypertrophied SLP should then be carefully contoured and reduced (Fig. 41.5C) to a more normal volume. This can be done by suctioning or by direct removal. Great care must be taken not to overreduce the SLP, which results in an inordinately stiff vocal fold (12). The vocal ligament should never be visualized directly. Overreduction of the SLP can result in a severely strained, harsh voice because these individuals generally employ high subglottal pressures to drive their floppy mass-loaded folds. To achieve an optimal vocal outcome, it is preferable to leave a larger fold than to create a visually pleasing smaller fold.

After the SLP has been reduced, the epithelium is redraped and trimmed appropriately (Fig. 41.5D). If there is keratotic or dysplastic epithelium, it should be excised and sent to the pathology department for histopathologic analysis. After an initial period of vocal rest (about 10 days), patients should receive vocal therapy and should be monitored closely. Preventing recurrence depends on modification of the predisposing factors, especially smoking.

## Respiratory Papillomatosis

Patients who have respiratory papillomatosis of the glottis most frequently present with hoarseness. Most commonly, the glottal disease is confined to the musculomembranous region (Fig. 41.6A), although it is not unusual to find extension into the ventricle and subglottis. Adult glottal papillomatosis tends to be more plaquelike than the juvenile variety. Because the disease is confined to the epithelium, great care should be taken to maximally preserve the underlying SLP. In all cases of initial presentation and in most recurrent cases,

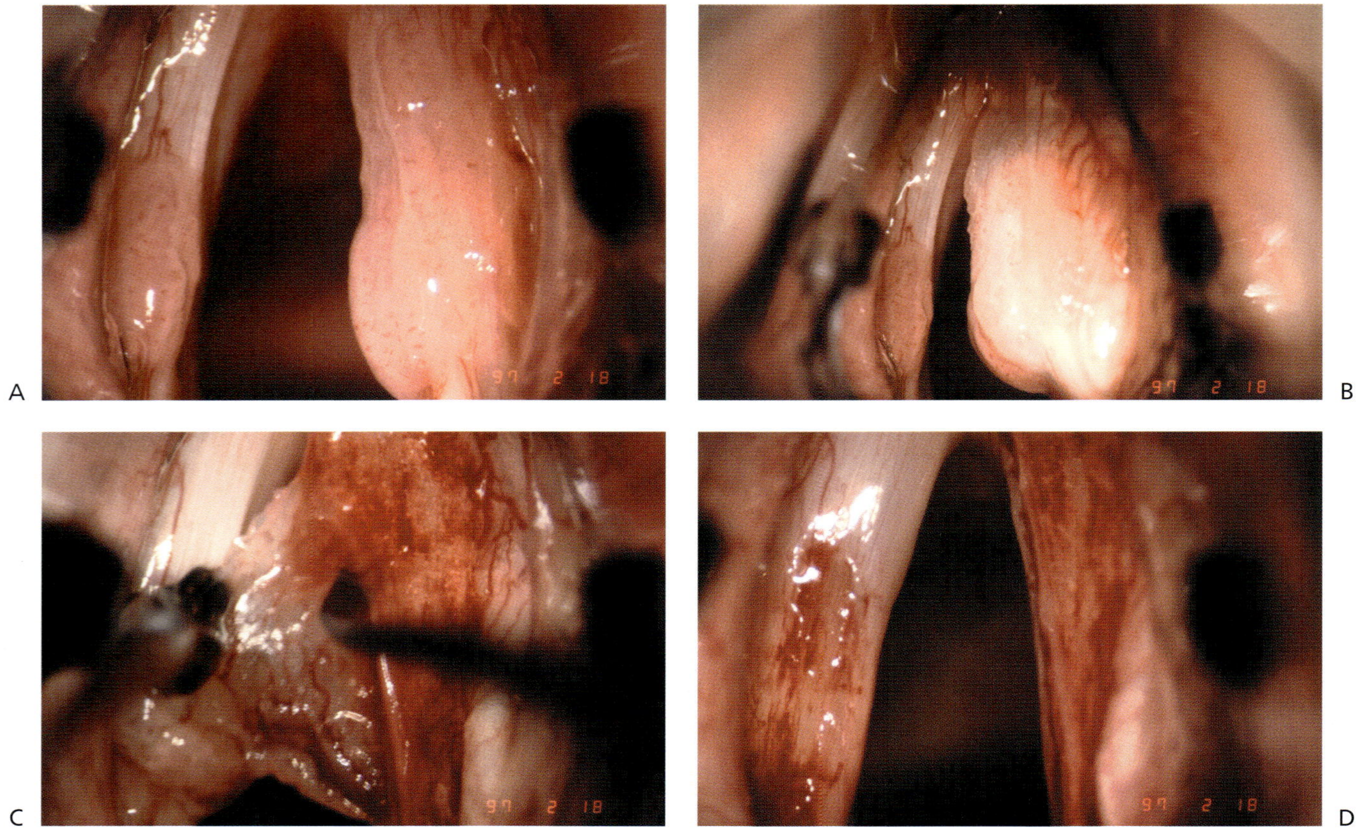


**FIGURE 41.6.** **A:** Papillomatosis of the right vocal fold and a smaller focus on the left. **B:** After subepithelial infusion of a 1:10,000 epinephrine and saline solution, there is distention of the superficial lamina propria (SLP) and vasoconstriction of the microvasculature. **C:** A curved dissector is used to dissect the epithelial microflap around the curving vocal fold to maximally preserve the SLP. **D:** There is maximal preservation of the normal SLP; a significant amount of the microvasculature of the SLP can be seen overlying the vocal ligament. (Courtesy of Endocraft LLC, Providence, RI.)

the subepithelial infusion technique (Fig. 41.6B) with cold instrument dissection (Fig. 41.6C) is best suited for this goal. An en bloc resection by means of a microflap can frequently be accomplished (Fig. 41.6D). Every attempt to perform a narrow-margin excision should be made, even if this includes serial procedures to preserve the integrity of the anterior commissure. Preliminary findings suggest that resecting this disease on initial presentation is likely to be curative (13) and that completely resecting previously recurrent disease is curative in about 30% of patients.

## INSTRUMENTATION

A well-designed direct laryngoscope is arguably the most critical single instrument because it provides the gateway to the larynx. For vocal fold surgery, a rigid glottiscope should have an examining tube that has a linear taper with a wide bore that provides binocular stereoscopic visualization at multiple magnifications (14). Ideally, the distal lumen should be triangular to accommodate the glottal aperture (14,15) and especially the anterior commissure (16). A universal modular glottiscope (Endocraft LLC, Providence, RI) is composed of a plurality of examining tubes that attach to a universal handle (17) (Fig. 41.7). This instrument has been designed to accommodate the spectrum of human anatomy, regardless of gender, age, or pathology.

Microlaryngeal hand instruments are used in routine classic sizes as designed by Jako and Kleinsasser, as well as the later and smaller pediatric phonomicrosurgical size (18). A specially designed infusion needle (Endocraft LLC) for injection into the SLP (6,7,19) is often helpful. The procedure may use a $CO_2$ laser with a microspot of about 0.3 mm.

An operating chair that is designed for microsurgery and has armrests to stabilize the hands for high-magnification (8× and 10×) cold instrument dissection is extremely helpful. If a one of these specially designed chairs is not available, the surgeon may use a stand to support the arms or place an extension on the table proximal to the patient's head.

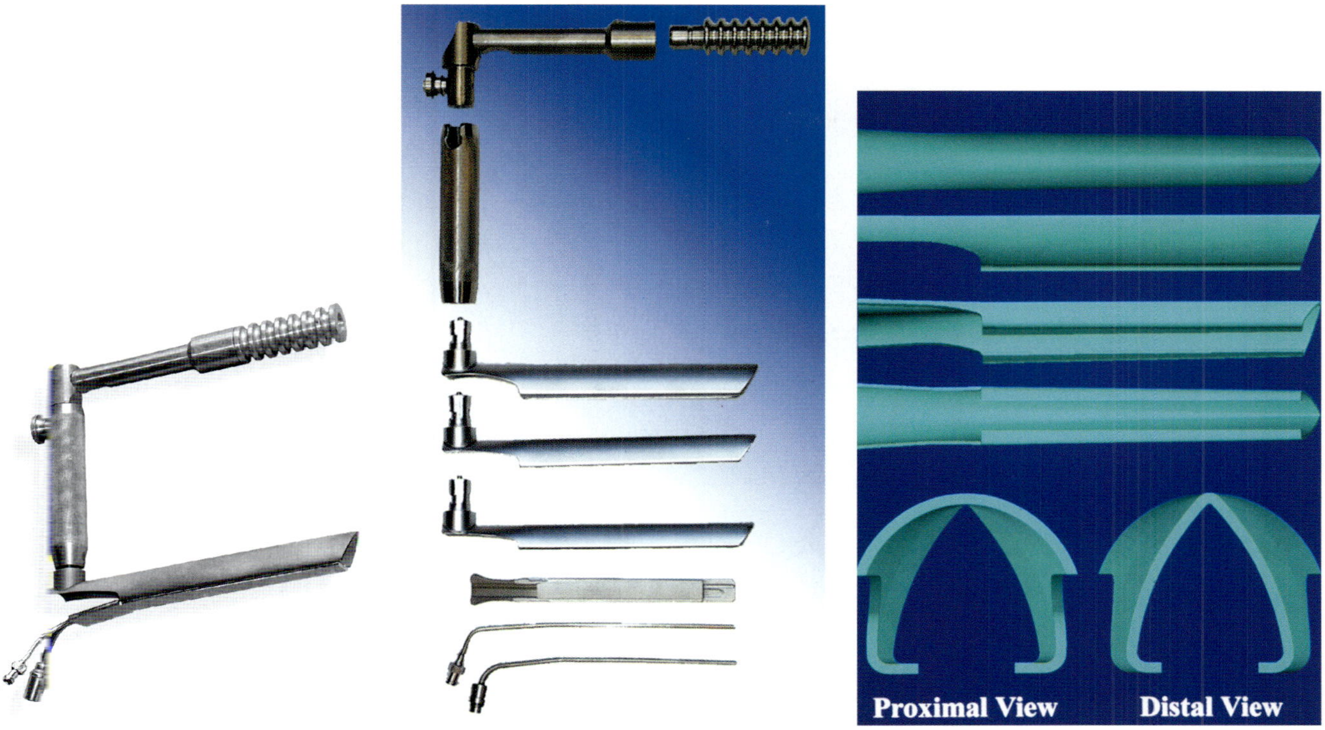


A,B C

**FIGURE 41.7. A:** Universal modular glottiscope. **B:** Detachable components of the universal modular glottiscope, including various sizes of the examining spatula. **C:** Schematic representation of the examining spatula-tube. (Courtesy of Endocraft LLC, Providence, RI.)

## ANESTHESIA

An orotracheal tube with the smallest diameter that can ventilate the patient adequately is selected. A laser-protected tube should be used when the $CO_2$ laser is employed. In selected cases, a jet ventilation catheter (Hunsaker catheter, Xomed, Jacksonville, FL) may be advantageous.

## OPERATIVE TECHNIQUE

Suspension microlaryngoscopy is performed with general endotracheal anesthesia and paralysis. *External counterpressure* (20) and *internal distention* (21,22) are employed routinely (23). An endotracheal tube provides a stable point from which the largest lumen laryngoscope is intercalated between the endotracheal tube and the infrapetiole region of the supraglottis (for glottal surgery) to internally distend the surgical field. Jet ventilation is not typically used by me, because it is not practical in treating many lesions and because it precludes adequate internal distention of the laryngeal introitus. The patient is placed in the classic Jackson position, with the neck flexed and the head extended at the atloid-occipital joint, and the position is maintained with a modified Killian gallows (24) (Pilling Co., Philadelphia, PA) in true elevated-vector suspension (4) (Fig. 41.8).

External laryngeal counterpressure is first applied manually to determine its value for improving exposure and then applied with a laryngeal cushion and overlying silk tape that is stretched from the lower laryngeal framework to the operating table. The magnitude of the pressure and vector of the force are adjusted to optimize the exposure of the lesion and the anterior glottis. If the $CO_2$ laser is to be used, the patient and a laser-safe endotracheal tube are protected in the appropriate fashion.

An operating microscope fitted with a 400-mm front lens is used to examine the glottal surgical field at magnifications of 4×, 8×, and 10×. In addition to the magnified visual examination, the lesion is palpated with a blunt probe to help assess the texture of the lesion and the depth of deep tissue involvement. Subepithelial infusion of saline and 1:10,000 epinephrine into the SLP is used for most benign glottal lesions.

During superficial glottal procedures, hemostasis is achieved by topical application of epinephrine-soaked cotton. For highly vascular glottal lesions, the laser can be employed with a defocused spot or electrocoagulation is used. When the surgery is completed, any residual blood or secretions that are in the laryngeal introitus or hypopharynx

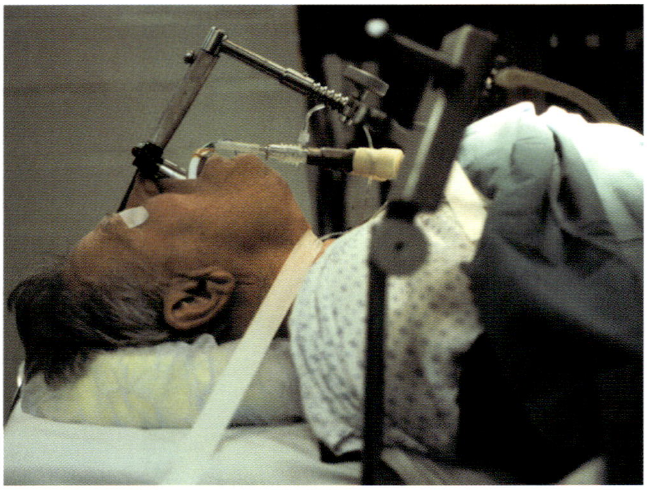

A

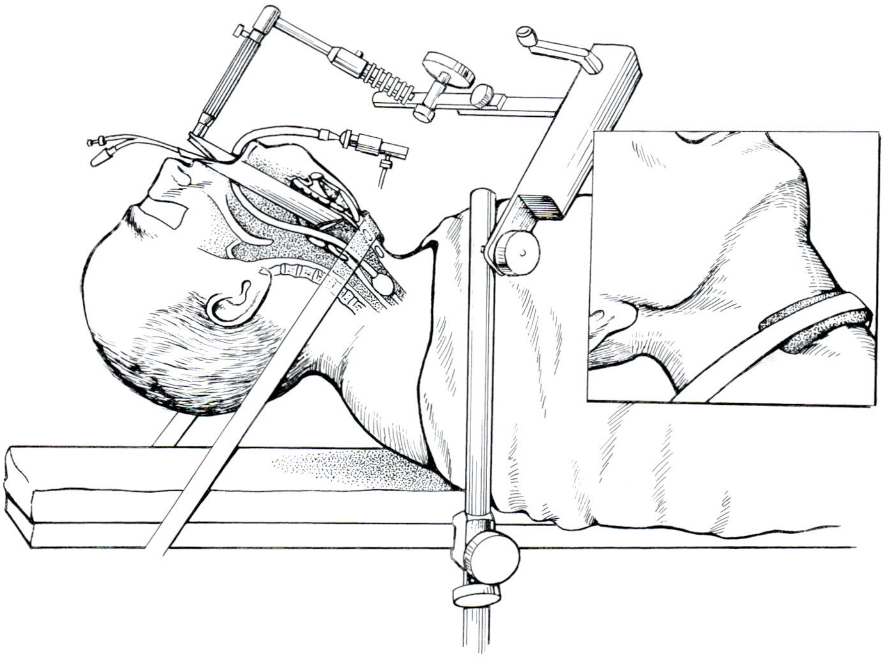

B

**FIGURE 41.8. A:** The patient is maintained in the Jackson position by the Boston University gallows (i.e., modified Killian suspension), which results in elevated-vector suspension. External counterpressure is applied with overlying silk adhesive tape. (Courtesy of Singular-Thomson Learning, San Diego, CA.) **B:** Artist's illustration of **A**.

are suctioned, and the larynx is sprayed with plain lidocaine to avoid laryngospasm during extubation.

## SPECIAL POINTS

Lesions along the glottal introitus impair entrained oscillation by creating stiffness in the diseased vocal fold and by preventing smooth closure of the vocal fold edge. These factors result in an aerodynamically inefficient glottal valve (25). Phonomicrosurgical procedures are designed to improve aerodynamic efficiency and vocal quality by creating a smooth vocal fold edge that is not excavated with overlying epithelium that is flexible.

Optimal phonomicrosurgical management of benign glottal lesions requires maximal preservation of normal laminae propria and epithelium. It is valuable to assess the microlayers of involvement of any lesion. This should involve high-magnification visual inspection and gentle retraction with palpation. Most procedures should be done with 8× or 10× magnification. Given the choice of sacrificing or disturbing normal SLP or normal epithelium, it is wiser to preserve normal SLP.

In my experience, there is little difficulty in the growth and regeneration of normal epithelium, as occurs after a cancer cordectomy that is left to heal secondarily; normal SLP does not regenerate if it has been removed. Postoperative stroboscopic findings further reveal that, if extensive dissection in normal SLP is performed to raise a wide microflap, stiffness is noticed in the field of dissection. Regenerated epithelium essentially reflects the viscoelastic properties and the oscillation characteristics of the tissue that it overlies. The location of epithelial incisions is not of great significance to vibratory function if the underlying SLP is preserved. This was demonstrated in a series of vocalists who underwent multiple epithelial incisions to resect traumatic varices and ectasias (26).

The glottiscope that provides the widest aperture for visualizing the glottal surgical field should be selected. Placing the largest tubular laryngoscope that can be admitted from the lips to the vocal folds can be hard work (23). It is not uncommon for the surgeon to avoid this struggle and resort to a smaller-lumen instrument that can be placed easily but that does not optimally expose the operative site. However, the precision of the procedure may be compromised because of limited exposure of the lesion and the limited ability to angulate hand instrumentation for tangential tissue dissection in the laminae propria. The use of a smaller-lumen glottiscope is less important when the laser is used, because only one hand instrument requires angulation. However, many laryngologists believe that precise microdissection is optimally performed by exclusive use of cold instruments for most glottal pathology. This requires a glottiscope that can accommodate angulation of two hand instruments.

The subepithelial infusion of saline and epinephrine into the SLP has further enhanced precision in microlaryngoscopic vocal fold surgery (4–7) with the use of the $CO_2$ laser and cold instruments. The infusion increases the depth of the SLP, which helps to preserve it. The saline with epinephrine infusion also enhances hemostasis (and therefore tissue visualization) by epinephrine-induced and hydrostatic-induced vasoconstriction of the microvasculature of the SLP.

In a recent report (9), 77% of 263 glottal procedures were done with cold instruments alone. The thermal trauma of the $CO_2$ laser may be detrimental to the delicate, loosely arranged, elastic tissue of the SLP. In my hands, the laser was used in more vascular lesions, because bleeding would otherwise obscure the operative site, and in larger lesions that could not be effectively retracted within the lumen of the laryngoscope.

Most endoscopic surgery in the glottis is done to treat benign processes. The most frequent presenting symptom for glottal disease is hoarseness. Benign lesions typically occur in vocal overdoers and seldom occur in individuals who are reticent and shy. Many of these individuals require preoperative and postoperative vocal therapy to undo habits that predisposed to the original lesion or to remove compensatory strategies that developed as a result of the lesion. Because the timing and decision about surgery is frequently linked to the response to vocal therapy, the surgeon must know the speech-language pathologist well to accurately assess the adequacy of therapy.

The preoperative workup should include flexible and rigid laryngeal stroboscopy as well as acoustic and aerodynamic assessment. Telescopic stroboscopy provides superior optics for analyzing the anatomy of the vocal folds, the details of the lesion, and the characteristics of the mucosal wave oscillation. Flexible stroboscopy is superior for analyzing generalized laryngeal configuration during sound production, which is necessary for assessing the magnitude of muscle tension that accompanies the lesion.

The aforementioned visual information and the acoustic and aerodynamic data provide the surgeon with objective information about laryngeal sound production. The acoustic and aerodynamic information should be obtained for normal and loud voice tasks. The aerodynamic efficiency (i.e., pressure, flow, and resistance) is an excellent indicator of a patient's work and effort of phonation. This factor is often overlooked in the preoperative history and postoperative discussions.

## POSTOPERATIVE CARE

Postoperatively, the patient is placed on humidified room air and is managed for laryngopharyngeal reflux as necessary. Antibiotics, steroids, and analgesics are prescribed selectively based on the surgeon's preference and the extent of the surgery.

After vocal fold surgery, I recommend complete voice rest for 10 to 14 days and modified voice use for 1 to 2 weeks. The patient should have preoperative and postoperative appointments with a speech pathologist for objective voice assessment and vocal hygiene discussion. Formal voice therapy is administered as is necessary. Diet restrictions are instituted after wide-field supraglottal resections because of concern about aspiration. Swallowing therapy is instituted as is necessary.

## COMPLICATIONS

Hoarseness or a worsening of vocal quality as a result of a phonomicrosurgical procedure is rare. It may be temporary or permanent and usually results from noncompliance with postoperative instructions.

Oral trauma is common from placement of large-bore laryngoscopes. This typically manifests as reversible mucosal abrasions, temporary taste alteration, or tongue numbness. Occasionally, dental trauma occurs, but these individuals usually have prior deterioration. Postoperative hemorrhage is also rare in patients with normal hemostasis. Temporomandibular joint dysfunction can occur in patients with a history of this difficulty.

## ADVANTAGES AND DISADVANTAGES OF THE ENDOSCOPIC TECHNIQUE

Procedures are well tolerated, and the patient is typically discharged several hours after the procedure if the airway is not at risk. The techniques and instrumentation are undergoing dynamic improvements such that the results are improving. Many patients can be restored vocally years after the onset of hoarseness.

Not all patients can be surgically exposed well enough to perform the procedure adequately. The procedures can be technically difficult under 10× magnification, especially manual control of the nondominant hand. Frequently, suboptimal results (e.g., scarring of the SLP) cannot be subsequently corrected.

## CONCLUSIONS

Endoscopic surgery of the larynx is one of the earliest examples of minimally invasive surgery. It has been just over a century since Kirstein formally introduced direct laryngoscopy, which paved the way for current endoscopic surgical approaches for laryngeal disease. Every substantive innovation in endoscopic surgery of the larynx enhanced precision and improved postoperative laryngeal function (i.e., airway, swallowing, and voice). Endoscopic glottal surgery has emerged as a physiologically based phonomicrosurgical approach. It has developed from the convergence of microlaryngoscopic surgical technique theory with mucosal wave theory of laryngeal sound production. Endoscopic glottal surgery will continue to evolve as a result of innovations in minimally invasive technology, as well as the interdependent collaboration of surgeons with voice scientists, speech pathologists, and other voice professionals.

## REFERENCES

1. Zeitels SM. *Atlas of phonomicrosurgery and other endolaryngeal procedures for benign and malignant disease*. San Diego, CA: Singular Publishing Group, 2001.
2. Mackenzie M. *Growths in the larynx*. London: J&A Churchill, 1871.
3. Solis-Cohen J. *Diseases of the throat: a guide to the diagnosis and treatment*. New York: William Wood, 1872.
4. Zeitels SM. Premalignant epithelium and microinvasive cancer of the vocal fold: the evolution of phonomicrosurgical management. *Laryngoscope* 1995;105:1–51.
5. Koufman JA. The otolaryngologic manifestations of gastroesophageal reflux disease (GERD). *Laryngoscope* 1991;101:1–78.
6. Zeitels SM, Vaughan CW. A submucosal vocal fold infusion needle. *Otolaryngol Head Neck Surg* 1991;105:478–479.
7. Kass ES, Hillman RE, Zeitels SM. The submucosal infusion technique in phonomicrosurgery. *Ann Otol Rhinol Laryngol* 1996;105:341–347.
8. Hochman II, Zeitels SM. Phonomicrosurgical management of vocal fold polyps. *J Voice* 2000;14:112–118.
9. Zeitels SM. Laser versus cold instruments for microlaryngoscopic surgery. *Laryngoscope* 1996;106:545–552.
10. Zeitels SM, Desloge R, Doyle P, et al. Phonomicrosurgery in singers and performing artists. Presented at the annual meeting of the American Laryngological, Rhinological and Otological Society, Palm Desert, CA, 1999.
11. Bouchayer M, Cornut G. Instrumental microscopy of benign lesions of the vocal folds. In: Ford C, Bless D, eds. *Phonosurgery*. New York: Raven, 1991:25–41.
12. Zeitels SM, Hillman RE, Bunting GW, et al. Reinke's edema: phonatory mechanisms and management strategies. *Ann Otol Rhinol Laryngol* 1996;106:533–543.
13. Zeitels SM, Sataloff RT. Phonomicrosurgical resection of glottal papillomatosis. *J Voice* 1999;13:123–127.
14. Zeitels SM. A universal modular glottiscope system: the evolution of a century of design and technique for direct laryngoscopy. *Ann Otol Rhinol Laryngol* 1999;108[Suppl 179]:1–24.
15. Vaughan CW. Vocal fold exposure in phonosurgery. *J Voice* 1993; 7:189–194.
16. Desloge RB, Zeitels SM. Endolaryngeal microsurgery at the anterior glottal commissure: controversies and observations. *Ann Otol Rhinol Laryngol* 2000;109:385–392.
17. Zeitels SM. Universal modular laryngoscope/glottiscope system. United States patent 5,893,830, 1999.
18. Shapshay SM, Healy GB. New microlaryngeal instruments for phonatory surgery and pediatric applications. *Ann Otol Rhinol Laryngol* 1990;98:821–823.
19. Hartig G, Zeitels SM. Phonosurgery. Part 1. Optimizing voice in conservation surgery for glottic cancer. *Otolaryngol Head Neck Surg* 1998;9:214–223.
20. Brunings W. Direct laryngoscopy: autoscopy by counter-pressure. In: *Direct laryngoscopy, bronchoscopy, and esophagoscopy*. London: Bailliere, Tindall, & Cox, 1912:110–115.
21. Israel S. The directoscope of Haslinger in diagnosis and surgery of the larynx. *Laryngoscope* 1923;33:945–948.
22. Jackson C, Tucker G, Clerf LH. Laryngostasis and the laryngostat. *Arch Otolaryngol* 1925;1:167–169.
23. Zeitels SM, Vaughan CW. "External counter-pressure" and "internal distension" for optimal laryngoscopic exposure of the anterior glottal commissure. *Ann Otol Rhinol Laryngol* 1994;103: 669–675.
24. Grundfast KM, Vaughan CW, Strong MS, et al. Suspension microlaryngoscopy in the Boyce position with a new suspension gallows. *Ann Otol Rhinol Laryngol* 1978;87:560–566.
25. Isshiki N. Vibration of the vocal folds. In: *Phonosurgery: theory and practice*. Tokyo: Springer-Verlag, 1989:7–11.
26. Hochman I, Sataloff RT, Hillman RE, et al. Ectasias and varices of the vocal folds: clearing the striking zone. *Ann Otol Rhinol Laryngol* 1998;108:10–16.

# 42

# TECHNIQUES FOR ENDOSCOPIC VOCAL FOLD AUGMENTATION

**CHARLES N. FORD**
**MARY J. SANDAGE**

Adequate exposure and proper patient selection are the most important factors in ensuring a satisfactory outcome for vocal fold augmentation. Direct microlaryngoscopy is the good standard for surgical exposure; however, limiting factors include the anatomic distortion introduced by suspending the larynx and the inability to functionally measure the effects of injection under general anesthesia. Consequently, the anatomic effects of vocal fold augmentation are difficult to assess in such a nonphysiologic setting. The advantages include the ability to view the larynx in a magnified and fixed position, and because of general anesthesia, it is not necessary for the patient to cooperate during the examination or the augmentation procedure. This is the approach most widely employed by otolaryngologists for injection of augmentation materials in the vocal fold.

Indirect laryngoscopy using a laryngeal mirror is technically more challenging, but it offers numerous advantages for augmentation injections. The most important of these is the ability to perform injections in an awake and cooperative patient. The injected material can be placed incrementally and the patient asked to phonate to determine the immediate effect on the voice. It is also possible to perform intermittent stroboscopy to determine the effect of the injection on vocal fold vibration. If the results are not optimal, the injected material can be redistributed by manipulating the vocal fold mucosal edge or injecting additional material. The obvious advantage of being able to perform the procedure under topical anesthesia is monitoring of the voice, but it also avoids the risks of general anesthesia.

## FIBEROPTIC LARYNGOSCOPY

The use of fiberoptic endoscopy for evaluation of the structure and function of vocal folds as an adjunct to the indirect mirror examination emerged in the early 1970s (1–3). This followed successful application of fiberoptic endoscopy in other areas such as the gastrointestinal tract and lower respiratory system. Several benefits of flexible fiberoptic endoscopy became apparent: videoendoscopy afforded an unhurried, dynamic view of the larynx and surrounding structures; accuracy of observations combined with stroboscopy to assess vibratory characteristics of the mucosal portion of the vocal folds (3); improved identification and staging of laryngeal cancer; and the ability to do such examinations in the office in an awake patient, obviating laryngoscopy under general anesthesia.

Early flexible fiberoptic laryngoscopes were designed for intubation during anesthesia, and they were of limited use because of the large diameter (6.25 mm) and inferior optics (4). Improvements were made in 1975, when Machida (Machida America, Closter, NJ) introduced a prototype with a smaller diameter (3.9 mm) suitable for adult and pediatric cases. Optics were improved by doubling the size of the optical bundle and reducing the length to 25 cm. Several instrument companies have introduced fiberscopes with superb optics and external diameters of only 3.7 mm.

Rigid telescopes allow for assessment of vocal fold structure and function while providing magnification of the laryngeal structures and excellent resolution for greater observation of mucosal changes, but they offer a narrow range of applications. With the increasing use of videostroboscopy in the assessment of vocal fold structure and function, rigid endoscopes are now an indispensable adjunct for laryngeal surgery. Although flexible endoscopes are useful in monitoring laryngeal surgery (5) and injection laryngoplasty (6), the rigid endoscope has superior optics. Rigid endoscopy is sufficiently versatile to allow a variety of procedures to be performed under videoendoscopic observation (7).

## ADVANTAGES AND LIMITATIONS OF ENDOSCOPIC VOCAL FOLD AUGMENTATION

Endoscopes are useful for providing exposure when direct laryngoscopy and indirect mirror laryngoscopy prove insufficient. Transnasal fiberoptic laryngoscopy affords visualiza-

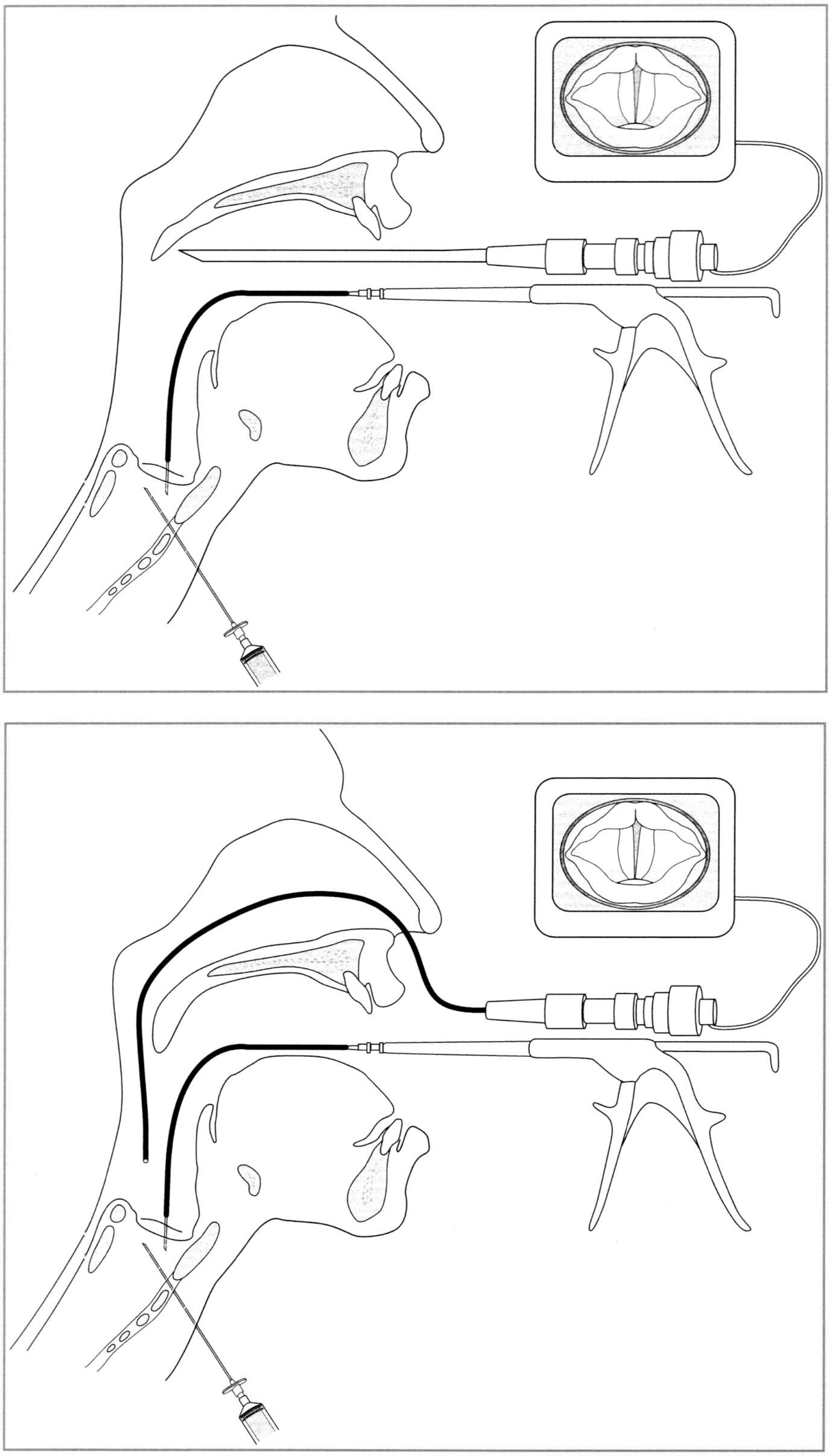

A

B

**FIGURE 42.1.** Four approaches to endoscopic injection of vocal folds for augmentation. **A:** The rigid endoscope is being used to monitor injection by transoral or cervical transcutaneous injection. **B:** The flexible endoscope is shown with the same two injection approaches.

**TABLE 42.1. ADVANTAGES AND LIMITATIONS OF FOUR APPROACHES TO ENDOSCOPIC VOCAL FOLD AUGMENTATION**

| Approach | Clarity on Magnification | Precision Placement | Anatomic Variations | | Patient with Strong Gag Reflex |
|---|---|---|---|---|---|
| | | | Larynx | Neck | |
| RIGID, PO | +++ | +++ | – | ++ | – |
| RIGID, TC | ++ | + | + | – | + |
| FLEX, PO | + | + | + | ++ | + |
| FLEX, TC | + | + | ++ | – | ++ |

PO, Per oral; TC, transcutaneous; Rigid, rigid endoscopic guidance; Flex, flexible nasolaryngoscopic guidance; +, favorable approach; –, unfavorable.

tion of the larynx in patients who have difficulty extending their necks, hyperactive gag reflexes, and various anatomic anomalies that preclude an adequate view of the larynx using per oral methods, such as patients with an omega-shaped epiglottis, prominent tongue-base, or supraglottic stenosis.

Rigid endoscopy is particularly useful where a clear magnified image is important such as in the slightly bowed vocal fold or one in which there is a focal defect. In these instances, the augmentation material to be injected can be placed with great precision, and the effects may be appreciated immediately.

Rigid (Fig. 42.1A) or flexible (Fig. 42.1B) instruments can be used for vocal fold augmentation, with the injection needle being passed transorally or percutaneously. There are four technical options for endoscopic vocal fold augmentation: rigid endoscopy for transorally guided peroral injection; flexible endoscopy for transnasally guided peroral injection; rigid endoscopy for transorally guided percutaneous injection; and flexible endoscopy for transnasally guided percutaneous injection. The percutaneous injection approach is useful in patients who present difficult exposure problems, such as patients with severe rheumatoid arthritis. All of these endoscopic approaches are usually preferable to direct microlaryngoscopic approaches in offering greater flexibility, less morbidity, and avoidance of general anesthesia. We think the rigid endoscopically guided transoral approach appears to be the most useful option (Table 42.1).

## INDICATIONS AND GOALS OF VOCAL FOLD AUGMENTATION

The most common goal of vocal fold augmentation injection is to resolve glottic insufficiency and restore more normal vocal fold oscillation to improve the voice. Restoration of glottic competence improves airway protection and swallowing, and it reduces aspiration. The medial edge of the affected vocal fold must be displaced medially with the augmentation injection. A smooth, free edge is the goal, and this should be along the length of the membranous vocal fold. Displacement should be in the vertical plane of the contralateral vocal fold. Failure to accomplish this can result in the illusion of closure when viewed from above, but aerodynamic and voice quality measures are suboptimal.

Excessive injection in the subglottis, supraglottis, or laryngeal ventricle can cause voice distortion and simultaneously fail to achieve effective glottic closure. Overcorrection anteriorly stiffens the injected side, compromises oscillation of the contralateral vocal fold, and exaggerates posterior glottic insufficiency. Because of this potential complication, a useful principle is to avoid overcorrecting the anterior third of the vocal fold.

## ANESTHESIA

With appropriate anesthesia, patients should not experience discomfort during vocal fold augmentation procedures. Any patient who can tolerate indirect laryngoscopy or endoscopic examination of the larynx should be considered a suitable candidate for awake, in-office vocal fold injection augmentation. The oral cavity and laryngopharynx can be anesthetized with topical 4% lidocaine (8). After spraying the oral cavity, the anesthetic solution is dripped on the tongue base, laryngeal surface of the epiglottis, and then the supraglottic larynx (Fig. 42.2), where it is allowed to run down onto the true vocal folds and distributed further by phonation—the vowel *e* works well. This is best done incrementally in three or four steps over 3 to 5 minutes. At each step, approximately 0.3 mL is dripped onto the mucosal surfaces of the larynx, resulting in a total of no more than 1.2 mL of 4% lidocaine for adequate topical anesthesia. In the event that a percutaneous approach is planned, it is not necessary to anesthetize the endolarynx. It may enhance patient comfort to inject a small amount of 1% lidocaine into the skin where the injection needle will be inserted. This step does not interfere with identification of landmarks or the augmentation injection.

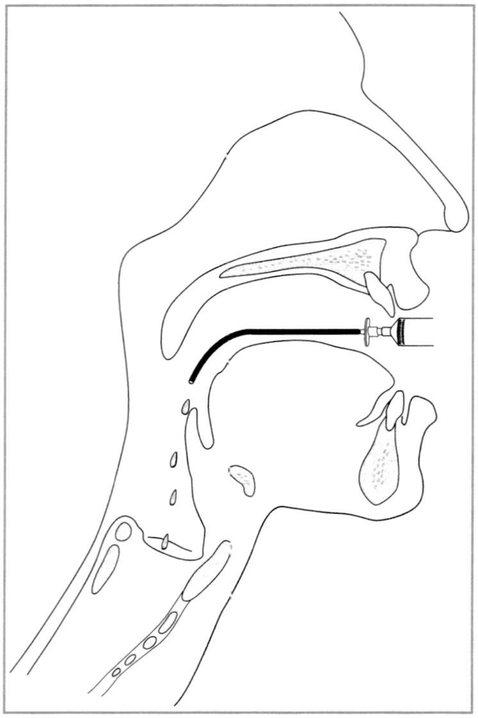

**FIGURE 42.2.** Topical anesthesia is rendered by dripping 4% lidocaine onto the mucosal surfaces of the tongue base, supraglottis, and true vocal folds. This activity can be monitored with a laryngeal mirror or either of the endoscopes shown in Figure 42.1.

## INSTRUMENTATION

For all transoral injections, it is necessary to use a curved-needle delivery device that follows the contour of the oropharyngeal cavity. Examples include the Bruening injector (Storz, St. Louis, MO) and the Laryngeal Injector (Xomed-Treace, Jacksonville, FL). For thicker injection materials, such as polytef (Teflon) or fat, the Bruening injector with its 19-gauge needle is appropriate. For other substances, such as botulinum toxin, collagen, and steroids, the Xomed-Treace orotracheal or laryngeal injector with its disposable 27-gauge needle is preferred (9). Prototypes of modified fiberoptic laryngoscopes have been used with needles attached to a delivery port for injecting vocal folds, and this is a possible alternative. Transcutaneous injections can be performed with any appropriately long needle while the endoscope is used to monitor placement of the needle and displacement of the vocal fold edge during injection.

## OPERATIVE TECHNIQUE

### Injection of Alloplastic Materials

Several alloplastic materials are available for injection laryngoplasty, including silicone, Bioplastique, and polytef paste. The latter has been maligned because of complications related to induced foreign body granuloma formation and migration, but it remains a useful material for injection augmentation in the elderly, infirm, or terminally ill patient with symptomatic glottic insufficiency due to vocal fold paralysis. It should not be injected into a mobile vocal fold.

Injection of polytef requires precise placement the first time because it is difficult to redistribute after it is injected. The goal is to place the material deep in the thyroarytenoid muscle and in the plane of the contralateral vocal fold (Fig. 42.3). Most practitioners have shunned the indirect laryngoscopic method of monitoring injections because of the coordination difficulty and limited visualization. With fiberoptic endoscopes, the technique still requires good hand-eye coordination to perform in the awake patient, but

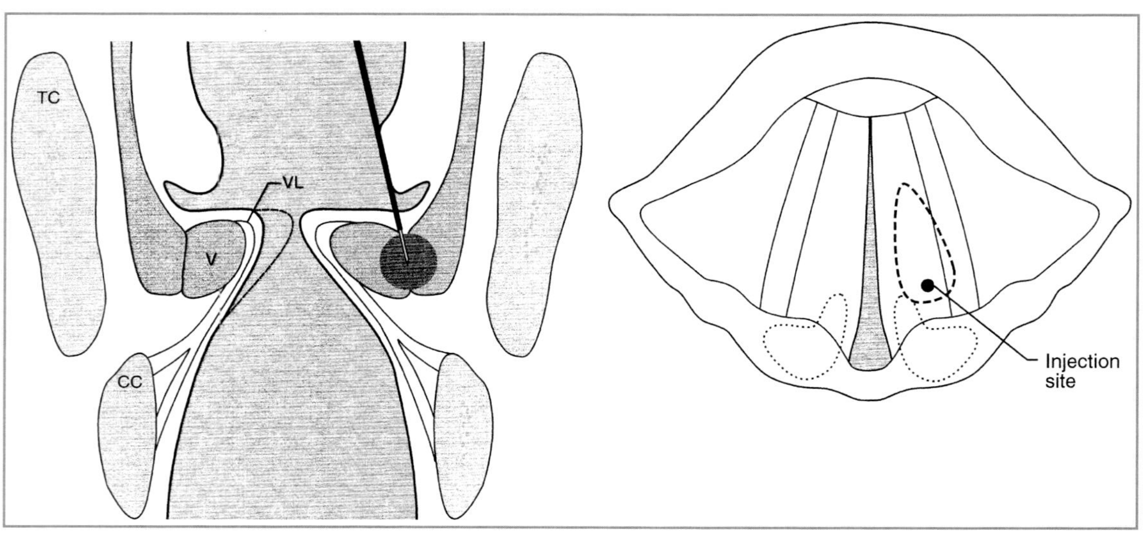


**FIGURE 42.3.** This diagram shows the preferred site for injecting substances such as Teflon (polytef paste) to achieve medialization of the vocal process of the arytenoid and augmentation of the vocal fold. The importance of the proper plane for injection is demonstrated in the coronal view. *TC,* thyroid cartilage; *VL,* vocal ligament; *V,* vocalis m.; *TA,* thyroid muscle; *CC,* cricoid cartilage.

visualization can be excellent for the surgeon and surgeons being trained to perform the technique.

***Step 1:*** The larynx is topically anesthetized, and the curved injector device is positioned to allow the needle to be inserted laterally in the thyroarytenoid muscle.

***Step 2:*** The level of injection is carefully set to correspond to the plane of the contralateral vocal fold.

***Step 3:*** The initial injection is usually just anterior and lateral to the tip of the vocal process of the arytenoid (Fig. 42.3). As the material is injected, the vocal fold edge is carefully monitored to ensure that there is displacement in the desired location.

***Step 4:*** If there is residual bowing or gaping of the midmembranous fold, an additional aliquot of material is injected there. Filling the anterior one third should be avoided.

***Step 5:*** If material is inadvertently injected subglottically or unevenly, it is possible to redistribute the injected material by rubbing the mucosal edge with the side of the injector needle or hub. It is best to underinject the tissue, test the voice, and then inject more as needed.

***Step 6:*** When in doubt, a stroboscopic examination can help to determine the effect of the injection on vocal fold vibration. Follow-up voice assessment should include videostroboscopic examination of the larynx to assess the effect of medialization on vocal fold oscillation and residual glottic configuration.

### Injection of Bioimplants

Bioimplants include collagen, fat, and fascia. There are various techniques described for injecting these materials, some of which are discussed in Chapter 43. Percutaneous injection technique is useful in patients with a strong gag reflex or those unable to extend their necks or open their mouths fully. This approach sometimes lacks precision because the needle is not directly observed, but its submucosal position is estimated by observing vocal fold displacement.

In most instances, collagen is injected into the superficial lamina propria (10,11), and fat is injected deeply and distributed through the entire vocal fold. The use of magnified rigid endoscopy with transoral injection is particularly valuable when a collagen is being used to treat adynamic segments (12). It is best to avoid placing the material too far anteriorly in the subglottic plane; in the event of inadvertent placements, it is possible to redistribute the injected material by gentle massage of the tissues with the edge of the injector device.

## POSTOPERATIVE ASSESSMENT AND FOLLOW-UP

The key to improving results is careful assessment and monitoring of results. Stroboscopic analysis of vibratory characteristics of each vocal fold and assessment of variation of vibration for different portions of the vocal fold are most useful for assessing postoperative results. Videostroboscopy is particularly useful in identifying focal adynamic areas that may not be seen with the naked eye (13). Stroboscopic evaluation of glottic closure and vibratory activity during the augmentation procedure is an application useful in refining technique and gaining optimal voice results.

## HIGHLIGHTS

- The use of endoscopes facilitates injection augmentation of vocal folds by improving visualization and precision of injection.
- Endoscopy is particularly useful for teaching residents and others learning the procedures, and it affords the patient an opportunity to see the procedure in real time and postoperatively.
- There are four endoscopic variations for injection augmentation: rigid endoscopy with transoral or transcutaneous injection and flexible fiberoptic endoscopy with transoral or transcutaneous injection. In a cooperative patient with normal anatomy, we prefer the rigid, transoral approach to injection augmentation. The use of stroboscopy allows a higher level of subtle optimization that should enhance results and facilitate surgeons in improving their technique.

## REFERENCES


1. Davidson TM, Bone RC, Nahum AM. Flexible fiberoptic laryngobronchoscopy. *Laryngoscope* 1974;84:1876–1882.
2. Dellon AL, Clifford AH, Chretien DB. Fiberoptic endoscopy in the head and neck region. *Plast Reconstr Surg* 1975;55:466–471.
3. Williams GT, Farquharson IM, Anthony J. Fiberoptic laryngoscopy in the assessment of laryngeal disorders. *J Laryngol Otol* 1975;89:299–316.
4. Silberman HD, Wilf H, Tucker JA. Flexible fiberoptic nasopharyngolaryngoscope. *Annals Otol Rhinol Laryngol* 1976;85:640–645.
5. Tai S, Chu P, Chang S. Transoral laryngeal surgery under flexible laryngovideostroboscopy. *J Voice* 1998;12:223–238.
6. Chu P, Chang S. Transoral Teflon injection under flexible laryngovideostroboscopy for unilateral vocal fold paralysis. *Ann Otol Rhinol Laryngol* 1997;106:783–786.
7. Ford CN, Roy N, Sandage M, et al. Rigid endoscopy for monitoring indirect vocal fold injection. *Laryngoscope* 1998;108:1584–1586.
8. Ford CN. Vocal cord injection for paralysis. In: Bailey BJ, Cal-

houn KH, Coffey AR, et al., eds. *Atlas of head and neck surgery–otolaryngology.* Philadelphia: Lippincott-Raven, 1996: 604–605.

9. Ford CN. A multipurpose laryngeal injector device. *Otolaryngol Head Neck Surg* 1990;103:135–137.
10. Ford CN, Bless DM. Clinical experience with injectable collagen for vocal fold augmentation. *Laryngoscope* 1986;96:863–869.
11. Ford CN, Bless DM, Loftus JM. Role of injectable collagen in the treatment of glottic insufficiency: a study of 119 patients. *Ann Otol Rhinol Laryngol* 1992;101:237–247.
12. Ford CN, Bless DM. Collagen injection in the scarred vocal fold. *J Voice* 1987;12:116–118.
13. Bless DM, Hirano M, Feder RJ. Videostroboscopic evaluation of the larynx. *Ear Nose Throat J* 1987;66:289–296.

43

# ENDOSCOPIC VOCAL FOLD AUGMENTATION

MILAN R. AMIN
GREGORY N. POSTMA
JAMES A. KOUFMAN

The concept of vocal fold augmentation by endoscopic injection technique was first described by Brunings in 1911 (1). Using a specially designed needle and syringe, he was able to improve glottal closure by injecting paraffin into the vocal fold. Unfortunately, the paraffin produced a brisk inflammatory reaction, and this technique did not become popular. Since Brunings' original description, many other substances have been used for injection augmentation of the vocal fold. One of the first to gain widespread acceptance was polytef (Teflon). Arnold (2) pioneered the use of this substance in the larynx, and it steadily gained popularity because of its ease of use. Although still in use today, polytef has largely been replaced by other substances because of its propensity for causing vocal fold stiffness and granuloma formation. Other substances that have been injected into the vocal folds include glycerine, sesame oil, cartilage paste, bone paste, silicone, Gelfoam, fat, collagen, and fascia. Of these, the latter four are the focus of this chapter because they are the most commonly used today.

## INDICATIONS AND CONTRAINDICATIONS

As an alternative to laryngoplastic surgery, vocal fold injection augmentation is used to treat many forms of glottal incompetence (Table 43.1). Glottal incompetence produces glottal closure symptoms such as breathy dysphonia, aphonia, vocal fatigue, effortful phonation, voice breaks, and even odynophonia (i.e., painful speaking). The most frequent clinical situations in which this technique is useful include unilateral vocal fold paralysis and unilateral or bilateral vocal fold paresis. Paralysis or paresis may be temporary or permanent; determination of prognosis often dictates the type of injectable material used.

Injection augmentation is also indicated for treatment of vocal fold atrophy and bowing (e.g., presbylaryngia). Such patients require bilateral injection augmentation to provide enough soft tissue bulk to allow vocal fold approximation for phonation. If atrophy is progressive, multiple injections may be necessary over a period of years to maintain optimal voice results.

Vocal fold injection may also be useful in certain situations to fill defects in the lamina propria layer caused by scarring or tissue loss. The results for this indication, however, have been relatively poor, although there is some evidence that collagen may soften scars (3).

Dysphonia resulting from certain movement disorders may also improve with the use of injection augmentation. Variable to poor results are seen in patients with parkinsonism (4). We have used this procedure in some patients with abductor-type spasmodic dysphonia, with excellent results in some cases.

In the pediatric population, injection augmentation (usually lipoinjection) has been successfully used to treat unilateral vocal fold paralysis. This technique is reserved for children with severe dysphonia and a large glottal gap (5,6).

Vocal fold augmentation is contraindicated in the patient with a marginal airway secondary to bilateral vocal fold immobility. The procedure may narrow the glottic airway and potentiate respiratory embarrassment. Because the injection augmentation is not easily or quickly reversible, care must be taken not to use this technique in patients who are at high risk for developing contralateral vocal fold paresis or paralysis (e.g., patients with bilateral head and neck chemodectomas).

Relative contraindications to injection augmentation include patients with amyotrophic lateral sclerosis, stroke, or cricoarytenoid joint fixation (with a wide posterior chink). It must be emphasized that the open posterior larynx cannot be closed by injection augmentation or by medialization laryngoplasty; only arytenoid adduction effectively closes the posterior larynx.

**TABLE 43.1. INDICATIONS AND CONTRAINDICATIONS FOR ENDOSCOPIC INJECTION AUGMENTATION**

| Indications | Relative Contraindications | Absolute Contraindications |
|---|---|---|
| Mild to moderate vocal fold atrophy (e.g., presbylaryngis)<br>Unilateral or bilateral vocal fold paresis<br>Unilateral vocal fold paralysis (when the posterior larynx is not open)<br>Soft tissue deficiency as a result of previous trauma<br>Soft tissue deficiency following irradiation for vocal fold carcinoma<br>Vocal fold scarring<br>Abductor-type spasmodic dysphonia (selected cases)<br>Vocal fold bowing due to Parkinson's disease (selected cases) | Unilateral paralysis with a wide-open posterior glottis (i.e., cadaveric position)<br>Arytenoid fixation with an open posterior larynx<br>Global neurologic laryngopharyngeal deficits (e.g., stroke, amyotrophic lateral sclerosis) | Bilateral vocal fold hypomobility with a narrow posterior glottal chink<br>Any marginal airway caused by any coexistent condition |

## PREOPERATIVE EVALUATION

In the assessment of candidates for vocal fold injection augmentation, it is important to define the cause of the glottal insufficiency. Correct diagnosis allows the physician to customize treatment for optimal results. In the patient with unilateral vocal fold immobility, it is essential to differentiate vocal fold paralysis from fixation. Fixation often results in a poor outcome, and paralysis is more treatable by vocal fold augmentation. Laryngeal electromyography (LEMG) is often helpful in distinguishing paralysis from fixation (7,8). LEMG may provide prognostic information that may be helpful in determining the type of injectable material to use. Preoperative videostroboscopy is routinely recommended, as well as acoustical analysis and counseling by a speech-language pathologist.

Other factors that are important to assess before surgery include vocal fold vibratory function, abnormal supraglottic compensatory vocal behaviors, and the status of the contralateral vocal fold. The contralateral vocal fold should be evaluated carefully to assess function and bulk. Undiagnosed paresis or bowing of the contralateral vocal fold may result in inadequate glottal closure despite optimal augmentation of the ipsilateral side. When the contralateral vocal fold is found to be weak or atrophic, bilateral vocal fold injection augmentation should be performed.

Another important consideration is the timing of the surgery. In patients with dysphagia and aspiration, the decision is simple—there should be little or no delay. Similarly, in patients with dysphonia from long-standing paralysis or paresis or in patients with presbylaryngis or other forms of atrophy, surgery may proceed as dictated by the patient's symptoms and vocal needs.

The difficulty is in deciding what to do in patients with paralysis or paresis of relatively recent onset or undetermined cause. In these circumstances, LEMG may be helpful in determining the prognosis. When electromyography is equivocal or indefinite, clinical judgment should be used in forming the treatment plan. If it is strongly suspected that function will return, the clinician may choose to use an injection substance that has a relatively high rate of resorption.

## SELECTION OF APPROPRIATE IMPLANT MATERIAL

During the preoperative evaluation, a decision is made regarding the choice of injected material. Table 43.2 shows the characteristics, properties, and uses of commonly employed injection augmentation substances. Although there are specific reasons to use particular substances in certain instances, the decision often is based on personal experience and preference of the surgeon. The most commonly employed injection augmentation material at our institution continues to be autologous fat. Autologous fat has been used for more than 100 years as a graft material (9) and has a proven record of reliability. Because of its ease of harvest, there is little associated morbidity. The only major disadvantage is the relatively unpredictable rate of resorption. This problem can, however, be overcome by overcorrecting defects or by repeat injections. In our hands, the estimated rate of long-term fat graft survival is about 40%.

Bovine collagen has been used extensively (10). Two different forms have been investigated: soluble bovine collagen and glutaraldehyde cross-linked collagen (GAX collagen). The potential advantage of these substances is that they do not need to be harvested, and therefore injections can be done more easily in the office setting. However, there

**TABLE 43.2. CHARACTERISTICS, PROPERTIES, AND USES OF COMMONLY EMPLOYED INJECTION AUGMENTATION SUBSTANCES**

| Property | Teflon | Collagen | Gelfoam | Fat | Fascia |
|---|---|---|---|---|---|
| Tissue consistency (match with vocal fold) | Poor | Good | Fair | Excellent | Poor |
| Reversibility | No | Yes | Yes | Yes | Yes |
| Potential antigenicity | Yes | Yes | Yes | No | No |
| In-office use | Yes | Yes | Yes | No | No |
| Recommended for unilat. paralysis | Rarely | Yes | Rarely | Yes | Yes |
| Recommended for small glottal gaps | No | Yes | No | Yes | Yes |
| Recommended for pediatric uses | No | Yes | Yes | Yes | No |
| Estimated long-term graft yield (%) | 100% | 20% | 0% | 50% | 40% |
| May be used at the free edge of the vocal fold | No | Yes | No | No | No |
| May be used in a mobile vocal fold | No | Yes | Yes | Yes | Yes |

remains a concern about the potential for inciting an immunologic reaction to the injected foreign material. To reduce this possibility, patients are skin tested before injection, but this does not eliminate the risk completely. In response to these concerns, a method of injecting *autologous* collagen was developed. This involves the harvest of a large piece of skin (30 cm$^2$), which is processed at an outside laboratory and returned in 8 weeks. At this time, the substance can be injected in the office setting. The obvious disadvantages are cost, the time delay involved in the processing, and the rather large piece of skin that is harvested.

As an alternative to these methods, there has been interest in injecting autologous fascia (11). Although somewhat burdensome to harvest and process in the operating room, the preliminary results have been encouraging (12).

Two substances that can be used in specific circumstances are polytef and Gelfoam. Polytef injected into the vocal folds can lead to long-term complications. However, it does have some advantages. It is easy to use, it is biocompatible in the short term, and there is no need to harvest. Polytef is indicated for use in patients who have multiple comorbidities or are terminally ill. In this setting, vocal fold augmentation can provide an immediate improvement in quality of life without taking the patient to the operating room. Polytef should never be injected into a mobile vocal fold.

Gelfoam was originally developed as a hemostatic material. Because of its record of biocompatibility, its use has been expanded. It is widely used as an absorbable implant in otology. Gelfoam was first used as an injectable material into the vocal folds in the late 1970s (13). Through continued use, it has been found that the augmentation provided by Gelfoam is temporary because the body absorbs the material. Because of this attribute, Gelfoam has been used as a temporizing measure, primarily in patients that are expected to regain vocal fold motion. Unfortunately, multiple injections may be necessary, because Gelfoam is usually absorbed within 2 to 8 weeks, and return of vocal fold function may take many months.

## INSTRUMENTATION

- Towel clips
- Tissue forceps (DeBakey and Adson)
- Liposuction cannulas (small and large) with handles
- Suction tubing with specimen trap
- Berkley VC-2 vacuum curettage system (cat. no. 6OHZ, Cabot Medical Corp., Langhorne, PA)
- Knife handles with no. 15 blades
- Retractors (Army-Navy, Richardson, and Weitlaner)
- Scissors (suture, tenotomy, and Metzenbaum)
- Needle holders (regular and Webster)
- Curved hemostats (regular and mosquito)
- Freer elevator
- Surgical microscope with a 400-mm lens
- Centra-CL2 centrifuge (cat. no. 42603159, International Equipment Company, Needham, MA)
- Test tubes
- Cutting block (metal or Teflon)
- Brunings syringe (cat. no. N7754, Karl Storz, Culver City, CA)
- Arnold-Bruening disposable, 19-gauge laryngeal needles (cat. no. N7757, Karl Storz, Culver City, CA)
- Laryngoscopes (Jako and Dedo) (cat. nos. 52-2200 and 52-2225, Pilling Surgical, Ft. Washington, PA)
- Suspension apparatus (Lewy arm or Boston University suspension) (cat. nos. 50-2248 and 50-2260, Pilling Surgical, Ft. Washington, PA)

For collagen, Gelfoam, or polytef injections performed in the office, the instrumentation required is much more limited. Depending on the choice of injection technique (transoral or transcervical), the surgeon requires a curved or straight Brunings syringe and a flexible fiberoptic or rigid 70° laryngoscope connected to a video monitor.

## OPERATING ROOM LAYOUT

The operating room layout for fat or fascia injection augmentation is similar to that for any microlaryngeal surgical procedure. The operating table is rotated 90° so that the surgeon has access to the airway. The microscope is positioned near the head of the patient, and the instrument table is positioned at foot, allowing room for the surgeon to harvest the fat.

Patients undergoing collagen, Gelfoam, or polytef augmentation are typically injected in the office setting. In these cases, the patient is seated in an examination chair, with a flexible fiberoptic laryngoscope passed transnasally. The video display unit is positioned to the side or behind the patient so the surgeon can watch the monitor while performing the procedure. Instruments are placed beside the surgeon.

## ANESTHESIA

Patients undergoing fat or fascia injection in the operating room typically require a general anesthetic. The patient must be paralyzed during the exposure of the larynx and injection of the vocal folds. Local anesthesia may be used for this procedure, but it is not our preference.

There is considerable variation in the type of airway used during this procedure. Our preference is to intubate the patient during the harvest of the fat. After the fat has been processed and placed in the syringe, the patient's larynx is exposed using a laryngoscope, and the endotracheal tube is removed. The patient is then ventilated using the Venturi jet technique (14). This allows unobstructed visualization of the vocal folds.

For patients undergoing injection augmentation in the office, there is a choice of anesthetic, depending on the type of injection planned. Transoral injection requires topical application of anesthetic solution (typically lidocaine) to the oral cavity, pharynx, and larynx. Anesthetic is usually delivered to the larynx from above using a curved applicator. Superior laryngeal nerve blocks may also be used. Patients undergoing percutaneous injection augmentation receive injectable lidocaine into the skin and subcutaneous tissues.

## OPERATIVE TECHNIQUE

### Injection Augmentation Techniques

Before surgery, patients receive intravenous dexamethasone, glycopyrrolate, and a systemic antibiotic. Patients are intubated by the surgeon using a small endotracheal tube (typically 4.0 to 5.5 mm internal diameter) before graft harvest. After graft preparation, the patient is placed in the standard position for direct laryngoscopy. The largest-bore laryngoscope is used to visualize the larynx.. The laryngoscope is inserted in such a way as to reflect the false vocal folds. The endotracheal tube is removed, and ventilation is performed using jet ventilation. An operating microscope fitted with a 400-mm lens is brought into position.

The Brunings syringe is used, and the injection is performed lateral to the vocal process in the plane of the glottis into the lateral aspect of the thyroarytenoid muscle. A disposable 19-gauge needle is employed. Occasionally, a second injection may be required in the anterior or midportion of the membranous vocal fold (Fig. 43.1). The vocal folds are always overcorrected by 100%—double the anticipated volume that is needed. Even when doing bilateral injections, significant airway compromise does not occur. If there appears to be any fat graft extrusion, the $CO_2$ laser is used to spot weld the injection hole shut. This is done by defocusing the beam at 2 to 4 W of power to seal the injection site. Lidocaine is then sprayed over the glottis to decrease the chance for laryngospasm, and the laryngoscope is removed. The patient is ventilated by mask and awakened.

Another technique using direct laryngoscopy is the use of a rigid telescope through the laryngoscope. This is particularly useful when performing direct laryngoscopy under local anesthesia with sedation (15). With this technique, a slotted laryngoscope is used. After exposure is attained, the assistant inserts a 0° endoscope, and the glottis is visualized on the television monitor. The surgeon then uses the Brunings syringe to perform the injection.

Advantages of using suspension laryngoscopy under general anesthesia are the outstanding visualization and the ease

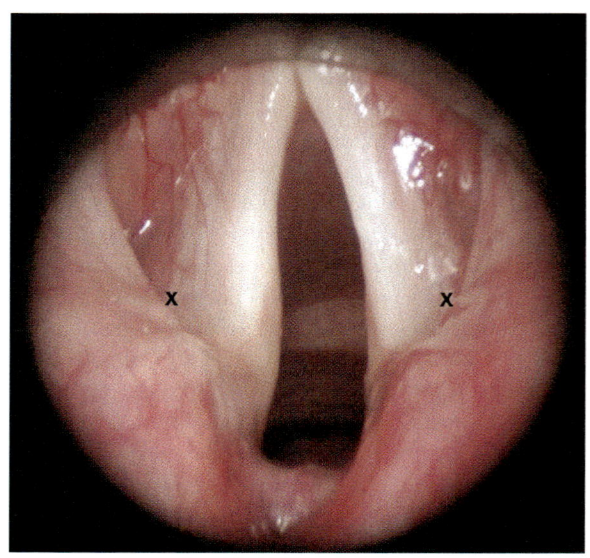


**FIGURE 43.1.** Vocal folds with marks showing ideal locations for injections *(x)*.

of injection. The disadvantage is the inability to directly monitor voice changes during the injection. This does not appear to be important with fat, Gelfoam, or fascia injections because they are routinely overcorrected.

In-office techniques performed with flexible laryngoscope are quite valuable. These injections may be done transorally or percutaneously. The transoral injection of vocal folds with polytef, Gelfoam, or collagen has been well described elsewhere (16,17). It has been our preference in the clinic to use percutaneous injections. Transnasal fiberoptic laryngoscopy is performed, and the injection procedure is observed on the monitor. A straight, 19-gauge needle attached to a Brunings syringe can then be inserted through the cricothyroid membrane and into the vocal fold from below. An incremental injection can then be performed while the patient is asked to phonate. The needle should be directed into the lateral portion of the thyroarytenoid muscle.

Collagen injections require a slightly different technique. It has been demonstrated that the absorption of collagen depends on its placement; the more superficially it is located, the longer the collagen seems to persist (18). Collagen injection is typically directed into the deep layer of the lamina propria (i.e., vocal ligament), where the greatest amount of dense collagen resides (16).

## Technique of Autologous Fat Harvest

For fat graft harvest, we usually employ the right lower quadrant of the abdomen. After sterile preparation, a local anesthetic with epinephrine for hemostasis is injected into

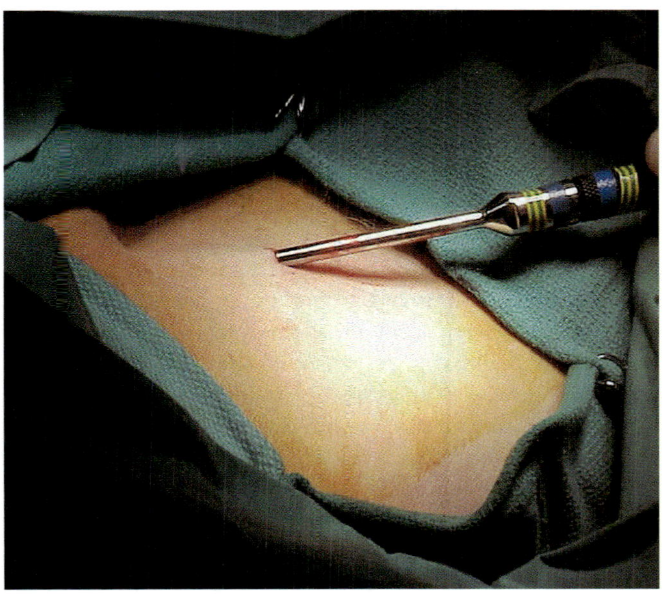

**FIGURE 43.2.** Liposuction procedure used to harvest fat for autologous fat augmentation.

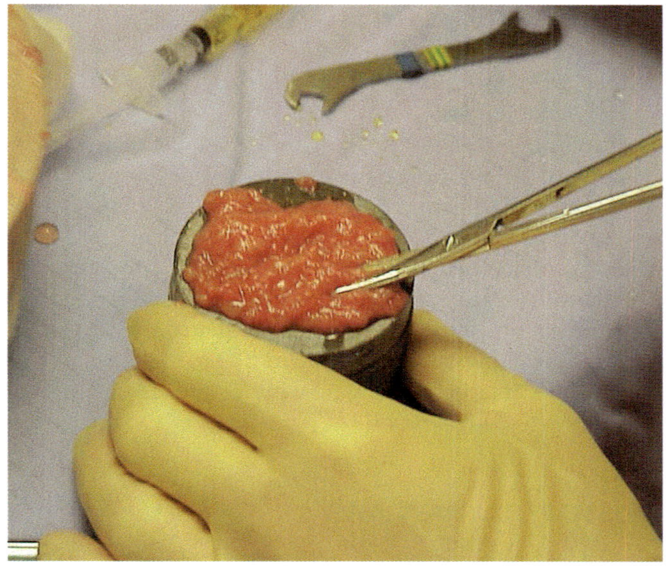

**FIGURE 43.3.** Chopping of fat with scissors.

the subcutaneous tissue. A 15.6-gauge liposuction cannula is used to remove 15 mL of fat through a stab incision (Fig. 43.2). We employ an abortion suction device for this because of the high vacuum pressures generated. Next, the fat is placed into the patient's own serum (obtained by centrifugation of 20 mL of blood). The fat-serum mixture is then centrifuged at 10,000 rpm for 10 minutes. After centrifugation, two layers are seen. The lower layer of serum and cellular debris is discarded. The top layer is the fat graft; it is placed into a Brunings syringe with a 19-gauge needle for injection.

As an alternative in very thin patients, the fat may be excised, gently minced using scissors, and then repeatedly irrigated with normal saline through mesh gauze to remove any blood, fatty acids, muscle fragments, or debris (Fig. 43.3). It is then centrifuged as previously described. The fat graft is then placed into the barrel of the syringe using a Freer elevator.

## Technique of Autologous Fascia Harvest

The patient's right leg is sterilely prepped and draped. Local anesthetic is injected in a longitudinal area approximately 4 cm below the greater trochanter of the hip and just anterior to the iliotibial tract. A 3- to 5-cm skin incision is made. This exposes the subcutaneous fat, which is harvested and set aside. Further dissection reveals the fascia lata. Using fine scissors, this layer is elevated off the muscle, and a 3 × 4 cm, oval portion of the fascia is excised. The fascia is then minced with scissors and mixed with serum to facilitate a smooth injection. It is then loaded into the Brunings syringe, followed by the fat. The fat serves to fill the remainder of the volume of the syringe. The wound is closed in layers, followed by the application of a pressure dressing.

## HIGHLIGHTS

- The selection of implant material determines the injection technique.
- Injection with fat or fascia typically is done in the operating room, with the patient under a general anesthetic.
- Collagen, Gelfoam, and polytef are typically injected in the office setting.
- Fat is harvested with liposuction and processed to remove free fatty acids, triglycerides, and cellular debris.
- Fascia is processed into a pastelike material and placed into a Brunings syringe, followed by fat.
- It is important to overcorrect with fat and fascia, because there is some resorption.

## POSTOPERATIVE CARE

After awakening the patient, we routinely place her or him on absolute voice rest for 48 hours. Patients are treated empirically with antireflux medication for at least 2 weeks, and antitussives are used as needed. Steroids and antibiotics are not routinely given after surgery. Routine postoperative care includes humidified oxygen in the initial period after surgery. Beginning 48 to 72 hours after surgery, the patient is allowed to speak in an unforced manner. Patients are told to avoid whispering, singing, or yelling for 4 to 6 weeks. Individuals undergoing unilateral vocal fold injections are discharged within a few hours of surgery, and those undergoing bilateral injections are usually observed overnight.

## COMPLICATIONS

For patients undergoing fat or fascia injection, potential problems may arise from hematoma formation or infection at the harvest site; this is rare. Because it is necessary to overinject the vocal folds, there is a theoretical risk of causing airway obstruction with bilateral injections. This has not occurred in our experience with more than 200 bilateral injections. There is generally minimal immediate risk with injection augmentation performed in the office. As covered elsewhere in this chapter, there are potential risks associated with specific injectable materials.

## ADVANTAGES AND LIMITATIONS OF THE ENDOSCOPIC TECHNIQUE

The advantages and limitations of these techniques depend on the method of injection used. Injection of fat or fascia typically requires a general anesthetic, which may be undesirable in some patients. However, in patients who cannot tolerate a procedure done under a local anesthetic (e.g., children), this may be an advantage. Another advantage is its technical ease when compared with the open technique of medialization laryngoplasty. Limitations of the specific injectable substances are highlighted in Table 43.2.

## LITERATURE REVIEW

Although several materials are used routinely for injection augmentation, there is relatively little literature directly comparing them. The most extensively studied injectable material is fat. The first description of its use in the human larynx appeared in 1991 (19). This was a rather modest report of three cases for which the investigators only had limited follow-up. In 1992, Brandenburg and colleagues (20) reported a series of 12 patients who underwent lipoinjection. All patients were reported to show marked improvement, with a follow-up ranging from 5 to 42 months. One patient required a repeat injection at 24 months for subsequent voice deterioration. In a larger study of 22 patients with a minimum 1-year follow-up, Shaw and coworkers (21) found statistically significant enhancement in most parameters tested (i.e., subjective and objective voice measures), with a persistence of improvement at 6 and 12 months. Other reports have demonstrated less impressive results. Shindo and associates (22) found that, despite excellent initial results, there was significant deterioration in the voice because of fat resorption over a period of 1 year. They were able to demonstrate this decrement on magnetic resonance imaging in seven patients.

Animal studies have similarly indicated that there is a significant rate of resorption when fat is injected into the vocal folds. Mikus and colleagues (23) reported fat survival rates of only 20% in dogs at 12 weeks. Zaretsky and coworkers (24) observed a decrease in the bulk of surviving fat between dog larynges examined 3 and 6 months after injection, although they did not quantify the results. In the longest follow-up animal study, Saccogna and associates (25) demonstrated that there was a significant drop-off of fat graft survival in cat larynges between 8 and 12 months.

It is uncertain whether this animal data is applicable to humans, who have a different histologic organization of the vocal fold. It is unclear whether fat is resorbed or replaced *in situ* by another material. There is some indication that, despite the loss of fat cells, there is a less significant loss of volume from a replacement of the injected fat by fibrosis (26). This could explain many of the conflicting results obtained clinically versus histologically.

Another controversy concerns the optimal method for harvesting and processing of the fat graft. Different methods have been reported, with none demonstrating clear superiority. Few controlled studies have been done comparing different methods directly, and only one focused on the larynx. Mikus and colleagues (23) compared liposuctioned fat injected without processing and traditionally excised fat processed by morselization and centrifugation. Significantly better graft take was found with the liposuctioned fat. Studies of fat transplantation in other sites in the human body have demonstrated variable results in long-term graft survival with a host of different techniques (27–30). Using the method of graft preparation (herein presented) in a canine model, Duke and colleagues (12) reported a mean long-term fat graft yield of 60%, with a range of 20% to 90%.

Collagen has also been extensively investigated. The first use of injected collagen in human larynges was reported by Ford and Bless (31) in the mid-1980s in the form of soluble bovine collagen. Many patients have been injected with this substance, with improvement in various outcomes (10). Patients undergoing bovine collagen injection are required to have a skin test before augmentation to ensure tolerance of the foreign material. Skin testing delays treatment by at least 4 weeks.

Relatively few patients have demonstrated positive skin tests (10). However, skin tests may not adequately predict long-term tolerance, and there is still some concern about injecting this substance. In response to this concern, a less antigenic form of bovine collagen was developed—GAX collagen. GAX collagen has essentially replaced soluble bovine collagen because of its better tissue tolerance and reportedly better long-term persistence (10,32,33). Despite the low incidence risk of clinical problems in humans, animal and human studies demonstrate a potential for the production of antibodies (34,35).

As an alternative, an injectable form of autologous collagen was developed. Preliminary studies of this substance have demonstrated good tissue tolerance in humans (36,37). However, histologic evaluation in canine vocal folds in one study has demonstrated an inflammatory reaction, with overlying ulceration of the vocal fold at 3 and 6 months (38). This was believed to result from improper processing, with inclusion of hair follicles in the preparation.

The persistence of collagen injected into the vocal folds has not been well studied, although clinical measures in patients injected with collagen are well maintained over the years (32). Animal studies have demonstrated persistence up to 1 year if collagen is injected superficial to the vocalis muscle. Rapid resorption occurred if the substance was injected into the muscle (18). Results of vocal fold injection with various forms of collagen are inconsistent with the results of studies of these same substances injected into subcutaneous tissues. In general, collagen injected under the skin has demonstrated considerably faster resorption (33). Long-term studies are needed to better evaluate the fate of injected collagen in the vocal folds.

Autologous fascia has not been studied as extensively in the larynx as fat and collagen. It has been used for other purposes (i.e., otologic, cosmetic, and reconstructive) with favorable results; fascia has demonstrated good long-term maintenance of graft volume (39). Preliminary results and our own experience with the use of autogenous fascia suggest that the long-term yield is similar to that of fat (11,12). It appears to be an alternative to fat in patients who appear to fail lipoinjection.

## CONCLUSIONS

Endoscopic vocal fold augmentation is valuable for providing improved glottal closure in patients with mild to moderate glottal incompetence. The techniques are varied and versatile, and they can be individualized depending on the specific needs and indications of each patient. Injection augmentation offers an excellent alternative to open procedures such as medialization laryngoplasty.

## REFERENCES


1. Brunings W. Uber eine neue Behandlungsmethode der Rekurrenslahmung. *Verh Ver Laryngol* 1911;18:151.
2. Arnold GE. Vocal rehabilitation of paralytic dysphonia. *Arch Otolaryngol* 1962;76:358–368.
3. Benninger MS, Alessi D, Archer S, et al. Vocal fold scarring: current concepts and management. *Otolaryngol Head Neck Surg* 1996;115:474–482.
4. Berke GS, Gerratt B, Kreiman J, et al. Treatment of Parkinson hypophonia with percutaneous collagen augmentation. *Laryngoscope* 1999;109:1295–1299.
5. Levine BA, Jacobs IN, Wetmore RF, et al. Vocal cord injection in children with unilateral vocal cord paralysis. *Arch Otolaryngol Head Neck Surg* 1995;121:116–119.
6. McGuirt WF Jr, Jacob SL, Puri SK, et al. Autologous fat injection in the pediatric larynx: indications and technique. *Arch Otolaryngol* 2001 (*in press*).
7. Koufman JA, Walker FO. Laryngeal electromyography in clinical practice. *Phonoscope* 1998;1:57–70.
8. Postma GN, Koufman JA. Laryngeal electromyography. *Curr Opin Otolaryngol Head Neck Surg* 1998;6:411–415.
9. Newman J. The biographical history of fat transplantation surgery. *Am J Cosmetic Surg* 1987;4:85–87.
10. Ford CN, Bless DM, Loftus JM. Role of injectable collagen in the treatment of glottic insufficiency: a study of 119 patients. *Ann Otol Rhinol Laryngol* 1992;101:237–247.
11. Rihkanen H. Vocal fold augmentation by injection of autologous fascia. *Laryngoscope* 1998;108:51–54.
12. Duke SG, Salmon J, Blalock PD, et al. Fascia augmentation of the vocal fold: graft yield in the canine and preliminary clinical experience. *Laryngoscope* 2001;111:759–764.
13. Schramm VL, May M, Lavorato AS. Gelfoam paste injection for vocal cord paralysis: temporary rehabilitation of glottic incompetence. *Laryngoscope* 1978;88:1268–1273.
14. Koufman JA, Little FB, Weeks DB. Proximal large-bore jet ventilation for laryngeal laser surgery. *Arch Otolaryngol Head Neck Surg* 1987;113:314–320.
15. Rosen CA. Phonosurgical vocal fold injection: indications and techniques. *Otolaryngol Head Neck Surg* 1998;9:1–8.
16. Ford CN. Laryngeal injection techniques. In: Ford CN, Bless DM, eds. *Phonosurgery: assessment and surgical management of voice disorders*. New York: Raven Press, 1991:123–141.
17. Dedo HH, Urrea RD, Lawson L. Intracordal injection of Teflon in the treatment of 135 patients with dysphonia. *Ann Otol Rhinol Laryngol* 1973;82:661–667.

18. Ford CN. Histologic studies on the fate of soluble collagen injected into canine vocal folds. *Laryngoscope* 1986;96: 1248–1257.
19. Mikaelian DO, Lowry LD, Sataloff RT. Lipoinjection for unilateral vocal cord paralysis. *Laryngoscope* 1991;101:465–468.
20. Brandenburg JH, Kirkham W, Koschkee D. Vocal cord augmentation with autogenous fat. *Laryngoscope* 1992;102: 495–500.
21. Shaw GY, Szewczyk MA, Searle J, et al. Autologous fat injection into the vocal folds: technical considerations and long-term follow-up. *Laryngoscope* 1997;107:177–186.
22. Shindo ML, Zaretsky LS, Rice DH. Autologous fat injection for unilateral vocal fold paralysis. *Ann Otol Rhinol Laryngol* 1996; 105:602–606.
23. Mikus JL, Koufman JA, Kilpatrick SE. Fate of liposuctioned and purified autologous fat injections in the canine vocal fold. *Laryngoscope* 1995;105:17–22.
24. Zaretsky LS, Shindo ML, Detar M, et al. Autologous fat injection for vocal fold paralysis: long-term histologic evaluation. *Ann Otol Rhinol Laryngol* 1995;104:1–4.
25. Saccogna PW, Werning JW, Setrakian S, et al. Lipoinjection in the paralyzed feline vocal fold: study of graft survival. *Otolaryngol Head Neck Surg* 1997;117:465–470.
26. Bartynski J, Marion MS, Wang TD. Histopathologic evaluation of adipose autografts in a rabbit ear model. *Otolaryngol Head Neck Surg* 1990;102:314–321.
27. Kononas TC, Bucky LP, Hurley C, et al. The fate of suctioned and surgically removed fat after reimplantation for soft tissue augmentation: a volumetric and histologic study in the rabbit. *Plast Reconstr Surg* 1993;91:763–768.
28. Moore JH Jr, Kolaczynski JW, Morales LM, et al. Viability of fat obtained by syringe suction lipectomy: effects of local anesthesia with lidocaine. *Aesthetic Plast Surg* 1995;19:335–339.
29. Marques A, Brenda E, Saldiva PH, et al. Autologous fat grafts: a quantitative and morphometric study in rabbits. *Scand J Plast Reconstr Surg Hand Surg* 1994;28:241–247.
30. Nguyen A, Pasyk KA, Bouvier TN, et al. Comparative study of survival of autologous adipose tissue taken and transplanted by different techniques. *Plast Reconstr Surg* 1990;85:378–386.
31. Ford CN, Bless DM. A preliminary study of injectable collagen in human vocal fold augmentation. *Otolaryngol Head Neck Surg* 1986;94:104–112.
32. Remacle M, Dujardin JM, Lawson G. Treatment of vocal fold immobility by glutaraldehyde-cross-linked collagen injection: long-term results. *Ann Otol Rhinol Laryngol* 1995;104:437–441.
33. Kligman AM, Armstrong RC. Histologic response to intradermal Zyderm and Zyplast (glutaraldehyde cross-linked) collagen in humans. *J Dermatol Surg Oncol* 1986;12:351–357.
34. Delustro F, Condell RA, Nguyen MA, et al. A comparative study of the biologic and immunologic response to medical devices derived from dermal collagen. *J Biomed Mater Res* 1986;20: 109–120.
35. Keefe J, Wauk L, Chu S, et al. Clinical use of injectable bovine collagen: a decade of experience. *Clin Mater* 1992;9:155–162.
36. Ford CN, Staskowski PA, Bless DM. Autologous collagen vocal fold injection: a preliminary clinical study. *Laryngoscope* 1995; 105:944–948.
37. Remacle M, Lawson G, Delos M, et al. Correcting vocal fold immobility by autologous collagen injection for voice rehabilitation: a short-term study. *Ann Otol Rhinol Laryngol* 1999;108: 788–793.
38. Staskowski PA, Ford CN, Inagi K. The histologic fate of autologous collagen injected into the canine vocal fold. *Otolaryngol Head Neck Surg* 1998;118:187–190.
39. Das SK, Davidson SF, Walker BL, et al. The fate of free autogenous fascial grafts in the rabbit. *Br J Plast Surg* 1990;43:315–317.

# 44

# PEDIATRIC LARYNGOLOGY AND BRONCHOESOPHAGOLOGY

MICHAEL A. ROTHSCHILD
MICHAEL J. RUTTER
ROBIN T. COTTON

Few procedures provide the setting for catastrophe as readily as instrumentation of the pediatric airway. The small laryngotracheal lumen combined with an obstructive disease process leaves little margin for error or faulty technique. The infant's pulmonary physiology results in precipitous desaturation if ventilation and/or oxygenation is even briefly compromised. The possibility of rapid oxygen desaturation has given rise to the adage that "babies drop like rocks."

Endoscopic evaluation of the pediatric airway must be performed in a safe, atraumatic fashion. The endoscopist must have the opportunity for a thorough examination, ideally allowing observation of dynamic changes and documentation of the findings. Because most children undergoing airway endoscopy are thought to have some underlying obstructive pathology, the surgeon must be prepared to secure a difficult airway at all times during the evaluation.

The study of diseases of the pediatric upper aerodigestive tract is complex, and many exhaustive works have been written on the subject (1,2). This chapter focuses on the details of endoscopic techniques as they are of use to the practicing surgeon in this setting. It is assumed that the reader is already familiar with the basics of pediatric otolaryngology as it pertains to the upper aerodigestive tract.

Before the advent of endoscopic visualization, the structures of the hypopharynx, laryngotracheal tree, and esophagus were only known through tracheotomy and autopsy. In the middle of the nineteenth century, the development of devices for the concentration of sunlight or candlelight allowed the first time the visualization of the living human larynx (3,4). In 1854, the voice teacher Manuel Garcia described the indirect observation of a larynx (his own!) using sunlight, a hand mirror, and a dental mirror. In the second half of the nineteenth century, several laryngoscopy clinics were established in Europe and the United States to deal with a variety of neoplastic, inflammatory, and infectious diseases that affected the larynx. The early laryngologists were able to achieve surprising success in diagnosis and intervention (e.g., polypectomy) despite the limited lighting and anesthesia available.

Direct laryngoscopy was not developed until the end of the nineteenth century and was made possible by further achievements in the field of illumination, including the invention of the electric light bulb by Thomas Edison in 1880. Kirstein described a device for direct laryngoscopy in 1895 (5), and over the next few decades, numerous refinements such as magnification (6) and suspension (7) were added. Perhaps one of the greatest therapeutic milestones in endoscopy is the retrieval of foreign bodies. The first successful case was reported by Killian in 1897, in which a soup bone was removed from the right mainstem bronchus in an adult using an open-tube bronchoscope, cocaine anesthesia, and a long forceps.

Before the advent of bronchoscopy, such an aspiration was frequently a death sentence because of airway obstruction, chronic pulmonary suppuration, or the high surgical mortality rate of thoracotomy. Although the technique of endoscopic foreign body removal was first described by Killian, it was Chevalier Jackson who fully developed this technique (8,9). Jackson was a brilliant innovator, whose early insights into bronchoscopic manipulation arose from his work maintaining the complex gas lines supplying his father's hotel. He manufactured many delicate grasping forceps and endoscopes, specifically tailoring the devices for the clinical problem at hand. In his hands, the mortality of foreign body aspiration fell to approximately 2%.

Chevalier Jackson saved thousands of children and adults with foreign body aspiration or esophageal impaction. Through his teaching clinics and animal laboratories, he was able to train a generation of endoscopists and establish the principles of this discipline, essentially unchanged to this day. Through his lobbying of Congress and other public health initiatives, he was able to prevent countless such injuries by ensuring adequate labeling of caustic substances and raising awareness of the dangers children pose to themselves: "More than 85% of foreign bodies in the air and food passages are there through carelessness, which is avoidable. . . . Over and over again, when a little baby came in with life in jeopardy from, for example, a safety pin, I have said: 'Why cannot such accidents be prevented? This baby could not have walked to get that pin' " (8).

Another major contribution to upper aerodigestive tract endoscopy and to all types of endoscopy was the development of the modern optical systems that carry light and images through rigid and flexible devices. These inventions produced a significant advance in the quality of images of the body's internal spaces. The development of teaching adapters allowed students to better observe difficult endoscopic procedures. Improved imaging techniques also enabled better documentation of endoscopic findings through still and motion photography.

In 1930, Lamm described the transmission of images through flexible strands of glass fiber (10). In 1954, the English physicist Harold Hopkins developed a system of fiber bundles that allowed transmission of images suitable for endoscopy (11), and the invention was applied to a number of clinical specialties over the next few years. In 1959, Hopkins developed another device, the glass rod-lens system. It used a series of glass rods in place of the traditional air spaces between the lenses in telescope systems. The resulting rigid telescope provided significantly better image and light transmission.

The final insight that produced the modern endoscopic telescope was by Karl Storz, a German instrument manufacturer. He was impressed with Hopkins' rod-lens system and with the flexible fiberoptic system used by Hirschowitz, a gastroenterologist. Storz wrapped a thin sheet of glass fibers around a rod-lens telescope (Fig. 44.1). The fibers were used for light transmission distally into the body cavity, while the telescope carried the magnified image back to the viewer. Because the fiber layer is quite thin but an excellent light carrier, it provides brilliant distal illumination without adding much bulk to the instrument (12). By adapting these telescopes to foreign body forceps, the retrieval of objects from the airway has been immeasurably facilitated and allowed major improvements in the ability to teach this surgical technique using video monitoring of endoscopic images.

One more invention that has revolutionized endoscopic surgery of the upper aerodigestive tract is the surgical laser. The development of better endoscopes with higher-quality illumination and optical transmission greatly improved diagnosis, but intervention was limited by the range of instruments that could be used. As it became apparent that the newly developed laser beam could be safely applied to human tissue, Geza J. Jako pioneered the use of the carbon dioxide ($CO_2$) laser in laryngology (13). Advantages cited for this particular type of laser beam included the ready energy absorption by soft tissue, the ease of focusing to allow precise incisions, and the ablation of diseased tissue with minimal damage to adjacent healthy structures. Jako realized the key concepts of using the operating microscope to provide a magnified stereoscopic view of the surgical field and using the micromanipulator to direct the coaxial laser beam in the field with precise, one-hand control.

Since the early 1970s, laser technology has been refined, with the development of smaller spot sizes, better micromanipulators, better alignment of the aiming and cutting beams, and reduced power requirements with less collateral tissue damage. The $CO_2$ laser has remained the most popular wavelength used in endoscopic procedures and has been used successfully for the removal of airway papillomas, carcinomas, and other neoplasia, as well as for scar revision, arytenoidectomy, and vocal cord lateralization. These procedures are discussed elsewhere in this textbook.

Although the $CO_2$ laser is in many ways ideal for use through a laryngoscope with a micromanipulator, it becomes more difficult to precisely deliver the beam into the more distal portions of the airway (i.e., subglottis, trachea, and bronchi). An elongated laryngoscope (i.e., sub-

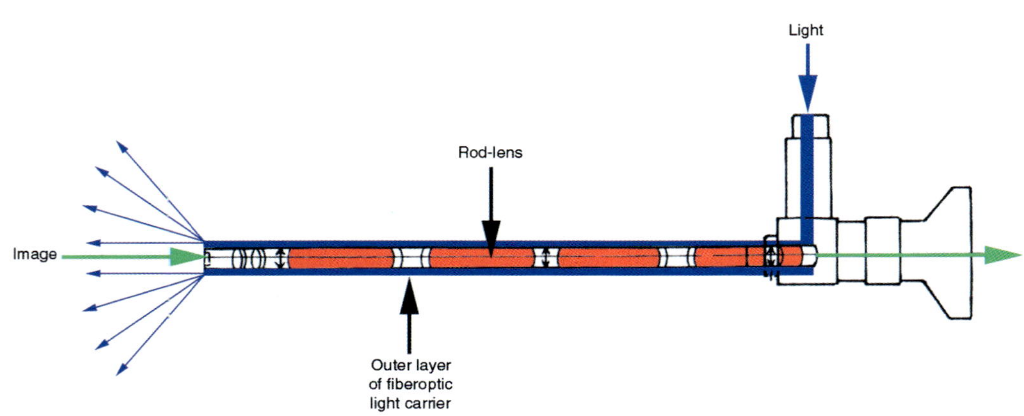


**FIGURE 44.1.** Rod-lens telescope with fiberoptic light carrier for distal illumination.

glottiscope may be used to visualize the upper trachea, but its necessarily narrow taper at the tip limits stereoscopic vision. $CO_2$ laser bronchoscopes have been devised, but they are cumbersome and not well adapted to fiberoptic telescopes. Use of a semi-flexible fiber enables delivery of a $CO_2$ beam through a ventilating bronchoscope alongside a telescope, but it is awkward and not usable in the smaller pediatric equipment.

Other types of lasers, such as the neodymium:yttrium-aluminum-garnet (Nd:YAG) and potassium-titanyl-phosphate (KTP) lasers, are well suited to bronchoscopic procedures, because the energy can be transmitted through flexible fiber systems more readily than the $CO_2$ beam. Flexible and rigid systems have been used to deliver these beams for distal obstruction from papillomatosis and neoplasia (14). The fiber can be used in contact or noncontact mode, depending on the desired effect. Touching the carrier to the tissue delivers more energy which may be useful in cutting scar tissue, whereas the noncontact mode provides better hemostasis and improved vaporization of neoplastic tissue (15).

Development of pediatric bronchoscopic applications for these beams has been slow because their energy is more widely scattered in tissue. Although this is better for coagulation of vascular lesions or granulation tissue, there is the potential risk of collateral tissue damage and obstructive airway edema (16). This is particularly troublesome in the smaller pediatric laryngotracheal complex. Nevertheless, some work suggests that non-$CO_2$ beams can be used safely to treat distal pediatric airway pathology, with the KTP beam having less depth of penetration and potential for injury of adjacent structures than the Nd:YAG (17).

## INDICATIONS

Unlike some of the other topics covered in this volume, there is no nonendoscopic surgical alternative to diagnostic laryngology and bronchoesophagology. Although radiographic procedures may provide useful structural and functional information about the upper aerodigestive tract, they are rarely a substitute for diagnostic esophagoscopy, and they almost never take the place of diagnostic laryngoscopy or bronchoscopy. The information gained by direct visualization of the airway is of primary importance in determining the functional effect of a variety of intrinsic and extrinsic disease processes that can affect the airway, such as stenosis, external compression, intraluminal neoplasia, collapse, and congenital structural anomalies.

Endoscopic techniques are indicated for a variety of therapeutic interventions in children, including foreign body retrieval, biopsy, tumor debulking, dilation, and stent placement in the airway and esophagus. Although some of these procedures do have open counterparts, endoscopy is generally the approach of choice. The common indications for endoscopy of the upper aerodigestive tract in infants and children are outlined in Table 44.1.

Endoscopy of the upper aerodigestive tract is most commonly done by otolaryngologists using rigid instruments. These have the advantage of larger working channels, better

**TABLE 44.1. SURGICAL INDICATIONS FOR AERODIGESTIVE TRACT ENDOSCOPY IN CHILDREN**

| | |
|---|---|
| *Flexible Laryngoscopy* | *Flexible Bronchoscopy* |
| Stridor | Stridor |
| Hoarseness or weak cry | Tracheotomy surveillance (e.g., distal granuloma) |
| Suspected pharyngeal foreign body | Difficult intubation |
| Unexplained sleep apnea | Persistent wheezing |
| Anticipated difficulty with intubation | Chronic cough |
| Evaluation of glottis and supraglottis before anesthesia | Extrinsic tracheobronchial compression |
| *Rigid Microlaryngoscopy and Bronchoscopy* | Mild hemoptysis |
| Stridor | Suspected endobronchial lung lesion |
| Tracheotomy surveillance (e.g., suprastomal granuloma) | Selective bronchography |
| Foreign body evaluation and management | Assessment of toxic inhalation or aspiration |
| Postoperative evaluation after airway reconstruction | Monitoring of lung transplant patients |
| Chronic cough | Confirmation of endotracheal tube position |
| Severe hemoptysis | Acute lobar atelectasis |
| Severe laryngotracheal infections (e.g., bacterial tracheitis) | Cystic fibrosis management |
| Airway trauma | Removal of mucus plugs |
| Extrinsic tracheobronchial compression | Pneumonia |
| Assessment of toxic inhalation, aspiration, or airway burns | Persistent |
| Laryngeal pathology (e.g., polyps, webs) | Recurrent |
| Airway mass lesions (e.g., papilloma) | Immunocompromised host (needing bronchoalveolar lavage) |
| Dilation of stenoses | Atypical |
| Placement of airway stents | |

optics, and the ability to ventilate past an area of airway obstruction. Flexible bronchoscopy certainly has a place in the evaluation of the pediatric airway, especially since technologic advances have provided for steerable endoscopes of small caliber with suction or instrument channels. Although few otolaryngologists use this technique, we are frequently called into consultation by pediatric pulmonologists to aid in the evaluation of structural pathology in the upper airway seen on flexible bronchoscopy.

The two main advantages of flexible bronchoscopy are the ability to examine the airway more peripherally (i.e., past the secondary bronchi) and the avoidance of general anesthesia. However, this technique is not appropriate in the presence of or in anticipation of significant hemorrhage, foreign body, or airway obstruction when surgical ventilation may be necessary. The area of most common interest to pediatric airway surgeons—the subglottis—is poorly visualized by flexible bronchoscopy. Typically, there is good visualization of the glottis, but the operator then rapidly "threads the needle" and passes into the upper trachea, without the opportunity to thoroughly examine the subglottis.

## PREOPERATIVE EVALUATION

Perhaps the most important assessment before airway endoscopy is the patient's clinical airway status. A decision must be made about whether the need for endoscopy is emergent, elective, or somewhere in between. The surgeon observes the child for signs of respiratory distress, such as tachypnea, obstructive-pattern chest wall motion, agitation, and stridor. Pallor, cyanosis, and lethargy are serious late signs of impending respiratory failure. In such cases, the preoperative evaluation may be quite limited. However, no matter what the clinical situation, it is important to preserve clear judgment and flexible thinking (18). As our residents are instructed, "If the patient is moving air, don't panic. But if the patient is *not* moving air . . . don't panic!"

The history, signs, and symptoms typically suggest the likely cause of airway disease and the most appropriate intervention. An experienced clinician can be quite accurate in a diagnosis based solely on the history and physical examination findings (19). It is important to differentiate conditions that present in early infancy (e.g., subglottic stenosis), later in infancy (e.g., subglottic hemangioma), and acutely during childhood (e.g., inflammatory conditions such as croup or epiglottitis). Although the ages of presentation for most childhood airway conditions are broad and overlapping, keeping in mind the typical setting for these conditions helps to exclude less likely diagnoses and to expedite the workup (Fig. 44.2).

The surgeon must never be coerced into proceeding to endoscopy without optimal conditions, equipment, and personnel, except in the most dire circumstances. The classic example of this situation is foreign body aspiration. Generally, objects that pass the glottis do not become impacted until after the carina, lodging in one of the

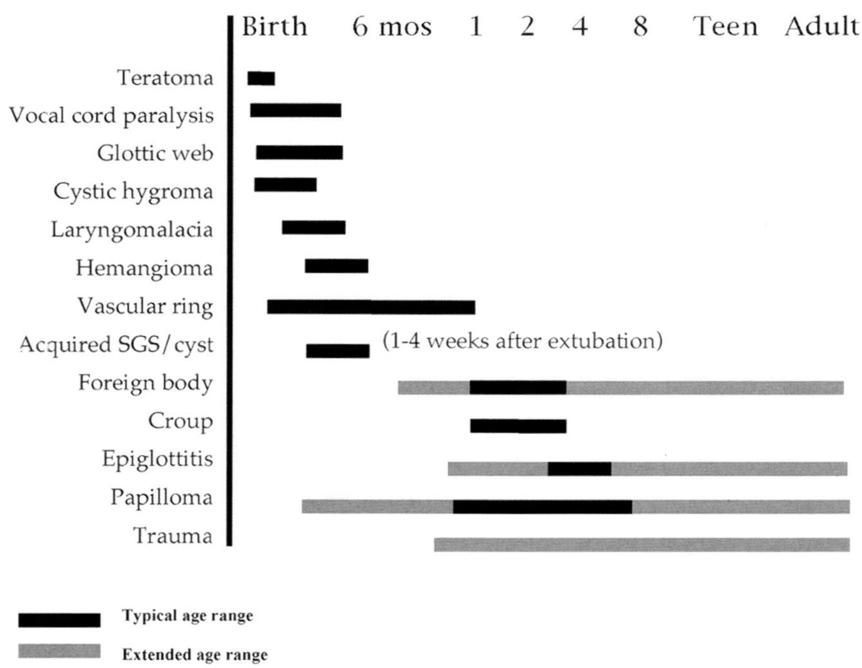


**FIGURE 44.2.** Typical age of presentation for a variety of conditions that affect the pediatric airway.

bronchi. These objects typically do not cause immediate respiratory distress, even if a mainstem bronchus is occluded. There are exceptions, such as conforming objects (e.g., balloon fragments, hot dogs, fruit skins), but in most cases, aspiration is not an airway emergency. The surgeon must be sure that all appropriate equipment is available, such as the full range of appropriate endoscopes, foreign body forceps, and a tracheotomy set. The contribution of an experienced anesthesiologist cannot be overstated. It may even be helpful to prepare the patient with a few days of intravenous steroid therapy if the foreign body has been impacted for any length of time and has induced an inflammatory reaction in the airway.

Inhaled anesthetic agents and instrumentation can exacerbate laryngotracheal edema and further compromise a narrow lumen. Care must be taken to avoid inappropriate endoscopy in a patient with suspected airway inflammation. Although some conditions require emergent therapeutic intervention (e.g., epiglottitis, bacterial tracheitis), the surgeon should resist the temptation to perform a diagnostic endoscopy when it is likely to contribute little to the overall management of the patient. Frequently, patients with laryngotracheal inflammation (i.e., croup) take weeks to improve and may require prolonged hospitalization. The surgeon may be encouraged by other physicians to "take a look down there" when there is frustration with the patient's slow progress. If the patient's presentation is typical, if there are no signs of underlying chronic airway problems, and if airway status is stable and slowly improving, it is extremely unlikely that endoscopy will uncover anything that will change the course of management. Rather, the procedure may worsen the situation, forcing the placement of an endotracheal tube into an inflamed airway with the associated risk of acquired subglottic stenosis.

Before proceeding with endoscopy, other conditions that may affect the procedure should be considered. Children with potential cervical spine instability, such as those with Down syndrome, should be assessed clinically and radiographically. Rigid esophagoscopy and bronchoscopy require significant neck extension and should be avoided if there is concern about stability of the spine. Flexible endoscopy can frequently be used in these patients, especially for diagnostic purposes. A lack of neurologic symptoms and full range of motion with active cervical flexion and extension while awake is a good indication of spinal stability, but neurosurgical consultation may be indicated.

Radiographic examination of the chest is also appropriate before performing endoscopy in a young infant, because long-segment tracheal stenosis may be present without obvious symptoms. If endoscopy is attempted in such a patient, the surgeon may encounter a highly lethal situation, with total inability to ventilate despite surgical access to the airway. Even if intubation is possible with an endotracheal tube or bronchoscope, it may not be possible to extubate the patient without formal transthoracic repair of the stenotic airway.

Chest radiographs are frequently obtained when foreign body aspiration is suspected. The classic signs of air trapping from a ball-valve–type lesion (i.e., ipsilateral hyperlucency and contralateral mediastinal shift) or consolidation from a chronic obstructing lesion (i.e., ipsilateral mediastinal shift, atelectasis, and collapse) may support the presence of a foreign body. Inspiratory and expiratory films or decubitus views may help demonstrate a subtle degree of obstruction or air trapping. However, a normal radiographic study is a common finding in cases of foreign body aspiration (20,21). If there is a strong clinical suspicion of a foreign body in the airway, a negative x-ray result should not preclude endoscopy.

Chest and neck radiographs frequently are used to determine the diagnosis of foreign body impaction in the esophagus. Coins are by far the most frequently ingested objects found in the upper esophagus (22). Some physicians observe children with impacted coins for spontaneous passage by serial radiographs, with or without the use of smooth muscle relaxants (e.g., glucagon). However, this is rarely successful in young children with upper esophageal coins, and there is some evidence that glucagon is no more effective than placebo in this setting (23). There is increasing concern about the corrosive potential of pennies minted after 1982, which have a zinc core (24). Esophagoscopy is done as soon as possible, although time is usually allowed for gastric emptying before the induction of anesthesia.

A lateral neck radiograph is also indicated in cases of coin ingestion, although not for the frequently quoted reason of determining whether the coin is in the airway or the esophagus. The teaching point is often made regarding sagittal orientation of coins in the airway versus coronal presentation in the esophagus, but a coin, given its size and shape, is an extremely rare airway foreign body in a child. Such an object would virtually never lodge in the larynx or mid-trachea and certainly not without inducing significant coughing or stridor. Respiratory symptoms occasionally occur in patients with esophageal impaction when a surrounding inflammatory reaction or the object itself impinges on the airway from behind. This airway narrowing may be demonstrated on lateral airway films. The main reason, however, that the lateral x-ray film is obtained is to ensure that there is not more than one coin present. Coins can stack and appear superimposed on anteroposterior films. Induction of anesthesia may induce relaxation, with distal passage of one coin into the lower esophagus. If, after retrieval of the first coin, no further endoscopy is performed, it would be possible to leave an unsuspected second coin in place.

Some upper airway obstructive conditions are dynamic and variable, especially those that manifest as sleep apnea. In such cases, full evaluation of the patient may require more than observing the anatomy of the airway under general anesthesia. Laryngomalacia, pharyngeal collapse, and vocal cord motion anomalies may be best demonstrated by awake fiberoptic nasopharyngoscopy. Tracheomalacia may not be apparent if positive-pressure ventilation and paralysis are used during rigid bronchoscopy. If flexible bronchoscopy is not appropriate, dynamic changes in the airway caliber may be demonstrated by awake videofluoroscopy, with or without esophageal contrast.

Patients who are suspected of having gastroesophageal reflux disease should be evaluated before endoscopy and certainly before any therapeutic intervention in a stenotic airway (25–27). This group includes patients with reflux symptoms, those with the characteristic appearance of reflux laryngitis on awake laryngoscopy (i.e., boggy, erythematous arytenoids), and new patients with laryngotracheal stenosis. Evaluation is typically done under the guidance of the pediatric gastroenterologist and generally includes a double-lumen pH probe. Gastric emptying scans and contrast esophagrams are also useful in assessing this condition. If reflux is detected, treatment should be instituted and optimized (medically or surgically) before proceeding with airway reconstruction.

## INSTRUMENTATION

It is the surgeon's responsibility to ensure that all necessary equipment is present in the operating room and functional

**TABLE 44.2. SUGGESTED EQUIPMENT FOR PEDIATRIC RIGID LARYNGOSCOPY AND BRONCHOSCOPY**

| | |
|---|---|
| *Storz Telescopes and Optical Forceps* | |
| 27005A[a] | 4 mm × 30 cm, used for diagnostic endoscopy without a ventilating bronchoscope sheath; good image; tends to obstruct the smaller ventilating bronchoscopes |
| 27020A | 2.9 mm × 30 cm, used in the longer (30-cm) bronchoscopes; image not as good as the 27005A and more fragile; occasionally used without a bronchoscope to traverse tight stenoses above a tracheotomy |
| 27018A | 2.7 mm × 18.5 cm, used in the shorter (20-cm) infant bronchoscopes; image similar to 27020A |
| 27017A | 1.9 mm × 18.5 cm, also may be used in the short infant bronchoscopes; image not very good; best reserved for very-small-caliber bronchoscopes (i.e., 2.5) when ventilation is critical |
| 10324A | 2.9 mm × 36 cm telescope, designed specifically for the 36-cm optical forceps (10378 series); forceps (barely) fit through the 3.5 bronchoscope tube |
| 10378H, K, L, U | 36-mm optical forceps: alligator, peanut, biopsy, upbiting |
| *Bronchoscope Tubes* | |
| Long (30-cm) tubes | 3.5, 4, 4.5, 5, 6 |
| Short (20-cm) tubes | 2.5, 3, 3.5 |

*Bronchoscopy Table Setup*[b]

- Ventilating bronchoscope setup for emergency use; infants may require smaller bronchoscope and telescope than listed here:
  - 3.5 × 30 cm bronchoscope tube
  - 27020A telescope
  - Locking adapter (to connect tube to telescope)
  - Prism adapter (to block side channel and allow ventilation; not for light input)
  - Suction adapter with rubber cap
  - FLUVOG adapter (for rapid switching between open tube and optical techniques)
- Appropriate-sized rigid suction (must fit *through* tube with telescope removed)
- Smallest-caliber (green-tipped) flexible suction and suction line tubing
- Glass window to fit over end of scope with locking adapter and telescope removed (for open tube bronchoscopy)
- Gray light cable
- Defogging solution
- Set of pediatric cuffless endotracheal tubes, 2.5–5.5 inclusive, with stylets
- Topical anesthesia, appropriate for patient's weight
- Pediatric tracheotomy set (if patient does not have tracheotomy tube in place)
- Straight-blade intubating laryngoscope of appropriate size, Miller or Wishipple

[a]The 0° scopes are used almost exclusively in bronchoscopy. The letter after the past number refers to the angle (e.g., A = 0°, B = 30°). Occasionally, angled telescopes may be useful, as when examining the undersurface of the vocal cords or the choanae.
[b]Standard, may vary with particular case.

before induction of anesthesia. This includes an open tracheotomy set when appropriate and any video or photographic apparatus needed for documentation. After the procedure has begun, a patient with an apparently stable airway may obstruct rapidly, and this is not the time to begin frantically searching for needed supplies. No amount of blame directed toward the operating room staff will improve the situation, and care must be taken to ensure that every possible need is anticipated. A suggested inventory for pediatric bronchoscopy is outlined in Table 44.2.

The equipment part numbers and sizes provided in this section correspond to the Karl Storz endoscopy product line. Although other companies also manufacture airway endoscopes, this equipment is of good quality and is the type most commonly available for use in the United States. The same basic concepts apply to other equipment, however, and the subsequent discussion should be generally useful to users of other brands of endoscopes.

Continuous video monitoring and recording of all endoscopic procedures is desirable. This greatly facilitates teaching and allows the anesthesiologist to better assist in managing the patient. Unusual findings may be only present briefly and later obscured by blood and edema. Although 35-mm endoscopic photography produces significantly better image resolution, by the time that this equipment is assembled, the image may no longer be obtainable. Images acceptable for publication and presentation may be obtained from the videotape if no other record is available.

The distinction should be made between telescopes and bronchoscopes. A *telescope* is the fiberoptic optical device that carries illumination distally and brings magnified images proximally. The use of a telescope justifies the qualified term *microlaryngoscopy*, despite the absence of a surgical microscope. The *bronchoscope* is the metal tube that may be used with the telescope in position or without the telescope (i.e., the open-tube approach). A modern ventilating bronchoscope appropriate for use with an optical telescope has ports for the telescope, the anesthesia circuit (standard 15-mm adapter), a flexible suction catheter (with rubber dam seal to prevent loss of ventilating pressure), and a prism (Fig. 44.3). The prism is used to direct light down the tube when no telescope is used. If the telescope is in place, the

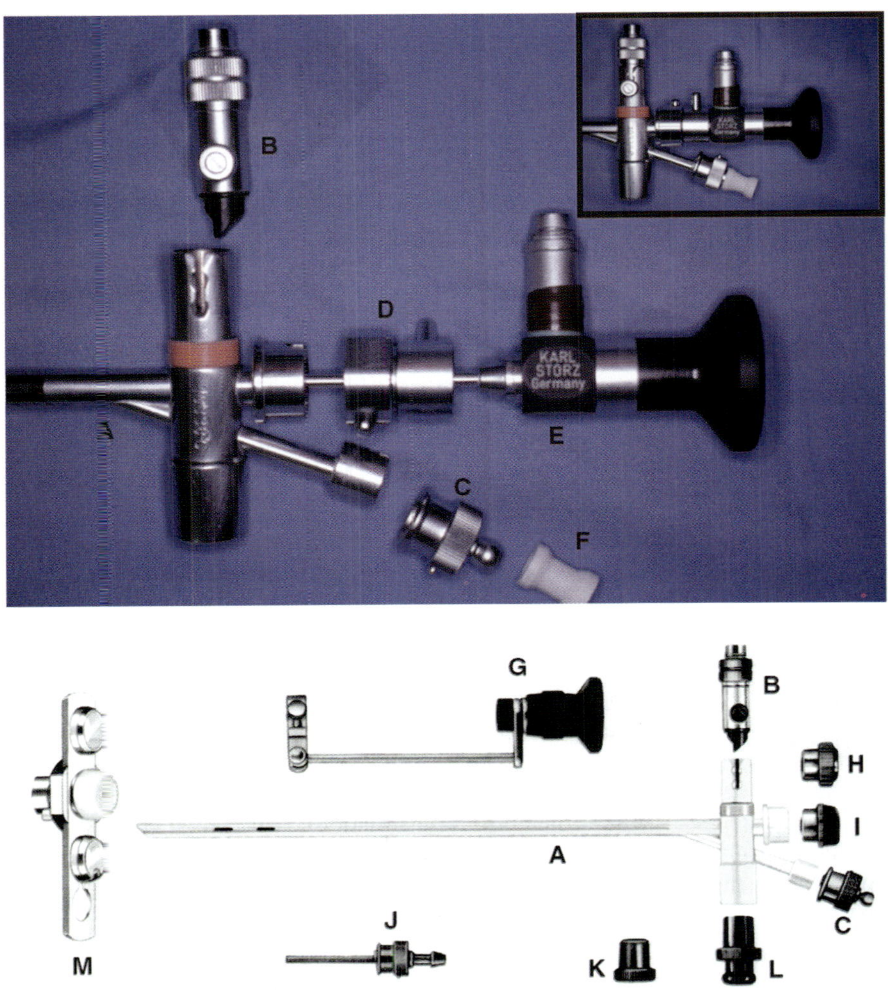


**FIGURE 44.3.** Typical assembly of the ventilating bronchoscope for optical and nonoptical (open-tube) use. *Inset:* The assembled apparatus. *A,* bronchoscope tube; *B,* prism, used to transmit light in open-tube use, is needed to maintain the airway seal when using the optical telescope; *C,* suction adapter for a side port; *D,* locking adapter for the telescope; *E,* optical telescope; *F,* rubber dam for the suction adapter maintains the seal and allows ventilation without a leak; *G,* magnification eyepiece for open-tube use; *H,* the glass port seal for open-tube use allows simultaneous visualization and ventilation; *I,* the rubber dam for the telescope allows use of a variety of telescope lengths in a bronchoscope without locking the adapter; *J,* jet ventilation adapter for a side port; *K,L,* ventilation adapter for circuits with other than 15 mm standard endpiece; *M,* a FLUVOG adapter enables rapid switching among the rubber dam, glass port, and open lumen during bronchoscopy. The keyhole slot allows an instrument to inserted through the open tube and then accepts a glass port to allow simultaneous visualization, ventilation, and manipulation. (Adapted from Karl Storz. Endoscopy catalog, with permission.)

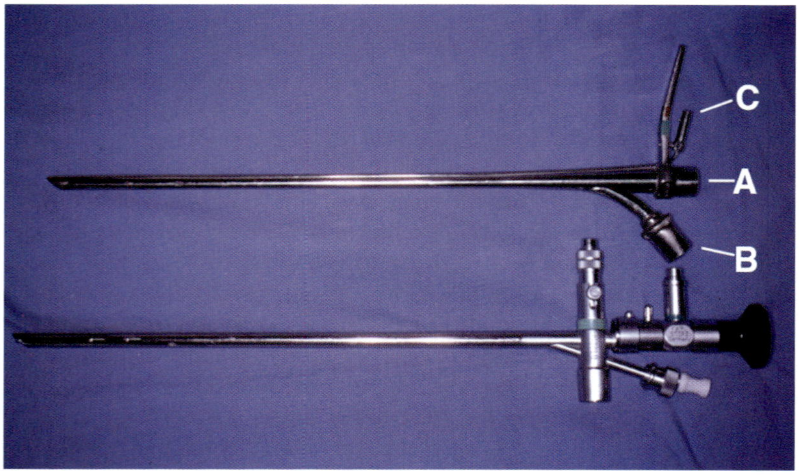


**FIGURE 44.4. Top:** Open-tube bronchoscope with proximal sites for visualization *(A)*, ventilation *(B)* and illumination *(C)*. **Bottom:** Modern ventilating bronchoscope with an attached optical telescope.

prism must still be partially inserted to maintain a seal and allow ventilation, but the light source is connected to the telescope. Older ventilating bronchoscopes were designed only for use as open-tube instruments, with illumination provided through a light carrier running the length of the tube (Fig. 44.4).

Although each clinical situation involves unique equipment needs, some general guidelines for equipment selection are appropriate. We prefer to use the insufflation technique for diagnostic laryngoscopy and bronchoscopy (see Table 44.3), but a ventilating bronchoscope of the appropriate size should be immediately available even if it is not used in the procedure. A smaller bronchoscope should also be available in case the airway lumen is not as large as anticipated. In general, this bronchoscope should be the smallest one that can practically be used to provide ventilation in an emergency. For most children 1 year of age or older, an appropriate tube is a 3.5 × 30 cm bronchoscope (or equivalent), which is the narrowest tube of sufficient length to reach the trachea. Younger infants may require a smaller tube, but the 2.5 × 20 cm bronchoscope is technically difficult to use, especially if suctioning is necessary during the procedure. A smaller telescope is required for this bronchoscope, which provides diminished image quality.

Although it is tempting to provide algorithms for equipment selection based on patient age and size, many children undergoing airway endoscopy have obstructive disease with reduced luminal diameters and therefore require devices that are smaller than anticipated. This problem is compounded by the lack of standardization in the sizing codes used for endotracheal tubes, bronchoscopic equipment, and tracheotomy tubes of different manufacturers. Figure 44.5 is a conversion scale that is useful for selecting equipment of the appropriate caliber (28).

Although the telescope provides far superior visualization, it may be necessary at times to work without the optical apparatus in place (i.e., open-tube bronchoscopy). When small-caliber bronchoscopes or foreign body forceps are necessary or when friable lesions result in the need for frequent suctioning, it may not be possible to work with the telescope in place, because it takes up a significant portion of the tube lumen. This problem may be partially overcome by using extra-small-caliber telescopes or *optical forceps*, which have a telescope built into the handle of the foreign body grasping device.

The bronchoscope has side slots cut into its distal end to allow for ventilation if the tip is occluded. This can be a problem when working high in the trachea, because the slots are above the glottis and prevent good pulmonary airflow. To overcome this problem, a variant on the bronchoscope known as a *tracheoscope* is available, with no slots in the wall of the tube. If such a device is not available, a Tegaderm occlusive dressing can be wrapped around the end of a bronchoscope to seal the side slots and provide ventilation only through the tip. Care must be taken that no excess dressing film is left loose, because it can easily become a source of airway obstruction.

Telescopes may also be fitted to rigid esophagoscopes for improved visualization during diagnostic endoscopy. These esophagoscopes are similar in design to the bronchoscopes, except for a flared, blunted tip to avoid mucosal injury and the lack of a ventilation port. A flexible suction catheter is useful for removing secretions from the esophagus and (carefully) as a seeker to guide passage of the rigid scope when the collapsed lumen is not readily apparent. Open-tube esophagoscopy (without the telescope) may be more appropriate in certain situations, especially if copious secretions are present.

Diagnostic laryngoscopy and bronchoscopy in children is preferentially done using an unsheathed telescope with spontaneous respiration. This quickly and easily provides a superb magnified view of the entire airway with minimal

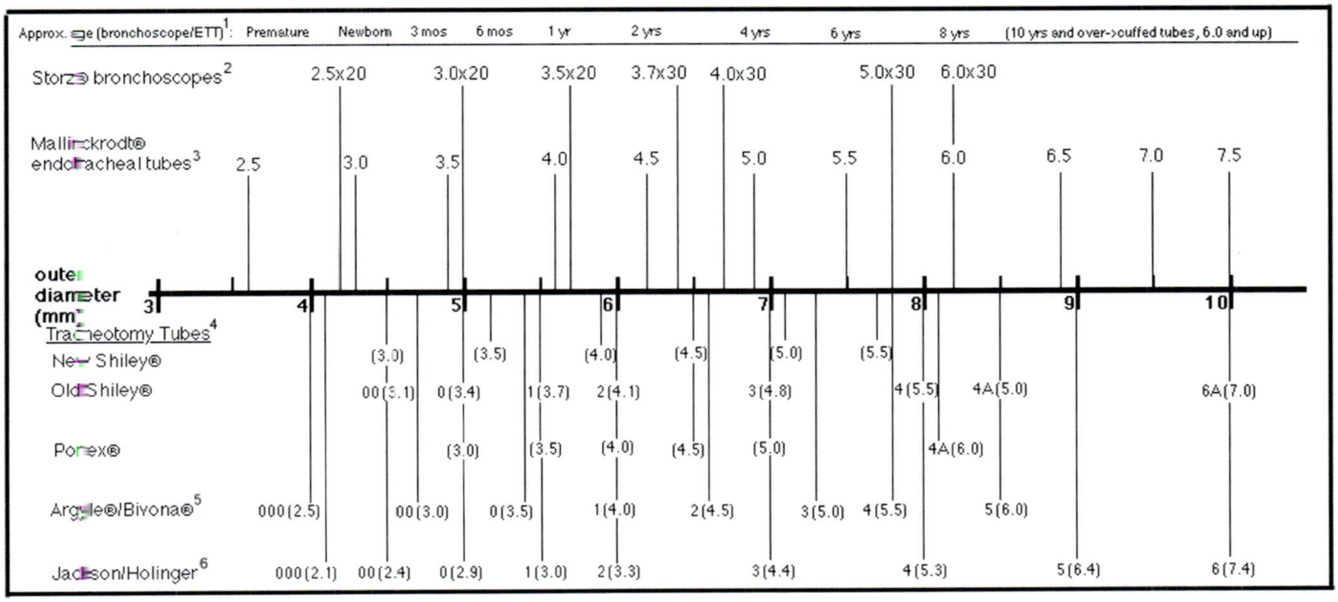


[1] Age ranges are approximate, and are presented as an initial guide to selecting a bronchoscope or endotracheal tube when the patient's subglottis is thought to be of normal caliber for the patient's age. Airway pathology may obviously reduce the lumen diameter, and therefore smaller tubes and endoscopes should always be immediately available. Furthermore, chronological age may not correlate well with overall somatic growth and development.

[2] Storz® bronchoscopes are sized as "X x Y", where X represents the caliber (although not the actual inner diameter) and Y represents the length in cm. The endoscopist may encounter some styles with a flared distal tip which may slightly raise the effective outer diameter.

[3] These numbers are the actual inner diameter in mm, and are the numbers used in referring to various sizes of endotracheal tubes. Wall thickness may vary between brands of endotracheal tube, therefore there may be some small variation in outer diameter if tubes other than Mallinckrodt® are used.

[4] The first numbers listed here are the "approximate Jackson numbers" as given by the manufacturers (except for Portex® and the new Shiley® series). Note that they may vary considerably from the inner and outer diameters of the corresponding Jackson tube. The second numbers in parentheses are the inner diameter in mm.

[5] The Argyle® and Bivona® series are within 1-2 mm for outer diameter with matching inner diameters. They are presented together for clarity.

[6] The Jackson and Holinger styles of metal tracheotomy tubes are made by a number of manufacturers. These measurements are from Pilling® brand tubes, and are within 1 mm of each other for corresponding inner diameters.

**FIGURE 44.5.** The Airway Scale. (Adapted from Rothschild MA. The Airway Scale: a simple device for estimating airway diameters. *Otolaryngol Head Neck Surg* 1994;111:847–848, with permission.)

instrumentation or incidental mucosal trauma. In some cases, however, other equipment may be necessary. Patients with voice disorders may require greater magnification to arrive at a correct diagnosis, and the operating microscope is needed. Similarly, endoscopic procedures such as the laser excision of laryngeal lesions, arytenoidectomy, cordotomy, and web division are done using two-handed techniques with the glottis visualized by suspension laryngoscopy. These techniques and the equipment used are discussed in detail in the sections on general laryngology and are not covered further in this chapter.

If a foreign body is suspected, all appropriate grasping forceps must be on hand. A wide variety of nonoptical grasping forceps were designed by Chevalier Jackson and others during the early 20th century. Foreign body aspiration was previously much more common before the widespread acknowledgment and management of its risk factors, such as small manufactured parts, age-inappropriate foods, and inadequate child supervision. Numerous tools are available to safely grasp, sheath, rotate, and extract foreign bodies that are sharp and dangerous or smooth and difficult to manipulate (Fig. 44.6). Although all optical forceps provide

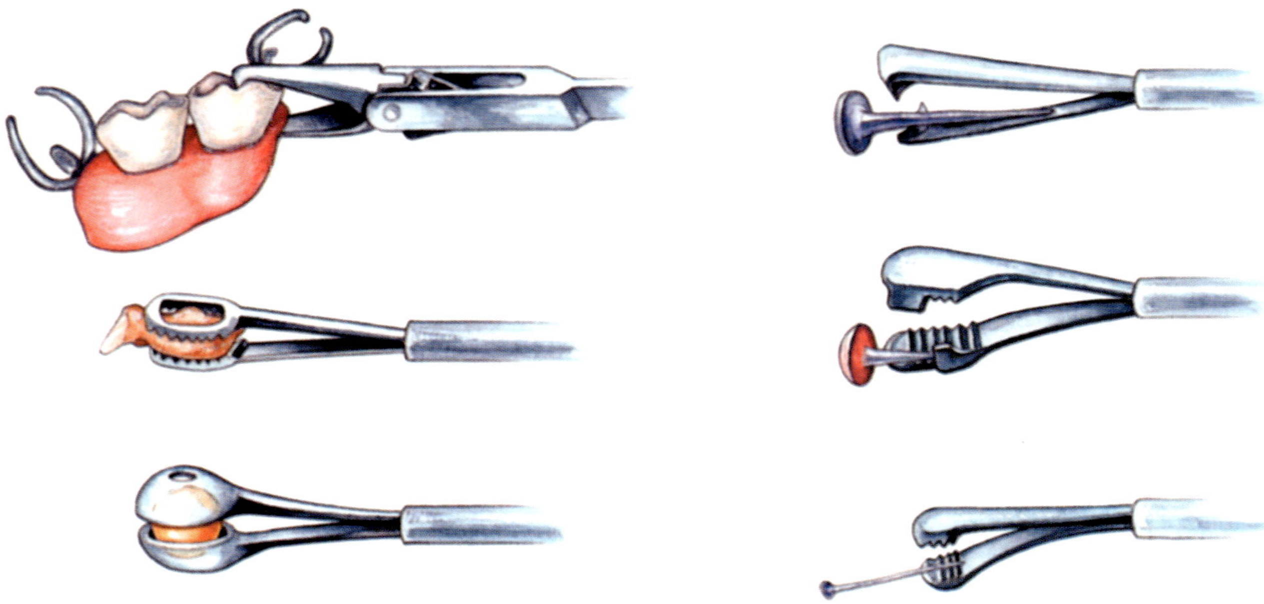

**FIGURE 44.6.** A variety of (nonoptical) grasping devices for the safe rotation, sheathing, and extraction of foreign bodies from the airway and the esophagus. (Adapted from Johns ME, Price JC, Mattox DE. *Atlas of head and neck surgery*, vol 1. Toronto: BC Decker, 1990, with permission.)

superb distal visualization by incorporating a long telescope into the forceps shaft, they are generally available in only a few designs (Fig. 44.7). They are quite delicate and may fracture during endoscopy, potentially resulting in a second foreign body (Fig. 44.8). Such equipment failure can happen with any device, however, and all endoscopic instrument should be inspected before use for signs of fatigue and wear (29).

Rigid and flexible suction catheters of appropriate caliber and length should be on the prep table. Flexible suction can keep the field clear while a telescope is in place, but the combination of the catheter and the telescope may cause unacceptable obstruction of the bronchoscope lumen, limiting ventilation. It may not be possible to pass the flexible suction and the telescope at the same time, and in this situation, the rigid suction can be used alternately with the telescope, switching quickly between optical and open-tube endoscopy with the sliding FLUVOG adapter (Fig. 44.3).

A tooth protector is used in suspension laryngoscopy, but it tends to be too bulky for the microlaryngoscopy and bronchoscopy technique described subsequently. Fog elimination solution or soapy water should be available for cleaning the telescope lens before and during the procedure. A complete set of uncuffed pediatric endotracheal tubes with stylets may be necessary for grading the caliber of airway stenosis, for emergency ventilation, and for safe dila-

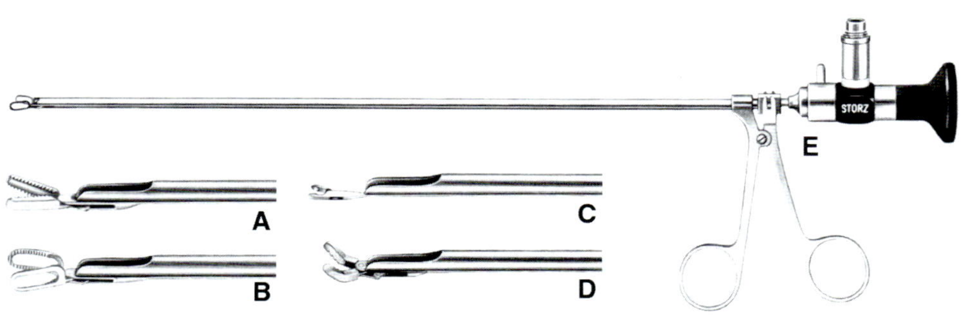


**FIGURE 44.7.** Optical forceps designed for foreign body retrieval. Notice the open channel in the shaft that accepts the telescope. **A:** Alligator forceps. **B:** peanut forceps. **C:** Biopsy forceps. **D:** Upbiting forceps. **E:** Assembled telescope and forceps. (Adapted from Karl Storz. Endoscopy catalog, with permission.)

lifted, and the epiglottis will prolapse over the larynx (Fig. 44.10). Correct technique provides an excellent panoramic view of the airway without excessive stimulation of laryngeal reflexes or injury to the epiglottis and laryngeal introitus.

The larynx and upper trachea are sprayed at this point with a topical anesthetic solution containing lidocaine. Although commercial prepackaged syringes in the form of a laryngotracheal applicator (LTA) may be used for this procedure, a simple syringe with a soft Angiocath catheter works as well. A 1% lidocaine solution may be used up to a total dose of 4 mg/kg (0.4 mL/kg of the 1% solution). After spraying the larynx, the mask is replaced, and a few breaths are given to allow the topical agent to take effect.

For purely diagnostic laryngoscopy and bronchoscopy, the larynx is again suspended with the intubating laryngoscope, and an unsheathed telescope is introduced into the airway. This provides a magnified view with good illumination from the proximal xenon light source. A video camera adapter allows teaching and documentation of endoscopic findings. Generally, the largest telescope that can atraumatically fit in the airway should be used, because the image quality of smaller instruments is limited. As a matter of course, the Storz no. 27005 is a good compromise in this situation, providing an excellent image but still being only 4 mm in diameter. This telescope is 30 cm long and is therefore long enough to visualize the carina in most children. Young infants or children with significant airway stenosis may require a smaller telescope, such as the Storz no. 27018 (2.7 mm diameter) or the no. 27020 (2.9 mm).

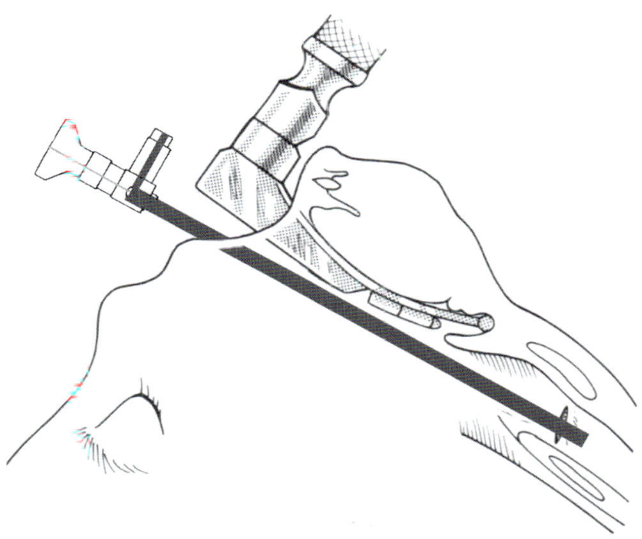

**FIGURE 44.10.** The correct position of the laryngoscope and the telescope for diagnostic microlaryngoscopy and bronchoscopy. The laryngoscope is deep in the vallecula, and the telescope is being passed from the "endoscopy gutter" along the upper right dental arch through the larynx. Care is taken not to direct the tip of the telescope posteriorly in the airway, which is a common mistake. (Adapted from Bluestone C, Stool S. *Atlas of pediatric otolaryngology*. Philadelphia: WB Saunders, 1995, with permission.)

The tongue and mandible are lifted with the intubating laryngoscope blade in the vallecula, providing a fairly straight line between the oral cavity and the carina. The telescope is passed down the "endoscopy gutter" lateral to the right upper molars. After the endoscopist has gained some practice with this technique, it should be possible to atraumatically pass the telescope through the glottis to the end of the trachea and into the proximal mainstem bronchi with minimal manipulation of the head and neck. No shoulder roll is used, and the head is maintained in the neutral position without excessive flexion or extension. Small babies have heads that are relatively large compared with their bodies, so some degree of flexion may be present even when lying supine. In this case, support of the shoulders may be necessary. Most of the work should be done with the left hand, which lifts the tongue base, and the telescope should not be bent or levered on the teeth. This is potentially injurious to the airway, and the optical fibers are easily broken if the shaft is stressed. If the image on the screen changes from a circle to a "half moon," chances are that the telescope is being bent somewhere along its length.

Typically, spontaneous inspiration of room air is sufficient to maintain oxygenation during brief procedures. The advent of intravenous anesthetic agents means that an appropriate plane of anesthesia can be maintained without relying on volatile agents that have unpredictable entrainment during insufflation technique endoscopy. Some patients, especially neonates or children with marginal pulmonary function, may quickly desaturate because of anesthesia-induced hypoventilation. The longer the procedure takes, the greater the chance is that this will occur. It may be advisable to use the pharynx as an oxygen reservoir, enriching the inspired oxygen concentration. The easiest way to do this is to place a small, uncuffed endotracheal tube through the nose into the upper pharynx and connect it to the anesthesia circuit. As long as no laser or cautery is used, this technique is quite safe. If for some reason intravenous anesthetic agents are not available, the pharyngeal reservoir can be flushed with inhalational anesthetic agent at a low flow rate, helping to maintain an appropriate depth of anesthesia.

All operating room personnel must treat the unsheathed telescopes with respect. Although the steel bronchoscope tubes protect the optical components well, the telescopes themselves are easily bent or broken when they are used alone. This usually happens when they are dropped, incorrectly sterilized (e.g., autoclaved), or picked up by the shaft, especially if a heavy camera is attached to the eyepiece.

It may become necessary to use the bronchoscope tube even with the insufflation technique. If it is not possible to maintain spontaneous respiration, the bronchoscope can allow further inspection of the airway with positive-pressure ventilation as needed. This may be the case for children who are overly sensitive to the respiratory suppression of anesthetic agents. If secretions or blood impede the endoscopist's vision, the bronchoscope provides an easy pathway for guiding a flexible suction catheter adjacent to the telescope. This takes up room in the tube lumen and may require a thinner telescope than would be otherwise appropriate. When working in the subglottis and upper trachea (or in the proximal portion of a tracheotomy tract), it may be necessary to occlude the side slots of the bronchoscope with a Tegaderm dressing or to use a tracheoscope as described previously.

When passing the ventilating bronchoscope or tracheoscope, the endoscopist must be aware of the position of the sharp leading edge of the instrument. This may not be visible through the telescope but can abrade the glottis during insertion. To compensate, the tube is rotated 90° in a clockwise fashion before insertion (i.e., leading edge to the right) and passed slightly off center toward the left vocal cord (Fig. 44.11).

We prefer to perform bronchoscopy using a video camera attached to a video tape recorder and printer. Although there is a slight degradation of image quality, this allows continuous documentation of findings that may be fleeting and provides safer monitoring of residents in training who are performing endoscopy. Frequently, the instructor can help the student perform a difficult maneuver by guiding his or her hands while watching the video screen. If time allows, higher-quality images may be taken through the optical telescope using the previously described 35-mm camera and flash synchronization cable.

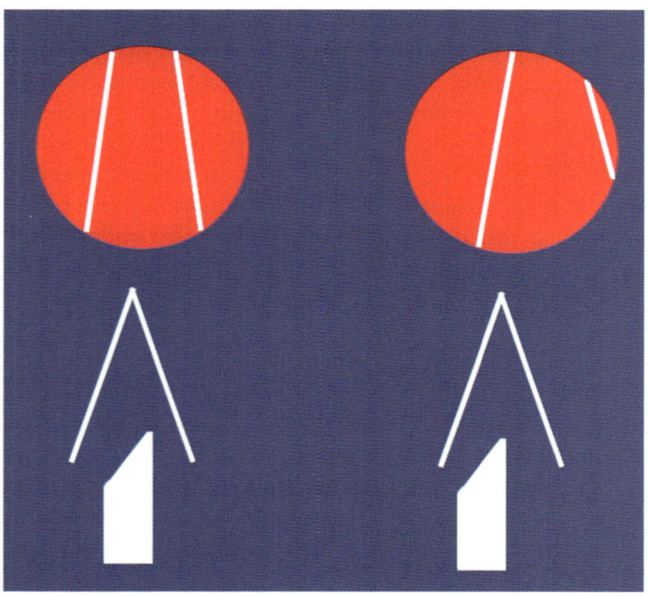
A B

**FIGURE 44.11.** The correct orientation for passing a bronchoscope into the glottis. The circle describes the endoscopic view, and the diagram below shows the orientation of the bronchoscope in relation to the vocal cords. The tube is rotated 90° clockwise, so that the leading tip is pointing to the right. **A:** The incorrect approach. As the telescope is centered on the glottis, the pointed tip of the bronchoscope abrades the right true vocal cord. **B:** The correct compensation. By visualizing the left vocal cord closer to the center of the endoscopic view, the tip passes between the cords and minimizes airway trauma.

## Tracheotomy Tube in Place

A tracheotomy tube clearly makes bronchoscopy much safer. The tube also provides a wider margin of safety with regard to titration of anesthetic agents. Laryngospasm due to an excessively light plane of anesthesia can still occur, but there is no risk of airway obstruction. Similarly, deeper planes of anesthesia causing apnea may easily be managed by supplemental positive-pressure ventilation while awaiting emergence, without disturbing the endoscopist. This does not usually require a cuff to seal the airway (as with adults) because infants and children typically have fairly high chest wall compliance, allowing ventilation at lower leak pressures. If the tube is in the way of the telescope, it may be partially or fully withdrawn from the tract to allow unimpeded examination of the lower airway.

## Subglottic and Tracheal Stenosis

One of the most common acquired forms of airway obstruction in children is stenosis, typically arising from prolonged endotracheal intubation for the respiratory distress syndrome of prematurity (30,31). In infants, this typically affects the subglottis, which is the bottleneck of the airway and a likely contact point between mucosa and the endotracheal tube. A similar phenomenon may be seen in older children and adults who have been intubated with cuffed endotracheal tubes, although in such cases, the affected area is usually in the upper trachea.

In preparation for the surgical management of laryngotracheal stenosis, the airway caliber must be assessed. The classic Cotton grading scale (described by and named for the senior author of this chapter) divided such patients into four groups. Grade I patients include all those with less than a 70% reduction in airway lumen. Symptoms are typically mild in these cases, possibly only manifesting during periods of upper respiratory tract infection. Grade IV represents a complete stenosis with no detectable lumen on endoscopy, no voice, and complete dependence on the tracheotomy tube for respiration. Grade III patients have a tiny lumen but more than 90% obstruction, and grade II represents patients with 70% to 90% obstruction. Although these groups have been prognostically useful and helpful in determining the most appropriate surgical approach to airway expansion, they are determined by subjective visual impression. They may not be appropriate for detecting more subtle changes, such as in individual patients after operative intervention or somatic growth. Furthermore, interobserver variability may result in inconstant grading of patients.

To provide a more reproducible and objective measure of airway caliber, the leak test is commonly used. This is done after visual inspection of the entire length of the stenosis, as described earlier. An appropriately sized, uncuffed endotracheal tube is placed through the stenotic area. Care is taken not to use an excessively large tube to avoid mucosal trauma. The tube is dipped in saline to lubricate the outer wall and passed in the usual fashion through the larynx. The anterior glottis is visualized with the telescope, and the pressure in the anesthesia circuit is slowly raised. The *leak point* is the pressure at which an air leak may be seen as bubbles around the tube or, alternatively, as auscultated over the larynx. If the leak is seen or heard at 10 cm $H_2O$ or less, the next larger tube is used, and the pressure is measured again. If the fit is tight or if the leak is at greater than 25 cm $H_2O$, the next smaller tube is used. The Cotton scale has been modified based on leak pressure and endotracheal tube size (32) (Fig. 44.12).

The management of significant pediatric airway stenosis is typically achieved through open surgical expansion (31,33) or resection (34,35) and is therefore outside the scope of this chapter. Endoscopic approaches may be appropriate for selected stenoses of the glottis, subglottis, or trachea as primary treatment (36,37) or as an adjuvant to open procedures. This is discussed elsewhere in this textbook and is not reviewed here separately. Tracheal stenoses may be dilated with a series of ventilating bronchoscopes or uncuffed styletted endotracheal tubes, although this is not recommended in place of tracheotomy if the narrowing is close to critical diameter. Recurrence is common after endoscopic treatment of tracheal stenoses by dilation, laser, or diathermy. It may be appropriate to initially dilate a tracheal stenosis to allow for safe anesthesia before definitive treatment (e.g., resection and anastomosis).

## Laryngeal and Tracheobronchial Papilloma

Human papillomavirus (HPV) infection may manifest in the pediatric laryngotracheal complex as chronic hoarseness or fulminant airway obstruction, depending on the extent and growth rate of the lesions. Although HPV infection can be seen in adults, the juvenile form is typically more aggressive, with multiple lesions requiring frequent treatment to maintain airway patency. Although several agents have shown promise as effective HPV chemotherapy (38–42), the primary treatment has remained serial endoscopic resection at appropriate intervals using the $CO_2$ laser (43). Although the $CO_2$ laser has the advantage of precise excision, it is limited by the well-known risks of laser surgery and the conventional delivery systems that make it hard to use in the distal airway. Investigations have explored the role of alternative laser beams (17), nonlaser coagulation beams (44), and mechanical debulking tools (45) for papilloma management.

**Classification of Stenosis With Actual Endotracheal Tube Size**

| Patient Age | | ID 2.0 | ID 2.5 | ID 3.0 | ID 3.5 | ID 4.0 | ID 4.5 | ID 5.0 | ID 5.5 | ID 6.0 |
|---|---|---|---|---|---|---|---|---|---|---|
| Premature | | | | | | | | | | |
| | | 40 | | | | | | | | |
| | | 58 | 30 | | | no obstruction | | | | |
| 0-3/12 | | 68 | 48 | 26 | | | | | | |
| 3/12-9/12 | No Detectable Lumen | 75 | 59 | 41 | 22 | | | | | |
| 9/12-2 | | 80 | 67 | 53 | 38 | 20 | | | | |
| 2 | | 84 | 74 | 62 | 50 | 35 | 19 | | | |
| 4 | | 86 | 78 | 68 | 57 | 45 | 32 | 17 | | |
| 6 | | 89 | 81 | 73 | 64 | 54 | 43 | 30 | 16 | |
| | Grade IV | Grade III | | | Grade II | | Grade I | | | |

**FIGURE 44.12.** Correlation of leak pressure for a given endotracheal tube, subglottic stenosis grade, and the expected diameters of the normal airway at different ages. (Adapted from Myer CM 3rd, O'Connor DM, Cotton RT. Proposed grading system for subglottic stenosis based on endotracheal tube sizes. *Ann Otol Rhinol Laryngol* 1994;103:319–323, with permission.)

Laser excision of laryngeal papillomas requires fine control of the beam, and suspension microlaryngoscopy is employed. The insufflation technique is preferred because there is no tube to catch fire or obstruct the field. Although laser-safe tubes are available, the smaller sizes are difficult to work with and may be traumatic to the airway, and they are to be avoided for this procedure if possible. Jet ventilation has the disadvantage of potentially seeding infectious particles from the mucosa or laser plume into the distal airway and even to the endoscopist (46–48). Barotrauma is also a risk when using jet ventilation in the face of partial airway obstruction. Apneic technique can be used with intermittent intubation and ventilation, but this is difficult to do without altering the microsurgical field, and repeated instrumentation may also potentially spread infection to previously unaffected areas of the airway.

To use the insufflation technique, the anesthesia circuit is attached to a side port of the Jako suspension laryngoscope. Care should be taken to avoid high concentrations of oxygen because of the risk of fire, and volatile agents should be replaced by intravenous anesthetic drugs to avoid contamination of the operating room. Perhaps the main drawback of the insufflation technique in this setting is that of insufficient relaxation without paralytic drugs, which may make suspension difficult. Fortunately, this is less of a problem in children than in adults. A deep plane of anesthesia is necessary—"just this side of apnea"— to avoid laryngospasm, maintain immobility of the laryngeal target, and allow adequate suspension and exposure. If there is an extensive carpet of papillomas with significant airway obstruction, it may be necessary to debulk the lesions before laser treatment. Despite an impressive appearance (Fig. 44.13), it is usually possible to intubate past the papilloma with a small endotracheal tube and use conventional microforceps to allow safe extubation and suspension for subsequent laser resection.

After the microscope is in position, the entire field outside of the laryngoscope lumen is draped with soaking-wet towels. A large syringe filled with saline is immediately available in case fire occurs despite precautions. Time is taken to ensure that the aiming beam is exactly coaxial with the cutting beam and that both are directed correctly along the long axis of the laryngoscope. The surgical field must be fully accessible to the beam without hitting the walls of the laryngoscope tube. Adequate depth of general anesthesia is ensured, as is appropriate topical anesthesia .

The $CO_2$ laser is used at 4 to 6 W in a pulsed mode with as small a spot size as possible using the micromanipulator. Large areas of papillomas may be treated in continuous mode, and the beam may be occasionally defocused to treat areas of hemorrhage. Care is taken not to be overly aggressive or to denude corresponding areas of the anterior glottis near the commissure to avoid scar and web formation (49,50). The laser is not curative; it is a temporizing measure while awaiting spontaneous remission of the disease.

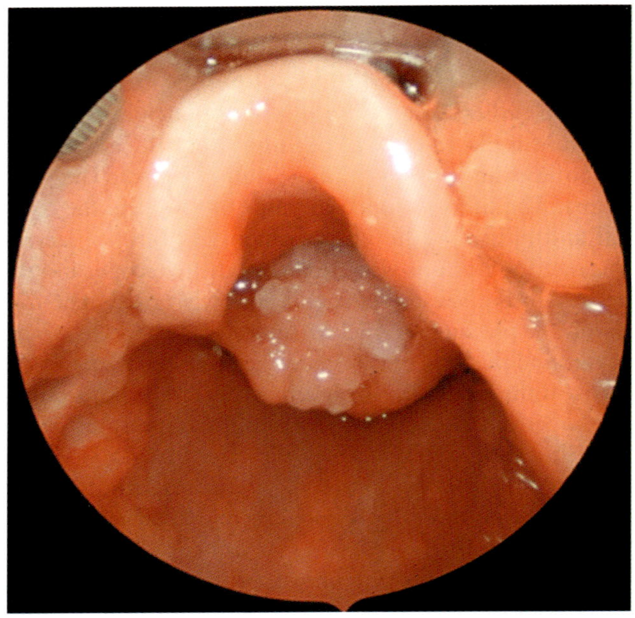

**FIGURE 44.13.** Extensive laryngeal papillomatosis obstructs the glottic lumen.

The goal should be a safe airway and a fairly good voice, not the complete eradication of all papillomas.

Distal papillomas present a serious surgical problem and are generally considered harbingers of advanced disease. The goal of treatment should be the maintenance of a safe airway. Overly aggressive laser surgery in the trachea can result in major complications (e.g., perforation, uncontrollable hemorrhage, worsening airway obstruction from edema and char). The Healy subglottiscope (Pilling Co., Philadelphia, PA) allows the use of a $CO_2$ laser and micromanipulator further into the airway than does the conventional microlaryngoscope, but at the cost of a constricted surgical field and frequent loss of binocular vision. This may be used through a tracheotomy site for disease near the carina. Because the subglottiscope passes into the airway itself, intermittent ventilation can be achieved by occluding the proximal end with the operator's thumb and ventilating through the anesthesia circuit adapted to the side port. Although not a perfect solution, this may be easier to use than the somewhat awkward adaptations of $CO_2$ lasers to ventilating bronchoscopes (51). Non-$CO_2$ lasers that may be delivered through flexible media (e.g., Nd:YAG and KTP) hold promise for this difficult situation (17).

## Airway Foreign Bodies

The techniques for retrieving airway foreign bodies have changed very little from the days of Chevalier Jackson in the early part of the 20th century. Perhaps the main advance since his time is the development of optical forceps, which bring the magnification and distal illumination of the surgical telescope to a variety of manipulation devices. This greatly facilitates the endoscopist's ability to work in small airways and to teach this procedure through video monitoring. The only disadvantage is that these instruments tend to be more delicate than their nonoptical counterparts and may occasionally fracture (Fig. 44.8). For this reason, they are generally not used for less delicate work, such as coin retrieval from the esophagus.

One of the most important principles in the management of airway foreign bodies is that they rarely manifest with acute airway obstruction. In the absence of such obstruction, no intervention should be undertaken unless conditions have been optimized, assembling the best possible endoscopist, anesthesiologist, and equipment. Children suspected of having chronically impacted foreign bodies in the airway may benefit from hospital admission and parenteral steroids for 1 to 2 days to reduce surrounding inflammation and granulation tissue (Fig. 44.14). Decadron is used at 0.6 mg/kg/day, divided into three daily doses. Cases of observed aspiration of dried peas or beans should not be delayed because of the likelihood of swelling in the airway. Similarly, known disc or "button" battery ingestion constitutes more of an emergency, because caustic leakage may result in esophageal wall injury in only a few hours (52).

Our preference for anesthetic management is the insufflation technique. Although many prefer to have complete relaxation of the patient with paralyzing agents, this requires the use of positive-pressure ventilation through a bronchoscope. Occasionally, this can result in distal impaction of a loose foreign body. An airway that the patient is maintaining by herself is often the safest, and paralysis may result in a situation in which ventilation is more difficult than with spontaneous respiration. This is especially true if prolonged instrumentation is necessary, resulting in edema or hematoma in the pharynx. With spontaneous respiration and topical anesthesia, it may be possible to retrieve a foreign body using only the unsheathed optical forceps, as described in the section on the General Approach to Diagnostic Rigid Laryngoscopy and Bronchoscopy.

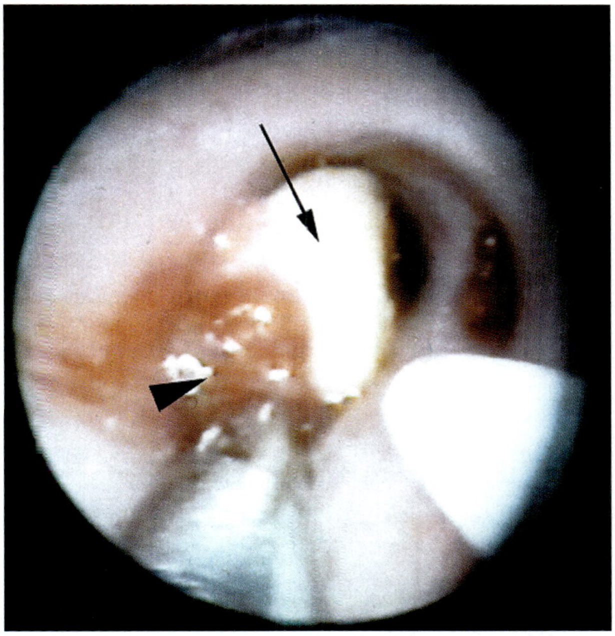

**FIGURE 44.14.** Granulation tissue *(arrowhead)* surrounding a chronically impacted peanut in the right mainstem bronchus *(arrow)*.

The bronchoscope tube may be needed if suctioning of blood or secretions is necessary. Patients with partial bronchial obstruction have a ventilation-perfusion mismatch and may quickly become hypoxic even if air movement in the remainder of the lungs is acceptable. In this situation, the bronchoscope allows the delivery of an oxygen-enriched gas mixture directly into the trachea through the anesthesia circuit while retrieving the foreign body.

After the object is well visualized and surrounding secretions have been cleaned, it should be grasped with an appropriate forceps. Care should be taken to grasp the object firmly but not to fragment it if it is fragile. If a bronchoscope is being used, the tube and forceps should be withdrawn as a unit to avoid "stripping off" the object at the end of the tube. Careful manipulation is necessary at the glottis, where the object may be stripped off into the trachea if it is sizable or has swelled considerably. Bronchoscopy should be repeated after extraction until the surgeon has ensured that no residual foreign bodies remain.

One of the major pitfalls in extracting airway foreign bodies is the worsening of airway obstruction during the procedure. Although a chronic foreign body past the carina rarely causes respiratory distress in an otherwise healthy patient, losing control of the object during extraction can have life-threatening results. If the foreign body is dropped in the trachea, it should be pushed down the same bronchus from which it was retrieved before another attempt is made. Significant edema and granulation tissue may result in airway obstruction even after the object is removed and may not resolve for days. If the contralateral mainstem bronchus is obstructed, ventilation and oxygenation may not be possible at all.

Occasionally, an organic foreign body swells so much after aspiration that it may not be possible to remove it through the glottis (Fig. 44.15). Two options remain: fragmentation or retrieval through a temporary tracheotomy. Although fragmentation appears less invasive, it should not be attempted by any but the most experienced operator, because multiple foreign bodies may then obstruct both lungs.

Sharp or pointed foreign bodies present a particular challenge to the endoscopist. Thankfully, this is becoming less

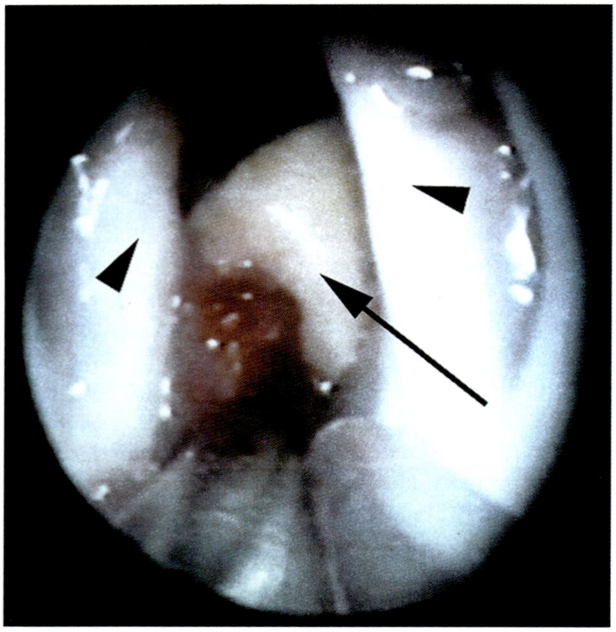

**FIGURE 44.15.** A large foreign body (i.e., a nut) in the airway *(arrow)* presents difficulty with extraction past the glottis *(arrowheads)*.

common as parents and manufacturing corporations have become more aware of the risks of small objects in the hands of young children. The best method for removing these objects is to sheath the point with the forceps or bronchoscope tube to protect the airway during extraction. If this is not possible, rotation forceps are available that allow the object to be removed with the point trailing. Each foreign body potentially requires a unique solution, and careful study before attempting extraction is vital, possibly with a duplicate of the object in question if available. This is not a skill that is easily acquired despite the advent of optical forceps and video monitoring. We are indebted to such dedicated and skilled surgeons such as Jackson and Holinger (1,9,53) for refining these techniques.

## Esophageal Foreign Bodies

When an object has been present in the esophagus for some time, a surrounding inflammatory reaction can result in a local mass effect (54) that can compress the airway from behind (Fig. 44.16). This can cause anything from a cough and stridor (55) to complete airway obstruction (56). Removal of the object usually results in resolution of the inflammation over the next few days if no full-thickness breakdown of the wall occurs. However, pulmonary edema has been reported in this setting (57), as is often seen in other situations in which airway obstruction is suddenly relieved.

Esophageal foreign bodies are commonly retrieved under general anesthesia with an endotracheal tube in place. Although some gastroenterologists have become proficient in the use of flexible esophagoscopy under mild sedation for this problem (58), such skill is not universal. Although there is no particular reason why many esophageal foreign bodies (e.g., coins) cannot be managed with flexible endoscopes, sharp objects or chronically retained objects with the possibility of complications are best managed by rigid techniques.

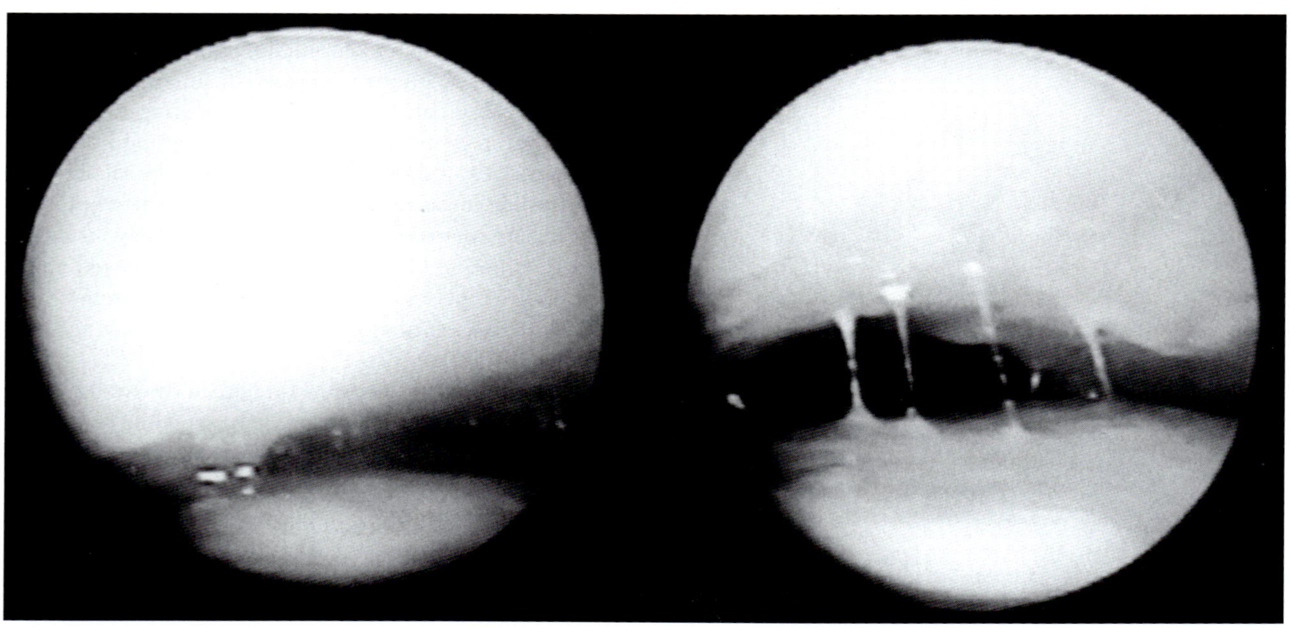

**FIGURE 44.16.** Tracheal compression from a chronically impacted coin in the upper esophagus at two levels in the airway.

Tracheal compression, airway obstruction, perforation, and fistulas between the esophagus and the trachea (59) or the aorta (60) have been reported in this setting. Similarly, the occasionally reported use of the fluoroscopy suite for Foley catheter extraction is discouraged because the lumen is not visualized, complications may be missed, and the clinical setting is often not conducive to rapid airway management or resuscitation if complications occur (61).

Most equipment manufacturers provide a range of pediatric esophagoscopes that can be fitted with the same telescopes used for the bronchoscopes. Although this provides excellent images of the esophageal wall, such optical devices are mainly of benefit in diagnostic esophagoscopy, in which subtle changes in the mucosa must be appreciated. The most common reason for rigid esophagoscopy in children—foreign body retrieval—usually does not require such equipment, and a simple open-tube esophagoscope may be easier to use. The entire range of grasping forceps should be available, especially if the foreign body is not the typical coin but is sharp or difficult to grasp (e.g., a smooth plastic bead). A flexible suction catheter may be kept in position during passage to keep the lumen clear of secretions, or careful, intermittent suctioning may be done with a rigid suction tube.

The technique for safe rigid esophagoscopy demands that the lumen be visualized at all times to avoid trauma to the esophageal wall. After the larynx has been visualized through the esophagoscope, the tip is passed posteriorly behind the arytenoids and cricoid plate to the esophageal inlet. This is found immediately posterior to the cricoid and slightly to the left. While the lumen is typically collapsed, the slit is usually well visualized, and secretions may be seen emanating from the lower esophagus. If there is any doubt, a soft suction catheter may be used as a probe to establish the site of the lumen, followed with the esophagoscope itself. When passing the upper portion of the esophagus, it is helpful to have an assistant raise the child's shoulders, easing the passage of the esophagoscope into the distal esophagus. Force should never be used, because an appropriately sized instrument should pass without difficulty through the entire length of the esophagus. Obstruction during passage usually represents incorrect positioning, although stenosis may be present in some patients. The fingers of the nondominant hand are used as a rest, as with a billiards cue, to support the tube and protect the upper teeth.

After the object is firmly grasped, the entire complex of the esophagoscope, the forceps, and the foreign body is withdrawn as a unit (as in bronchoscopy). No attempt should be made to pull the object into the lumen of the esophagoscope, with the exception of a sharp point that may need to be sheathed before withdrawal. After passing the upper esophageal sphincter, the operator should stand and change the direction of pull from superiorly to anteriorly, moving the equipment and foreign body smoothly out of the mouth. Care should be taken to avoid dropping the object in the mouth or dislodging the endotracheal tube. If visualization was incomplete during extraction or if the foreign body had fragmented, esophagoscopy should be repeated to thoroughly examine the esophagus for injury or a retained second foreign body.

## FLEXIBLE BRONCHOSCOPY

Flexible fiberoptic bronchoscopy has become an integral component of pediatric pulmonology over the past few decades. Significant technologic advances have resulted in better illumination, better optics, and instruments of increasingly smaller diameter. All but the smallest (2.2 mm) have suction channels. However, pediatric flexible bronchoscopes with an outer diameter of less than 4 mm usually do not accommodate instrumentation down the suction channel.

Although rigid bronchoscopes are generally used by otolaryngologists and other airway surgeons, flexible bronchoscopes are typically used by pulmonologists. These tools each have their own indications and limitations, with a significant degree of overlap between the personnel involved. Flexible instruments have the advantage of maneuverability in the bronchial tree past the mainstem bronchi, including retroflexion to examine branches of the airway that turn superiorly toward the endoscopist that are essentially inaccessible to rigid techniques. Rigid bronchoscopy requires general anesthesia, whereas flexible bronchoscopy can be performed with topical anesthesia and light sedation while maintaining spontaneous respiration. This avoids general anesthesia and enables a better assessment of airway motion and dynamic pathology (e.g., tracheomalacia). In some children, however, such an approach may be difficult because of a tenuous and/or hyperreactive airway or limited cooperation, making deeper levels of anesthesia more appropriate.

If general anesthesia is necessary and spontaneous ventilation is not possible, a flexible bronchoscope can be introduced through an endotracheal tube, tracheotomy tube, or laryngeal mask airway. A proximal seal valve allows the instrument to be introduced into the circuit without a large air leak, maintaining good ventilation. The smallest (2.2-mm) flexible bronchoscope can theoretically fit through a 2.5-mm endotracheal tube or a 3.0-mm tracheotomy tube. However the lumens of such small tubes can be significantly obstructed by the bronchoscope.

For transoral or transnasal introduction without mechanical ventilation, the cords are visualized and a local anesthetic solution is introduced down the suction channel and sprayed over the larynx into the lower airway. After a few seconds, the bronchoscope can be placed through the cords. The suction channel may be used to clear secretions and provide supplemental oxygen (although not ventilation). In experienced hands, it is possible to examine all segmental bronchi within 1 to 2 minutes using flexible bronchoscopy.

A flexible bronchoscope may provide valuable assistance in securing a "difficult airway" in which routine direct laryngoscopy and orotracheal intubation is compromised by the anatomy of the jaw, pharynx, or larynx. An appropriate endotracheal tube is threaded over the bronchoscope, and the instrument is passed into the airway under direct vision through the nose or mouth. The endotracheal tube is then advanced into the trachea over the bronchoscope. Such cases imply difficulty in visualizing the larynx on direct laryngoscopy, and are not to be confused with a "difficult airway" caused by stenosis. In the latter case, visualization is easy but intubation is not. Flexible laryngoscopy should not be used in this situation.

The maneuverability of the tip of the flexible bronchoscope permits easy access to the upper lobes of either lung. The suction channel allows subsegmental bronchoalveolar lavage to be performed with more accuracy than can be provided by a rigid bronchoscope. Even large mucus plugs may be removed with a flexible bronchoscope using a slow suction and withdrawal technique, despite the seemingly small suction channel.

The flexible bronchoscope does have several limitations compared with rigid endoscopy. It is not the best method for evaluation of the posterior glottis or posterior tracheal wall. Visualization of the subglottis is usually limited, because the transition between the view of the vocal cords and the upper trachea tends to be fairly rapid as the operator "threads the needle." Cases in which significant bleeding is anticipated are best handled with rigid telescopes that permit better suctioning. It is also generally not appropriate to remove foreign bodies using a flexible bronchoscope, given the lesser degree of airway control, the limited range of grasping instruments, and the small suction channel. However, flexible and rigid bronchoscopy should be considered complementary modalities for the investigation and treatment of pediatric airway disease.

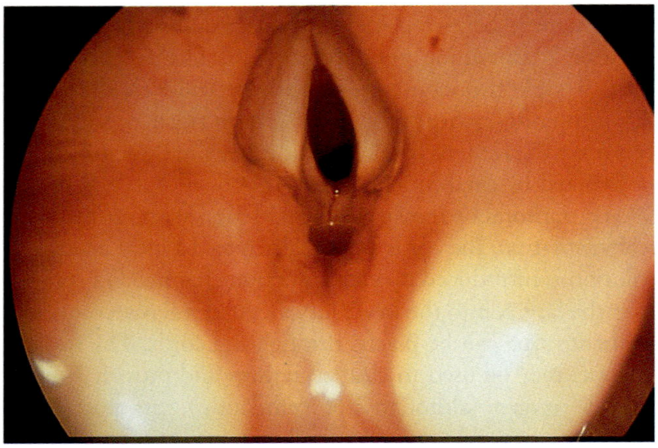

**FIGURE 44.17.** Case 1: An interarytenoid scar band.

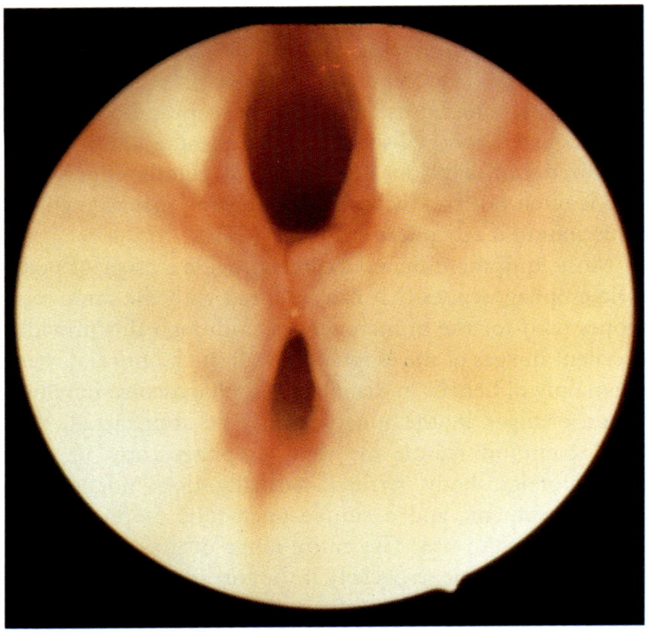

**FIGURE 44.18.** Case 1: An interarytenoid scar band.

## CASE EXAMPLES

### Case 1

A 6-year-old girl was to undergo general anesthesia for a dental procedure. Difficulty was encountered at intubation, and otolaryngologic consultation was requested. Her medical history included a prolonged intubation for external and inhalation burns 3 years earlier. Mild exercise intolerance had been observed since that time.

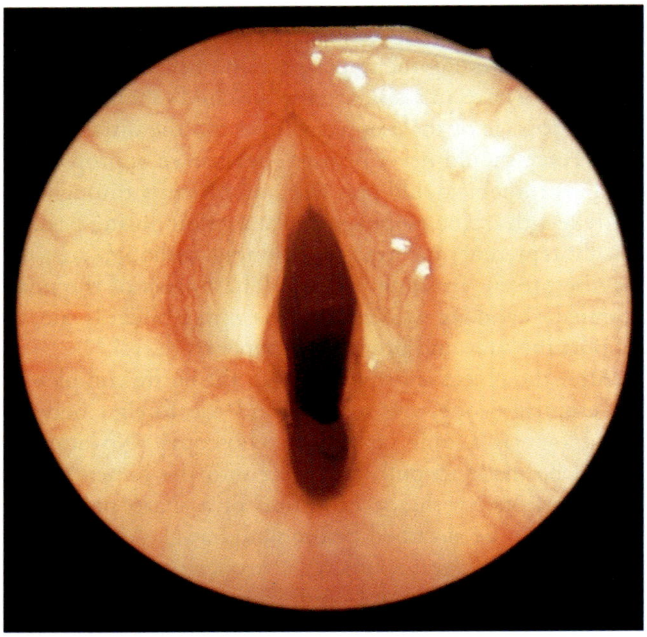

**FIGURE 44.19.** Case 1: Excision of an interarytenoid scar band.

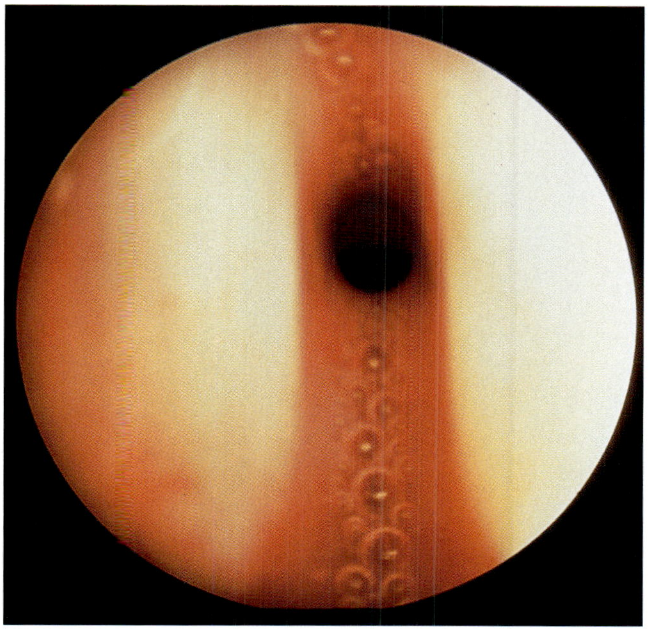

FIGURE 44.20. Case 2: Grade III congenital subglottic stenosis.

Examination confirmed an interarytenoid scar band (Figs. 44.17 and 44.18), which was excised using microlaryngeal instruments (Fig. 44.19). The patient has had no further symptoms.

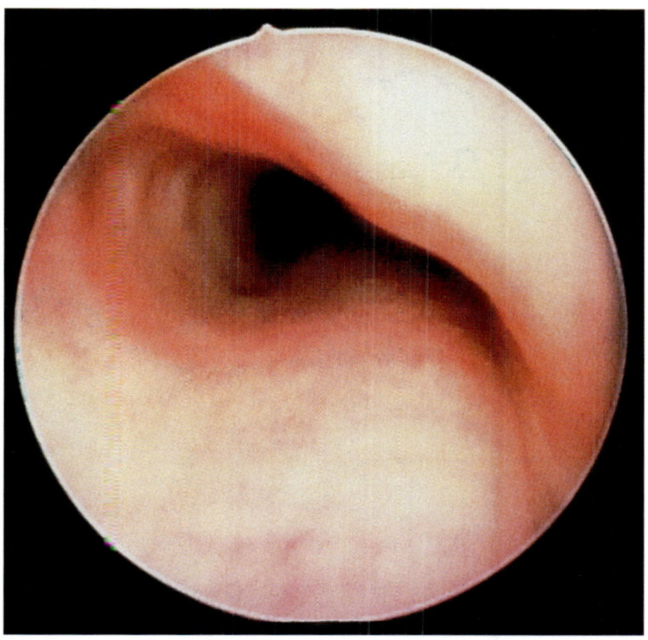

FIGURE 44.21. Case 2: Tracheal compression by the innominate artery.

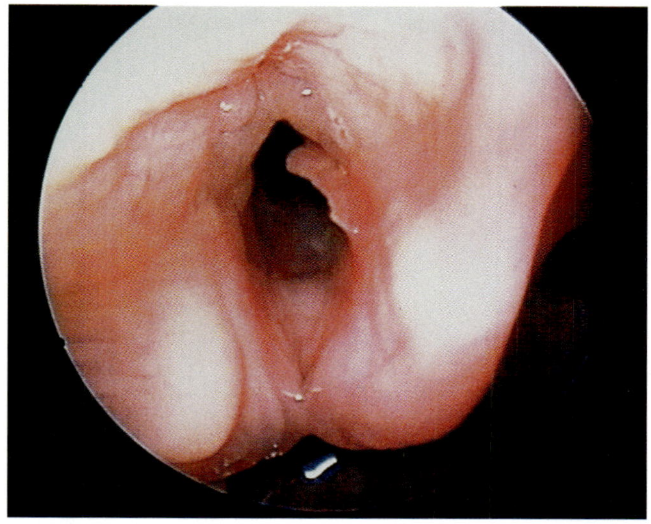

FIGURE 44.22. Case 2: Granulation tissue after single-stage laryngotracheoplasty and extubation.

## Case 2

A girl presented at the age of 2.5 years with Down syndrome and long-standing, mild inspiratory stridor at rest. Endoscopy confirmed a grade III congenital subglottic stenosis (Fig. 44.20) and significant innominate artery compression of the trachea (Fig. 44.21). She had gastroesophageal reflux disease that was controlled by medication.

Because of the prominence of the innominate artery, it was felt that a tracheotomy was undesirable. Magnetic resonance imaging (MRI) showed insufficient room to perform an aortopexy. A single-stage laryngotracheoplasty with ante-

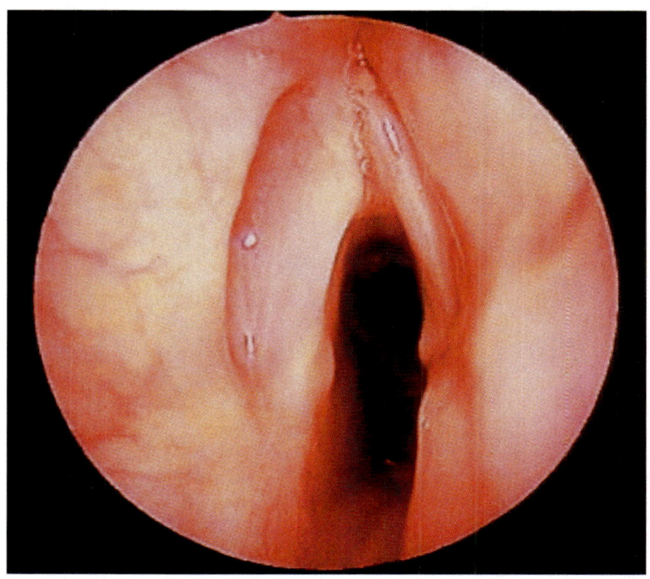

FIGURE 44.23. Case 2: 1-year follow-up examination after laryngotracheoplasty.

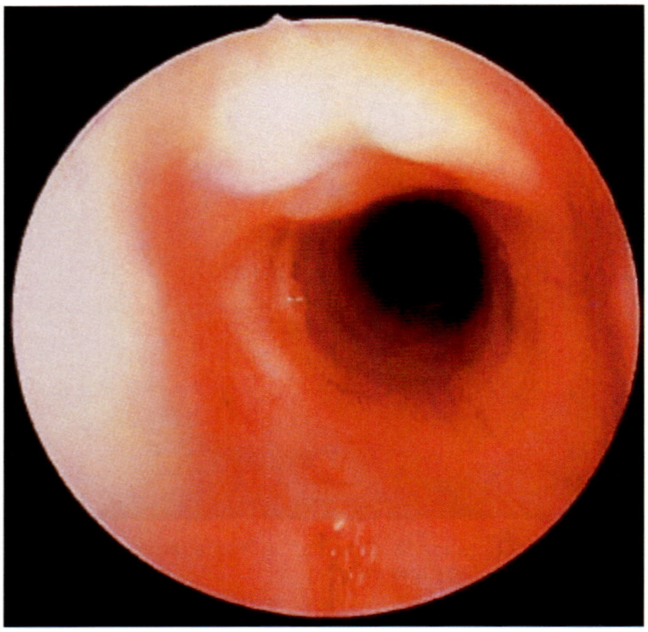

FIGURE 44.24. Case 2: 1-year follow-up examination after laryngotracheoplasty.

rior and posterior costal cartilage grafting was performed. The patient was kept intubated for 12 days. On extubation, the airway was greatly improved, although some granulation tissue was present (Fig. 44.22). At 1-year follow-up, the patient was symptom free (Figs. 44.23 and 44.24).

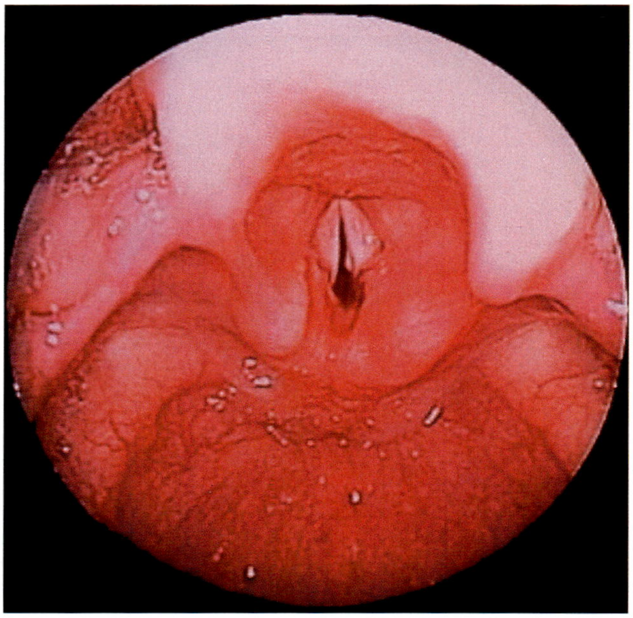

FIGURE 44.25. Case 3: Posterior glottic stenosis was misdiagnosed initially as bilateral vocal cord paralysis.

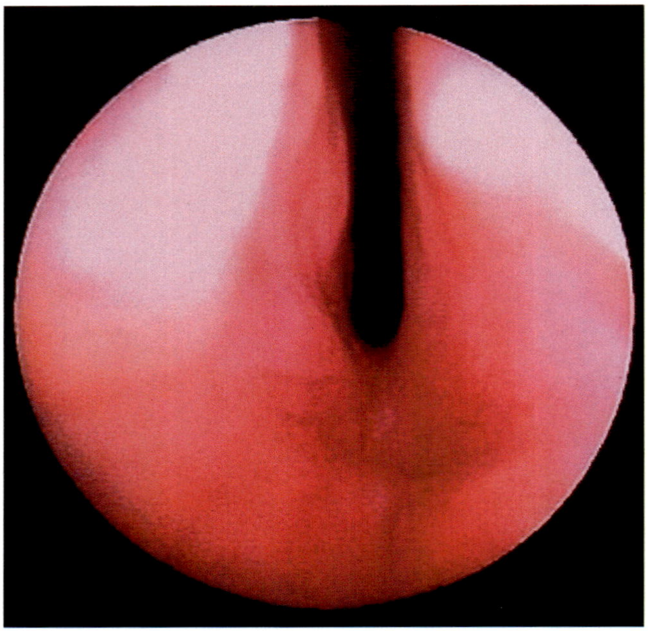

FIGURE 44.26. Case 3: Posterior glottic stenosis was misdiagnosed initially as bilateral vocal cord paralysis.

## Case 3

A boy presented at the age of 3 years, at which time he was tracheotomy dependent and had a diagnosis of bilateral vocal cord paralysis. He had been born at term with panhypopituitarism and required prolonged intubation because of neonatal

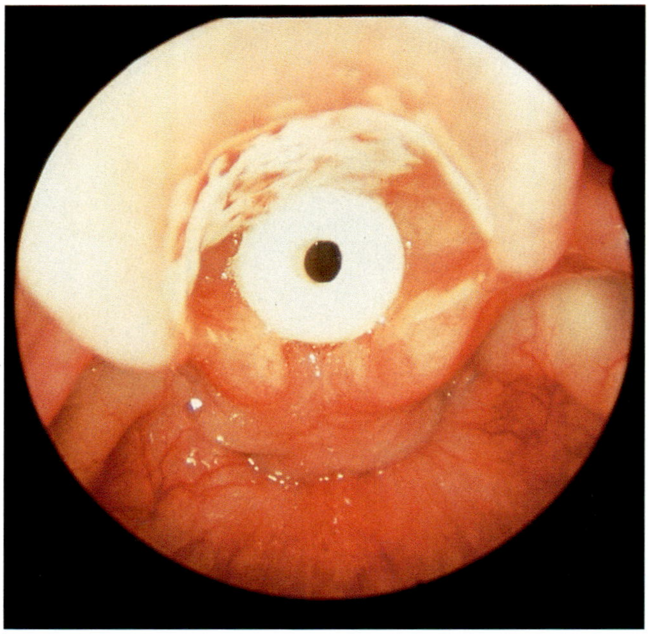

FIGURE 44.27. Case 3: Suprastomal stent used in the repair of posterior glottic stenosis.

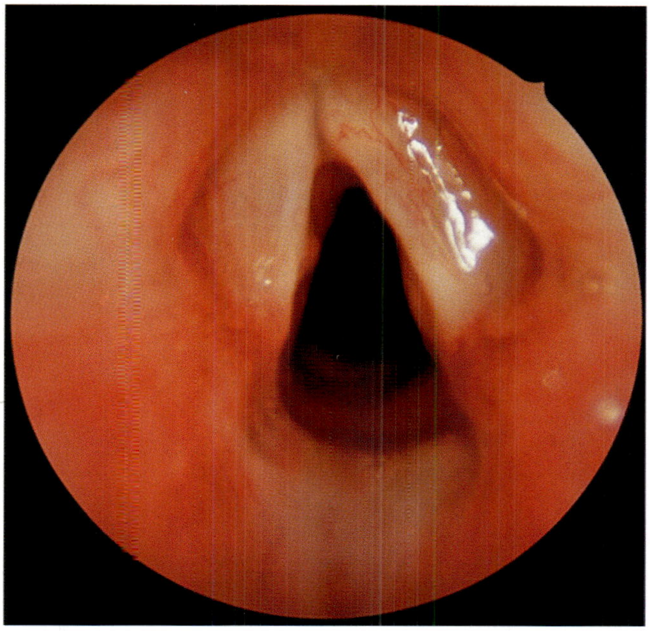

**FIGURE 44.28.** Case 3: Postoperative appearance of the posterior glottic stenosis repair with a costal cartilage graft.

sepsis. He could not be extubated, and a tracheotomy had been performed. Rigid endoscopy demonstrated a marked posterior glottic stenosis (Figs. 44.25 and 44.26). Flexible nasopharyngoscopy confirmed mobile but tethered vocal cords.

A two-stage laryngotracheal reconstruction using a posterior costal cartilage graft was performed. The graft was stabilized with a suprastomal stent (Fig. 44.27). The stent

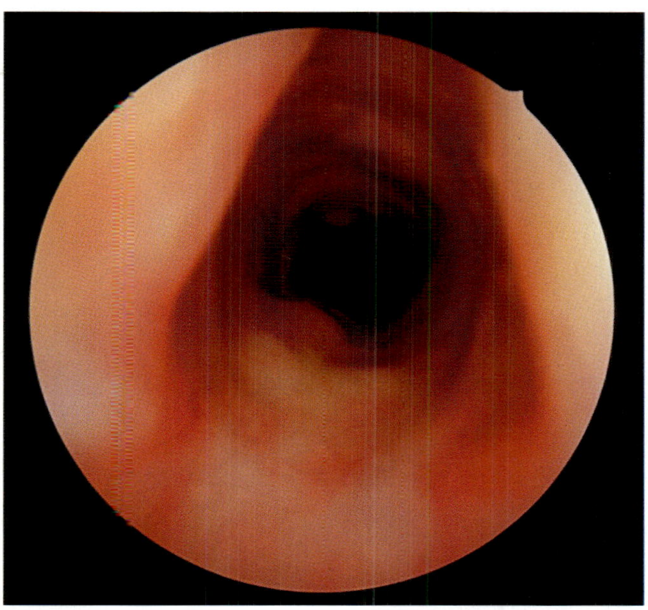

**FIGURE 44.29.** Case 3: Postoperative appearance of the posterior glottic stenosis repair with a costal cartilage graft.

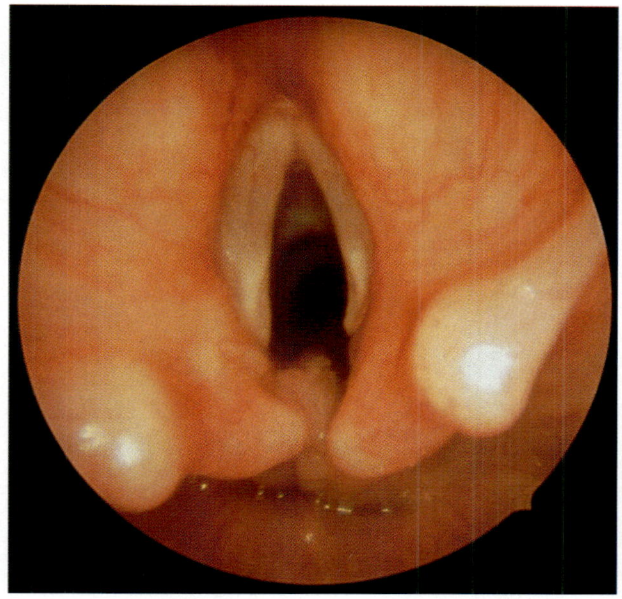

**FIGURE 44.30.** Case 4: Type III laryngotracheoesophageal cleft.

was removed at 6 weeks, and the tracheotomy tube removed 6 weeks later. The posterior costal cartilage graft was well mucosalized, and the child remains symptom free 2 years after the procedure (Figs. 44.28 and 44.29).

## Case 4

A 2-year-old girl presented with a previously diagnosed laryngotracheoesophageal cleft. She primarily relied on gas-

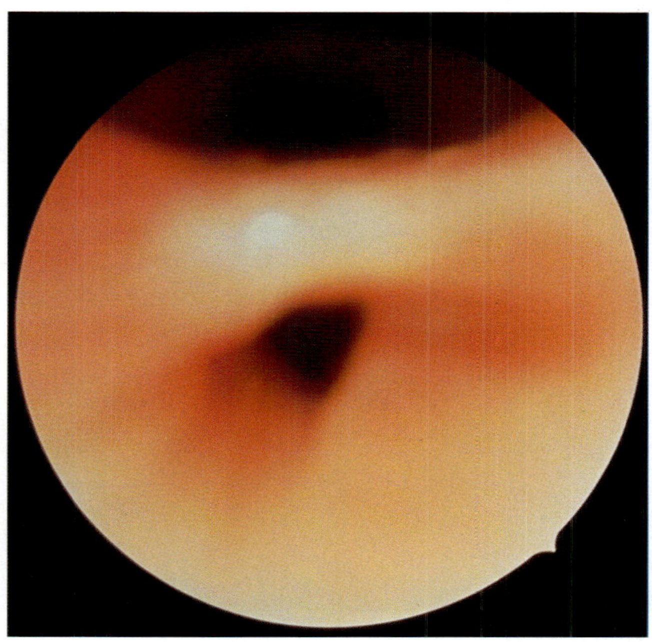

**FIGURE 44.31.** Case 4: Type III laryngotracheoesophageal cleft.

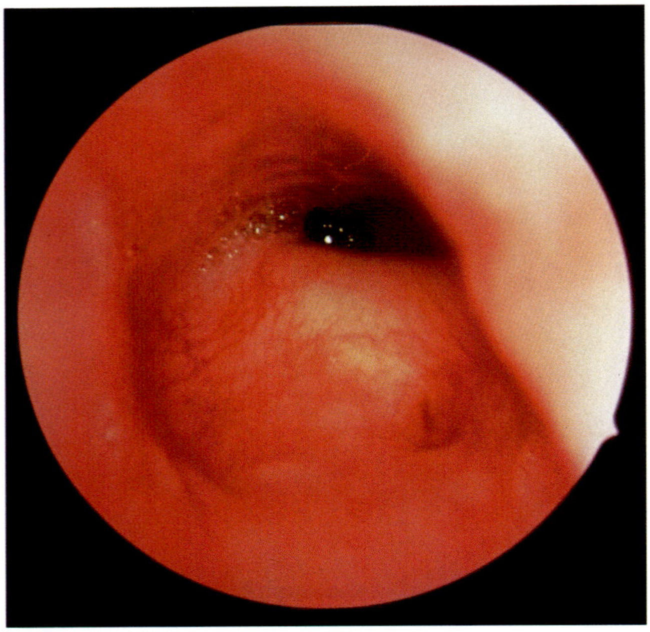

**FIGURE 44.32.** Case 4: Retroesophageal subclavian artery.

trostomy tube feedings but was receiving oral supplementation despite minor aspiration. She did not have a tracheotomy. Endoscopy confirmed a type III cleft (Fig. 44.30), and endoscopic probing clearly showed the common-party wall between the trachea and esophagus at the cleft apex below the cricoid (Fig. 44.31). Esophagoscopy confirmed the incidental finding of a retroesophageal subclavian artery (Fig. 44.32).

The patient had a single-stage repair of the cleft through an anterior laryngofissure and was successfully extubated on

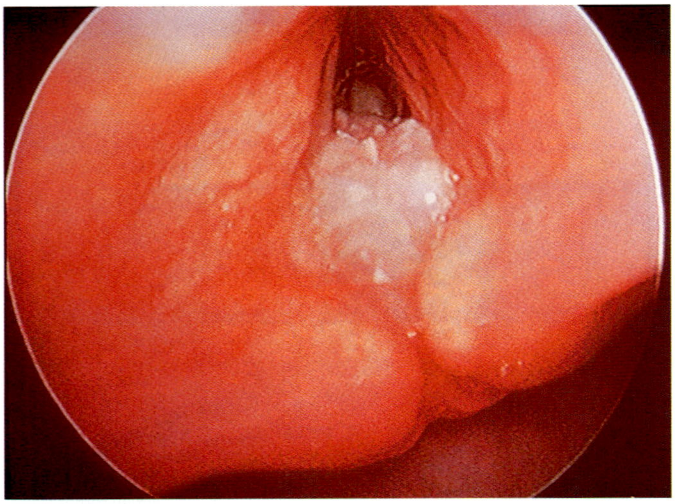

**FIGURE 44.33.** Case 4: Redundant mucosa after repair of a posterior laryngeal cleft.

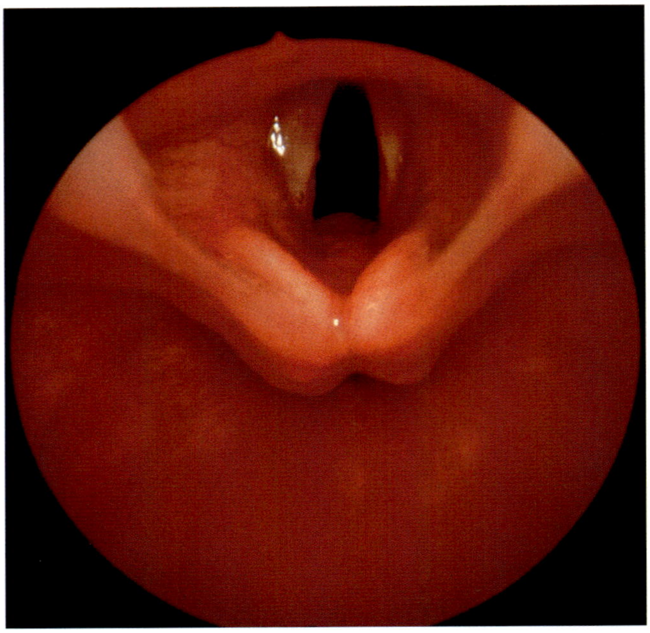

**FIGURE 44.34.** Case 4: Postoperative view.

the sixth postoperative day. There was initially some degree of mild stridor associated with redundant mucosa in the posterior glottis (Fig. 44.33), which required laser excision.

At follow-up, her airway was excellent, and she had no symptoms except for minimal dysphagia associated with the retroesophageal subclavian artery (Fig. 44.34).

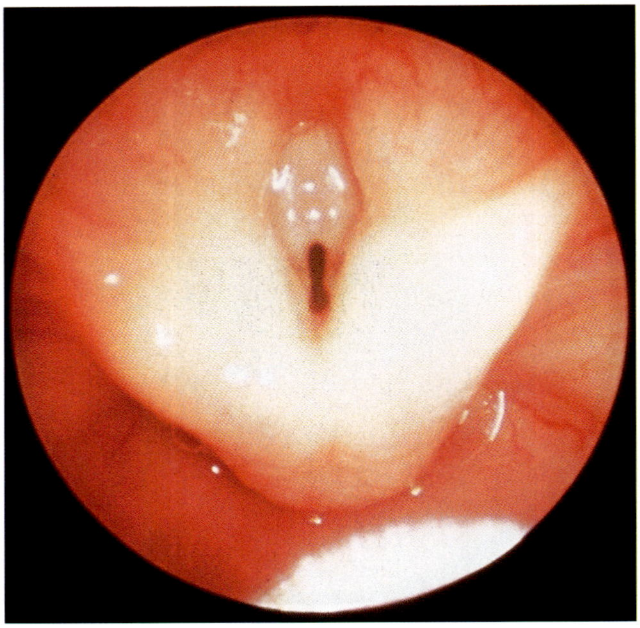

**FIGURE 44.35.** Case 5: Anterior glottic web.

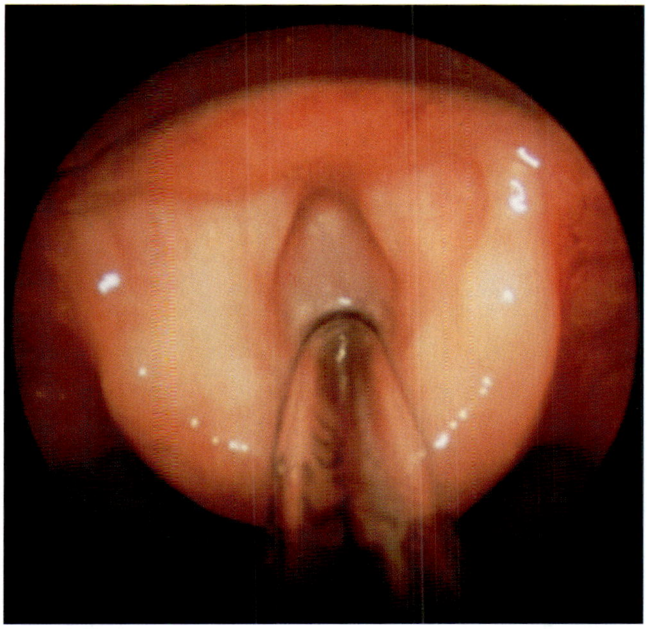

**FIGURE 44.36.** Case 5: Narrow airway associated with a glottic web.

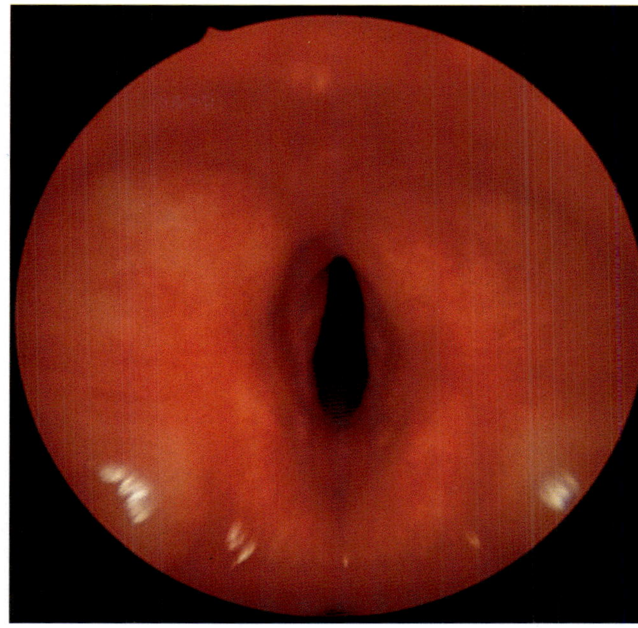

**FIGURE 44.38.** Case 5: 1-year postoperative view after repair of an anterior glottic web.

## Case 5

A 1-month-old girl was referred with mild inspiratory stridor at rest. She was found to have a partial laryngeal atresia with a thick anterior glottic web. Her sibling had died at birth because of complete laryngeal atresia. Endoscopy confirmed the web (Fig. 44.35), and no leak was found around a 2.0 endotracheal tube despite a subglottic pressure of 40 cm $H_2O$ (Fig. 44.36).

The patient did not have a tracheotomy, and it was elected to repair her larynx as a single-stage procedure with an anterior cricoid split and reconstruction of the anterior commissure through a laryngofissure. The laryngofissure was performed with endoscopic guidance, and the web can be seen stretched in Figure 44.37 just before division. The patient was left intubated for 10 days, and follow-up 1 year later showed an excellent anterior commissure with normal vocalization for her age (Fig. 44.38).

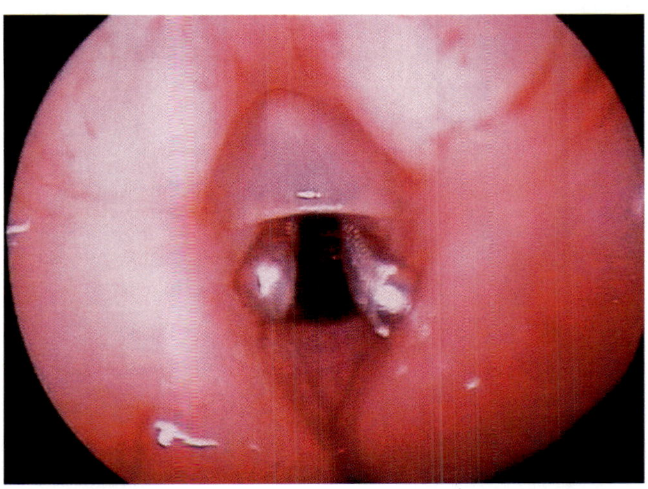

**FIGURE 44.37.** Case 5: Glottic web stretched just before division.

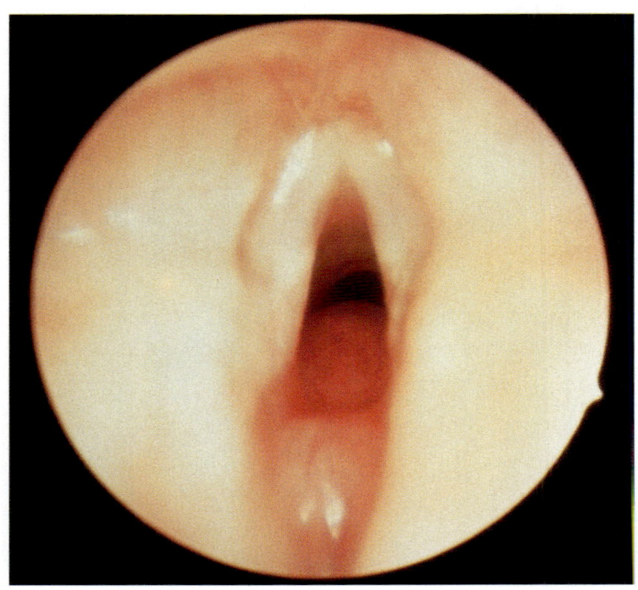

**FIGURE 44.39.** Case 6: Posteriorly based subglottic hemangioma.

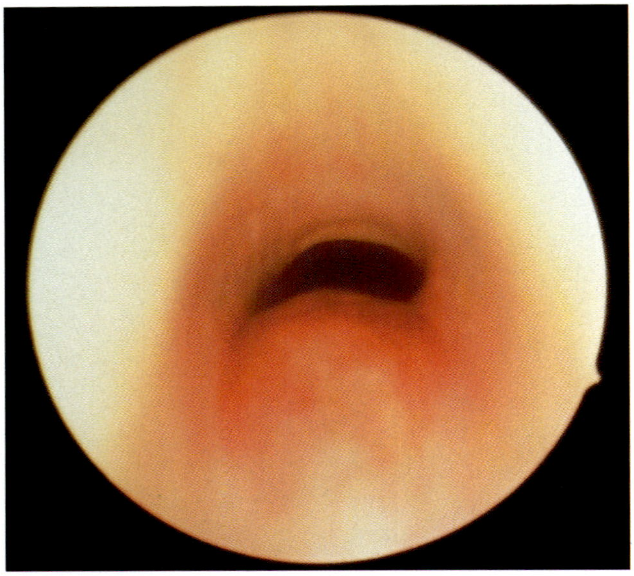

**FIGURE 44.40.** Case 6: Posteriorly based subglottic hemangioma.

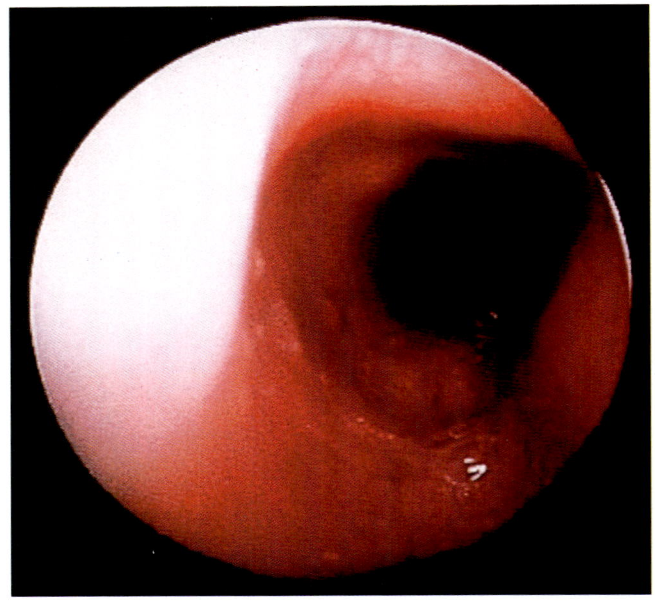

**FIGURE 44.42.** Case 6: Appearance after open excision of a posteriorly based subglottic hemangioma.

## Case 6

The child was referred at the age of 6 weeks with airway obstruction due to a subglottic hemangioma despite high-dose steroids. Rigid endoscopy confirmed a large, posteriorly based subglottic hemangioma (Figs. 44.39 and 44.40).

The options were tracheotomy, laser surgery, and excision. The parents wished to avoid a tracheotomy, and it was felt that serial laser excision in this area would risk formation of posterior glottic stenosis. The hemangioma was excised through an anterior laryngofissure as a single-stage procedure, and follow-up at 6 weeks showed a marked improvement to the airway (Figs. 44.41 and 44.42).

## Case 7

A girl was referred at the age of 14 months with extensive recurrent respiratory papillomatosis. By 18 months of age,

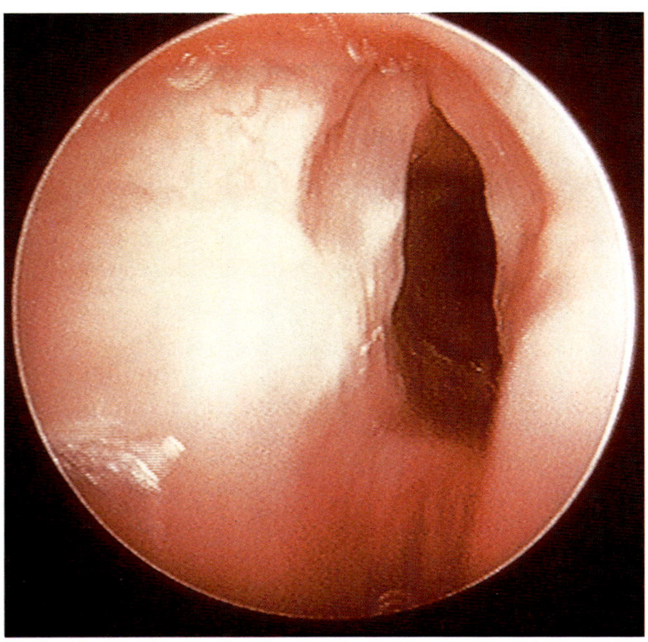

**FIGURE 44.41.** Case 6: Appearance after open excision of a posteriorly based subglottic hemangioma.

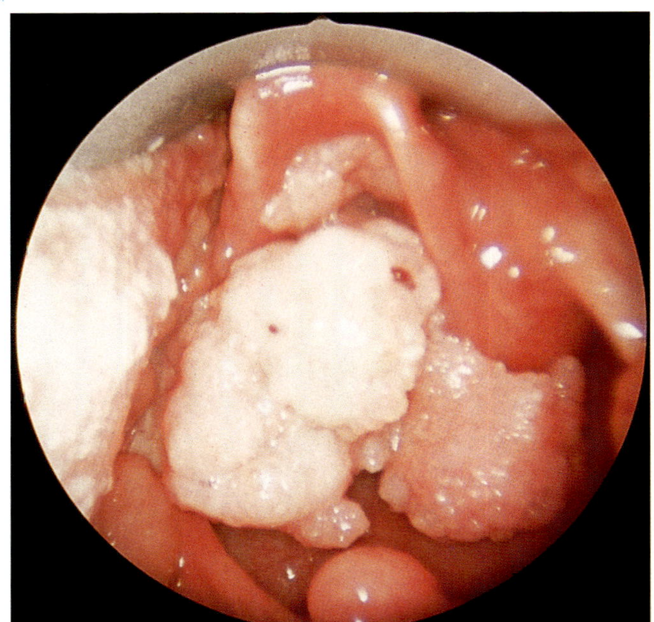

**FIGURE 44.43.** Case 7: Extensive papillomatosis.

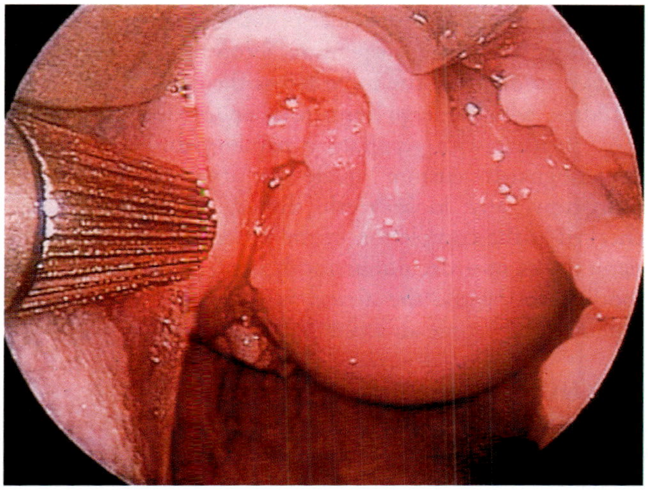

**FIGURE 44.44.** Case 7: Internal laryngocele associated with an obstructing papilloma of the airway.

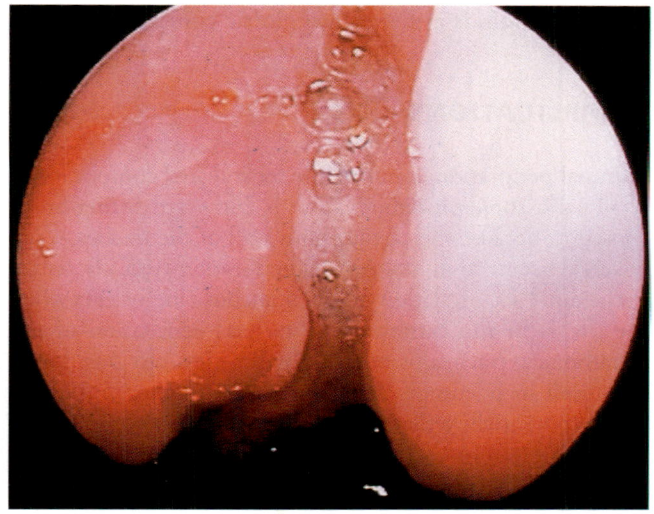

**FIGURE 44.46.** Case 7: Recent quiescence of a papilloma after excision of an internal laryngocele.

the papillomatosis was extensive enough to require placement of a tracheotomy. At this time, there was already disease in the subglottis, but the worst papillomas remained in the glottic and supraglottic regions (Fig. 44.43). The disease continued to progress, with papillomas affecting the trachea, glottis, supraglottis, pharynx, and nasopharynx.

At 5 years of age, she developed an internal laryngocele because of obstruction of her ventricle (Fig. 44.44). By 8 years of age, the papillomas were improving, but decannulation could not be considered because of the obstructing saccular cyst. The cyst was excised through an open approach, with dissection achieved through the thyrohyoid membrane, staying external to the pharyngeal mucosa. A large cyst was removed, with the neck completely occluded by papillomas. Postoperatively, access to the larynx was greatly improved by removal of this lesion, but there was an initial resurgence in papilloma activity (Fig. 44.45). Subsequently, the papillomatosis rapidly became quiescent (Fig. 44.46), and decannulation is being contemplated.

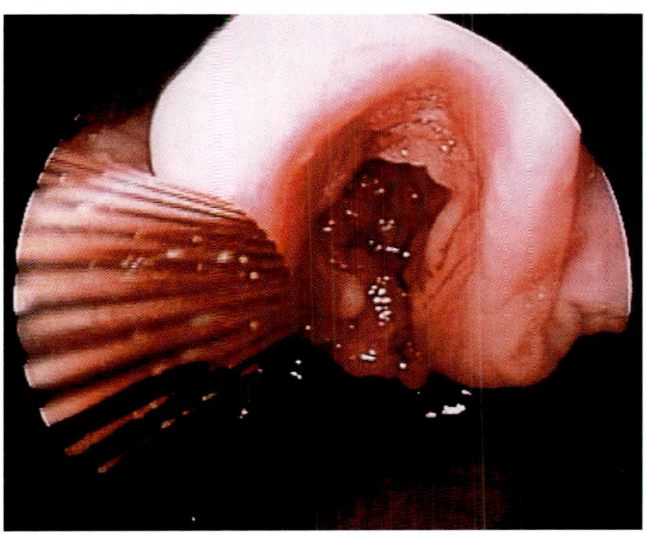

**FIGURE 44.45.** Case 7: Resurgence of a papilloma after excision of an internal laryngocele.

## POSTOPERATIVE CARE

Little intervention is necessary after uncomplicated diagnostic endoscopy of the upper aerodigestive tract in children. If iatrogenic trauma to the airway or esophagus is suspected, a chest radiograph should be obtained before discharge from the recovery room to rule out the presence of pneumothorax or mediastinal changes due to the presence of air or bleeding. Patients who have undergone extraction of chronic esophageal foreign bodies with mucosal injury should undergo contrast esophagography before feeding. After removal of a chronic airway foreign body, the patient should be observed at least overnight, and a follow-up chest x-ray film should be obtained the morning after to ensure improvement in any pulmonary pathology. Patients who have undergone therapeutic bronchoscopy or laryngoscopy for any mass lesions (e.g., papillomas, cysts, polyps) should be observed before discharge to ensure no airway obstruction is incipient. All such patients generally receive intravenous Decadron intraoperatively (1 mg/kg, up to a total dose of 12 mg).

Patients who are expected to have significant crusting or mucosal defects (e.g., children with papillomas undergoing laser laryngoscopy), should be treated with humidification, hydration, and systemic antibiotics, especially if there is potential for cartilage exposure. Diet is generally unrestricted, but patients at risk for temporary aspiration (e.g., after laser cordotomy for vocal cord paralysis) should avoid thin liquids at first, until glottic competence is certain.

## COMPLICATIONS

Luminal perforation is among the most feared complications of all endoscopic procedures. This is fairly rare during bronchoscopy, because the cartilaginous wall of the trachea is relatively resistant to injury. Airway perforation typically results in the rapid accumulation of subcutaneous emphysema when the site is in the extrathoracic trachea. Perforation of the intrathoracic trachea or bronchi may be less obvious, but it can result in pneumomediastinum, pneumothorax (including the potentially lethal tension pneumothorax), or injury to a major intrathoracic blood vessel. Extravasation of air is exacerbated by positive-pressure ventilation, but minor perforations usually heal spontaneously after appropriate drainage has been achieved. Perforation of the esophagus is more common but may be less obvious initially. Signs of crepitus, deep neck infection, or mediastinitis (e.g., fever, tachycardia) may develop over the next 1 or 2 days. Contrast esophagography is indicated if transmural injury is suspected. Management of significant esophageal perforation usually involves open draining and may require surgical repair.

Laryngoscopy and bronchoscopy can result in laryngospasm if the patient is not appropriately anesthetized topically and systemically. Although laryngospasm should eventually break spontaneously, complications such as arrhythmias, postobstructive pulmonary edema, and hypoxic brain injury can occur. Infants are especially vulnerable because their airway reflexes may be immature and hyperreactive and because their pulmonary functional residual capacity is low, resulting in more rapid desaturation than in adults. Laryngospasm is treated with positive-pressure mask ventilation, followed by paralyzing agents if necessary. These can be given by the intramuscular route if no intravenous line is available. Frantic attempts at endotracheal intubation should be discouraged, because trauma from the tube can result in edema or hematoma in the airway. Although laryngospasm eventually resolves and can be treated with paralyzing agents, edema or hematoma may result in life-threatening airway obstruction.

Patients with reactive airway disease are especially at risk for developing bronchospasm, because the inhalational agents used for anesthesia cause various degrees of airway irritation. This effect is compounded if inflammation is present in the airway, as in cases of upper respiratory tract infection. Given the additive effect of inflammation and anesthetic gasses, all elective endoscopy should be deferred until any acute infection has resolved.

The surgeon should be aware of the potential for dental trauma during endoscopy. Bronchoscopes, laryngoscopes, and esophagoscopes can rest on the upper teeth if care is not taken. Chipping or displacement of the central incisors can easily occur, and cosmetic dental work is at risk for fracture if undue pressure is placed on the upper teeth.

Dental injury is a particular problem during suspension laryngoscopy. During suspension, a tooth protector should be used to dissipate the force across the entire dental arch. Children who undergo numerous endoscopic procedures (i.e., patients with respiratory papillomatosis) may have dental guards custom made for their teeth. Before endoscopy, any loose teeth should be identified and checked at the completion of the procedure. Although the natural loss of a deciduous tooth is of no concern, if the tooth is lost while the airway is unprotected, it has the potential to become an aspirated foreign body.

## ACKNOWLEDGMENT

We would like to thank Francine Yudkowitz, M.D., Director of Pediatric Anesthesia at Mount Sinai Hospital, for her assistance with this chapter.

## REFERENCES

1. Holinger LD, Lusk RP, Green CG. *Pediatric laryngology and bronchoesophagology*. Philadelphia: Lippincott–Raven Publishers, 1997.
2. Myer CM, Cotton RT, Shott SR. *The pediatric airway: an interdisciplinary approach*. Philadelphia: JB Lippincott, 1995.
3. Alberti PW. The history of laryngology: a centennial celebration. *Otolaryngol Head Neck Surg* 1996;14:345–354.
4. Bailey B. Laryngoscopy and laryngoscopes—who's first? The forefathers/four fathers of laryngology. *Laryngoscope* 1996;106: 939–943.
5. Kirstein A. Autoskopie des Larynx und der Trachea. Laryngoscopia direeta, Euthyskopie, Besichtigung ohne Spiegel. *Arch Laryngol Rhinol* 1895;3:156–164.
6. Brunings W. *Direct laryngoscopy, bronchoscopy, and oesophagoscopy* [translated by WG Howarth]. London: Bailliere, Tindall & Cox, 1912.
7. Killian G. Die Schwebelaryngoscopie. *Arch Laryngol Rhinol* 1912;26:277–317.
8. Jackson C. *The life of Chevalier Jackson: an autobiography*. New York: Macmillan, 1938.
9. Jackson C, Jackson CL. Diseases of the air and food passage of foreign body origin. Philadelphia: WB Saunders, 1936.
10. Lamm H. Biegsame optische Gerate. *Z Instrumentenkd* 1930;50: 579–581.
11. Hopkins HH, Kapany NS. A flexible fiberscope. *Nature* 1954; 173:39–41.
12. Linder TE, Simmen D, Stool SE. Revolutionary inventions in the 20th century: the history of endoscopy [See comments]. *Arch Otolaryngol Head Neck Surg* 1997;123:1161–1163.
13. Jako GJ. Laser surgery of the vocal cords: an experimental study with carbon dioxide lasers on dogs. *Laryngoscope* 1972;82: 2204–2216.
14. Rebeiz EE, Shapsay SM, Ingrams DR. Laser applications in the tracheobronchial tree. *Otolaryngol Clin North Am* 1996;29: 987–1003.
15. Shapshay SM. Laser applications in the trachea and bronchi: a comparative study of the soft tissue effects using contact and noncontact delivery systems. *Laryngoscope* 1987;97:1–26.
16. Werkhaven J. Laser applications in pediatric laryngeal surgery. *Otolaryngol Clin North Am* 1996;29:1005–1010.
17. Rimell FL, Shapiro AM, Mitskavich MT, et al. Pediatric fiberoptic laser rigid bronchoscopy. *Otolaryngol Head Neck Surg* 1996; 114:413–417.

18. Lusk RP. Decision making. In: Holinger LD, Lusk RP, Green CG, eds. *Pediatric laryngology and bronchoesophagology*. Philadelphia: Lippincott-Raven, 1997:35–39.
19. Wiseman NE, Sanchez I, Powell RE. Rigid bronchoscopy in the pediatric age group: diagnostic effectiveness. *J Pediatr Surg* 1992; 27:1294–1297.
20. Silva AB, Muntz HR, Clary R. Utility of conventional radiography in the diagnosis and management of pediatric airway foreign bodies. *Ann Otol Rhinol Laryngol* 1998;107:834–838.
21. Zerella JT, Dimler M, McGill LC, et al. Foreign body aspiration in children: value of radiography and complications of bronchoscopy. *J Pediatr Surg* 1998;33:1651–1654.
22. Darrow DH, Holinger LD. Aerodigestive tract foreign bodies in the older child and adolescent. *Ann Otol Rhinol Laryngol* 1996; 105:267–271.
23. Tibbling L, Bjorkhoel A, Jansson E, et al. Effect of spasmolytic drugs on esophageal foreign bodies. *Dysphagia* 1995;10: 126–127.
24. O'Hara SM, Donnelly LF, Chuang EM, et al. Radiographic appearance and hazards of gastric retention of zinc based pennies. Presented at the Radiologic Society of North America, 84th Scientific Assembly and Annual Meeting, Chicago, IL. *Radiol Soc North Am* 1998;209[Suppl]:249.
25. Halstead LA. Gastroesophageal reflux: a critical factor in pediatric subglottic stenosis. *Otolaryngol Head Neck Surg* 1999;120: 683–688.
26. Halstead LA. Role of gastroesophageal reflux in pediatric upper airway disorders. *Otolaryngol Head Neck Surg* 1999;120: 208–214.
27. Walner DL, Stern Y, Gerber ME, et al. Gastroesophageal reflux in patients with subglottic stenosis. *Arch Otolaryngol Head Neck Surg* 1998;124:551–555.
28. Rothschild MA. The airway scale: a simple tool for comparing calibers of airway devices. *Otolaryngol Head Neck Surg* 1994;111: 847–848.
29. Roach JM, Ripple G, Dillard TA. Inadvertent loss of bronchoscopy instruments in the tracheobronchial tree. *Chest* 1992; 101:568–569.
30. McDonald I. Prolonged nasotracheal intubation. *Br J Anaesth* 1965;37:161.
31. Cotton RT. The problem of pediatric laryngotracheal stenosis: a clinical and experimental study on the efficacy of autogenous cartilaginous grafts placed between the vertically divided halves of the posterior lamina of the cricoid cartilage. *Laryngoscope* 1991; 101:1–34.
32. Myer CM 3rd, O'Connor DM, Cotton RT. Proposed grading system for subglottic stenosis based on endotracheal tube sizes. *Ann Otol Rhinol Laryngol* 1994;103:319–323.
33. Cotton RT, Myer CM, O'Connor DM, et al. Pediatric laryngotracheal reconstruction with cartilage grafts and endotracheal tube stenting: the single-stage approach. *Laryngoscope* 1995;105: 818–821.
34. Molter DW, Cotton RT. Management of tracheal stenosis in children. *Acta Otorhinolaryngol Belg* 1995;49:383–387.
35. Stern Y, Gerber ME, Walner DL, et al. Partial cricotracheal resection with primary anastomosis in the pediatric age group. *Ann Otol Rhinol Laryngol* 1997;106:891–896.
36. Rimell FL, Dohar JE. Endoscopic management of pediatric posterior glottic stenosis. *Ann Otol Rhinol Laryngol* 1998;107: 285–290.
37. Shapshay SM, Beamis JF Jr, Hybels RL, et al. Endoscopic treatment of subglottic and tracheal stenosis by radial laser incision and dilation. *Ann Otol Rhinol Laryngol* 1987;96:661–664.
38. Snoeck R, Wellens W, Desloovere C, et al. Treatment of severe laryngeal papillomatosis with intralesional injections of cidofovir [(S)-1-(3-hydroxy-2-phosphonylmethoxypropyl)cytosine]. *J Med Virol* 1998;54:219–225.
39. Rosen CA, Woodson GE, Thompson JW, et al. Preliminary results of the use of indole-3-carbinol for recurrent respiratory papillomatosis. *Otolaryngol Head Neck Surg* 1998;118:810–815.
40. Kashima H, Leventhal B, Clark K, et al. Interferon alfa-n1 (Wellferon) in juvenile onset recurrent respiratory papillomatosis: results of a randomized study in twelve collaborative institutions. *Laryngoscope* 1988;98:334–340.
41. Healy GB, Gelber RD, Trowbridge AL, et al. Treatment of recurrent respiratory papillomatosis with human leukocyte interferon: results of a multicenter randomized clinical trial. *N Engl J Med* 1988;319:401–407.
42. Abramson AL, Waner M, Brandsma J. The clinical treatment of laryngeal papillomas with hematoporphyrin therapy. *Arch Otolaryngol Head Neck Surg* 1988;114:795–800.
43. Strong MS, Vaughan CW, Cooperband SR, et al. Recurrent respiratory papillomatosis: management with the $CO_2$ laser. *Ann Otol Rhinol Laryngol* 1976;85:508–516.
44. Bergler W, Honig M, Gotte K, et al. Treatment of recurrent respiratory papillomatosis with argon plasma coagulation. *J Laryngol Otol* 1997;111:381–384.
45. Myer CM 3rd, Willging JP, McMurray S, et al. Use of a laryngeal micro resector system. *Laryngoscope* 1999;109:1165–1166.
46. Abramson AL, DiLorenzo TP, Steinberg BM. Is papillomavirus detectable in the plume of laser-treated laryngeal papilloma? *Arch Otolaryngol Head Neck Surg* 1990;116:604–607.
47. Hallmo P, Naess O. Laryngeal papillomatosis with human papillomavirus DNA contracted by a laser surgeon. *Eur Arch Otorhinolaryngol* 1991;248:425–427.
48. Kashima HK, Kessis T, Mounts P, et al. Polymerase chain reaction identification of human papillomavirus DNA in $CO_2$ laser plume from recurrent respiratory papillomatosis. *Otolaryngol Head Neck Surg* 1991;104:191–195.
49. Crockett DM, McCabe BF, Shive CJ. Complications of laser surgery for recurrent respiratory papillomatosis. *Ann Otol Rhinol Laryngol* 1987;96:639–644.
50. Wetmore SJ, Key JM, Suen JY. Complications of laser surgery for laryngeal papillomatosis. *Laryngoscope* 1985;95:798–801.
51. Ossoff RH, Duncavage JA, Toohill RJ, et al. Limitations of bronchoscopic carbon dioxide laser surgery. *Ann Otol Rhinol Laryngol* 1985;94:498–501.
52. Litovitz T, Schmitz BF. Ingestion of cylindrical and button batteries: an analysis of 2382 cases [See comments]. *Pediatrics* 1992; 89:747–757.
53. Holinger LD. Management of sharp and penetrating foreign bodies of the upper aerodigestive tract. *Ann Otol Rhinol Laryngol* 1990;99:684–688.
54. Fernandes ET, Hollabaugh RS, Boulden T. Mediastinal mass and radiolucent esophageal foreign body. *J Pediatr Surg* 1989;24: 1135–1136.
55. Kirks DR, Merten DF. Stridor in infants and children due to esophageal inflammatory disease. *Gastrointest Radiol* 1980;5:321–323.
56. Byard RW, Moore L, Bourne AJ. Sudden and unexpected death—a late effect of occult intraesophageal foreign body. *Pediatr Pathol* 1990;10:837–841.
57. Rao CC, McNiece WL, Krishna G. Acute pulmonary edema after removal of an esophageal foreign body in an infant. *Crit Care Med* 1986;14:988–989.
58. Webb WA. Management of foreign bodies of the upper gastrointestinal tract: update [See comments]. *Gastrointest Endosc* 1995; 41:39–51.
59. Obiako MN. Tracheoesophageal fistula: a complication of foreign body. *Ann Otol Rhinol Laryngol* 1982;91:325–327.
60. McComas BC, van Miles P, Katz BE. Successful salvage of an 8-month-old child with an aortoesophageal fistula. *J Pediatr Surg* 1991;26:1394–1395.
61. Stool SE, Deitch M. Potential danger of catheter removal of foreign body. *Pediatrics* 1973;51:313–314.

# 45

# ENDOSCOPIC MANAGEMENT OF TRACHEAL AND ESOPHAGEAL DISEASES

ELIE E. REBEIZ
STANLEY M. SHAPSHAY

Since the introduction of bronchoscopy at the end of the nineteenth century, significant improvements in instrumentation and technology have taken place. Gustav Killian is credited with the first successful use of bronchoscopy in 1896 to remove a bronchial foreign body (1). Since that time, rigid and flexible endoscopy have become increasingly valuable in the diagnosis and treatment of airway and lung disease.

In 1902, Chevalier Jackson designed a bronchoscope, which was illuminated distally by a small lamp and a separate aspirating channel (2). By 1912, the bronchoscope had become an accepted instrument for evaluation of the trachea and bronchi and for removal of foreign bodies. In the 1960s and 1970s, the role of the bronchoscope was extended for transbronchial biopsies (3).

Esophageal endoscopy has become more popular with the development of rigid and flexible telescopic optic systems. Previously, barium radiography and esophageal manometry were the only available means for evaluating esophageal pathology. In the past 15 years, esophageal endoscopy has become the principal diagnostic and therapeutic procedure for esophageal pathology. The use of outpatient esophagoscopy has been extended as an important tool for the evaluation of swallowing disorders.

This chapter reviews the surgical anatomy of the trachea and esophagus and describes techniques for diagnostic and therapeutic endoscopy, including their indications, limitations, and potential complications. We also discuss diagnostic and therapeutic advances such as lasers and the use of flexible endoscopes in the office setting.

## TRACHEA

### Anatomy

Every bronchoscopist should have solid knowledge of the tracheobronchial and chest anatomy, the relationship of the tracheobronchial tree to the surrounding structures in the chest, and the possible anatomic variations. Knowledge of the pulmonary vascular anatomy is essential to avoid complications. The airway endoscopist should also know the endoscopic anatomy of the tracheobronchial tree and its relationship to the esophagus and the major blood vessels of the mediastinum. Distortion of the anatomy can occur because of pathologic conditions such as tracheobronchial cancer or by previous surgery or radiation therapy (4).

From a vascular point of view, the cervical trachea is relatively safe. The thoracic trachea, however, descends through the upper third of the thorax, where it has multiple, close relationships with the large blood vessels of the mediastinum.

The trachea varies in length and angulation from infancy to adulthood. The adult trachea is 9 to 15 cm long and is 13 to 22 mm wide (Fig. 45.1). The angle between the trachea and the main stem bronchi varies. The angle of the right main bronchus is 10° to 15° less than that of the left bronchus. The right main stem bronchus is approximately 1.5 cm long and gives rise to the upper lobe bronchus, which divides into three segmental bronchi. The right bronchus then continues as the bronchus intermedius, which gives rise to the middle lobe bronchus anteriorly, the superior segment of the right lower lobe posteriorly, and the right lower lobe bronchus (Fig. 45.2).

The right main bronchus branches off at a 20° to 30° angle from the trachea, and the left main bronchus lies at a 40° to 50° angle. The right main bronchus is more vertical and easier to intubate with a rigid bronchoscope. Laser applications in the left main bronchus are often more difficult because it is longer than the right bronchus (5 versus 2.5 cm), more acutely angled, and smaller in diameter (11 versus 15 mm) than the right.

The left main bronchus has more anatomic danger zones than the right main bronchus. The esophagus adheres to the first 2 cm of the left bronchus on its posterior aspect;

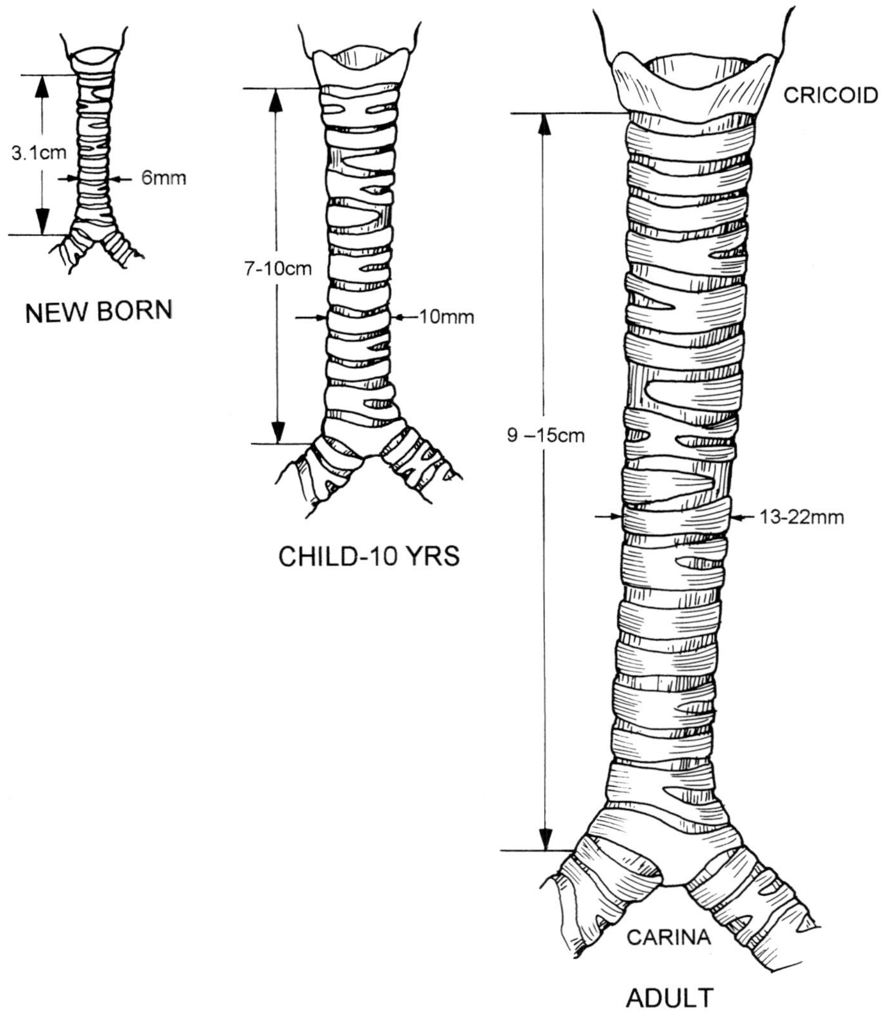


**FIGURE 45.1.** Developmental changes in tracheal anatomy from birth to adulthood.

the arch of the aorta drapes over it at the front, and in the back, the bifurcation of the right and left pulmonary arteries is closely situated. The pulmonary vein makes contact at the root of the left upper lobar bronchus. The right main bronchus has the right pulmonary artery crossing above it at the level of the right upper lobar bronchus.

The left main stem bronchus is longer than the right. It is 4 to 4.5 cm long and points posteriorly and laterally. It terminates in a bifurcation between the left upper lobe and left lower lobe bronchi. The left upper bronchus gives rise to the lingular orifice. After giving rise to the superior segment of the lower lobe, which descends posteriorly, the left lower bronchus continues for approximately 1 cm before dividing into the terminal bronchi. Treatment of patients with lesions of the left upper pulmonary lobe is risky. Because of its nearly vertical position, the lobe is difficult to intubate with a bronchoscope. The pulmonary vein wraps around the back and sides of the left upper lobar bronchus, and the pulmonary artery passes over the front.

The arch of the aorta passes on the left anterior aspect of the trachea, making a definite imprint. From the curvature of the arch arises the innominate artery, tightly pressed onto the trachea and passing from left to right toward the base of the neck. The azygos vein winds around the right side of the distal trachea before joining the superior vena cava. The esophagus lies in continual close contact with the posterior aspect of the cervical and thoracic tracheal segments. The left recurrent laryngeal nerve originates under the arch of the aorta and runs up to the cricoid cartilage in the tracheoesophageal groove. The right recurrent laryngeal nerve meets the trachea in the cervical region at the level of the sixth cartilaginous ring.

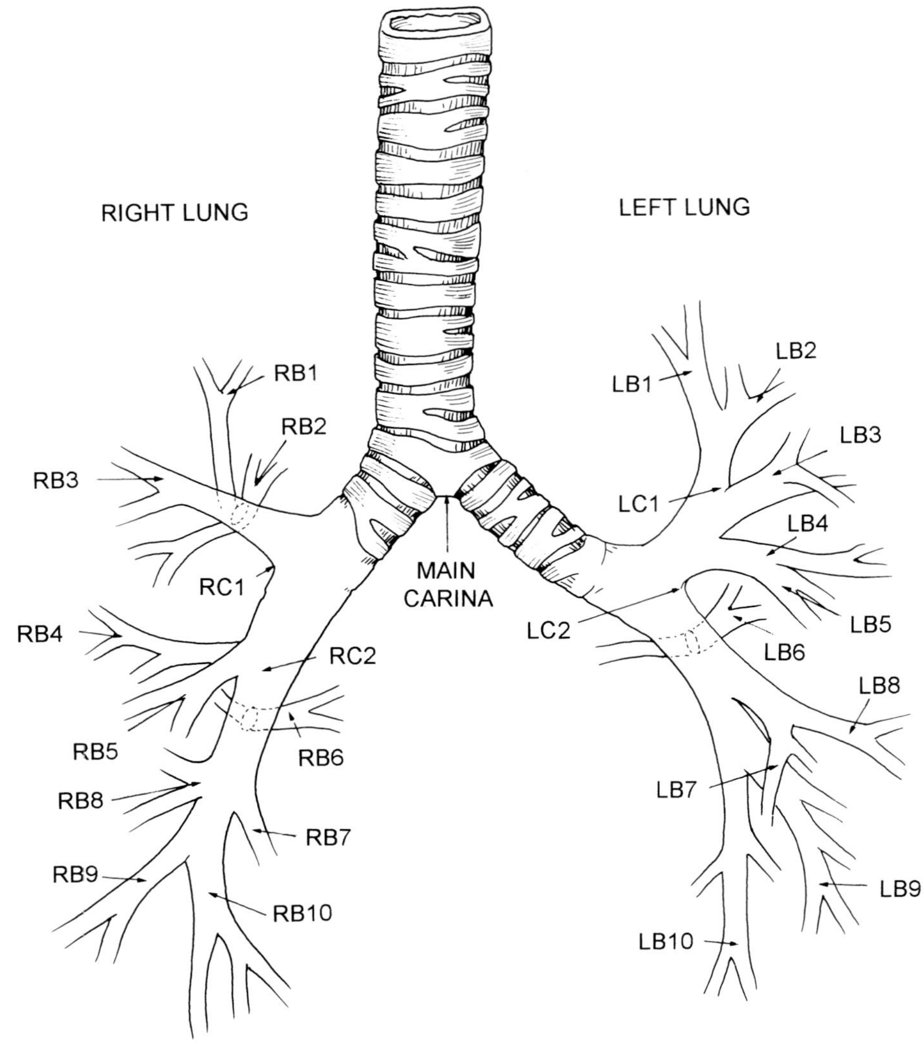


RB1 APICAL
RB2 POSTERIOR } UPPER LOBE
RB3 ANTERIOR
RB4 LATERAL } MIDDLE LOBE
RB5 MEDIAL
RB6 SUPERIOR
RB7 MEDIAL BASAL
RB8 ANTERIOR BASAL } LOWER LOBE
RB9 LATERAL BASAL
RB10 POSTERIOR BASAL
RC1 CARINA BETWEEN BRONCHUS TO RIGHT UPPER LOBE AND BRANCHUS INTERMEDIUS
RC2 CARINA BETWEEN BRANCHUS TO RIGHT MIDDLE LOBE AND LOWER LOBE BRANCHUS

LB1 & 2 APICAL POSTERIOR } UPPER LOBE
LB3 ANTERIOR
LB4 SUPERIOR } LINGULA
LB5 INFERIOR
LB6 SUPERIOR
LB7 & 8 ANTEROMEDIAL BASAL } LOWER LOBE
LB9 LATERAL BASAL
LB10 POSTERIOR BASAL
LC1 CARINA BETWEEN BRONCHUS TO ANTERIOR SEGMENT OF LEFT UPPER LOBE AND LINGULAR BRONCHUS
LC2 CARINA BETWEEN BRONCHUS TO LINGULAR SEGMENT OF LEFT UPPER LOBE AND LEFT LOWER LOBE BRONCHUS

**FIGURE 45.2.** Anatomy of the adult trachea.

## Laser Bronchoscopy

Strong and colleagues introduced laser bronchoscopy in the late 1960s (5). The carbon dioxide ($CO_2$) laser was the first laser applied in bronchology, but because of its cumbersome mirror delivery system, it was not easy to use in the tracheobronchial tree. This laser is ideal for cutting because of its superficial effect on tissue, and its energy is almost fully absorbed at the impact site, which makes it a poor laser for deep vaporization and coagulation.

The neodymium:yttrium aluminum garnet (Nd:YAG) laser is very useful in therapeutic bronchoscopy. Its beam is delivered through an optical quartz fiber, and its energy can achieve levels high enough for resection, vaporization, or coagulation of tissue. Its wavelength (1.06 μm) is ideal for heating large volumes of vascularized tissue to induce hemostasis, deep tissue coagulation, and necrosis. It can be used to coagulate tissue into a friable consistency, allowing easy and immediate removal by suction or by delayed necrosis. Laser users should be warned about the soft tissue effects of the Nd:YAG laser wavelength. Caution is required, because it is extremely difficult to judge the depth of penetration of the laser energy into biologic tissue, especially when treating pale, whitish tissue. The Nd:YAG laser wavelength absorption by tissue is very poor and is somewhat color dependent. This laser is a tissue coagulator and is not useful for precise tissue removal. The surface appearance of the laser-irradiated tissue does not usually indicate the status of the underlying tissue. The second important outcome to avoid is the "popcorn effect," which results from overheating of the underlying tissue and causes formation of an air pocket below the surface that ultimately explodes, leaving a large cavity and causing splatter of tissue. This effect can produce tracheal or vascular perforation.

Another important wavelength for laser bronchoscopy is available in the potassium-titanyl-phosphate (KTP-532) laser. The 532-nm wavelength is very close to the spectrum of the argon laser; therefore, the same type of tissue interaction is expected. Like the argon laser wavelength, the 532-nm wavelength can be passed through a very small quartz fiber (200 μm), which increases power density to permit cutting as well as coagulation. This wavelength is a compromise between the more precise cutting effects of the $CO_2$ laser and the superior coagulating properties of the noncontact Nd:YAG laser. The argon and KTP-532 laser wavelengths are best absorbed by pigment, especially red, which delays their initial absorption by light-colored lesions until desiccation and charring take place.

The role of laser technology in the management of airway obstruction is well-established (6). Obstruction due to malignant lesions is palliated more effectively with the Nd:YAG laser, which has some distinct advantages over other lasers in regard to hemostasis and deep penetration. Benign stenotic lesions of the airways and recurrent respiratory papillomatosis involving the larynx and the trachea are treated more effectively with the $CO_2$ laser. Whenever possible, the $CO_2$ laser is delivered using a microspot microdelivery system through a subglottic place laryngoscope to access the subglottis and upper trachea. A semiflexible waveguide type of technology is useful for laser energy delivery in the trachea, and this is described later in this chapter. The hemostatic capability of the $CO_2$ laser is limited to blood vessels not larger than capillaries. This is generally not a problem in the treatment of benign stenosis because these areas are fibrous and poorly vascularized. Treatment of benign subglottic stenosis with the $CO_2$ laser is one of its earliest endoscopic applications, and this technique is still well accepted as the first approach to the problem of benign upper airway stenosis. The best indication for laser treatment is a stenosis that is fibrous, not larger than 1 cm in its vertical length, and not associated with cartilage malacia or narrowing. The $CO_2$ laser still has an important role in tracheobronchial laser therapy because it remains ideal therapy for patients with benign stenosis and tracheobronchial papillomatosis. The excellent cutting and vaporization qualities of the $CO_2$ laser energy permit discrete resection of benign stenosis with minimal damage to the airway wall. Central airway papillomas can undergo vaporization with the $CO_2$ laser with minimal bleeding. We prefer to use the more convenient Nd:YAG laser with its flexible fiber delivery system to coagulate the papillomas and mechanically remove them with suction or forceps.

Until the mid-1980s, the only option for application of the $CO_2$ laser was to use a bronchoscopic coupler. The coupling device permitted marriage of the articulating arm of the $CO_2$ laser to a specially modified rigid bronchoscopic system. In 1982, Ossoff and Karlan (7) described their clinical experience using a universal endoscopic coupler for $CO_2$ laser surgery. This instrument provided direct coaxial vision because the invisible $CO_2$ laser beam permitted simultaneous transmission of the helium-neon aiming light down the lumen of the bronchoscope with minimal distortion. Surgeons were able to visualize the precise area of tissue to be vaporized by the invisible wavelength. Included with this was a continuous variable defocused lens system for laser incision, vaporization, and coagulation. With this system, surgeons could vary the spot size of the laser beam as needed. A quick on-off centering screw was designed to facilitate coaxial alignment and disengagement of the bronchoscope from the coupler. Because it weighed only 1 pound, the surgeon was able to grasp the coupler and the attached bronchoscope easily in one hand and perform the bronchoscopic laser procedure in the same fashion as conventional bronchoscopy. A set of custom-designed laser bronchoscopes was used with the universal endoscopic coupler.

Waveguides able to transmit the $CO_2$ laser beam have been used to eliminate the bronchoscopic coupling system. An advantage of the waveguide transmission is the ability to use an open rigid bronchoscopic system rather than a closed-coupled system. An open bronchoscopic system gives the surgeon excellent visualization associated with rigid telescopes and permits the simultaneous use of flexible suction catheters to maintain a dry operative field.

With the Nd:YAG laser, a flexible quartz fiber approximately 2 mm in diameter can be passed through a flexible or rigid bronchoscope. Rigid bronchoscopes of various designs have been specialized for laser fiber application, permitting simultaneous use of flexible suction catheters, laser fibers, and a rigid telescope with an open or closed ventilating system.

There are many advantages to using a rigid bronchoscope:

1. Secure ventilation with the side channel connector or with Venturi jet ventilation attachment
2. Rapid evacuation of blood clots and secretions through the use of one or two suction catheters
3. It is a nonflammable system.
4. Palpation of the tracheal wall and determination of the cartilage-tumor interface
5. Tamponade of a bleeding tumor
6. Use of a débriding device after photocoagulation of the tumors
7. Use of telescopic optics

The disadvantages of the rigid bronchoscope compared with flexible fiberoptic bronchoscopes are limited access to the bronchi of the left main, distal, and upper lobe and the need for general anesthesia.

The advantages of a flexible fiberoptic bronchoscopic system include the ability to perform operations easily with patients under local anesthesia and ready access to upper lobar and distal endobronchial tumors. There are also several disadvantages:

1. Lack of ventilatory control of the compromised airway
2. Minimal suction capability simultaneous with laser use
3. Inability to palpate the tumor at the cartilaginous interface
4. Inefficient evacuation of tumor fragments and debris compared with the open rigid bronchoscopic system
5. Inability to tamponade bleeding tumors
6. Risk of igniting the plastic covering of the bronchoscope (8)

## Instrumentation and Anesthetic Techniques

The choice of instrumentation to be used depends on the site and the nature of the pathologic condition in the airway. Whenever possible, a "ventilating laryngoscope" is used so that the operating microscope and $CO_2$ laser can be used to remove tumor in the immediate glottic and subglottic airway. A Venturi jet ventilation system with a needle attached to the proximal lip of the operating laryngoscope is the preferred method of ventilation. When the tumor obstruction occurs in the cervical trachea beyond the reach of the laryngoscope, a ventilating tracheoscope specially prepared for laser application is the best choice. This tracheoscope does not have the ventilation holes of the rigid bronchoscope, and ventilation is not lost at the glottic level. The Nd:YAG laser fiber is inserted through the tracheoscope along with a flexible suction catheter for rapid removal of bloody secretions and maintenance of a dry field. A shorter telescope than that used with the rigid bronchoscope provides good optic control. For tumors in the middle to distal trachea and main bronchi, the ventilating bronchoscope is the instrument of choice. When tumors are located in the upper lobe with obstruction and subsequent atelectasis and infection, the flexible bronchoscope with a suction channel large enough to accommodate the Nd:YAG laser fiber is used to approach them. The ventilating bronchoscope is used as a conduit for the flexible bronchoscope, providing ventilation and the ability to extract tumor fragments and secretions rapidly. In general, however, the flexible bronchoscope is used more as an instrument for tracheobronchial toilet than for actual laser application.

The anesthetic management of patients who require laser bronchoscopy is challenging to the anesthesiologist and the endoscopist. Multiple anesthetic techniques are available for use with rigid bronchoscopy. The choice of anesthetic and ventilation technique depends on the site and the nature of the obstruction. Use of topical anesthetics is preferred, with some intravenous sedation and spontaneous ventilation for patients with high obstructing cervical tracheal lesions. In high-risk patients or in elderly patients, we usually attempt to perform the procedure with topical lidocaine, intravenous sedation, and assisted ventilation. However, with this topical technique, control of cough is often impossible.

For more distal tracheobronchial obstruction, particularly near the carina in a patient with a very sensitive cough reflex, general anesthesia is preferred, employing an inhalation technique or intravenous narcotics. We prefer muscle relaxation for complete control of the airway. Muscle paralysis reverses rapidly, and reintubation is rarely necessary at the end of the procedure. Anesthesia is periodically reinforced with topical application of 4% lidocaine.

## Treatment of Benign Conditions

### *Trauma*

Prolonged or traumatic tracheal intubation, tracheostomy, penetrating or blunt tracheal trauma, and inflammatory diseases usually cause stenosis. Stenosis is usually cicatricial or weblike, and patients present with dyspnea as the chief complaint. A complete physical examination, diagnostic fiberoptic bronchoscopy, chest radiography, computed tomography, electrocardiography, and routine blood tests, including arterial blood gas determinations, should be done during the preoperative evaluation.

The surgical procedure is performed in an operating room especially equipped for laser bronchoscopy. The patient's eyes are carefully covered with moist gauze pads, and the operating room personnel should wear protective glasses. General intravenous anesthesia with muscle relaxation is used. A manually driven Venturi jet attached to the side arm of a ventilating Storz bronchoscope (Karl Storz, Culver City, CA) can adequately administer ventilation. Topical anesthesia with intravenous sedation can be employed and allows spontaneous ventilation.

The $CO_2$ laser beam is delivered through flexible waveguides. If the stenosis is proximal, laser incisions can be achieved using an Ossoff subglottiscope, with a microscope coupled to a micromanipulator. Alternatively, a diagnostic Dedo laryngoscope (Pilling, Philadelphia, PA) can be used between the cords as a subglottic laryngoscope. If the stenosis is distal beyond the reach of a laryngoscope, a ventilating bronchoscope is used. After induction of general intravenous anesthesia, patients are intubated with the open-tube rigid bronchoscope, and Venturi jet ventilation is administered. The waveguide and a suction catheter for smoke evacuation are introduced through the rigid bronchoscope. Using the Helium-Neon aiming beam, the stenotic tracheal band is targeted and is easily vaporized using the technique of laser radial incisions, followed by gentle dilation.

This method proved to be effective in opening the cicatricial formation without causing a circumferential defect. Preservation of intact islands of mucosa prevents circumferential scarring and allows rapid re-epithelialization of the denuded areas. Gradual gentle dilation of the trachea is achieved by increasing the size of the rigid ventilating bronchoscope. This technique permits retention of epithelial areas between incisions and promotes rapid re-epithelialization of the area. Patients are usually extubated in the operating room and are transferred to a recovery room for observation. They are discharged on the first postoperative day. The relief of dyspnea is usually immediate and significant.

The use of the waveguide delivery system allows accurate delivery of laser energy to the targeted tissue, with minimal thermal damage to the healthy tracheal mucosa and cartilage. Continuous suction with a flexible catheter for removal of smoke is extremely important and ensures visibility for the operator.

Treatment of benign stenosis of the airway is challenging. Laser treatment can be safe and effective and should be tried as the first line of therapy before more aggressive surgery. In cases of restenosis, an open surgical procedure (i.e., tracheal resection) can still be performed. Healy and coworkers reported successful management of 177 pediatric patients with benign tracheal stenosis, tracheal granulomas, and papillomas (9). They recommended a trial of endoscopic laser therapy in patients with acquired tracheal stenosis before performing an open procedure, which is often associated with higher morbidity. Grillo (10) analyzed the complications of tracheal reconstruction performed on a series of 279 patients with tracheal stenosis after intubation. Granulations at the anastomosis site developed in 28 patients (10%) and partial or complete restenosis in 21 patients (7.5%). Koufman and associates (11) reported a 77% success rate when treating 13 patients with subglottic stenosis with the $CO_2$ laser. Dedo and Sooy (12) described another approach for the treatment of posterior glottic stenosis, in which the $CO_2$ laser was used to raise a mucosal flap and to vaporize submucosal scar tissue, with subsequent repositioning of the flap in place.

Technical limitations in the delivery systems have been evident since the early application of the $CO_2$ laser in the trachea and bronchi. The main problem is the difficulty in delivering the $CO_2$ laser beam through commonly available quartz fibers because of its long wavelength (10.6 μm) and its absorption by this material. The Nd:YAG and argon lasers, with much shorter wavelengths (1.06 and 0.5 μm, respectively), can be delivered through fibers. The holmium:YAG laser is another laser being tested for incising tracheal stenotic bands. This laser can be transmitted through quartz fibers and can achieve incisions as precisely as the $CO_2$ laser with minimal thermal damage. This is a pulsed laser, and tissue splatter on impact can be problematic because the optic telescope lens is easily soiled impairing visualization.

### *Recurrent Respiratory Papillomatosis*

Recurrent respiratory papillomatosis is a condition that affects mucous membranes of the respiratory tract. It is characterized by multiple and recurrent squamous papillomas, most commonly involving the larynx, but other areas of the upper and lower respiratory tract may be involved, causing hoarseness and respiratory obstruction. It is less common and usually less troublesome in adults. Histologic, ultrastructural, and immunohistochemical studies implicate the human papillomavirus (HPV) as the cause of this disease. No treatment has been successful in curing this disease, but spontaneous remissions can occur. Frequent excisions are recommended to try to avoid a tracheotomy and to allow the child to develop good phonation, preserving normal vocal cord anatomy as much as possible. The $CO_2$ laser has been very helpful in the treatment of these lesions in the larynx, pharynx, upper trachea, and nasal and oral cavities, allowing longer periods of disease-free intervals than with cold instruments.

Airway management of the patient with laryngotracheal papillomas is a critical consideration before treatment. Patients often present with insidious onset of biphasic stridor and airway distress. Endotracheal intubation must be performed with great care, using a 5- to 6-mm, laser-safe tube. Intubation is generally done with relaxation-type (e.g., succinylcholine chloride) induction anesthesia. A rigid ventilating bronchoscope and a tracheotomy set should be prepared in the event that intubation is not possible. In adult patients, the airway is best intubated with the head flexed forward in the "sniffing position." A suitable-sized (Dedo-Jako–type) laryngoscope is placed in position and suspended. Our preference is to use the Boston University (BU) suspension system (Pilling Co., Philadelphia, PA) which is attached to a holder on the operating table.

After the glottic papillomas are cleared using the $CO_2$ laser, the endotracheal tube is removed, and Venturi jet ventilation is used. It is attached to the proximal part of the laryngoscope with a 16-gauge, blunt needle screw that is clamped in place or placed in one of the fiberoptic cable side ports on the laryngoscope. A very useful clamp-on Venturi device is available from Karl Storz Endoscopy (Culver City, CA). It is extremely important that the patient has good muscle relaxation before removal of the endotracheal tube because vocal cord adduction makes ventilation very difficult. The tip of the laryngoscope is insinuated into the immediate subglottic region to provide a clear path for ventilation. The oxygen blender is set at 75%, but the mixture of air drawn in by the jet insufflation system provides an approximately 50% oxygen mixture. Ventilation is achieved by manual injection ventilation while chest movement is watched as an indication of adequate ventilation. The $CO_2$ laser used with a microspot micromanipulator coupled to the operating microscope is used to remove the posterior glottic and immediate subglottic-obstructing papillomas.

The surgeon and the anesthesiologist should coordinate the laser firing with the Venturi jet cycles. The anesthetic jet ventilates three to five cycles for every 1 second of laser exposure. Care must also be taken to keep the operating field dry because insufflation blows secretions and blood into the distal tracheobronchial tree, impairing ventilation. Close monitoring of arterial oxygen saturation is necessary throughout the procedure.

The technique for tracheobronchial removal of papillomas depends on their location and growth pattern. If the growth is relatively isolated to the upper cervical trachea, a ventilating tracheoscope (Karl Storz, Culver City, CA) is inserted, allowing simultaneous use of a rigid 0° telescope; a heat-resistant, semi-flexible polyethylene suction catheter; and a 2.3-mm Nd:YAG laser noncontact fiber. The papillomas can be removed mechanically after the tumor mass is photocoagulated, vaporized, or both. Laser power settings of 30 to 40 W at 0.5- to 1-second exposures are used. The laser fiber tip is about 1 cm from the target tissue, creating a 1-mm spot size. The tracheoscope is particularly valuable in this location because this shortened version of the ventilating laser bronchoscope does not have any ventilating holes on the side of the instrument to prevent loss of ventilation at the glottic level. The shorter instrument is also easier for the endoscopist to handle, especially when working in the upper third of the trachea. Papillomatous growth is often sessile and has a cobblestone appearance. The Nd:YAG laser is particularly useful for this type of growth because the endoscopist can essentially "paint" this diffuse growth pattern for photodestruction rather than vaporization. Laser power is reduced to approximately 30 W at 1-second exposures. Care is taken not to overtreat the underlying tracheobronchial wall, always using the laser parallel to the wall. Use of the $CO_2$ laser in this situation can be dangerous because vaporization of tissue can lead to tracheobronchial ulceration and perforation.

For more distal tracheobronchial involvement, a specially prepared laser bronchoscope is used. In general, we prefer to use the Storz ventilating laser bronchoscope for laser fiber application with Venturi jet ventilation. This permits use of an open system for rapid insertion of suction catheters and bronchoscopic forceps if necessary. Anesthesia is accomplished with intravenous narcotics, muscle relaxation, and topical 4% lidocaine (Xylocaine) to supplement the anesthesia. Care should be taken to use frequent suctioning of the distal tracheobronchial tree to prevent retention of secretions and resulting hypoxemia.

After a satisfactory airway is obtained, the bronchoscope is removed, and the patient is reintubated with a no. 7 standard endotracheal tube. Reintubation is performed at this time to allow postoperative suctioning and return of respiratory musculature strength. The patient is usually extubated in the operating room. Complete removal of all tracheobronchial papillomas is not the end point of treatment, because this is usually impossible and does not change the natural history of the disease process; the goal is a safe, patent airway.

Recurrence of papillomatosis is the rule rather than the exception. Spontaneous remission in these patients, although hoped for within the age range of puberty, is less common in the adult patient. Repeated treatment is usually planned at the sixth postoperative month, depending on the growth rate of the individual papillomas and symptoms.

Repeated applications of the $CO_2$ and Nd:YAG laser are safe because ionizing radiation is not associated with laser application and does not lead to cumulative risk for the patient. The major danger is scarring from excessive heat and collateral damage as well as perforation. An open bronchoscopic system is preferable to a closed, coupled $CO_2$ laser and rigid bronchoscopic setup. The open system permits simultaneous use of suction catheters for evacuation of secretions, use of a rigid 0° telescope for excellent optic control of the airway, and rapid insertion of instruments, such as forceps and open, rigid suction tubes.

## Treatment of Tumors

Primary or metastatic malignant lesions are responsible for tracheobronchial obstruction in 90% of patients (13). Most patients have severe obstruction and require urgent intervention. Squamous cell carcinoma, which often arises at the level of the lobar bronchi, is the most common primary lung neoplasm that causes airway obstruction. Endobronchial metastatic renal cell carcinoma is the most common metastatic tumor, followed by carcinoma of the esophagus. Esophageal cancer produces obstruction of the central airways by direct extension from the primary tumor or from local mediastinal nodes rather than by hematogenous spread, as seen with the other metastatic cancers.

Patients presenting with obstruction of the main airways are usually critically sick, with profound dyspnea, hemoptysis, or postobstructive sepsis. Most patients have inoperable tumors, with mediastinal involvement or large, unresectable primary lesions. Chemotherapy has proved inadequate for the treatment of such patients, and external beam radiotherapy has been the classic treatment for control of endobronchial disease.

The introduction of laser technology in bronchology has proved to be an important addition to the management of patients with endobronchial obstruction. Unlike radiation therapy, laser photocoagulation may be used repeatedly for the palliation of malignant tracheobronchial obstruction. The technique of Nd:YAG laser resection of malignant endobronchial lesions obstructing the airways has been well described (13) and attests to the safety and effectiveness of this therapy. Brutinel reported that the quality and duration of life were improved for 116 patients with obstructing carcinoma who were treated with Nd:YAG laser applications (14).

Although the $CO_2$ laser was the initial laser employed for tracheobronchial laser therapy, its use in the treatment of patients with malignant obstruction has largely been abandoned because of poor hemostatic properties. Although effective for hemostasis, the argon and KTP lasers tissue effects are too superficial to effectively coagulate and vaporize bulky tumors. The hypervascularity of many malignant endobronchial neoplasms is best treated with the Nd:YAG laser because of its excellent coagulation properties (13). One of the most serious and sometimes fatal complications of resection of tracheal tumors is bleeding. The Nd:YAG laser is the preferred wavelength for malignant neoplasms because these tumors have a greater propensity for hemorrhage.

The goal of laser bronchoscopy, particularly for malignant tumors, is palliation of airway obstruction, relief of pneumonitis resulting from obstruction, and control of tracheobronchial hemorrhage. Palliation is the main goal, because patients with early and potentially curable carcinoma of the airway should be treated with open resection or radiation therapy. Intermediate tumors, such as carcinoid and adenoid cystic carcinoma, are also good indications for endoscopic laser application, especially with the Nd:YAG laser. Both of these tumors, when resectable, should be removed by sleeve resection rather than endoscopic laser therapy.

The use of the rigid bronchoscope offers a number of advantages over the flexible bronchoscope. It permits better control of bleeding by using large suction catheters, more effective ventilation with the Venturi jet, excellent visualization because of the high-quality optics of the telescope, and rapid removal of tumor through the open tube with large biopsy forceps. The flexible bronchoscope is sometimes used through the rigid bronchoscope to visualize and treat upper lobe segmental bronchi that cannot be reached with the rigid endoscope. It may also be useful in the outpatient bronchoscopy suite for the treatment of patients with limited disease, such as a small, noncritically obstructing tumor requiring photocoagulation for hemoptysis or for benign lesions such as papillomas or suture granulomas. The flexible bronchoscope should not be used for the treatment of patients with highly vascular and bulky tumors. If bleeding or obstruction occur, a rigid bronchoscope allows better control while maintaining good ventilation.

Life-threatening operative complications leading to morbidity and mortality occur. These include tension pneumothorax and hemorrhage. Survival data are difficult to interpret in this group of patients with advanced carcinoma, and a prospective, controlled study would be difficult to perform.

## Complications

In our series of more than 300 laser bronchoscopies performed between 1982 and 1988, only one operative death occurred because of tension pneumothorax and pericardial tamponade (13). No major hemorrhage, airway fire, or postoperative septicemia occurred. Two patients with severe coronary artery disease died of myocardial infarction in the postoperative period. The risk of complications was also analyzed in a large combined series of patients from four medical centers in the United States and Europe (15). A total of 1,503 laser bronchoscopic treatments were performed in 1,156 patients. Six deaths occurred in this large series, all of which were attributable to hypoxemia resulting from excessive anesthesia, bleeding, or retained secretions. No perforation, fire, or catastrophic arterial hemorrhage occurred.

## Management of Complications

Although the Nd:YAG laser has had a remarkably safe record for more than 10 years, it remains the most powerful and perhaps the most dangerous of available medical lasers. The power density of the Nd:YAG laser is concentrated below the surface of the tissue, as opposed to the surface effect of the $CO_2$ laser, necessitating intermittent exposure settings of 1 second or less at a power setting of less than 50 W (usually 40 to 45 W).

### *Risk of Combustion with Endotracheal Tubes*

In general, the use of endotracheal tubes in bronchoscopic surgery should be avoided because of the risk of combustion, particularly in an oxygen-rich environment. A polyvinyl chloride tube should never be used because the $CO_2$ and Nd:YAG lasers beam can cause combustion and production of toxic fumes, as well as a potential blowtorch effect. External taping of the polyvinyl chloride endotracheal tube does not protect the internal wall from combustion when the Nd:YAG laser is used inside the tube.

### Bronchoscopic Fire

Ignition of the sheath of the flexible bronchoscope can cause fire. It is extremely important to be able to see the laser fiber at all times before activating the laser. However, combustion of the flexible bronchoscope most often occurs from ignition of charred tumor fragments or flammable material such as the endotracheal tube. Environmental oxygen should be kept at less than 50% when possible. The first response to an endobronchial fire is prompt removal of all flammable materials, including the endotracheal tube. When this occurs, the airway should be reestablished, and endoscopic inspection for tracheobronchial burns should follow. The patient should be treated with antibiotics and steroids to diminish the inflammatory response and decrease the possibility of subsequent scarring. Flammable materials within the rigid bronchoscopic system include the laser fiber itself and the plastic suction materials. The laser fiber should be kept free of debris at all times, and plastic material should be kept proximal to the laser tip when possible.

### Perforation of the Tracheobronchial Tree

The risk of tracheobronchial perforation with the Nd:YAG laser is much greater than with the $CO_2$ or argon laser. Depth of penetration and scatter are also considerably greater with this wavelength, and its soft tissue interaction is less predictable. Cautious, intermittent Nd:YAG laser irradiation using less than 50 W of power is highly advisable during endoscopy. The Nd:YAG laser fiber should always be used parallel with and never perpendicular to the tracheobronchial wall. The tip of the rigid bronchoscope can be used as a palpating device to help determine the interface of the tumor and the tracheal cartilage. Laser irradiation at continued high power of greater than 40 W with exposure times of more than 1 second may cause explosive rupture of the tissues—the so-called popcorn effect. The surgeon may see blanching of the surface of the tissue followed by charring before explosion of tissue.

### Hemorrhage

The most common hemorrhagic situation is persistent, uncontrolled bleeding of the tracheobronchial tree. Massive hemorrhage is usually caused by perforation of a major pulmonary blood vessel and, fortunately, is a rare complication. However, life-threatening hypoxemia may occur from the accumulation of distal tracheobronchial hemorrhagic secretions. Cessation of tumor resection with immediate tracheobronchial toilet and hemostasis is imperative. Two semi-rigid suction catheters passed through the rigid bronchoscope are used to maintain a dry operative field. The laser is applied at a coagulating power of 30 to 40 W with the fiber approximately 2 cm from the target tissue. Coagulation should begin circumferentially around the bleeding site and end at the area itself. Massive bronchial hemorrhage necessitates placing the patient in the lateral safety position with the healthy lung above the affected lung. With the patient in this position, the ventilating bronchoscope is used to evacuate blood and secretions and to achieve patency of the airway. Heroic measures should not be taken when hemorrhage from perforation of a pulmonary artery or other great vessel occurs. These patients usually do not respond to resuscitative measures.

### Hypoxemia

The major cause of death during and after laser resection is hypoxemia. Hypoxemia can arise from distal collection of secretions and debris and from induced respiratory depression caused by anesthetic medications. Uncontrolled hypoxemia leads to cardiovascular complications such as arrhythmia and bradycardia, as well as myocardial infarction and subsequent cardiac arrest. Constant monitoring of oxygen saturation using a finger pulse oximeter and frequent monitoring of blood gases are important when treating high-risk patients. Adequate ventilation and frequent tracheobronchial toilet should be the constant preoccupation of the endoscopist during the laser procedure.

# ESOPHAGUS

## Anatomy

The esophagus is a distensible muscular tube arising from the hypopharynx and connecting to the stomach inferiorly. Superiorly, it starts as a slitlike opening of the cricopharyngeus muscle, approximately 20 cm from the incisor teeth, at the level of the cricoid cartilage (C6). It then traverses the neck into the mediastinum between the trachea and the vertebral column. It remains just anterior to the spine superiorly and then follows the contour of the left atrium, anteriorly and to the left, toward the diaphragmatic hiatus. The length of the esophagus changes with age and sex, and it varies between 23 and 25 cm.

The cricopharyngeus and the lower esophageal sphincter are in constant contraction and usually open during peristalsis resulting from swallowing. Other sites of narrowing are at the thoracic inlet (T1), the aortic arch (T4), and the tracheal bifurcation (T6), where the left bronchus crosses anteriorly.

Branches of the inferior thyroid arteries, the thyrocervical trunk, and the subclavian arteries richly supply the cervical esophagus. In the upper thorax, the blood supply comes from the bronchial artery branches and esophageal branches coming directly from the aorta. Other arterial blood supply includes intercostals, left gastric artery, and the right and left inferior phrenic arteries.

## Esophagoscopy

Esophagoscopy is performed for diagnostic and therapeutic reasons. There are two basic methods of endoscopy using rigid and flexible esophagoscopes. Rigid esophagoscopy, usually done under general anesthesia, allows direct visualization and operative manipulation for removal of foreign bodies, dilatation, and biopsy. The flexible scope provides comfort for the patient and allows visualization and biopsy under local anesthesia with sedation. Biopsies are easily done, and gastric and duodenal examination can be done at the same sitting.

For the otolaryngologist, interest in esophageal endoscopy is mainly in the diagnosis and treatment of a number of conditions of the cervical and upper thoracic esophagus. These conditions include foreign bodies, strictures, caustic injury, benign and malignant tumors, and diverticula. Other conditions are usually evaluated and treated by gastroenterologists, and these include esophageal varices, hiatal hernia, Barrett's esophagus, esophagitis (viral and bacterial), achalasia, scleroderma, and Crohn's disease.

Significant advances have been made in the evaluation of the esophagus in the office setting. The work of Aviv and colleagues has greatly improved our understanding of the swallowing mechanism, as well as the pathophysiology of aspiration and the associated anomalies of the larynx, hypopharynx, and cervical esophagus. In 1998, he introduced an office procedure to evaluate the motor and sensory components of swallowing called fiberoptic endoscopic evaluation of swallowing with sensory testing (FEESST). FEESST allows the clinician to obtain a comprehensive bedside assessment of swallowing that is performed as the initial swallowing evaluation for the patient with dysphagia. The technique combines the established endoscopic evaluation of swallowing with a technique that determines laryngopharyngeal sensory discrimination thresholds by endoscopically delivering air pulse stimuli to the mucosa innervated by the superior laryngeal nerve (16).

Aviv and coworkers extensively studied the laryngopharyngeal sensory discrimination and the laryngeal adductor reflex by endoscopically administering air pulse stimuli to the mucosa innervated by the superior laryngeal nerve and asking the patient if he or she could feel the stimulus. They observed that the laryngeal adductor reflex was evoked at stimulus intensities similar to those capable of eliciting the psychophysical or perceptual response and that it could be used as an objective clinical method of endoscopically assessing laryngopharyngeal sensory capacity (17).

## Foreign Bodies

The esophagus is the most common site for foreign body obstruction. The most common sites of foreign body lodging are at the cricopharyngeus muscle, the level of the aortic arch, the level of the left main stem bronchus, the gastroesophageal junction, and any site of pathologic narrowing such as a web or a tumor. Pathologic narrowing should be suspected in patients with recurrent esophageal foreign bodies, and further evaluation by endoscopy and barium swallow should be done. Chest radiography is routinely performed before and after the endoscopy.

Several important facts must be known: the type of object ingested (i.e., food, metal, sharp or blunt item); the location of the impaction; time elapsed since the ingestion; presence of partial or complete obstruction; and presence of potential complications at the time of the presentation such as dehydration or esophageal perforation with mediastinal involvement.

Endoscopy is the primary method for treating foreign body obstruction. We prefer rigid endoscopy done in the operating room because the rigid scope allows distention of the esophagus, better visualization, and safer removal of the foreign body with large optical grasping forceps. After the diagnosis is made on the basis of the history and radiographs, general anesthesia is administered with orotracheal intubation, especially if the foreign body is proximal at the cricopharyngeal inlet, to prevent aspiration and to protect the airway. If endoscopy is done early (ideally within 12 hours), it allows removal of the foreign body before swelling and further obstruction occurs and provides prompt relief of symptoms. The esophagoscope is inserted down to the level of the foreign body, and the object is then grasped with a large forceps specially designed for that particular type of foreign body. In most instances the object may be larger than the bore of the esophagoscope, necessitating removal of the endoscope while the object is being withdrawn. If a piece of meat has been lodged in the esophagus for several days, it may be friable and difficult to grasp. In selected cases, it is acceptable to push it into the stomach if its withdrawal is impossible. Special care should be taken when removing sharp objects such as pins, razor blades, bone, or glass because of the potential for perforation.

In some cases, it is preferable not to perform a complete esophagoscopy after removal of a foreign body, because the mucosa may be inflamed and friable, and the risk of perforation is high. Two rules must be respected while extracting foreign bodies from the esophagus: protect the patient's airway, and maintain control of the object at all times as it is being removed to avoid accidental aspiration into the airway.

## Stenosis

Esophageal stenosis may be caused by webs or rings, or it can occur after surgery or irradiation for esophageal and laryngopharyngeal cancer. Therapy is most effectively achieved by endoscopic dilatation. Rarely is open surgery required for excision or repair. Most patients, especially those with acquired stenosis, require serial dilatations.

Dilatation is most commonly done using bougies. Newer flexible esophagoscopy techniques using endoscopically placed guide wires, over-the-wire dilators, and dilatation balloons have made dilatation easier and safer.

Dilatation can be performed with the push dilators (i.e., Maloney, Eder-Puestow, Savary-Gilliard, and the American Endoscopy dilators) or with balloon dilators. The Maloney dilators are made of mercury-filled bougies, and the Eder-Puestow dilators have a metal olive tip. The Savary-Gilliard dilators consist of a guide wire with a flexible tip that is placed endoscopically. Flexible, soft dilators are then passed over the guide wire in a graded, stepwise fashion to dilate the stricture to the desired width. The American Endoscopy dilators are similar to the Savary-Gilliard type, but they are shorter and radiopaque.

Balloon dilators are relatively new. The balloon is made of a special polymer that can dilate to a specific size, beyond which the balloon ruptures. They can be used through the scope or under fluoroscopy.

If the stricture is a moderate size and soft, proximal dilatation can be done using a Maloney dilator. For complicated strictures, a wire-guided dilator or a balloon dilator should be used.

## Zenker's Diverticulum

Management of Zenker's diverticulum is surgical. Surgical options include an open approach for diverticulectomy, diverticulopexy, cricopharyngeal myotomy, or endoscopic diverticuloplasty and myotomy. Endoscopic management of Zenker's diverticulum was performed by Dohlman in 1960 (18) and popularized by van Overbeek in 1982 (19).

The advantages of the endoscopic approach are a shorter operating time, a shorter hospital stay, a faster recovery with oral intake, and fewer complications. Recurrence, however, is more common, and this technique is somewhat dependent on the surgeon's expertise. In general, it is reserved for older or sicker patients who cannot undergo or refuse an open approach and for patients who have recurrence of their diverticulum after open resection because of cricopharyngeal muscle hypertrophy. This technique has been gaining in popularity because of the excellent results reported by van Overbeek (19).

A specially designed scope is used for this procedure (Fig. 45.3). It is double lipped and longer than a standard laryngoscope (Karl Storz, Culver City, CA). The scope is inserted so that the longer (anterior) blade penetrates the cervical esophagus, and the shorter (posterior) blade is introduced into the sac. This allows the tissue containing the cricopharyngeal muscle to go between the two blades, and it is then easily incised using a $CO_2$ laser (Fig. 45.4). The use of the operating microscope allows visualization of the muscle fibers, and cutting is terminated when the last muscle fibers are cut. Division of the wall of the diverticulum can also be done with diathermy or stapling technique. A chest radiograph is routinely obtained after surgery, which may reveal air in the mediastinum. Patients are observed for signs and symptoms of mediastinitis. Patients are allowed to eat 48 hours later and are then discharged home.

## Complications

Tears and perforation of the esophageal wall can occur after blunt or sharp trauma, most commonly surgical manipulation. The incidence of iatrogenic perforation is 0.1% to 1.5% (20). A water-soluble contrast study confirms the diagnosis. Surgical therapy includes immediate drainage and adequate nutritional support.

Iatrogenic hemorrhage is a rare but a very serious complication. It can occur during dilatation or laser debulking

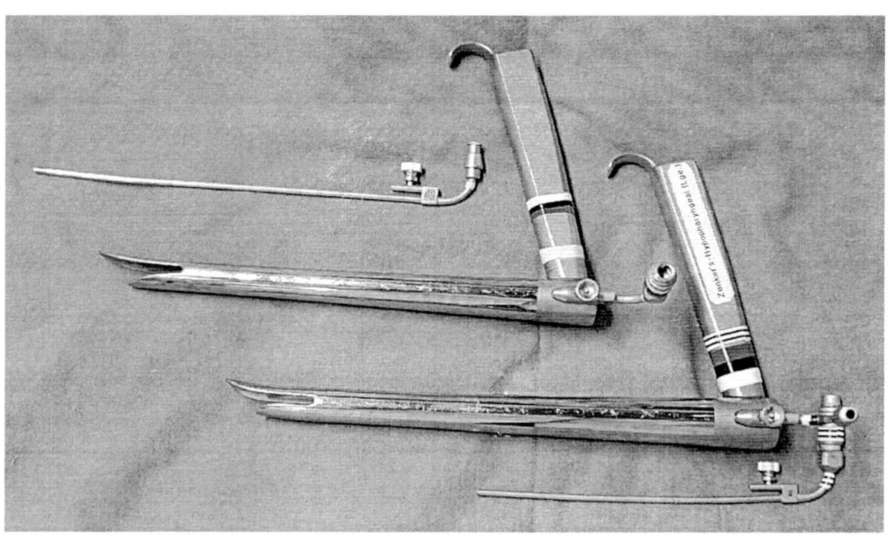

**FIGURE 45.3.** Zenker's diverticuloscope.

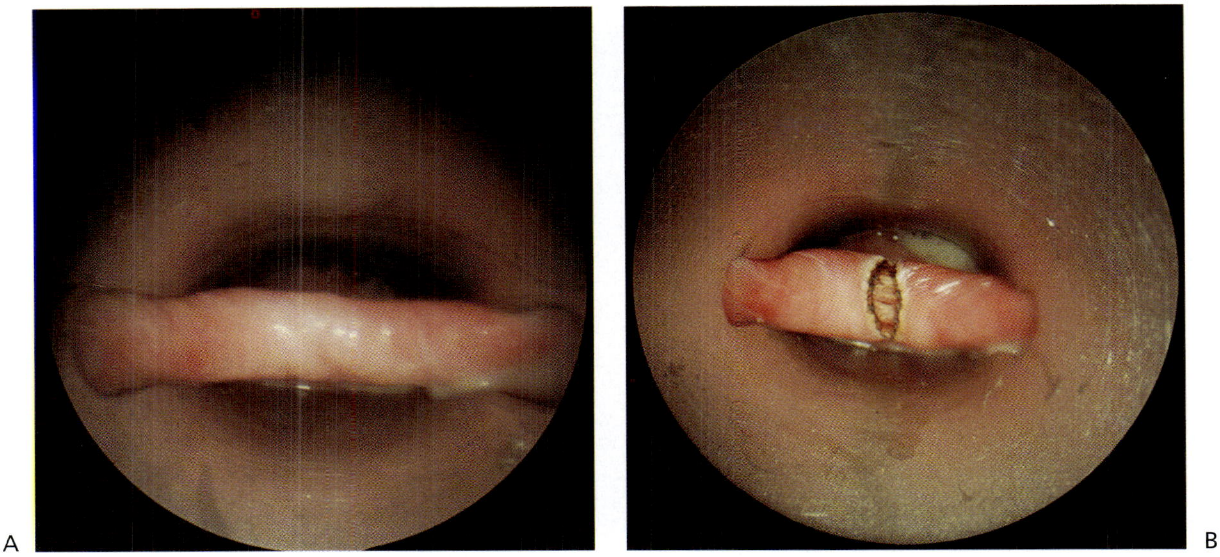

FIGURE 45.4. A: The anterior blade of the scope is inserted in the esophageal lumen and the posterior blade in the diverticulum. B: The laser incisions are made in the cricopharyngeus, which is held between the two blades of the scope.

of carcinoma. It is important to recognize the presence of varices and avoid trauma.

Mediastinitis is an uncommon but potentially life-threatening complication. It results from a tear and a leakage of fluid from the esophageal lumen into the chest. Its course may be rapid, and early recognition and treatment are key to a favorable outcome. Typical symptoms include chest pain, shoulder and back pain (interscapular), tachycardia, fever, tachypnea, and dysphagia. Water-soluble, thin contrast radiographs can be helpful, and plain chest radiographs show widening of the mediastinum. Management depends on the extent of the tear. Thoracotomy may be indicated for drainage and repair of the tear.

## REFERENCES


1. von Eiken C. The clinical application of the method of direct examination of the respiratory passes and the upper alimentary tract. *Arch Laryngol Rhinol* 1904;Nov:15.
2. Jackson C. Foreign bodies in the trachea, bronchi and esophagus. *Laryngoscope* 1905;15:527–539.
3. Andersen HA, Fontana RS. Transbronchoscopic lung biopsy for diffuse pulmonary diseases: technique and results in 450 cases. *Chest* 1972;62:125–128.
4. Dumon J-F. *YAG laser bronchoscopy*. New York: Praeger Publishers, 1985:9–19
5. Strong MS, Vaughan CW, Polanyi T, et al. Bronchoscopic carbon dioxide laser surgery. *Ann Otol Rhinol Laryngol* 1974;83:769–776.
6. Dumon JF, Shapshay S, Bourcereau J, et al. Principles of safety in application of neodymium-YAG laser in bronchology. *Chest* 1984;86:163–168.
7. Ossoff RH, Karlan MS. Universal endoscopic coupler for carbon dioxide laser surgery. *Ann Otol Rhinol Laryngol* 1982;91[Pt 1]: 608–609.
8. Casey KR, Fairfax WR, Smith SJ, et al. Intratracheal fire ignited by the Nd:YAG laser during treatment of tracheal stenosis. *Chest* 1983;84:295–296.
9. Healy GB, McGill T, Simpson GT, Strong MS. The use of the carbon dioxide laser in the pediatric airway. *J Pediatr Surg* 1979;14:735–740.
10. Grillo HC, Zannini P, Michelassi F. Complications of tracheal reconstruction. *J Thorac Cardiovasc Surg* 1986;91:322–328.
11. Koufman JA, Thompson JN, Kohut RI. Endoscopic management of subglottic stenosis with the $CO_2$ surgical laser. *Otolaryngol Head Neck Surg* 1981;89:215–220.
12. Dedo HH, Sooy CD. Endoscopic laser repair of posterior glottic, subglottic and tracheal stenosis by division or micro-trapdoor flap. *Laryngoscope* 1984;94:445–450.
13. Beamis JF, Rebeiz EE, Vergos K, Shapshay SM. Endoscopic laser therapy for obstructing tracheobronchial lesions. *Ann Otol Rhinol Laryngol* 1991;100:413–419.
14. Brutinel WM, Cortese DA, McDougall JC, et al. A two-year experience with the neodymium-YAG laser in endobronchial obstruction. *Chest* 1987;91:159–165.
15. Dumon JF, Shapshay S, Bourcereau J, et al. Principles of safety in application of neodymium-YAG laser in bronchology. *Chest* 1984;86:163–168.
16. Aviv JE, Kim T, Sacco RL, et al. FEESST: a new bedside endoscopic test of the motor and sensory components of swallowing. *Ann Otol Rhinol Laryngol* 1998;107[Pt 1]:378–387.
17. Aviv JE, Martin JH, Kim T, et al. Laryngopharyngeal sensory discrimination testing and the laryngeal adductor reflex. *Ann Otol Rhinol Laryngol* 1999;108:725–730.
18. Dohlman G, Mattsson O. The endoscopic operation for hypopharyngeal diverticula. *Arch Otolaryngol* 1960;71:744.
19. van Overbeek JJ, Hoeksema PE. Endoscopic treatment of the hypopharyngeal diverticulum: 211 cases. *Laryngoscope* 1982;92: 88–91.
20. Mercer CD, Hill LD. Perforation, rupture and injury the esophagus. In: Hill L, Kozarek R, McCallum R, Mercer CD, eds. *The esophagus: medical and surgical management*. Philadelphia: WB Saunders, 1988:211.

# SUBJECT INDEX

## M

**Q**



**R**

**T**



**U**



**V**

## W



## Z